OPERATIVE
PEDIATRIC ORTHOPAEDICS

OPERATIVE
PEDIATRIC ORTHOPAEDICS

Edited by

S. TERRY CANALE, M.D.

Associate Professor
Department of Orthopaedic Surgery
University of Tennessee;
Chief of Pediatric Orthopaedics
Le Bonheur Children's Medical Center;
Active Staff, The Campbell Clinic, Inc., Baptist Memorial
Hospital and Regional Medical Center
Memphis, Tennessee

JAMES H. BEATY, M.D.

Assistant Professor
Department of Orthopaedic Surgery
University of Tennessee;
Chief of Tennessee Crippled Children's Service;
Associate Chief of Pediatric Orthopaedics
Le Bonheur Children's Medical Center;
Active Staff, The Campbell Clinic, Inc., Baptist Memorial
Hospital and Regional Medical Center
Memphis, Tennessee

With over **1800** *illustrations*

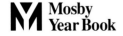
Mosby
Year Book

St. Louis Baltimore Boston Chicago London Philadelphia Sydney Toronto

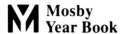

**Mosby
Year Book**

Dedicated to Publishing Excellence

Editor: Eugenia A. Klein
Senior developmental editor: Kathryn H. Falk
Project manager: Patricia Tannian
Production editor: Stephen Dierkes
Book and cover design: Gail Morey Hudson

Mosby–Year Book, Inc.
11830 Westline Industrial Drive, St. Louis, Missouri 63146

Library of Congress Cataloging in Publication Data

Pediatric operative orthopaedics / edited by S. Terry Canale, James H. Beaty.
    p. cm.
    Includes bibliographical references.
    Includes index.
    ISBN 0-8016-0392-7
    1. Pediatric orthopedics. 2. Surgery, Operative. I. Canale, S.
T. (S. Terry)
    [DNLM: 1. Orthopedics—in infancy & childhood. WS 270 P3709]
RD732.3.C48P424 1991
617.3′0083—dc20
DNLM/DLC
for Library of Congress
                                   90-6665
                                    CIP

CL/MY/MY 9 8 7 6 5 4 3 2 1

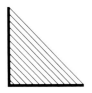

Contributors

JAMES H. BEATY, M.D.

Assistant Professor
Department of Orthopaedic Surgery
University of Tennessee;
Chief of Tennessee Crippled Children's Service;
Associate Chief of Pediatric Orthopaedics
Le Bonheur Children's Medical Center;
Active Staff, The Campbell Clinic, Inc.
Baptist Memorial Hospital and Regional Medical Center
Memphis, Tennessee

S. TERRY CANALE, M.D.

Associate Professor
Department of Orthopaedic Surgery
University of Tennessee;
Chief of Pediatric Orthopaedics
Le Bonheur Children's Medical Center;
Active Staff, The Campbell Clinic, Inc.
Baptist Memorial Hospital and Regional Medical Center
Memphis, Tennessee

ALVIN H. CRAWFORD, M.D.

Professor of Orthopaedic Surgery and Pediatrics
University of Cincinnati College of Medicine;
Director of Pediatric Orthopaedics
Children's Hospital Medical Center
Cincinnati, Ohio

LUCIANO S. DIAS, M.D.

Associate Professor
Department of Orthopaedic Surgery
Northwestern University Medical School;
Chief, Orthopaedic Section, Spinabifida Clinic
Children's Memorial Hospital
Chicago, Illinois

BARNEY L. FREEMAN III, M.D.

Clinical Assistant Professor of Orthopaedic Surgery
University of Tennessee, Memphis;

Active Staff, Le Bonheur Children's Medical Center;
Active Staff, The Campbell Clinic, Inc.
Memphis, Tennessee

NEIL E. GREEN, M.D.

Professor and Vice Chairman
Department of Orthopaedics and Rehabilitation
Vanderbilt University
Head, Pediatric Orthopaedics
Vanderbilt University Medical Center
Nashville, Tennessee

JOHN E. HERZENBERG, M.D.

Assistant Professor, Department of Surgery
Section of Orthopaedic Surgery
University of Michigan Medical Center
Consultant Surgeon, Veterans Administration Hospital
Ann Arbor, Michigan

F. STIG JACOBSEN, M.D.

Pediatric Orthopaedic Surgeon
Marshfield Clinic
Marshfield, Wisconsin

MARK T. JOBE, M.D.

Clinical Instructor of Orthopaedic Surgery
University of Tennessee, Memphis;
Associate Chief of Hand Surgery
Le Bonheur Children's Medical Center;
Active Staff, The Campbell Clinic, Inc.
Memphis, Tennessee

JAMES R. KASSER, M.D.

Assistant Professor, Orthopaedic Surgery
Harvard Medical School;
Associate Chief, Orthopaedic Surgery
Boston Children's Hospital
Boston, Massachusetts

CHARLES T. PRICE, M.D.

Pediatric Orthopaedic Surgeon
Arnold Palmer Hospital for Children and Women
Orlando, Florida

DEMPSEY S. SPRINGFIELD, M.D.

Associate Professor, Department of Orthopaedics
Harvard Medical School;
Visiting Orthopaedic Surgeon,
Massachusetts General Hospital
Boston, Massachusetts

WILLIAM C. WARNER, JR., M.D.

Clinical Instructor of Orthopaedic Surgery
   University of Tennessee, Memphis;
Chief, Mississippi Crippled Children's Service;
Active Staff, The Campbell Clinic, Inc.
Memphis, Tennessee

PHILLIP E. WRIGHT II, M.D.

Associate Professor of Orthopaedic Surgery
   University of Tennessee, Memphis;
Chief of Hand Surgery Service
Le Bonheur Children's Medical Center;
Active Staff, The Campbell Clinic, Inc.
Memphis, Tennessee

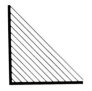

Preface

Although many orthopaedic conditions in children are best treated nonoperatively, when surgery is required for a musculoskeletal problem in a child, the choice, timing, and technique of the procedure are critical because the outcome will affect the child's whole life. The unique characteristics of the child's skeleton have inspired a multitude of techniques. In this text we have attempted to describe those procedures most commonly used for orthopaedic conditions in children. Also included are brief discussions of the etiology and prognosis of various orthopaedic conditions, nonoperative treatment, indications for operative treatment, and complications that may be encountered. This text is intended to be a concise guide to the *surgical* treatment of orthopaedic problems in children and to provide operative descriptions of appropriate techniques. Some of the most commonly performed procedures, applicable to musculoskeletal problems from a variety of causes, are collected in Chapter 1, "Special Techniques," for easy reference. Other techniques are described in chapters discussing the conditions for which they are commonly performed. This book would of course have been impossible without the expertise and experience of our distinguished contributors. They bring to the material a wealth of knowledge and advice and expand the viewpoint beyond a single institution.

We hope that this condensation of information will be helpful to medical students, interns, orthopaedic residents, and practicing orthopaedists and that it will ultimately benefit the children, who are the reason for this undertaking.

We would like to thank Kay Daugherty for her editorial assistance with this undertaking. We also appreciate the efforts of Richard Fritzler, artist; the Campbell Foundation Staff; Joan Crowson, Librarian; and Eugenia Klein and Kathy Falk of Mosby–Year Book, Inc.

In addition to all those who actually had a hand in the preparation of this book, we owe a great debt to our families for their patience and support. Our thanks, too, to our colleagues and partners for their suggestions and encouragement, and to Dr. Alvin Ingram and Dr. Fred P. Sage who, by example and instruction, inspired us always to consider the care of children a special privilege and obligation.

S. Terry Canale, M.D.   **James H. Beaty, M.D.**

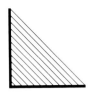

Contents

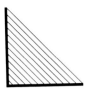

Detailed Contents

11 Cerebral Palsy, 611

Neil E. Green

12 Myelomeningocele, 683

Luciano S. Dias

13 Neuromuscular Disorders, 717

James H. Beaty

14 Osteochondroses, 743

S. Terry Canale

15 Sports Medicine, 777

S. Terry Canale

1

Special Techniques

S. TERRY CANALE

The orthopaedic treatment of children differs in many ways from that of adults because of the differences in musculoskeletal characteristics and the potential for growth in children. Many surgical procedures have been devised or modified especially for treatment of orthopaedic conditions in children, and many are applicable to deformities caused by very different disease processes. To avoid repetition, some of these commonly used special techniques have been collected in this chapter and are referred to in other chapters.

OSTEOTOMIES FOR ANGULAR AND ROTATIONAL DEFORMITIES
General Indications for Osteotomy and Complications of Osteotomy

Angular deformity and shortening of the lower extremity may be caused by congenital, developmental, or traumatic factors. Osteotomy, along with bony bar resection, epiphysiodesis, and bone lengthening and shortening procedures, have long been used to correct these deformities. There are, however, no standard guidelines as to the severity of deformity that requires osteotomy. Commonly cited indications include a significant, progressive, angular deformity that cannot be corrected by bracing, pain, knee or ankle malalignment, and progressive ligamentous laxity about the knee or ankle. The definition of *significant* angulation, however, is imprecise. The amount of true angulation should be determined by comparing standing roentgenograms of both extremities. Leg lengths should be determined by leg length scanograms or by computed tomography (CT). The normal physiologic valgus of 4 to 6 degrees in boys and 5 to 7 degrees in girls should be subtracted from any valgus deformity and added to any varus deformity. Whether the deformity is static or progressive also must be determined. Angulation caused by developmental conditions usually remains static, but physeal growth arrest or retardation usually is progressive.

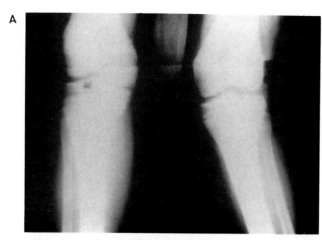

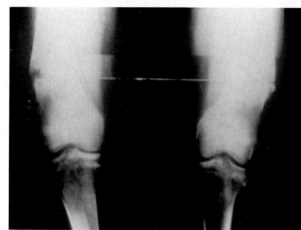

Fig. 1-1 A, Bilateral genu valgum. On left knee *(above)* deformity is in tibia and knee is parallel to floor; on right knee *(below)* deformity appears to be in femur and knee is not parallel to floor. **B,** After supracondylar femoral osteotomy, right knee is parallel to floor. Tibial osteotomy should have been performed on left knee because it is not parallel to floor.

OSTEOTOMIES FOR ANGULAR AND ROTATIONAL DEFORMITIES
General Indications for Osteotomy and Complications of Osteotomy

Angular deformity and shortening of the lower extremity may be caused by congenital, developmental, or traumatic factors. Osteotomy, along with bony bar resection, epiphysiodesis, and bone lengthening and shortening procedures, have long been used to correct these deformities. There are, however, no standard guidelines as to the severity of deformity that requires osteotomy. Commonly cited indications include a significant, progressive, angular deformity that cannot be corrected by bracing, pain, knee or ankle malalignment, and progressive ligamentous laxity about the knee or ankle. The definition of *significant* angulation, however, is imprecise. The amount of true angulation should be determined by comparing standing roentgenograms of both extremities. Leg lengths should be determined by leg length scanograms or by computed tomography (CT). The normal physiologic valgus of 4 to 6 degrees in boys and 5 to 7 degrees in girls should be subtracted from any valgus deformity and added to any varus deformity. Whether the deformity is static or progressive also must be determined. Angulation caused by developmental conditions usually remains static, but physeal growth arrest or retardation usually is progressive. More correction, and perhaps even overcorrection, is required for progressive deformity. Finally, the deformity should present a significant physical or cosmetic problem before osteotomy is considered. The risks of a major surgical procedure should be carefully weighed against the advantage of correcting mild deformity.

The indications for tibial or femoral osteotomy, with a closing or opening wedge, also are not definitive. In general, if a roentgenogram taken with the patient standing shows that the knee is parallel to the floor, tibial osteotomy is indicated; if the knee is not parallel to the floor, supracondylar femoral osteotomy is indicated (Fig. 1-1). One exception to this general rule is the deformity that occurs in Blount's disease in which the tibial plateau and knee joint are angulated, but the major deformity is in the tibial metaphysis, which requires a proximal tibial osteotomy.

The efficacy of corrective osteotomy as prophylaxis against the early development of arthritis caused by physiologic genu varum and genu valgum has not been substantiated. In some young adults with significant physiologic genu varum, osteotomy may be required for pain relief and for narrowing of the medial joint line (Fig. 1-2).

Neurovascular complications are the most serious sequelae of osteotomy. Some neurovascular complications associated with tibial osteotomy may be avoided by the performance of fasciotomy at the time of osteotomy. If a neurovascular problem develops after surgery, it must be determined whether the cause is a compartment syndrome, kinking of the artery at the trification near the proximal tibia as described by Steel et al, or peroneal nerve palsy. Compartment syndrome usually produces severe, unrelenting pain that increases steadily over a 12- to 24-hour period; passive motion of the toes causes severe pain. All circumferential bandages should be removed, and compartment pressures should be measured. Kinking of the artery or arterial occlusion near the knee (trification), in contrast, usually causes sudden, severe pain immediately after surgery. This is an emergency situation, and prompt action is mandatory. All bandages should be removed and an arteriogram taken. If osteotomy has been performed and the arteriogram confirms kinking or occlusion, the leg should be immediately returned to its original position. Peroneal nerve palsy frequently is painless. The toes may be moved passively but not actively. All constricting bandages should be removed and pressure promptly relieved at the fibular head. Neurovascular compromise must be avoided at all costs. A markedly angulated but functional extremity is superior to a straight but functionless extremity.

A 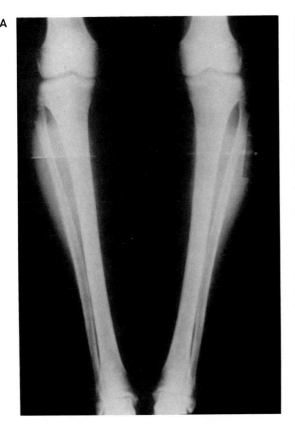 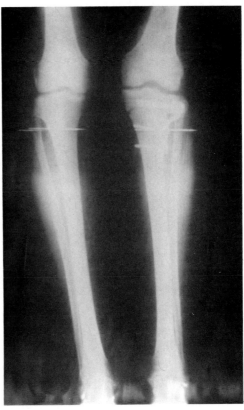 B

Fig. 1-2 **A,** Bilateral genu varum in young adult. **B,** After valgus osteotomy, which was performed when the patient was 23 years old, because of severe pain and narrowing of medial joint line.

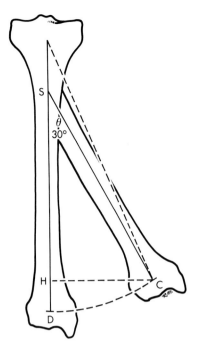

Fig. 1-3 Model and equation proving gain in length if angulated bone is straightened, regardless of type of osteotomy. S, Maximum point of 30-degree angulation (φ); SC = angulated bone, corrected to SD; thus HD = absolute gain in length from osteotomy. (From Canale ST and Harper MC. In The American Academy of Orthopaedic Surgeons: Instructional course lectures, vol 30, St. Louis, 1981, The CV Mosby Co.)

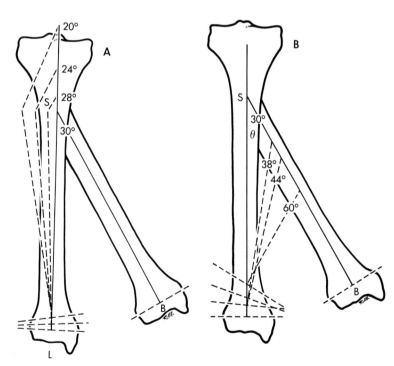

Biotrigonometric Principles

Although osteotomies have been performed for centuries, much of the information about this procedure has been gained empirically, with techniques and principles handed down from one generation of orthopaedists to the next, without exactness or objectivity. Milch made a significant contribution to the science of osteotomy with his 1947 description of pelvic osteotomy and review of other osteotomies. The effects of the size, shape, and location of the osteotomy determine the choice and timing of procedure. These effects can be determined mathematically if certain basic biomechanical principles are kept in mind.

First, any straightening of an angulated bone results in lengthening of that bone. Although this point seems obvious, the gain in length often is overlooked in calculations for osteotomy. The gain in length actually occurs through an arc and can be computed with the following formula that uses the cosine of the angle of the deformity and the length of the angulated segment:

$$HD = SD \times \text{Cosine of the deformity angle}$$

where
HD = Length gained
SD = Length of the angulated segment

As an example, consider a tibia 15 inches long with a 30-degree angulation deformity 3 inches below the knee (Fig. 1-3). In this instance the cosine of the deformity angle is 0.134, and the length of the angulated segment is 12 inches. Thus:

$$HD = 0.134 \times 12 \text{ inches} =$$
$$1.6 \text{ inches (length gained by osteotomy)}$$

Fig. 1-4 **A,** Model showing 30-degree angulation deformity and computation of compensatory osteotomies progressively proximal to maximum deformity (S). At one fourth the distance proximal to S, 24-degree wedge is required to correct to midline; at one half the distance, a 20-degree wedge is required. **B,** Same model as **A,** and computation of compensatory osteotomies is progressively distal to maximum deformity (S). At one fourth the distance from S, 38-degree osteotomy is required; at one half the distance, 60-degree osteotomy is required. Note that loss of anticipated gain in length is greater when osteotomy is moved distally than when moved proximally to S. (From Canale ST and Harper MC. In The American Academy of Orthopaedic Surgeons: Instructional course lectures, vol 30, St. Louis, 1981, The CV Mosby Co.)

Although the optimal location for osteotomy is at the site of maximum angulation, this area often must be avoided because of scar formation, infection, sclerosis, or poor skin condition. Often the choice for osteotomy location must be the *next* best site. Moving distally to the site of maximum angulation requires increasingly greater degrees of correction and, conversely, moving proximally to the site of angulation requires increasingly fewer degrees of correction. In either case the expected gain in length progressively decreases the farther the osteotomy is removed from the site of angulation (Fig. 1-4).

The size of the wedge of bone removed at osteotomy generally has been determined empirically or with a preoperative "cut-out"; however, a general rule of thumb has been that for every degree of correction required 1 mm of wedge should be removed. This rule is reasonably accurate for high tibial osteotomies in a tibia approximately 6 to 7 cm in diameter (the average adult tibia measures 9 cm). In a child with a tibial diameter of 4 cm or less, the calculation may be in error by as much as 40%. If the angle of correction needed is measured before surgery and the diameter of the bone (in centimeters) is measured during surgery, the appropriate size of the wedge can be determined by means of the following formula (Fig. 1-5):

$$W = D \times 0.02 \times \text{Angle of correction}$$

where
W = Size of wedge
D = Diameter

The exact trigonometric formula multiplies the diameter of the bone by the tangent of the angle of correction; however, because this information must be obtained from a tangent table, this formula has little practical application. The simpler formula has been proved to have only a 10% margin of error when compared with the more complex formula; it is sufficiently accurate for tibial osteotomies between 15 and 40 degrees and is much more useful clinically.

The amount of lengthening or shortening produced by an opening or closing wedge osteotomy equals one half the base of the wedge (W/2) (Fig. 1-6). This gain or loss or length should be combined with the earlier estimate of length gained by straightening the angulated bone.

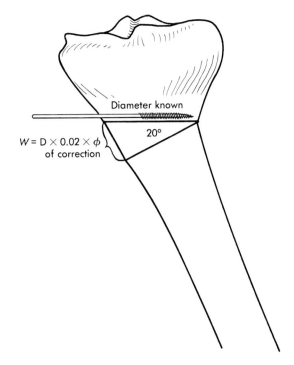

Fig. 1-5 Method of determining length of wedge *(W)* to be removed when desired angle of correction (20 degrees) is known before surgery and diameter of bone is determined at surgery. (From Canale ST and Harper MC. In The American Academy of Orthopaedic Surgeons: Instructional course lectures, vol 30, St. Louis, 1981, The CV Mosby Co.)

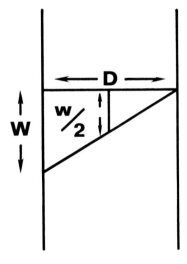

Fig. 1-6 Length lost or gained is equal to one half the base *(W)* of the osteotomy. *D,* Diameter. (From Canale ST and Harper MC. In The American Academy of Orthopaedic Surgeons: Instructional course lectures, vol 30, St. Louis, 1981, The CV Mosby Co.)

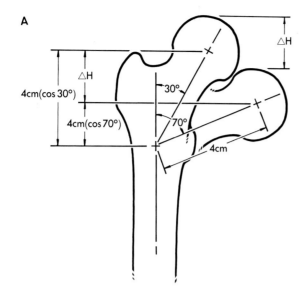

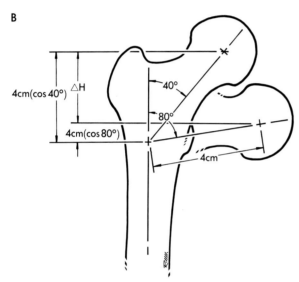

In proximal femoral osteotomies, the rule of thumb has been that varus osteotomy decreases length and valgus osteotomy increases length. Because the distance from the center of the femoral head to the varus or valgus osteotomy site does not change, any change in length is due to the change in angle of the deformity (Fig. 1-7). The exact amount of length gained or lost can be determined with the following formula:

$$\Delta H = L \times (\cos \phi_1 - \cos \phi_2)$$

where

ΔH = Change in length

L = Constant distance from the femoral head to the osteotomy site

cos = Cosine of angle of deformity (ϕ_1) and angle of correction (ϕ)

Table 1-1 gives estimates of the leg length change for a variety of angulation changes, in both varus and valgus positions. The effect of the opening or closing wedge (W/2) also must be added or subtracted from the change listed in the table.

Fig. 1-7 **A,** Change in height for varus osteotomy. **B,** Change in height for valgus osteotomy. (From Harper MC, Canale ST, and Cobb RM: J Pediatr Orthop 3:431, 1983.)

Table 1-1 Estimates of leg length change for a variety of angulation changes

L, original angle (degrees)	Desired angle (degrees)								
	90	100	110	120	130	135	140	150	160
2 cm									
90	0	0.3	0.6	1.0	1.3	1.4	1.5	1.7	1.9
100	−0.3	0	0.3	0.7	0.9	1.1	1.2	1.4	1.5
110	−0.6	−0.3	0	0.3	0.6	0.7	0.9	1.0	1.2
120	−1.0	−0.7	−0.3	0	0.3	0.4	0.5	0.7	0.9
130	−1.3	−0.9	−0.6	−0.3	0	0.1	0.2	0.4	0.6
135	−1.4	−1.1	−0.7	−0.4	−0.1	0	0.1	0.3	0.5
140	−1.5	−1.2	−0.9	−0.5	−0.2	−0.1	0	0.2	0.3
150	−1.7	−1.4	−1.0	−0.7	−0.4	−0.3	−0.2	0	0.1
160	−1.9	−1.5	−1.2	−0.9	−0.6	−0.5	−0.3	−0.1	0
3 cm									
90	0	0.5	1.0	1.5	1.9	2.1	2.3	2.6	2.8
100	−0.5	0	0.5	1.0	1.4	1.6	1.8	2.1	2.3
110	−1.0	−0.5	0	0.5	0.9	1.1	1.3	1.6	1.8
120	−1.5	−1.0	−0.5	0	0.4	0.6	0.8	1.1	1.3
130	−1.9	−1.4	−0.9	−0.4	0	0.2	0.4	0.7	0.9
135	−2.1	−1.6	−1.1	−0.6	−0.2	0	0.2	0.5	0.7
140	−2.3	−1.8	−1.3	−0.8	−0.4	−0.2	0	0.3	0.5
150	−2.6	−2.1	−1.6	−1.1	−0.7	−0.5	−0.3	0	0.2
160	−2.8	−2.3	−1.8	−1.3	−0.9	−0.7	−0.5	−0.2	0
4 cm									
90	0	0.7	1.4	2.0	2.6	2.8	3.1	3.5	3.8
100	−0.7	0	0.7	1.3	1.9	2.1	2.4	2.8	3.1
110	−1.4	−0.7	0	0.6	1.2	1.5	1.7	2.1	2.4
120	−2.0	−1.3	−0.6	0	0.6	0.8	1.1	1.5	1.8
130	−2.6	−1.9	−1.2	−0.6	0	0.3	0.5	0.9	1.2
135	−2.8	−2.1	−1.5	−0.8	−0.3	0	0.2	0.6	0.9
140	−3.1	−2.4	−1.7	−1.1	−0.5	−0.2	0	0.4	0.7
150	−3.5	−2.8	−2.1	−1.5	−0.9	−0.6	−0.4	0	0.3
160	−3.8	−3.1	−2.4	−1.8	−1.2	−0.9	−0.7	−0.3	0
5 cm									
90	0	0.9	1.7	2.5	3.2	3.5	3.8	4.3	4.7
100	−0.9	0	0.8	1.6	2.3	2.7	3.0	3.5	3.8
110	−1.7	−0.8	0.8	1.5	1.8	2.2	2.6	3.0	
120	−2.5	−1.6	−0.8	0	0.7	1.0	1.3	1.8	2.2
130	−3.2	−2.3	−1.5	−0.7	0	0.3	0.6	1.1	1.5
135	−3.5	−2.7	−1.8	−1.0	−0.3	0	0.3	0.8	1.2
140	−3.8	−3.0	−2.2	−1.3	−0.6	−0.3	0	0.5	0.9
150	−4.3	−3.5	−2.6	−1.8	−1.1	−0.8	−0.5	0	0.4
160	−4.7	−3.8	−3.0	−2.2	−1.5	−1.2	−0.9	−0.4	0
6 cm									
90	0	1.0	2.1	3.0	3.9	4.2	4.6	5.2	5.6
100	−1.0	0	1.0	2.0	2.8	3.2	3.6	4.2	4.6
110	−2.1	−1.0	0	0.9	1.8	2.2	2.5	3.1	3.6
120	−3.0	−2.0	−0.9	0	0.9	1.2	1.6	2.2	2.6
130	−3.9	−2.8	−1.8	−0.9	0	0.4	0.7	1.3	1.8
135	−4.2	−3.2	−2.2	−1.2	−0.4	0	0.4	1.0	1.4
140	−4.6	−3.6	−2.5	−1.6	−0.7	−0.4	0	0.6	1.0
150	−5.2	−4.2	−3.1	−2.2	−1.3	−1.0	−0.6	0	0.4
160	−5.6	−4.6	−3.6	−2.6	−1.8	−1.4	−1.0	−0.4	0

From Harper MC, Canale ST, and Cobb RM: J Pediatr Orthop 3:431-434, 1983.
Left hand column is different angles, with L (the length of the neck to the center of the head) being 2 cm, 3 cm, 4 cm, 5 cm, and 6 cm, going from the original angle in the left-hand column to the desired angle in the right-hand column, and the change in relative height noted in centimeters.

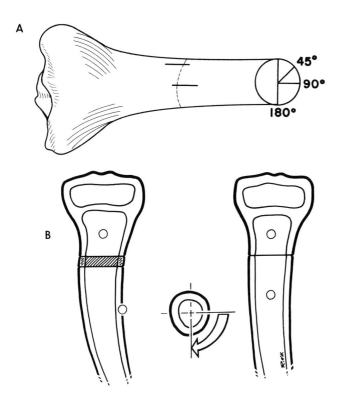

Fig. 1-8 **A,** Rotation of femur from one orientation mark to another through an arc of 360 degrees. **B,** Orientation marks with pins or drill holes to determine limits of rotation. (From Canale ST and Harper MC. In The American Academy of Orthopaedic Surgeons: Instructional course lectures, vol 30, St. Louis, 1981, The CV Mosby Co.)

In addition to the effect of straightening an angulated bone, the effect of rotation during the osteotomy must be considered. The bone should be considered as a 360-degree circle even if the contours are not perfectly round. Thus a change of 45 degrees requires very slight rotation of the bone (Fig. 1-8, *A*). Pins inserted into the bone fragments at the correct degree of rotation and then brought parallel are helpful (Fig. 1-8, *B*). A string may be used to measure the circumference of the bone and, determining the degrees of rotation needed as a percentage of 360, the correct percentage of the string can be determined and used as a guide for rotation. Crider and Leber described a formula in which the amount of rotation can be determined easily and accurately (Fig. 1-9):

$$L = (0.017)(Q)(R)$$

where

Q = Desired angle of correction in degrees
R = Radius of the bone as measured on standard
   roentgenograms (or by direct measurement at surgery)
L = Distance between marks on the two rotated segments
   of the bone

A longitudinal line is drawn on the femoral shaft in the area selected for the osteotomy. After osteotomy the femoral shaft is rotated so that the distance between the displaced marks equals the *L* calculated previously.

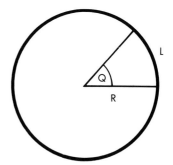

Fig. 1-9 Measurement of surface distance *(L)* of rotation using amount of rotation in degrees *(Q)* and radius *(R)* in formula—*L* = (0.017) (Q) (R). (From Crider RJ and Leber C: J Pediatr Orthop 7:468, 1987.)

To determine the total effect of osteotomy, all the various aspects must be considered, including straightening, location of osteotomy, type of wedge, and rotation. As an example that combines the various calculations, consider a patient with a right leg 3.4 cm shorter than the left, an 8-degree normal valgus on the left, and a 17-degree varus deformity on the right, thus requiring 25 degrees of correction (Fig. 1-10). With the use of the previously cited formula, HD = SD (cos angle of deformity), HD = 0.1

(3.3) = 3.3 cm of length gained by straightening the angulated bone. When the size of the closing wedge is determined (W = 0.2 × 6 cm × 25 degrees = 3 cm), half its base, 1.5 cm, is subtracted from the expected gain in length, giving a realistic estimate of length gained of 1.7 cm. For an opening wedge osteotomy in the same patient, the length gained would be 4.8 cm, since the opening wedge would gain an additional 1.5 cm (Fig. 1-11).

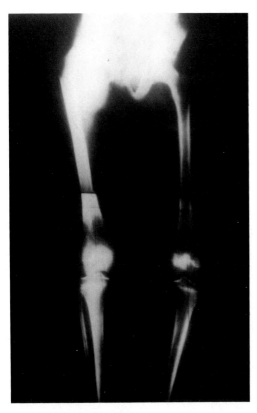

Fig. 1-10 Varus deformity of 17 degrees on right with valgus deformity of 8 degrees on left; right extremity is 3.4 cm shorter than left.

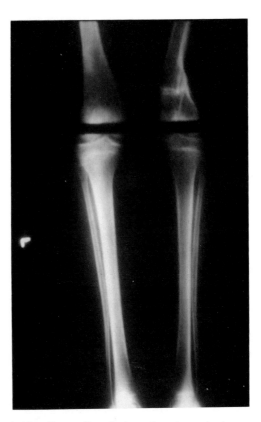

Fig. 1-11 Even after closing of wedge osteotomy, gain in length is 1.7 cm on right extremity.

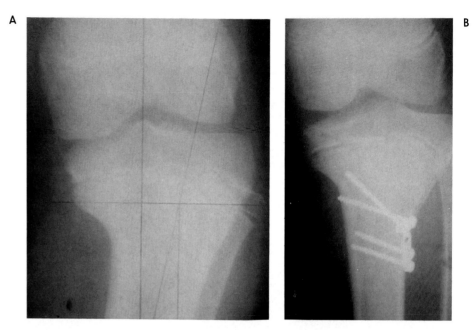

Fig. 1-12 **A,** Varus deformity of proximal tibia. **B,** After closing wedge tibial osteotomy with the use of small plate and screws for fixation.

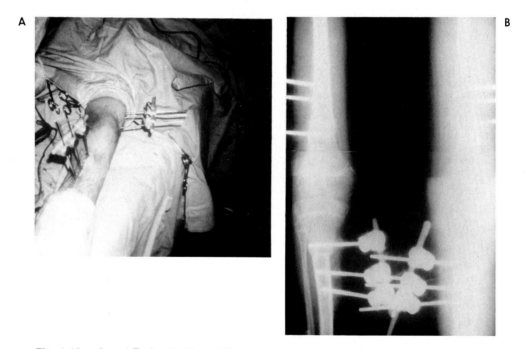

Fig. 1-13 **A** and **B,** Application of Roger Anderson external fixator after bilateral femoral and tibial osteotomies.

General Surgical Principles

Fixation of the osteotomy, either internally or externally, may be achieved by several different methods, depending on the type and location of the osteotomy and the stability of the fragments. Fixation may include pins and plaster, screws and plates (Fig. 1-12), Kirschner wires, tension band wires, Knowles pins, intramedullary nails, and external fixators (Fig. 1-13). Whatever method is chosen, the goal of the fixation is to provide splinting, compression, and buttressing.

Two other fixation devices for intertrochanteric osteotomies have been recommended in the European literature: the AO fixed angle blade plates described by Müller and the Altdorf hip clamp, which is a modification of the Becker angled plate developed by Wagner.

If screws and plates are used, they must be placed to achieve maximum biomechanical efficiency in relation to the osteotomy site. If rigid compression is desired, the screws should be placed at right angles to the axis of the bone, with the plate perpendicular to the osteotomy site. Lag screws can be used for additional security. Plates placed on the side of the bone should neutralize shearing and bending stresses and add to intrafragmentary compression by axial tension. Compression plates are used to compress the osteotomy fragments. The dynamic compression principle described by Perren and Allgöwer in 1970 combines both neutralization and tension band plating. Long side plates of any type should not be used in the metaphyseal area because of the danger of crossing the physis with the fixation screws (Fig. 1-14).

External fixation has become increasingly popular, but these devices are expensive, complex, and time-consuming to apply. Often the position and angulation of the osteotomy are determined by the external fixation device used (Fig. 1-15). Too rigid fixation inhibits callus formation and too elastic fixation deforms under loading. Dynamic axial external fixation (Fig. 1-16) has been reported to allow axial loading and callus formation while decreasing stress at the pin-bone interface. It also can be left in place until healing is complete. Early reports in the English literature indicate good results with the Ilizarov external fixation system, but this system is especially complex and requires extensive training and experience to be used effectively.

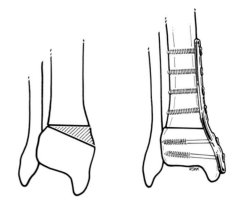

Fig. 1-14 Fixation of osteotomy of distal tibia with plate at right angles to osteotomy site and screws at right angle on axis of bone. Distal screws and plate should not cross physis.

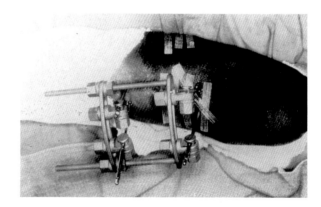

Fig. 1-15 External fixation of tibial osteotomy.

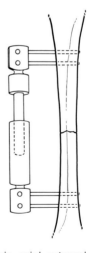

Fig. 1-16 Dynamic axial external fixation allows rigid fixation, axial loading, and callus formation and may be left in place until osteotomy heals. (From Songer JE, Kendra JC, and Price CT: Scientific exhibit, presented at the 55th annual meeting of the American Academy of Orthopaedic Surgeons, Atlanta, Feb 4-9, 1988.)

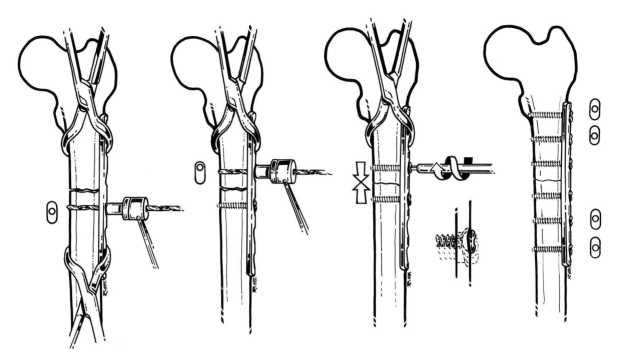

Fig. 1-17 Axial compression accomplished by screws inserted in the axial and transverse planes. (Redrawn from Heim U and Pfeiffer KM: Internal fixation of small fractures, technique recommended by the AO-ASIF Group, ed 3, Berlin, 1988, Springer-Verlag.)

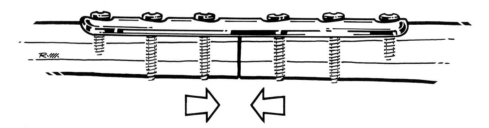

Fig. 1-18 Compression plates with screws crossing five or six cortices. (Redrawn from Heim U and Pfeiffer KM: Internal fixation of small fractures, technique recommended by the AO-ASIF Group, ed 3, Berlin, 1988, Springer-Verlag.)

The ASIF small fragment set is especially suited for fixation of osteotomies and fractures in children. Heim and Pfeiffer described three rules of stabilization for the use of the ASIF small fragment set:

1. Fixation of spiral or long oblique osteotomies or fractures can be accomplished only with two or more screws placed in different planes, preferably with a plate (Fig. 1-17). Resistance to tensile and shearing forces is considerably greater when two screws are used rather than a single screw in the center of the osteotomy or fracture line.

2. Plates with screws that cross three or four cortices may be adequate in the distal bones of the hand or foot, but in larger proximal bones, plates with screws that cross five or six cortices in each fragment are required (Fig. 1-18).

3. The dominant side of an osteotomy should be reduced and held by a "load-bearing" beam (usually a large plate) to prevent displacement. The application of this plate will effect reduction of the smaller fragments (vasal portion) of the osteotomy or fracture, which may be fixed by the simplest means possible, such as with a single screw (Fig. 1-19).

Heim and Pfeiffer recommend removal of all metal implants when the osteotomy or fracture has united. They maintain that large implants in the extremities may limit movement of the displaced surrounding soft tissues, may promote adhesions between gliding soft tissue layers, cause irritation, produce bursa, hinder rehabilitation, or cause implant intolerance as a result of corrosion or allergy. Especially in children, the implant may cause alterations in the structure of the bone. Although individual screws may be left in place, plates should be removed because of their propensity for causing rarefaction of the underlying cortex and for acting as stress risers. Plates should be removed within 1 year of union of the osteotomy before the bone-screw interface becomes so hard as to make removal difficult.

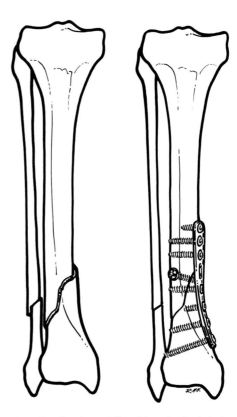

Fig. 1-19   Application of "load-bearing" plate to dominant side of osteotomy site or fracture effects reduction of smaller fragments. (Redrawn from Heim U and Pfeiffer KM: Internal fixation of small fractures, technique recommended by the AO-ASIF Group, ed 3, Berlin, 1988, Springer-Verlag.)

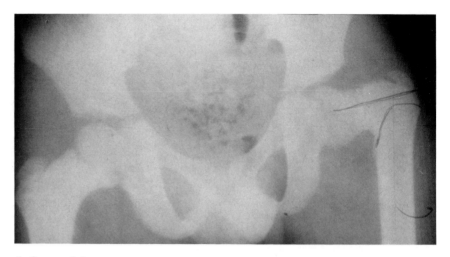

A, Congenital coxa vara.

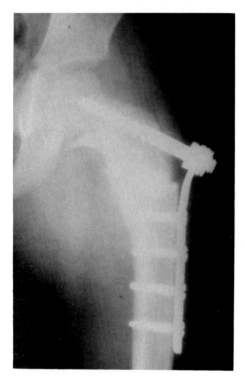

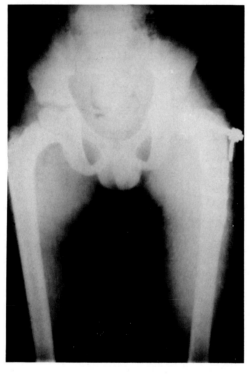

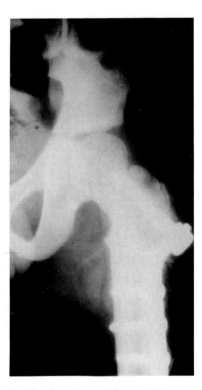

B, After valgus subtrochanteric osteotomy with the use of Coventry lag screw.

C, One year after surgery Coventry lag screw has broken at most proximal screw hole.

D, After insertion of Campbell screw.

Fig. 1-20

Hip

Most deformities in the hip area can be classified as coxa valga, coxa vara, or rotational deformity. Coxa valga deformity is more prevalent in congenital, developmental, and neuromuscular conditions such as cerebral palsy; coxa vara deformity may develop after trauma, asymmetric closure of the capital femoral physis, or osteotomy. Most technical problems associated with osteotomies in the hip area occur because of inadequate correction or failure to calculate accurately the effect of the trochanteric physis. Osteotomies in the hip area generally are performed in the trochanteric or subtrochanteric area and are fixed with a side plate and screw system, such as the Coventry or Campbell pediatric screw systems. Reported complications of the Coventry system include nonunion, malunion, premature physeal closure, loss of fixation, plate failure, and fracture of the femur (Fig. 1-20). Although some complications are due to technical errors and some are unavoidable, many seem attributable to deficiencies in the system. The Campbell cannulated system has the advantages of a larger screw with larger cutting flutes and reverse cutting flutes for ease of removal, a small hexagonal screw attachment, and pre-bent, thicker side plates of various sizes (Fig. 1-21). Instrumentation includes an inserter/extractor wrench, calibrated to assist alignment of the screw and plate, and a tap to facilitate screw insertion over a guide pin. Schmidt also has developed a similar pediatric lag screw with the same basic features. These systems provide a positive hexagonal fit between the plate and screw with broader screw threads to engage the cortical wall of the femoral neck, which reduces the chance of screw disengagement. Regardless of the fixation system used, preoperative planning is important to determine the required angular and rotational alignment of the proximal femur, the type of osteotomy, and the position of the fixation device relative to the osteotomy site. In patients younger than 9 years, special effort should be taken to avoid crossing the physis with the fixation screws.

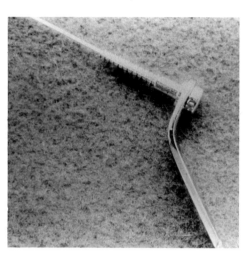

Fig. 1-21 Campbell cannulated pediatric hip screw with large cutting flutes, heavy side plate, and holding screw attaching side plate and cannulated screw.

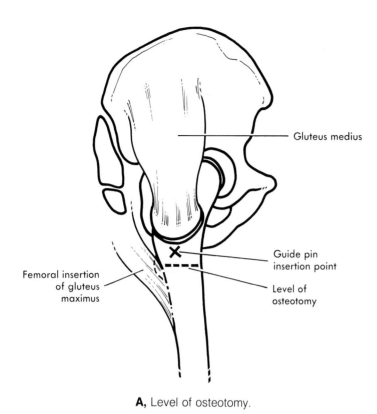

A, Level of osteotomy.

Varus Derotational Osteotomy with Campbell Screw Fixation

▶ *Technique.* Place the patient supine on the operating table with a roentgen cassette holder beneath the patient. Image intensification, positioned in the anteroposterior projection, is desirable. Prepare and drape the affected extremity, leaving it free to allow for intraoperative roentgenograms or imaging.

Make a lateral incision from the greater trochanter distally 8 to 12 cm, and reflect the vastus lateralis to expose the lateral aspect of the femur. Identify the femoral insertion of the gluteus maximus, and make a transverse line in the femoral cortex with an osteotome to mark the level of the osteotomy at the level of the lesser trochanter or slightly distal (Fig. 1-22, *A*). Correct positioning of the osteotomy site may be verified with image intensification. Now make a longitudinal orientation line in the femoral cortex to determine correct rotation; position this line so that it can be seen through the plate holes or around the plate. Position the plate on the femur with the osteotomy site located between the hexagonal opening and the first screw hole to determine the site of guide pin insertion, or use an angle guide in the standard manner. Insert the guide pin into the midline of the femoral neck, taking care not to penetrate the proximal femoral physis plate (Fig. 1-22, *B*). Confirm correct

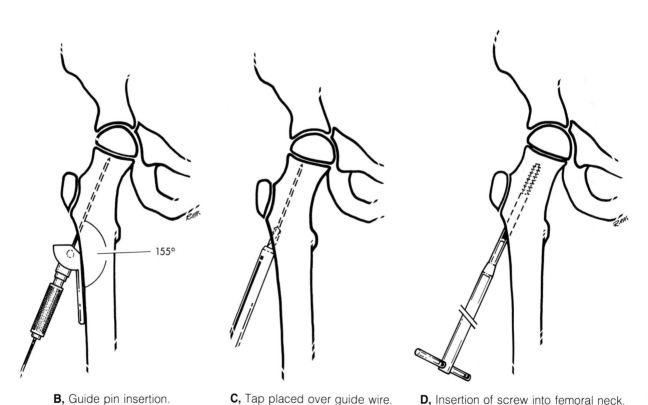

B, Guide pin insertion.   **C,** Tap placed over guide wire.   **D,** Insertion of screw into femoral neck.

Fig. 1-22   Varus derotational osteotomy (see text).

guide pin position at the level of or slightly proximal to the lesser trochanter with roentgenograms or image intensification.

Measure the proper length of the guide wire to determine the needed screw length, and with a cortical reamer, ream the outer cortex over the guide wire for approximately 0.5 inch, taking care not to extend the reaming into the underlying cancellous bone. Place the tap over the guide wire (Fig. 1-22, *C*) and tap the appropriate length for ease of insertion of the screw into the femoral neck; it is not necessary to tap the entire length of the screw. Before the osteotomy cut is made, insert the proper size screw into the femoral neck with the use of the inserter/extractor wrench (Fig. 1-22, *D*), but do not tighten it completely. One apex of the screw should be parallel to the shaft of the femur. Now make the osteotomy cut at the transverse line in the cortex in a transverse or oblique direction, depending on the correction desired. If rotational, in addition to angular, correction is desired, complete the osteotomy through the medial cortex. By means of longitudinal mark in the femoral cortex as a guide, rotate the femur as needed to correct femoral anteversion (generally 30 to 45 degrees). To achieve varus angulation, remove an appropriate wedge of bone from the medial cortex to achieve a neck-shaft angle of 120 to 135 degrees (Fig. 1-22, *E*).

Next attach the side plate to the base of the screw. When properly aligned with the hexagonal head of the screw, the side plate should fit flush to the proximal femoral shaft (Fig. 1-22, *F*). If not, adjust it slightly with a bending instrument or with a plate with a different angle. Secure the side plate with the screw with the use of either the T-holder or securing bolt. Insert the securing bolt through the hexagonal hole in the side plate and into the hexagonal head of the screw. Tighten it completely to firmly join the proximal and distal fragments. Secure the plate to the femoral shaft with a bone clamp if desired. Confirm the position of the fixation device and the proximal and distal fragments with anteroposterior roentgenogram or image intensification. Then firmly fix the side plate to the femoral shaft with 4.5 mm bone screws and a hexagonal-head screwdriver (Fig. 1-22, *G*). Irrigate the wound and close in layers, inserting a suction drain if needed. Apply a one and a half spica cast.

▶ *Postoperative management.* The spica cast is worn for 8 to 12 weeks, until union is effected. The internal fixation may be removed 12 to 24 months after the osteotomy if desired.

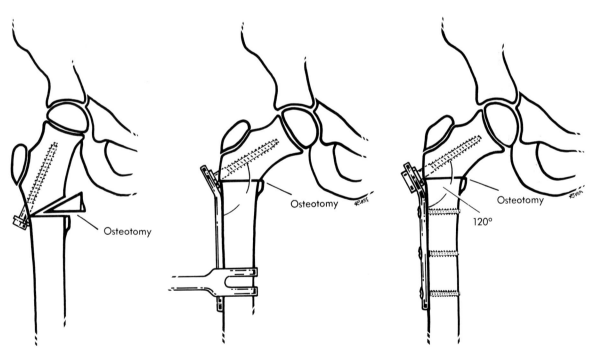

E, Removal of wedge. **F,** Attachment of side plate. **G,** Final attachment of side plate.

Varus Derotational Osteotomy with AO Fixation

The Müller system includes a seating chisel, seating chisel guide, flag triangles, and a slotted hammer. Plate variations include a 90-degree plate for adults, adolescents, and children; a 120-degree double-angle plate; a 95-degree condylar blade plate; and a 130-degree plate (Fig. 1-23). The 90-degree plate generally is used for varus and valgus osteotomies that require up to 25 degrees of correction (Fig. 1-24, *A*); for more than 25 degrees of correction the 120-degree double-angle plate is recommended (Fig. 1-24, *B*). An essential feature of the Müller technique is a subtrochanteric transverse osteotomy, which allows for both rotation and displacement of the fragments. According to Müller, in children younger than 15 years, resection of wedges is unnecessary; the fragments are simply tilted to form an opening wedge osteotomy that, despite the gap created, will unite rapidly (Fig. 1-25). Because of the stability of fixation, Müller does not recommend postoperative immobilization in a spica cast and reports that union usually occurs within 5 to 8 weeks. The 90-degree plate or condylar plate can be placed under tension with a tensioning device to achieve axial compression.

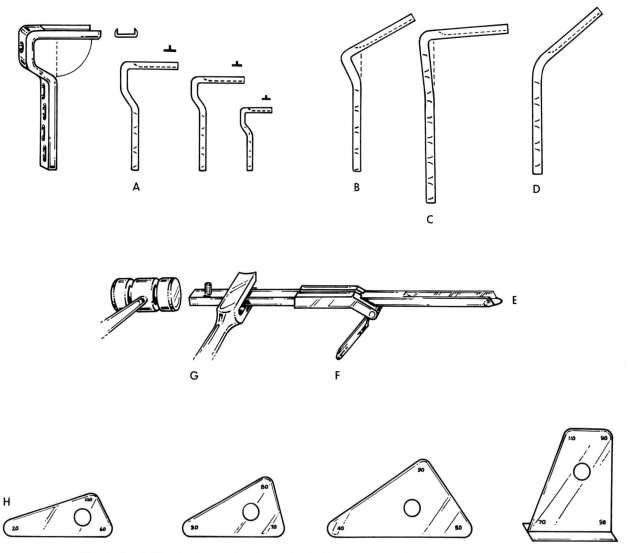

Fig. 1-23 Müller fixation system for pediatric hip osteotomy. **A,** 90-degree plate for adolescents, children, and small children. **B,** Double-angled, 120-degree plate. **C,** Condylar blade plate. **D,** 130-degree blade plate. **E,** U-shaped seating chisel. **F,** Seating chisel guide. **G,** Slotted hammer. **H,** Triangles used to determine angles. (Redrawn from Müller ME. In Schatzker J, editor: The intertrochanteric osteotomy, Berlin, 1984, Springer-Verlag.)

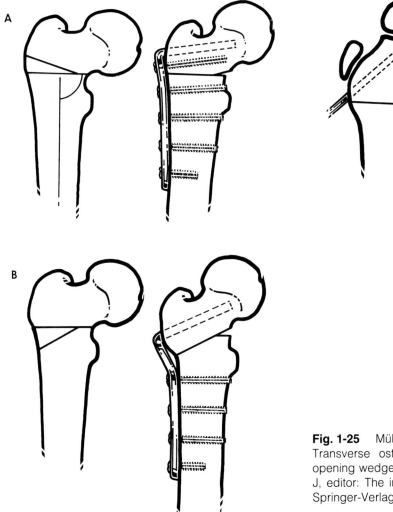

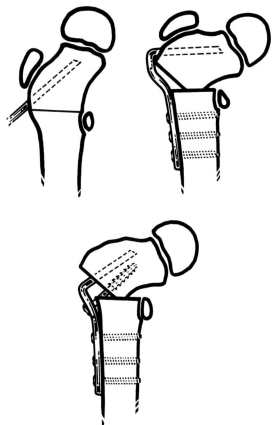

Fig. 1-25 Müller intertrochanteric osteotomy (see text). Transverse osteotomy with fragments tilted to form opening wedge. (Redrawn from Müller ME. In Schatzker J, editor: The intertrochanteric osteotomy, Berlin, 1984, Springer-Verlag.)

Fig. 1-24 **A,** 90-degree plate used for osteotomies requiring up to 25 degrees correction. **B,** 120-degree double-angle plate used for more than 25 degrees correction. (Redrawn from Müller ME. In Schatzker J, editor: The intertrochanteric osteotomy, Berlin, 1984, Springer-Verlag.)

▲*Technique (Müller)*. Make a straight lateral incision, approximately 15 to 20 cm long. Open the fascia in line with the skin incision, and reflect the vastus lateralis muscle anteriorly and medially. Insert a reverse retractor medially around the calcar and another just medial to the tip of the greater trochanter. Insert a Kirschner wire parallel to the femoral neck and to the upper edge of the 60-degree angle guide (Fig. 1-26, *A*), taking care not to place the wire in the greater trochanter apophysis. In an older child a second wire may be used to determine the angle of insertion for the seating chisel. Place a transverse Kirschner wire in the subtrochanteric area just distal to the level of the osteotomy site (Fig. 1-26, *B*). Insert the seating chisel parallel and adjacent to the first Kirschner wire (Fig. 1-26, *C*). The chisel should be aimed at the center of the femoral neck and inserted to a depth of approximately 3.5 to 4.5 cm; it should not violate the trochanteric epiphysis or capital femoral epiphysis in the young child. The angle formed by the seating chisel and the transverse pin represents the amount of varus tilting necessary through the osteotomy site. Now place a reverse retractor medially and subperiosteally to the lesser trochanter, and with an oscillating saw transect the femur at right angles to its long axis (Fig. 1-26, *D*). Using the seating chisel as

a lever, tilt the proximal fragments into varus and, with the oscillating saw, cut a small wedge medially, starting in the middle of the osteotomy site parallel to the seating chisel (Fig. 1-26, *E*). Remove the seating chisel and insert the blade of the right-angle osteotomy plate carefully into the precut channel. With the plate engaged, reduce the osteotomy, and clamp the plate to the shaft. Check for any rotational component, and confirm the proper length of the proximal portion of the plate with image intensification (Fig. 1-26, *F*).

If necessary, now fix the tensioning device on the femur, and place the osteotomy under axial compression by tightening the device (Fig. 1-26, *G*). If alignment is satisfactory, fix the plate to the femoral shaft with screws and remove the tensioning device. Note that the last screw traverses only one cortex so that it will not act as a stress riser (Fig. 1-26, *H*).

▲*Postoperative management*. If the child is younger than 7 years or if fixation is not secure, a hip spica cast is used after surgery. In the older, more compliant child, the cast is not used and nonweight-bearing crutch ambulation is allowed as soon as tolerated. The osteotomy site generally heals within 6 to 8 weeks.

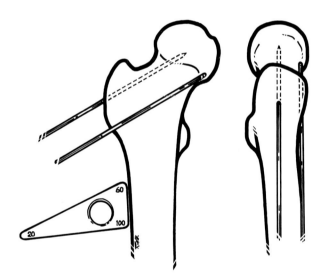

A, Insertion of guide wire with use of angle guide.

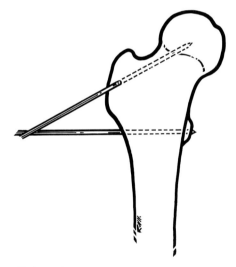

B, Insertion of second guide wire distal to osteotomy level.

Fig. 1-26   Müller intertrochanteric osteotomy (see text). (**A** to **H** redrawn from Müller ME. In Schatzker J, editor: The intertrochanteric osteotomy, Berlin, 1984, Springer-Verlag.)

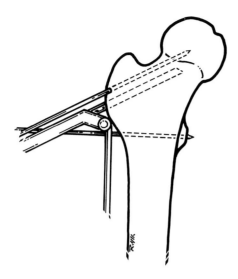

C, Insertion of seating chisel.

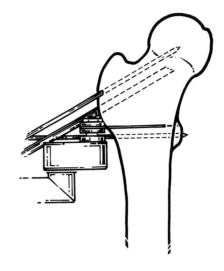

D, Transection of femur.

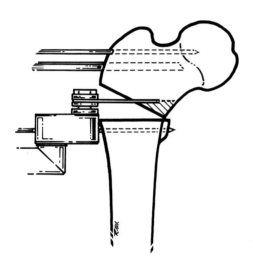

E, Removal of wedge.

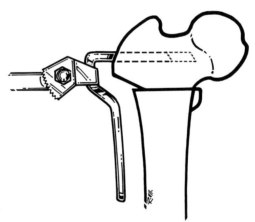

F, Reduction of osteotomy.

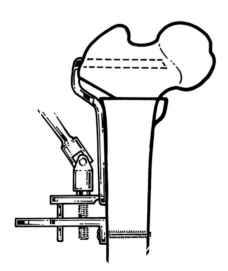

G, Use of tensioning device.

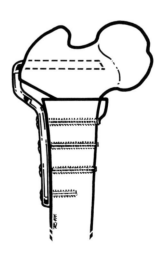

H, Screw placement.

Varus Derotational Osteotomy with Altdorf Clamp

The Altdorf hip clamp is a modification of the Becker angled clamp developed by Wagner and is available in three sizes. The proximal end of the clamp is bifurcated and forms an angle of 130 degrees with the rest of the plate. The device is malleable so that it can be adjusted with bending irons (Fig. 1-27, *A*). The plate has two flat screw holes to allow shift during compression; the most proximal hole is round to allow insertion of a lag screw into the proximal fragment (Fig. 1-27, *B*). Alonso, Lovell, and Lovejoy reported good results with this device and list as advantages a decrease in complications, especially of lateral prominence, because the device is inserted at the osteotomy site; a decrease in the risk of injury to the trochanteric physis; and the prevention of rotation. They did find, however, more complications in children older than 8 years and recommend the device for children younger than 8 years.

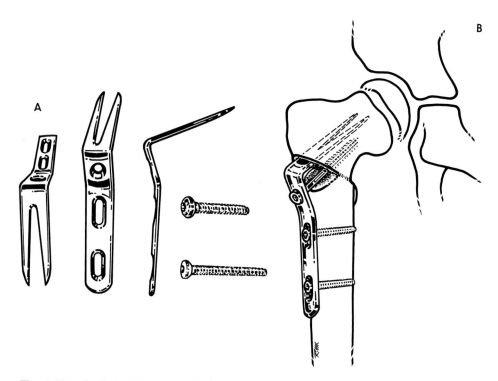

Fig. 1-27   A, Altdorf hip clamp. **B,** Note round proximal hole for insertion of lag screw. (Redrawn from Alonso JE, Lovell WW, and Lovejoy JF: J Pediatr Orthop 6:399, 1986.)

▲*Technique (Alonso et al)*. Place the patient supine on a fracture table with the involved extremity draped free. A conventional operating table may be used with an extension to allow the use of an image intensifier. Approach the hip through a lateral incision to expose the proximal end of the femoral shaft and distal portion of the greater trochanter. Use two 3-mm Steinmann pins as guide pins, placing the first in the soft tissue anterior to the femoral neck to identify the calcar and to determine anteversion. Place the second pin in the bone below the greater trochanteric physis, making certain it is parallel to the first pin. Score the anterior cortex of the femur at this level to monitor rotation (Fig. 1-28, *A*). Using roentgenograms or image intensification for orientation, make the intertrochanteric osteotomy at the level of the first guide pin. Make a second cut in the distal femur, and remove a medial wedge approximately one third the width of the femoral shaft (Fig. 1-28, *B*). Insert the bifurcated blade of the hip clamp into the osteotomy surface of the proximal fragment. The further medially the bifurcated blade is inserted, the more medial the displacement of the distal fragment. Place a screw in the distal hole of the plate, adjacent to the lateral cortex of the femoral shaft (Fig. 1-28, *C*). Insert a second screw to pull the shaft to the plate, and place the proximal fragment into the varus position (Fig. 1-28, *D*). Insert an interfragmentary screw through the round proximal hole into the proximal fragment (Fig. 1-28, *E*). A 3.5 or 4.0 mm cancellous malleolar screw can be used.

▲*Postoperative management*. Postoperative spica cast immobilization is not routinely recommended; however, immobilization may be indicated in the young, noncompliant child or in the child with spasticity.

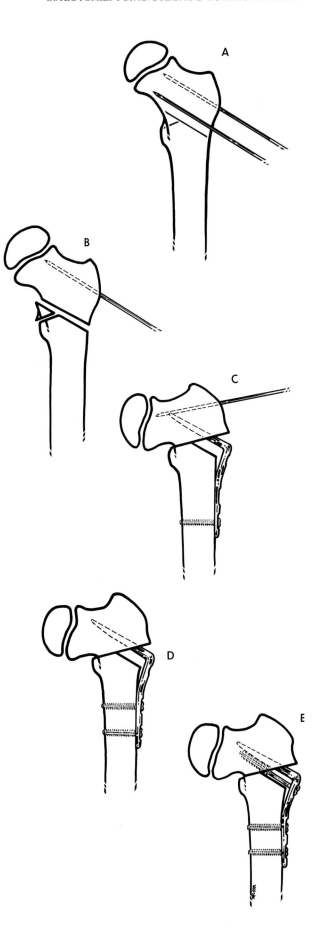

Fig. 1-28 Varus derotational osteotomy with Altdorf hip clamp (see text). **A,** Placement of guide pins. **B,** Removal of medial wedge. **C,** Attachment of plate. **D,** Insertion of second screw for compression. **E,** Use of malleolar screw. (Redrawn from Alonso JE, Lovell WW, and Lovejoy JF: J Pediatr Orthop 6:399, 1986.)

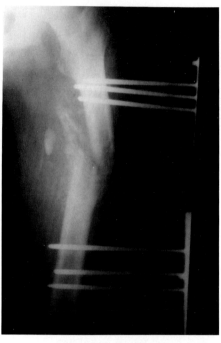

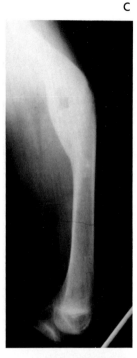

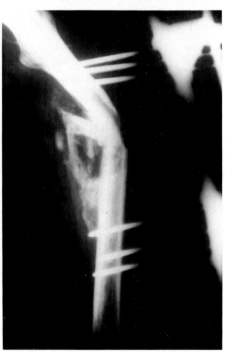

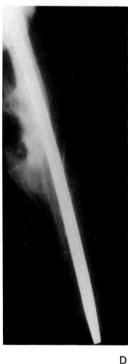

A

B

C

D

Femur

Most angular deformities of the femoral shaft are varus deformities and may occur because of developmental, congenital, or acquired conditions (malunion of fractures). Most anterior angulation deformities of the femur are well tolerated and require no treatment, as are most rotational deformities. Varus deformities, however, are unsightly and may cause functional disability. Compensatory osteotomies for midshaft angular deformities include conventional subtrochanteric and supracondylar osteotomies, as well as more recent techniques for "closed" osteotomies fixed with intramedullary rods.

Diaphyseal osteotomies fixed with standard plates and screws applied at right angles to the osteotomy have produced frequent complications, particularly fracture below the plate or through the weakened bone after plate removal. The closed technique of intramedullary fixation avoids this complication. Basically, a guide pin first is passed down the intramedullary canal to the site of maximum angulation. Then, through a small lateral incision or by closed intramedullary method, an osteotomy is made to allow straightening of the angulation and passage of the intramedullary rod (Fig. 1-29, *A* to *D*). Frequently, multiple-level osteotomies in different planes are required to correct the deformity and allow smooth passage of the guide pin and rod, and shortening of the femur may be required to avoid stretching the neurovascular structures. The intramedullary rod is inserted after gentle reaming of the femoral canal. In older children postoperative immobilization generally is not required and results are satisfactory. The technique generally should not be used in young children because of the size of the intramedullary rods and the risk of violating the proximal greater trochanteric apophysis and distal femoral physis. In young children with multiple angular deformities as a result of osteogenesis imperfecta or myelomeningocele, however, intramedullary rodding is beneficial because it serves as an internal splint and corrects the deformity. Steinmann pins, Rush rods, and Bailey-Dubow telescoping rods are all smooth and pass through the physis, causing only minimal or no damage.

Fig. 1-29   A, Femoral fracture initially treated with external fixation. **B,** Healing in varus, flexed position. **C,** Malunion in anteroposterior and lateral planes. **D,** After osteotomy and intramedullary rodding to correct malalignment.

Closed Femoral Osteotomy with Intramedullary Fixation

More recently, the Russell-Taylor interlocking nail system has proved effective for correction of angular deformity of the femur, as well as for femoral fractures and limb length equalization procedures. Proximal and distal locking transfixing screws permit fixation of osteotomy sites between the distal fifth of the femur and just distal to the lesser trochanter. Osteotomies at the isthmus can be treated by conventional unlocked methods, especially if the osteotomy is stable. Osteotomies proximal to the isthmus require proximal locking screws, and more distal osteotomies should be locked with one or two distal screws. Grossly unstable osteotomies should be locked both distally and proximally to maintain length and prevent rotation. Preoperative roentgenograms should be used to determine the site of the osteotomy, the amount of resection required to realign the femur, the proper nail size, the amount of reaming required,

and the appropriate length of the nail. Overlapping of the angulated femur requires a limited transverse osteotomy followed by either traction or external fixation to distract the femur out to length; this usually requires 5 to 6 days with external fixation. Once maximum length has been achieved, the external fixator is removed and closed osteotomy is performed (Fig. 1-30). Nail length should allow the proximal end to lie flush with the tip of the greater trochanter and the distal end to lie between the proximal pole of the patella and the distal femoral physis. In the growing child the distal femoral physis and greater trochanteric apophysis should be avoided; because this is not always possible, intramedullary fixation generally should be used only near the end of growth. The proximal and distal locking screws should be removed only if the osteotomy site is not healing or is distracted; removal of the locking screws allows "dynamization" of the fragments with weight bearing.

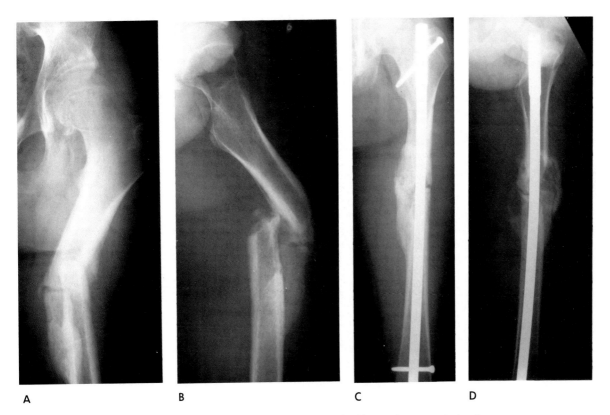

A B C D

Fig. 1-30 **A** and **B,** Proximal femoral fracture initially treated with traction at early healing shows excessive valgus and flexion.**C** and **D,** After osteotomy at fracture site and closed intramedullary rodding.

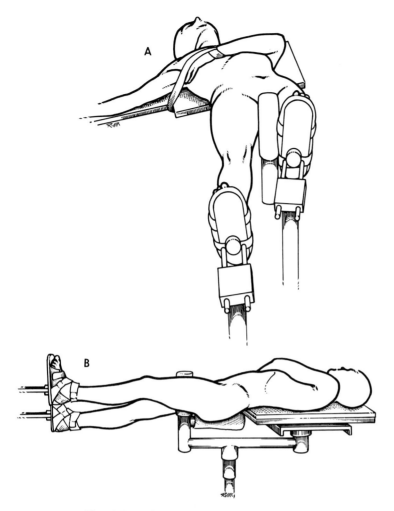

Fig. 1-31 Closed femoral osteotomy with intramedullary fixation with Russell-Taylor interlocking nail (see text). **A,** Position of patient. **B,** Traction applied through footplate. (Redrawn from Russell TA, Taylor JC, and LaVelle DG: Russell-Taylor interlocking intramedullary nails, technique manual, Memphis, 1985, Richards Manufacturing Co.)

Fig. 1-32 Closed femoral osteotomy with intramedullary fixation with Russell-Taylor interlocking nail (see text). (**A to D** and **F to I,** redrawn from Russell TA, Taylor JC, and LaVelle DG: Russell-Taylor interlocking intramedullary nails, technique manual, Memphis, 1985, Richards Manufacturing Co.)

▶ *Technique.* Place the patient supine with the trunk and affected extremity adducted (Fig. 1-31, *A*); the lateral decubitus position may be used if the angulation deformity is severe. Flex the affected hip to 15 degrees, and apply traction through the footplate if necessary (Fig. 1-31, *B*). Prepare and drape the buttocks, ipsilateral thigh, and involved extremity down to the popliteal crease, and cover the image intensifier with sterile isolation drapes.

Make an oblique incision 2 cm distal to the proximal tip of the greater trochanter, and continue it proximally and medially for 3 to 10 cm (Fig. 1-32, *A*). Incise the fascia of the gluteus maximus in line with the skin incision, and divide the gluteus maximus in line with its fibers. Identify the subfascial plane of the gluteus maximus, and palpate the trochanteric fossa. Use self-retaining retractors on the gluteus muscle. Trafton et al recommend using a percutaneous guide pin inserted manually at the entrance site and enlarging the site with a cannulated reamer (Fig. 1-32, *B*); this method is particularly efficient when the patient is supine. Alternatively, introduce a curved awl at the trochanteric fossa, with the straight portion parallel to the floor and in line with the femoral shaft (Fig. 1-32, *C*). Make the opening directly in the midplane of the femur, verifying position with anteroposterior and lateral image intensification. Use the awl to further enlarge the entry portal, and insert the blunt tip of a

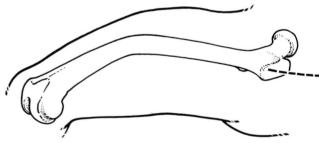

A, Incision.

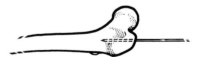

B, Percutaneous guide pin as recommended by Trafton et al.

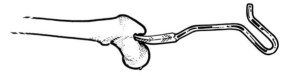

C, Introduction of curved awl.

tapered T-handle reamer to enlarge the metaphyseal canal, taking care to avoid the greater trochanteric physis. Introduce the ball-guide rod to the level of maximum angulation or until its passage is impeded (Fig. 1-32, *D*); verify position with image intensification. Then make a short lateral incision approximately 5 to 7 cm long over this area. Carry dissection down to the lateral aspect of the femur, retracting the vastus lateralis anteriorly. Using an oscillating saw, a Midas Rex drill, or other appropriate cutting instrument, make an osteotomy at the site of maximum angulation. Take an appropriate wedge at this site, or shorten the femur, to allow the ball-tip guide rod to be passed into the intramedullary canal and straighten the angulation (Fig. 1-32, *E*). If angulation is severe and the ball-tip guide is impeded more than once, additional osteotomies may be necessary. Pass the rod distal to the osteotomy site and, using the cannulated reamer, ream the canal of the proximal femur to the appropriate diameter. Using progressively larger reamers in 0.5-mm increments, ream the proximal femur to 1.5 mm larger than the planned nail size (rods are available in sizes from 9 to 16 mm). Use the skin protector during reaming. If the osteotomy cannot be reduced and the ball-tip guide

passed easily, the internal fracture alignment device may be used (Fig. 1-32, *F*). Once alignment is attained, advance the guide pin distally just proximal to the physis. Remove the alignment device if used. Verify containment and appropriate length of the guide rod with image intensification and the nail length gauge (Fig. 1-32, *G*). Verify reaming with the reamer template; reaming to 1.5 mm larger than nail size is mandatory to prevent nail incarceration (Fig. 1-32, *H*). Hold the proximal drill guide with its cylindrical handle pointed upward (outward when the patient is supine). Hold the locking nail horizontally so that its curve matches that of the femur. Attach the key on the guide with the keyway on the nail and screw, and insert the attachment bolt through the guide into the nail. Attach the sliding hammer (or supine position driver) to the hexagonal bolt of the guide and, using the handle to control nail rotation, insert the nail (Fig. 1-32, *I*). Tighten the handle of the proximal drill guide assembly as needed before final seating of the nail. Withdraw the curved ball-tip guide wire after the rod has entered the distal fragment by several centimeters. Then drive the nail until the proximal end is flush with the tip of the greater trochanter and remove the sliding hammer.

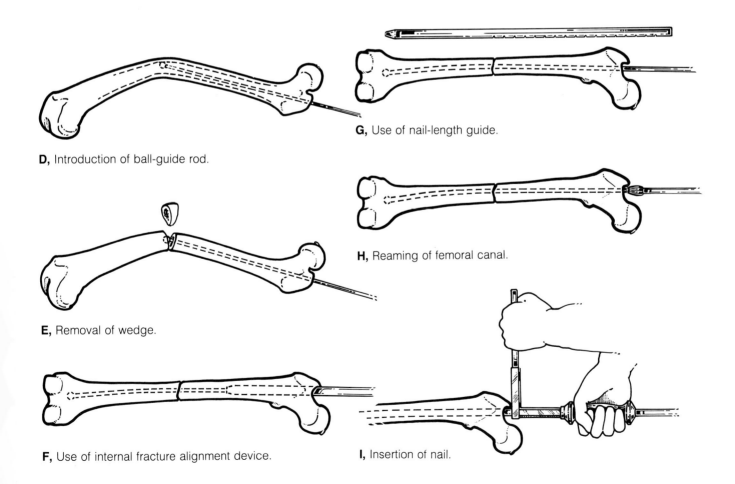

D, Introduction of ball-guide rod.

E, Removal of wedge.

F, Use of internal fracture alignment device.

G, Use of nail-length guide.

H, Reaming of femoral canal.

I, Insertion of nail.

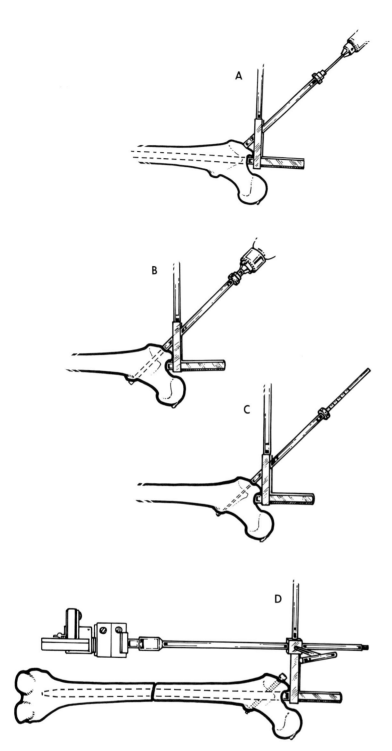

For proximal interlocking, make sure the hexagonal bolt is tightened, and then place a set of three stacking drill sleeves (green, 8 mm; blue, 4.8 mm; and red, 3.2 mm) within the proximal drill guide. Using the 3.2-mm threaded guide pin, dimple the bone for the drill bit (Fig. 1-33, *A*). Remove the guide pin and the red sleeve. Insert the 4.8-mm drill bit (blue), and drill through both cortices; make a measurement using the 4.8-mm drill calibration and record the length against the top of the blue drill sleeve (Fig. 1-33, *B*). Remove the blue drill sleeve. Using the depth gauge, confirm the proper locking screw by reading the length against the top of the green drill sleeve (Fig. 1-33, *C*). The drill sleeve must be against the cortex for accurate reading. Insert the selected self-tapping diagonal locking screw through the drill sleeve with the T-handle hexagonal driver, then remove the hexagonal driver and drill sleeve.

Before attaching the distal targeting device, confirm with image intensification that the distal hole of the nail appears perfectly centered on the screen (perfect circle). Allow the maximum distance between the lateral thigh and image intensifier. Make a distal incision holding the knife handle with a ring forceps to ascertain incision position with image intensification. Position the C-arm of the image intensifier high enough above the thigh to allow the drill sleeve to be inserted through the device. Attach the adapter block to the handle of the drill guide so that proper identification (left or right) is facing the ceiling (Fig. 1-33, *D*) or facing laterally if the patient is supine. Insert the shaft to the distal targeting device through the adapter block until the shaft calibration (read from the proximal side of the block) equals the nail length. Adjust the height of the adapter block and distal targeting device assembly so that the target platform is far enough from the skin to allow a 10- to 15-

Fig. 1-33 Closed femoral osteotomy with intramedullary fixation with Russell-Taylor interlocking nail (see text). **A,** Locating site for drilling. **B,** Drilling proximal hole. **C,** Use of depth gauge. **D,** Attachment of adapter block. (Redrawn from Russell TA, Taylor JC, and LaVelle DG: Russell-Taylor interlocking intramedullary nails, technique manual, Memphis, 1985, Richards Manufacturing Co.)

degree tilt, but close enough so that the 6-inch-long green drill sleeve touches the lateral cortex. Lock the assembly by tightening the hexagonal screw with the hexagonal driver. The distal targeting device allows control of four separate axes along the anteroposterior, cephalad-caudad, transverse, and coronal planes. Using the adjustment instrument, rotate gear No. 1 to move the distal targeting device along the anteroposterior axis until the cross hair bisects the more proximal hole (Fig. 1-34, *A*). To make adjustments in the cephalad-caudad axis, rotate adjustment knob No. 2 on the shaft of the distal targeting device until the other cross hair bisects the same hole (Fig. 1-34, *A*).

Insert the target bead, and gently tighten the thumb screw. Rotate gear No. 4 to move the bead into view. Then rotate gear No. 3 to move the bead into the coronal plane and center it over the cross hair (Fig. 1-34, *B*). Rotate gear No. 4 to move the bead into the transverse plane and center it perfectly with the hole (Fig. 1-34, *C*). The axis of the distal targeting device should now be the same as the screw hole axis.

Remove the target bead and insert the green drill sleeve through the plastic locating block to the cortex. A final check with the image intensifier is mandatory; a near-perfect circle should be visible. If not, repeat the distal targeting. Insert the blue and red drill sleeves (Fig. 1-34, *D*), and drill through both cortices with a threaded–tip guide pin, and confirm by image intensification that the guide pin is centered within the nail hole. Remove the guide pin and the red drill sleeve. Use the 4.8-mm drill in the blue sleeve, and drill through the lateral cortex, nail hole, and medial cortex; make a depth measurement using the 4.8-mm drill calibration and read the length against the top of the blue drill sleeve. Remove the drill and blue drill sleeve.

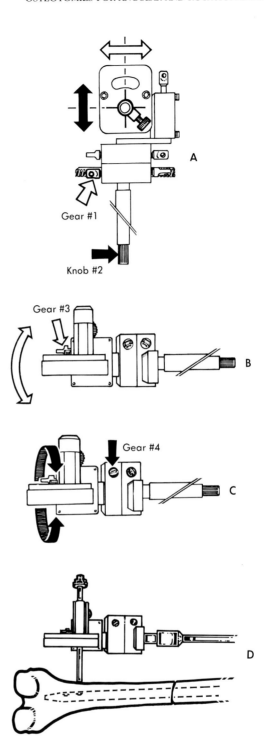

Fig. 1-34 Closed femoral osteotomy with intramedullary fixation with Russell-Taylor interlocking nail (see text). **A** to **D,** Use of distal targeting device. (Redrawn from Russell TA, Taylor JC, and LaVelle DG: Russell-Taylor interlocking intramedullary nails, technique manual, Memphis, 1985, Richards Manufacturing Co.)

To confirm proper locking screw length, use the depth gauge and read the length against the top of the green drill sleeve. Then insert the selected self-tapping screw through the green drill sleeve with a T-handle hexagonal driver. Place the second screw into the distal hole by repeating the targeting procedure, or if there is no valgus tilt in the first screw, use the dual drill sleeve to locate the second hole (Fig. 1-35). If the latter method is chosen, insert the drill sleeve through the incision to the cortex and insert the screw as described. Remove the drill sleeve, and disassemble the distal targeting device.

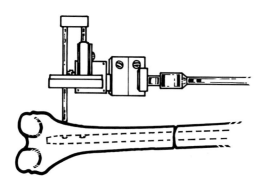

Fig. 1-35 Closed femoral osteotomy with intramedullary fixation with Russell-Taylor interlocking nail (see text). Insertion of second distal screw. (Redrawn from Russell TA, Taylor JC, and LaVelle DG: Russell-Taylor interlocking intramedullary nails, technique manual, Memphis, 1985, Richards Manufacturing Co.)

An alternate method to the distal targeting device is a freehand technique described by Hall. Place the image intensifier in the lateral position over the distal area; a true lateral image should be produced and the screw holes should appear circular. Otherwise, adjust leg rotation to obtain a true lateral image of the rod. When the holes are completely circular, center a ring forceps over the proximal hole on the lateral side of the leg. Then introduce a No. 15 blade within the confines of the ring forceps. Make a longitudinal incision along the midline axis of the leg, and carry this incision down to the bone. Repeat the procedure at the distal screw hole, and connect the two incisions with an incision approximately 3 cm in length, also carried down to the bone. Using image intensification, adjust the awl until the point is centered over the screw hole. Return the image intensifier to the anteroposterior view, and maintain constant pressure on the awl to prevent skidding. Swing the awl perpendicular to the axis of the bone, and adjust the angle of the anteroposterior image so that the awl is directed toward the hole and the nail, aligning the awl in both the lateral and anteroposterior planes. Using a mallet, drive the awl to the lateral side of the rod. Remove the handle of the awl, and obtain a lateral image of the femur. The awl should point directly at the center of the hole within the rod. If not, make necessary adjustments. Once proper alignment has been obtained, withdraw the awl, place the drill in the hole, and drill through the rod and opposite cortex. Determine the length of the screw, using the depth gauge, and insert the appropriate screw in the proper position. Repeat the procedure on the distal screw hole if necessary.

Obtain a final image to confirm satisfactory placement of the screws. Close all incisions in a routine manner, and apply a sterile dressing.

▶*Postoperative management.* Touchdown weight bearing with crutches is allowed 2 to 3 days after surgery. Non–weight-bearing and spica cast immobilization are used only for noncompliant patients. Full weight bearing usually is allowed by 8 to 10 weeks after surgery. Dynamization (removal of either the proximal or distal locking screws to allow axial loading of the femur) is not always indicated and should be considered only if delayed union is determined 3 to 6 weeks after surgery.

Supracondylar Femoral Osteotomy

Most angular deformities in the supracondylar area of the femur are varus deformities as a result of developmental or congenital anomalies or of malunion. A lateral closing wedge osteotomy is the simplest means of correction of these deformities, although some length of the femur is lost. For more complex deformities, which include rotational malalignment or flexion contracture of the knee, multiplane or extension osteotomies can be performed. Extension osteotomy may place extreme pressure on the posterior neurovascular bundle, and shortening of the femur may be required. Closing wedge osteotomies are preferable because of their inherent stability, but opening wedge osteotomies may be performed in this area. A lateral approach allows placement of the wedge laterally or medially. Resection of bony bridges at the distal femoral physis also can be done in conjunction with the opening wedge osteotomy. Correction of femoral anteversion usually is better accomplished with intertrochanteric osteotomy because this is closer to the actual deformity. Internal fixation generally is not recommended in this area, except in the older child, because of the necessity of crossing the physis with the fixation devices. Therefore pins and plaster and external fixation usually are better choices for fixation of supracondylar osteotomies.

Preoperative and intraoperative planning is essential for complex, multiplane, supracondylar osteotomies. Tracings and cut-outs made from preoperative roentenograms should be used to determine osteotomy sites and appropriate wedge resection (Fig. 1-36). Draping both extremities free allows comparison of the affected limb to the contralateral side to confirm proper alignment. Orientation marks placed on the bone sufficiently proximal and distal to the planned osteotomy site remain in place for reference after the osteotomy incision is made. The cut may be made in two planes and derotated in the third plane. This frequently leaves a rough, uneven area of bone at the osteotomy site. Derotation may be done first and then a single or multidirectional wedge taken to leave flat, smooth osteotomy surfaces for apposition (Fig. 1-37).

▶ *Technique (pins and plaster).* Place the patient supine on an operating table with an extension to allow image intensification. Prepare and drape the extremity in the usual fashion. Expose the femur from the lateral side through a straight lateral incision, reflecting the vastus lateralis, lateral intermuscular septum, and iliotibial band anteriorly. Locate the physis by exposure or image intensification. If necessary, ligate branches of the perforating arteries as they ascend through the lateral intermuscular

septum. Incise the periosteum at the linea aspera femoris and reflect all muscle mass anteriorly with the periosteum. Use a hemostat or guide wire in the soft tissue, and note its placement relative to the distal femoral plate as shown on image intensification; select an osteotomy site proximal to the physis. Incise the periosteum proximal to the physis, and place reverse retractors subperiosteally around the distal femur. Place longitudinal orientation marks in the femur, make the appropriate single or multidirectional osteotomy, and derotate the femur. Place two pins proximal and one or two distal to the osteotomy site, making certain the distal pins avoid the physis. If external fixation is to be used, use the appropriate threaded pins. Place the pins at an oblique angle corresponding to the angle of correction desired. After osteotomy, bring the pins horizontally until parallel. Close the soft tissues and apply a sterile dressing; then apply a plaster cast incorporating the pins or an external fixator.

▶ *Postoperative management.* Frequent neurovascular evaluation is imperative. Any loss of function should be determined to be due to either ischemic or neurovascular compromise. All constricting bandages should be removed, and arteriography or returning the extremity to the deformed position should be considered. Pins are removed at approximately 6 weeks after surgery. Weight bearing usually is not allowed for 12 weeks.

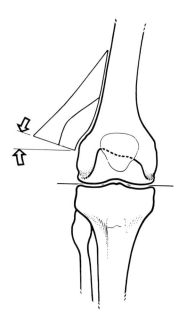

Fig. 1-36 Determination of osteotomy site and appropriate wedge to be resected. (Redrawn from Holz U. In Hierholzerg G and Muller KH, editors: Corrective osteotomies of the lower extremity after trauma, Berlin, 1985, Springer-Verlag.)

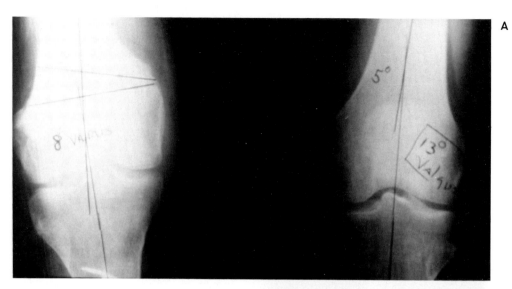

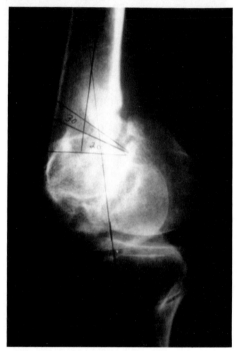

Fig. 1-37 After treatment of femoral fracture in skeletal traction, young patient has malunion with 8 degrees of varus (**A**), 30 degrees of flexion (**B**), and severe internal rotation (**C**). **D** and **E,** Correction obtained by multiplane osteotomy fixed with right-angle blade plate.

C

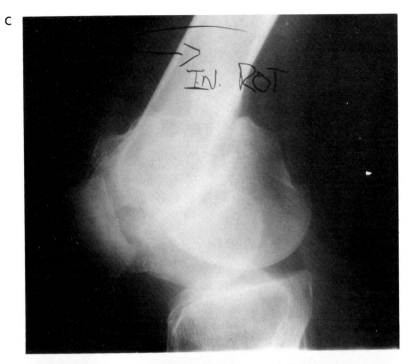

D

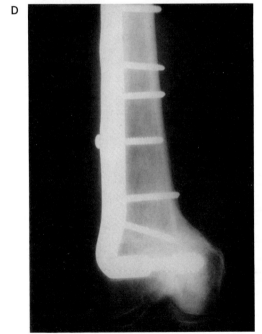

E

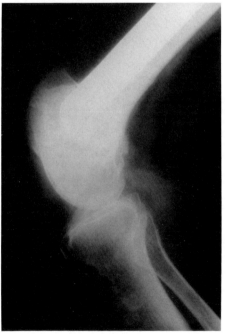

Lateral Supracondylar Femoral Osteotomy

Right angle plates have been used successfully in the correction of distal femoral deformities in adults, and they may be used in older children in whom the physes have closed or have been destroyed.

▲ *Technique (Holz)*. Make a longitudinal incision on the lateral aspect of the distal femur, following an imaginary line that connects the greater trochanter to the lateral femoral condyle and then curves slightly to cross the tibial tubercle. Release the vastus lateralis, and retract it anteriorly. With reverse retractors, expose the lateral femoral cortex. Apply the condylar plate guide to the lateral cortex (Fig. 1-38, *A*), and place a triangular angle guide against the lower edge to mark the desired angle of correction. Insert a Kirschner wire into the femoral condyle parallel to the condyles, normally parallel to the joint line of the knee. Drive the seating chisel into the condyles parallel to the guide wire, and attach the chisel guide so that it is aligned with the axis of the femoral shaft (Fig. 1-38, *B*). If a flexion or recurvatum deformity is

to be corrected, as well as the varus deformity, the chisel guide should be diverged posteriorly or anteriorly by the desired angle of correction (Fig. 1-38, *C*). Loosen the seating chisel, and make a transverse osteotomy with an oscillating saw (use a chisel in osteoporotic bone). Resect the corrective wedge, and replace the seating chisel with the selected condylar plate. Insert a cancellous screw through the hole next to the plate to secure the plate to the distal femur. If axial compression is desired, use the tensioning device (Fig. 1-38, *D*). Then fix the plate to the femoral shaft with cortex screws (Fig. 1-38, *E* and *F*). Close the wounds in a routine manner, and apply a long leg cast with the knee bent 50 degrees.

Varus osteotomy can be performed in the same manner through a lateral incision. The valgus osteotomy is best fixed with a condylar plate and the varus osteotomy with the right angle plate.

▲ *Postoperative management*. If the osteotomy is stable, the long leg cast can be changed to a cast brace and range of motion exercises begun during the second week.

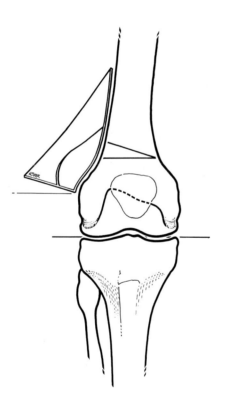

A, Use of triangular angle guide.

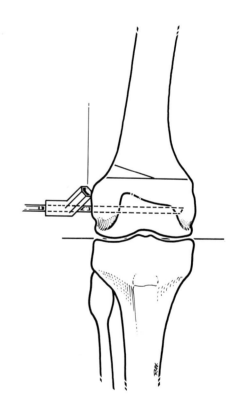

B, Use of seating chisel.

Fig. 1-38   Holz supracondylar femoral osteotomy (see text). (**A** to **F** redrawn from Holz U. In Hierholzerg G and Muller KH, editors: Corrective osteotomies of the lower extremity after trauma, Berlin, 1985, Springer-Verlag.)

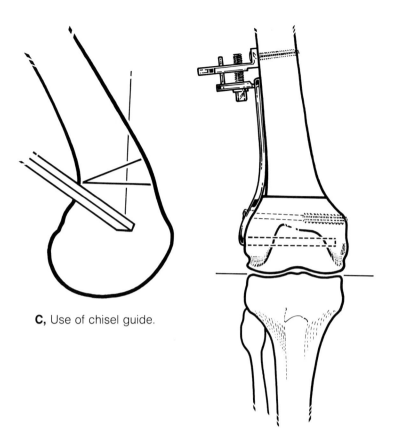

C, Use of chisel guide.

D, Use of tensioning device.

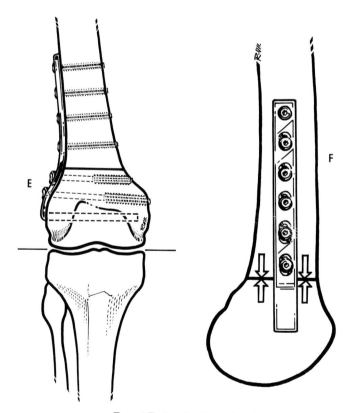

E and **F,** Application of plate.

Tibia

Tibial osteotomies may be performed in the area of the knee joint, in the midshaft of the tibia, or in the distal tibia. Some special considerations must be observed in tibial osteotomies. (1) Neurovascular complications are frequent, usually involving the posterior tibial artery (the artery at risk) at the trifurcation (kinking of the artery). (2) Most tibial osteotomies should be performed below the insertion of the patellar tendon on the tibial tuberosity because more proximal osteotomy may damage the physis. (3) The proximal tibial physis is wavy rather than straight, and this configuration requires careful roentgenographic or image intensification control to be sure osteotomy is not performed through a portion of the physis. (4)

Osteotomies of the midshaft of the tibia have a higher incidence of nonunion than more proximal or distal osteotomies.

The basic deformity for which tibial osteotomy is indicated is varus and valgus hyperextension. Hyperextension deformities generally occur after trauma that causes closure of the anterior portion of the proximal physis, allowing posterior growth and hyperextension deformity of the tibia and knee. Salter-Harris types III and IV fractures of the proximal tibial epiphysis are frequent precursors of this deformity (Fig. 1-39). Varus and valgus deformities also may occur after trauma caused by premature physeal closure, or they may result from developmental or congenital deformities.

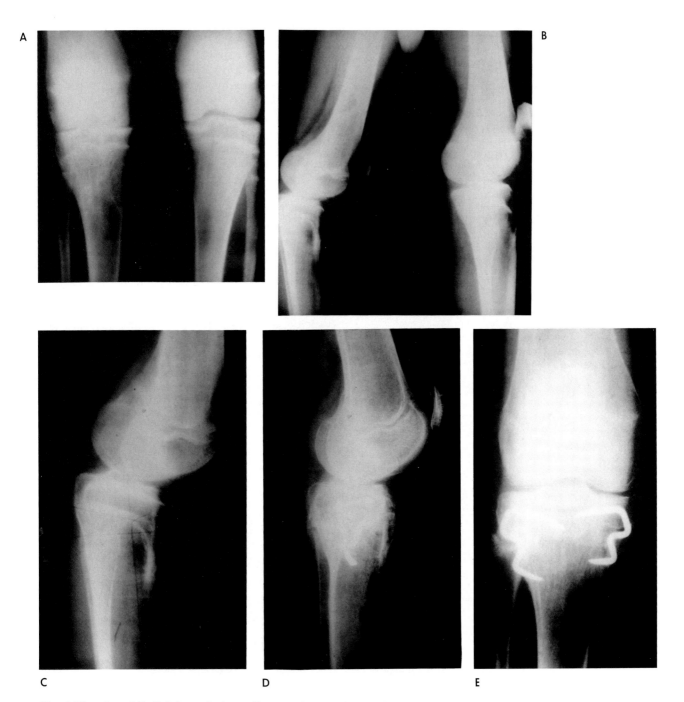

Fig. 1-39 **A** and **B,** Epiphyseal plate still open after proximal tibial epiphyseal fracture; premature fusion and hyperextension are evident on lateral view. **C,** Weight-bearing view shows 16 degrees of hyperextension deformity as a result of proximal phyeal arrest anteriorly and continuation of growth posteriorly. **D** and **E,** High tibial osteotomy performed at skeletal maturity.

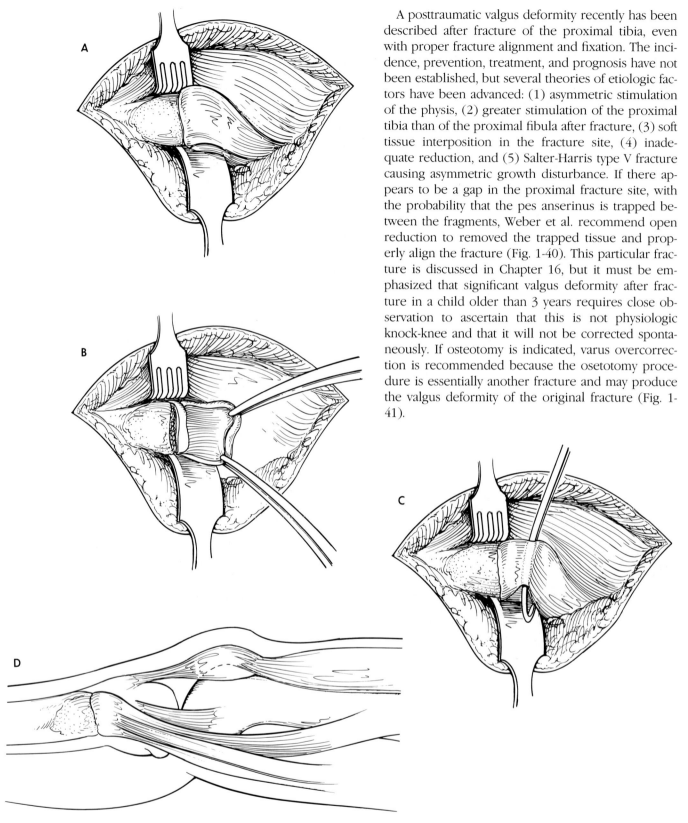

A posttraumatic valgus deformity recently has been described after fracture of the proximal tibia, even with proper fracture alignment and fixation. The incidence, prevention, treatment, and prognosis have not been established, but several theories of etiologic factors have been advanced: (1) asymmetric stimulation of the physis, (2) greater stimulation of the proximal tibia than of the proximal fibula after fracture, (3) soft tissue interposition in the fracture site, (4) inadequate reduction, and (5) Salter-Harris type V fracture causing asymmetric growth disturbance. If there appears to be a gap in the proximal fracture site, with the probability that the pes anserinus is trapped between the fragments, Weber et al. recommend open reduction to removed the trapped tissue and properly align the fracture (Fig. 1-40). This particular fracture is discussed in Chapter 16, but it must be emphasized that significant valgus deformity after fracture in a child older than 3 years requires close observation to ascertain that this is not physiologic knock-knee and that it will not be corrected spontaneously. If osteotomy is indicated, varus overcorrection is recommended because the osetotomy procedure is essentially another fracture and may produce the valgus deformity of the original fracture (Fig. 1-41).

Fig. 1-40 **A** to **D,** Pes anserinus trapped in proximal tibial metaphyseal fracture site; at open reduction the soft tissue interposition is removed. (Redrawn from Weber BG. In Weber BG, Brunner C, and Freuler F, editors: Treatment of fractures in children and adolescents, New York, 1980, Springer-Verlag.)

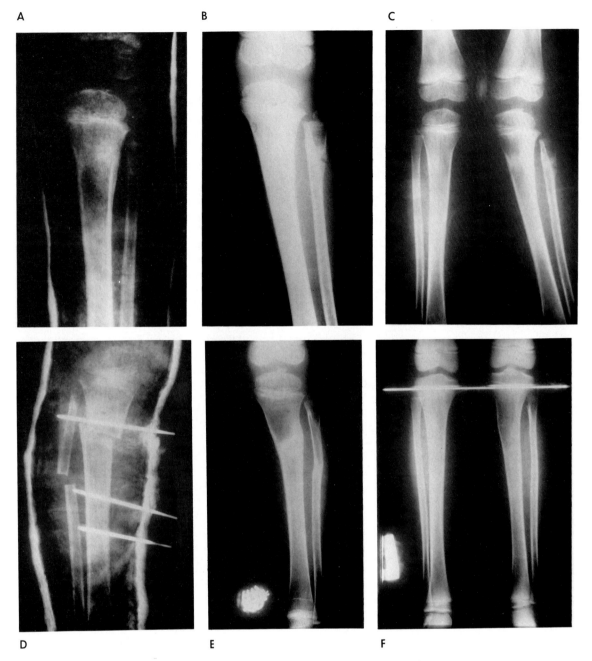

Fig. 1-41 **A,** Fracture of proximal tibial metaphysis in 4-year-old child. **B,** Obvious valgus deformity 8 weeks after fracture. **C,** Progression of valgus deformity 6 months after fracture. **D,** After varus osteotomy of tibia and fibula held with pins in plaster. **E,** Early healing of osteotomy with mild varus overcorrection. **F,** Three years after osteotomy, slight valgus deformity has recurred, but result is functionally and cosmetically good.

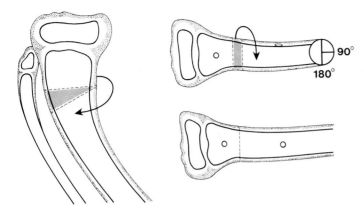

Fig. 1-42   Closing wedge and derotation osteotomy.

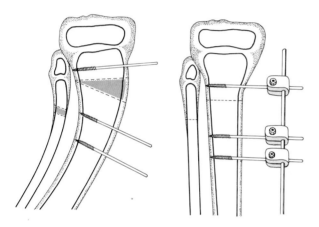

Fig. 1-43   Closing wedge osteotomy.

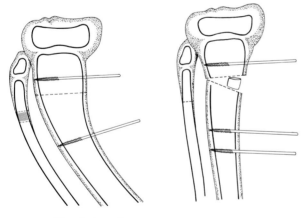

Fig. 1-44   Opening wedge osteotomy.

General principles of tibial osteotomy include careful examination to determine any ligamentous laxity in the knee area before surgery, especially in varus or valgus deformity. A segment of the fibula almost always should be resected at the time of tibial osteotomy to facilitate correction of the tibial deformity. Generally, a segment of 1 to 2 cm, depending on the length of the fibula, should be resected to prevent the fibula's acting as a limiting hinge. This fibular osteotomy may be performed through a separate incision just distal to the proximal third of the fibula, through muscles, thus avoiding the risk of injury to the main sensorimotor branch of the peroneal nerve.

A variety of techniques and fixation devices are used in tibial osteotomies. The *closing wedge osteotomy* (Fig. 1-42) is the most inherently stable, but it has the disadvantage of shortening the tibia. Plate and screw fixation is difficult to position so that it avoids the patellar tendon and physis; if used, the plate should be fixed on the lateral side of the tibia. External fixators or pins in plaster may be used effectively to hold the osteotomy, with the pins placed parallel (Fig. 1-43) or crossing the osteotomy site. The *opening wedge osteotomy* is unstable and usually requires a fibular graft inserted in the open wedge (Fig. 1-44) and rigid internal or external fixation. Slipping of the graft may cause delayed union of the osteotomy site (Fig. 1-45). The opening wedge osteotomy has the advantage of gaining some length in the tibia (one half the base of the opening wedge). *Broomstick or ball-and-socket osteotomy* (Fig. 1-46) is relatively stable but sacrifices some length of the tibia. Pins-in-plaster fixation usually is adequate. An advantage of the broomstick osteotomy is that it allows postoperative manipulation for necessary alignment (Fig. 1-47). *Hinge or offset osteotomy* is most useful when neither internal nor external fixation is appropriate, as in patients with hemophilia, infection, or scarring (Fig. 1-49, *A*) because the "ledge" or "hinge" stabilizes the osteotomy (Fig. 1-48). *Flexion osteotomy,* removal of a large posterior wedge with or without a hinge, may be required for extension deformity (Fig. 1-49, *B*). Because of the vessels in the area of trifurcation, extreme care must be taken to avoid neurovascular injury; adequate exposure is mandatory. Ingram, Siffert, and Storen have described combined epiphyseal and metaphyseal osteotomies (Figs. 1-50 and 1-51) for severe deformity in Blount's disease (pp. 43 and 44), and Beck et al, as well as others, reported good results when osteotomy was combined with bony bar resection (pp. 47 to 51).

A

B

C

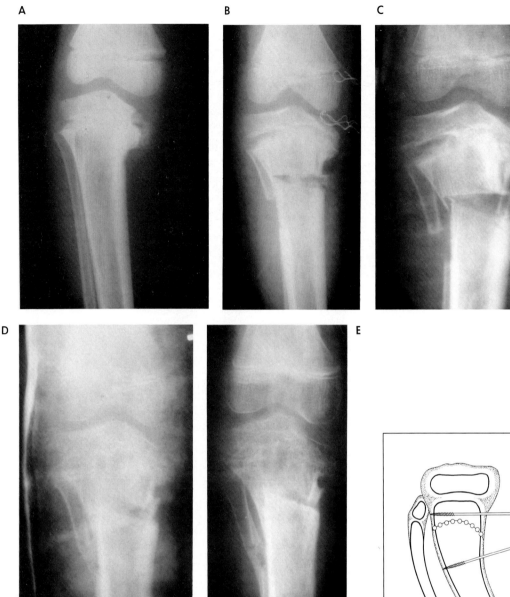

D

E

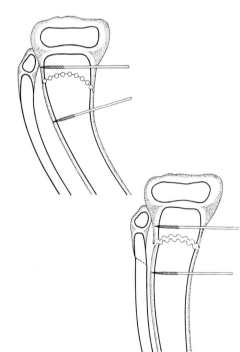

Fig. 1-45   **A,** Severe varus deformity from Blount's disease. **B,** Opening wedge osteotomy with fibular graft. **C,** Graft turned on end to produce larger opening wedge. **D,** In plaster cast immobilization without internal fixation, graft slipped. **E,** Deformity was corrected despite unstable graft, although correction was less than anticipated.

Fig. 1-46   Broomstick, ball-and-socket, or dome osteotomy.

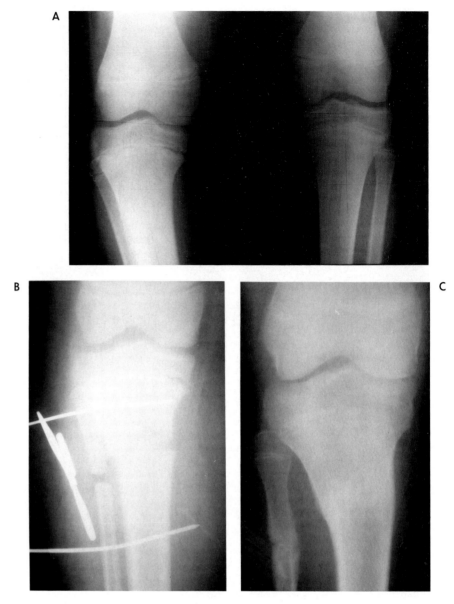

Fig. 1-47 **A,** Varus deformity of left tibia. **B,** Broomstick osteotomy fixed with pins in plaster. **C,** Correction of varus deformity.

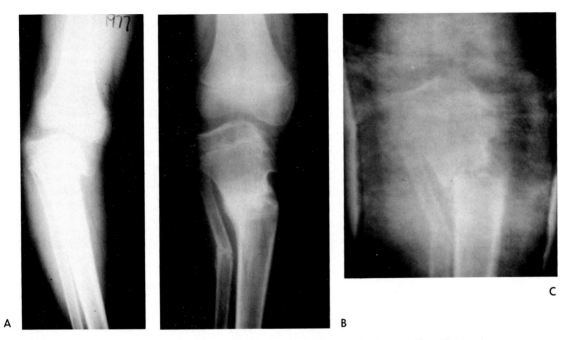

A

B

C

Fig. 1-48   A, Severe Blount's disease. **B,** After valgus hinge osteotomy without internal fixation. **C,** Excellent correction of varus deformity 1 year after surgery.

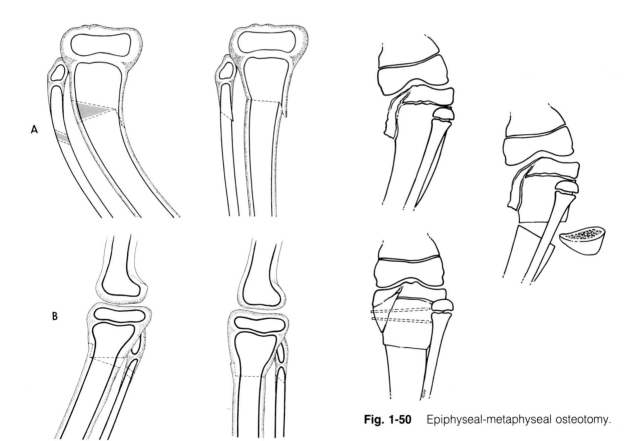

A

B

Fig. 1-49   A, Hinge or offset osteotomy. **B,** Flexion or extension osteotomy.

Fig. 1-50   Epiphyseal-metaphyseal osteotomy.

A

B

Fig. 1-51 **A,** Epiphyseal-metaphyseal osteotomy. **B,** Severe Blount's disease, Langenskiöld type IV deformity. **C,** Closing wedge metaphyseal osteotomy. **D,** Epiphyseal elevation. **E,** At follow-up.

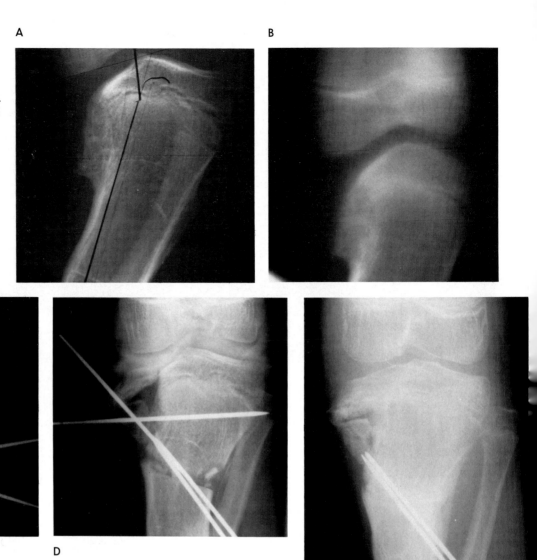

C

D

E

High Tibial Osteotomy

▶ *Technique.* The size of wedge to be removed and the amount of correction needed should be determined before surgery, as should the type of internal fixation to be used.

Prepare and drape the patient in the routine manner, and apply and inflate a tourniquet. The contralateral extremity may be draped free if comparison for alignment is anticipated. Make a vertical incision approximately 7 to 10 cm long at the lateral border of the proximal tibia, distal to the physis and the insertion of the tibial tubercle. Take care in soft tissue dissection and subperiosteal exposure to avoid the physis. Place reverse retractors medially and laterally about the tibial shaft. With long scissors, perform a closed fasciotomy of the anterior compartment for the length of the tibia (as an alternative, perform the fasciotomy through the small incision for fibular osteotomy). Make a small incision at the junction of the middle and distal thirds of the fibula. Carry soft tissue dissection through the peroneal musculature down to the fibular shaft. Place a small reverse retractor around the fibular shaft, and, with bone-biting forceps or oscillating saw, remove approximately 1 to 2 cm of the fibula. Removal of the segment rather than simple osteotomy is required for adequate correction of the tibia.

Now place a smooth Steinmann pin through the tibial shaft to measure its diameter so that the size of the opening or closing wedge can be computed. Score vertical marks on the tibial shaft for rotational orientation. Choose a level for the osteotomy that is distal enough to allow the placement of two parallel pins proximal to the osteotomy site but distal to the physis. Place these pins, and then with an oscillating saw make the osteotomy parallel to the pins; cut only the transverse limb of the osteotomy with the saw and complete it by manual "greensticking" of the posterior cortex or use a flat osteotome. After correction of the deformity, place the two distal pins parallel to the proximal pins (the distal pins may be placed before the osteotomy is made and then aligned parallel to the proximal pins). Confirm alignment of the osteotomy site with image intensification, and ma~~k~~ ~~y~~ rotational corrections, referring to th~~e~~ tation marks on the tibial s~~h~~ ally only slight r~~ osteot~~

~~b~~ ~~weeks.~~

~~tomy~~

D~~ ~~ osteotomies do not heal as readily as metaphyseal osteotomies, but many deformities in children involve the diaphysis, such as those in pseudarthrosis of the tibia, osteogenesis imperfecta, myelomeningocele, and other congenital and paralytic disorders, and these require diaphyseal osteotomy. In older children, single or multiple osteotomies may be held with a closed intramedullary nail, such as the Russell-Taylor Delta nail. If the bone is small, however, this method may not be appropriate because the smallest-diameter nail is 9 mm and damage to the proximal or distal physis is a risk. Other osteotomy techniques and intramedullary fixation may be more appropriate, such as the Sofield multilevel osteotomy or Bailey-Dubow telescoping rods (p. 25).

The Russell-Taylor Delta tibial nail allows proximal and distal locking to prevent rotation and maintain length in multiple and unstable osteotomies; stable osteotomies of the isthmus may be fixed with conventional unlocked methods. The 9- or 10-mm nail may be inserted with or without reaming. In older children with larger medullary canals, the standard Russell-Taylor tibial nail with diameters of 11 to 14 mm may be inserted without reaming. Preoperative roentgenograms should be used to determine proper nail size, amount of reaming necessary, and estimated final length after osteotomy. Proper nail length allows the proximal end to be countersunk and the distal end to be centered in the tibia just proximal to the distal physis, which should be avoided if still open (Fig. 1-52), or the procedure should be delayed until physeal closure.

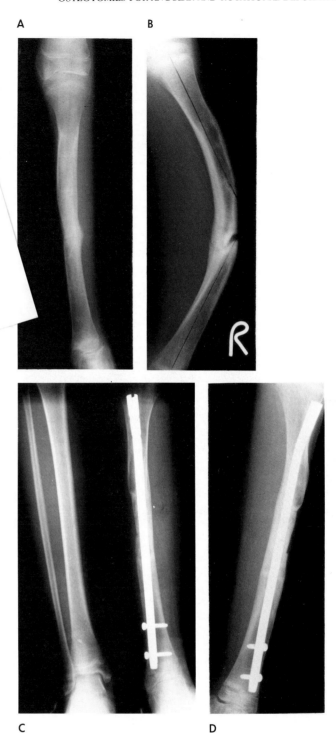

Fig. 1-52 **A** and **B,** Six years after tibial lengthening in child with fibular hemimelia there are multiple fractures through the lengthened area and gross angular deformity. **C** and **D,** Diaphyseal tibial osteotomy with intramedullary rod fixation, which avoids proximal and distal physes.

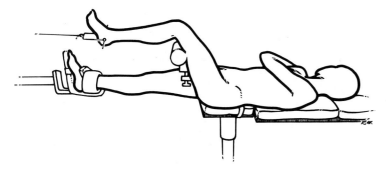

Fig. 1-53   Positioning for diaphyseal tibial osteotomy, Russell-Taylor technique (see text). (Redrawn from Russell TA, Taylor JC, and LaVelle DG: Russell-Taylor interlocking intramedullary tibial nail, technique manual, Memphis, 1986, Richards Manufacturing Co.)

▶ *Technique (Russell-Taylor).* Place the patient supine on the fracture table, with a well-padded bar beneath the distal thigh. Flex the hips and knees approximately 90 degrees. Align the iliac crest, patella, and second ray of the foot for correct rotational alignment. Apply traction through either a calcaneal pin or special foot holder, or arrange the C-arm of the image intensifier in the appropriate position (Fig. 1-53). Prepare and drape the patient in the standard manner, and cover the image intensifier arm with a sterile isolation drape.

Make a 5-cm incision either through or medial to the patellar ligament. Using a curved awl, open the medullary canal proximal to the tibial tuberosity in the midline behind or slightly medial to the patellar ligament (Fig. 1-54, *A*). Avoid the proximal physis, but do not make the entry site too distal as this may

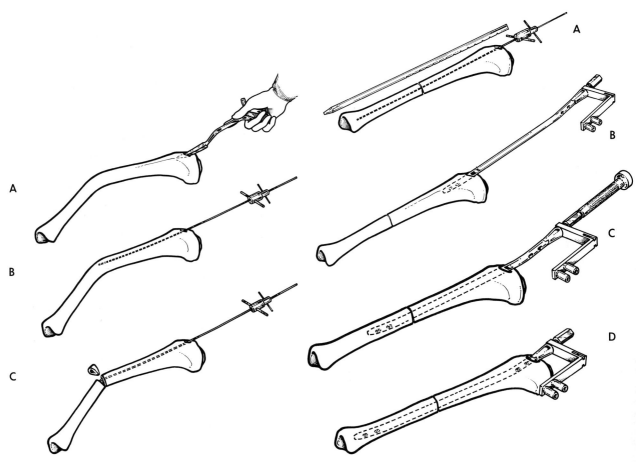

Fig. 1-54   Diaphyseal tibial osteotomy, Russell-Taylor technique (see text). **A,** Opening the medullary canal. **B,** Ball-tip guide impeded at site of maximum angulation. **C,** Osteotomy at apex of deformity. (**A** and **B** redrawn from Russell TA, Taylor JC, and LaVelle DG: Russell-Taylor interlocking intramedullary tibial nail, technique manual, Memphis, 1986, Richards Manufacturing Co.)

Fig. 1-55   Diaphyseal tibial osteotomy, Russell-Taylor technique (see text). **A,** Determining proper nail size. **B,** Matching key guide to nail keyway. **C** and **D,** Proper nail position. (Redrawn from Russell TA, Taylor JC, and LaVelle DG: Russell-Taylor interlocking intramedullary tibial nail, technique manual, Memphis, 1986, Richards Manufacturing Co.)

cause the nail to enter the cortex at too steep an angle and split the tibia. Ream the proximal 4 to 6 cm of the tibia to 12 mm in diameter. Again, take care not to involve the physis or apophysis of the tibial tubercle.

Pass the ball-tip guide until it is impeded and can be advanced no further, usually at the site of maximum angulation (Fig. 1-54, *B*). Make a 4-cm incision over this area, verified by image intensification, and carry the soft tissue dissection down to the tibia. With an oscillating saw, Midas-Rex drill, or osteotome, perform an osteotomy at the level of the ball-tip guide (Fig. 1-54, *C*). Cut the appropriate wedge or shorten the bone to allow the ball-tip guide to proceed down the canal in the proper alignment of the tibia. Severe angulation or angulation in multiple planes may require more than one osteotomy. Now ensure that the osteotomy is properly aligned, and determine the proper nail length, using the nail length gauge (Fig. 1-55, *A*). If reaming is not done, "sounds" can be used to determine canal size.

Attach the selected nail to the proximal drill guide. Hold the proximal drill guide with its handle pointed medially. Match the key guide to the keyway on the nail, and screw the attachment bolt through the guide into the nail (Fig. 1-55, *B*). Then attach the supine driver to the hexagonal bolt of the guide, and drive the nail to the osteotomy site. Confirm reduction of the osteotomy, and continue driving the nail until the proximal tip is flush with the tibial entry portal (Fig. 1-55, *C* and *D*). Usually the nail can be inserted without a guide rod, but if necessary the nail may be driven over a 3-mm guide rod.

Proximal locking is similar to that in the femur (pp. 26 to 27), although there are two proximal locking holes in the tibial nail and the guide is slightly different (Fig. 1-56). Distal locking is also similar to that in the femur (Fig. 1-57), and either the distal targeting guide or the freehand technique is used (pp. 30 to 32).

Close the wounds in the usual manner. Apply a sterile dressing and a long leg, bent knee cast.

▶*Postoperative management.* A patellar tendon-bearing brace is fitted 2 weeks after surgery and touchdown weight bearing is allowed; weight bearing is gradually increased over 6 to 8 weeks depending on healing. Dynamization (removal of one set of locking screws, usually distal) should be considered only if there appears to be delayed union 3 to 6 months after osteotomy, and weight bearing should be instituted after dynamization.

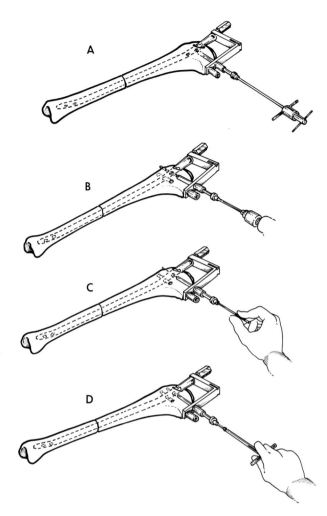

Fig. 1-56 **A** to **D,** Proximal locking, diaphyseal tibial osteotomy, Russell-Taylor technique (see text). (Redrawn from Russell TA, Taylor JC, and LaVelle DG: Russell-Taylor interlocking intramedullary tibial nail, technique manual, Memphis, 1986, Richards Manufacturing Co.)

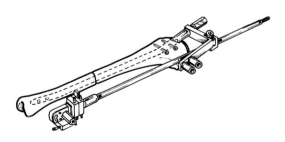

Fig. 1-57 Distal locking, diaphyseal tibial osteotomy, Russell-Taylor technique (see text). (Redrawn from Russell TA, Taylor JC, and LaVelle DG: Russell-Taylor interlocking intramedullary tibial nail, technique manual, Memphis, 1986, Richards Manufacturing Co.)

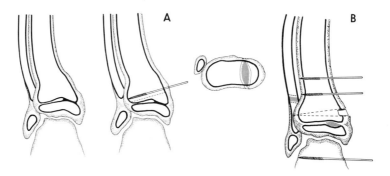

Fig. 1-58   **A** and **B,** Supramalleolar osteotomy with bony bar resection.

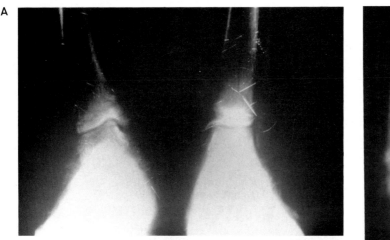

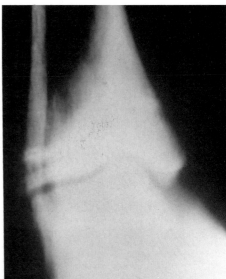

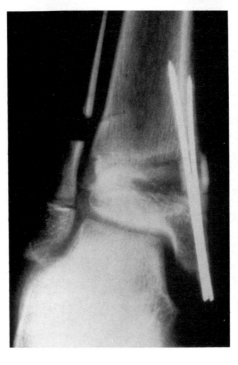

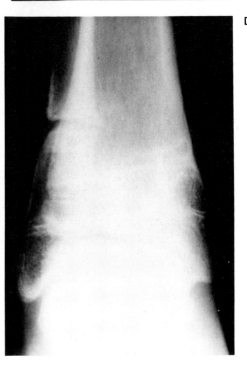

Fig. 1-59   **A,** Varus deformity of ankle caused by premature physeal closure and angulation deformity after fracture. **B,** Tomogram shows bony bar on medial side of physis. **C,** Opening wedge osteotomy alone with fibular graft held with pins in plaster. Note slight valgus overcorrection. **D,** Good correction at 2-year follow up.

Supramalleolar Osteotomy and Bony Bar Resection

Osteotomies immediately above the ankle joint should be reserved for angulation in the tibia itself; their use for correction of foot deformities generally are unsuccessful, and osteotomy of the talar, subtalar, midtarsal, or distal portion of the foot should be done instead. A varus position of the foot causes abnormal stresses on the ankle and lateral border of the foot and is poorly tolerated; overcorrection into the valgus position at osteotomy is acceptable, but varus overcorrection is not. Bony bar resection alone in this area may allow correction of a slight deformity, but significant deformity requires osteotomy and bony bar resection (Fig. 1-58).

Pins and plaster or external fixation is preferred to plate fixation in the distal tibia (Fig. 1-59) because of the risk of damaging the physis with the screws and the subcutaneous location of a plate on the medial tibia, which may cause discomfort or skin and wound breakdown; the interosseous membrane limits plate application on the lateral tibia. Simple screw fixation with AO or cancellous screws usually is not adequate.

▶ *Technique*. Expose the ankle joint through an approximately 10 cm long anteromedial incision. Carry soft tissue dissection down to the physis, and expose the tibia by subperiosteal dissection. If there is medial physeal arrest, place a smooth guide pin parallel to the open lateral portion of the physis (Fig. 1-60), and make an osteotomy adjacent and parallel to the guide pin. Then make a short incision over the distal fibula, and with a rongeur, bone cutting forceps, or power saw, remove a 1.5- to 2-cm opening wedge graft. Open the tibial osteotomy site with a lamina spreader and locate the bony bar; it usually is completely distal and its hard sclerotic bone is obvious in comparison to cancellous bone (Fig. 1-61). Remove the entire bony bar down to and through the physis and into the epiphysis, leaving only cancellous bone at the margins of the crater. Obtain a fat graft from the posterior tibia, and place it in the defect (Fig. 1-62). Insert two pins above the osetotomy site and two below. Hold the incision open with the fibular strut graft, which has been cut to the appropriate size. Place the graft on the cortical shell of bone and not in the area of bony resection (Fig. 1-63). Verify resection of the bony bar and configuration of the osteotomy with image intensification. If the entire physis is closed, bony bar resection is not indicated, and the osteotomy alone may correct the deformity. Close the wound in the usual manner and apply a long leg, bent knee cast incorporating the pins (Fig. 1-63).

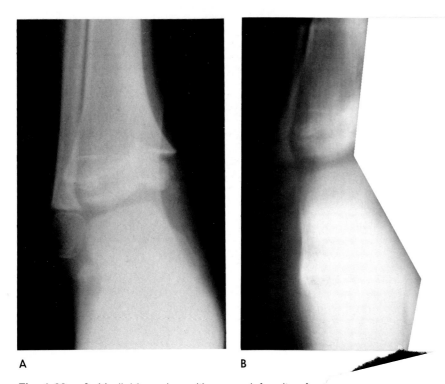

A   B

Fig. 1-60 **A,** Medial bony bar with varus deformity after trauma. **B,** Tomogram shows location of bony bridge. **C,** Guide pins placed parallel to open physis.

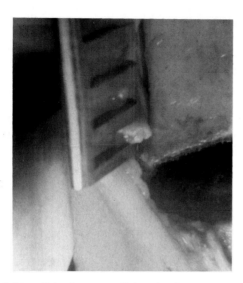

Fig. 1-61 Osteotomy parallel and adjacent to proximal pin opened with lamina spreader to expose sclerotic bony bar.

Postoperative management. Non–weight-bearing immobilization is continued for 8 to 12 weeks depending on the age of the child and the amount of callus formation. The pins are removed 6 weeks after surgery (Fig. 1-64).

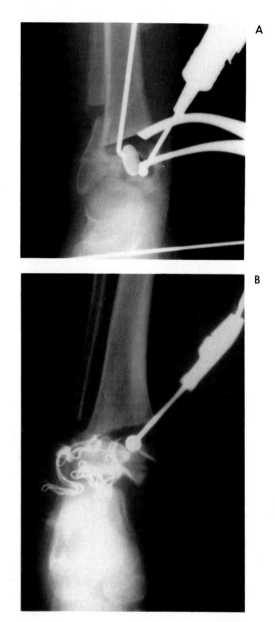

Fig. 1-62 **A,** Power dental burr and dental mirror used to resect bony bar. **B,** Defect filled with autogenous fat.

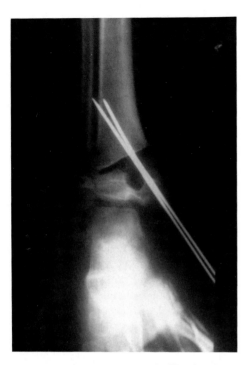

Fig. 1-63   Internal fixation of graft. Pins in plaster used to hold graft and osteotomy in place.

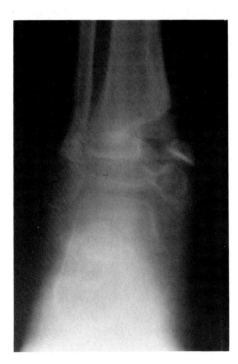

Fig. 1-64   After pin removal, excellent alignment of ankle joint in mild valgus position.

BONY BAR RESECTION
Etiology

Bony bars result from premature partial arrest of growth of a physis and produce angular and length abnormalities of involved bones. Any injury to physeal cells may cause formation of a bony bar; the most common cause is fracture, although infection, tumors, irradiation, thermal burns, and metal implants across the physis all may result in bony bars. Other suggested etiologic factors include neural and vascular abnormalities, reduced vascular supply from any cause, frostbite, electric burns, and metabolic abnormalities. Some bony bars have no apparent cause and are called "developmental," such as in Blount's disease. Because bony bars result from damage to the physeal cells, they usually cannot be prevented; the exception is the bony bar caused by the use of metal pins and screws across the physis. Small-diameter, smooth pins placed perpendicularly across the center of the physis for a short time (2 to 3 weeks) rarely cause growth arrest; threaded wires of any diameter placed obliquely across the physis for a few weeks usually result in a bony bar. The most common sites of bony bars are the proximal tibial and distal femoral physes, which account for 60% to 70% of the growth of their respective bones.

Evaluation

Clinical signs of a bony bar usually are angular deformity or shortening of the involved extremity. In addition to routine roentgenograms, scanograms should be obtained to document lengths of the extremities. Bone age must be determined to assess the potential for remaining growth, usually by roentgenogram of the hand that is compared with the atlas of Gruelich and Pyle. Computed tomography is of little value because of the irregularity of the physis. Hypocycloidal tomograms are helpful to determine the configuration and area involved by the bony bar and to delineate the configuration and area of the remaining normal physis because the small cuts in this technique (as small as 1 mm in thickness) give sharp focus.

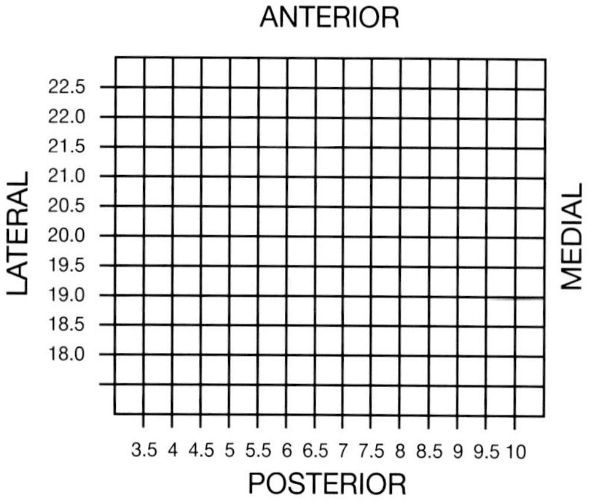

Fig. 1-65 Graph paper labeled for orientation and tomographic levels. (Redrawn from Carlson WO and Wenger DR: J Pediatr Orthop 4:232, 1984.)

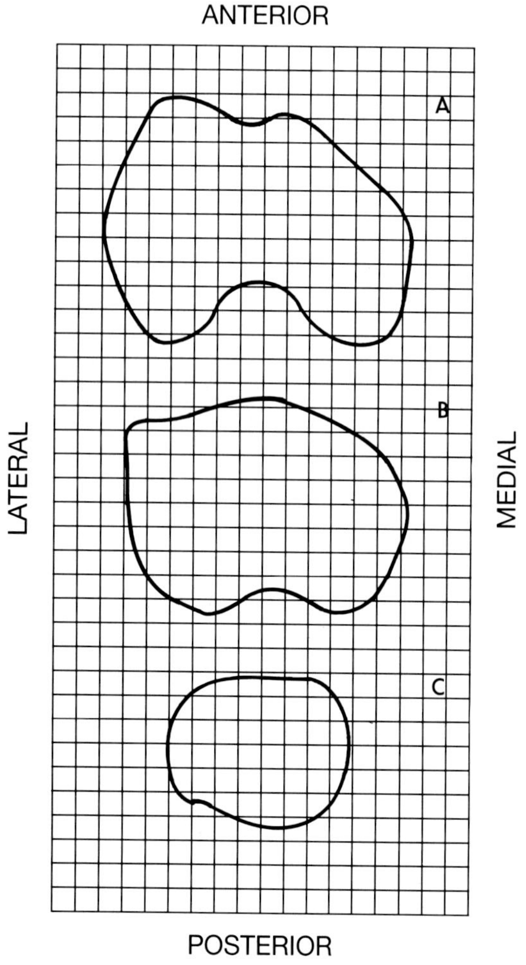

Fig. 1-66 Outlines for mapping physeal bar. **A,** Distal femoral physis. **B,** Proximal tibial physis. **C,** Distal tibial physis. (Redrawn from Carlson WO and Wenger DR: J Pediatr Orthop 4:232, 1984.)

Preoperative Tomogram Mapping

Carlson and Wenger have described a method for producing a schematic cross-sectional map on graph paper from the data obtained from biplane polytomography. They report that this map helps to identify lesions that should be treated surgically and aids in planning the surgical approach and resection. Their criteria for surgical excision are the age of the patient and the size of the bony bar as a percentage of the total cross-sectional area, noting that optimal correction results when 2 years of longitudinal growth remain and the physeal bar involves less than 50% of the physes.

◣ *Technique (Carlson and Wenger).* After obtaining the appropriate anteroposterior and lateral tomograms, prepare a piece of graph paper by labeling it for anterior, posterior, medial, and lateral orientation to avoid confusion. Label the numerical levels of each tomographic cut along the side and bottom of the graph in both anteroposterior and lateral projections. Starting with the lowest numbered cut, divide the remainder of the graph into equal sections so that all levels can be easily transferred to the diagram (Fig. 1-65). To outline the cross-sectional shape of the physis, make a tracing using the cross section of a plastic model bone at the level of the growth plate (a cadaveric bone also can be used). Outlines of the distal femoral, proximal tibial, and distal tibial physes superimposed on graph paper are illustrated in Fig. 1-66. Starting with either the anteroposterior or lateral tomograms, analyze the extent of the bony bridge on each cut, proceeding from the lowest to the highest numbered cut, making certain to maintain orientation. Determine the extent of the bony bridge at each level, and plot it as a thick, straight line on the outline (Fig. 1-67); repeat this process for all the anteroposterior tomographic cuts (Fig. 1-68). Use the same technique to plot the lateral tomographic cuts (Fig. 1-69, *A*) to obtain the actual cross-sectional anatomy of the physeal bar (Fig. 1-69, *B*).

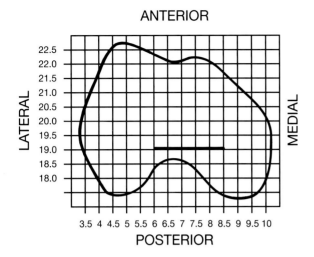

Fig. 1-67 Anteroposterior projection level indicated on graph with thick, straight line. (Redrawn from Carlson WO and Wenger DR: J Pediatr Orthop 4:232, 1984.)

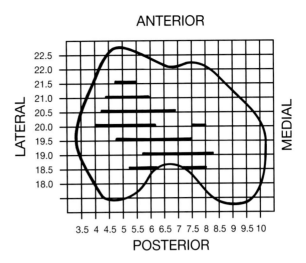

Fig. 1-68 All anteroposterior levels plotted from tomograms. (Redrawn from Carlson WO and Wenger DR: J Pediatr Orthop 4:232, 1984.)

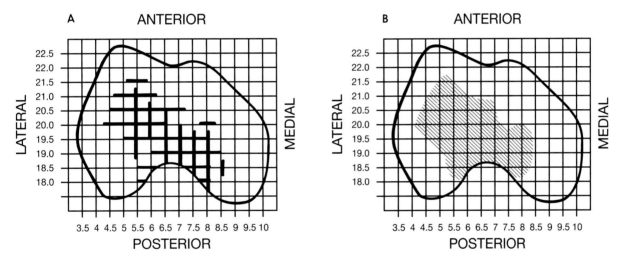

Fig. 1-69 **A,** Lateral projection levels plotted on graph. **B,** Final cross-sectional map of the physeal bar. (Redrawn from Carlson WO and Wenger DR: J Pediatr Orthop 4:232, 1984.)

Treatment

The treatment of bony bars ranges from observation in the adolescent with little remaining growth to a combination of surgical modalities in the young patient with significant remaining growth. The surgical options include (1) arrest of the remaining growth of the injured physis, which should be considered in the older child with mild angular deformity and expected minor limb length discrepancy, (2) arrest of the remaining growth of the injured physis and of the physis of the adjacent bone, (3) arrest of the remaining growth of the injured physis, the physis of the adjacent bone, and the corresponding physes of the contralateral bones, (4) combinations of physeal ar-

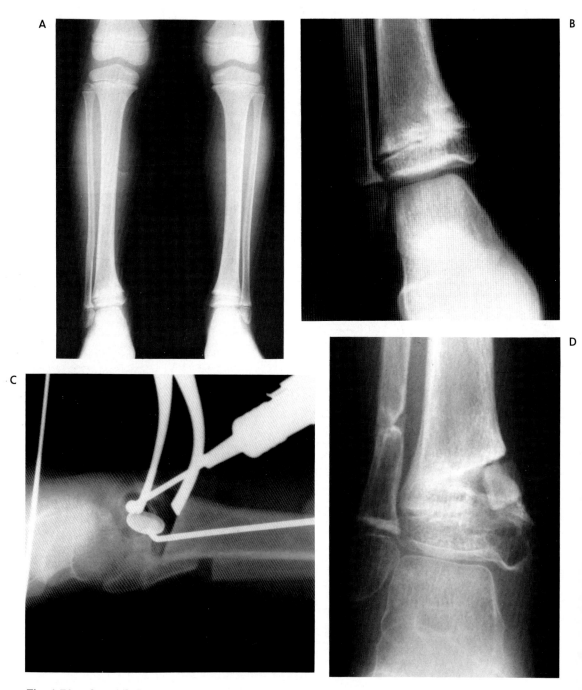

Fig. 1-70 **A** and **B,** Bony bar on medial third of tibial physis causing varus deformity. **C,** Open wedge osteotomy and bony bar resection; dental mirror is used to determine circumferential limits of physis and dental burr for resection. **D,** At follow-up with good correction into neutral position.

rests with opening or closing wedge osteotomy to correct angular deformity, (5) opening or closing wedge osteotomy without physeal arrests, which may require several osteotomies because of recurrence of the deformity, (6) lengthening or shortening of the involved bone (bone shortening should be considered only for the femur), (7) resection of the physeal bar and insertion of interposition material, (8) resection of the bony bar and osteotomy for correction of angular deformity (Fig. 1-70), and (9) various combinations of these techniques.

Resection with Interposition Material

Early advocates of resection of the bony bar, with and without interposition material, include Langenskiöld and Bright in both experimental and clinical reports. Peterson, in a review of physeal bar treatment, listed several interposition materials used experimentally to prevent bony bar formation, including gold leaf, rubber film, gelfoam, bone wax, methyl methacrylate, muscle, fat, and cartilage. These materials were tested in defects created by the removal of a portion of the physis from the periphery or production of a type IV Salter-Harris injury by osteotomy. Results of these experimental studies have been varied, but evidence suggests that formation of the bony bar can be prevented or inhibited; conversely, when no interposition material is inserted, bar formation occurs consistently. Of the interposition material used, fat, bone wax, polymeric silicone (Silastic), and methyl methacrylate are the most frequently reported. Peterson reported the successful use of methyl methacrylate without barium (Cranioplast) as interposition material in 68 patients. He lists the following advantages of this material: it is easily available; there is no control by the Food and Drug Administration (FDA) (as there is for Silastic); no second incision is needed (as for fat); it is easy to handle and mold; it is sterile; it provides hemostasis (by occupying the entire desired portion of the cavity); it is strong so that postoperative immobilization is not necessary; and there are no apparent side effects. Like Carlson and Wenger, Peterson recommends bar resection only if the area of the bar is 50% or less of the entire physis; he notes that osteotomy usually is required, in addition to bony bar resection and insertion of the Cranioplast plug, if angular deformity is greater than 20 degrees.

▲ *Technique (Peterson).* Approach peripherally located bars directly from the periphery (Fig. 1-71). Excise any periosteum overlying the bar. Under direct vision and using a motorized burr, remove the bar from inside out until normal physis can be seen on all sides of the cavity.

For bars extending completely across the physis, evaluate tomographic maps to determine surgical approach and ensure complete removal (Fig. 1-72).

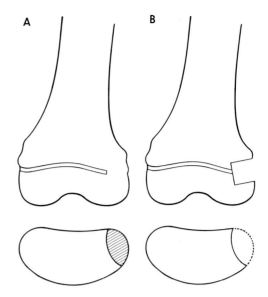

Fig. 1-71 **A** and **B,** Peripheral bar in anteroposterior view (see text). (Redrawn from Peterson HA: J Pediatr Orthop 4:246, 1984.)

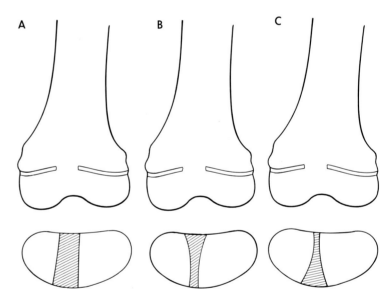

Fig. 1-72 **A** to **C,** Elongated bar extending from anterior to posterior surfaces. Although all three have same appearance on anteroposterior view *(above),* they have different contours on the transverse sections *(below)* (see text). (Redrawn from Peterson, HA: J Pediatr Orthop 4:246, 1984.)

Approach centrally located bars (Fig. 1-73, *A*) through the metaphysis or epiphysis. Because the bar is not readily accessible through the transepiphyseal approach and because it usually requires traversing the joint, the transmetaphyseal approach is preferable, although it requires removal of a window of cortical bone and some cancellous metaphyseal bone to reach the bony bar (Fig. 1-73, *B*). After removal of the entire bar, inspect the normal physis with a small dental mirror (Fig. 1-73, *C*).

Place metal markers, such as surgical clips, in the metaphysis and epiphysis to aid in accurate measurement of subsequent growth of the involved physis. Place these markers in cancellous bone, not in contact with the cavity, and in the same longitudinal plane proximally and distally to the defect.

In a large cavity that is gravity dependent, pour liquid Cranioplast into the defect. If the cavity is not gravity dependent, place the Cranioplast in a syringe and push it into the defect through a short polyethylene tube (Fig. 1-74, *A*), or allow the Cranioplast to partially set and push it like putty into the defect. Allow as little Cranioplast as possible to remain in the metaphysis. After the Cranioplast has set, fill the remainder of the metaphyseal cavity with cancellous bone (Fig. 1-74, *B*).

The sides of the cavity should be flat and smooth (Fig. 1-75). The contour of the cavity also is important. Bar formation is less likely when the interposition material remains in the epiphysis (Fig. 1-76, *A*) than when the epiphysis grows away from it (Fig. 1-76, *B*). Methods of keeping the plug in the epiphysis include drilling holes in the cavity (Fig. 1-77) and enlarging the cavity (Fig. 1-78).

▶ *Postoperative management.* Joint motion is begun immediately. If osteotomy has not been performed, no cast or other immobilization is necessary. Weight bearing is encouraged on the day of surgery or as soon as comfort permits. Follow-up with scanograms continues until maturity.

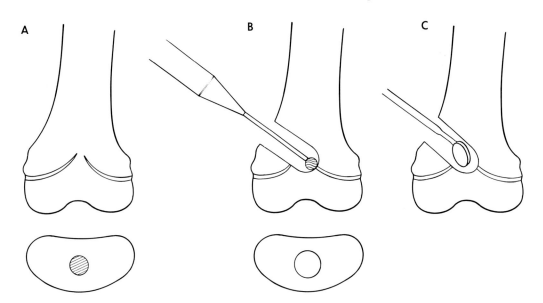

Fig. 1-73 **A,** Central bar with peripheral growth results in "tenting" or "cupping" of the physis (see text). **B,** Excision of central bar through window in metaphysis (see text). **C,** Examination of entire physis with dental mirror (see text). (Redrawn from Peterson HA: J Pediatr Orthop 4:246, 1984.)

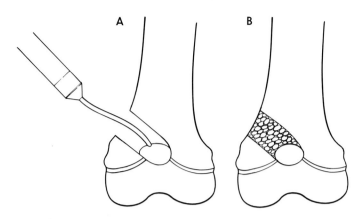

Fig. 1-74   A, Insertion of Cranioplast with syringe (see text). **B,** Bone graft filling remainder of defect (see text). (Redrawn from Peterson HA: J Pediatr Orthop 4:246, 1984.)

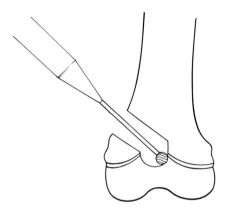

Fig. 1-75   Smoothing metaphyseal bone surface (see text). (Redrawn from Peterson HA: J Pediatr Orthop 4:246, 1984.)

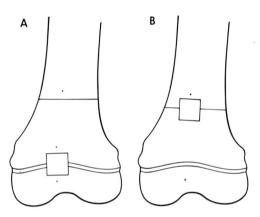

Fig. 1-76   A, Plug growing away from proximal marker and growth arrest line (see text). **B,** Plug remaining with metaphysis as epiphysis grows (see text). (Redrawn from Peterson HA: J Pediatr Orthop 4:246, 1984.)

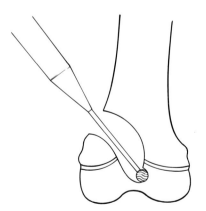

Fig. 1-77   Undermining of epiphysis (see text). (Redrawn from Peterson HA: J Pediatr Orthop 4:246, 1984.)

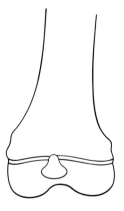

Fig. 1-78   "Collar button" contour of plug to act as anchor (see text). (Redrawn from Peterson HA: J Pediatr Orthop 4:246, 1984.)

ARTHRODESIS OF THE LOWER EXTREMITY

Because arthrodesis, or fusion, of a joint implies joint stiffness, it generally is not recommended for children. Sometimes, however, arthrodesis is necessary to relieve pain, halt progression of disease, or provide stability. Arthrodesis may be appropriate in some adolescents and children who will be active for many years and in whom total joint arthroplasty is not feasible. If at all possible, intraarticular arthrodesis should be performed to preserve the physes proximal and distal to the fused joint. When anatomically practical, compression principles should be used. The knee and ankle are more stable and therefore more suitable for compression arthrodesis than are other major joints.

Ankle

Ankle arthrodesis usually is cosmetically and functionally satisfactory in young patients. Talonavicular motion of 18 to 20 degrees generally compensates for the lack of dorsiflexion and plantarflexion of the ankle. The most commonly used techniques of ankle arthrodesis are the Charnley technique (with a Calandruccio triangular compression device [Fig. 1-79], Charnley compression clamps, or external fixator), and the Chiunard-Peterson technique, which is especially appropriate for children because it does not damage the distal tibial physis and preserves length of the extremity (Fig. 1-80). The Chiunard-Peterson technique also can be used with compression devices such as the Charnley or Calandruccio clamp.

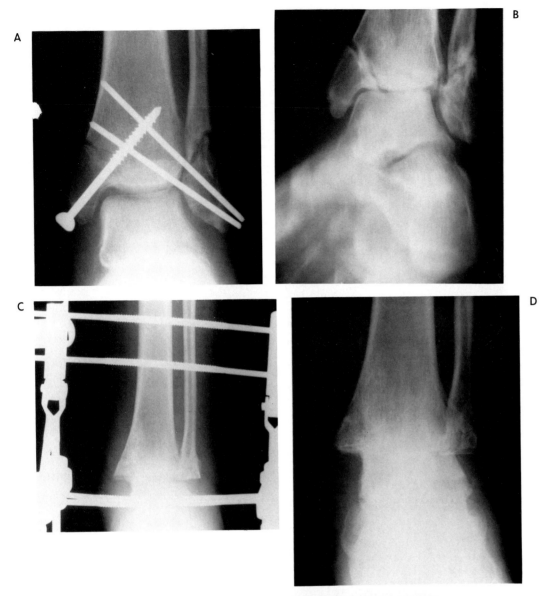

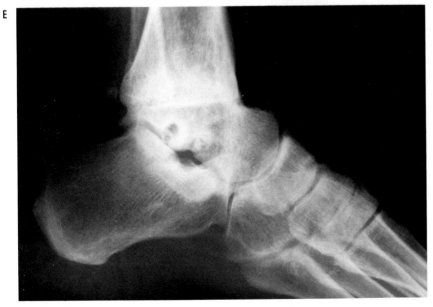

Fig. 1-79   A, Bimalleolar ankle fracture after open reduction and internal fixation in adolescent with closed epiphyses. **B,** After removal of internal fixation, narrowed and painful ankle joint as a result of nonunion of fracture. **C,** Charnley compression arthrodesis with Calandruccio clamp; note slight bowing of parallel compression pins. **D** and **E,** Excellent fusion and alignment 1 year after ankle fusion.

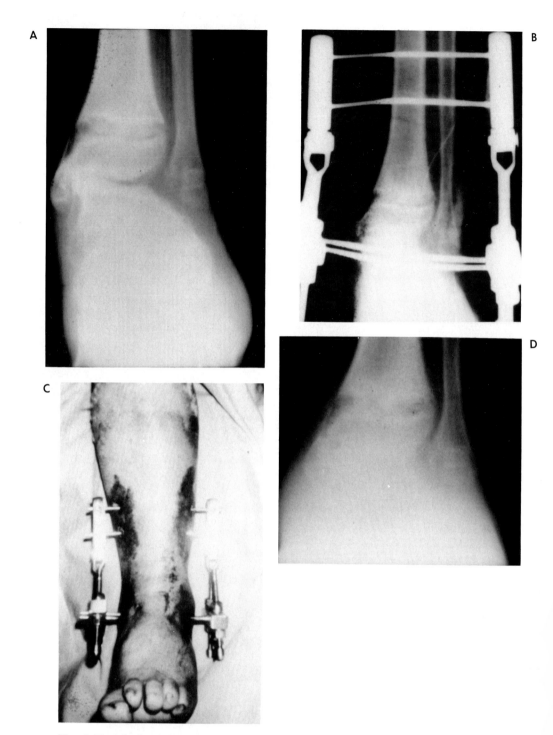

Fig. 1-80   **A,** Severe traumatic disruption of ankle joint from lawnmower injury caused pain and deformity. **B,** Chuinard ankle fusion with the use of Calandruccio compression clamp; note open physes. **C,** Clamp in place. **D,** Successful fusion with physes still open after removal of compression clamp.

Charnley Arthrodesis, Calandruccio Compression Clamp

▶ *Technique.* Make an anterolateral incision approximately 5 cm above the ankle joint extending down over the dorsum of the foot, taking care to preserve the extensor tendons. Expose the distal tibia and posterolateral side of the lateral malleolus. If necessary for complete examination of the entire medial malleolus, make a second incision medially over the anteromedial aspect of the joint. Carry soft tissue dissection down to the medial malleolus and to the anteromedial joint line, taking care to preserve the anterior tibialis tendon and the neurovascular bundle. Carry out subperiosteal dissection to expose both malleoli. Place periosteal elevators or reverse retractors behind each malleolus. Remove all soft tissue, including the synovium and anterior joint capsule, to adequately expose the entire dome of the talus and the distal tibia. Divide the tibial and fibular collateral ligaments, and plantarflex the foot. With an oscillating saw, cut the distal ends of the tibia and fibula horizontally (6 mm or more proximal to the joint), and complete the osteotomy with an osteotome. Remove a corresponding section of bone approximately 6 mm thick from the superior surface of the talus, parallel to the distal tibia. Remove the distal portion of the fibula at the level of the osteotomy. Appose the talus and tibia in the correct position, correcting any rotary or tilt deformity (Fig. 1-81). Select pins that are threaded in the center but not on each end, and make sure they will fit over the proximal portion of the Calandruccio clamp. Pass these pins through the distal tibia vertically. Now pass two similar pins through the talus, one anterior to the axis of the bone and one posterior, using the Calandruccio clamp as a guide. Be careful not to pierce the subtalar joint with the distal pin. Apply the triangular compression clamp, and tighten the clamp (Fig. 1-82) until there is some bowing of the proximal and distal pins. Obtain roentgenograms to evaluate the position of fragments from the osteotomy, and correct any offset or displacement. Apply a posterior splint incorporating the triangular clamp.

▶ *Postoperative management.* A short leg cast incorporating the entire Calandruccio apparatus is applied 72 hours after surgery. The cast, clamps, and sutures are removed 6 to 10 weeks after surgery and a walking cast is applied and worn another 6 weeks; weight-bearing ambulation is allowed in this cast. A patellar tendon-bearing brace with limited or no ankle motion is worn for an additional 9 months.

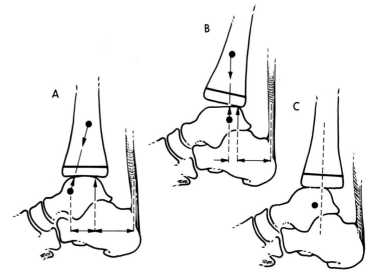

Fig. 1-81 Compression arthrodesis of ankle. **A,** Distal pin inserted anterior to transverse axis of body of talus to counteract pull of tendo Achilles. **B,** If pin is inserted through or posterior to axis, force of tendo Achilles will separate osseous surfaces. **C,** Osseous surfaces should not be flush anteriorly as shown; rather talus should be displaced as far posteriorly as possible to preserve heel prominence. (Redrawn from Russell TA. In Crenshaw AH, editor: Campbell's operative orthopedics, ed 7, St Louis, 1987, The CV Mosby Co.)

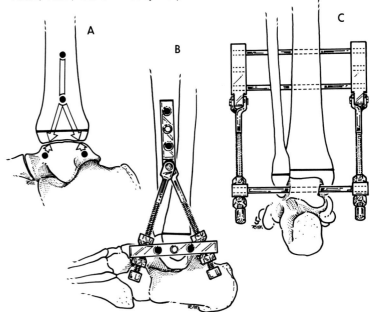

Fig. 1-82 Calandruccio triangular compression device. **A,** Two pins are inserted through talus and two through tibia for additional compression and more rigid fixation. Device allows for some correction of talipes equinus or dorsiflexion and varus or valgus angulation. **B** and **C,** Lateral and posterior views of ankle with device in place. (Redrawn from Russell TA. In Crenshaw AH, editor: Campbell's operative orthopedics, ed 7, St Louis, 1987, The CV Mosby Co.)

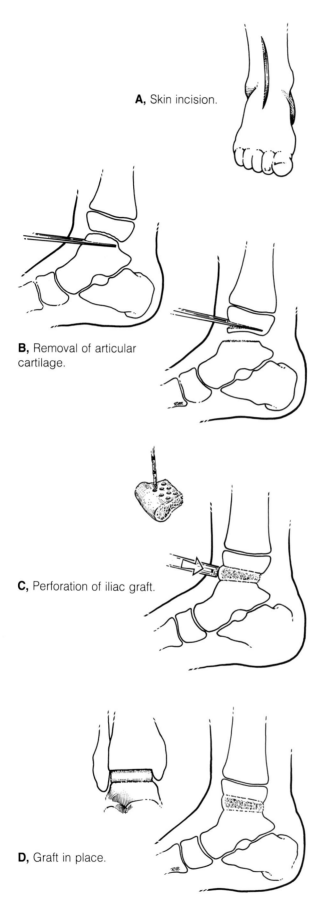

A, Skin incision.

B, Removal of articular cartilage.

C, Perforation of iliac graft.

D, Graft in place.

Chinuard and Peterson Arthrodesis

▶ *Technique.* Make an anterior longitudinal incision over the ankle joint, and develop the approach between the extensor hallucis longus and extensor digitorum longus tendons (Fig. 1-83, *A*). Retract medially the anterior tibial vessels and nerve, and detach the capsule of the ankle joint from the anterior margin of the tibia. With an osteotome and mallet, remove the articular cartilage from the horizontal surface of the tibia and talus but not from the vertical surfaces of these bones or the fibula (Fig. 1-83, *B*). Correct any deformity by removing appropriate wedges of bone. Take care to avoid injury to the distal tibial physis. With an osteotome the same width as the ankle mortise, remove a full-thickness bone graft from the anterior iliac crest as wide as the ankle mortise and as long as the anteroposterior dimension of the ankle. Do not include the cartilage of the anterosuperior iliac spine. Now tailor the graft to fit the mortise, and perforate it with a drill (Fig. 1-83, *C*). Manually distract the ankle joint and tap the graft into place with the wide rim facing anteriorly and the surface of the graft firmly apposed to the surfaces of the tibia and talus (Fig. 1-83, *D*). Check the position of the foot and adjust it to neutral. Fill any remaining recesses with cancellous bone from the ilium. Close the wound, and apply a cast from the base of the toes to the proximal thigh with the knee flexed 15 degrees.

▶ *Postoperative management.* Two weeks after surgery, the cast is either windowed or changed and the sutures are removed. After 6 weeks a cast is applied from the base of the toes to below the knee. After 2 to 3 months a walking cast is applied, and after 3 to 4 months a short leg brace with a rigid ankle joint is fitted and worn until roentgenograms show solid fusion.

Fig. 1-83 Chuinard and Peterson technique of ankle arthrodesis (see text). (**A** to **D** redrawn from Chuinard EG and Peterson RE: J Bone Joint Surg [Am] 45:481, 1963.)

Knee

Arthrodesis of the knee usually is reserved as a salvage procedure, even in adults; however, total knee arthroplasty, despite improvements in design and performance of components, is not a viable alternative in children or adolescents because of the potential loosening of the prosthesis during a lifetime. Arthrodesis of the knee is indicated for progressive posttraumatic arthritis, suppurative arthritis, recurrent infection, some congenital anomalies (such as proximal femoral focal deficiency), or tumorous conditions that require significant ablation of the knee joint. Besides the stiff knee joint after arthrodesis, the fused extremity invariably is shorter, the physis may be damaged by the fusion, and later conversion to total knee arthroplasty is difficult. Knee arthrodesis should be the last resort in the growing child, and bracing until skeletal maturity or osteotomy to "unload" the painful compartment should be considered.

Flexion contractures, especially with rheumatoid or traumatic arthritis and hemophilic arthropathy, are common. Because the joint should be fused in full extension or minimal flexion, sufficient bone must be removed to prevent neurovascular compromise when the extremity is extended for fusion. The peroneal and posterior tibial nerves and popliteal vessels are especially vulnerable to damage from stretching.

The three basic techniques of intraarticular fusion of the knee joint include the use of bone grafts alone, compression by external fixation, and internal fixation with medullary nails or plates and screws. The use of bone grafts alone, as described by Hibbs and Key in the early 1900s, generally is not successful in children, and the use of plates and screws or intramedullary rods may damage the physis; therefore compression arthrodesis with external fixation is recommended when knee fusion is required in the growing child. Various types of external fixation may be used, including the Charnley compression clamp, Calandruccio compression clamp, and Hoffman and Ace-Fischer external fixators. Charnley and Lowe reported satisfactory union in 98.5% of 67 patients with this device. An advantage of the Calandruccio clamp is that it allows easy alignment of the two fragments in the apparatus (Fig. 1-84).

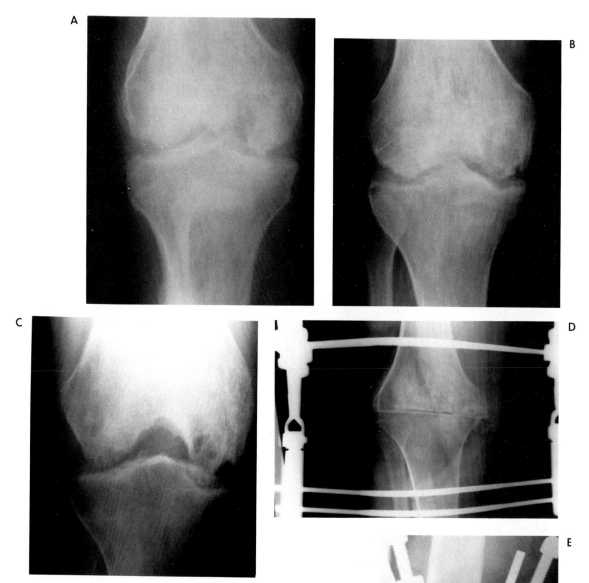

Fig. 1-84 **A,** Knee joint of adolescent after arthroscopy and subsequent bacterial infection. **B,** One year after active infection with persistent drainage for which irrigation and debridement were performed; knee joint is destroyed by septic necrosis. **C,** Eighteen months after arthroscopy, drainage ceased but patient had severe pain and limitation of motion. **D,** and **E,** Charnley compression arthrodesis with Calandruccio clamps applied upside down to match configuration of femur and tibia better. **F** and **G,** Solid fusion 9 months after surgery.

F

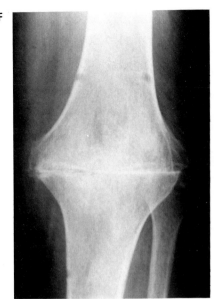

G

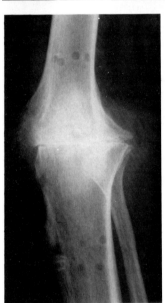

Compression Arthrodesis of the Knee

▶ *Technique.* Make a long medial parapatellar incision close to the midline. Expose and excise the patella. Free the anterior portion of the knee extensively, resecting the collateral ligaments, patellar tendon, and anterior joint capsule to expose completely both the medial and lateral femoral condyles and the tibial plateau. This should allow complete flexion of the knee, with the anterior structures falling posteriorly. Excise the synovium, menisci, anterior cruciate ligament, and patellar fat pad. Pull the tibia anteriorly to examine the posterior structures in the intercondylar notch. Remove the proximal 1 cm of the tibia and the proximal 1 cm of the femur to allow alignment in full extension. If there is significant flexion contracture, remove more than 1 cm of bone from the tibia and femur to prevent stretching of the neurovascular structures posteriorly. After removal of these wafers of bone, appose the two cancellous bone surfaces with the joint in full extension. Insert the appropriate pins for either the Charnley or the Calandruccio clamp parallel to the osteotomy and perpendicular to the femur and tibia. Correct any varus or valgus deformity by appropriately wedged osteotomy. Compress the two cut surfaces tightly until there is mild bowing of the pins in the clamp. Close the wound in layers anteriorly.

▶ *Postoperative management.* A stiff or rigid bandage is applied the first day after surgery until swelling subsides and neurovascular status is evaluated. Then a long leg cast is applied, incorporating the external fixator, Charnley clamp, or Calandruccio clamp. The pins and external fixation device or clamp are removed 6 weeks after surgery. Cast immobilization is continued for another 6 to 8 weeks.

Hip

Hip arthrodesis most often is indicated for significant deformity caused by avascular necrosis or chondrolysis after Legg-Calvé-Perthes disease, slipped capital femoral epiphysis, infection, or rheumatoid arthritis. Total hip arthroplasty generally is not feasible in the young child, and hip arthrodesis may be indicated to alleviate pain and improve ambulation. Both intraarticular and extraarticular techniques of hip fusion have been advocated, but intraarticular arthrodesis, with or without muscle pedicle graft, using some form of intramedullary fixation across the joint into the ilium, most frequently is recommended at the present time (Fig. 1-85). Dislocation of the hip to remove all cartilage from the head and neck of the femur and from the acetabulum is controversial. Anterior dislocation of the head of the femur is difficult on a standard fracture table, and removal of too much of the femoral head and acetabulum makes apposition of convex and concave surfaces difficult. The value of subtrochanteric osteotomy in association with the hip fusion also is controversial. Some authors report that subtrochanteric osteotomy allows better alignment of the extremity and relieves tension across the hip joint by preventing the leg from acting as a lever arm. The recommended position for fusion of the hip joint is 30 degrees of flexion, neutral abduction and adduction, and 5 to 15 degrees of external rotation. The use of the fracture table facilitates positioning, especially flexion, because the normal lumbar lordosis is 30 degrees and keeping the operated extremity horizontal achieves the correct flexion of the hip.

Fig. 1-85 **A** and **B,** 15-year-old adolescent with idiopathic avascular necrosis, pain, and limitation of motion. **C** and **D,** Arthrodesis with the use of compression screw into pelvis and iliac bone graft. **E** and **F,** Movement at fusion site and breakage of metal at screw-plate interface; however, joint has fused; at long-term follow-up, patient was free of symptoms.

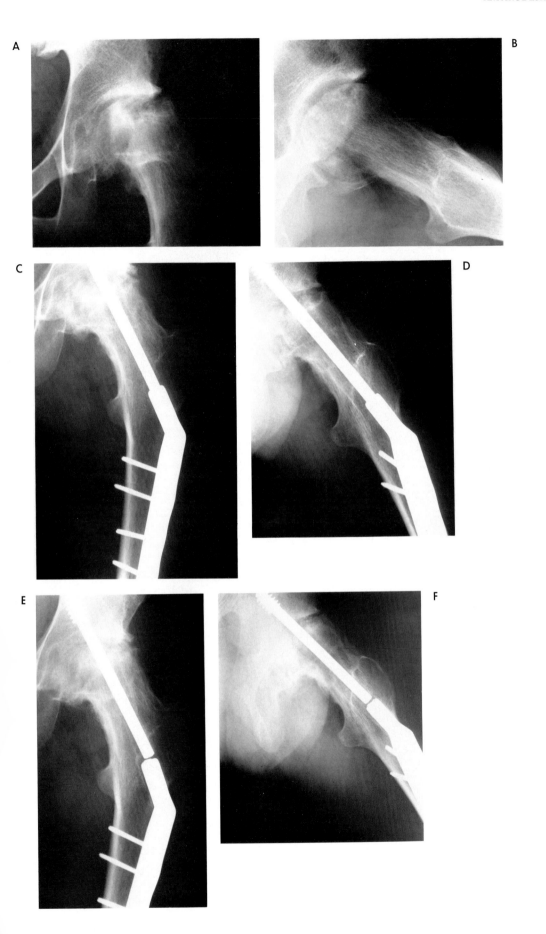

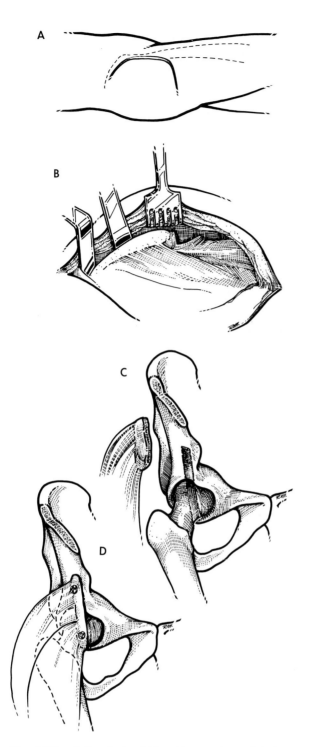

Fig. 1-86 Arthrodesis of hip with muscle pedicle bone graft (see text). **A,** Skin incision. **B,** Osteotome placed medial to iliac crest in preparation for resection of graft. **C,** Slot made in ilium and femoral head and neck. **D,** Graft fixed to ilium and femoral neck with screws. (Redrawn from Davis JB: J Bone Joint Surg [Am] 36:790, 1954.)

Compression Arthrodesis of the Hip

▲ *Technique.* Place the patient supine on a fracture table. Prepare and drape the hip in the usual manner. Through an anterior iliofemoral approach, expose the hip capsule, the greater trochanter, the head of the femur, and the rim of the acetabulum (Fig. 1-86, *A* and *B*). With a curet and osteotome, remove the cartilaginous surface of the anterior aspect and most of the middle and posterior aspects of the head of the femur, as well as part of the acetabulum. Femoral head exposure can be improved by flexing and rotating the extremity on the fracture table, but if adequate exposure cannot be obtained, dislocate the hip joint anteriorly. Approximate the osseous surfaces by reducing the joint or compressing the femoral head into the acetabulum. Remove any soft tissue or synovium that may impede union. Insert three or more long-threaded intramedullary pins, such as Knowles pins, through the femoral neck and head across the joint well into the ilium. Alternatively, use an adult compression hip screw and side plate across the joint and into the pelvis.

Make a slot in the ilium above the acetabulum and in the anterior part of the femoral head and neck to receive a graft (Fig. 1-86, *C* and *D*). Determine the location of the slot by placing the graft over the area it is to cover. Place the graft in the slot, and secure it with one screw in the ilium and one in the femoral neck or intertrochanteric area. Alternatively, place the wide, free surface of the graft on a flat bed prepared on the ilium and the femoral head and neck, and fix the graft as already described. Intertrochanteric osteotomy, as recommended by Davis, may be performed at this time if desired. Close the wounds in the usual manner, and apply a one and a half hip spica cast.

▲ *Postoperative management.* Cast immobilization is continued until roentgenographic evidence of solid fusion. Depending on the security of fixation, weight bearing is allowed at 12 weeks. Internal fixation should be removed approximately 1 year after solid fusion to help prevent pathologic fracture, which occurs in as many as 15% of patients, especially in the subtrochanteric area.

REFERENCES

General

Birch JG, Herring JA, and Wenger DR: Surgical anatomy of selected physes, J Pediatr Orthop 4:224, 1984.

Blount WP: Unequal leg length. In the American Academy of Orthopaedic Surgeons: Instructional course lectures, vol 17, St Louis, 1960, The CV Mosby Co.

Bright RW: Operative correction of partial epiphyseal plate closure by osseous bridge resection and silicone rubber implant, J Bone Joint Surg 56A:655-664, June 1974.

Carlson WO and Wenger DR: A mapping method to prepare for surgical excision of a partial physeal arrest, J Pediatr Orthop 4:232, 1984.

Charnley J: Compression arthrodesis, Edinburgh, 1953, E & S, Livingstone, Ltd.

Clawson RS and McKay DW: Arthrodesis in the presence of infection, Clin Orthop 114:209, 1976.

Crenshaw AH, editor: Campbell's operative orthopaedics, ed 6, St Louis, 1987, The CV Mosby Co.

Engel GM and Staheli LT: The natural history of torsion and other factors influencing gait in childhood, Clin Orthop 99:12, March-April 1974.

Evans FG: Mechanical properties of bone, Springfield, Ill, 1973, Charles C Thomas, Publisher.

Gruelich WW and Pyle SI: Radiographic atlas of skeletal development of the hand and wrist, ed 2, Palo Alto, Calif, 1959, Stanford University Press.

Harper MC and Canale ST: Angulation osteotomy: a trigonometric analysis. Clin Orthop 166:173, 1982.

Heim U and Pfeiffer KM: Internal fixation of small fractures, technique recommended by the AO-ASIF Group, ed 3, Berlin, 1988, Springer-Verlag.

Langenskiöld A: An operation for partial closure of an epiphysial plate in children, and its experimental basis, J Bone Joint Surg 57B:325, 1975.

Mayer A: Historische and statistische Notizen. Die von Dr. Mayer verrichtete Osteotomien, Deutsche Klinik von Göschen 8:119, 1856. Cited in Milch H: Osteotomy of the long bones, Springfield, Ill, 1947, Charles C Thomas, Publisher.

Milch H: Osteotomy of the long bones, Springfield, Ill, 1947, Charles C Thomas, Publisher.

Perren SM and Allgöwer M: Biomechanik der Frakturheilung nach Osteosynthesen, Nova Acta Leopold 44, 223:61, 1976.

Perren SM et al: The reaction of cortical bone to compression, Acta Orthop Scand [Suppl] 125:19, 1969.

Perren SM et al: Biomechanics of fracture healing after internal fixation, Surg Annu 7:361, 1975.

Peterson HA: Partial growth plate arrest and its treatment, J Pediatr Orthop 4:246, 1984.

Poss R: Valgus-extension osteotomy for primary protrusio acetabuli and coxa vara, Strat Orthop Surg 5(2):1, 1986.

Putti V: Arthrodesis for tuberculosis of the knee and of the shoulder, Chir Organi Mov 18:217, 1933.

Songer JE, Kendra JC, and Price CT: Pediatric applications of a dynamic axial external fixator, Scientific exhibit presented at the 55th Annual Meeting of the American Academy of Orthopaedic Surgeons, Atlanta, Feb 4-9, 1988.

Wagner H: Prophylaktische und therapeutische Moglichkeiten bei Alenkdysplasien. Therapiewoche 27:1244, 1977.

Ankle

Barr JS and Record EE: Arthrodesis of the ankle joint: indications, operative technic, and clinical experience, N Engl J Med 248:53, 1953.

Boyd HB: Indications for fusion of the ankle, Orthop Clin North Am 5(1):191, 1974.

Bratberg JJ and Scheer GE: Extraarticular arthrodesis of the subtalar joint: a clinical study and review, Clin Orthop 126:220, 1977.

Calandruccio RA: Personal communication, 1988.

Campbell CJ, Rinehart WT, and Kalenak A: Arthrodesis of the ankle: deep autogenous inlay grafts with maximum cancellous-bone apposition, J Bone Joint Surg 56A:63, 1974.

Campbell WC: An operation for the induction of osseous fusion in the ankle joint, Am J Surg 6:588, 1929.

Charnley J: Compression arthrodesis of the ankle and shoulder. J Bone Joint Surg 33B:180, 1951.

Chuinard EG and Peterson RE: Distraction-compression bone-graft arthrodesis of the ankle: a method especially applicable in children, J Bone Joint Surg 45A:481, 1963.

Davis RJ and Mills MB: Ankle arthrodesis in the management of traumatic ankle arthrosis: a long-term retrospective study. J Trauma 20:674, 1980.

Hetti FL, Baumann JU, and Morscher EW: Ankle joint fusion: determination of optimal position by gait analysis, Arch Orthop Trauma Surg 96:187, 1980.

King HA, Watkins TB Jr, and Samuelson KM: Analysis of foot position in ankle arthrodesis and its influence on gait, Foot Ankle 1:44, 1980.

Lance EM et al: Arthrodesis of the ankle joint: a follow-up study. Clin Orthop 142:146, 1979.

Lloyd-Roberts GC, Swann M, and Catterall A: Medial rotation osteotomy for severe residual deformity in clubfoot, J Bone Joint Surg 56B:37, Feb 1974.

Marcus RE, Balourdas GM, and Heiple KG: Ankle arthrodesis by chevron fusion with internal fixation and bone-grafting. J Bone Joint Surg 65A:833, 1983.

Morrey BF and Wiedeman GP Jr: Complications and long-term results of ankle arthrodesis following trauma, J Bone Joint Surg 62A:777, 1980.

Ratliff AH: Compression arthrodesis of the ankle, J Bone Joint Surg 41B:524, 1959.

Speed JS and Boyd HB: Operative reconstruction of malunited fractures about the ankle joint, J Bone Joint Surg 18:270, 1936.

Stewart MJ, Beeler TC, and McConnell JC: Compression arthrodesis of the ankle: evaluation of a cosmetic modification, J. Bone Joint Surg 65A:219, 1983.

White AA III: A precision posterior ankle fusion, Clin Orthop 98:239, 1974.

Femur

Canario AT et al: A controlled study of results of femoral osteotomy in severe Perthes' disease. J Bone Joint Surg 62B:438, 1980.

Compere EL, Garrison M, and Fahey JJ. Deformities of the femur resulting from arrestment of the growth of the capital and greater trochanteric epiphyses, J Bone Joint Surg 22:909, 1940.

Crider RJ and Leber C: Accurate correction in rotational osteotomies, J Pediatr Orthop 7:468, 1987.

Eilert RE and MacEwen GD. Varus derotational osteotomy of the femur in cerebral palsy, Clin Orthop 125:168, 1977.

Hall RF Jr: Freehand technique for inserting distal nail. In Russell TA, Taylor JC, and LaVelle DG: Russell-Taylor interlocking intramedullary nails, technique manual, Memphis, 1985, Richards Manufacturing Co.

Harper MC, Canale ST, and Cobb RM: Proximal femoral osteotomy: a trigonometric analysis of effect on leg length, J Pediatr Orthop 3:431, 1983.

Heikkinen E and Puranen J. Evaluation of femoral osteotomy in Legg-Calvé-Perthes disease, Clin Orthop 150:60, 1980.

Holz U: Form and function of supracondylar osteotomy. In Hierholzerg G and Muller KH, editors: Corrective osteotomies of the lower extremity after trauma, Berlin, 1985, Springer-Verlag.

Lloyd-Roberts GC, Catterall A, and Salamon PB. A controlled study of the indications for and the results of femoral osteotomy in Perthes' disease, J Bone Joint Surg 58B:31, 1976.

Milch H: Osteotomy at the upper end of the femur, Baltimore, 1965, The Williams & Wilkins Co.

Monticelli G: Intertrochanteric femoral osteotomy with concentric reduction of the femoral head in treatment of residual congenital acetabular dysplasia, Clin Orthop 119:48, 1976.

Russell TA, Taylor JC, and LaVelle DG: Russell-Taylor interlocking intramedullary nails, technique manual, Memphis, 1985, Richards Manufacturing Co.

Southwick WO: Compression fixation after biplane intertrochanteric osteotomy for slipped capital femoral epiphysis, J Bone Joint Surg 55A:1218, 1973.

Weighill FJ: The treatment of developmental coxa vara by abduction subtrochanteric and intertrochanteric femoral osteotomy with special reference to the role of adductor tenotomy, Clin Orthop 116:116, 1976.

Trafton PG et al: A comparative study of compression hip screw and condylocephalic nail for intertrochanteric fractures of the femur, Orthop Trans 8:391, 1984 (abstract).

Hip

Alonso JE, Lovell WW, and Lovejoy JF: The Altdorf hip clamp, J Pediatr Orthop 6:399, 1986.

Axer A: Compression arthrodesis of the hip joint, J Bone Joint Surg 43A:492, 1961.

Brackett EG: A study of the different approaches to the hip-joint, with special reference to the operations for curved trochanteric osteotomy and for arthrodesis, Boston Med Surg J 166:235, 1912.

Calandruccio RA: Personal communication, 1977.

Canale ST: Campbell pediatric cannulated hip screw, technique manual, Zimmer

Canale ST and Holand RW: Coventry screw fixation of osteotomies about the pediatric hip, J Pediatr Orthop 3:592, 1983.

Carnesale PG: Arthrodesis of the hip: a long-term study, Orthop Digest 4:12, 1976.

Chapchal GJ: The intertrochanteric osteotomy in the treatment of congenital dysplasia of the hip, Clin Orthop 119:54, 1976.

Charnley J: Stabilisation of the hip by central dislocation. In Proceedings of the British Orthopaedic Association, May 1955, J Bone Joint Surg 37B:514, 1955 (abstract).

Chuinard EG and Logan ND: Varus producing and derotational subtrochanteric osteotomy in the treatment of congenital dislocation of the hip, J Bone Joint Surg 45A:1397, 1963.

Coleman SS: Congenital dysplasia and dyslocation of the hip, St Louis, 1978, The CV Mosby Co.

Crenshaw AH: Muscle pedicle bone graft in arthrodesis of the hip, South Med J 50:169, 1957.

Curtis BH: The hip in the myelomeningocele child, Clin Orthop 90:11, 1973.

Davis JB: The muscle-pedicle bone graft in hip fusion, J Bone Joint Surg 36A:790, 1954.

Davis JB, Fagan TE, and Beals RK: Follow-up notes on articles previously published in the journal, Muscle-pedicle bone graft in hip fusion, J Bone Joint Surg 53A:1645, 1971.

DePalma AF and Fenlin JM Jr: Arthrodesis of the hip with intramedullary fixation, Clin Orthop 48:191, 1966.

Dickson JA and Willien LJ: Arthrodesis of the hip joint in degenerative arthritis: a modified one-stage procedure with internal fixation, J Bone Joint Surg 29:687, 1947.

Fulkerson JP: Arthrodesis for disabling hip pain in children and adolescents. Clin Orthop 128:296, 1977.

Ghormley RK: Use of the anterior superior spine and crest of ilium in surgery of the hip joint, J Bone Joint Surg 13:784, 1931.

Makley JT et al: Varus-medial displacement osteotomy of the hip for control of valgus instability in children, J Bone Joint Surg 57A:1172, 1975.

McKee GK: Arthrodesis of the hip with a lagscrew, J Bone Joint Surg 39B:477, 1957.

Mowery CA et al: A simple method of hip arthrodesis, J Pediatr Orthop 6:7, 1986.

Müller ME: Arthrodesis of the hip using the cross-plate. In Hip surgery: twelve hip procedures, AO Bulletin (Official periodical of the Association for the Study of the Problems of Internal Fixation), Sept 1967, p 48.

Müller ME: Allgower M, and Willenegger H. Manual of internal fixation, New York: 1970, Springer-Verlag.

Müller ME et al: Manual of internal fixation, techniques recommended by the AO Group, ed 2, Berlin, 1977, Springer-Verlag.

Onji Y, Kurata Y, and Kido H: A new method of hip fusion using an intramedullary nail: preliminary report, J Bone Joint Surg 47B:690, 1965.

Pease CN: Fusion of the hip in children: the Chandler method, J Bone Joint Surg 29:874, 1947.

Price CT and Lovell WW: Thompson arthrodesis of the hip in children. J Bone Joint Surg 62A:1118, 1980.

Ranawat CS, Jordan LR, and Wilson PD Jr: A technique of muscle-pedicle bone graft in hip arthrodesis: a report of its use in ten cases, J Bone Joint Surg 53A:925, 1971.

Root L and Siegal T: Osteotomy of the hip in children: posterior approach, J Bone Joint Surg 62A:571, 1980.

Samilson RL et al: Dislocation and subluxation of the hip in cerebral palsy. Pathogenesis, natural history and management, J Bone Joint Surg 54A:863, 1972.

Schatzker J, editor: The intertrochanteric osteotomy, Berlin, 1984, Springer-Verlag.

Stewart MJ and Coker TP Jr: Arthrodesis of the hip: a review of 109 patients, Clin Orthop 62:136, 1969.

Tronzo RG, editor: Surgery of the hip joint, Philadelphia, 1973, Lea & Febiger.

Wagner H: Osteotomies for congenital hip dislocations. In The hip: proceedings of the Fourth Scientific Meeting of the Hip Society, St Louis, 1976, The CV Mosby Co.

Knee

Charnley J and Baker SL: Compression arthrodesis of the knee: a clinical and histological study, J Bone Joint Surg 34B:187, 1952.

Charnley J and Lowe HB: A study of the end-results of compression arthrodesis of the knee, J Bone Joint Surg 40B:633, 1958.

Clawson, RS and McKay, DW: Arthrodesis in the presence of infection, Clin Orthop 114:207, 1976.

Coventry MB: Osteotomy about the knee for degenerative and rheumatoid arthritis: indications, operative technique and results, J Bone Joint Surg 55A:23, 1973.

Drennan DB, Fahey JJ, and Maylahn DJ: Important factors in achieving arthrodesis of the Charcot knee, J Bone Joint Surg 53A:1180, 1971.

Hibbs RA: An operation for stiffening the knee joint with report of four cases from the service of the New York Orthopedic Hospital, Ann Surg 53:404, 1911.

Hibbs RA and von Lackum HL: End-results in treatment of knee joint tuberculosis, JAMA 85:1289, 1925.

Kaplan CJ: Compression arthrodesis of the knee joint: a case report, J Bone Joint Surg 35A:781, 1953.

Key JA: Arthrodesis of the knee with a large central autogenous bone peg, South Med J 30:574, 1937.

Mazet R Jr and Urist MR: Arthrodesis of the knee with intramedullary nail fixation, Clin Orthop 18:43, 1960.

McKeever FM: Tuberculosis of the knee in infancy and childhood, JAMA 113:1293, 1939.

Morley AJM: Knock knee in children, Br Med J 11:976, 1957.

Morris HD and Mosiman RS: Arthrodesis of the knee: a comparison of the compression method with the non-compression method, J Bone Joint Surg 33A:982, 1951.

Peterson LFA and Bryan RS: Arthrodesis of the knee, Orthop Clin North Am 2:729, 1971.

Stewart MJ and Bland WG: Compression in arthrodesis: a comparative study of methods of fusion of the knee in ninety-three cases, J Bone Joint Surg 40A:585, 1958.

Velazco A and Fleming LL: Compression arthrodesis of the knee and ankle with the Hoffman external fixator, South Med J 76:1393, 1983.

Zuege RC, Kempken TG, and Blount WP: Epiphyseal stapling for angular deformity of the knee, J Bone Joint Surg 61A:320, 1979.

Tibia

Bauer GCH, Insall J, and Koshino T: Tibial osteotomy in gonarthrosis, J Bone Joint Surg 51A:1545, 1969.

Beck CL et al: Physeal bridge resection in infantile Blount disease, J Pediatr Orthop 7:161, 1987.

Blount WP: Tibia vara (osteochondrosis deformans tibiae). In Adams JP, editor: Current practice in orthopaedic surgery, vol 3, St Louis, 1966, The CV Mosby Co.

Canale ST and Harper MC: Biometric analysis and practical applications of osteotomies of tibia in children. The American Academy of Orthopaedic Surgeons: Instructional course lectures, vol 30, St. Louis, 1981, The CV Mosby Co.

Coventry MB: Osteotomy of the upper portion of the tibia for degenerative arthritis of the knee: a preliminary report, J Bone Joint Surg 47A:984, 1965.

Harris WR and Kostuik JP: High tibial osteotomy for osteo-arthritis of the knee, J Bone Joint Surg 52A:330, 1970.

Ingram AJ: Personal communication, Memphis, 1980.

Insall J, Shoji H, and Mayer V: High tibial osteotomy, J Bone Joint Surg 56A:1397, 1974.

Jackson JP, Waugh W, and Green JP: High tibial osteotomy for osteoarthritis of the knee, J Bone Joint Surg 51B:88, 1969.

Langenskiöld A and Riska EB: Tibia vara (osteochondrosis deformans tibiae), J Bone Joint Surg 46A:1405, 1964.

Salenius P and Vankka E: Development of the tibiofemoral angle in children, J Bone Joint Surg [Am] 57:259, 1975.

Siffert RS: Intraepiphyseal osteotomy for progressive tibia vara: case report and rationale of management, J Pediatr Orthop 2:81, 1982.

Steel HH, Sandrow RE, and Sullivan PD: Complications of tibial osteotomy in children for genu varum or valgum, J Bone Joint Surg 53A:1629, 1971.

Støren H: Operative evaluation of the medial tibial joint surface in Blount's disease—one case observed for 18 years after surgery. Acta Orthop Scand 40:788, 1970.

Weber BG: Fractures of the proximal tibial metaphysis. In Weber BG, Brunner C, and Freuler, F, editors: Treatment of fractures in children and adolescents, New York, 1980, Springer-Verlag.

2 Congenital Anomalies of the Lower and Upper Extremities

JAMES H. BEATY

Congenital anomalies of the foot, lower extremity, hip, pelvis, trunk, and upper extremity are described in this chapter. Congenital anomalies of the hand and the spine are discussed in Chapters 4 and 9, respectively. Many of the operative techniques described here are useful for other conditions and are referenced in other chapters.

Foot and Lower Extremity

ANOMALIES OF FOOT
Congenital Metatarsus Adductus

Metatarsus adductus, which consists of adduction of the forefoot in relation to the midfoot and hindfoot, is a fairly common anomaly, often causing intoeing in children. It may occur as an isolated anomaly or in association with clubfoot. Of those with metatarsus adductus, 1% to 5% may also have congenital hip dislocation or acetabular dysplasia.

Clinically, metatarsus adductus may be classified as mild, moderate, or severe as described by Bleck. In the mild form the forefoot can be clinically abducted to the midline of the foot and beyond. The moderate form has enough flexibility to allow abduction of the forefoot to the midline, but usually not beyond. In rigid metatarsus adductus the forefoot cannot be abducted at all. There also may be a transverse crease on the medial border of the foot or an enlargement of the web space between the great and second toes (Fig. 2-1). In general, mild metatarsus adductus will resolve without treatment. Moderate or severe metatarsus adductus is best treated initially by serial stretching and casting until the foot is clinically flexible.

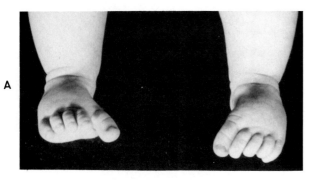
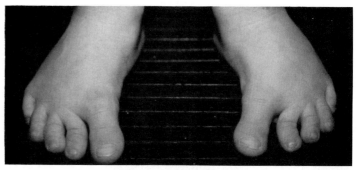
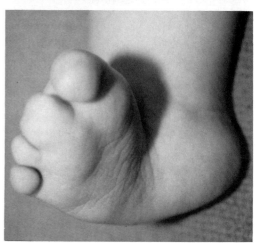

Fig. 2-1 Congenital metatarsus adductus. **A,** Mild. **B,** Moderate. **C,** Severe.

Metatarsus adductus may be seen as a residual deformity in patients previously treated for congenital clubfoot, either surgically or nonsurgically. This residual metatarsus adductus may be rigid, indicating a fixed positioning of the forefoot on the midfoot and hindfoot, or it may be dynamic, caused by imbalance of the tibialis anterior tendon during gait. The rigidity or flexibility of the forefoot should be determined before any surgical correction in the older child is undertaken.

Surgical Treatment

In the young child surgery is not indicated until conservative treatment has failed. Once a child passes the appropriate age for serial stretching and casting, surgery becomes a reasonable option. The indications for surgery include pain, objectional appearance, or difficulty in fitting shoes because of residual forefoot adduction.

Numerous soft tissue and bony procedures have been described for correction of metatarsus adductus; the choice of procedure depends on the age and deformity of the particular child.

Lichtblau described division of the abductor hallucis tendon for early correction of metatarsus adductus, especially after treatment for clubfoot. This procedure is indicated infrequently because one rarely can be confident that release of the tendon will correct the deformity. Heyman and Herndon described mobilization of the tarsometatarsal and intermetatarsal joints by capsular release for correction of metatarsus adductus. This is the procedure of choice in a child of preschool age with severe, symptomatic, metatarsus adductus. Potential complications include dorsal subluxation of the bases of the metatarsals and injury to the small joints of the midfoot and forefoot.

In children 5 years old and older with residual rigid metatarsus adductus, metatarsal osteotomy is the preferred procedure. Berman and Gartland described dome-shaped osteotomies made at the bases of the metatarsals for this situation. Full correction also may require small lateral closing wedge osteotomies.

Rarely, in children with dynamic metatarsus adductus from imbalance of the tibialis anterior tendon, especially after treatment for congenital clubfoot, either a split transfer of the tibialis anterior tendon or transfer of the entire tendon to the middle cuneiform is appropriate if symptoms are sufficient to require surgery. This is infrequently indicated in neurologically normal children.

• • •

In 1970 Kendrick et al reviewed 80 feet treated by capsular releases at the metatarsal bases (Heyman-Herndon procedure), and the result was good or excellent in 92%. They recommend the operation for children 3 to 8 years of age. Stark, Johanson, and Winter reviewed results in 32 patients and found a 41% overall failure rate and a 51% incidence of painful dorsal prominence at the surgical scar. The procedure is included for completeness.

▶ *Technique (Heyman-Herndon).* Make two straight incisions, one between the first and second metatarsals and the second in line with the fourth metatarsal (Fig. 2-2, *A*). A curved dorsal incision across the full width of the foot just distal to the tarsometatarsal joints may be used instead, but two incisions are preferable. With gentle care for the skin edges, free the extensor hallucis longus and the extensor digitorum longus muscles of the second toe and retract them medially and laterally, respectively. Protect the neurovascular bundle between the bases of the first and second metatarsals. Now identify the intermetatarsal space by probing with a small hemostat, and sharply divide the intermetatarsal ligament between the first and second metatarsals from distally to proximally. Locate and divide the dorsal capsule of the first tarsometatarsal joint, avoiding damage to the articular surfaces of the

bones. Protect the tibialis anterior tendon, and divide sharply the medial capsule of the first tarsometatarsal joint, leaving only the plantar capsule of this joint intact (Fig. 2-2, *B*). Next identify the second tarsometatarsal joint a little proximal to the first and divide its dorsal capsule. Dissect longitudinally over the third metatarsal, protecting the neurovascular bundles and the extensor tendons, to reach the intermetatarsal space between the second and third metatarsals. Divide the intermetatarsal ligament here also, and incise the dorsal capsule of the third tarsometatarsal joint. By similar incisions free the bases of the other metatarsals, leaving the plantar capsules intact (Fig. 2-2, *C*). Preserve the lateral capsule of the fifth tarsometatarsal joint to serve as a hinge and to prevent lateral displacement of the base of the fifth metatarsal. While plantar flexing each metatarsal and apply-

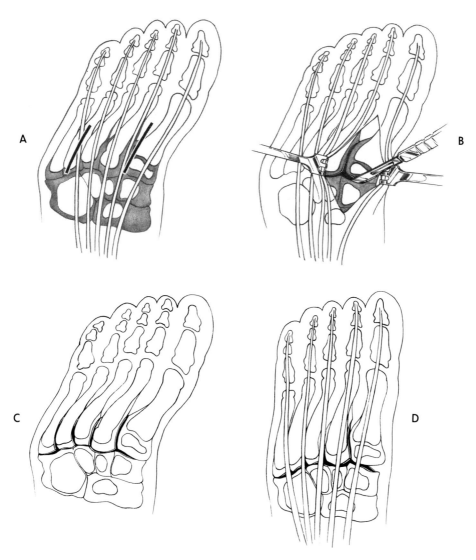

Fig. 2-2 Heyman-Herndon procedure for correcting congenital metatarsus adductus (see text). (Redrawn from Kendrick RE et al: J Bone Joint Surg 52A:61, 1970.)

ing traction, and using care not to damage the articular surfaces, divide the medial two thirds of the plantar capsule of each joint, leaving the lateral one third intact. Enough stability should be retained to prevent displacement of the metatarsal bases when the bones are properly aligned. Now abduct the metatarsals to their normal positions (Fig. 2-2, *D*), but do not be concerned that the articular surfaces are irregular because they will remodel with time. Next secure hemostasis and close the incision. Apply a well-molded short leg cast with the foot in the corrected position. When the metatarsal bases are unstable, Kirschner wires can be used to fix the first metatarsal base to the first cuneiform and the fifth to the cuboid. Thus position will not be lost during changes of the cast.

▶ *Postoperative management.* At 3 weeks when the wound has healed, the cast is changed and the sutures are removed. A carefully molded short leg cast should be worn for about 3 months and then removed along with the Kirschner wires. Occasionally there is slight dorsal subluxation of the proximal end of the first metatarsal or lateral prominence of the base of the fifth metatarsal. Preservation of one third of each plantar capsule should prevent these deformities. Damage to the articular surfaces should be avoided to minimize early stiffening of the forefoot and osteoarthritis in later life.

• • •

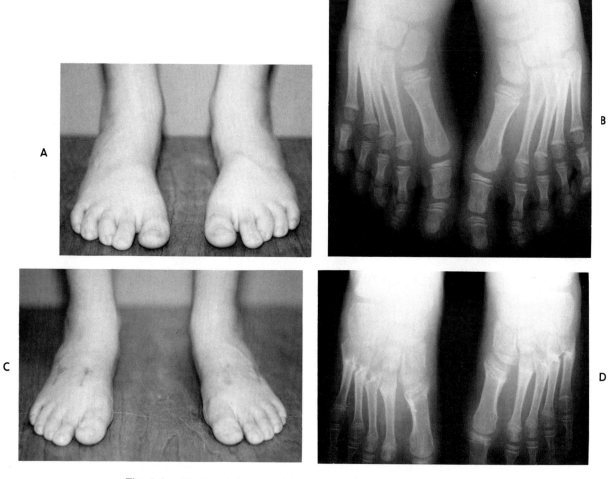

Fig. 2-3 Rigid metatarsus adductus in 8-year-old child before (**A** and **B**) and after (**C** and **D**) metatarsal osteotomies.

Berman and Gartland have recommended dome-shaped osteotomies of all five metatarsal bases for resistant forefoot adduction in children 5 years of age or older (Fig. 2-3).

For the mature foot with uncorrected metatarsus varus, because all the medial structures are shortened, Berman and Gartland recommend a laterally based closing wedge osteotomy through the bases of the metatarsals and through the cuneiforms and the cuboid. Correcting the alignment without shortening the lateral border of the foot may cause excessive tension on the skin on the medial border or on the neurovascular bundle posterior to the medial malleolus. Steinmann pins inserted parallel to the medial and lateral borders of the foot usually are necessary to hold the foot in the corrected position until the osteotomy has healed. Without internal fixation the tight structures on the medial side may cause recurrence of deformity and nonunion of the osteotomy.

▶ *Technique (Berman and Gartland).* Approach all five metatarsal bases dorsally. Make two longitudinal dorsal incisions, one between the first and second metatarsals and the other overlying the fourth. Protect the extensor tendons and superficial nerves, and preserve the superficial veins as much as possible. Next expose subperiosteally the proximal metaphysis of each metatarsal, and with a small power drill make a dome-shaped osteotomy in each with the apex of the dome proximally (Fig. 2-4). Avoid the physis at the base of the first metatarsal. When adequate correction cannot be obtained by these osteotomies, resect small wedges of bone based laterally at the osteotomies as needed. Align the metatarsals, and transfix the foot in the corrected position with small smooth Steinmann pins inserted proximally through the shafts of the first and fifth metatarsals and across the osteotomies in these bones. Prevent dorsal or volar angulation and overriding of the fragments. Before closing the wound, check the placement of the pins and position of the osteotomies by roentgenograms. The talo–first metatarsal angle should be corrected 0 to plus-10 degrees.

▶ *Postoperative management.* A short leg cast is applied with the foot in the corrected position. At 6 weeks the cast and pins are removed and weight bearing is begun, commonly in a walking cast for a few weeks. Complications from this operation have been few. Exposure is better through a single curved incision, but small skin sloughs occasionally occur, so two dorsal longitudinal incisions are preferred.

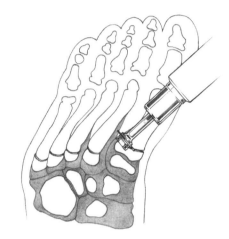

Fig. 2-4 Berman and Gartland technique for metatarsal osteotomy. Dome-shaped osteotomy is being completed at base of each metatarsal.

Clubfoot

The incidence of congenital clubfoot is approximately 1 in every 1000 live births. Although most cases occur sporadically, cases of families with clubfoot as an autosomal dominant trait with incomplete penetrance have been reported. Bilateral deformities occur in 50% of children.

Several theories have been proposed regarding the cause of clubfoot. One is that a primary germ plasm defect in the talus causes continued plantar flexion and inversion of this bone with subsequent soft tissue changes in the joints and musculotendinous complexes. Another theory is that primary soft tissue abnormalities within the neuromuscular units cause secondary bony changes. Clinically children with clubfoot have a hypotrophic anterior tibial artery, in addition to the obvious atrophy of the musculature around the calf. The abnormal foot may be as much as a half to one size smaller in both length and width.

The pathologic changes caused by congenital clubfoot must be understood if the anomaly is to be treated effectively. The three basic components of clubfoot are equinus, varus, and adduction deformities, but the deformity varies in severity from one in which the entire foot is in an equinus and varus position, the forefoot is in adduction, and there is a cavus deformity to one much less severe in which the foot is in only a mild equinus and varus position (Fig. 2-5, *A* and *B*). Clubfoot often is accompanied by internal tibial torsion. The ankle, midtarsal, and subtalar joints all are involved in the pathologic process.

Turco attributes the deformity to medial displacement of the navicular and calcaneus around the talus, and his observations at surgery have helped to delineate more clearly the bony deformities in the clubfoot. According to Turco the talus is forced into equinus position by the underlying calcaneus and navicular, whereas the talar head and neck of the talus are deviated medially. The calcaneus is inverted under the talus, with the posterior end displaced upward and the anterior end displaced downward and medially.

McKay added an awareness of the three-dimensional aspect of bony deformity of the subtalar complex in clubfoot. According to his description, the relationship of the calcaneus to the talus is characterized by abnormal rotation in the sagittal, coronal, and horizontal planes. As the calcaneus rotates horizontally while pivoting on the interosseous ligament, it slips beneath the head and neck of the talus anterior to the ankle joint, and the calcaneal tuberosity moves toward the fibular malleolus posteriorly. Thus the proximity of the calcaneus to the fibula is due primarily to horizontal rotation of the talocalcaneal joint rather than to equinus. The heel appears to be in varus because the calcaneus rotates through the talocalcaneal joint in a coronal plane as well as horizontally. The talonavicular joint is in an extreme position of inversion as the navicular moves around the head of the talus. The cuboid is displaced medially on the calcaneus.

Herzenberg et al demonstrated with three-dimensional computer modeling that in the clubfoot the talar neck is rotated internally relative to the ankle mortise, but the talar body is externally rotated in the mortise. They also showed the calcaneus to be significantly internally rotated with the sloped articular facet of the calcaneocuboid joint, causing additional internal rotation of the midfoot.

Contractures or anomalies of the soft tissues exert further deforming forces and resist correction of bony deformity and realignment of the joints. Talocalcaneal joint realignment is opposed by the calcaneo fibular ligament, the superior peroneal retinaculum (calcaneofibular retinaculum), peroneal tendon sheaths, and posterior talocalcaneal ligament. Resisting realignment of the talonavicular joint are the posterior tibial tendon, deltoid ligament (tibial navicular), calcaneonavicular ligament (spring ligament), the entire talonavicular capsule, dorsal talonavicular ligament, bifurcated (Y) ligament, inferior extensor retinaculum and, occasionally, the cubonavicular oblique ligament. Internal rotation of the calcaneocuboid joint causes contracture of the bifurcated (Y) ligament, the long plantar ligament, plantar calcaneocuboid ligament, navicular cuboid ligament, inferior extensor retinaculum (cruciate ligament), dorsal calcaneocuboid ligament, and occasionally the cubonavicular ligament.

The metatarsals often are also deformed. They may deviate at their tarsometatarsal joints, or these joints may be normal and the shafts of the metatarsals themselves may be adducted.

If the clubfoot is allowed to remain deformed, many other late adaptive changes occur in the bones. These changes depend on the severity of the soft tissue contractures and the effects of walking. At skeletal maturity some of the joints may spontaneously fuse, or they may develop degenerative changes as a result of the contractures.

The initial examination of the foot and the progress of treatment should depend on both clinical judgment and roentgenographic examination. A standard roentgenographic technique is essential, and the technician should be carefully instructed in its use.

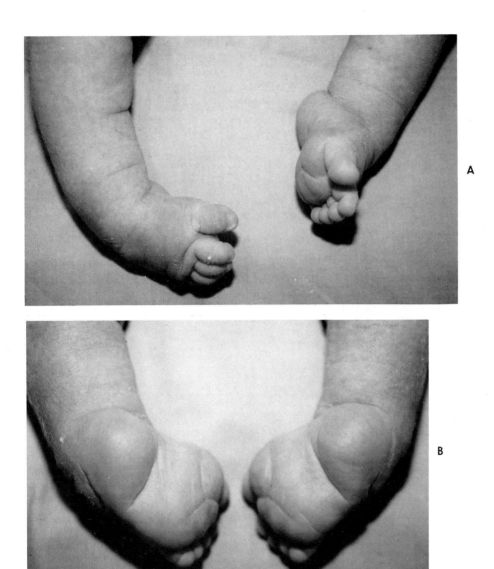

A

B

Fig. 2-5   Bilateral congenital clubfoot in newborn. **A,** On anterior view, note adduction and supination of forefoot and equinus of hindfoot. **B,** On posterior view, note inversion, plantar flexion, and internal rotation of calcaneus, as well as associated cavus deformity with transverse plantar crease.

Roentgenographic Evaluation

Roentgenograms should be included as part of the evaluation of clubfoot, before, during, and after treatment. In the nonambulatory child, standard roentgenograms include anteroposterior and dorsiflexion lateral stress views of both feet. Anteroposterior and lateral standing roentgenograms may be obtained for the older child.

Fig. 2-6 Roentgenographic evaluation of clubfoot. **A,** Anteroposterior view of right clubfoot with decrease in talocalcaneal angle and negative talo–first metatarsal angle. **B,** Talocalcaneal angle on anteroposterior view of normal left foot. **C,** Talocalcaneal angle of zero and negative tibiocalcaneal angle on dorsiflexion lateral view of right clubfoot. **D,** Talocalcaneal and tibiocalcaneal angles on dorsiflexion lateral view of normal left foot.

Important angles to consider in the evaluation of clubfoot are the talocalcaneal angle on the anteroposterior roentgenogram, the talocalcaneal angle on the lateral roentgenogram, the tibiocalcaneal angle on the lateral roentgenogram, and the talometatarsal angle (Fig. 2-6). The anteroposterior talocalcaneal angle in the normal child ranges from 30 to 55 degrees. In clubfoot, this angle progressively decreases with increasing heel varus. On the dorsiflexion lateral roentgenogram the talocalcaneal angle in the normal foot varies from 25 to 50 degrees; in clubfoot, this angle progressively decreases with the severity of the deformity to an angle of zero. The tibiocalcaneal angle on the stress lateral roentgenogram is 10 to 40 degrees in the normal foot. In clubfoot this angle generally is negative, indicating equinus of the calcaneus in relation to the tibia. Finally, the talo–first metatarsal angle is a roentgenographic measurement of forefoot adduction. This is useful in the treatment of metatarsus

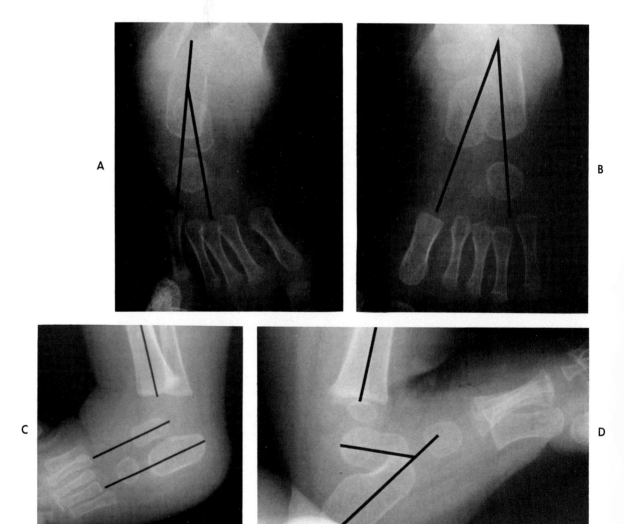

adductus alone, but it is equally important in the treatment of clubfoot to evaluate the position of the forefoot. In a normal foot this angle is 0 to 20 degrees; in clubfoot, it usually is negative, indicating adduction of the forefoot.

The importance of the roentgenographic findings and the measurement of angles in clubfoot cannot be overstated. The angles correlate well with the clinical appearance of the foot and with the result after nonsurgical and surgical treatment. Adequate roentgenograms should be obtained during treatment to be certain that the foot is corrected not only clinically but roentgenographically. If the deformity is unilateral, the normal foot can be used as a control to determine roentgenographic correction.

Nonsurgical Treatment

The initial treatment of clubfoot is nonsurgical. Various treatment regimens have been proposed, including the use of corrective splinting, taping, and casting. Treatment consists of weekly serial manipulation and casting during the first 6 weeks of life, followed by manipulation and casting every other week until the foot is clinically and roentgenographically corrected.

With experience, the clinician is able to predict which feet will respond to nonsurgical treatment. The more rigid the initial deformity, the more likely it is that surgical treatment will be required.

The order of correction by serial manipulation and casting should be as follows: first, correction of forefoot adduction; next, correction of heel varus; and finally, correction of hindfoot equinus. Correction should be pursued in this order so that a rocker-bottom deformity will be prevented by dorsiflexing the foot through the hindfoot rather than the midfoot (Fig. 2-7). The casting program initially outlined by Kite and modified by Lovell has been successful. The success rate of serial manipulation and casting, as reported in the literature, ranges from 15% to 80%. The experience at the Campbell Clinic has been that correction occurs in approximately 20% of children with serial casting alone. If a rocker-bottom deformity does occur, the forefoot may be placed back in plantar flexion and casting resumed. Surgery frequently is necessary in this situation.

If the clubfoot is corrected by the time the child is 6 months of age, this should be documented both by the clinical appearance and by repeated anteroposterior and dorsiflexion lateral stress roentgenograms.

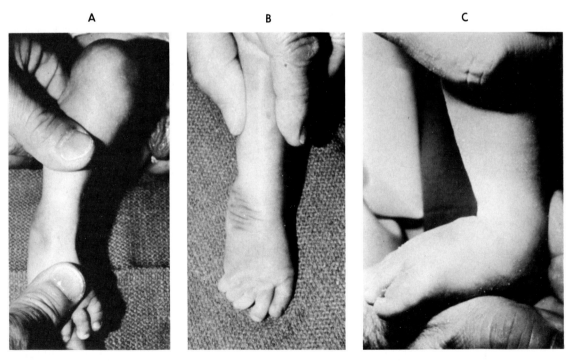

Fig. 2-7 Serial manipulation and stretching of clubfoot in newborn. **A,** Initial stretching for correction of metatarsus adductus. **B,** Forefoot stretched to corrected position at initial examination. Note redundant skin on anterolateral border of foot and ankle. **C,** Initial manipulation of hindfoot to correct heel valgus. Note placement of palm under hindfoot rather than at midfoot or forefoot level. (Courtesy Dr. Wood Lovell.)

Then the foot may be placed in a series of holding casts that can be used part-time on children with compliant families. Continued casting or bracing is an effort to prevent recurrence. The first sign of recurrence usually is progressive contracture of the tendo Achilles. In children between 6 and 18 months of age, a Phelps brace fitted with an inside bar and outside T-strap on a hightop shoe or an ankle-foot orthosis may be used as a holding device.

Surgical Treatment

Surgery in clubfoot is indicated for deformities that do not respond to conservative treatment by serial manipulation and casting. Often in children with a significant rigid clubfoot deformity the forefoot has been corrected by conservative treatment, but the hindfoot remains fixed in both varus and equinus or deformity has recurred. Surgery in the treatment of clubfoot must be tailored to the age of the child and to the deformity to be corrected.

For the mild deformity without severe internal rotation deformity of the calcaneus that does not require extensive posterolateral release, the treatment of choice is a one-stage surgical release, such as the posteromedial release described by Turco. A more extensive release, including the posterolateral ligament complex, is required for severe deformity. The procedure described by McKay takes into consideration the three-dimensional deformity of the subtalar joint and allows correction of the internal rotation deformity of the calcaneus and release of the contractures of the posterolateral and posteromedial foot. A modified McKay procedure through a transverse Cincinnati incision is preferred for the initial surgical management of most cases of clubfoot. General principles for any one-stage extensile clubfoot release include (1) release of the tourniquet at the completion of the procedure, obtaining hemostasis by electrocautery, and (2) careful subcutaneous and skin closure with the foot in plantar flexion if necessary to prevent tension on the skin. The foot may be placed in a fully corrected position 2 weeks after surgery at the first postoperative cast change. Surgery may be performed with the child supine or prone at the discretion of the surgeon.

▶ *Technique of posteromedial release (Turco).* Make a medial incision 8 to 9 cm long extending from the base of the first metatarsal to the tendo Achilles, curving it slightly just inferior to the medial malleolus (Fig. 2-8, *A*). Do not undermine the skin. Next expose and mobilize by careful dissection the tendons of the tibialis posterior, flexor digitorum longus, and flexor hallucis longus and the posterior tibial neurovascular bundle; also expose the tendo Achilles (Fig. 2-8, *B*). Incise the sheaths of the tendons as they are exposed.

Next free the posterior tibial neurovascular bundle, and retract it posteriorly. Now by continuing the incision in the sheaths of the flexor digitorum longus and flexor hallucis longus, divide the master knot of Henry beneath the navicular. Divide the calcaneonavicular (spring) ligament and the abnormal origin of the abductor hallucis.

Of the remaining contractures, release the posterior ones first. Lengthen the tendo Achilles by Z-plasty technique, detaching the medial half of its tendinous insertion on the calcaneus (Fig. 2-8, *C*). Now retract the neurovascular bundle and the flexor hallucis longus anteriorly, and expose the posterior aspect of the ankle and subtalar joints. Incise the posterior capsule of the ankle joint under direct vision (Fig. 2-8, *D*). If necessary divide the posterior talofibular ligament at this time. Next identify the posterior capsule of the subtalar joint and divide this along with the calcaneofibular ligament. This ligament usually is contracted in older children.

Retract the neurovascular bundle posteriorly, and divide the tibiocalcaneal part of the deltoid ligament. Do this by merely extending the incision in the posterior capsule of the subtalar joint medially and anteriorly. Next release the deep medial structures. Retract the neurovascular bundle and lengthen by Z-plasty the tibialis posterior tendon just proximal to the medial malleolus. Use its distal end as a retractor of the navicular. Now pull on the distal end of the tendon, and mobilize the navicular by opening the talonavicular joint and excising that part of the deltoid ligament that inserts on this bone. Incise the talonavicular capsule but avoid damaging any articular surfaces. Next free the tibialis posterior attachment to the sustentaculum tali and the spring ligament, and detach the spring ligament from the sustentaculum.

Now return to the posterior part of the incision and evert the foot. Release the superficial layer of the deltoid ligament from the calcaneus posteriorly under direct vision. Do not incise the deep layer of this ligament that extends from the body of the talus to the medial malleolus because this would cause a flatfoot deformity. The only remaining structures to be released are the subtalar ligaments. Evert the foot, expose the talocalcaneal interosseous ligament, and cut the ligament under direct vision (Fig. 2-8, *E*). Now divide the bifurcated (Y) ligament that extends from the calcaneus to the lateral border of the navicular and to the medial border of the cuboid. This completes the mobilization of the navicular.

Reduce the navicular onto the head of the talus, which will properly align the other tarsal bones. Avoid pushing the navicular too far laterally on the head of the talus. Make sure that the relationship of the calcaneus and the navicular to the talus is correct.

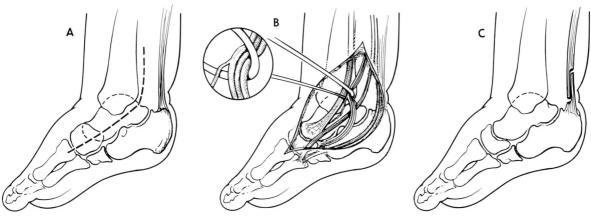

Fig. 2-8 Turco procedure for posteromedial clubfoot release (see text).

Next insert a Kirschner wire percutaneously from the dorsum of the first metatarsal shaft across the medial cuneiform and the navicular and into the talus, transfixing the talonavicular joint. A second plantar Kirschner wire may be used to fix the subtalar joint. The foot now should remain corrected without external force. Intraoperative roentgenograms may be obtained to assess correction.

Repair the tendo Achilles with one or two interrupted sutures after it has been lengthened enough to allow dorsiflexion of the ankle to a right angle. Do not lengthen the tendon too much. Suture the tibialis posterior tendon. Now close the subcutaneous tissues and skin with interrupted sutures. Bend the wire as it lies just outside the skin so that it does not migrate, and place a sterile piece of felt between the wire and the skin for protection. Apply a well-padded long leg cast with the knee in slight flexion and the ankle dorsiflexed only to the neutral position. Excessive dorsiflexion will cause too much tension on the skin and subcutaneous tissues (Fig. 2-9).

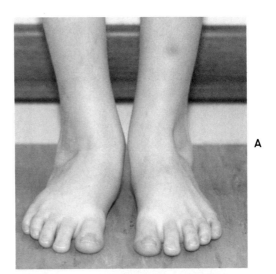

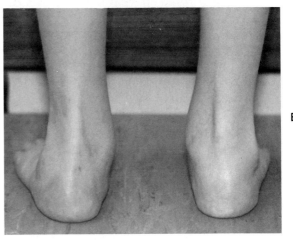

Fig. 2-9 Six-year-old child had Turco procedure at 12 months of age. **A,** Anterior view. **B,** Posterior view.

▲ *Postoperative management.* At 2 weeks the cast is changed with the patient under general anesthesia. A new long leg cast is applied with the foot in greater dorsiflexion. At 6 weeks the cast and the Kirschner wire are removed. A new long leg cast is applied with the foot held in full correction. This cast is worn until 4 months after surgery. Bracing with either a Phelps brace or polypropylene ankle-foot orthosis may be used full-time or part-time for an additional 6 to 9 months.

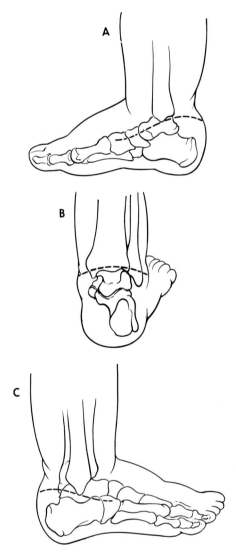

Fig. 2-10 Transverse or Cincinnati incision as described by Crawford et al. **A,** Medial view. **B,** Posterior view. **C,** Lateral view. (Redrawn from Crawford AH, Marxen JL, and Osterfeld DL: J Bone Joint Surg 64A:1355, 1982.)

▲ *Technique of Cincinnati incision (Crawford et al).* One option available in performing posteromedial or posterolateral release is the use of the transverse, or Cincinnati, incision. This incision provides excellent exposure of the subtalar joint and is useful in patients with a severe internal rotational deformity of the calcaneus. One potential problem with this incision is tension on the suture line when the surgeon attempts to place the foot in dorsiflexion to apply the postoperative cast. To avoid this, the foot may be placed in plantar flexion in the immediate postoperative cast and then in dorsiflexion to the corrected position at the first cast change when the wound has healed at 2 weeks after surgery. This cast change frequently requires sedation or general anesthesia on an outpatient basis.

Begin the incision on the medial aspect of the foot in the region of the naviculocuneiform joint (Fig. 2-10, *A*). Carry the incision posteriorly, gently curving beneath the distal end of the medial malleolus and then ascending slightly to pass transversely over the tendo Achilles approximately at the level of the tibiotalar joint (Fig. 2-10, *B*). Continue the incision in a gentle curve over the lateral malleolus, and end it just distal and slightly medial to the sinus tarsi (Fig. 2-10, *C*). Extend the incision distally either medially or laterally, depending on the requirements of the operation.

▲ *Extensile posteromedial and posterolateral release (modified McKay)* (Fig. 2-11). Incise the skin through a Cincinnati incision, preserving if possible the veins on the lateral side and protecting the sural nerve. Then dissect the subcutaneous tissue up and down the tendo Achilles to lengthen the tendon at least 2.5 cm in the coronal plane. Incise the superior peroneal retinaculum off the calcaneus at the point where it blends with the sheath of the tendo Achilles. Dissecting carefully, separate the calcaneofibular and posterior calcaneotalar ligaments, the thickened superior peroneal retinaculum, and the peroneal tendon sheath. Cut off the calcaneofibular ligament close to the calcaneus (this ligament is short and thick and attached very close to the apophysis). Elevate the peroneal tendon sheaths and the superior peroneal retinaculum from the lateral side of the calcaneus, using sharp dissection but being careful not to cut the peroneal tendons.

Incise the lateral talocalcaneal ligament and the lateral capsule of the talocalcaneal joint from their attachment to the calcaneocuboid joint to the point where they enter the sheath of the flexor hallucis longus tendon posteriorly. In the more resistant clubfoot the origin of the extensor digitorum brevis, cruciate crural ligament (inferior extensor retinaculum), dorsal calcaneocuboid ligament, and, occasionally, cu-

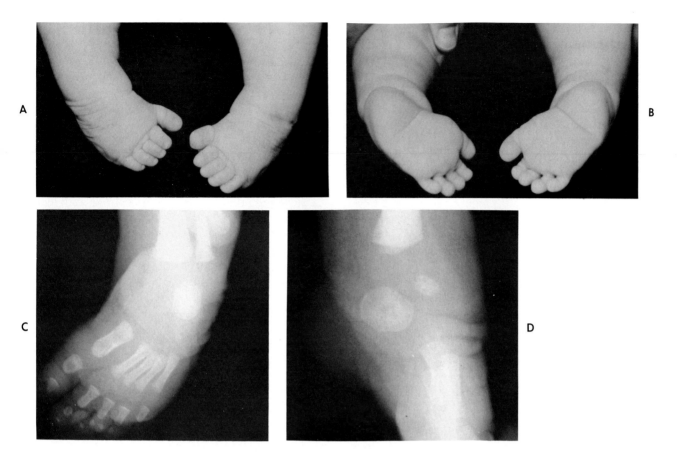

Fig. 2-11 Bilateral clubfoot deformities before modified McKay procedure. **A** and **B,** Clinical appearance. **C,** Roentgenographic appearance on anteroposterior view. **D,** Dorsiflexion lateral view.

bonavicular oblique ligament must be dissected off the calcaneus to allow the anterior portion of the calcaneus to move laterally.

On the medial side, dissect free the neurovascular bundle (medial and lateral plantar nerves and associated vascular components) into the arch of the foot, taking particular care to preserve the medial calcaneal branch of the lateral plantar nerve. Protect and retract the neurovascular bundle with a small Penrose drain. Complete dissection of the medial and lateral neurovascular bundle throughout the arch of the foot, being careful not to enter the sheath of the flexor hallucis longus and flexor digitorum longus tendons or the posterior tibial tendon.

Enter the compartment of the medial plantar neurovascular bundle, and follow it into the arch of the foot well beyond the cuneiforms, taking down the master knot of Henry. Elevate the abductor hallucis muscle and the sheaths of the posterior tibial tendon and the flexor hallucis longus and flexor digitorum longus tendons. Section the narrow strip of fascia be-

tween the medial and lateral branches of the plantar nerve to allow the abductor hallucis to slide distally.

Enter the sheath of the posterior tibial tendon just posterior to and above the medial malleolus. Split the sheath and superficial deltoid ligament up the tibia until the muscle can be identified. Then lengthen the tendon by Z-plasty at least 2.5 cm proximal from the medial malleolus to the maximum distance allowed by the incision. Starting from the point at which the flexor digitorum longus and the flexor hallucis longus tendons cross, sharply dissect both sheaths from the sustentaculum tali, moving in a proximal direction until the talocalcaneal joint is entered.

Continue the dissection down and around the navicular, holding the distal segment of the lengthened posterior tibial tendon attached to the bone. Open the talonavicular joint by pulling on the remaining posterior tibial tendon attachment, and carefully cut the deltoid ligament (medial tibial navicular ligament), talonavicular capsule, dorsal talonavicular ligament, and plantar calcaneonavicular (spring) ligament close to the navicular. Enter and carefully expose by blunt dissection and retraction the interval between the dorsal aspect of the talonavicular joint and the extensor tendons and neurovascular bundle on the dorsum of the foot. Take special care not to dissect or disturb the blood supply to the dorsal aspect of the talus.

Follow through with the dissection, incising the capsule of the talonavicular joint all the way around medially, inferiorly, superiorly, and laterally. Inferior and lateral to the joint is the bifurcated (Y) ligament; incise both ends of this ligament to correct the horizontal rotation of the calcaneus. Complete the release of the talocalcaneal joint ligaments and capsule by incising the remaining medial and posteromedial capsule and superficial deltoid ligament attached to the sustentaculum tali. Do not incise the three talocalcaneal ligaments (interosseous ligament) at this point.

Using a periosteal elevator, gently remove the quadratus plantae muscle origin on the medial inferior surface of the calcaneus and expose the long plantar ligament over the plantar calcaneocuboid ligament and the peroneus longus tendons.

The posterior ankle capsule is identified and divided from the posterior tibialis tendon sheath to the lateral aspect of the tibiofibular articulation. At this point, the talus should roll back into the ankle joint, exposing at least 1.5 cm of hyaline cartilage on its body. If this does not happen, incise the posterior talofibular ligament. If the talus still does not roll back into the ankle joint, cut the posterior portion only of the deep deltoid ligament.

Now the decision must be made as to the necessity of cutting the interosseous talocalcaneal ligament to correct the horizontal rotational abnormality through the talocalcaneal joint. This decision depends on the completeness of the correction and the mobility of the subtalar complex, as determined by the position of the foot. Line up the medial side of the head and neck of the talus with the medial side of the cuneiforms, and medially push the calcaneus posterior to the ankle joint while pushing the foot as a whole in a posterior direction. Then examine the angle made by the intersection of the bimalleolar ankle plane with the horizontal plane of the foot; if the angle is 85 to 90 degrees, there is no need to cut the ligament. In children older than 1 year, however, such an incision generally is necessary because the ligament usually has become broad and thick, preventing derotation of the talocalcaneal joint.

After the foot has been satisfactorily corrected, pass a smooth Kirschner wire through the talus from the posterior aspect to the middle of the head. Positioning the pin in a slightly lateral direction in the head of the talus is beneficial in the older child with more pronounced medial deviation of the talar head and

neck because it allows for lateral displacement of the navicular and cuneiforms on the head of the talus to eliminate forefoot adduction. Pass the pin through the talonavicular joint and cuneiforms and out the forefoot on either the medial or lateral side of the first metatarsal. While an assistant is inserting the pin, mold the forefoot out of adduction. Cut off the end of the pin close to the body of the talus, and use a drill anteriorly to advance the pin out the forefoot until it is buried in the posterior body of the talus.

To correct rotation of the calcaneus beneath the talus, push the calcaneocuboid joint anterior to the ankle joint in a lateral direction while pushing the calcaneus posterior to the ankle joint in a medial and plantar direction. Check for proper positioning of the foot: the longitudinal plane of the foot is 85 to 90 degrees to the bimalleolar ankle plane and the heel under the tibia is in slight valgus. Then insert a pin through the calcaneus, burying it deep in the talus from the plantar surface. Be careful not to penetrate the ankle joint.

Suture all tendons snugly with the foot in a maximum of 20 degrees of dorsiflexion. After suturing the tendons, pull the sheath of the flexor hallucis longus and flexor digitorum longus tendons down over them. With the fibrofatty tissue left attached to the calcaneus anterior to the tendo Achilles, cover the lateral aspect of the ankle joint. Keep the peroneal tendons and sheath from subluxating around the fibula by suturing the sheath of the peroneal tendons to the fibrofatty flap. Close the subcutaneous tissue and skin with interrupted sutures.

Apply nonadherent dressing and then, very loosely, one or two layers of cast padding. With the knee bent approximately 90 degrees, roll strips of pound cotton 3 to 4 inches wide around the foot, up the calf, and over the thigh. Apply light pressure with loosely woven gauze, and roll on another layer of cast padding. Holding the foot in a neutral or slightly plantar-flexed position, apply a few rolls of plaster from the toes to midthigh (Fig. 2-12).

▶ *Postoperative management.* McKay recommends a detailed regimen for postoperative management. The postoperative cast is changed to a hinged cast 7 to 10 days after surgery, depending on the age of the child, so that ankle motion can begin. To construct a hinged cast, first apply a boot cast incorporating the foot and pins. Next, with the knee bent to 90 degrees, apply a long-leg cylinder cast just proximal to the ankle. Align the foot in the proper position, and push in a slightly posterior direction. Holding the foot properly aligned, have an assistant incorporate a U-shaped 14- or 16-gauge stranded electric wire into the cylinder cast and then the boot cast, aligning it with the bimalleolar plane. The parents are instructed to move the foot daily into maximum plantar flexion and dorsi-

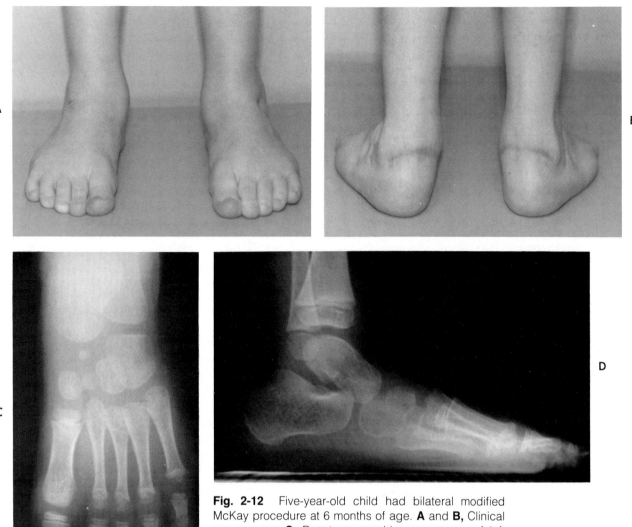

Fig. 2-12 Five-year-old child had bilateral modified McKay procedure at 6 months of age. **A** and **B,** Clinical appearance. **C,** Roentgenographic appearance of left foot on standing anteroposterior view. **D,** Lateral view.

flexion; in about 2 to 3 weeks the child will move the foot voluntarily. Six weeks after surgery the cast and pins are removed and a short-leg cast is applied. This cast is worn until the wounds have healed and swelling has disappeared; in the walking child older than 1 year of age, the cast should be left on for at least 6 weeks. A postoperative regimen similar to that after the Turco procedure also may be followed with satisfactory results.

• • •

Special attention should be given to two specific problems in clubfoot. The first is residual hindfoot equinus in children aged 6 to 12 months who have obtained adequate correction of forefoot adduction and hindfoot varus. This equinus can be corrected adequately by tendo Achilles lengthening and posterior capsulotomy of the ankle and subtalar joints without an extensive one-stage release. The roentgenograms must be reviewed carefully to be certain that a more extensive release is not required instead of a limited procedure that corrects only hindfoot equinus. The heel varus and internal rotation must have been corrected adequately if tendo Achilles lengthening and posterior capsulotomy alone are to be used.

The second specific problem is dynamic metatarsus adductus caused by overpull of the tibialis anterior tendon in older children who have had correction of clubfoot. In the rare child with symptoms, the treatment of choice is transfer of the tibialis anterior tendon, either as a split transfer or as a transfer of the entire tendon to the middle cuneiform. The forefoot must be flexible for a tendon transfer to succeed. This treatment is rarely indicated in neurologically normal children.

Tendo Achilles Lengthening and Posterior Capsulotomy

▲ *Technique.* Make a straight longitudinal incision over the medial aspect of the tendo Achilles, beginning at its most distal point and extending proximally to 3 cm above the medial malleolus at the level of the ankle joint. Carry sharp dissection through the subcutaneous tissue. Identify the tendo Achilles, and make an incision through the peritenon medially. Dissect the tendo Achilles circumferentially to expose it for a length of 3 to 4 cm. Perform a tenotomy of the plantaris tendon if it is present. Identify medially the tendon of the flexor hallucis longus, flexor digitorum communis, posterior tibialis, and the neurovascular bundle; protect these with Penrose drains. Perform Z-plasty to lengthen the tendo Achilles by releasing the medial half distally and the lateral half proximally for a distance of 2.5 to 4 cm (Fig. 2-13). Gently debride pericapsular fat at the level of the subtalar joint. Identify the posterior aspect of the ankle joint by gentle plantarflexion and dorsiflexion of the foot. If the ankle joint cannot be easily identified, make a small vertical incision in the midline until synovial fluid exudes from the joint. Then perform a transverse capsulotomy at the most medial aspect, stopping at the sheath of the posterior tibial tendon and the most lateral articulation of the tibiofibular joint. Take care not to divide the posterior tibial tendon sheath and its underlying deep deltoid ligament. If posterior subtalar capsulotomy is required, enter the subtalar joint at the most proximal aspect of the sheath of the flexor

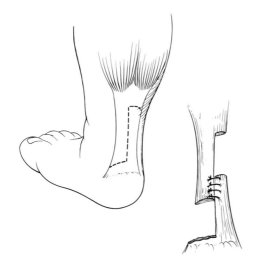

Fig. 2-13 Posterior tendo Achilles lengthening.

hallucis longus tendon and extend the capsulotomy medially and laterally as necessary. Place the foot in 10 degrees of dorsiflexion, and approximate the tendo Achilles to assess tension. Then place the foot in plantar flexion, and repair the tendo Achilles at the appropriate length. Deflate the tourniquet, obtain hemostasis with electrocautery, and close the wound in layers. Apply a long-leg, bent-knee cast with the foot in 5 degrees of dorsiflexion.

▲ *Postoperative management.* The cast is removed 6 weeks after surgery. Postoperative bracing with either an ankle-foot orthosis or short-leg Phelps brace should be continued for an additional 6 to 9 months.

Resistant Clubfoot

Treatment of residual or resistant clubfoot in the older child is one of the most difficult problems in pediatric orthopaedics. The deformity may take many forms, and there are no clear-cut guidelines for treatment. Each child must be carefully evaluated to determine what treatment will best correct the particular functional impairment. Thorough physical examination should include careful assessment of the forefoot and hindfoot. Residual forefoot deformity should be determined to be either dynamic (with a flexible forefoot) or rigid. The amount of inversion and eversion of the calcaneus should be determined, as well as dorsiflexion and plantar flexion of the ankle. Any prior surgical procedures that have caused significant scarring of the foot or loss of motion should be noted. Anteroposterior and lateral roentgenograms of the standing child should be obtained to assess anatomic measurements; if the clubfoot deformity is unilateral, the opposite foot may be used as a control for measurements. All possible etiologic factors of the persistent deformity, including underlying neuropathy, abnormal growth of the bones, and muscle imbalance, should be investigated. The uncorrected clubfoot by clinical and roentgenographic evaluation may not always require surgery. The functional ability of the child, the severity of symptoms associated with the deformity, and the likelihood of progression of the deformity if left untreated must be considered before a recommendation of surgery.

The basic surgical correction of resistant clubfoot includes both soft tissue release and osteotomies. The appropriate procedures and combination of procedures depend on the age of the child, the severity of the deformity, and the pathologic processes involved. General guidelines for use in decision making are outlined in Table 2-1.

Table 2-1 Treatment of resistant clubfoot

Deformity	Treatment
Metatarsus adductus	>5 yr: metatarsal osteotomy
Hindfoot varus	<2-3 yr: modified McKay procedure
	3-10 yr:
	Dwyer osteotomy (isolated heel varus)
	Dillwyn-Evans procedure (short medial column)
	Lichtblau procedure (short medial column)
	10-12 yr: triple arthrodesis
Equinus	Tendo Achilles lengthening plus posterior capsulotomy of the subtalar joint, ankle joint (mild to moderate deformity)
	Lambrinudi procedure (severe deformity, skeletally mature)
All three deformities	>10 yr: triple arthrodesis

In general, the older the child, the more likely that combined procedures will be required. Children aged 12 to 36 months may be candidates for the modified McKay procedure, but if prior soft tissue release has caused stiffness of the subtalar joint, avascular necrosis of the talus, or severe skin contractures, osteotomies probably will be required. Children older than 5 years almost always require osteotomies for correction of resistant deformity. It is those children between the ages of 1 year and 5 years who constitute a "gray area" in which treatment guidelines are unclear and careful judgment is required. The separate components of the residual deformity must be accurately assessed and treatment directed appropriately.

Common components of resistant clubfoot deformity are adduction and/or supination of the forefoot, a short medial column or long lateral column of the foot, internal rotation and varus of the hindfoot, and equinus.

Correction of the forefoot with residual adduction and/or supination is similar to that of isolated metatarsus adductus by metatarsal osteotomies.

Evaluation of the hindfoot should determine whether the deformity is caused by isolated heel varus, a long lateral column of the foot, or a short medial column. In children younger than 2 or 3 years of age, residual heel varus may be corrected by extensive subtalar release, but children aged 3 to 10 years with residual soft tissue and bony deformity usually require combined procedures.

For isolated heel varus with mild supination of the forefoot, Dwyer osteotomy with a lateral closing wedge of the calcaneus may performed.

If the hindfoot deformity includes heel varus and residual internal rotation of the calcaneus with a long lateral column of the foot, either the Dillwyn-Evans or Lichtblau procedure may be appropriate. The Dillwyn-Evans procedure is indicated for children 6 years old or older. It includes wedge resection of the calcaneocuboid joint to shorten the lateral column of the foot. The disadvantage of this procedure is that it may produce stiffness in the hindfoot and occasional pronation of the forefoot. The Lichtblau procedure corrects the long lateral column of the foot by a closing wedge osteotomy of the lateral aspect of the calcaneus. Best results with this procedure are obtained in children aged 3 years or older in whom the calcaneus and lateral column are long relative to the medial column. Potential complications include the development of a "Z"-foot or "skew"-foot deformity.

Correction of residual heel equinus may be obtained by tendo Achilles lengthening and posterior ankle and subtalar capsulotomies in the younger child with a mild deformity. Rarely, an isolated, fixed equinus deformity in an older child will require Lambrinudi arthrodesis.

If all three deformities are present in a child older than 10 years of age, triple arthrodesis may be appropriate. Internal tibial torsion occasionally is associated with resistant clubfoot deformity but only rarely requires derotational osteotomy. That the pathologic condition is confined to the tibia and is not a resistant deformity in the foot must be determined absolutely before tibial osteotomy is considered.

Opening wedge osteotomy of the calcaneus occasionally is followed by sloughing of tight skin along the incision over the calcaneus. Consequently, although some height of the calcaneus is lost after a lateral closing wedge osteotomy, this is preferable.

Osteotomy of calcaneus for persistent varus deformity of heel. In 1963 Dwyer reported osteotomy of the calcaneus for relapsed clubfoot using an opening wedge osteotomy medially to increase the length and height of the calcaneus. The osteotomy is held open by a wedge of bone taken from the tibia. The ideal age for the operation is 3 to 4 years, but there is really no upper age limit.

▲ *Technique (Dwyer, modified).* Expose the calcaneus through a lateral incision over the calcaneus, cuboid, and base of the fifth metatarsal (Fig. 2-14). Strip the lateral surface of the bone subperiosteally, and with a wide osteotome resect a wedge of bone based laterally large enough, when removed, to permit correction of the heel varus (Fig. 2-15, *B*). Take care not to injure the peroneal tendons. Remove the wedge of bone, pull the heel into the corrected position (Fig. 2-15, *B*), and close the incision with interrupted sutures. If necessary, fix the osteotomy with a Kirschner wire. Apply a short leg cast with the foot in a corrected position.

▲ *Postoperative management.* The Kirschner wire is removed 6 weeks after surgery, and casting is discontinued at 3 months.

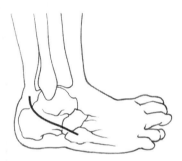

Fig. 2-14 Modified Dwyer osteotomy. Laterally based incision beginning posterior to fibula and ending at base of fifth metatarsal.

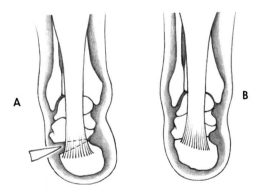

Fig. 2-15 Modified Dwyer osteotomy. **A** Closing wedge removed from lateral aspect of calcaneus. **B**, Osteotomy is closed with calcaneus placed in "mild valgus."

Resection and arthrodesis of calcaneocuboid joint. Dillwyn-Evans believes that in congenital clubfoot the basic deformity is at the midtarsal joints, that all other deformities are adaptive, and that fully correcting the deformity at the midtarsal joints and releasing all contracted soft structures medially will result in a reasonably normal foot. He devised an operation that shortens the lateral side of the foot by resecting a wedge of bone including the calcaneocuboid joint and releases the medial side by dividing the contracted soft structures. The navicular then can be placed in its normal relation with the talus so that the longitudinal axis of the first metatarsal is in line with that of the talus. The calcaneus then is allowed to fuse with the cuboid to hold the foot in the corrected position. The Dillwyn-Evans procedure and the Lichtblau procedure may be performed with their respective soft tissue releases or as isolated bony procedures after previous soft tissue release.

In 1979 Tayton and Thompson reported good results with this procedure in 78% of 118 cases of resistant clubfoot; however, 93% of patients had stiffness of the subtalar joint after surgery. In 1983 Addison et al. reported a modified Dillwyn-Evans procedure for severe relapsed clubfoot after which 93% of their patients had unrestricted activity. Both reports stress the importance—and the difficulty—of anatomic reduction of the navicular on the talus (Fig. 2-16, *A* to *C*).

▲ *Technique (Dillwyn-Evans).* Make a posteromedial incision beginning at the medial cuneiform and extending posteriorly along the course of the posterior tibial tendon, inferior to the medial malleolus, and then proximally up the leg along the anterior border of the tendo Achilles for a distance of 7.5 cm. Perform Z-plasty of the tendo Achilles and capsulotomy of the posterior parts of the ankle and subtalar joints to correct the equinus deformity. Dorsiflex the foot to at least neutral. Identify the neurovascular bundle and protect it. Perform Z-plasty of the posterior tibial tendon. Expose the talonavicular joint, and divide the capsule on the superior, medial, and inferior aspects. If necessary, also divide the tight plantar structures.

Make a lateral incision 4 cm in length centered over the calcaneocuboid joint, parallel with the tendon of the peroneus brevis. Divide the subcutaneous tissue and retract the skin flaps. Retract the peroneus brevis tendon plantarward to fully expose the calcaneocuboid joint. Resect a laterally based wedge of the calcaneocuboid joint. If there is associated equinus distortion of the forefoot, make the wedge thicker dorsally; if the foot is rocker-shaped, make the wedge thicker on the plantar surface. With a periosteal elevator connect the resected area of the calcaneocuboid and the mobile talonavicular joint, ensuring free motion of Chopart's joint as a unit. Now manipulate the foot, shifting the middle and forepart of the foot laterally and aligning the axes of the first metatarsal and talus. Insert a Kirschner wire to hold the calcaneus and cuboid securely together. A second longitudinal Kirschner wire may be inserted across the talonavicular joint if needed. Suture the enlongated tendons, close the incisions, and apply a long-leg cast with the foot in the corrected position.

▶ *Postoperative management.* The Kirschner wires are removed 6 weeks after surgery, and cast immobilization is discontinued at 3 months.

• • •

An alternative to calcaneocuboid arthrodesis is lateral closing wedge osteotomy of the calcaneus as described by Lichtblau. This procedure may decrease the long-term stiffness of the hindfoot seen with the Dillwyn-Evans procedure.

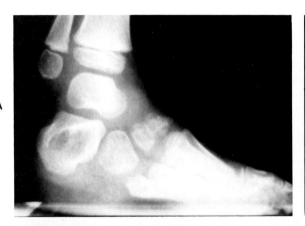

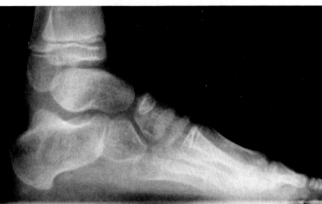

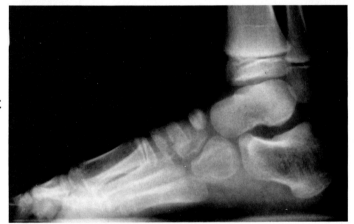

Fig. 2-16 **A,** Severe residual clubfoot deformity, left foot in 5-year-old child. **B,** After Dillwyn-Evans procedure. **C,** Compared with normal right foot. **D,** Technique of Dillwyn-Evans procedure.

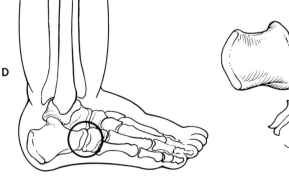
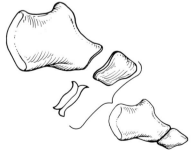

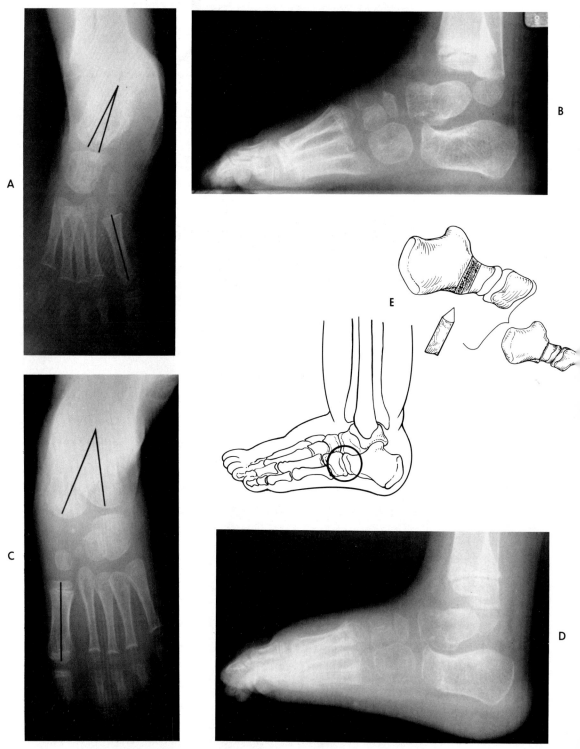

Fig. 2-17 Severe residual clubfoot deformity in 5-year-old child on anteroposterior **(A)** and lateral roentgenograms **(B)**. **C** and **D,** After Lichtblau procedure. **E,** Technique of Lichtblau procedure.

▶ *Technique of medial release with osteotomy of distal calcaneus (Lichtblau)* (Fig. 2-17). Make an incision on the medial aspect of the foot, beginning about 1 cm below the medial malleolus, crossing the tuberosity of the navicular, and sloping downward to the base of the first metatarsal. Identify and free the superior border of the abductor hallucis muscle, and reflect it plantarward. Isolate the posterior tibial tendon at its insertion on the beak of the navicular, dissect it from its sheath, and perform Z-plasty about 1 cm from its insertion. Allow the proximal end of the tendon to retract, while using the distal end as a guide to the talonavicular joint. Resect the tendon sheath overlying the joint, and open it generously on its medial, dorsal, and plantar aspects. Open the flexor tendon sheaths and lengthen them by Z-plasty technique.

Now make a lateral incision, 4 cm long, centered over the calcaneocuboid joint. Dissect the origin of the extensor digitorum brevis muscle from the calcaneus, and reflect it distally to permit exposure and opening of the calcaneocuboid joint. Identify the distal end of the calcaneus, and perform a wedge-shaped osteotomy, removing about 1 cm of the distal and lateral border of the calcaneus and 2 mm of the distal and medial border. Take care to leave the articular surface of the calcaneus intact. Bring the cuboid into contact with the distal end of the calcaneus that has undergone osteotomy, and evaluate the amount of correction of the varus deformity. If the cuboid cannot be closely approximated to the calcaneus, resect more of the calcaneus. A smooth Kirschner wire may be inserted across the calcaneocuboid joint to fix the osteotomy. Repair the posterior tibial tendon, attach the origin of the extensor digitorum brevis muscle to the surrounding soft tissues, and close the subcutaneous tissue and skin. Apply a long-leg cast with the foot in the corrected position.

▶ *Postoperative management.* Three weeks after surgery the long leg cast is changed to a short leg cast that is worn an additional 12 weeks. The pin is removed at 6 weeks.

Triple arthrodesis and talectomy for uncorrected clubfoot. Triple arthrodesis and talectomy generally are salvage operations for uncorrected clubfoot in older children and adolescents. Galdino et al, however, reported excellent or good results in 68% of 19 triple arthrodeses in children aged 10 years or younger (average age at surgery, 8.4 years) with severe hindfoot deformity after failure of soft tissue release (Fig. 2-18). Nonunion occurred in 7% of joints, and fair and poor results primarily were due to residual rather than to recurrent deformity. They believe that triple arthrodesis is functionally and cosmetically superior to talectomy. Triple arthrodesis corrects the severely deformed foot by a lateral closing wedge osteotomy through the subtalar and midtarsal joints. Functional results are generally improved despite postoperative joint stiffness. Talectomy should be reserved for severe, untreated clubfoot or previously treated clubfoot that is uncorrectable by any other surgical procedures.

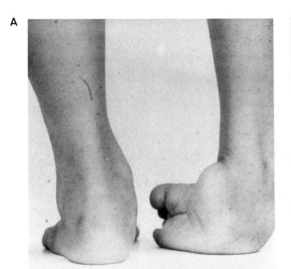 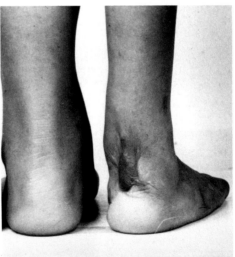

Fig. 2-18 **A,** Uncorrected clubfoot in 10-year-old female. **B,** After posteromedial release and triple arthrodesis. (From Galindo MJ Jr et al: Foot Ankle 7:319, 1987.)

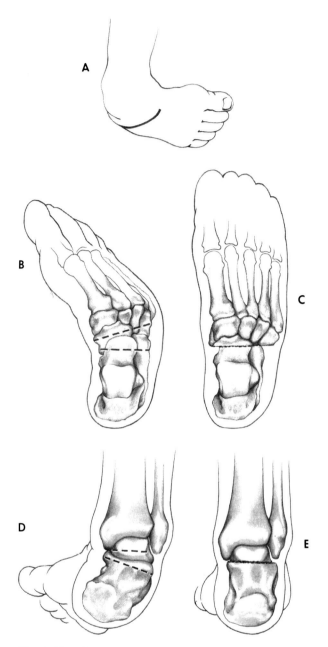

Fig. 2-19 Arthrodesis for persistent or untreated clubfoot. *Between broken lines,* Amount of bone removed from midtarsal region and subtalar joint in moderate, fixed deformity. In severe deformity, wedge may include large part of talus and calcaneus and even part of cuneiforms.

▶ *Technique (triple arthrodesis for clubfoot).* Make an incision along the medial side of the foot parallel to the inferior border of the calcaneus. Free the attachments of the plantar fascia and of the short flexors of the toes from the plantar aspect of the calcaneus. Now by manipulation correct the cavus deformity as much as possible. Next through an oblique anterolateral approach expose the midtarsal and subtalar joints (Fig. 2-19). Then resect a laterally based wedge of bone to include the midtarsal joints. Resect enough bone to correct the varus and adduction deformities of the forefoot.

Next through the same incision resect a wedge of bone, again laterally based, to include the subtalar joint. Resect enough bone to correct the varus deformity of the calcaneus. If necessary include in the first wedge the navicular and most of the cuboid and the lateral cuneiform, as well as the anterior part of the talus and calcaneus, and in the second wedge much of the superior part of the calcaneus and the inferior part of the talus. Finally lengthen the tendo Achilles by Z-plasty, and perform a posterior capsulotomy of the ankle joint. Then by manipulating the ankle, correct the equinus deformity. Hold the corrected position with a Kirschner wire inserted through the calcaneocuboid and talonavicular joints.

▶ *Postoperative management.* With the foot in the corrected position and the knee flexed 30 degrees, a long leg cast is applied from the base of the toes to the groin. The Kirschner wires and cast are removed 6 weeks after surgery. A short leg walking cast is worn an additional 4 weeks.

▶ *Technique (talectomy—Whitman and Thompson).* Expose the talus through a long anterolateral incision (Fig. 2-20, *A*) and divide the tendons of the peroneus longus and brevis. Incise the calcaneofibular ligament of the ankle, and turn the foot medially to permit easy delivery of the talus. Excise the talus, preferably in one piece; allow no fragments to remain (Fig. 2-20, *B*). Strip the ligaments from both malleoli and from the distal 1.3 cm of the tibial metaphysis so that the foot may be easily displaced posteriorly. After the foot is displaced posteriorly, the medial malleolus should lie against the navicular and the lateral malleolus against the calcaneocuboid joint. To place the foot in this position rotate it externally on the leg; often 30 or 40 degrees of rotation are necessary because the foot must be aligned with the ankle mortise rather than with the patella. Thus the new transverse axis will extend between the malleoli at a right angle to the long axis of the foot. When the tibialis anterior is contracted, either lengthen its tendon or transfer it to the middle cuneiform. Now suture the peroneal tendons. The calcaneus tends to migrate proximally and anteriorly after talectomy. If this is allowed, the normal contour of the heel is lost. A transverse pin may be placed in the calcaneus and incorporated in the cast to hold the hindfoot in the corrected position. An axial plantar pin may be added if alignment is difficult to control (Fig. 2-20, *C*).

▶ *Postoperative management.* A long leg cast is applied, with the knee in flexion and with the foot displaced well posteriorly and in equinus and valgus position. Any attempt to correct external rotation of the foot will produce a varus deformity. At 2 or 3 weeks the cast is changed, the position of the foot is observed, and if necessary minor changes in position are made. A snug short leg cast is applied, with the foot still in mild equinus, slight valgus, and external rotation. Twelve weeks after the operation the cast and pins are removed, and a shoe is fitted. The heel of the shoe is raised 2.5 to 4 cm, and a lateral wedge is applied if there has been or is the slightest tendency toward varus deformity. When necessary, a short leg brace with an ankle stop and an outside T-strap or an ankle-foot orthosis to hold the foot in a mild valgus position is used temporarily. If the patient cannot compensate for the external rotation of the foot by internal rotation of the entire extremity, a tibial derotation osteotomy may be done later.

Correction of Tibial Torsion in Clubfoot

After a clubfoot has been corrected, any severe internal tibial torsion also should be corrected. Otherwise as the patient walks, the internally rotated foot is dynamically adducted and inverted, and adduction of the forefoot, inversion of the heel, and cavus deformity all may recur. For the rare patient with symptoms, correction by derotational osteotomy of the tibia occasionally is performed (p. 366).

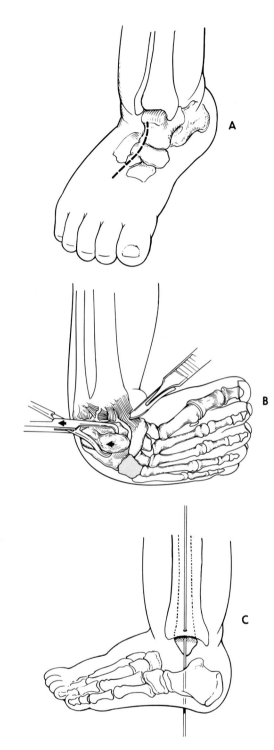

Fig. 2-20 Technique of talectomy. **A,** Anterolateral skin incision. **B,** Total talectomy. **C,** Axial plantar pin to control position.

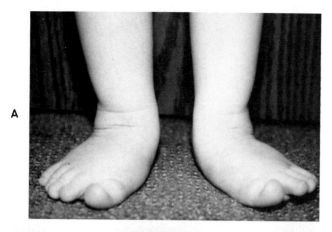

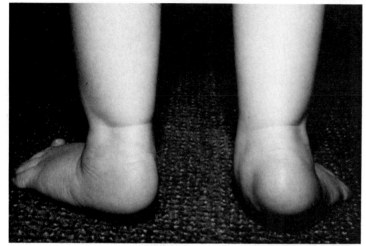

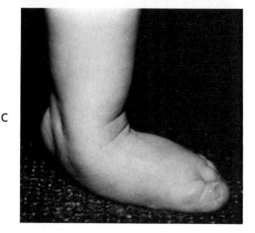

Congenital Vertical Talus

Congenital vertical talus, rocker-bottom flatfoot, or congenital rigid flatfoot must be distinguished from flexible pes planus commonly seen in infants and children. Many neuromuscular disorders often are associated with congenital vertical talus, including arthrogryposis and myelomeningocele. It may occur as an isolated congenital anomaly.

Congenital vertical talus usually can be detected at birth by the presence of a rounded prominence of the medial and plantar surfaces of the foot produced by the abnormal location of the head of the talus (Fig. 2-21). The talus is so distorted plantarward and medially as to be almost vertical. The calcaneus is in an equinus position also but to a lesser degree. The forefoot shows dorsiflexion at the midtarsal joints, and the navicular lies on the dorsal aspect of the head of the talus. The sole is convex, and there are deep creases on the dorsolateral aspect of the foot anterior and inferior to the lateral malleolus. As the foot develops and weight bearing is begun, adaptive changes occur in the tarsal bones. The talus becomes shaped like an hourglass but remains in so marked an equinus position that its longitudinal axis is almost the same as that of the tibia, and only the posterior one third of its superior articular surface articulates with the tibia. The calcaneus remains in an equinus position also and becomes displaced posteriorly, and the anterior part of its plantar surface becomes rounded. Callosities develop beneath the anterior end of the calcaneus and along the medial border of the foot superficial to the head of the talus. When full weight is borne, the forefoot becomes severely abducted and the heel does not touch the floor. Adaptive changes, of course, also occur in the soft tissues. All of the capsules, ligaments, and tendons on the dorsum of the foot become contracted. The tendons of the tibialis posterior and peroneus longus and brevis may come to lie anterior to the malleoli and act as dorsiflexors rather than plantarflexors.

Fig. 2-21 Bilateral congenital vertical talus in 18-month-old child. **A,** On anterior view, note weight bearing on medial aspect of feet. **B,** On posterior view, note contracture of tendo Achilles and peroneal musculature. **C,** Medial view with plantar prominence of talar head.

Congenital vertical talus may be difficult to distinguish from severe pes planus. This can be accomplished by the use of appropriate roentgenograms. Routine roentgenograms should include anteroposterior and plantar flexion lateral stress views; the latter will confirm the diagnosis of congenital vertical talus (Fig. 2-22).

Congenital vertical talus is difficult to correct and tends to recur. Gentle manipulations, however, followed by immobilization in casts is beneficial in that the skin, the fibrous tissue structures, and the tendons on the anterior aspect of the foot and ankle are stretched. Reduction of the talonavicular joint rarely is possible by conservative means alone, and consequently an open reduction usually is necessary.

The exact surgery indicated is determined by the age of the child and the severity of the deformity. Children 1 to 4 years old generally are best treated by open reduction and realignment of the talonavicular and subtalar joints. Occasionally in children aged 3 years or older with severe deformity, the navicular may require excision at the time of open reduction. Children 4 to 8 years old may be treated by open reduction and soft tissue procedures combined with extraarticular subtalar arthrodesis. Children 12 years old and older are best treated by triple arthrodesis for permanent correction of resistant deformity.

For a young child with a mild or moderate deformity the technique of Kumar et al is recommended. For an older child with a more severe deformity or recurrent deformity, open reduction and a Grice extraarticular subtalar fusion is recommended by Coleman. For the older child (12 years old or older) with symptoms a triple arthrodesis is preferred.

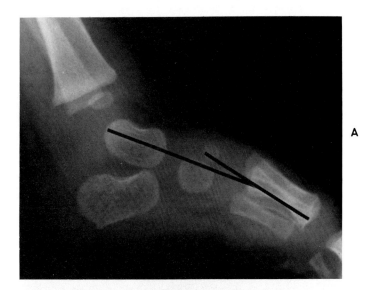

A

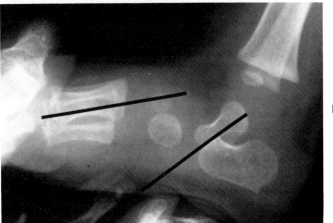

B

Fig. 2-22 Plantar flexion lateral stress roentgenogram in diagnosis of congenital vertical talus. **A,** In normal foot, long axis of first metatarsal passes plantarward to long axis of talus. **B,** In congenital vertical talus, long axis of first metatarsal remains dorsal to long axis of talus, indicating dorsal dislocation of midfoot and forefoot. Note equinus deformity of calcaneus.

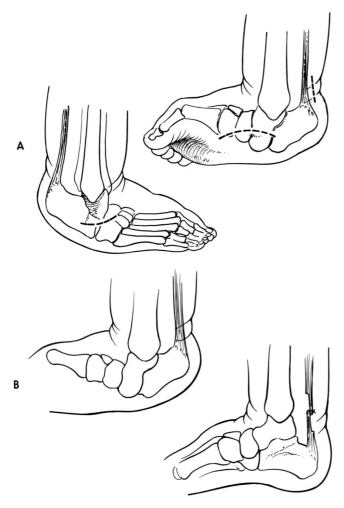

Fig. 2-23 Technique for correction of congenital vertical talus. **A,** Three skin incisions placed medially, posteriorly, and laterally. Single Cincinnati incision may be used instead. **B,** Corrected position of foot after tendon lengthening, capsular release, and reduction of navicular on talus.

■ *Technique (Kumar, Cowell, and Ramsey).* Make the first of three incisions on the lateral side of the foot centered over the sinus tarsi (Fig. 2-23, *A*), or use the Cincinnati approach (p. 84). Avoid entering the sinus tarsi laterally. Expose the extensor digitorum brevis, and reflect it distally to expose the anterior part of the talocalcaneal joint. Next, identify the calcaneocuboid joint, and release all tight structures around it, including the calcaneocuboid ligament. Next, make the second incision on the medial side of the foot centered over the prominent head of the talus (Fig. 2-23, *A*). This exposes the head of the talus and medial part of the navicular. The tibialis anterior tendon also is exposed. Release all tight structures on the medial and dorsal aspects of the head of the talus and the navicular. Free also the anterior part of the talus from its ligamentous attachments to the navicular and calcaneus. This includes releasing the dorsal talonavicular ligament, the plantar calcaneonavicular ligament, and the anterior part of the superficial deltoid ligament. If necessary, divide part of the talocalcaneal interosseous ligament so that the talus can be easily maneuvered into position by a blunt instrument. If the peroneal, extensor hallucis longus, and extensor digitorum longus tendons remain contracted, expose and lengthen them by Z-plasty.

Next, make a third incision, two inches (5 cm) long on the medial side of the tendo Achilles. Lengthen this tendon by Z-plasty, and if necessary, carry out a capsulotomy of the posterior ankle and subtalar joints (Fig. 2-23, *B*). The talus and calcaneus now can be placed in the corrected position and the forefoot reduced on the hindfoot. In the older child, if the tibialis anterior is to be transferred, drill a small hole in the neck of the talus from the superior surface to the inferior surface. Release two thirds of the tibialis anterior tendon from its insertion, and thread it through this hole and suture it to itself. This forms a sling to hold the talus in the reduced position. Now pass a smooth Steinmann pin through the navicular and into the neck of the talus to maintain the reduction. Obtain anteroposterior and lateral roentgenograms to confirm reduction of the vertical talus (Fig. 2-24). Make an attempt to reconstruct the talonavicular ligament, and close the wound in layers. Apply a long-leg cast with the knee flexed and the foot in proper position.

▲ *Postoperative management.* At 8 weeks the cast and Steinmann pin are removed. A new long-leg cast is applied, and this type of cast is worn for 1 month. A short leg cast is worn for an additional month. Then the foot is supported in an ankle-foot orthosis for another 6 months.

• • •

Coleman described open reduction and extraarticular subtalar fusion in the older child with severe deformity. The technique combines the procedure of Kumar et al with a Grice-Green fusion performed 6 to 8 weeks afterward.

A
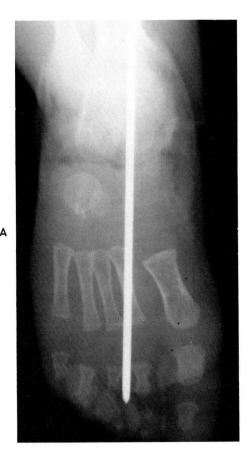
B
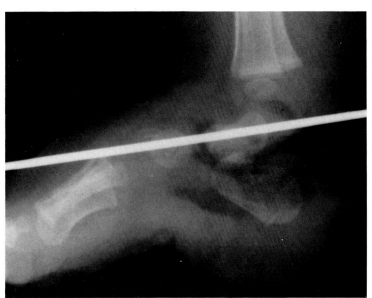

Fig. 2-24 Intraoperative roentgenograms after correction of congenital vertical talus through Cincinnati approach. **A,** Anteroposterior view shows correction of talocalcaneal angle and talo–first metatarsal angle. **B,** Lateral view shows corrected position of talus and reduction of navicular and forefoot and fixation with single Steinmann pin.

▲ *Technique (Grice-Green).* Make a short curvilinear incision on the lateral aspect of the foot directly over the subtalar joint. Carry the incision down through the soft tissues to expose the cruciate ligament overlying the joint. Split this ligament in the direction of its fibers, and dissect the fatty and ligamentous tissues from the sinus tarsi. Dissect the short toe extensors from the calcaneus and reflect them distally. The relationship of the calcaneus to the talus now can be determined and the mechanism of the deformity demonstrated. Place the foot in equinus, and then invert it to position the calcaneus beneath the talus. A severe, long-standing deformity may require division of the posterior capsule of the subtalar joint or removal of a small piece of bone laterally from beneath the anterosuperior articular surface of the calcaneus. Insert an osteotome or broad periosteal elevator into the sinus tarsi, and block the subtalar joint to evaluate stability of the graft and its proper size and position. Prepare the graft beds by removing a thin layer of cortical bone from the inferior surface of the talus and superior surface of the calcaneus (Fig. 2-25).

Now make a linear incision over the anteromedial surface of the proximal tibial metaphysis, incise the periosteum, and take a block of bone large enough for two grafts (usually 3.5 to 4.5 cm long and 1.5 cm wide). As alternatives to tibial bone, take a short segment of the distal fibula or a circular segment of the iliac crest. Cut the tibial grafts to fit the prepared beds. Use a rongeur to shape the grafts so that they

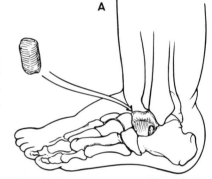

Fig. 2-25 Grice-Green subtalar fusion. **A,** Preparation of graft bed and placement of graft in lateral aspect of subtalar joint. **B,** Lateral view of 10-year-old patient who had open reduction and Grice-Green fusion for congenital vertical talus at 3 years of age.

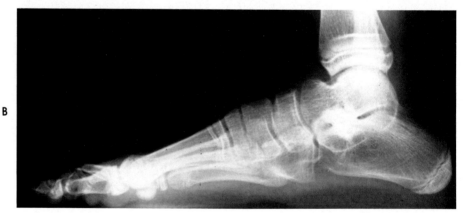

can be countersunk into cancellous bone to prevent lateral displacement. With the foot held in a slightly overcorrected position, place the grafts in the sinus tarsi. Evert the foot to lock the grafts in place. If a segment of the fibula or iliac crest is used, a smooth Kirschner wire may be used to hold the graft in place for 12 weeks. A screw may be inserted anteriorly from the talar neck into the calcaneus for rigid fixation (Fig. 2-26). The foot now should be stable enough to allow correction of equinus deformity by tendo Achilles lengthening if necessary. Apply a long-leg cast with the knee flexed, the ankle in maximum dorsiflexion, and the foot in the corrected position.

▶ *Postoperative management.* The long-leg cast is worn for 12 weeks, and weight bearing is not allowed. A short-leg walking cast then is worn for an additional 4 weeks.

• • •

The older child with an uncorrected congenital vertical talus with pain or difficulty with shoe wear may be treated with a triple arthrodesis. The procedure generally requires medial and lateral incisions and adequate osteotomies to place the foot in a plantigrade position, similar to that used for correction of a severe tarsal coalition deformity (see p. 102).

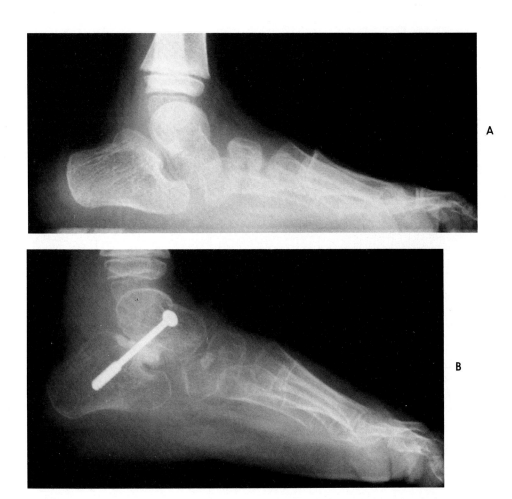

Fig. 2-26   **A,** Congenital vertical talus in 6-year-old child. **B,** Corrected position of talus fixed with screw through neck of talus into calcaneus. Bone graft in middle and posterior aspects of subtalar joint.

Tarsal Coalition

The cause of tarsal coalition is believed to be a failure of primitive mesenchyme to segment and produce a normal peritalar joint complex. Several authors have noted a hereditary tendency for tarsal coalition and have suggested that calcaneonavicular coalition may be caused by a specific gene mutation behaving as an autosomal dominant gene with reduced penetrance. The most common symptomatic coalitions are calcaneonavicular and talocalcaneal. Rare other coalitions include talonavicular, calcaneocuboid, naviculocuboid, and naviculocuneiform.

Tarsal coalition, rigid pes planus, and peroneal muscle spasm frequently are discussed together as essential components of peroneal spastic flatfoot. It is important to clarify that peroneal muscle spasm actually is an acquired or adaptive shortening of the muscle-tendon units of the peroneal muscles. Inversion stress by the examiner, producing unsustained clonus of the peroneal muscles, is the stretch reflex of a shortened muscle-tendon unit. Peroneal muscle tightness is seen in clinical disorders other than tarsal coalition. Common differential diagnoses include juvenile rheumatoid arthritis, osteochondral fracture, infection in the subtalar joint, and neoplasm adjacent to the subtalar joint in the talus or calcaneus.

Some patients with tarsal coalitions, especially calcaneonavicular coalitions, have little deformity suggestive of pes planus. Heel valgus may be slight and loss of the longitudinal arch minimal; however, most patients with tarsal coalition have some rather fixed hindfoot valgus or more significant loss of the normal longitudinal arch and loss of subtalar motion (Fig. 2-27).

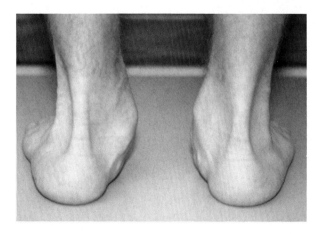

Fig. 2-27   Left tarsal coalition in 15-year-old male. Note valgus position of hindfoot, loss of longitudinal arch, and prominence of peroneal tendons laterally.

Calcaneonavicular Coalition

The calcaneonavicular coalition probably is present at birth; however, it does not ossify until the child is approximately 8 to 14 years old. Before this age, because of the flexibility of the cartilage surrounding the primary ossification centers, significant symptoms are rare. It is believed that as the coalition ossifies, hindfoot stiffness results and the ability to withstand the stress of vigorous activity declines.

The coalition may be bony (synostosis), cartilaginous (synchondrosis), or fibrous (syndesmosis). The incomplete coalitions, those that are cartilaginous or fibrous, usually produce symptoms, which generally are vague dorsolateral foot pain and, occasionally, difficulty walking on uneven surfaces. The symptoms usually worsen with increasing age. The physical examination may or may not show significant loss of subtalar motion. If the condition is unilateral, careful examination of subtalar motion shows a difference between the two feet. Roentgenographic diagnosis generally is made by a 45-degree lateral oblique view (Fig. 2-28). The abnormal coalition usually runs from the anterior process of the calcaneus just lateral to the anterior facet dorsally and medially to the lateral and dorsolateral extraarticular surface of the navicular. It usually is 1 to 2 cm long and 1 to 2 cm wide. In a coalition with cartilaginous or fibrous interface the adjacent bony margins are irregular and indistinct. Beaking of the dorsal articular margin of the head of the talus, which is common in talocalcaneal coalition, is uncommon in calcaneonavicular coalition.

Treatment of calcaneonavicular coalition depends on the age of the child and the severity of symptoms. Generally, children who have symptoms between the ages of 8 and 12 years will become worse as the cartilaginous coalition ossifies. The family should be educated regarding the congenital nature of the lesion, the reason for delay in symptoms to adolescence, and the fact that some coalitions never cause symptoms. Initially, reduced activity or cast immobilization may be used. Cast immobilization for 4 to 6 weeks often alleviates symptoms for varying lengths of time. If a trial of casting or modifications in shoe wear or activities does not relieve symptoms, then surgical treatment is recommended.

The two most commonly performed surgical procedures for calcaneonavicular coalition are (1) resection of the coalition with interposition of muscle or fat and (2) triple arthrodesis. Kumar, Cowell, and Ramsey reported that 23 of 26 feet in their patients were symptom free after excision of the calcaneonavicular coalition. Swiotkowski et al reported that 35 of 39 calcaneonavicular resections successfully restored some subtalar motion and relieved symptoms in their patients. Resection of the calcaneonavicular coalition

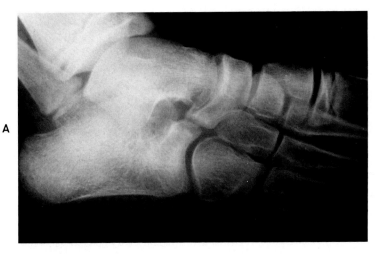

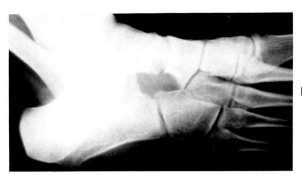

Fig. 2-28   A, Fibrous calcaneonavicular coalition on oblique view of right foot. **B,** One year after resection.

is indicated in the young adolescent with an incompletely ossified bar who does not respond to casting or any other conservative treatment. It is contraindicated in the patient with severe beaking of the neck of the talus, indicative of early degenerative changes in the subtalar joint complex. Although subtalar motion improves, it usually does not equal that of the uninvolved side in unilateral cases, and 50% of normal is considered a good result.

▶ *Technique of calcaneonavicular bar resection.* Make a lateral oblique (Ollier) incision, being careful to preserve the branches of the intermediate dorsal cutaneous branch of the superficial peroneal nerve that crosses the incision and attempting to preserve the sheaths of the extensor digitorum longus and peroneus tertius tendons anteriorly and the peroneal tendons posteriorly. Identify the muscle belly of the extensor digitorum brevis. Now raise the muscle by sharp dissection from the confines of the tarsal sinus in a proximal to distal direction until the entire tarsal sinus and anterior process of the calcaneus are identified.

Identify the talonavicular and calcaneocuboid joints by manually rocking the forefoot-midfoot segment on the hindfoot. The bar runs from the anterior process of the calcaneus just lateral to the anterior facet anteriorly and medially to the lateral and dorsolateral margin of the navicular (Fig. 2-29, *A*). If the exact location of the articular margins of the calcaneocuboid or talonavicular joints is questionable, open the capsules of these joints just enough to identify the articular surfaces.

Use small Hohmann retractors around the waist of the bar to enhance exposure. At the calcaneal origin of the bar, place a ¼- or a ½-inch osteotome parallel

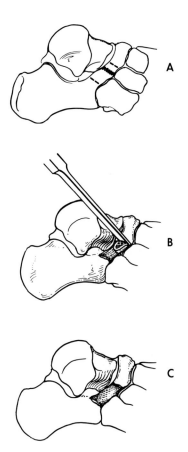

Fig. 2-29 Calcaneonavicular coalition resection. **A,** Outline of coalition at margins of calcaneus and navicular. **B,** Completion of osteotomy through medial aspect of coalition at articular surface of navicular. **C,** Resected coalition.

to the floor of the tarsal sinus, and cut up to but not through the medial cortex of the bar. Direct the upper cut at the dorsolateral aspect of the navicular medially, plantarward, and obliquely at about 30 degrees from the vertical plane. Complete this osteotomy through the bar. Then, by placing the osteotome in the inferior cut, fracture the bar through its medial cortex and smooth it with a rongeur (Fig. 2-29, *B*). In this manner the chance of damaging the anterior facet of the subtalar joint or the inferior aspect of the head and neck of the talus is decreased (Fig. 2-29, *C*).

Generous resection of the bar is recommended (Fig. 2-29, *C*). Because the tendency is to remove less than an optimal amount of bone, a lateral oblique roentgenographic examination on the operating table after resection is recommended. Usually, a 1.5 to 2.5 cm segment of bar is removed. Leave the lateral fourth of the articular surface of the talar head uncovered by navicular to ensure adequate removal.

Using an absorbable suture woven through the proximal margin of the extensor digitorum brevis muscle, interpose the muscle in the depths of the defect by passing small, straight needles medially through the defect, carrying the suture and therefore the muscle with it into the defect. Bring the ends of the suture out through the skin medially beneath the talonavicular joint, pass them through a broad felt pad, and tie them firmly. Deflate the tourniquet, secure hemostasis, and close the skin with absorbable sutures. Apply a well-padded, short-leg cast in the operating room.

▶ *Postoperative management.* The initial cast (nonwalking) remains in place 3 weeks. At 3 weeks the cast is removed and active plus gentle, active-assisted, inversion-eversion exercises are begun. Weight bearing to tolerance with the aid of crutches is begun and the crutches are discontinued when full weight bearing is comfortable.

In the older adolescent or young adult, resection of a complete calcaneonavicular coalition may not improve subtalar motion or completely relieve symptoms, especially if there is roentgenographic evidence of degenerative arthritis in the subtalar or talonavicular joint. Although excision is preferred if possible, triple arthrodesis is recommended for these patients. If the hindfoot is in an acceptable position, a standard triple arthrodesis is performed; however, if the position of the forefoot must be changed, the bony bar is removed and appropriate resection of the articular surface of the subtalar joint is made to reposition the hindfoot. Occasionally, a separate medial incision may be required for surgical correction and fusion of the talonavicular joint at the time of triple arthrodesis.

Talocalcaneal Coalition

Harris and Beath in 1948 published an extensive description of talocalcaneal coalition in which they attributed the difficulty in diagnosis to the fact that the coalition may be bony, fibrous, or cartilaginous and is not ordinarily seen on standard roentgenographic views of the foot. Talocalcaneal coalition ossifies ei-

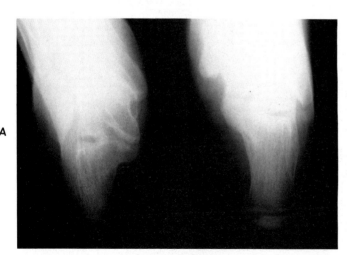
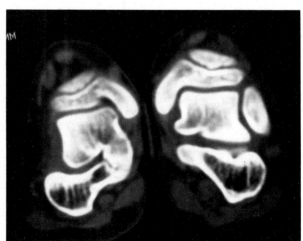

Fig. 2-30 Middle facet talocalcaneal coalition. **A,** Axial or coalition view. Note sloping and obliquity of middle facet of left foot compared with normal right foot. **B,** CT scan demonstrates obliquity and sloping of middle facet coalition on left foot compared with normal right foot.

ther completely or incompletely between 12 years of age and adulthood. It generally occurs in patients older than those with calcaneonavicular coalitions. The symptoms are similar for both groups, including foot fatigue and pain along the hindfoot, with occasional loss of the longitudinal arch. Peroneal muscle spasm frequently is present, but the classic physical finding is marked reduction or complete absence of subtalar motion.

Normal variations in the osseous anatomy of the hindfoot make roentgenographic standarization difficult for diagnosis of talocalcaneal coalition. Normally the medial and posterior subtalar joint facets lie in planes at approximately 35 to 60 degrees relative to the long axis of the calcaneus, but this is extremely variable. In addition, the anterior facet is more horizontal and the rare coalition of this facet cannot be seen on a coalition view. Conway and Cowell recommend lateral tomograms made in sections of 1 cm depth from the lateral to medial aspect of the foot.

Kumar and Cowell recommend that a standing lateral roentgenogram of the foot be obtained, from which angles made by the posterior and medial facets with the floor can be measured and, from these, the angle of inclination can be determined for the "coalition" view. The coalition view then is made with the patient standing on the cassette with the knees flexed enough to remove the calf shadow from the beam. The roentgen cone is directed toward the heel at the previously determined angle to the cassette. A medial facet coalition appears narrowed and sloped compared with the normal facet. Other roentgenographic findings include beaking of the head of the talus at the dorsal articular margin, broadening or rounding of the lateral process of the talus, narrowing of the posterior talocalcaneal joint space, and loss of the medial subtalar joint. Herzenberg et al outlined the use of computed tomography (CT) for the diagnosis of talocalcaneal coalition (Fig. 2-30). They recommend positioning the feet in plantar flexion and obtaining coronal CT sections from the posterior aspect of the talus through the navicular in 5-mm widths. Coronal cuts taken at greater than 5-mm intervals may give a false-positive result because of the changing anatomy of this facet, and overlapping 5-mm images are recommended.

Conservative therapy, including reduced activities, a walking cast, or shoe modification may be tried initially, but if conservative treatment fails, operative treatment is indicated. Surgical options for the treatment of talocalcaneal coalition include excision of the middle facet talocalcaneal coalition and triple arthrodesis. Limited series in the literature show encouraging results with excision of the coalition, but no large series with long-term follow-up have been reported (Fig. 2-31). The current recommendations are for excision of early, small, fibrocartilaginous coalitions. When the foot is in severe, fixed valgus, and the coalition is large and ossified, triple arthrodesis is recommended. Danielsson reported successful treatment of three patients with resection of the talocalcaneal coalition, and the technique is described.

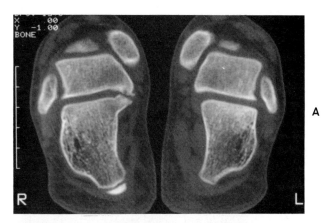

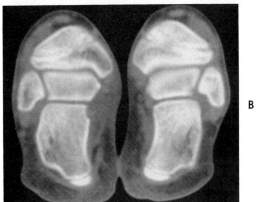

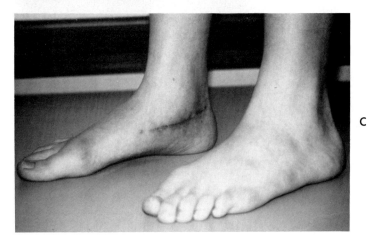

Fig. 2-31 Excision of talocalcaneal middle facet coalition. **A,** Preoperative CT scan shows fibrocartilaginous coalition. **B,** CT scan after resection of middle facet coalition. **C,** Postoperative clinical appearance.

◣ *Technique for resection of talocalcaneal coalition.* Make a curvilinear incision beginning at the base of the first cuneiform and extending posteriorly over the tarsal tunnel to the area between the tendo Achilles and the medial malleolus. Explore the coalition through the tarsal tunnel. Identify and protect the structures in the tarsal tunnel, and then explore the medial talocalcaneal joint. To identify the anterior and posterior edges of the coalition, the talocalcaneal joint must be explored distally and proximally to the bar. When the bony bar is extensive, the anterior talocalcaneal joint can be identified by exposure of the talonavicular joint. Subperiosteally, a thin cartilaginous disk may reveal the exact location of the talocalcaneal joint and the bony bar. When the limits of the bar, as well as the cartilaginous disk, have been carefully determined, resect the bar, using a chisel and bone rongeur. After resection of the bar, cover the bleeding bone surfaces with bone wax, and interpose subcutaneous fat in the resected area. Apply a short-leg walking cast.

◣ *Postoperative management.* Weight bearing to tolerance is allowed in the short-leg cast. The cast is removed 3 weeks after surgery, and range of motion exercises are begun.

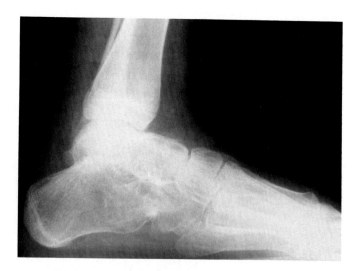

Fig. 2-32 Triple arthrodesis for middle facet talocalcaneal coalition.

◣ *Technique of arthrodesis (Harris and Beath).* Begin a medial, gently curved incision at the base of the first cuneiform, and end it 2 cm inferior and posterior to the tip of the medial malleolus. Take care to avoid sensory branches of the medial calcaneal and posterior tibial nerves. Open the sheath of the tibialis posterior tendon and retract the tendon inferiorly. The medial facet lies deep to the floor of the tunnel for the tibialis posterior tendon. Do not disturb the flexor hallucis longus muscle immediately plantar to the sustentaculum tali. Incise the medial capsule overlying the talonavicular and medial subtalar joints longitudinally to clearly expose both articulations. The bar frequently is toward the posterior aspect of the sustentaculum. Harris reports "rudimentary talocalcaneal bridges" that are bony projections originating from the sustentaculum (most commonly) or from the talus. By crossing the medial aspect of the subtalar joint these projections block subtalar motion even though they are incompletely united to either the talus or calcaneus. The articular side of these projections may be covered by articular cartilage.

In the presence of complete bony union of the subtalar joint at the medial facet with the hindfoot in acceptable valgus, only a talonavicular fusion is needed (Harris). If, however, the hindfoot valgus is unacceptable, the subtalar fusion must be taken down, the articular cartilage is removed, and the subtalar joint is repositioned and fused along with the talonavicular and calcaneocuboid joints.

Using a ½- to ¾-inch osteotome, denude the head of the talus and the proximal articular surface of the navicular. Be careful to reach only subchondral bone because removal of too much bone will increase the chance of nonunion at this joint. Remove the articular cartilage of the calcaneocuboid joint to expose subchondral bone. If the subtalar joint requires fusion, remove the obstructing bridge with an osteotome or rongeur, and continue the medial capsular incision posteriorly to identify the posterior talocalcaneal facet. Denude this facet, removing slightly more bone medially to correct the valgus of the hindfoot. Be careful, however, not to remove excess bone to produce varus (Fig. 2-32). Kirschner wire fixation may be used to fix the talonavicular and calcaneocuboid joints.

Close the capsule and skin with absorbable sutures after the tourniquet is deflated and hemostasis is secured. A deep suction drain may be inserted. Apply a well-padded, short-leg nonwalking cast.

◣ *Postoperative management.* The nonwalking cast is worn for 6 weeks. The pins are removed and a short-leg walking cast is worn for an additional 6 weeks.

Accessory Navicular

Kidner in 1929 stated that the support of the medial longitudinal arch offered by the tibialis posterior tendon was compromised by the tendon's insertion into an accessory navicular. He devised a procedure intended to correct the loss of suspension by the tibialis posterior tendon. Whether excision of the accessory navicular and advancement of the tibialis posterior tendon alters the medial longitudinal arch is doubtful; however, the efficacy of simple excision of the accessory navicular in the child who has symptoms, with or without pes planus, is affirmed by several reports. The true accessory navicular must be differentiated from a sesamoid within the tibialis posterior tibial tendon. A prominent medial navicular tuberosity caused by fusion of an accessory to the main navicular produces local symptoms that may warrant surgery (Fig. 2-33, A). Excising this medial beak of the navicular flush with the medial border of the first cuneiform usually relieves the symptoms. The Kidner procedure is recommended for the adolescent patient who has an accessory navicular with symptoms unresponsive to conservative treatment.

▶ *Technique (Kidner).* Beginning 1 to 1.5 cm inferior and distal to the tip of the medial malleolus, arch the skin incision slightly dorsalward, peaking at the medial prominence of the accessory navicular, and sloping distally to the base of the first metatarsal. After ligating the plantar communicating branches of the saphenous system, identify the tibialis posterior tendon as it approaches the accessory navicular. Identify the dorsal and plantar margins of the tendon 2 cm proximal to the accessory navicular, and expose the tendon distally, ending at the bone. By this means the entire tendon can be exposed and the part extending plantarward toward its multiple insertions will not be disturbed.

Using sharp dissection, shell the accessory navicular from the tibialis posterior tendon, attempting to leave a small sliver of bone within the tendon if transposition of the tendon is planned. Resect the medial prominence of the main navicular flush with the medial border of the first cuneiform using a rongeur and rasp (Fig. 2-33, B). Remove that portion of the tendon inserting into the navicular tuberosity and first cuneiform using sharp dissection and shift it plantarward and laterally as far as possible. Suture the tendon to the apex of the medial longitudinal arch, using periosteum and ligamentous tissue to secure the transposed tendon slip or by passing the sutures through holes drilled in the center of the navicular and tying them dorsally. Try to advance this slip of tendon while the talonavicular joint is reduced and the medial longitudinal arch is reestablished by holding the midfoot and forefoot in a cavovarus position.

Close the skin and subcutaneous tissue with absorbable sutures or adhesive skin strips so that the postoperative cast can remain in place for 4 weeks. Apply a short-leg nonwalking cast. The cast is well padded and gently molded into the longitudinal arch with the talonavicular joint reduced and the foot inverted.

▶ *Postoperative management.* The cast is left on for 4 weeks. A walking cast then is applied with the foot plantigrade and is worn for 2 additional weeks; weight bearing to tolerance is allowed with crutches.

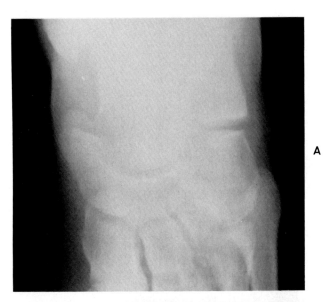

A

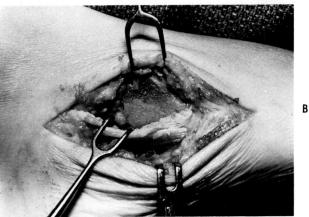

B

Fig. 2-33 **A,** Accessory tarsal navicular on oblique view. **B,** After removal of tuberosity of navicular.

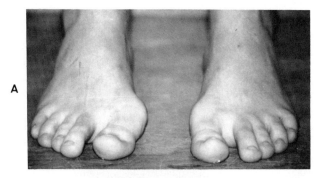

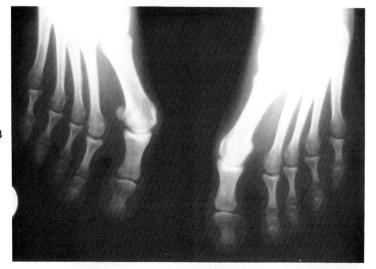

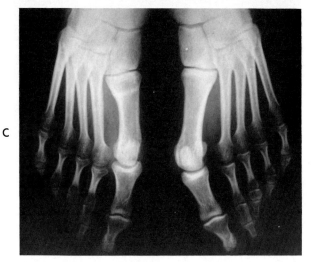

Adolescent Hallux Valgus

The indications for surgical correction of adolescent hallux valgus are neither rigid nor clearly defined, nor is there agreement on the timing of surgery during adolescence. Several well-documented series recommend operative correction only for painful progressive deformity in adolescents older than 16 years whose physes are closed. Other reports, however, indicate that surgery performed before the adolescent is 15 years old yields the best long-term results with or without the presence of open physes.

Any adolescent between the ages of 10 and 16 years with progressive, cosmetically unacceptable hallux valgus and a family history that is positive for hallux valgus is considered a candidate for surgery. Pain and difficulty with shoe wear are even stronger indications for operative correction of the deformity. The patient and family should be informed of the chance of recurrence of the deformity and that pain may recur in adulthood. Hallux valgus and metatarsus primus varus in the adolescent usually are progressive, and surgical treatment is the best means of correcting the deformity with reasonable certainty in the patient who has symptoms (Fig. 2-34).

Adolescent hallux valgus differs from that in adults in that (1) cosmetic correction frequently is desired; (2) pain is not the primary complaint in many instances; (3) prominence of the medial eminence and bursal hypertrophy usually are minor; (4) there generally is varus of the first metatarsal with a widened first-second intermetatarsal angle; (5) pes planus with pronation of the forefoot is frequent; (6) there is an increased risk of recurrence of the deformity; (7) hallux valgus interphalangeus may be present and may require correction in addition to the hallux valgus; (8) the family history generally is positive for hallux valgus; (9) soft tissue procedures alone are unlikely to result in permanent correction; and (10) osteotomy of the first metatarsal or proximal phalanx, or both, almost always is required if surgical correction is undertaken.

Fig. 2-34 A and **B,** Adolescent hallux valgus of right foot in 16-year-old girl. **C,** After surgical correction of hallux valgus, right foot, with modified Simmons-Menelaus technique.

The medial eminence of the first metatarsal head may or may not require excision, depending on its size. Any first-second intermetarsal angle of 10 degrees or greater requires metatarsal osteotomy, and hallux valgus greater than 25 degrees requires an additional adductor tenotomy, medial capsulorrhaphy, and lateral capsulotomy at the metatarsophalangeal joint. If the intermetatarsal angle is corrected to 5 degrees or less and the hallux valgus angle to 15 degrees or less, recurrence of unacceptable deformity is rare. Pronation of the great toe in early adolescence is uncommon but, if present, may be the result of pronation of the first ray and not simply the hallux. If so, then derotation to a neutral position should be done at the time the varus position of the metatarsal is corrected.

Any surgical procedure that relieves symptoms, retains a functional range of motion of the metatarsophalangeal joint, corrects the valgus posture of the hallux, and narrows the forefoot probably will be successful. Many surgical alternatives are available for correction of hallux valgus, but the following are most often recommended for the deformity in adolescents:

1. Proximal metatarsal osteotomy. If the first metatarsal physis is growing in an immature foot, a medial opening wedge osteotomy distal to the physis is recommended, with the use of the resected medial eminence for a graft. In the younger adolescent, if the medial eminence is not prominent, bone bank or autogenous bone may be substituted, or a "dome," or lateral closing wedge osteotomy, may be performed.
2. Adductor tenotomy, lateral capsulotomy, medial eminence removal, and medial capsulorrhaphy.
3. Osteotomy of the proximal phalanx. If the deformity at the interphalangeal joint is prominent, once the metatarsus primus varus and hallux have been corrected, a proximal phalangeal osteotomy may be required. The osteotomy can be performed near the base of the proximal phalanx if the physis is closed or, if the physis is open, at the neck. If a phalangeal osteotomy is required, the pronation, as well as the valgus, should be corrected at the distal hallux.

▲ *Technique (modified Simmonds and Menelaus).* Apply a tourniquet, and prepare and drape the extremity in the usual manner. Two incisions are used; the first is a long medial incision from the base of the first metatarsal to the middle of the proximal phalanx of the hallux, and the second is a short incision lateral to the first metatarsophalangeal joint. Through the medial incision, define the medial capsule of the metatarsophalangeal joint. Make a longitudinal capsular incision with the plantar capsular flap to be imbricated later over the dorsal flap. Remove the underlying medial eminence with an osteotome, and save it for later use. Through the lateral incision, define the tendon of the adductor hallucis and detach it from the proximal phalanx and lateral sesamoid. Divide the lateral capsule of the metatarsophalangeal joint. Perform an osteotomy at the base of the first metatarsal approximately one-half inch distal to the physis. Then insert the previously removed medial eminence on the medial aspect of the osteotomy to obtain an opening wedge. Kirschner wire fixation may be used to fix the osteotomy if necessary. Kirschner wires may be placed longitudinally across the first metatarsophalangeal joint to hold the hallux in 5 degrees of valgus. With the hallux held in a slight varus position, imbricate the medial capsule, suturing the plantar capsule over the dorsal capsule. Confirm correction with roentgenograms. The ideal intermetatarsal angle is approximately 5 degrees, and the hallux valgus should be corrected to 10 to 15 degrees. Deflate the tourniquet and obtain hemostasis. Close the incisions in a routine manner.

▲ *Postoperative management.* A short-leg cast that extends distal to the toes is worn for 6 weeks, nonweight bearing for the first 4 weeks. The pins may be removed at 6 weeks. A night splint that holds the hallux in neutral or slight valgus is worn for 6 additional weeks while active toe exercises are encouraged.

Cleft Foot (Partial Adactylia)

Cleft foot (lobster foot) is an anomaly in which a single cleft usually extends proximally into the foot, sometimes even as far as the midfoot. Generally, one or more toes and parts of their metatarsals are absent, and often the tarsals are abnormal. Although the deformity varies in degree and type, the first and fifth rays usually are present (Fig. 2-35). If a metatarsal is partially or completely absent, its respective toe always is absent.

Any surgery for cleft foot should improve function; improving appearance is of secondary importance. When the cleft extends proximally between the metatarsals, the skin of the apposing surfaces within the cleft is excised, but dorsal and plantar flaps are left that will close the cleft when sutured together. If a metatarsal has no corresponding toe, it is resected and the cleft is closed as just described (Fig. 2-36). Any bony or joint deformity of the first or fifth ray should be corrected at the time of surgery. This may require capsulotomies and osteotomies of any retained rays. If pin fixation is used, the pins and short-leg cast are removed 6 weeks after surgery.

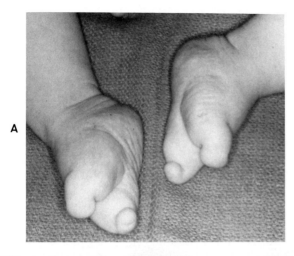
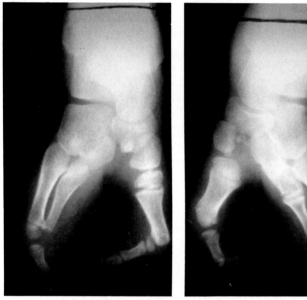

Fig. 2-35   Bilateral cleft foot in, **A,** newborn and, **B,** 4-year-old child.

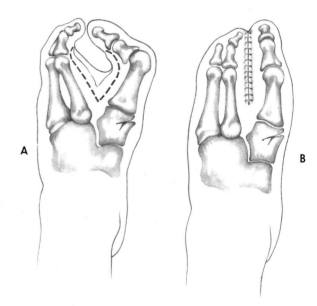

Fig. 2-36   Correction of cleft foot. **A,** Outlines of skin incisions along cleft between abnormal rays of foot. **B,** Artificial syndactyly created after excision of skin cleft and apposition of rays.

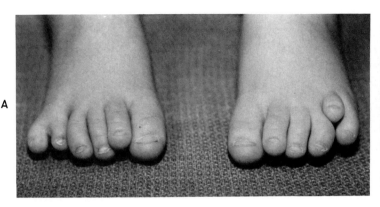 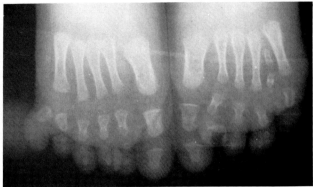

Fig. 2-37 **A,** Bilateral polydactyly in 6-month-old child. **B,** Accessory metatarsal of left foot can be seen on roentgenogram.

ANOMALIES OF TOES

The most common anomaly of the toes is polydactyly, the presence of supernumerary digits; others are syndactyly (webbed toes), macrodactyly (enlarged toes), congenital hallux varus, and congenital contracture or angulation. Any of these may require surgery.

When surgery is being contemplated for anomalies of the toes, several factors must be considered, including cosmesis, pain, and difficulty in fitting shoes. A satisfactory clinical result should correct all these problems.

Polydactyly

Polydactyly of the toes may occur in established genetic syndromes, but it occurs most commonly as an isolated trait with an autosomal dominant inheritance pattern and variable expression. The overall incidence of polydactyly is approximately two cases per 1000 live births.

Surgical treatment of polydactyly is amputation of the accessory digit. Preoperative roentgenograms should be obtained to detect any extra metatarsal articulating with the digit, which should be amputated with its associated digit (Fig. 2-37).

Venn-Watson classified polydactyly and directed attention to the difference between preaxial and postaxial types. In preaxial polydactyly the medial great toe usually is excised. The remaining great toe should have a careful repair of the capsule and, if necessary to prevent residual hallux varus, Kirschner wire fixation for 4 to 6 weeks. The technique for postaxial polydactyly is described.

▶ *Technique of amputating extra toe.* At the base of the toe to be amputated make an oval or racquet-shaped incision through the skin and fascia (Fig. 2-38). Draw the tendons distally as far as possible and divide them. Incise the capsule of the metatarsophalangeal joint transversely, dissect it from the metatarsal, and disarticulate the joint. With an osteotome or bone-cutting forceps resect any bone that may have protruded from the metatarsal head to support the articular surface of the amputated phalanx. If the roentgenogram has revealed an accessory metatarsal, resect it after continuing the incision proximally on the lateral or dorsal aspect of the foot.

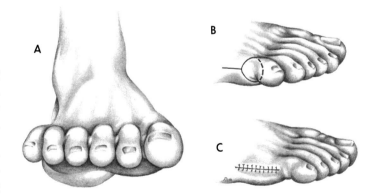

Fig. 2-38 Polydactyly. **A,** Frontal view of foot with polydactyly. **B,** Outline of incision passing through web space between fifth and sixth toes and extending in racquet-shaped incision along lateral border of foot. **C,** Surgical excision of supernumerary digit completed.

Syndactyly

Syndactyly of the toes rarely interferes with function, and surgery is indicated for cosmetic reasons only. The same technique is used as for the fingers (p. 292).

Macrodactyly

Macrodactyly occurs when one or more toes or fingers have hypertrophied and are significantly larger than the surrounding toes or fingers. The most common associated conditions are neurofibromatosis and hemangiomatosis. Surgery is indicated to relieve functional symptoms, primarily pain or difficulty in fitting shoes. The cosmetic goal is to alter the grotesque appearance of the toes and foot and to achieve a foot similar in size to the opposite foot (Fig. 2-39).

Many operative procedures have been described for the treatment of macrodactyly, including reduction syndactyly, soft tissue debulking combined with ostectomy or epiphysiodesis, toe amputation, and ray amputation. Reduction syndactyly may be used as a primary surgical procedure when macrodactyly involves the great toe and second toe. Soft tissue debulking combined with ostectomy or epiphysiodesis may be used in the initial treatment of a single digit with macrodactyly. Unfortunately, recurrence following this technique is virtually 100%. Ray amputation is indicated in patients with massive enlargement of the bone and soft tissues. Ray amputation also is the procedure of choice for recurrence after reduction syndactyly or soft tissue debulking. Hallux valgus may occur after ray resection and occasionally requires surgical correction during adolescence.

A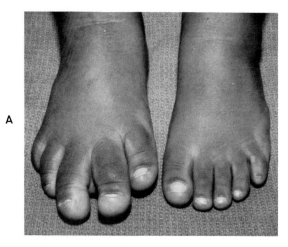

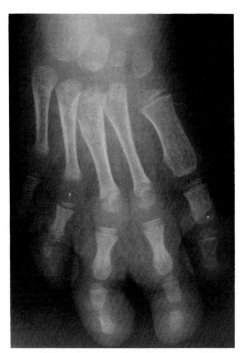 B

Fig. 2-39 **A,** Macrodactyly of right foot secondary to hemangiomatosis. **B,** Note enlargement of second and third metatarsals, phalanges, and associated soft tissues.

■ *Technique of reduction syndactyly (Diamond and Gould)*. With their apices at the bases of the first and second metatarsals, make identical V-shaped incisions on the dorsal and plantar aspects of the foot and extend them distally in the midsagittal plane of the great and second toes (Fig. 2-40). Now deepen the incisions and remove a central wedge of tissue as a block, including the skin and the underlying parts of the phalanges and metatarsals that are in line with the incisions. If necessary realign the first metatarsal by a distal osteotomy to decrease the space between the first and second rays; transfix the osteotomy with a Kirschner wire. Next excise any bony prominences along the remainder of both metatarsals. Appose the bone and soft tissue surfaces with deep interrupted sutures. Also suture together the adjacent capsules of the metatarsophalangeal joints. Excise any nail beds that interfere with skin closure or that might cause pressure on an adjoining toe. Next secure hemostasis and close the skin and subcutaneous tissues with interrupted sutures. Apply a bulky dressing and a heavy plaster splint.

■ *Postoperative management.* After the skin has healed, a short-leg cast is applied and is worn for 6 to 12 weeks until any osteotomy has healed.

■ *Technique of ray amputation.* Outline the ray to be amputated with skin flaps to include amputation from the tip of the toe to the base of the metatarsal. Make dorsal and plantar incisions starting over the metatarsophalangeal joint, with connecting incisions in the web space of adjacent toes. Continue the incisions proximally, both dorsally and plantarward, to the base of the metatarsal to be resected (Fig. 2-41). Amputate the metatarsal and its associated phalanges, as well as any surrounding hypertrophied soft tissue. Take care to protect the neurovascular bundles that supply adjacent toes. After adequate resection of tissue, close the wound with interrupted sutures in the usual manner, from deep to superficial.

■ *Postoperative management.* A short-leg cast is applied to protect the wound until healing occurs at 6 weeks.

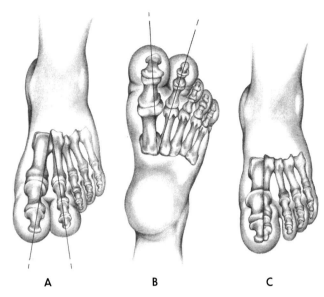

Fig. 2-40 Diamond and Gould reduction syndactyly technique to decrease size of great and second toes. **A** and **B,** Dorsal and plantar views of foot showing identical V-shaped incisions (see text). **C,** Dorsal view after reduction syndactyly operation. (Redrawn from Diamond LS and Gould VE: South Med J 67:645, 1974.)

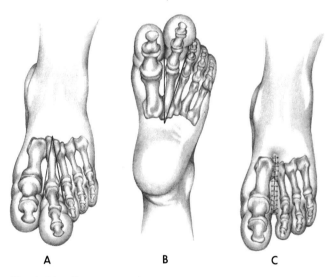

Fig. 2-41 Ray amputation for macrodactyly. **A,** Outline of incision on dorsal surface of foot. **B,** Plantar incision. **C,** Closed incision after amputation.

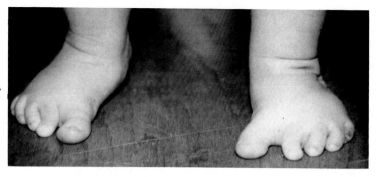

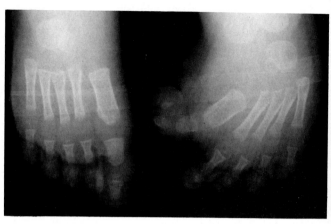

Fig. 2-42 **A,** Congenital hallux varus of left foot. Note varus position of great toe with increased web space between great and second toes. **B,** Anteroposterior roentgenogram; note short first metatarsal and accessory distal phalanx.

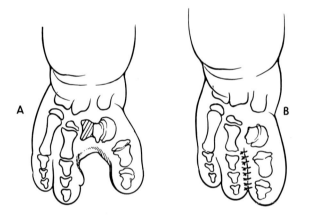

Fig. 2-43 Kelikian procedure for congenital hallux varus. **A,** Preoperative appearance of foot. **B,** After artificial syndactyly.

Congenital Hallux Varus

Hallux varus is a deformity in which the great toe is angulated medially at the metatarsophalangeal joint. It should not be confused with varus deformity of the first metatarsal (metatarsus primus varus) in which the metatarsophalangeal joint is not deformed. The varus deformity of the toe varies in severity from only a few degrees to as much as 90 degrees.

Hallux varus usually is unilateral and is associated with one or more of the following: (1) a short, thick first metatarsal, (2) accessory metatarsals and phalanges, (3) varus deformity of one or more of the four lateral metatarsals, and (4) a firm fibrous band that extends from the medial side of the great toe to the base of the first metatarsal (Fig. 2-42).

The explanation for this anomaly is that two great toes originate in utero but the medial or accessory one fails to develop. Later the rudimentary medial toe, together with the band of fibrous tissue, acts like a taut bowstring and gradually pulls the more fully developed great toe into a varus position.

The proper treatment for congenital hallux varus depends on the severity of the deformity and the rigidity of the contracted soft structures. The Farmer technique is effective in correcting mild or moderate deformity. The operation of Kelikian et al also is satisfactory for the severe deformity with an excessively short first metatarsal (Fig. 2-43). When the deformity is complicated by traumatic arthritis of the metatarsophalangeal joint, arthrodesis of this joint as described by McKeever is indicated (see p. 676). Rarely, when the deformity is too severe to be either corrected or fused, amputation is indicated.

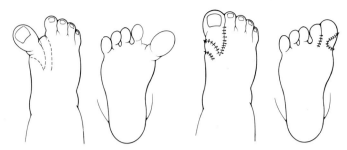

Fig. 2-44 Farmer procedure for congenital hallux varus (see text).

▶ *Technique (Farmer).* Raise a broad Y-shaped flap of skin and subcutaneous tissue from the dorsal surface of the web between the first and second toes (Fig. 2-44); base the flap dorsally in the space between the first and second metatarsals and include in it the skin contiguous with the web distally along the two toes for one third their length. From the medial edge of the base of the flap curve the incision medially and slightly distally across the medial aspect of the first metatarsophalangeal joint. Deepen this incision transversely through the medial part of the capsule of the first metatarsophalangeal joint. Then move the great toe laterally against the second toe, and create a syndactyly between these two toes by suturing the apposing skin edges together. Excise any accessory phalanx or hypertrophic soft tissue from the great toe through a separate dorsomedial incision. Now swing the Y-shaped flap of skin and subcutaneous tissue medially, and suture it in place to cover the defect in the skin on the dorsal and medial aspects of the first metatarsophalangeal joint.

Farmer described an alternative technique in which the Y-shaped flap of skin and subcutaneous tissue is raised from the plantar surface of the foot (Fig. 2-45); the same procedure then is performed, the flap being swung medially to cover the defect in the skin at the first metatarsophalangeal joint. Any defect that cannot be closed by the flap either is left open to heal secondarily or is covered by a full-thickness skin graft.

▶ *Postoperative management.* The foot is immobilized in a cast. At 6 weeks the cast is removed, and full activities are allowed.

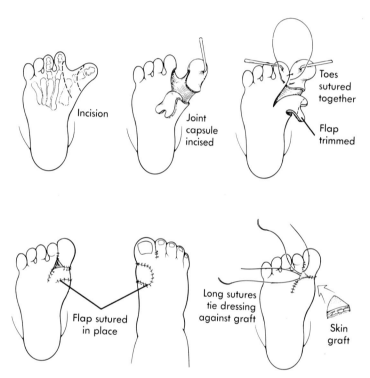

Fig. 2-45 Alternative Farmer procedure for congenital hallux varus (see text).

Contracture or Angulation

Congenital contracture, angulation, or subluxation of the fifth toe is a fairly common familial deformity but rarely causes symptoms. The anomaly rarely is disabling, and surgery usually is indicated only to improve function of the foot. The direction of angulation of the fifth toe determines the operative procedure (Fig. 2-46).

Lapidus described an operation for correction of hyperextension of the fifth toe when it is either in neutral position or overlapping the fourth toe.

◤ *Technique (Lapidus)*. Make a longitudinal bayonet-shaped incision, coursing first along the dorsomedial aspect of the fifth toe from the distal interphalangeal joint to the web between the fifth and the fourth toes, then laterally over the dorsum of the fifth metatarsophalangeal joint, and then proximally along the lateral aspect of the head of the fifth metatarsal. Flex the toe to tighten its long extensor tendon. Now make a second incision dorsally and transversely 1 cm long over the middle of the fifth metatarsal. Through this second incision identify the long extensor tendon, cut it transversely, and retract its distal part through the first incision. Then completely free this part of the tendon distally to its insertion on the distal phalanx.

By blunt dissection expose the capsule of the fifth metatarsophalangeal joint, and incise it transversely on its dorsal and medial aspects to relieve the contracture of the capsule and of the medial collateral ligament. Now make a channel through the soft tissues; start it near the distal interphalangeal joint on the dorsomedial aspect of the fifth toe, wind it around the plantar aspect of the toe proximally and laterally, and end it on the plantar lateral aspect of the fifth metatarsophalangeal joint. Pass the end of the freed tendon proximally through this tunnel. Split the abductor and short flexor of the fifth toe longitudinally, and then suture the long extensor tendon through these two tendons under enough tension to correct all components of the deformity. Close the skin with interrupted sutures, shifting its edges as necessary to correct any severe contracture.

◤ *Postoperative management*. The toe is immobilized for 4 weeks. Walking is allowed in a shoe cut out over the fifth toe.

• • •

Kelikian et al also reported successful correction of contracture and angulation of central toes in adolescents and young adults with a similar surgical syndactyly.

◤ *Technique (Kelikian et al)*. Fashion cruciate incisions between the two toes to undergo syndactyly. Begin the first incision on the dorsal surface of the web proximal to the base of the toes, and carry it between the toes over the middle of the web and then proximally on the plantar surface of the foot to the level of the metatarsal heads. Then on the adjacent surfaces of the two toes make longitudinal incisions that bisect the first incision. Carry these incisions to the tips of the toes if the deformity to be corrected involves the distal interphalangeal joints. Now resect triangular flaps of plantar skin from the adjacent surfaces of each toe. Excise as much of the base of the proximal phalanx of the deformed toe or of both toes as is necessary for easy closure. Secure hemostasis, and suture the dorsal and plantar skin margins to produce an artificial syndactyly.

◤ *Postoperative management*. A pressure dressing is applied. At 2 weeks the sutures are removed, and 2 or 3 days later weight bearing is allowed.

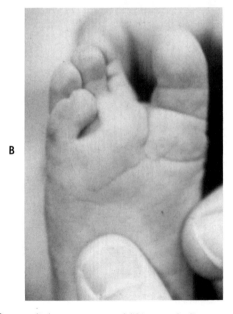

Fig. 2-46 Congenital contracture of fifth toe. **A,** Dorsal overlapping of fifth toe over fourth toe. **B,** Fifth toe shows plantar flexion and medial contracture beneath fourth toe.

The fifth toe may be fixed in plantar flexion and adducted beneath the fourth toe. For the severe fixed deformity the procedure described by Ruiz-Mora or Thompson may be used.

▲ *Technique (Ruiz-Mora).* Excise an elliptic segment of skin and subcutaneous tissue from the plantar surface of the fifth toe and the adjacent metatarsal area as shown in Fig. 2-47. Curving the proximal end of the ellipse medially makes the fifth toe approximate the fourth more closely after surgery. Now excise the proximal phalanx and close the deep tissues by two subcutaneous sutures. Then close the skin by three interrupted sutures.

For fifth toe plantar constrictures, Thompson recommends making a Z-plasty skin incision over the dorsal aspect of the fifth toe, excising the proximal phalanx, and rotating and closing the skin flaps (Fig. 2-48).

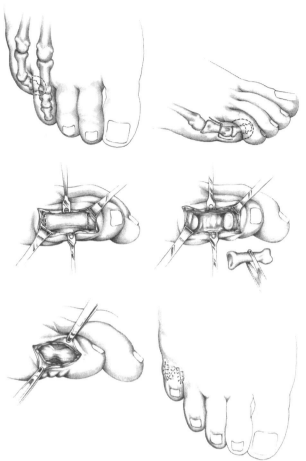

Fig. 2-48 Thompson technique for congenital contracture of fifth toe in young adult. Z-plasty incision is made over dorsal aspect of toe, proximal phalanx is excised, and skin flaps are rotated and closed. (Redrawn from Thompson TC: J Bone Joint Surg 46A:1117, 1964.)

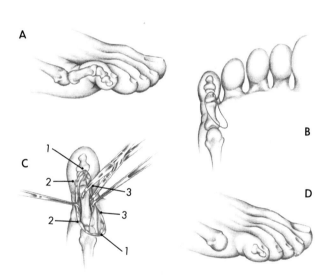

Fig. 2-47 Ruiz-Mora operation for correction of congenital contracture of fifth toe in young adult. **A,** Deformity. **B,** Ellipse of skin has been excised from plantar surface of toe and foot. **C,** Proximal phalanx of toe is being excised. In closing skin, point *1* is sutured to point *1*, *2* to *2*, and *3* to *3*. **D,** Appearance of toe after surgery. (Redrawn from Straub LR. In Cecil RL, editor: The specialties in general practice, Philadelphia, 1951, WB Saunders Co.)

CONGENITAL ANGULAR DEFORMITIES OF LEG

Congenital angular deformities of the leg are primarily of two kinds: those in which the apex of the angulation is anterior and those in which it is posterior. In both, the tibia often is bowed not only anteriorly or posteriorly but also medially or laterally; Badgley et al suggested the term *congenital kyphoscoliotic tibia* for both these deformities. Anterior bowing of the tibia commonly is associated with neurofibromatosis, but there is not an absolutely established causal relationship between the two.

Posterior angular deformities of the tibia usually tend to improve with growth (Fig. 2-49). A limb length discrepancy also may be present, which can range from several millimeters to several centimeters. Children with these deformities should be examined yearly for any potential limb length discrepancy that may require limb equalization, usually by an appropriately timed epiphysiodesis.

In contrast, anterior angular deformities of the tibia are more worrisome because of their potential association with congenital pseudarthrosis of the tibia. Occasionally these tibias maintain a normal medullary canal and show no evidence of narrowing or the sclerotic "high-risk tibia." If any indication of narrowing of the medullary canal is present or develops in an anteriorly bowed tibia, the limb should be braced until skeletal maturity.

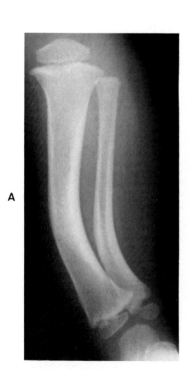
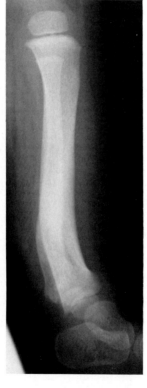

Fig. 2-49 Congenital posteromedial bowing of left tibia. **A,** Anteroposterior view. **B,** Lateral view.

CONGENITAL PSEUDARTHROSIS

Congenital pseudarthrosis is a specific type of nonunion that at birth is either present or incipient. Its cause is unknown, but it occurs often enough in patients with either neurofibromatosis or related stigmata to suggest that neurofibromatosis, if not the cause, is closely related to congenital pseudarthrosis. Congenital pseudarthrosis most commonly involves the distal half of the tibia and often that of the fibula in the same limb, as well as the clavicle, the humerus, the radius, the ulna, and the femur.

Fibula

Congenital pseudarthrosis of the fibula often precedes or accompanies the same condition in the ipsilateral tibia. Several grades of severity of this pseudarthrosis are seen: bowing of the fibula without pseudarthrosis, fibular pseudarthrosis without ankle deformity, fibular pseudarthrosis with ankle deformity, and fibular pseudarthrosis with latent pseudarthrosis of the tibia. Sometimes it even develops between the time of successful bone grafting of a pseudarthrosis of the tibia and skeletal maturity. Then, because the lateral malleolus becomes displaced proximally, a progressive valgus deformity of the ankle develops.

Until skeletal maturity is reached, the ankle can be stabilized by an ankle-foot orthosis. At maturity any significant deformity can be treated by supramalleolar osteotomy made through essentially normal bone, and union of the osteotomy can be expected. Langenskiöld, however, has devised an operation for children to prevent this valgus deformity or to halt its progression. He creates a synostosis between the distal tibial and fibular metaphyses. Because in congenital pseudarthrosis securing union by bone grafting may be as difficult in the fibula as in the tibia, an operation that prevents the ankle deformity without grafting the fibular pseudarthrosis is useful (Fig. 2-50).

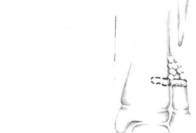

Fig. 2-50 Langenskiöld technique of creating synostosis between distal tibial and fibular metaphyses to prevent valgus deformity of ankle in congenital pseudarthrosis of fibula (see text). (Redrawn from Langenskiöld A: J Bone Joint Surg 49A:463, 1967.)

▲ *Technique (Langenskiöld).* Make a longitudinal incision anteriorly over the distal fibula. Then divide the fibula 1 to 2 cm proximal to the level of the distal tibial physis, and excise the cone-shaped part of the distal fibular shaft. In the lateral surface of the tibia at the level of the cut surface of the fibula and at the attachment of the interosseous membrane, make a hole as wide as the diameter of the fibula. Then proximal to the hole remove the periosteum and interosseous membrane from the tibia over an area of several square centimeters. From the ilium obtain a bone graft the same width as that of the hole in the tibia and long enough to extend from the lateral surface of the fibula into the spongy bone of the tibial metaphysis. Insert the graft perpendicular to the long axis of the limb so it rests on the cut surface of the fibula and extends into the slot in the tibial cortex. Then pack spongy iliac bone in the angle between the proximal surface of the graft and the lateral surface of the tibia. Apply a cast from below the knee to the base of the toes.

▲ *Postoperative management.* At 2 months full weight bearing in the cast is allowed, and at 4 months the cast is removed.

Tibia

Congenital pseudarthrosis of the tibia is rare, with an incidence of approximately 1 in 250,000 live births. Most large series report 50% to 90% association of this disorder with the stigmata of neurofibromatosis, including skin and osseous lesions.

Congenital pseudarthrosis of the tibia has been classified by Boyd into six different types.

Type I pseudarthrosis occurs with anterior bowing and a defect in the tibia that are present at birth. Other congenital deformities also may be present, and these may affect the management of the pseudarthrosis.

Type II pseudarthrosis occurs with anterior bowing and an hourglass constriction of the tibia that are present at birth. Spontaneous fracture, or fracture after minor trauma, commonly occurs before the child is 2 years old. This is the so-called high-risk tibia. The tibia is tapered, rounded, and sclerotic, and the medullary canal is obliterated. This type is the most frequent, is often associated with neurofibromatosis, and has the poorest prognosis. Recurrence of the fracture is common during the growth period but decreases in frequency with age and generally ceases to occur after skeletal maturation (Fig. 2-51).

Type III pseudarthrosis develops in a congenital cyst, usually near the junction of the middle and distal thirds of the tibia. Anterior bowing may precede or follow the development of a fracture. Recurrence of the fracture after treatment is less frequent than in type II, and excellent results after only one operation have been reported to last well into adulthood (Fig. 2-52).

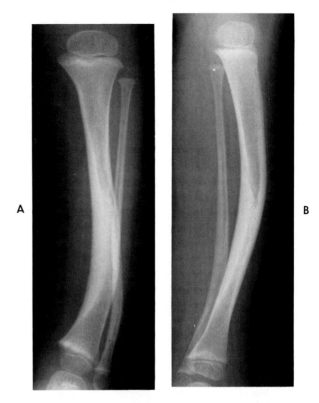

Fig. 2-51 Type II congenital pseudarthrosis of tibia. **A,** Anteroposterior view of left tibia. **B,** Lateral view. Note anterior bowing and narrow sclerotic medullary canal.

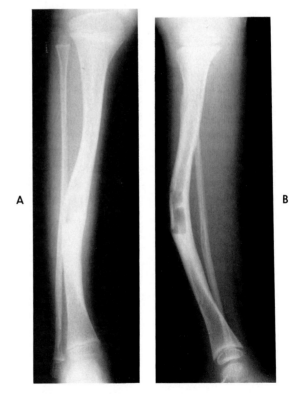

Fig. 2-52 Type III congenital pseudarthrosis of tibia. **A,** Anteroposterior view of right tibia. **B,** Lateral view. Note cyst formation in middle third of tibia with anterior bowing and narrow medullary canal distal to cyst.

Type IV pseudarthrosis originates in a sclerotic segment of bone in the classic location without narrowing of the tibia. The medullary canal is partially or completely obliterated. An "insufficiency" or "march" fracture develops in the cortex of the tibia and gradually extends through the sclerotic bone. With completion of the fracture, healing fails to occur, and the fracture site widens and becomes a pseudarthrosis. The prognosis for this type is generally good, especially when treated before the insufficiency fracture becomes complete (Fig. 2-53).

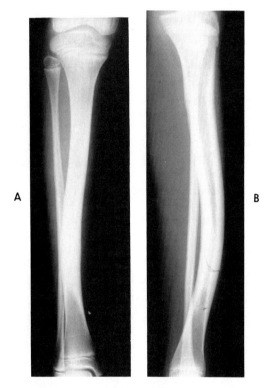

Fig. 2-53 Type IV congenital pseudarthrosis of tibia. **A,** Anteroposterior view of right tibia. **B,** Lateral view. Note fracture in anterior cortex distal third of tibia.

Type V pseudarthrosis of the tibia occurs with a dysplastic fibula. A pseudarthrosis of the fibula or tibia, or both, may develop. The prognosis is good if the lesion is confined to the fibula. If the lesion progresses to a tibial pseudarthrosis, the natural history usually resembles that of type II.

Type VI pseudarthrosis occurs as an intraosseous neurofibroma or schwannoma that results in a pseudarthrosis. This is extremely rare. The prognosis depends on the aggressiveness and treatment of the intraosseous lesion.

Treatment of congenital pseudarthrosis of the tibia depends on the age of the patient and the type of pseudarthrosis. A true congenital pseudarthrosis of the tibia will not heal when treated by casting alone. Initially, the decision must be made whether to attempt to secure union or to amputate. Factors that favor amputation include anticipated shortening of more than 2 or 3 inches (5 to 7.5 cm), a history of multiple failed surgical procedures, and stiffness and decreased function of a limb that would be more useful after an amputation and fitting with a prosthesis.

For the tibia with a cyst in the medullary canal, prophylactic curettage and autogenous iliac bone grafting are recommended. The limb is immobilized in plaster until the grafts have united, and then a brace, preferably of the patellar tendon–bearing type, is worn until skeletal maturity.

A tibia with anterior bowing and the narrow sclerotic canal of the high-risk tibia often will fracture during the first 2 years of life. Initially, bracing may be beneficial for an anterolaterally bowed tibia with a narrow canal in which a fracture has not developed. Once a fracture does occur, the treatment usually is surgical.

Treatment of Established Pseudarthrosis

Established congenital pseudarthrosis of the tibia has been treated by a variety of methods, primarily bone grafting or amputation. Osseous union probably is more difficult to obtain in this condition than in any other. Boyd and Sage in 1958 reviewed the English literature and found primary union obtained in approximately 56% of 91 patients treated with 23 different surgical procedures. More recently, Morrissy et al reported union in fewer than 50% of 40 patients treated with 172 bone grafting procedures, and Murray and Lovell reported successful treatment in only 31% of 36 pseudarthroses after a total of 85 grafting procedures. In a long-term follow-up study, Crossett et al reported good or fair results in 52% of 25 patients treated with 96 surgical procedures.

The age of the patient, the difficulty in obtaining union, and should union be obtained, the anticipated residual shortening and other deformities of the tibia all must be considered in determining proper treatment. In an infant or a young child bone grafting is indicated as early as feasible. Even though the likelihood of obtaining union increases with increasing age, especially after puberty, the longer grafting is delayed, the shorter and more poorly developed the leg will be and the more deformed and smaller the foot will be. When union is obtained in a young child, weight bearing in a brace may result in more normal development of the limb. The child's parents should be told that treatment often consists of several operations and that even then amputation may be necessary later because of failure to obtain union. If grafting is indicated but for some reason must be delayed, the limb should be braced to prevent increase in angulation at the pseudarthrosis. In an older child bone grafting is indicated unless shortness or other deformity of the limb is such that function would be better after amputation and fitting with a prosthesis.

Several newer treatment modalities for congenital pseudarthrosis of the tibia currently are being evaluated, but the number of cases is too small and the follow-up period too short to recommend these as standard treatment. A recent technique is the free vascularized bone graft by means of either fibular or iliac crest grafts (Fig. 2-54). Weiland reported successful treatment of six pseudarthroses of the tibia with free fibular grafts; only one of his seven patients required a second procedure after fracture distal to the graft. Other authors have reported good results in small series of patients with this technique. The procedure, however, requires experience with microvascular techniques and is technically demanding. Pulsating electromagnetic fields externally and constant direct current implanted internally have been reported to enhance union of bone grafting of the

pseudarthroses, but the indications for their applications are narrow. Ilizarov has reported successful bridging of large pseudarthroses without loss of limb length with the use of his external fixation system, but the technique has not been used long enough or in enough patients in the United States for adequate evaluation.

Bone grafting procedures remain the mainstay of treatment for congenital pseudarthrosis of the tibia. Although many techniques have been described, those commonly used in recent years include the Boyd dual onlay graft, the dual intramedullary rodding technique of Umber et al, and the Paterson modification of the Sofield technique to include an intramedullary rod, bone grafting, and the implantation of an electrical stimulation device in the medullary canal. McElvenny first called attention to the heavy cuff of tissue surrounding the bone at the pseudarthrosis and reasoned that the presence of this tissue, whether congenital or a result of the fracture, may decrease bone production and consequently healing. Any operation for congenital pseudarthrosis should include complete excision of this tissue.

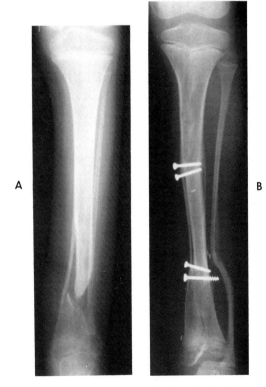

Fig. 2-54 Congenital pseudarthrosis of tibia treated with vascularized fibular bone graft. **A,** Preoperative roentgenogram of tibia with established distal pseudarthrosis after multiple failed surgical procedures. **B,** Three years after vascularized fibular graft.

Surgical technique. The Boyd dual onlay graft is the treatment of choice in patients with stress fractures that proceed to pseudarthrosis but that do not have a wide gap between the bone ends. Intramedullary nailing with bone grafting, with or without electrical stimulation, is the recommended treatment for established pseudarthrosis. The vascularized graft may be useful in patients in whom standard bone grafting procedures fail.

▶ *Technique of applying dual grafts (Boyd).* Prepare two cortical tibial grafts 11 cm long and 2 cm wide, and remove the endosteal bone from each. As an alternative, a full-thickness iliac graft may be used for both cortical and cancellous bone. Have available an ample supply of cancellous bone in addition to that removed for the onlay grafts.

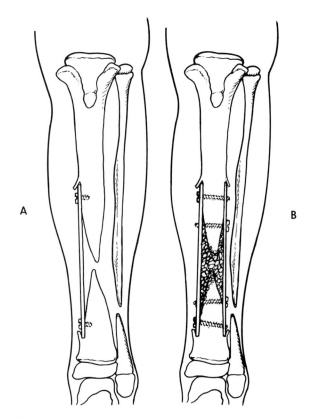

Fig. 2-55   Boyd dual onlay bone graft for congenital pseudarthrosis of tibia. **A,** First graft temporarily held in position by two short screws. **B,** Medial and lateral grafts fixed with transfixing screws. Resected pseudarthrosis filled with cancellous graft.

Expose the pseudarthrosis through a long anterior longitudinal incision. Excise all thickened periosteum and constricting fibrous tissue to healthy muscle and subcutaneous tissue. Resect all sclerotic bone from the ends of the fragments, but take care to preserve as much length of the bone as possible. Then with a drill open the medullary canal of each fragment. If the proximal and distal fragments of the tibia are opposed and the tendo Achilles is under excessive tension, lengthen the tendo Achilles through a small posterior incision. Osteotomy of the fibula usually is unnecessary because apposition of the tibial fragments is not needed and the intact fibula adds stability to the grafted tibia.

Next prepare beds for the grafts on the medial and lateral surfaces of the tibial fragments. Shave away enough bone from each side to create a flat surface for maximum contact between the grafts and the tibia. Remove more bone from the expanded areas of the tibia proximally and distally than from the region of pseudarthrosis. In fact, considerable space may remain between the tibia and the grafts near the pseudarthrosis, especially if the ends of the fragments are conical. This is not a disadvantage if the space is filled with cancellous bone. Place the graft as far distally on the tibia as possible without damaging the distal tibial physis and also as far proximally as possible—the longer the graft the better. In small children it may extend to the proximal tibial physis. Begin applying the grafts by placing one on the medial or lateral surface of the tibia and temporarily fixing it in position (Fig. 2-55). Then apply the second graft on the opposite side of the bone, and transfix both grafts and the proximal and distal tibial fragments by two screws. Place the screws as far as practical from the pseudarthrosis because they may predispose the tibia to fracture later.

Finally pack the space between the two grafts and around the pseudarthrosis with cancellous bone. Completely fill these areas both anteriorly and posteriorly. With interrupted sutures close only the skin and subcutaneous tissues.

▶ *Postoperative management.* Apply a long-leg cast or, if needed for adequate immobilization in a small child, a spica cast. At 10 to 14 days the cast usually is changed and should be changed again thereafter as often as necessary to ensure immobilization until the bone has united. A cast usually is necessary for a total of 4 to 6 months or more. After the last cast has been discarded, a long-leg brace or a patellar tendon-bearing brace is fitted and is worn until maturity. If union is obtained, follow-up is recommended at 6- to 12-month intervals with serial roentgenograms and brace modifications.

Paterson technique. For patients with an established pseudarthrosis of the tibia, the tibia must be straightened and held in position with a medullary rod; the use of a large quantity of autogenous iliac cancellous bone also is necessary to obtain union. Paterson reported a 75% union rate with his technique, and Umber et al obtained union in four of six patients with their technique (Fig. 2-56).

▶ *Technique (Paterson).* Calculate preoperatively the amount of diseased bone to be excised from tracings made of recent anteroposterior and lateral roentgenograms. Approach the fibula through a lateral incision, and perform an osteotomy to allow correction of the tibial deformity. Then approach the tibia through an anterior longitudinal incision. The exact amount of bone to be removed varies, but union is most likely when the whole sclerotic segment is excised and good quality bone is left in contact at each end. Such extensive excision, however, often leaves an unacceptable shortening (leg-length discrepancy of up to 8 cm is acceptable). Sometimes the sclerotic segment is so long that some of it must be left in place, but union still occurs in most instances. Remove all abnormal, thick, fibrous tissue, including the

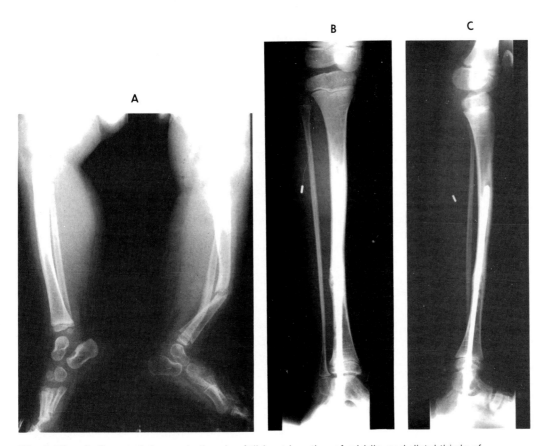

Fig. 2-56   A, Congenital pseudarthrosis of tibia at junction of middle and distal thirds of shaft. **B** and **C,** Anteroposterior and lateral roentgenograms after union of pseudarthrosis. (Courtesy Sir Dennis Paterson.)

periosteum from the area of the defect. Choose a medullary rod, a Steinmann pin in the young child, or an intramedullary interlocking nail in the adolescent near skeletal maturity. If the tibial medullary canal is quite small, a Rush nail can be used. Insert the rod in a retrograde fashion, beginning at the defect and proceeding through the tibia, ankle joint, the talus, and the calcaneus to emerge through a small incision on the bottom of the heel. As an alternative, the intramedullary device chosen may be inserted from proximal to distal in an antegrade manner to remain in the tibia only. Take care to avoid any inversion, eversion, or equinus deformity of the foot. Then hammer the rod upward into the proximal tibia to just below the physis (Fig. 2-57, *A*). Cut off the distal end of the rod at the base of the calcaneus. Then insert the electrical bone growth stimulator according to the manufacturer's instructions (Fig. 2-57, *B* and *C*). Pack the area with cancellous bone grafts from the iliac crest, close the wound with absorbable sutures, and apply a long-leg cast.

▶ *Postoperative management.* The cast is changed at 2 weeks, and weight bearing is encouraged once the skin has healed. The patient is examined every 2 months, and at 6 months the cast is removed if roentgenographic union has occurred. It is important to test for rotation of the distal tibial fragment around the intramedullary rod.

When union of the tibial pseudarthrosis is obtained after surgery, bracing should be continued until skeletal maturity. Initially a long-leg brace with a patellar tendon–bearing lower component should be used and converted to a patellar tendon–bearing brace when the child is approximately 6 years of age. These patients should be evaluated at 6- to 12-month intervals with careful examination for problems that may follow surgery: (1) recurrent fracture with pseudarthrosis, (2) limb length discrepancy, which if progressive should be treated, and (3) valgus deformity of the ankle that may require treatment by a Langenskiöld procedure or osteotomy at skeletal maturity.

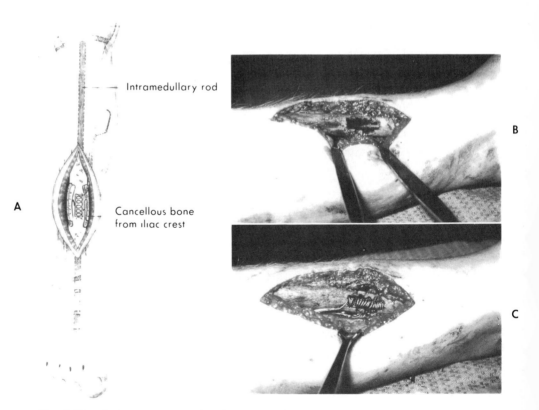

Fig. 2-57   **A,** Paterson procedure for congenital pseudarthrosis of tibia consisting of insertion of intramedullary nail, cancellous bone grafts, and constant direct current stimulation. **B,** Pseudarthrosis of tibia with intramedullary nail in canal and defect in cortical bone. **C,** Constant direct current stimulator placed in medullary canal. (Courtesy Sir Dennis Paterson.)

CONSTRICTURES OF LEG

A congenital circumferential constricture or Streeter band of the soft tissues of the leg is rare. It is seen at birth as a depression in the soft tissues, completely encircling the limb (Fig. 2-58). Often the foot also is deformed. The skin, subcutaneous tissue, and deep fascia all may be affected, and usually the lymphatic vessels and superficial circulation are partially obstructed. Distal to the constricture is a persistent pitting edema that can be cured only by excising the constricture and in most instances the edematous tissues distal to it. Fractures of the tibia and fibula at the level of the constricture have been reported. In marked contrast to congenital pseudarthrosis, after successful treatment of the constricture, the fractures heal promptly without surgery.

An operation to eliminate a constricture must include a Z-plasty; if it is simply excised, the constricture usually recurs. The technique of Cozen and Brockway is recommended for a severe constricture to be corrected in stages. The technique of Peet is appropriate for mild and moderate constrictures.

▲ *Technique (from Cozen and Brockway).* Lengthen the constricted tissues in stages; at least three Z-plasty operations usually are required. In each, first make the middle limb of the Z in the cleft of the constricture. Then make the superior and inferior limbs of the Z each at an angle of 60 degrees to the middle limb. Deepen all three incisions through the subcutaneous tissue and fascia, and undermine widely the two triangular flaps thus created. Transpose each flap to the original bed of the opposite flap, and suture the free edges of the skin.

Repeat the operation two or more times, allowing the wound to heal after each, until the area of constricture has been lengthened throughout its circumference.

▲ *Technique (Peet).* Remove the entire constricture by circumferential excision of the skin and subcutaneous tissue down to the deep fascia (Fig. 2-59). If the limb tapers, curve the distal incision in a serpentine line so that its length is about the same as that of the proximal one. Then undermine the skin and subcutaneous tissue on each side of the excised area. Approximate the deep tissues with interrupted sutures. Approximate the skin edges with interrupted mattress sutures except in one area; in this area lengthen the edges of the skin with one or more Z-plasty procedures, the limbs of which are approximately 2 cm long. Raise and transpose the triangular flaps, and suture them in position with small interrupted sutures.

▲ *Postoperative management.* A pressure bandage is applied from proximal to the area of surgery to the distal end of the limb. With young children a cast or plaster splint is applied and worn until the incision has healed.

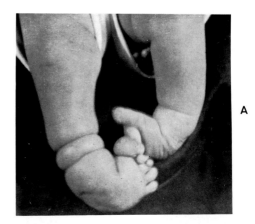

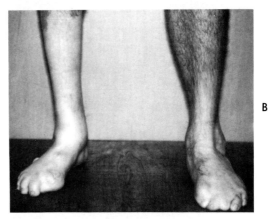

Fig. 2-58 **A,** Congenital constricture of right leg and great toe and bilateral clubfoot. **B,** Adult with loss of several toes caused by congenital constrictures.

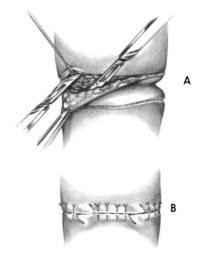

Fig. 2-59 Congenital constricture. **A,** Excision of constricture and undermining of skin edges. **B,** Skin edges have been sutured except in two areas in which Z-plasty incisions have been made. (Redrawn from Peet EW. In Rob C and Smith R, editors: Operative surgery, part 10, London, 1959, Butterworth & Co, Ltd.)

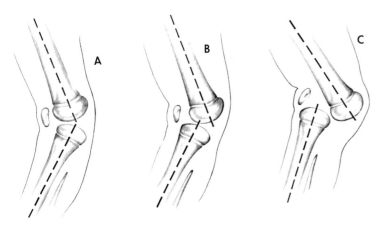

Fig. 2-60 Stages of congenital hyperextension, subluxation, and dislocation of knee. **A,** Hyperextension. **B,** Subluxation. **C,** Dislocation. (Redrawn from Curtis BH and Fisher RL: J Bone Joint Surg 51A:225, 1969.)

CONGENITAL HYPEREXTENSION AND DISLOCATION OF KNEE

Congenital hyperextension of the knee is only the first of three degrees of severity of a single abnormality. These are (1) congenital hyperextension, (2) congenital hyperextension with anterior subluxation of the tibia on the femur, and (3) congenital hyperextension with anterior dislocation of the tibia on the femur (Fig. 2-60).

Congenital hyperextension or dislocation of the knee usually is associated with skeletal abnormalities elsewhere in the extremity. Katz et al, in a study of 155 children with congenital dislocation of the knee, found other musculoskeletal abnormalities in 82%; 45% had congenital dislocation of the hip. Curtis and Fisher in a study of 15 knees with congenital hyperextension and anterior subluxation of the tibia in 11 patients found an abnormality of the hip in each. Johnson et al found other abnormalities in 88% of their 17 patients, and Nogi and MacEwen reported congenital hip dysplasia in 8 of 17 patients (Fig. 2-61).

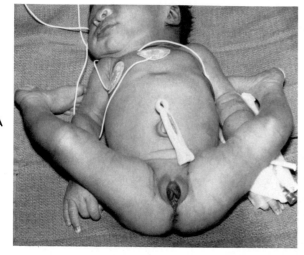

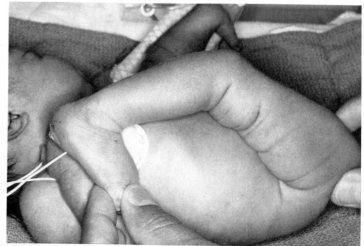

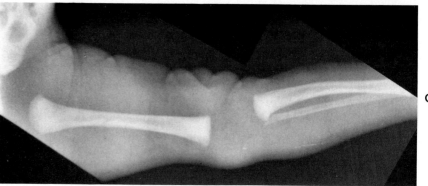

Fig. 2-61 Congenital dislocation of knee. **A,** Newborn with bilateral congenital dislocation of knee. **B,** Note prominence of femoral condyles posterior to anteriorly dislocated tibia and fibula. **C,** Anterior displacement of tibia and fibula is evident on lateral roentgenogram. (Courtesy Dr. Jay Cummings.)

Katz et al found the cruciate ligaments in five knees to be either markedly attenuated or absent and postulated that the basic defect in congenital dislocation of the knee is absence or hypoplasia of these ligaments. Other investigators, however, consider these findings a result of the dislocation.

The pathology usually varies with the severity of the deformity, but always the anterior capsule of the knee and the quadriceps mechanism are contracted. As the severity of the anterior displacement of the tibia increases, other findings include intraarticular adhesions and other abnormalities within the joint and hypoplasia or absence of the patella. Curtis and Fisher noted fibrosis and loss of bulk of the vastus lateralis muscle. Furthermore, the suprapatellar pouch was obliterated by the adherent quadriceps tendon, and in more than half the knees the patella was displaced laterally. In severe anterior dislocation the collateral ligaments coursed anteriorly from their femoral attachments, and the hamstring muscles in some patients were subluxated anteriorly to function as extensors of the knee in the deformed position.

The treatment of congenital hyperextension of the knee depends on the severity of the subluxation or dislocation and the age of the patient. In the newborn with mild to moderate hyperextension or subluxation, conservative treatment methods such as the use of the Pavlik harness for posturing of the knee in a continued position or serial casting to increase knee flexion is most likely to succeed. In children who do not respond to conservative measures the use of skeletal traction for correction is an option, but the deformity is difficult to correct by this method. In older children with a moderate to severe subluxation or dislocation, surgery is indicated. In a child with both congenital dislocation of the knee and congenital dislocation of the hip, surgical correction of the knee first is advisable.

Curtis and Fisher described a procedure for correction of congenital dislocation of the knee. The operation is recommended for children between the ages of 6 and 18 months. The technique combines anterior capsular release, lengthening of the quadriceps mechanism, and release of intraarticular adhesions.

Occasionally, the articular surfaces of the knee remain abnormal if the deformity recurs. Ideally, a functional range of motion can be obtained. Rarely osteotomy of the femur or tibia may be required in the older child.

▶ *Technique (Curtis and Fisher).* Make a long anterior incision starting superomedially at the level of the lesser trochanter and extending inferolaterally to the tibial tuberosity. Expose the anterior thigh muscles, and divide the quadriceps mechanism superior to the

patella by either an inverted V-shaped incision or a Z-plasty (Fig. 2-62). The former incision provides a tongue of tissue superior to the patella suitable for attachment of the proximal muscle mass after the extensor mechanism has been lengthened. Next divide the anterior capsule transversely, and extend the incision posteriorly to the tibial and fibular collateral ligaments. Mobilize and displace these ligaments posteriorly as the knee is flexed. If the patella is displaced laterally, release the lateral part of the patellar tendon so that the patella may be moved to its proper location on the femoral condyles. Now release any tight iliotibial band, and lengthen the fibular collateral ligament if needed. Mobilize all normal-appearing quadriceps muscle, and align it in the long axis of the femur to exert a direct pull on the patella. Suture the lengthened quadriceps mechanism with repair of the vastus medialis muscle to the lengthened rectus femoris. Evaluate tracking of the patella from extension to 90 degrees of flexion. Close the wound and apply a long-leg cast with the knee flexed 30 degrees.

▶ *Postoperative management.* At 4 to 6 weeks the cast is removed, and active and passive exercises are begun. In older patients to prevent hyperextension of the knee, a long-leg brace is worn for 6 to 12 months.

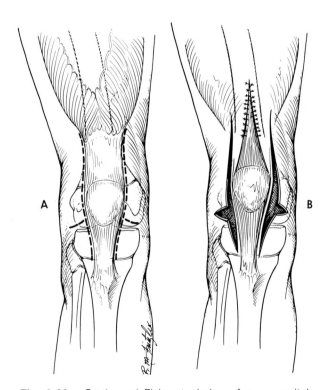

Fig. 2-62   Curtis and Fisher technique for congenital dislocation of knee. **A,** Lines of incision to release anterior capsule medially and laterally, as well as medial and lateral retinaculum of quadriceps mechanism. **B,** Correction after soft tissue release and lengthening of rectus femoris muscle.

CONGENITAL DISLOCATION OF PATELLA

Congenital dislocation of the patella often is familial and bilateral. Occasionally it is accompanied by other abnormalities, especially arthrogryposis multiplex congenita and Down syndrome. It is persistent and irreducible, and there usually are abnormalities of the quadriceps mechanism; the vastus lateralis muscle may be absent, and the patella may be attached to the anterior aspect of the iliotibial band. Often the patella is small and misshapen and in an abnormal location in the quadriceps mechanism. Genu valgum and external rotation of the tibia on the femur commonly develop. The capsule on the medial side of the knee is stretched, the lateral femoral condyle is flattened, or the insertion of the patellar tendon is located more laterally than normally.

The diagnosis of congenital dislocation of the patella sometimes is difficult to make before the patient is 3 to 4 years old because of lack of ossification of the patella. Because the severity of the deformity is directly related to the length of time that the deformity is allowed to remain uncorrected, surgery may be performed as soon as the diagnosis is made (Fig. 2-63).

Stanisavljevic et al described an operation to correct malrotation of the quadriceps muscle by medially rotating the muscle mass, the patella, and the lateral half of the patellar tendon.

▶ *Technique (Stanisavljevic et al).* Make a skin incision along the lateral aspect of the thigh, beginning proximally 4 cm inferior to the greater trochanter, curving anteriorly over the lateral femoral condyle, and ending 4 or 5 cm inferior to the medial tibial condyle.

Incise the subcutaneous tissues, and expose the fascia lata and the anterior and medial aspects of the knee, including the pes anserinus. Next excise as much of the fascia lata from the lateral aspect of the thigh as possible and preserve it in a saline solution. Separate the vastus lateralis muscle from the lateral intermuscular septum, and expose the periosteum on the lateral aspect of the femur. Now incise the periosteum of the femur longitudinally 1 to 2 cm anterior to the lateral intermuscular septum. Incise the lateral capsule of the knee joint distally alongside the dislocated patella and the patellar tendon to the tibial tuberosity. Next elevate the periosteum and the quadriceps muscle from the lateral and anterior aspects of the femur, and rotate them medially, carrying with them the patella. If necessary for adequate rotation of the soft tissues, incise the periosteum along the anterior aspect of the knee just proximal to the distal femoral physis. Next expose the knee joint and correct any other pathologic conditions found. Make a medial parapatellar incision in the capsule to allow anatomic reduction of the patella. Next divide the patellar tendon longitudinally, detach its lateral half from the tibial tuberosity, carry this half beneath the remaining medial half, and suture it to the tibia near the insertion of the tibial collateral ligament. Now place the patella in normal position beneath the thickened medial capsule, and suture its medial border to this structure. Draw the remaining flap of medial capsule anteriorly and laterally over the patella and suture it to the lateral edge of the bone. To prevent a synovial fistula cover the defect in the lateral retinaculum between the biceps femoris and the patella with the fas-

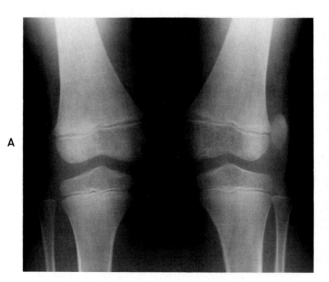
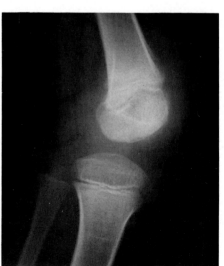

Fig. 2-63 Congenital dislocation of left patella in untreated 5-year-old boy. **A,** Anteroposterior view shows fixed lateral dislocation. **B,** On lateral view patella appears absent because of superimposed femoral condyles.

cia lata that was previously excised. Close the incision, and apply a long-leg cast with the knee flexed 5 to 10 degrees.

▶ *Postoperative management.* At 5 to 6 weeks the long-leg cast is removed, and active and passive exercises are started.

Another surgical option for the treatment of congenital dislocation of the patella is the combination of extensive lateral release with medial imbrication of the vastus medialis obliquus muscle. This procedure is similar to that used for recurrent dislocation of the patella, but it must be modified to correct more severe congenital soft tissue anomalies.

▶ *Technique.* Make a medial parapatellar incision from the distal aspect of the femur to the tibial tubercle. Perform full-thickness skin dissection over the patella to expose the medial and lateral aspects of the knee joint and the quadratus femoris muscle. Release the vastus lateralis from its most proximal muscle origin in the quadratus femoris to the level of the joint. This may require release of the iliotibial band laterally to the intermuscular septum. Occasionally the rectus femoris must be dissected and lengthened by a Z-plasty. Incise the vastus medialis obliquus from its origin proximally and distally from the patella, the medial capsule, and the patellar tendon. Reduce the patella into the femoral groove. Reattach laterally and distally the vastus medialis obliquus to the rectus femoris to secure the patella in the femoral groove. Once the initial suture is placed, move the knee through a gentle range of motion to assess reduction and tracking of the patella in the femoral groove. If the tension is too tight on the vastus medialis obliquus, remove the suture and transfer the muscle slightly proximally. If the tension is too lax, attach the vastus medialis obliquus farther distally and medially. Then suture the vastus medialis obliquus to the remaining retinaculum of the patella and the quadratus femoris. Continue the repair of the vastus medialis obliquus proximally and distally. Move the knee again through a range of motion to ensure reduction of the patella in the femoral groove and normal tracking during flexion and extension. Deflate the tourniquet, and obtain hemostasis with electrocautery. Insert a drain deep into the wound, and close the subcutaneous tissue and skin. Apply a long-leg cast with the knee in 30 degrees of flexion.

▶ *Postoperative management.* The cast is removed approximately 6 weeks after surgery, and both active and passive range of motion exercises are begun.

Hip and Pelvis

CONGENITAL AND DEVELOPMENTAL DISLOCATION OF HIP

Congenital dislocation of the hip usually includes subluxation (partial dislocation) of the femoral head, acetabular dysplasia, and complete dislocation of the femoral head from the true acetabulum. In the newborn with true congenital dislocation of the hip, the femoral head can be dislocated and reduced in and out of the true acetabulum; in the older child the femoral head remains dislocated and secondary changes in the femoral head and acetabulum develop.

The incidence of congenital dislocation of the hip is approximately 1 in 1000 births. The left hip is more commonly involved than the right, and bilateral involvement is more common than involvement of the right hip alone. Several risk factors should arouse suspicion of congenital dislocation of the hip. The disorder is more common in girls than in boys, in many series as much as five times more common. Breech deliveries comprise approximately 3% to 4% of all deliveries, and the incidence of congenital dislocation of the hip is significantly increased in this patient population. MacEwen and Ramsey in a study of 25,000 infants found the combination of female infants and breech presentation to result in congenital dislocation of the hip in 1 of 35 births. Congenital dislocation of the hip is more common in firstborn children than in subsequent siblings. A family history of congenital dislocation of the hip increases the likelihood of this condition to approximately 10%. Ethnic background plays some role in that congenital dislocation of the hip is more common in white children than in black children. Other reported examples include the high incidence among the Navajo Indians and the relatively low incidence among the Chinese. A strong association also exists between congenital dislocation of the hip and other musculoskeletal abnormalities, such as skull and facial abnormalities, congenital torticollis, metatarsus adductus, and talipes calcaneovalgus.

Several theories regarding the cause of congenital dislocation of the hip have been proposed, including mechanical factors, hormone-induced joint laxity, primary acetabular dysplasia, and genetic inheritance. Breech delivery, with the mechanical forces of abnormal flexion of the hips, easily can be seen as a cause of posterior dislocation of the femoral head.

Several authors have proposed ligamentous laxity as a contributing factor in congenital dislocation of the hip. The theory is that the influence of the maternal hormones that produce relaxation of the pelvis during delivery may cause enough ligamentous laxity in the child in utero and during the neonatal period to allow dislocation of the femoral head.

Wynne-Davies described a familial occurrence of shallow acetabulum, defined as a *dysplasia trait,* in proposing primary acetabular dysplasia as one of the risk factors for congenital dislocation of the hip. The risk of a genetic influence was noted by Ortolani, who reported a 70% incidence of a positive family history for congenital dislocation of the hip.

Diagnosis and Clinical Presentation

The clinical presentation of congenital dislocation of the hip varies according to the age of the child. In the newborn (up to 6 months) it is especially important to perform a careful clinical examination because roentgenograms are not absolutely reliable in making the diagnosis of congenital dislocation of the hip in this age-group.

Several recent reports have evaluated the use of ultrasound screening of neonates for early diagnosis of congenital dislocation of the hip. The most comprehensive accounts of the anatomy of the infant hip by ultrasound are by Graf in Austria, who has devised

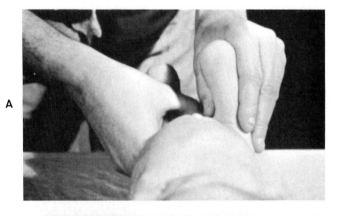

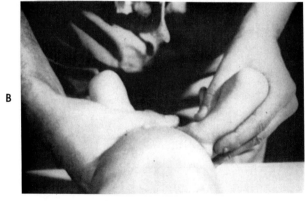

Fig. 2-64   A, Barlow and, **B,** Ortolani maneuvers for routine screening of congenital dislocation of hip. Note that examiner stabilizes infant's left hip and lower extremity and places left hand around right thigh and index and middle fingers over greater trochanter.

an ultrasonographic classification for hip dysplasias.

Routine clinical screening should include both the Ortolani test and the provocative maneuver of Barlow. The Ortolani test is performed by gently abducting and adducting the flexed hip to detect any reduction into or dislocation of the femoral head from the true acetabulum. The provocative maneuver of Barlow detects any potential subluxation or posterior dislocation of the femoral head by direct pressure on the longitudinal axis of the femur while the hip is in adduction. Both these tests require a relaxed and pacified child (Fig. 2-64). However, a child may be born with acetabular dysplasia without dislocation of the hip, and the latter may develop weeks or months later. Westin et al reported the late development of dislocation of the hip in children with normal neonatal clinical and roentgenographic examinations; they termed this *developmental dislocation* as opposed to congenital dislocation of the hip.

As the child reaches the age of 6 to 18 months, several factors in the clinical presentation change. Once the femoral head is dislocated and the ability to reduce it by abduction has disappeared, several other clinical signs become obvious. The first and most reliable is a decrease in the ability to abduct the dislocated hip because of a contracture of the adductor musculature. Asymmetric skin folds commonly are mentioned as a sign to look for, but unfortunately, this sign is not reliable in that normal children may have asymmetric skin folds, and children with a dislocated hip may have symmetric folds. The Galeazzi sign is noted when the femoral head becomes displaced not only laterally but proximally as well, causing an apparent shortening of the femur on the side of the dislocated hip. Bilateral dislocations may appear symmetrically abnormal (Fig. 2-65).

In the child of walking age with an undetected dislocated hip, families describe a "waddling" type of gait, indicating dislocation of the femoral head and a Trendelenburg gait pattern. Mothers also may describe difficulty in abducting the hip during diaper changes.

Although roentgenograms are not always reliable in making the diagnosis of congenital dislocation of the hip in the newborn, screening roentgenograms may reveal any acetabular dysplasia or teratologic dislocation. As the child with a dislocated hip ages and the soft tissues become contracted, the roentgenograms become more reliable and helpful in the diagnosis and treatment (Fig. 2-66). The most commonly used lines of reference are Perkins' vertical line and Hilgenreiner's horizontal line, both used to assess the position of the femoral head. In addition, Shenton's line will be disrupted in the older child with a dislocated hip. Reference lines for the evaluation of the acetabulum include the acetabular index and the center

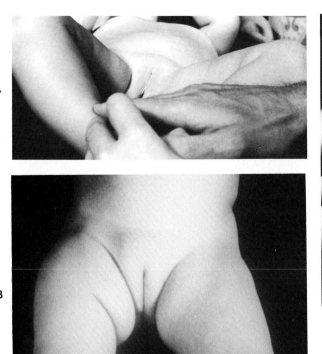

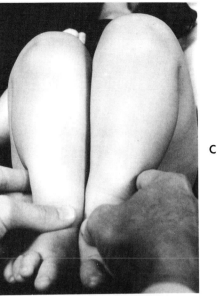

Fig. 2-65   Clinical signs of congenital dislocation of hip in 13-month-old girl. **A,** Decrease in abduction of right hip with adduction contracture. **B,** Asymmetric skin fold of right thigh. **C,** Positive Galeazzi sign with apparent shortening of right lower extremity.

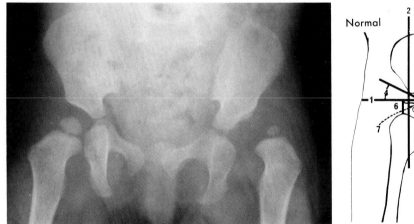

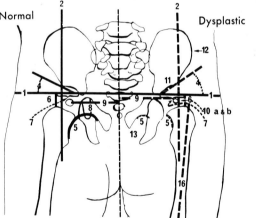

Fig. 2-66   **A,** Congenital dislocation of left hip in 13-month-old child. **B,** Roentgenographic signs of congenital hip dislocation. *1,* Horizontal Y line (Hilgenreiner's line). *2,* Vertical line (Perkins' line). *3,* Quadrants (formed by lines *1* and *2*). *4,* Acetabular index (Kleinberg and Lieberman). *5,* Shenton's line. *6,* Upward displacement of femoral head. *7,* Lateral displacement of femoral head. *8,* U figure of teardrop shadow (Kohler). *9,* Y coordinate (Ponseti). *10,* Capital epiphyseal dysplasia: *a,* delayed appearance of center of ossification of femoral head; *b,* irregular maturation of center of ossification. *11,* Bifurcation (furrowing) of acetabular roof in late infancy (Ponseti). *12,* Hypoplasia of pelvis (ilium). *13,* Delayed fusion (ischiopubic juncture). *14,* Absence of shapely, defined, well-ossified acetabular margin, caused by delayed ossification of cartilage of roof of socket. *15,* Femoral shaft-neck angle. *16,* Adduction attitude of extremity. (**B** from Hart V: Congenital dysplasia of the hip joint and sequelae, Springfield, Ill, 1952, Charles C Thomas.)

edge (CE) angle of Wiberg. Normally, the metaphyseal beak of the proximal femur will lie within the inner lower quadrant of the reference lines noted by Perkins and Hilgenreiner. The acetabular index in a newborn generally is 30 degrees or less. Any significant increase in this measurement may be a sign of acetabular dysplasia.

Treatment

The treatment of congenital dislocation of the hip is age-related and tailored to the specific pathologic condition. Five treatment groups related to age have been designated: (1) newborn, birth to 6 months of age, (2) infant, 6 to 18 months of age, (3) toddler, 18 to 36 months of age, (4) child and juvenile, 3 to 8 years of age, and (5) adolescent and young adult, beyond 8 years of age.

Newborn (Birth to 6 Months of Age)

From birth to approximately 6 months of age, treatment is directed at stabilizing the hip that has a positive Ortolani or Barlow test or reducing the dislocated hip with a mild to moderate adduction contracture. Both the Pavlik harness and von Rosen splint have been used in this age-group, but the Pavlik harness is most commonly used. A success rate of 85% to 95% has been reported in children treated in the Pavlik harness during the first few months of life. A multicenter study by Grill et al for the European Paediatric Orthopaedic Society evaluated Pavlik harness treatment of 3611 hips in 2636 patients. They reported a reduction rate of 92% overall and 95% in dysplastic hips. As the child ages and soft tissue contractures develop, along with secondary changes in the acetabulum, the success rate of the Pavlik harness decreases. Attention to detail is required in the use of this harness because the potential complications include avascular necrosis of the femoral head.

When properly applied and maintained, the Pavlik harness is a dynamic flexion, abduction orthosis that can produce excellent results in the treatment of dysplastic and dislocated hips in infants up to approximately 6 months of age. Once the diagnosis has been made, either clinically or roentgenographically, it is essential to carefully evaluate the direction of dislocation, the stability, and the reducibility of the hip before treatment. If a teratologic dislocation is present, the Pavlik harness should not be used.

The Pavlik harness consists of a chest strap, two shoulder straps, and two stirrups. Each stirrup has an anteromedial flexion strap and a posterolateral abduction strap.

The harness is applied with the child supine in a comfortable undershirt. The chest strap is fastened first, allowing enough room for a hand to be placed between the chest and the harness. The shoulder straps are buckled to maintain the chest straps at the nipple line. The feet then are placed in the stirrups one at a time. The hip is placed in flexion (90 to 110 degrees), and the anterior flexion strap is tightened to maintain this position. Finally, the lateral strap is loosely fastened to limit adduction—not to force abduction. Excessive abduction to ensure stability is not acceptable. The knees should be 3 to 5 cm apart at full adduction in the harness (Fig. 2-67).

The Barlow test should be performed within the limits of the harness to ensure adequate stability. The child then is placed in the prone position and the greater trochanters are palpated; if asymmetry is

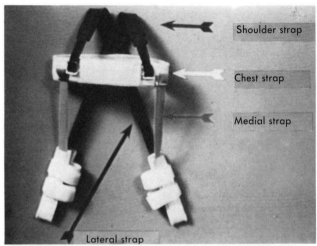

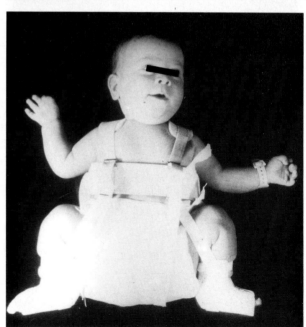

B

Fig. 2-67   A, Pavlik harness. **B,** Fitted on infant. (Courtesy Alfred I duPont Institute.)

noted, a persistent dislocation is present. A roentgenogram of the patient in the harness may be obtained to confirm that the hip has been reduced or the femoral neck is directed toward the triradiate cartilage (Fig. 2-68).

Four basic patterns of persistent dislocation have been observed after application of the Pavlik harness: superior, inferior, lateral, and posterior. If the dislocation is superior, additional flexion of the hip is indicated. If the dislocation is inferior, a decrease in flexion is indicated. A lateral dislocation in the Pavlik harness should be observed initially. As long as the femoral neck is directed toward the triradiate cartilage, the head may gradually reduce into the acetabulum. A persistent posterior dislocation is difficult to treat and usually is accompanied by tight hip adductor muscles. This type of dislocation may be diagnosed by palpation of the greater trochanter posteriorly.

If any of these patterns of dislocation or subluxation persist for more than 6 to 8 weeks, treatment in the Pavlik harness should be discontinued and a new program initiated; in most patients this consists of traction, closed or open reduction, and casting. The Pavlik harness should be worn full-time until stability is attained, as determined by negative Barlow and Ortolani test results. During this time the patient is examined every week, and the harness straps are adjusted to accommodate growth. The family is instructed in care of the child in the harness, including bathing, diapering, and dressing.

The duration of treatment depends on the patient's age at diagnosis and the degree of hip instability. For example, the duration of full-time harness wear for a patient with a dislocated hip is approximately equal to the age at which stability is attained plus 2 months. Weaning then is started by removing the harness for 2 hours each day. This time is doubled every 2 to 4 weeks until the device is worn only at night. Night bracing may be continued until the hip is roentgenographically normal. Roentgenographic documentation may be used throughout the treatment period to verify the position of the hip. Roentgenograms are useful at the following times: immediately after the initiation of treatment, after any major adjustment in the harness, 1 month after weaning begins, at 6 months of age, and at 1 year of age.

Viere et al reported that of 128 dislocations in 110 patients treated with the Pavlik harness, stable reduction was not obtained in 30 hips in 25 patients. Their statistically significant risk factors for Pavlik harness failure included absent Ortolani sign at initial evaluation (irreducible dislocations), bilateral hip dislocations, and delay of Pavlik harness treatment beyond 7 weeks of age. They concluded that failure of Pavlik harness management of congenital hip dislocation indicates a frequent need for open reduction and a more dysplastic acetabulum, which may lead to redislocation after closed reduction.

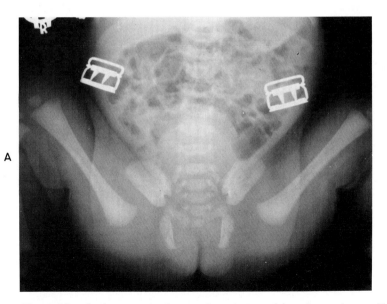
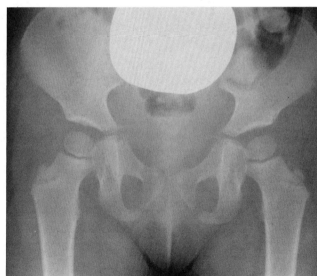

Fig. 2-68   **A,** Anteroposterior roentgenogram of female newborn with bilateral congenital dislocation of hip positioned in Pavlik harness. **B,** At 5 years of age after successful treatment.

Infant (6 to 18 Months of Age)

Once a child reaches crawling age (approximately 6 months), success with the Pavlik harness decreases significantly. The child aged 6 to 18 months with a dislocated hip will probably require either closed manipulation or open reduction.

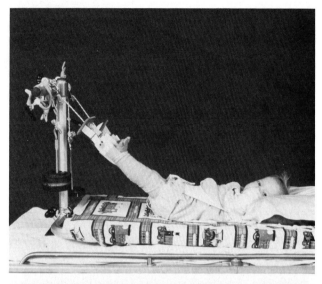

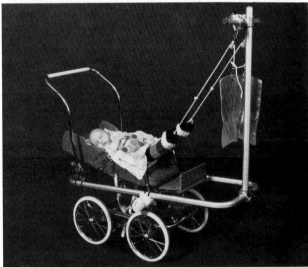

Fig. 2-69 Home skin traction program for 14-month-old girl. (Courtesy Alfred I duPont Institute.)

Children in this age-group often are seen initially with a shortened extremity, limited passive abduction, and a positive Galeazzi sign. If the child is walking, a Trendelenburg gait will be present. Roentgenographic changes include delayed ossification of the femoral head, lateral and proximal displacement of the femoral head, and a shallow acetabulum.

With persistent dysplasia, the femoral head eventually moves superiorly and laterally with weight bearing. The capsule becomes permanently elongated, and anteriorly the psoas tendon may obstruct reduction of the femoral head into the true acetabulum. The acetabular limbus may fold and invert into the acetabulum, and the ligamentum teres hypertrophies and elongates. The femoral head becomes reduced in size with a posteromedial flattening, and coxa valga and excessive anteversion are noted. The true acetabulum is characteristically shallow and at surgery appears small because of the anterior capsular constriction and the inverted limbus.

Treatment in this age-group should follow a detailed regimen, which includes adequate preoperative traction, adductor tenotomy, closed reduction and arthrogram, or open reduction in children with a failed closed reduction. Adequate preoperative traction, adductor tenotomy, and gentle reduction are especially helpful in the prevention of avascular necrosis of the femoral head.

Preoperative traction. In children with compliant and educated parents the use of a home skin traction program spares the expense of hospitalization and allows the child to stay in traction in a home environment (Fig. 2-69). Skeletal traction in the hospital is used if home traction is impossible. The objectives of traction are to bring the laterally and proximally displaced femoral head down to and below the level of the true acetabulum to permit a more gentle reduction.

Adductor tenotomy. A percutaneous adductor tenotomy under sterile conditions may be performed for a mild adduction contracture. For an adduction contracture of long duration, an open adductor tenotomy through a small transverse incision is preferable.

CLOSED REDUCTION

Gentle closed reduction is accomplished with the child under general anesthesia.

The interposition of soft tissue in the acetabulum may be suggested by lateralization of the femoral head. Because the roentgenogram of the hip in an infant or young child cannot yield all the information desired in diagnosing or treating congenital dysplasia, arthrography often is helpful in determining (1) whether mild dysplasia is present, (2) whether the femoral head is subluxated or dislocated, (3) whether manipulative reduction has been or can be successful, (4) to what extent any soft structures within the acetabulum may interfere with complete reduction of the dislocation, (5) what is the condition and position of the acetabular labrum (the limbus), and (6) whether the acetabulum and femoral head are developing normally. Because arthrograms are not always easy to interpret, the surgeon must be thoroughly familiar with the normal and abnormal signs they may reveal and with the technique of making arthrograms (Fig. 2-70).

An arthrogram of the hip should be made in all children, regardless of age, who are given a general anesthetic for closed reduction. It is most helpful when manipulative reduction is unstable or when the femoral head is not concentrically seated within the acetabulum. Race and Herring emphasized the importance of confirming reduction by arthrography in 59 hips treated with closed reduction. Their results confirm that the most important factor that determines outcome of closed treatment of congenital hip dislocation is the quality of the initial reduction. In hips with good or adequate reduction, 94% had good or acceptable results. Conversely, in those hips with poor reductions and those in which the quality of reduction could not be determined, only 21% had acceptable results. They also noted that as the quality of reduction declined, treatment time increased. Their criteria for accepting a reduction are a medial dye pool of 7 mm or less and maintenance of reduction in an acceptable "safe zone."

The use of image intensification makes placement of the needle much easier. The danger of damaging the articular surfaces by the needle is decreased, and the possibility of injecting the contrast medium directly into the ossific nucleus or the physis is prevented. When such equipment is not available, brief but careful use of an ordinary fluoroscope can aid in centering the needle properly.

The findings of the clinical examination and of arthrography at the time of attempted closed reduction determine if the hip will be stable or may require open reduction.

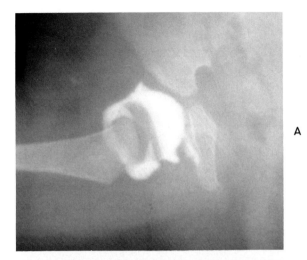
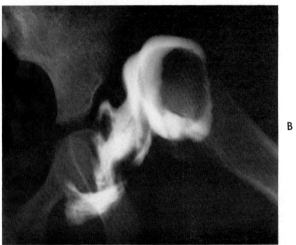
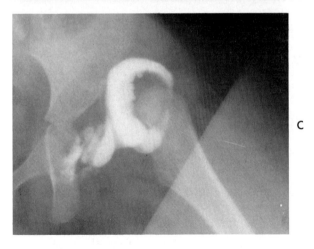

Fig. 2-70 Arthrography in evaluation of congenital dislocation of hip. **A,** Normal hip at necropsy. Note positive "thorn" sign outlining normal labrum, cartilaginous anlage of normal acetabulum, and small amount of dye pooling medially. **B,** Dislocated left hip shows inverted, hypertrophied labrum and obstructed reduction with large pool of dye medially. **C,** Nonconcentric closed reduction with hourglass capsular constricture preventing reduction.

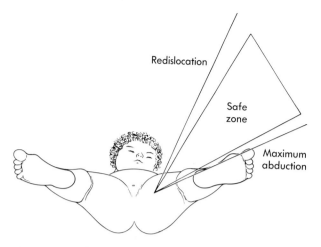

Fig. 2-71 "Safe zone" used to determine acceptability of closed reduction of congenital dislocation of hip.

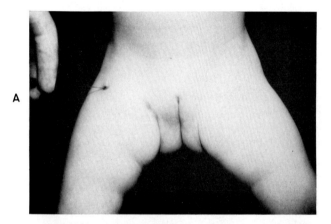

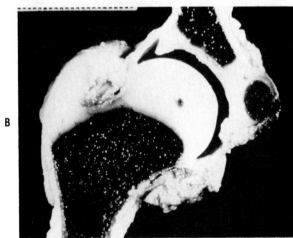

Fig. 2-72 **A,** Insertion of 22-gauge spinal needle one fingerbreadth lateral to femoral artery and immediately inferior to anterosuperior iliac spine for arthrography. **B,** In necropsy specimen, areas of hip in which dye may be easily injected: beneath acetabular labrum, in medial or lateral capsular pouch, and at junction of ossified and cartilaginous portion of femoral head. (Courtesy Dr. John Ogden.)

Clinical findings that usually result in an acceptable closed reduction include the sensation of a "clunk" as the femoral head reduces in the true acetabulum. The "safe zone" concept of Ramsey et al can be used in determining the zone of abduction and adduction in which the femoral head remains reduced in the acetabulum. A wide safe zone (minimum of 20 degrees, preferably 45 degrees) (Fig. 2-71) is desirable, and a narrow safe zone implies an unstable or unacceptable closed reduction. A careful clinical evaluation of the reduction should be made before an arthrogram, because once the hip capsule is distended with dye, clinical examination becomes difficult.

Arthrography permits analysis of the cartilaginous anlage of the femoral head and acetabulum. Roentgenographic factors that help determine the success or failure of closed reduction include the amount of dye pooling in the medial joint space, inversion of the acetabular limbus, or an "hourglass" constriction obstructing reduction.

▶ *Technique.* Place the child supine after general anesthesia has been administered. Then perform sterile preparation and draping of the hip or hips. With a gloved fingertip locate the hip joint immediately inferior to the middle of the inguinal ligament and one fingerbreadth lateral to the pulsating femoral artery (Fig. 2-72). As an alternative, the needle may be inserted medially anterior to the adductor musculature. With the assistance of image intensification insert a 22-gauge needle, to which is attached a 5-ml syringe filled with normal saline solution, until it enters the hip joint; resistance will be met as the needle passes through the joint capsule. Then inject the saline solution into the joint; this is easy at first but becomes more difficult as the joint becomes distended. Release the plunger of the syringe; if the joint has been successfully entered, the saline solution that is under pressure in it will reverse the plunger and fluid will escape into the syringe. Then aspirate the saline solution from the joint and remove the syringe from the needle. Next fill the syringe with 5 ml of a 25% strength Hypaque solution and inject 3.5 to 5 ml through the needle into the joint with image intensification. Then rapidly withdraw the needle, and while the hip is still unreduced, have an arthrogram made. Before it is developed, gently reduce the hip into a stable position and have a second arthrogram made. Maintain reduction until both arthrograms have been developed and studied.

When arthrograms are to be made of both hips, insert a needle into each, being sure that both are within the joints before either joint is injected. Then inject both hips as described here, and make arthrograms of both on the same cassette.

Application of hip spica. After confirmation of a stable reduction, a hip spica cast is applied. The desired position of the hip joint is 95 degrees of flexion and 40 to 45 degrees of abduction. Studies have indicated that the "human position" is best for maintaining hip stability and minimizing the risk of avascular necrosis. Kumar has described an easily reproducible and simple technique for applying a hip spica cast. Fiberglass may be used in place of plaster, but the technique is described in its original form.

▲ *Technique (Kumar).* Place the anesthesized child on the spica frame. Abduct the hip to 40 to 45 degrees, and flex it to about 95 degrees (Fig. 2-73, *A*). The amount of hip flexion and abduction required to keep the hip in the most stable position should be determined clinically and checked by roentgenograms.

After the correct position of flexion and abduction for stability is determined, place a small towel in front of the abdomen. Then roll 2-inch (5 cm) Webril from the level of the nipples down to the ankles (Fig. 2-73, *B*). Pad around the bony points with 2-inch (5 cm) standard felt. Apply the first pad over the proximal end of the spica, near the nipple line (Fig. 2-73, *C*). Start a second piece of the same sized felt at the level of the right groin, and carry it posteriorly across the gluteal fold, over the right iliac crest, in front of the abdomen, over the lateral aspect of the left thigh, and then to the left inguinal area (Fig. 2-73, *C*). Apply a third piece of felt over the knee (Fig. 2-73, *D*) and a fourth piece above the ankle over the distal leg (Fig. 2-73, *D*). Place similar pieces of felt over the opposite knee and leg.

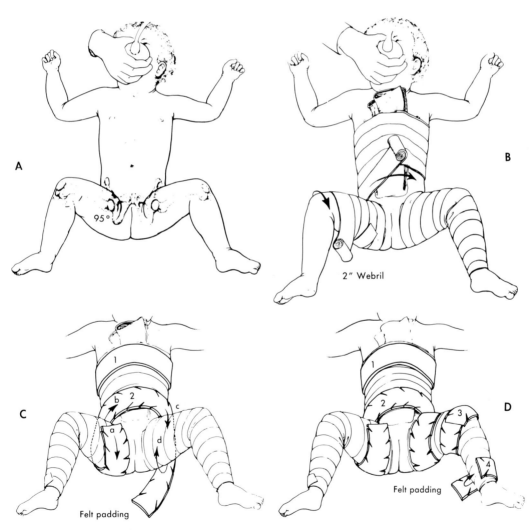

Fig. 2-73 Technique of application of spica cast for congenital dislocation of hip. Note positioning of patient in "human" position (see text). (From Kumar SJ: J Pediatr Orthop 1:97, 1981.)

Apply the plaster in two sections: a proximal section from the nipple line to the knees and a distal section from the knees to the ankles. Apply a single layer of 4-inch (10 cm) plaster roll from the nipple line to the level of the knees on both sides. Apply four or five plaster splints back to front from the nipple line to the back of the sacrum to reinforce the back of the cast. At the same time apply a short, thick splint over the anterolateral aspect of the inguinal area (Fig. 2-73, *E*). Apply another splint: starting from the right inguinal area, carry it posteriorly across the gluteal region, the iliac crest, the front of the abdomen, and back the same way on the opposite thigh (Fig. 2-73, *E*). This is a reinforcing splint that attaches the thigh to the upper segment. Apply another long splint from the level of the knee across the anterolateral aspect of the inguinal area and up the chest wall (Fig. 2-73, *F*). This splint is one of the main anchors of the thigh to the body segment. Follow this by a roll of 4-inch (10 cm) plaster from the nipple line to the knees. This completes the proximal section of the spica.

Then complete the cast from the knees down to the ankles. Do this by applying on both sides a single roll of 3-inch (7.5 cm) plaster from the knee to the ankle level, and reinforce this by two splints over the medial and lateral aspects of the thigh, knee, and leg. Follow this by another roll of 3 inch (7.5 cm) plaster. Then apply shoulder straps to prevent pistoning of the child in the cast (Fig. 2-73, *G*).

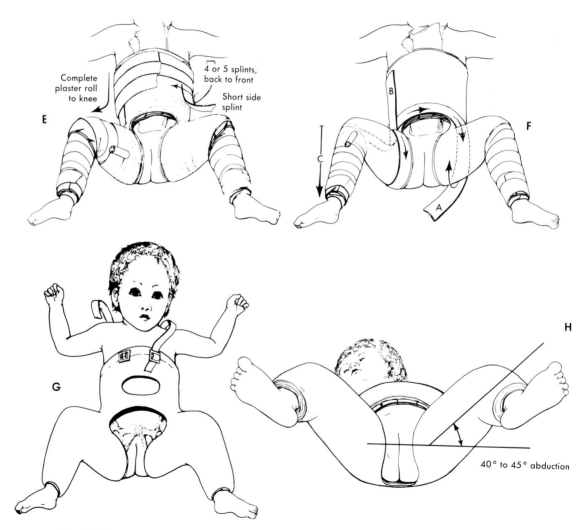

Fig. 2-73, cont'd   Technique of application of spica cast for congenital dislocation of hip.

Since the cast is reinforced laterally around the hips, a wide segment can be removed from the front of the hips without weakening the cast. This permits easier care of the child and better roentgenograms of the hips (Fig. 2-73, *G*).

The final view of the spica from an inferior aspect should appear as shown in Fig. 2-73, *H,* with about 40 to 45 degrees of abduction. The amount of abduction is determined by the position of hip stability. Once again it is emphasized that excessive abduction should be avoided.

◤*Postoperative management.* Spica cast immobilization is continued for 4 months. The cast is changed with the patient under general anesthesia at 2 months. Roentgenograms or arthrograms are indicated to be sure that the femoral head is reduced anatomically into the acetabulum. Clinical and roentgenographic follow-up is essential until the hip is considered normal. CT is useful in the postoperative assessment of reduction. In contrast to routine roentgenography the presence of a cast does not alter the image of the CT scan (Fig. 2-74).

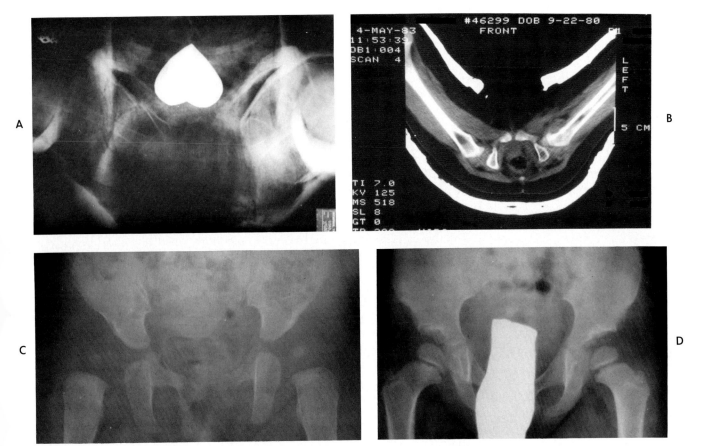

Fig. 2-74 **A,** Anteroposterior roentgenogram of pelvis obtained with patient in spica cast after closed reduction. Note difficulty in assessing position of femoral head. **B,** CT scan of pelvis to document reduction of femoral head into true acetabulum. **C,** Bilateral dislocated hips in 6-month-old child before closed reduction. **D,** At age 6 years, normal development of femoral head and acetabulum.

OPEN REDUCTION

In a child younger than 18 months of age in whom efforts to reduce a dislocation without force have failed, open reduction is indicated to "correct" the offending soft tissue structures and to reduce the femoral head concentrically in the acetabulum. Open reduction may be performed through an anterior, an anteromedial, or a medial approach; the choice depends on the experience of the surgeon and the particular dislocation. The anterior approach (Somerville) requires more anatomic dissection but provides greater versatility because the pathologic condition in the anterior and lateral aspects is easily reached and pelvic osteotomy may be performed through this approach if necessary. The infero medial aspect of the acetabulum is not easily seen through this approach. The anteromedial approach described by Weinstein and Ponseti actually is an anterior approach to the hip through an anteromedial incision. The hip is approached in the interval between the pectineus muscle and the femoral neurovascular bundle. Weinstein and Ponseti recommend this approach for children up to the age of 24 months, but it should be done by an experienced pediatric hip surgeon. Access to the lateral structures for dissection or osteotomy is not possible with this approach. The medial (Ludloff) approach, although it is simpler and involves less dissection, places the medial circumflex vessels at a higher risk and has been reported to be associated with a higher incidence of avascular necrosis.

▲ *Technique of anterior open reduction.* Make an anterior bikini incision from the midaspect of the iliac crest to a point midway between the anterosuperior iliac spine and the midline of the pelvis. The anterosuperior iliac crest should be at the midpoint of the incision, which may be placed 1 cm below the iliac crest (Fig. 2-75, *A*). Carry sharp dissection through the subcutaneous tissue to the deep fascia. Identify and enter the interval between the sartorius and tensor fasciae latae muscles. Take care to protect the lateral femoral cutaneous nerve by retraction with a Penrose drain during the entire procedure. Detach the iliac apophysis from the ilium, beginning at the anterosuperior iliac spine and extending 4 cm posteriorly along the ilium. Subperiosteally dissect the tensor fasciae latae laterally to expose the ilium and the full extent of the anterolateral capsule. Identify the origin of the sartorius muscle at the anterosuperior iliac crest, divide it, and allow it to retract distally. Now dissect the tensor fasciae latae origin to the anteroinferior iliac spine. Place a retractor along the medial aspect of the anteroinferior spine onto the superior pubic ramus. Identify the psoas tendon in its groove on the superior pubic ramus, and perform a tenotomy to facilitate placement of a right angle retractor in the groove on the superior pubic ramus in the normal groove for the iliopsoas tendon. This retractor will protect the psoas muscle and neurovascular bundle anteriorly. Identify the origins of both the direct and oblique heads of the rectus femoris muscle, and perform a tenotomy approximately 1 cm distal to the anteroinferior iliac spine (Fig. 2-75, *B*). Tag the distal segment, and allow the tendon to retract distally.

Identify the capsule of the hip joint anteriorly, medially, and laterally. Usually there is a large amount of redundant capsule laterally in the region of the false acetabulum. Make a T-shaped incision from the most medial aspect of the capsule to the most lateral, and continue the incision along the anterior border of the head and neck of the femur (Fig. 2-75, *C*). For more exposure, use Kocher clamps to retract the capsule. Identify the femoral head and the ligamentum teres; detach the ligamentum teres from the femoral head and place on it a Kocher clamp. Trace the ligamentum teres to the true acetabulum, and excise with a rongeur or sharp dissection any pulvinar in the true acetabulum (Fig. 2-75, *D*). Gently expose the bony articular surface of the acetabulum with its circumferential cartilage. If an inverted, hypertrophied labrum is present, make several radial, T-shaped incisions laterally and superiorly to facilitate enlargement of the true acetabulum (Fig. 2-75, *E*). Expose the acetabulum laterally, superiorly, medially, and inferiorly to the level of the deep transverse acetabular ligament, which can be divided to enlarge the inferiormost aspect of the acetabulum. Enlarge the entrance to the acetabulum with sequential incisions in the labrum or excision of the fat from the innermost aspect of the acetabulum until the entrance is large enough to allow reduction of the femoral head without difficulty. After reducing the femoral head into the acetabulum, move the hip through a complete range of motion, including flexion, extension, adduction, and abduction, to determine the "safe zone" of reduction. If the reduction is concentric and stable, reduce the femoral head and close the capsule, suturing the lateral flap of the T-shaped incision as far medially as possible to eliminate any redundant capsule in the region of the false acetabulum. An adequate capsulorrhaphy will significantly enhance stability of the hip when weight bearing is resumed. Place sutures in the tips of the "T" and along the superior border of the acetabulum. When capsulorrhaphy is completed, suture the rectus femoris tendon to its origin, the sartorius to its origin, and the iliac apophysis to the fascia of the tensor fasciae latae along the iliac crest. Close the superficial fascial layers, the subcutaneous tissues, and the skin. Apply a double spica cast with the hips in 90 to 100 degrees of flexion and 40 to 55 degrees of abduction.

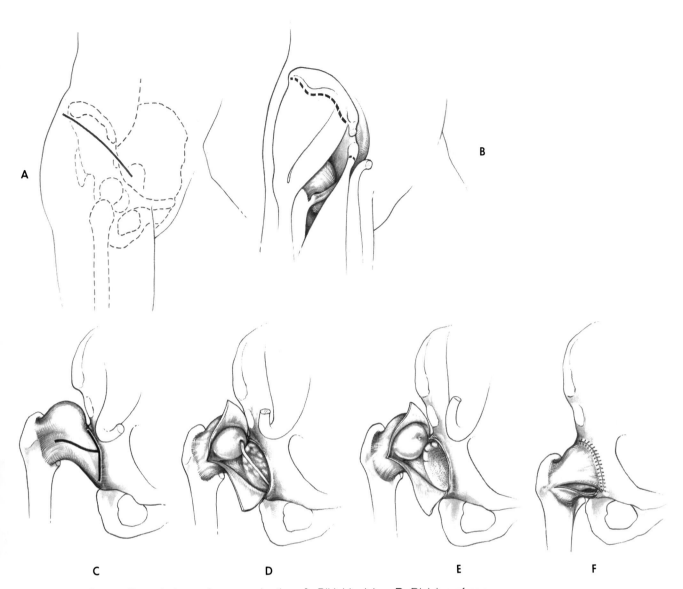

Fig. 2-75 Somerville technique of open reduction. **A,** Bikini incision. **B,** Division of sartorius and rectus femoris tendons and iliac apophysis. **C,** T-shaped incision of capsule. **D,** Capsulotomy of hip and use of ligamentum teres to find true acetabulum. **E,** Radial incisions in acetabular labrum and removal of all tissue from depth of true acetabulum. **F,** Capsulorrhaphy after excision of redundant capsule.

▲ *Postoperative management.* Roentgenograms or CT scans may be used to confirm reduction of the femoral head in the acetabulum. The spica cast is removed 10 to 12 weeks after surgery. Sequential roentgenograms are used to assess the development of the femoral head and acetabulum.

▸ *Technique of open reduction by anteromedial approach (Weinstein and Ponseti).* With the patient supine, prepare and drape the affected extremity and hemipelvis free to allow full motion of the hip and knee. With the hip flexed to 70 degrees in unforced abduction, identify the neurovascular bundle and the superior and inferior borders of the adductor longus muscle. Make an incision from the inferior border of the adductor longus to just inferior to the femoral neurovascular bundle in the groin crease. Incise the skin and subcutaneous tissues down to the deep fascia, and incise the fascia over the adductor longus in the direction of the muscle fibers. Isolate the adductor longus, section it at its origin, and allow it to retract. Follow the anterior branch of the obturator nerve proximally to its entrance into the thigh under the pectineus muscle. Gently retract the neurovascular bundle superiorly. Keep the anterior branch of the obturator nerve in sight, open the sheath overlying the pectineus muscle, and identify its superior and inferior borders. Identify and bluntly dissect the interval between the pectineus muscle and the femoral neurovascular bundle. Isolate the iliopsoas tendon in the inferior aspect of the wound, section it sharply, and allow it to retract. With gentle retraction of the femoral neurovascular bundle superiorly and the pectineus muscle inferiorly, isolate the hip joint capsule by blunt dissection. Make a small incision in the anteromedial capsule parallel to the anterior acetabular margin. Grasp the ligamentum teres with a Graham hook and bring it into the wound. Extend the capsular incision along the ligamentum teres to its insertion on the femoral head. Rotate the leg to bring this attachment into view. If the ligamentum teres is hypertrophied or elongated, excise it to facilitate reduction. Grasp the stump of the ligamentum teres with a Kocher clamp, and identify the interval between the ligament and the anteroinferomedial aspect of the joint capsule; mark this interval with a pair of scissors. Retract the pectineus muscle, and sharply incise the anteromedial margin of the capsule. Section the ligamentum teres at its base along with the transverse acetabular ligament to open up the "horseshoe" of the acetabulum and increase its diameter. Remove all pulvinar with a pituitary rongeur. Now reduce the femoral head into the acetabulum, and move the hip through a range of motion to assess stability of the reduction. Irrigate the wound copiously, leave the joint capsule open, and approximate the deep fascia with running absorbable sutures. Close the subcutaneous tissues and skin with absorbable sutures. Apply a 1½ spica cast with the hip in a position of maximum stability (Fig. 2-76).

▸ *Postoperative management.* The cast is worn for 10 to 12 weeks. If roentgenograms show satisfactory position of the hip 4 to 6 weeks after surgery, the portion of the cast below the knee is removed to allow knee motion and some hip rotation. After total cast removal, an abduction brace is worn full-time for 4 to 8 weeks, then at night and during naps for 1 to 2 years, until normal acetabular development is evident.

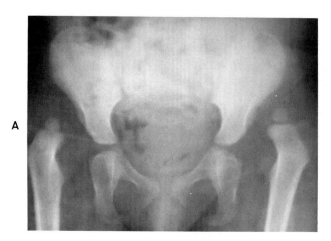
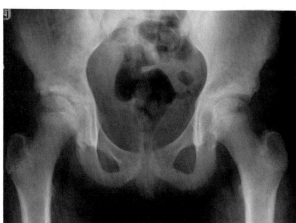

Fig. 2-76   A, Anteromedial open reduction of bilateral congenital dislocation of hip in 32-month-old female. **B,** At age 12 years, normal development of femoral head and acetabulum bilaterally. (Courtesy Dr. Stuart Weinstein.)

▲ *Technique by medial approach (Ferguson)*. Preliminary traction in an infant younger than 2 years old is not necessary. Place the patient supine with the affected hip abducted and flexed 90 degrees. Make a straight incision along the posterior margin of the adductor longus muscle beginning at its origin and extending distally. Incise the deep fascia in line with the skin incision, and by blunt dissection with the finger separate the adductor longus anteriorly from the adductor magnus and gracilis muscles posteriorly. Extend the dissection posterior to the adductor brevis muscle, and palpate the lesser trochanter. Next push the pericapsular fat medially so that the psoas tendon can be seen. With a curved hemostat isolate this tendon and divide it transversely. As the tendon retracts superiorly, push the fat from the anterior capsule of the hip joint. This exposes an hourglass constriction of the capsule that has been formed by the taut psoas tendon. Now pass a retractor over the capsule superior to the femoral head. Incise the capsule in line with the femoral neck, and extend the incision anteriorly as far as necessary to permit the femoral head to enter the acetabulum with ease. After the dislocation has been reduced, the capsular incision spreads and cannot be closed. Suturing the adductors is unnecessary. Close the skin in a routine manner.

▲ *Postoperative management.* A spica cast is applied with both hips in 10 degrees of flexion, 30 degrees of abduction, and 10 to 20 degrees of internal rotation. The cast is molded posterior to the affected hip to press anteriorly on the greater trochanter, thus preventing redislocation. A spica cast with the hips in this position is worn for 4 months after surgery.

Special Problems

Teratologic dislocations. A teratologic dislocation of the hip is one that occurs sometime before birth, resulting in significant anatomic distortion and resistance to treatment. Teratologic dislocations also are called *antenatal, prenatal,* and *atypical.* They often occur with other conditions such as arthrogryposis, Larsen syndrome, myelomeningocele, and diastrophic dwarfism. The anatomic changes are much more advanced than those in a typical congenital hip dislocation in a child of the same age. The acetabulum is small, with an oblique or flattened roof, the ligamentum teres is thickened, and the femoral head is of variable size and may be flattened on the medial side (Fig. 2-77). The hip joint is stiff and irreducible, and roentgenograms show superolateral displacement. Most authors agree that closed reduction is not effective and that open reduction is necessary, but indications for treatment are not clear. Most agree that unilateral dislocations should be treated more aggressively than bilateral. Gruel et al list the ambulatory potential of the patient as the most important consideration in deciding whether to treat bilateral dislocations. The difficulty of treating teratologic dislocations is reflected in their results: of the 27 hips in their series 44% had poor results and 70% had complications. Avascular necrosis occurred in 48% of hips, redislocation in 19%, and subluxation in 22%. Anterior open reduction and femoral shortening produced the best results with the fewest complications, whereas the worst results and most complications occurred in those hips treated by closed reduction. Although multiple procedures may be required, regardless of the procedure chosen, good results can be obtained and a stable hip usually can be achieved in properly selected patients.

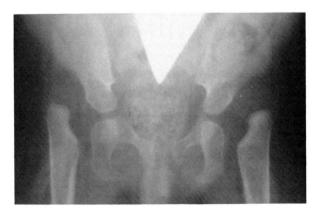

Fig. 2-77 Bilateral teratologic dislocation of hip in 3-month-old female infant with arthrogryposis.

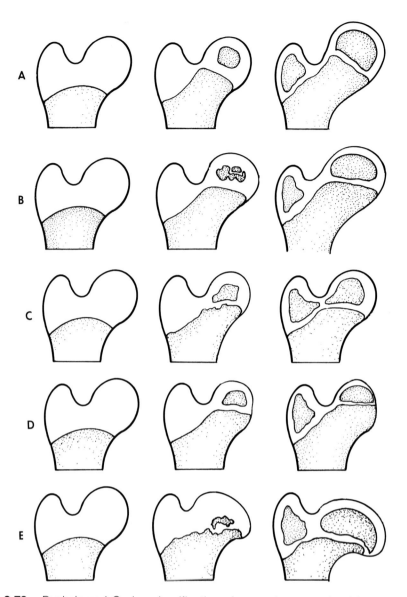

Fig. 2-78 Bucholz and Ogden classification of avascular necrosis of femoral head in congenital dislocation of hip. **A,** Normal femoral head at 2 months, 1 year, and 9 years of age. **B,** Type I: *a,* sites of temporary vascular occlusion; *b,* irregular ossification in secondary center; *c,* normal physeal contour, slight decrease in height of capital femoral ossification center. **C,** Type II: *a,* probable primary site of vascular occlusion; *b,* metaphyseal and epiphyseal irregularities; *c,* premature fusion of lateral metaphysis and epiphysis. **D,** Type III: *a,* sites of temporary vascular occlusion; *b,* impaired longitudinal growth of capital femoral epiphysis; *c,* irregularly shaped femoral head. **E,** Type IV: *a,* sites of temporary vascular occlusion; *b,* impaired longitudinal and latitudinal growth, *c,* premature epiphyseal closure. (Redrawn from Bucholz RW and Ogden JA. In The hip, St Louis, 1978, The CV Mosby Co.)

Avascular necrosis. The most serious complication associated with the treatment of congenital dislocation of the hip in early infancy is the development of avascular necrosis. Potential sequelae of avascular necrosis include femoral head deformity, acetabular dysplasia, lateral subluxation of the femoral head, relative overgrowth of the greater trochanter, and limb-length inequalities; osteoarthritis is a common late complication. Bucholz and Ogden, as well as Kalamchi and MacEwen, have proposed classification systems based on morphologic changes in the capital femoral epiphysis, the physis, and the proximal femoral metaphysis (Fig. 2-78). These classifications are useful in determining proper treatment and prognosis for a particular patient, and the proper classification should be identifiable on roentgenograms within 2 years of treatment of the congenitally dislocated hip. Treatment should be directed toward the clinical problems associated with each roentgenographic classification group. A large percentage of patients will not require any treatment during adolescence and young adulthood. In a small percentage of patients, femoral head deformity and acetabular dysplasia predisposing the hip joint to incongruity and persistent subluxation can be treated with either femoral osteotomy or appropriate acetabuloplasty, or both. Children with avascular necrosis after treatment of congenital dislocation of the hip should be observed to maturity with serial orthoroentgenograms. Significant limb-length inequality can be corrected by appropriate techniques. Symptomatic overgrowth of the greater trochanter can be treated in older patients with greater trochanteric advancement, which will increase the abductor muscle resting length and increase the abductor lever arm (Fig. 2-79).

▲ ***Technique of trochanteric advancement (Lloyd-Roberts and Swann).*** Approach the trochanter through a long lateral incision. Place a Gigli saw deep to the gluteus medius and minimus muscles, and divide the trochanter at its base. Then mobilize the glutei anteriorly and posteriorly as they are dissected off the joint capsule and strip them for a short distance from the ilium above. Displace the detached trochanter with its attached muscles distally to the lateral cortex of the femur while the hip is abducted. Bevel the femoral cortex to help reduce tension and improve placement of the trochanter. Secure the trochanter to the femur with screws, and suture the femoral periosteum and vastus lateralis muscle. The top of the greater trochanter now should be positioned at the level of the center of the femoral head on anteroposterior roentgenogram. The trochanter usually requires advancement anteriorly as well as distally.

▲ ***Postoperative management.*** The hip is protected by a spica cast in abduction for 6 to 8 weeks.

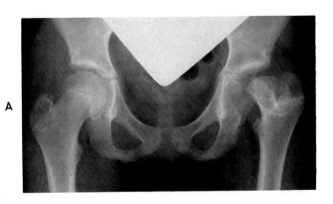
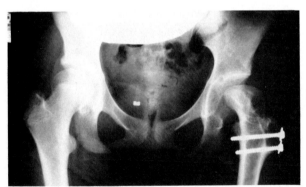

Fig. 2-79   **A,** Avascular necrosis of left femoral head and apparent trochanteric overgrowth in 10-year-old girl after treatment of congenital dislocation of hip. **B,** After transfer of greater trochanter distally and anteriorly.

Toddler (18 to 36 Months of Age)

Because of widespread screening of newborns, it is becoming uncommon for congenital dislocation of the hip to be undetected beyond the age of 1 year. The older child with this condition has a wide perineum, shortened lower extremity, and hyperlordosis of the lower spine as a result of femoropelvic instability. For these children with well-established hip dysplasia, open reduction with femoral or pelvic osteotomy, or both, often is required. Persistent dysplasia can be corrected by a redirectional proximal femoral osteotomy. If the primary dysplasia is acetabular, pelvic redirectional osteotomy alone is more appropriate. Some patients, however, will require both femoral and pelvic osteotomies if significant deformity is present on both sides of the joint.

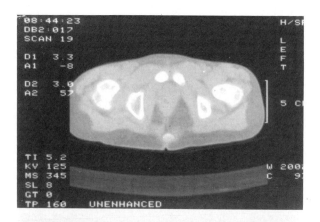

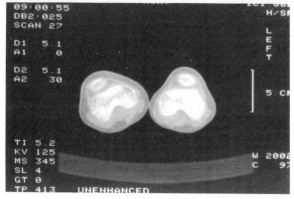

Fig. 2-80   CT for assessment of femoral anteversion. Note scan of right and left hips to determine anatomic angles through femoral necks and intertrochanteric regions, as well as transverse plane of femoral condyles.

Femoral osteotomy in dysplasia of hip. Most surgeons who recommend femoral osteotomies advise an operation on the pelvic side of the joint only after the femoral head has been concentrically seated in the dysplastic acetabulum by such an osteotomy, the joint has failed to develop satisfactorily, and the growth potential of the acetabulum no longer exists. Opinions differ widely as to the age at which the acetabulum loses its ability to develop satisfactorily over a femoral head concentrically located; Kasser et al reported consistently good results in patients younger than 4 years old at the time of femoral osteotomy. Remodeling of the acetabulum occurred through the age of 8 years, but 4 of 13 hips in patients between the ages of 4 and 8 years showed persistent dysplasia despite the operation. The results were less predictable as the patients approached the age of 8 years. No benefit was derived from femoral osteotomy alone in 10 of 11 hips in patients older than 8 years of age.

The degree of femoral anteversion and the amount of derotation to be performed surgically traditionally have been measured by the method described by Magilligan in 1956 by means of anteroposterior and lateral roentgenographic views. More recently, CT scanning has been shown to give a more accurate assessment of femoral anteversion without the use of special leg-holding devices or computation tables. Only three scanning slices are necessary if localized precisely through the superior, middle, and inferior regions of the acetabulum. The angle of femoral neck anteversion can be measured directly if the orientation of the knee is known. If precise determination of anteversion is desired, a fourth slice through the patellae and femoral condyles is made, with care taken not to let the legs rotate between exposures. By the construction of a line through the femoral head and neck and another through the transcondylar plane of the distal portion of the femur, the exact angle of anteversion can be obtained (Fig. 2-80).

▶ *Technique (varus derotational osteotomy of the femur in hip dysplasia, with Campbell screw fixation).* Place the patient supine on the operating table, with a roentgen cassette holder beneath the patient. Image intensification in the anteroposterior projection is desirable. Prepare and drape the affected extremity, leaving the unaffected leg draped free to allow for intraoperative roentgenograms or imaging.

Make a lateral incision from the greater trochanter distally 8 to 12 cm, incise the iliotibial band, and reflect the vastus lateralis muscle to expose the lateral aspect of the femur. Make a transverse line in the femoral cortex with an osteotome to mark the level of the osteotomy at the level of the lesser trochanter or slightly distal. Correct positioning of the osteotomy may be verified with image intensification. Now make a longitudinal orientation line in the femoral cortex to determine correct rotation; position this line so that it can be seen through the plate holes or around the plate. Position the plate on the femur with the osteotomy site located between the hexagonal opening and the first screw hole to determine the site of guide pin insertion, or use an angle guide in the standard manner. Insert the guide pin into the midline of the femoral neck, taking care not to penetrate the proximal femoral physis. Confirm correct guide pin position at the level of or slightly proximal to the lesser trochanter with roentgenograms or image intensification on both anteroposterior and lateral views.

Measure the proper length of the guide wire to determine the needed screw length, and with a cortical reamer, ream the outer cortex over the guide wire for approximately 0.5 inch, taking care not to extend the reaming into the underlying cancellous bone. Place the tap over the guide wire, and tap the appropriate length for ease of insertion of the screw into the femoral neck; it is not necessary to tap the entire length of the screw. Before the osteotomy cut is made, insert the proper sized screw into the femoral neck with the use of the inserter/extractor wrench. One apex of the hex screw should be parallel to the shaft of the femur. Now make the osteotomy cut at the transverse line in the cortex in a transverse or oblique direction, depending on the correction desired. If rotational, in addition to angular, correction is desired, complete the osteotomy through the medial cortex. Using the longitudinal mark in the femoral cortex as a guide, rotate the femur as needed to correct femoral anteversion (generally 15 to 30 degrees). Because the deformity is more rotational than angulatory, evaluate the position of the femur with roentgenograms or image intensification before continuing with varus correction. To achieve varus angulation, remove an appropriate wedge of bone from the medial cortex to achieve a neck-shaft angle of 120 to 135 degrees.

Now attach the side plate to the base of the screw. When properly aligned with the hex head of the screw, the side plate should fit flush to the proximal femoral shaft. If not, adjust it slightly with a bending instrument or use a plate with a different angle. Secure the side plate with the screw, using either the T-holder or securing bolt. Insert the securing bolt through the hexagonal hole in the side plate and into the hex head of the screw. Tighten it completely to firmly join the proximal and distal fragments. Secure the plate to the femoral shaft with a bone clamp if desired. Confirm the position of the fixation device and the proximal and distal fragments with anteropos-

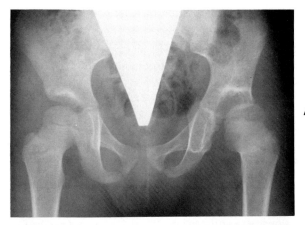

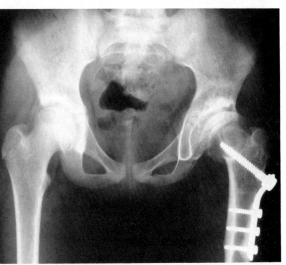

Fig. 2-81   Femoral varus derotational osteotomy in congenital dislocation of hip. **A,** Four-year-old girl with residual acetabular dysplasia and subluxation of left hip after closed reduction at 12 months of age. **B,** Six years after femoral varus derotational osteotomy fixed with Campbell hip screw.

rior roentgenogram or image intensification. Then firmly fix the side plate to the femoral shaft with 4.5-mm bone screws and a hex-head screwdriver. Irrigate the wound and close in layers, inserting a suction drain if needed. Apply a 1½ spica cast.

▶ *Postoperative management.* The spica cast is worn for 8 to 12 weeks, until union of the osteotomy. The internal fixation may be removed 12 to 24 months after surgery if desired (Fig. 2-81).

Juvenile (3 to 8 Years of Age)

The management of untreated congenital dislocation of the hip in the child older than 3 years of age is difficult. By this age adaptive shortening of the periarticular structures and structural alterations in both the femoral head and the acetabulum have occurred. Most dislocated hips in this age-group require open reduction. Preoperative skeletal traction should not be used. Schoenecker and Strecker reported a 54% incidence of avascular necrosis and a 31% incidence of redislocation after the use of skeletal traction in patients older than 3 years. Open reduction combined with femoral shortening resulted in no avascular necrosis and only an 8% incidence of redislocation. Coleman reported an 8% incidence of avascular necrosis in his series of femoral shortening. Although femoral shortening aids in the reduction and decreases the potential for complications, it is technically difficult.

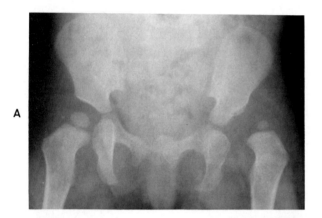

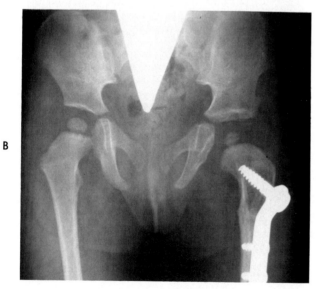

Fig. 2-82 Primary femoral shortening for congenital dislocation of hip. **A,** Undetected congenital dislocation of left hip in 3-year-old female. **B,** After open reduction, primary femoral shortening, and Salter osteotomy.

Primary femoral shortening. During the last decade the combination of primary open reduction and femoral shortening, with or without pelvic osteotomy, has become an accepted method of treatment of congenital hip dislocation in older children. This approach avoids expensive in-hospital traction, obtains predictable reduction, and produces a low rate of avascular necrosis.

Klisic and Jankovic reported the use of combined procedures in both unilateral and bilateral dislocations, combining open reduction and femoral shortening with acetabular procedures as indicated (Fig. 2-82). In a long-term follow-up study Klisic et al noted that their late subjective results were significantly better with the Pemberton osteotomy than with either the Salter or Chiari osteotomy.

Wenger, in a report of his experience with this technique in the treatment of congenital hip dislocation in the older child, recommends primary femoral shortening, anterior open reduction, and capsulorrhaphy, with or without pelvic osteotomy as indicated, in children aged 3 years or older. He also emphasizes the importance of correcting soft tissue deformity, as well as bony deformity, to prevent redislocation. Certain circumstances, such as teratologic hip dislocation or a failed traction program, may make the procedure appropriate for younger children. The completely dislocated hip in the older child becomes fixed in a position superior to the true acetabulum. The degree of this superior migration ranges from severe subluxation (inferior head still adjacent to labrum), to dislocation with formation of a false acetabulum just superior to the true acetabulum, to severe dislocation with the femoral head high in the abductor musculature without formation of a false acetabulum. The extent of proximal migration determines the degree of deformation of the capsule and the extent of soft tissue reconstruction required to correct the deformity.

The capsular abnormality in the congenitally dislocated hip must be recognized and corrected to achieve successful open reduction. The methods for bony correction are well defined, perhaps because the techniques can be clearly illustrated and documented roentgenographically, but the soft tissue abnormalities and methods for their correction are not well described. As a result a hip that appears reduced immediately after surgery may subluxate or redislocate with weight bearing even though the bony procedure appears roentgenographically faultless. The dislocation of the hip leads to adaptive enlargement of the hip capsule, with the capsule becoming nearly twice the normal size in the completely dislocated hip. The ligamentum teres hypertrophies and often becomes a partial weight-bearing structure. In older children this ligament occasionally avulses from the femoral head, retracting and reattaching to the inferior capsule and forming a mass of tissue in the inferior capsule that may impede reduction. The fibrocartilaginous labrum is flattened superolaterally, with the attached, hypertrophied capsule protruding into the overlying abductor muscle mass, which adheres to the displaced capsule. If the capsule is not separated adequately from the adherent overlying muscles, reduction is difficult and the chance of postoperative redislocation is increased. In a high, severe dislocation the abductor muscles have contracted, and occasionally, despite prior traction or femoral shortening, these contracted muscles and fascia make it difficult to pull the proximal femur distal enough to fully reduce the femoral head (Fig. 2-83). In rare instances this requires release of the piriformis insertion and/or release of the anteriormost gluteus mini-

mus fibers to allow adequate distal movement of the femoral head after femoral shortening. The middle and inferior portions of the capsule predictably are constricted by the overlying psoas tendon. The transverse acetabular ligament, crossing the base of the horseshoe-shaped true acetabulum, is contracted and thickened.

• • •

The following description of the technique for primary femoral shortening is a modification of the techniques described both by Klisic and by Wenger and includes anterior open reduction and varus derotational osteotomy. These techniques are described on p. 140 and p. 16, respectively, and should be reviewed carefully before performing primary femoral shortening (Fig. 2-84).

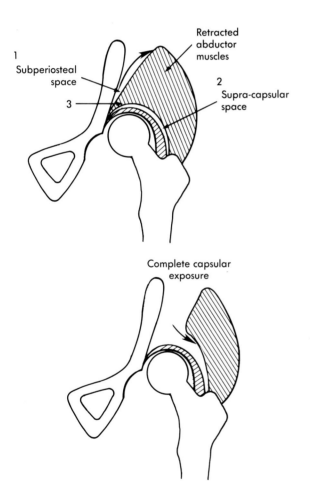

Fig. 2-83 Complete capsular exposure occasionally required in severe, high dislocation of hip. (Redrawn from Wenger DR. In The American Academy of Orthopaedic Surgeons: Instructional course lectures, 38:343, 1989.)

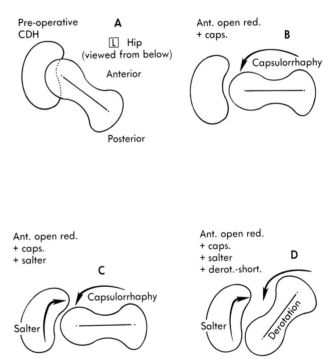

Fig. 2-84 **A,** Anteverted femur and acetabulum in untreated congenital dislocation of hip. **B,** Redirection of femoral neck by snug anterior capsulorrhaphy. **C,** Capsulorrhaphy and Salter innominate osteotomy. **D,** Capsulorrhaphy, Salter innominate osteotomy, and full femoral derotation. Combined in excess, this sequence can produce posterior dislocation. (Redrawn from Wenger DR. In The American Academy of Orthopaedic Surgeons: Instructional course lectures, 38:343, 1989.)

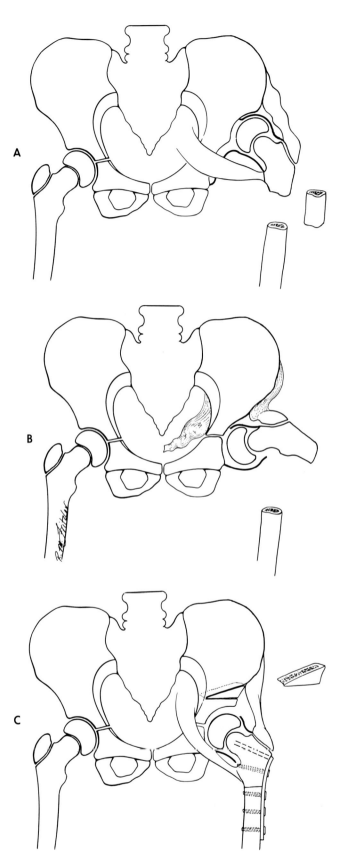

▲ *Technique.* Place the patient supine on the operating table with a small radiolucent pad beneath the affected hip. Prepare and drape the extremity in the usual manner to allow exposure of the pelvis and femur. Two incisions are used, an anterior ilioinguinal incision and a straight lateral incision as previously described both for anterior open reduction (p. 140) and for femoral osteotomy (p. 16).

Through the anterior ilioinguinal incision, perform anterior open reduction as previously described (p. 140), continuing the dissection to the point where capsulorrhaphy normally would be performed. Now turn attention to the femoral shortening. Make a straight lateral incision from the tip of the greater trochanter to the distal third of the femoral shaft. Expose the femoral shaft by dissection through the tensor fascia lata muscle, iliotibial band, and vastus lateralis muscle. Make a transverse mark on the femoral shaft at the level of the lesser trochanter to indicate the osteotomy site and a longitudinal mark on the anterior border of the proximal femoral shaft to orient derotation of the femur. Insert a lag screw into the femoral neck in the usual manner. Estimate the amount of shortening that will be necessary from preoperative roentgenograms, measuring from the most proximal aspect of the femoral head to the triradiate cartilage. The amount of shortening generally required varies from 1 to 3 cm. Perform an osteotomy of the femur slightly distal to the lag screw in the femoral neck. Make a second osteotomy at the appropriate distance distal to the first osteotomy. Angle this osteotomy to allow varus and derotation of the femur as necessary.

Fig. 2-85 Technique for open reduction, primary femoral shortening, and Salter osteotomy. **A,** Femoral head is dislocated. Gluteal muscles *(a)* are retracted and slightly shortened. Ilipsoas muscle *(b)* is intact. Capsule *(c)* is interposed between femoral head and ilium. Segment of femur is resected. **B,** Proximal femur is abducted. Iliopsoas tendon *(b)* is divided. Capsule (d) is incised on inferior surface parallel to femoral neck. **C,** Operation is complete. Gluteal muscles *(a)* are tight. Iliopsoas muscle *(b)* is reattached. Salter osteotomy completed with graft in place. Femoral fragments are fixed with hip screw.

Remove the measured segment of femoral shaft (Fig. 2-85). Carefully incise subperiosteally the iliopsoas attachment to the lesser trochanter and the capsule attached to the medial femoral neck, avoiding the medial circumflex artery. Then gently reduce the femoral head into the acetabulum, using the lag screw in the femoral neck as a lever. Derotation of the proximal fragment of approximately 15 to 45 degrees usually is required. Now appose the two segments of the femur, and attach a side plate to the screw in the femoral neck and fix it to the distal femoral shaft. Use roentgenograms or image intensification to assess the femoral shortening and reduction of the femoral head. At this point, if indicated to correct acetabular dysplasia, Salter or Pemberton osteotomy may be performed. A thorough and meticulous capsulorrhaphy should be performed as previously described. The most lateral flap of capsule should be transposed medially to eliminate the redundant capsule of the false acetabulum (Fig. 2-86).

Irrigate both wounds and close them in the usual manner. Suction drains may be inserted if necessary. Apply a spica cast with the extremity in neutral rotation and slight flexion and abduction.

▶ *Postoperative management.* The drains are removed 24 to 48 hours after surgery. The spica cast is removed 8 to 12 weeks after surgery. Sequential roentgenograms are obtained to assess development of the femoral head and acetabulum. Although uncommon, limb length discrepancy should be assessed annually by roentgenographic evaluation.

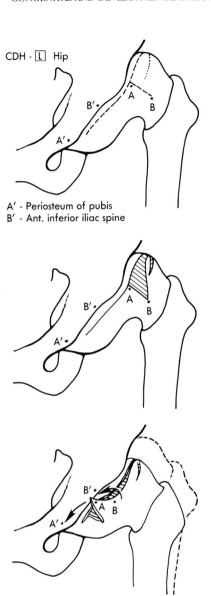

A' - Periosteum of pubis
B' - Ant. inferior iliac spine

Fig. 2-86 Technique of capsulorrhaphy during open reduction of congenital dislocation of hip. *CDH,* Congenital dysplasia of hip. (Redrawn from Wenger DR. In The American Academy of Orthopaedic Surgeons: Instructional course lectures, 38:343, 1989.)

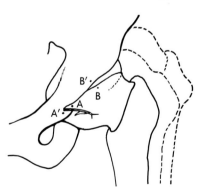

PELVIC OSTEOTOMY IN CONGENITAL DISLOCATION OF HIP

Operations on the pelvis, either alone or combined with open reduction, are useful in congenital dysplasia or dislocation of the hip to ensure or to increase stability of the joint. Those most often used are (1) osteotomy of the innominate bone, (2) acetabuloplasty, (3) osteotomies that free the acetabulum (triple innominate osteotomy or dial acetabular osteotomy), (4) shelf operation, and (5) innominate osteotomy with medial displacement of the acetabulum. In an older child one of these operations may be combined with femoral osteotomy to correct femoral and acetabular pathology.

Osteotomy of the innominate bone, an operation devised by Salter, is useful only when any subluxation or dislocation has been reduced or can be reduced by open reduction at the time of osteotomy in a child 18 months to 6 years of age. The entire acetabulum together with the pubis and ischium is rotated as a unit, the symphysis pubis acting as a hinge. The osteotomy is held open anterolaterally by a wedge of bone, and thus the roof of the acetabulum is shifted more anteriorly and laterally.

Acetabuloplasty is also useful only when any subluxation or dislocation has been reduced or can be reduced by open reduction at the time of operation in children at least 1 year old. In it the inclination of the acetabular roof is decreased by an osteotomy of the ilium made superior to the acetabulum. Pemberton described a *pericapsular osteotomy of the ilium* in which the osteotomy is made through the full thickness of the bone from just superior to the anteroinferior iliac spine anteriorly to the triradiate cartilage posteriorly; the triradiate cartilage acts as a hinge on which the acetabular roof is rotated anteriorly and laterally.

Osteotomies that free the acetabulum have been devised by Steel and by Eppright. These operations free part of the pelvis, creating a movable segment of bone that includes the acetabulum. They are indicated in older adolescents and skeletally mature adults with residual dysplasia and subluxation in whom remodeling of the acetabulum can no longer be anticipated. They are useful because they place articular cartilage over the femoral head. On the other hand, the shelf operations and the operation of Chiari interpose capsular fibrous tissue between the femoral head and the reconstructed acetabulum. In the triple innominate osteotomy (Steel), the ischium, the superior pubic ramus, and the ilium superior to the acetabulum all are divided, and the acetabulum is repositioned and stabilized by a bone graft and metal pins. In the dial osteotomy of the acetabulum (Eppright) the entire acetabulum superiorly, posteriorly, inferiorly, and anteriorly is freed by osteotomy and, as a single segment of bone, is redirected to appropriately cover the femoral head.

The *shelf procedure* is useful for subluxations and dislocations that have been reduced and in which no other osteotomy will establish a congruous joint with apposition of the articular cartilage of the acetabulum on the femoral head. In a classic shelf operation the acetabular roof is extended laterally, posteriorly, or anteriorly, either by a graft or by turning distally over the femoral head the acetabular roof and part of the lateral cortex of the ilium superior to it.

Innominate osteotomy with medial displacement of the acetabulum, an operation devised by Chiari for patients older than 4 years, is a modified shelf operation that places the femoral head beneath a surface of bone and joint capsule and corrects the pathologic lateral displacement of the femur. An osteotomy is made at the level of the acetabulum, and the femur and the acetabulum are displaced medially. The inferior surface of the proximal fragment forms a roof over the femoral head.

General recommendations for these osteotomies are summarized in Table 2-2.

Table 2-2   Recommended osteotomies for congenital dislocation of the hip

Osteotomy	Age	Indications
Salter innominate osteotomy	18 mo–6 yr	Congruous hip reduction; <10-15 degrees correction of acetabular index required
Pemberton acetabuloplasty	18 mo–10 yr	>10-15 degrees correction of acetabular index required; small femoral head, large acetabulum
Dial or Steel osteotomy	Skeletal maturity	Residual acetabular dysplasia; symptoms; congruous joint
Shelf procedure or Chiari osteotomy	Skeletal maturity	Incongruous joint; symptoms; other osteotomy not possible

INNOMINATE OSTEOTOMY (SALTER)

During open reduction of congenital dislocations of the hip, Salter observed that the entire acetabulum faces more anterolaterally than it should. Thus when the hip is extended, the femoral head is insufficiently covered anteriorly, and when it is adducted, there is insufficient cover superiorly. Salter's osteotomy of the innominate bone redirects the entire acetabulum so that its roof covers the head both anteriorly and superiorly. Any dislocation or subluxation must have been reduced concentrically before this operation is performed, or if not, then open reduction is carried out at the time of osteotomy. During the operation any contractures of the adductor or iliopsoas muscles are released by tenotomy, and in dislocations in which the capsule is elongated, a capsulorrhaphy is carried out. Salter recommends his osteotomy in the primary treatment of congenital dislocation of the hip in children between the ages of 18 months and 6 years and of congenital subluxation as late as early adulthood. He also recommends it in the secondary treatment of any residual or recurrent dislocation or subluxation after other methods of treatment within the age limits described (Fig. 2-87).

The following prerequisites are necessary for the success of this operation:

1. The femoral head must be pulled inferiorly to the level of the acetabulum. This may require a period of traction before surgery or primary femoral shortening.
2. Any contractures of the iliopsoas and adductor muscles must be released. This is indicated in subluxations as well as dislocations.
3. The femoral head must be reduced into the depth of the true acetabulum completely and concentrically. This generally requires careful open reduction and excision of any debris, exclusive of the labrum, from the acetabulum.
4. The joint must be reasonably congruous.
5. The range of motion of the hip must be good, especially in abduction, internal rotation, and flexion.

▶ *Technique, including open reduction (Salter)*. Place the patient supine on the operating table with the thorax on the affected side elevated by a sandbag. Drape the trunk on the affected side to the midline anteriorly and posteriorly and to the lower rib cage superiorly. Drape the lower extremity so that it can be moved freely during the operation. Now release the adductor muscles by subcutaneous tenotomy. Then make a skin incision beginning just inferior to the middle of the iliac crest, extending anteriorly to just inferior to the anterosuperior iliac spine and continuing to about the middle of the inguinal ligament. Decrease bleeding by applying pressure with sponges to the wound edges. Bluntly dissect between the tensor fasciae latae muscle laterally and the sartorius and rectus femoris muscles medially, and expose the anterosuperior iliac spine. Release the origins of the sartorius and the direct head of the rectus femoris. Next dissect the rectus femoris from the underlying joint capsule, and release its reflected head. Make a deep incision that splits the iliac epiphysis along the crest from the posterior end of the skin incision to the anterosuperior iliac spine anteriorly and then turns distally to the anteroinferior iliac spine.

Reflect the lateral part of the iliac epiphysis and the periosteum from the lateral surface of the iliac wing in a continuous sheet inferiorly to the superior edge of the acetabulum and posteriorly to the greater sciatic notch. Free any adhesions of the joint capsule from the lateral surface of the ilium and from any false acetabulum. Expose the capsule anteriorly and laterally by dissecting bluntly the interval between it and the abductor muscles.

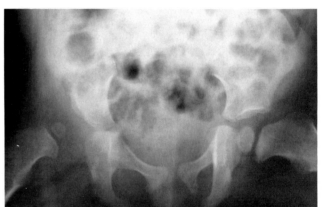

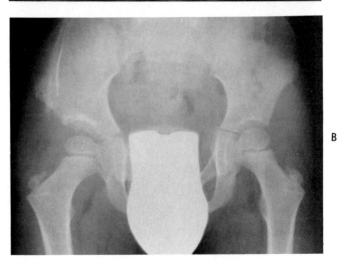

Fig. 2-87 Salter osteotomy for congenital dislocation of hip. **A,** Residual acetabular dysplasia and subluxation of right hip in 2-year-old boy. **B,** At age 10 years after prior open reduction and Salter osteotomy.

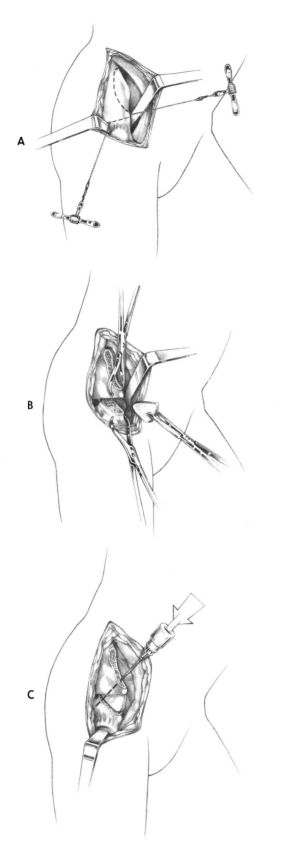

Fig. 2-88 Salter technique of osteotomy of innominate bone, including open reduction (see text). (Redrawn from Salter RB: J Bone Joint Surg 43B:518, 1961.)

Now pack the dissected spaces with large sponges to control bleeding and to increase the interval between the reflected periosteum and the sciatic notch. If concentric reduction of the femoral head into the acetabulum is impossible, open the capsule superiorly and anteriorly, parallel with and about 1 cm distal to the rim of the acetabulum.

Excise the ligamentum teres only if it is hypertrophied. Now gently reduce the femoral head into the acetabulum. Never excise the limbus. Now incise the distal flap of capsule at right angles to the first incision, thus creating a T-shaped incision, and resect the inferolateral triangular flap so created. Now test the stability of the joint; if the head becomes displaced superiorly from the acetabulum when the hip is adducted or anteriorly when it is extended or externally rotated, then osteotomy of the innominate bone is indicated.

Next allow the hip to redislocate. Then strip the medial half of the iliac epiphysis from the anterior half of the iliac crest and the periosteum from the medial surface of the ilium posteriorly and inferiorly to expose the entire medial aspect of the bone to the sciatic notch. Pack the surfaces thus exposed with sponges, again to control the loss of blood and to enlarge the interval between the periosteum and the bone. Next expose the tendinous part of the iliopsoas muscle at the level of the pelvic brim. With scissors separate the tendinous part from the muscular part and divide the former while protecting the muscle. Then pass a curved forceps subperiosteally medial to the ilium into the sciatic notch, and with it grasp one end of a Gigli saw. Then gently retract the curved forceps to pass the Gigli saw into the sciatic notch.

Retract the tissues medially and laterally from the ilium, and divide the bone with the saw in a straight line from the sciatic notch to the anteroinferior spine. Now remove a full-thickness graft from the anterior part of the iliac crest (Fig. 2-88, *A*), and trim it to the shape of a wedge. Make the base of the wedge about as wide as the distance between the anterosuperior and anteroinferior iliac spines. With towel clips grasp each fragment of the ilium that underwent osteotomy. Next insert a curved elevator into the sciatic notch, and by levering it anteriorly and exerting traction on the towel clip that grasps the inferior fragment, shift this fragment anteriorly, inferiorly, and laterally to open the osteotomy anterolaterally. Be sure that the osteotomy remains closed posteriorly (Fig. 2-88, *B*).

Do not apply traction in a cephalad direction on the proximal fragment because this may dislocate the sacroiliac joint. Now insert the bone graft into the osteotomy site, and release the traction on the inferior fragment. Drill a strong Kirschner wire through the remaining superior part of the ilium, through the graft, and into the inferior fragment (Fig. 2-88, *C*). Be sure that the Kirschner wire does not enter the acetabulum but that it does traverse all three fragments. Now drill a second Kirschner wire parallel with the first, using the same precautions. Next reduce the femoral head again into the acetabulum and reevaluate its stability. Reduction now should be stable with the hip either in adduction or in slight external rotation. While closing the wound, have an assistant hold the knee flexed and the hip slightly abducted, flexed, and internally rotated. Next obliterate any residual pocket of capsule by performing a capsulorrhaphy.

Move the distal half of the lateral flap of capsule medially beyond the anteroinferior iliac spine. This brings the capsular edges together and increases the stability of reduction by keeping the hip internally rotated. Now repair the capsule with interrupted sutures. Suture the sartorius and rectus femoris tendons to their origins. Suture together over the iliac crest the two halves of the iliac epiphysis. Cut the Kirschner wires so that their anterior ends lie within the subcutaneous fat. Now close the skin with a continuous subcuticular suture. With the hip held in the same position as during closure, apply a single spica cast.

▶ *Postoperative management.* At 8 to 12 weeks the spica cast is removed, and with the patient under general or local anesthesia, the Kirschner wires also are removed. The position of the osteotomy and of the hip is checked by roentgenograms.

Pemberton acetabuloplasty. The term *acetabuloplasty* designates operations that redirect the inclination of the acetabular roof by an osteotomy of the ilium superior to the acetabulum followed by levering of the roof inferiorly.

Pemberton devised an acetabuloplasty that he called *pericapsular osteotomy of the ilium,* in which an osteotomy is made through the full thickness of the ilium, using the triradiate cartilage as the hinge about which the acetabular roof is rotated anteriorly and laterally (Fig. 2-89). After a review of 115 hips in 91 patients observed for at least 2 years after surgery, he recommends it for any dysplastic hip in patients between the age of 1 year and the age when the triradiate cartilage becomes too inflexible to serve as a hinge (about 12 years of age in girls and 14 years in boys), provided that any subluxation or dislocation has been reduced or can be reduced at the time of osteotomy. In Pemberton's experience anteversion of the femoral neck is not a threat to continued stability after surgery.

Coleman, in a review of pericapsular and innominate osteotomies, noted that one advantage of the former operation is the lack of need for internal fixation, and thus a second operation, although minor, is avoided. Furthermore, a greater degree of correction can be achieved with less rotation of the acetabulum in the pericapsular osteotomy because the fulcrum, the triradiate cartilage, is nearer the site of desired correction. According to Coleman, however, Pemberton's operation is technically more difficult to perform. In addition, it alters the configuration and capacity of the acetabulum and may result in an incongruous relationship between it and the femoral head; consequently some remodeling of the acetabulum may be required.

A
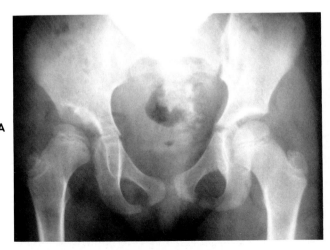

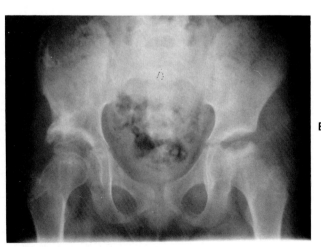
B

Fig. 2-89 Pemberton osteotomy. **A,** Symptomatic residual acetabular dysplasia in 8-year-old girl after treatment of congenital dislocation of right hip. **B,** After Pemberton acetabuloplasty.

▲ *Technique (Pemberton).* Place the patient supine with a small radiolucent pad beneath the affected hip, and expose the hip joint through an anterior iliofemoral approach. Make the superior part of the incision distal to and parallel with the iliac crest, and extend it from the anterosuperior spine anteriorly to the middle of the crest posteriorly. Extend the distal part of the incision from the anterosuperior spine inferiorly for 5 to 7 cm parallel to the inguinal crease. Beginning at the crest, strip the gluteus and the tensor fasciae latae muscles subperiosteally from the anterior third of the ilium distally to the joint capsule and posteriorly until the greater sciatic notch is exposed. Now with a sharp elevator separate the iliac apophysis, with its attached abdominal muscles, from the anterior third of the iliac crest. Then strip the muscles subperiosteally from the medial aspect of the ilium until the sciatic notch again is exposed. At this point open the capsule of the hip and remove any soft tissue that restricts reduction. Reduce the hip under direct vision and be sure that it is well seated; then redislocate it until the osteotomy has been made and propped open with a graft.

Now insert two flat retractors subperiosteally into the sciatic notch, one along the medial surface of the ilium and one along the lateral to keep the anterior third of the ilium exposed both medially and laterally. With a narrow curved osteotome cut through the lateral cortex of the ilium as follows. First start slightly superior to the anteroinferior iliac spine, and curve the osteotomy posteriorly about 1 cm proximal to and parallel with the joint capsule until the osteotome is seen to be well anterior to the retractor resting in the sciatic notch. Image intensification will aid in confirming correct placement of the osteotomy.

From this point when driven farther, the blade of the osteotome disappears from sight, and it is therefore important to direct its tip sufficiently inferiorly so that it does not enter the sciatic notch but instead enters the ilioischial rim of the triradiate cartilage at its midpoint. After directing the osteotome properly, drive it 1.5 cm farther to complete the osteotomy of the lateral cortex of the ilium. With the same osteotome make a corresponding cut in the medial cortex of the ilium, starting anteriorly at the same point just superior to the anteroinferior iliac spine. Direct this cut posteriorly parallel with that in the lateral cortex until it reaches the triradiate cartilage (Fig. 2-90).

The direction in which the acetabular roof becomes displaced after the osteotomy is controlled by varying the position of the posterior part of the osteotomy of the medial cortex. The more anterior this part of the osteotomy the less the acetabular roof rotates anteriorly; conversely, the more posterior this part of the osteotomy the more the acetabular roof rotates anteriorly. After completing the osteotomy of the two cortices, insert a wide curved osteotome into the anterior part of the osteotomy, and lever the distal fragment distally until the anterior edges of the two fragments are at least 2.5 to 3 cm apart.

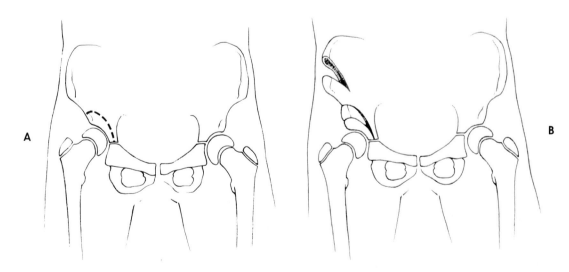

Fig. 2-90 Pemberton pericapsular osteotomy. **A,** Line of osteotomy beginning slightly superior to anterosuperior iliac spine and curving into triradiate cartilage. **B,** Completed osteotomy with acetabular roof in corrected position and wedge of bone impacted into open osteotomy site.

The acetabular roof should be turned inferiorly far enough to result in an estimated acetabular index of zero degrees. Next cut a narrow groove in the antero-posterior direction in each raw surface of the ilium. Resect a wedge of bone from the anterior part of the iliac wing, including the anterosuperior spine. Then with a laminar spreader separate the fragments and place the wedge of bone in the grooves made in the surfaces of the ilium; drive the wedge into place and impact it firmly. The acetabular roof then should remain fixed in the corrected position. Hold the correction with a Kirschner wire, if necessary. If the hip has remained dislocated during the osteotomy, reduce it at this time. Perform a meticulous capsulorrhaphy for additional soft tissue stability. Suture the iliac apophysis over the remaining ilium and close the wound.

▶ *Postoperative management.* With the hip in neutral position (or in slight abduction and internal rotation if this has been found the most favorable position for closure of the wound), a spica cast is applied from the nipple line to the toes on the affected side and to above the knee on the opposite side. At 2 months the cast is removed, and the osteotomy is checked by roentgenograms.

Steel osteotomy. The Pemberton pericapsular osteotomy is limited by the mobility of the triradiate cartilage and, by hinging on this cartilage, may cause premature physeal closure. Although the Salter innominate osteotomy may be used in older patients, its results depend on the mobility of the symphysis pubis, and the amount of femoral head coverage is limited. Other, more complex osteotomies, such as those of Steel and of Eppright, can provide more correction and improve femoral head coverage.

In the *triple innominate osteotomy* developed by Steel, the ischium, the superior pubic ramus, and the ilium superior to the acetabulum all are divided, and the acetabulum is repositioned and stabilized by a bone graft and pins. Its goal is to establish a stable hip in anatomic position in older children with dislocation or subluxation of the hip when this is impossible by any one of the other osteotomies (Fig. 2-91). For the operation to be successful the articular surfaces of the joint must be congruous or become so once the acetabulum has been redirected so that a functional, painless range of motion will be achieved and a Trendelenburg gait will be absent. Steel reviewed 45 patients in whom 52 of his operations had been performed. The results were satisfactory in 40 hips and unsatisfactory in 12. The unsatisfactory hips were painful and easily fatigued; in two results of the Trendelenburg test were positive, and in one significant motion had been lost.

Before surgery skeletal traction must be used until the femoral head is brought distally to the level of the acetabulum or femoral shortening must be performed; if necessary any contracted muscles about the hip are released surgically.

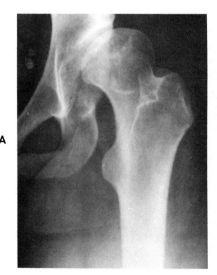 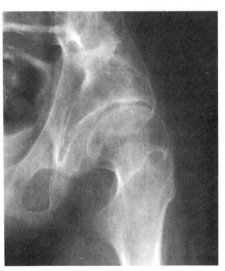

A   B

Fig. 2-91 **A,** Primary acetabular dysplasia in 16-year-old girl before Steel osteotomy. **B,** One year after osteotomy. (Courtesy Drs. H. Steel and R. Betz.)

▶ *Technique (Steel).* Place the patient supine on the operating table, and flex the hip and knee 90 degrees. Keep the hip in neutral abduction, adduction, and rotation. First drape the posterior aspect of the proximal thigh and the buttock, leaving the ischial tuberosity exposed. Make a transverse incision perpendicular to the long axis of the femoral shaft 1 cm proximal to the gluteal crease. Retract the gluteus maximus muscle laterally, and expose the hamstring muscles at their ischial origin. By sharp dissection

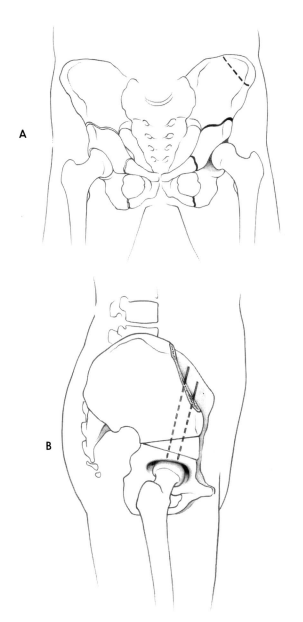

Fig. 2-92 Steel triple innominate osteotomy. **A,** Osteotomies to be performed in iliac wing and superior and inferior pubic rami. Note wedge of bone to be taken as graft from most superior portion of ilium. **B,** Lateral view showing graft in place and fixation with two Kirschner wires.

free the biceps femoris, the most superficial muscle in the area, from the ischium and expose the interval between the semimembranosus and the semitendinosus muscles. The sciatic nerve lies far enough laterally not be endangered. Now pass a curved hemostat in the interval between the origins of the semimembranosus and the semitendinosus deep to the ischium and into the obturator foramen. Elevate the origins of the obturator internus and externus, and bring the tip of the hemostat out at the inferior margin of the ischial ramus. Be sure the hemostat remains in contact with the bone during its passage deep to the ramus. Now with an osteotome directed posterolaterally and 45 degrees from the perpendicular divide the ischial ramus completely. Allow the origin of the biceps femoris to fall into place. Next suture the gluteus maximus to the deep fascia and close the skin.

Change gowns, gloves, and instruments, and in the iliopubic area begin the second stage of operation. As an alternative, the superior and inferior pubic rami may be dissected and divided through a medial adductor approach. If a posterior incision was chosen, proceed with a full skin preparation medially to the midline and superiorly to the costal margin and drape the extremity free. Through an anterior iliofemoral approach reflect the iliac and gluteal muscles from the wing of the ilium. Detach the sartorius and the lateral attachments of the inguinal ligament from the anterosuperior iliac spine and reflect them medially. Now reflect the iliacus and psoas muscles subperiosteally from the inner surface of the pelvis; this protects the femoral neurovascular bundle. Next divide the tendinous part of the origin of the iliopsoas, and expose the pectineal tubercle. Detach the pectineus muscle superiosteally from the superior pubic ramus, and expose the bone 1 cm medial to the pubic tubercle. Pass a curved hemostat superior to the superior pubic ramus into the obturator foramen near the bone. With it penetrate the obturator fascia so that its tip is brought out inferior to the ramus. If the bone is especially thick, pass a second hemostat inferior to the ramus and direct it superiorly to contact the first one. Now direct an osteotome posteromedially and 15 degrees from the perpendicular, and perform an osteotomy of the pubic ramus.

The obturator artery, vein, and nerve are protected by the hemostat. Now using the technique described by Salter for innominate osteotomy, divide the ilium with a Gigli saw. When this osteotomy has been completed, free the periosteum and fascia from the medial wall of the pelvis to free the acetabular segment (Fig. 2-92). If the femoral head is subluxated or dislocated, open the capsule at this time and remove any tissue obstructing reduction. Reduce the femoral head as near as possible to the center of the triradiate cartilage and close the capsule.

Next with a towel clip grasp the anteroinferior iliac spine and rotate the acetabular segment in the desired direction, usually anteriorly and laterally, until the femoral head is covered. In an older child use a laminar spreader to open the osteotomy because the sacroiliac joint usually is more stable in this age-group and is not likely to be damaged. With the acetabular fragment in proper position, stabilize it with a triangular bone graft removed from the superior rim of the ilium. Transfix the graft with two pins that penetrate the inner wall of the ilium. Now allow the pectineus and iliopsoas muscles to fall into place. Reattach the sartorius muscle and the lateral end of the inguinal ligament to the anterosuperior iliac spine, and close the wound in layers.

▸ *Postoperative management.* A spica cast is applied with the hip in 20 degrees of abduction, 5 degrees of flexion, and neutral rotation. At 8 to 10 weeks the cast and pins are removed, and active and passive motion of the hip is started. All three osteotomies probably will unite by 12 weeks after surgery. At 12 to 14 weeks, when the osteotomies have united, weight bearing on crutches is started.

Dial osteotomy. In the *dial osteotomy* of the acetabulum, developed by Eppright, the entire acetabulum superiorly, posteriorly, inferiorly, and anteriorly is freed by osteotomy and, as a single segment of bone, is redirected to appropriately cover the femoral head. It was devised to treat residual dysplasia in older children or young adults in whom the hip is painful, is easily fatigued, and feels unstable and in whom the results of the Trendelenburg test are positive. It is indicated only in a truly dysplastic hip in which the head is concentrically located but the CE angle of Wiberg is less than 15 to 20 degrees. In addition, the thickness of the cartilaginous surfaces should be almost normal, and motion in the hip should be normal except for some limitation of external rotation. Eppright reported the use of this operation in 178 patients, none of whom developed avascular necrosis of the acetabular fragment or femoral head (Fig. 2-93).

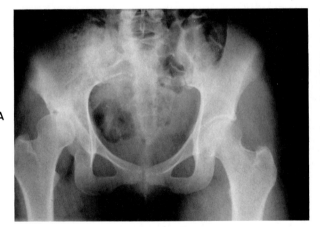

A

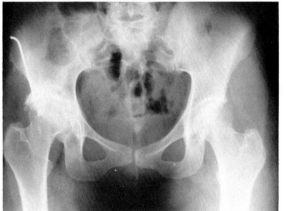

B

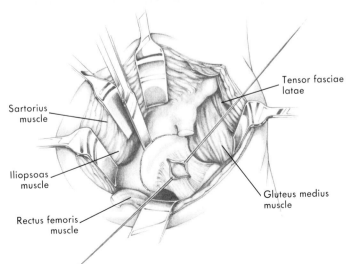

Sartorius muscle

Iliopsoas muscle

Rectus femoris muscle

Tensor fasciae latae

Gluteus medius muscle

Fig. 2-93 Eppright dial osteotomy. **A,** Acetabular dysplasia in 16-year-old female before operation. **B,** After dial osteotomy. **C,** Line of osteotomy for rotation of acetabular fragment. (**A** and **B** courtesy Dr. R.H. Eppright.)

▶ *Technique (Eppright).* Place the patient supine on the operating table over a roentgenographic cassette holder to allow roentgenograms to be made in the anteroposterior direction if needed during surgery, or use an image intensifier. Drape the lower limb so that it can be moved freely during the operation. Now expose the hip through an anterior iliofemoral incision, modifying it slightly by extending it farther distally. Now divide proximally the lateral femoral cutaneous nerve, and separate the sartorius muscle from the tensor fasciae latae muscle. Reflect the muscles from the lateral aspect of the iliac crest subperiosteally. Next reflect the iliac apophysis, if present, medially from the anterior half of the iliac crest, and strip the periosteum from the medial wall of the ilium. Divide the tendon of the rectus femoris muscle at the anteroinferior iliac spine, and reflect it medially and distally. Expose the capsule of the hip joint adjacent to the acetabulum over as much of its circumference as possible.

Now with a curved periosteal elevator carefully remove the periosteum from the posterior aspect of the ilium and the acetabulum down to the ischium. The sciatic nerve commonly lies near the ilium posteriorly. Consequently strip the periosteum posteriorly, and when indicated during the operation, place a finger posterior to the acetabulum to protect the nerve. Now flex the hip slightly and remove the iliopsoas tendon and muscle from the lesser trochanter. This allows additional medial retraction so that the iliopubic eminence can be exposed medially and inferiorly. To prevent injuring the femoral nerve and artery keep the knee and hip flexed 20 degrees or more while retracting the iliopsoas muscle. Next incise the capsule of the hip joint in line with the femoral neck. Retract the capsule superiorly and inferiorly, locate precisely the acetabular margins, and determine the condition of the cartilage on the femoral head.

With a 1.3 cm osteotome outline the osteotomy anteriorly. Start it at the anteroinferior iliac spine, extend it medially and inferiorly as close as possible to the iliopectineal line, and then curve it inferiorly and laterally. Ideally take 1 cm of bone with the acetabular cartilage to avoid a fracture into the articular surface. Now continue the osteotomy straight posteriorly until it approaches the posterior surface of the ilium. Place a finger posterior to the acetabulum to protect the sciatic nerve, and continue the osteotomy through the posterior cortex of the ilium until the point of the osteotome can be felt. Now dissect inferior to the capsule of the hip. Retract the obturator externus muscle posteriorly and inferiorly, and extend the osteotomy through the posterior aspect of the ischium. After the osteotomy has been completed, place gentle traction on the leg to allow the acetabular fragment to be dialed to the desired position over the femoral head. If the anterior part of the acetabulum is deficient, take a bone graft from the exposed ilium and wedge it in anteriorly, thus tilting the entire acetabulum posteriorly. Now abduct the hip and release the traction; the acetabulum now should be held in place by the tension of the soft structures. If, however, better fixation is needed, transfix the fragment with a Steinmann pin.

Now hold the hip in slight abduction through the rest of the procedure. Close the capsule and attach the iliopsoas tendon to the periosteum on the medial side of the proximal femur. Reattach the tendon of the rectus femoris muscle proximal to the osteotomy on the anteroinferior iliac spine, and replace the iliac epiphysis. Close the subcutaneous tissues with interrupted absorbable sutures and the skin with a continuous subcuticular suture. With the hip in slight abduction, 10 degrees of flexion, and neutral rotation, apply a spica cast to the toes on the affected side and to above the knee on the opposite side.

▶ *Postoperative management.* At 6 weeks the spica cast is removed, and roentgenograms are made. Active motion of the hip and knee is encouraged. As soon as the patient has active control of the limb and passive flexion of the hip allows sitting, crutch walking with partial weight bearing is started. Full weight bearing is not permitted until active abduction of the hip can be carried out against gravity; this usually occurs at 4 to 6 weeks after the cast has been removed.

SHELF OPERATIONS

Shelf procedures commonly have been performed by enlarging the volume of the acetabulum; however, pelvic redirectional and displacement osteotomies have largely replaced this operation. The redirectional osteotomies are inappropriate in hips in which the femoral head and acetabulum are misshapen but still congruent because redirection may cause incongruity.

Staheli shelf procedure. Staheli has described a slotted acetabular augmentation procedure to create a congruous acetabular extension in which the size and position of the augmentation can be easily controlled. A deficient acetabulum that cannot be corrected by redirectional pelvic osteotomy is the primary indication for this operation. Contraindications include dysplastic hips with spherical congruity suitable for redirectional osteotomy, hips requiring concurrent open reduction that must have supplementary stability, and patients unsuited for spica cast immobilization.

▲ *Technique (Staheli).* Before surgery the CE angle of Wiberg is determined from anteroposterior pelvic roentgenograms of the standing child, and a normal CE angle (about 35 degrees) is drawn on the film. The additional width necessary to extend the existing acetabulum to achieve the normal angle is measured (Fig. 2-94). This determines the width of the augmentation; this measurement added to the depth of the slot gives the total graft length. If the patient is small or easily moved, the procedure is performed on a standard operating table with the affected side elevated 15 degrees on a pad. For heavier patients a fracture table is used and the involved limb is draped free.

Make a straight "bikini" skin incision 2 cm below and parallel to the iliac crest. Expose the hip joint through a standard iliofemoral approach. Divide the tendon of the reflected head of the rectus femoris muscle anteriorly and displace it posteriorly. If the capsule is abnormally thick (greater than 6 to 7 mm), thin it by "filleting" with a scalpel.

The placement of the acetabular slot is the most critical part of the procedure; the slot must be created *exactly* at the acetabular margin. Determine the position of the slot by placing a probe into the joint to palpate the position of the acetabulum. Next place a drill in the selected site, and make an anteroposterior roentgenogram to verify correct position. The floor of the slot should be acetabular articular cartilage and little bone; the end and roof of the slot should be cancellous bone. The slot should be 1 cm deep.

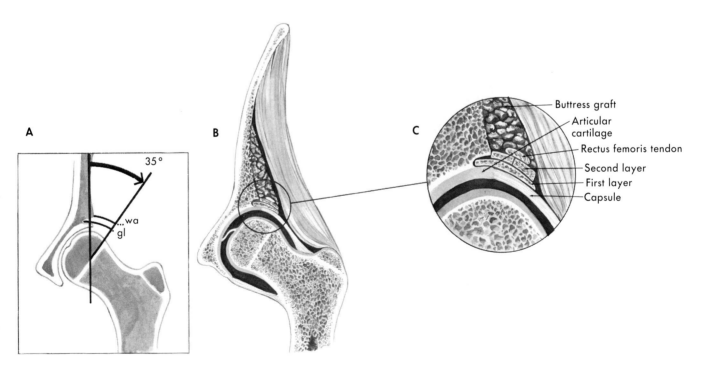

Fig. 2-94   Slotted acetabular augmentation of Staheli. **A,** Width of augmentation *(wa)* is determined preoperatively from standing anteroposterior roentgenogram of pelvis. CE angle and 35-degree angle are drawn. Graft length *(gl)* is sum of *wa* and slot depth. **B,** Objective of procedure is to provide congruous extension of acetabulum. **C,** Details of extension. (From Staheli LT: J Pediatr Orthop 1:321, 1981.)

Make the slot by drilling a series of holes with a ⁵⁄₃₂-inch (4.5 mm) bit, and join them with a narrow rongeur. Determine the length of the slot intraoperatively by the need for coverage. If excessive femoral anteversion is present, extend the slot anteriorly. If the acetabulum is deficient posteriorly, extend the slot in that direction.

Take thin strips of cortical and cancellous bone from the lateral surface of the ilium; cut these as long as possible. Extend the shallow decortication inferiorly from the iliac crest to the superior margin of the slot to ensure rapid fusion of the graft to the ilium. Do not remove the inner table of the ilium because this may change the contour of the pelvis.

Now measure the depth of the slot, and add this to the width of the augmentation as determined before surgery. Select thin strips (1 mm) of cancellous bone, and cut them into rectangles about 1 cm wide and of the appropriate length. Assemble these rectangular pieces on a moist sponge, cutting enough to provide a single layer the length of the augumentation. Apply the first layer radially from the slot with the concave side down to provide a congruous extension.

Select longer cancellous strips for the second layer, and cut them to the length of the extension. Place these at right angles to the first layer and parallel to the acetabulum. They may be a little thicker (2 mm), especially the most lateral strip, to provide a well-defined lateral margin of the extension. Both layers must be of appropriate width and length. To avoid blocking hip flexion the augmentation should not extend too far anteriorly.

Secure these two layers of cancellous grafts by bringing the reflected head of the rectus femoris muscle forward over the graft and suturing it back in its original position. A capsular flap may be substituted if this tendon is not available. Cut the remaining grafts into small pieces, and pack them above but not beyond the initial layer. They are held in place by the reattached abductor muscles. Confirm the position and width of the graft by roentgenograms. After closure, apply a single hip spica cast with the hip in 15 degrees of abduction, 20 degrees of flexion, and neutral rotation (Fig. 2-95).

▲ *Postoperative management.* The cast is removed after 6 weeks, and crutch walking is permitted with partial weight bearing on the affected side until the graft is incorporated, usually at 3 to 4 months.

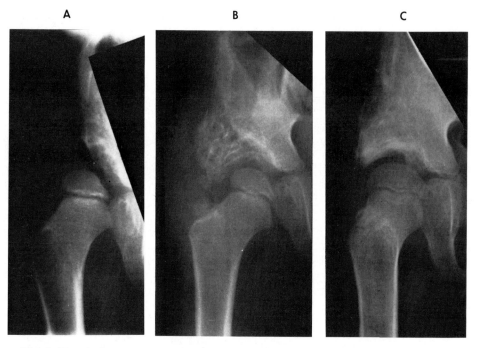

Fig. 2-95   A, Severe congenital acetabular dysplasia in 4-year-old girl. **B,** Immediately after slotted acetabular augmentation. **C,** Six months after operation. (From Staheli LT: J Pediatr Orthop 1:321, 1981.)

Chiari osteotomy . The Chiari osteotomy is a capsular interposition arthroplasty and should be considered only in those instances in which other reconstructions are impossible: when the femoral head cannot be concentrically reduced in the acetabulum or in painfully subluxated hips with early signs of osteoarthritis. This procedure deepens the deficient acetabulum by medial displacement of the distal pelvic fragment and improves superolateral femoral coverage.

The Chiari procedure is an operation that uses no bone grafts, places the femoral head beneath a surface of spongy bone with the capacity for regeneration, and corrects the lateral pathologic displacement of the femur. An osteotomy of the pelvis is performed at the superior margin of the acetabulum, and the pelvis inferior to the osteotomy along with the femur is displaced medially (Fig. 2-96). The superior fragment of the osteotomy then becomes a shelf, and the capsule is interposed between it and the femoral head. After using this operation on more than 600 patients, 400 of whom have been observed for more than 2 years, Chiari recommends the following criteria for the operation:

1. For all congenital subluxations in patients 4 to 6 years old or older, including adults. These include subluxations persisting after conservative treatment of dislocations and those never treated before.
2. For untreated congenital dislocations in patients older than 4 years, soon after open or closed reduction.
3. For dysplastic hips with osteoarthritis, including those with severe involvement.
4. For paralytic dislocations caused by muscular weakness or spasticity.
5. For coxa magna after Perthes disease or avascular necrosis with congenital dislocation, forced orthopaedic treatment of congenital dislocation with resultant avascular necrosis.

These indications are broader than those usually accepted in this country. For a child younger than 10 years of age, the osteotomy is not recommended in subluxations or in dislocations that can be reduced either surgically or conservatively and in which osteotomy of the innominate bone, acetabuloplasty, or osteotomies that free the acetabulum would result in a competent acetabulum. Some surgeons recommend the operation for patients in the second and later decades who have symptomatic early sublux-

ation of the hip with acetabular dysplasia too severe to be treated by other pelvic osteotomies; for them innominate osteotomy with medial displacement is preferred to a shelf operation. The procedure also has been used in older children with underlying neuromuscular disorders and acetabular dysplasia.

Chiari's operation is a capsular arthroplasty because the capsule is interposed between the newly formed acetabular roof and the femoral head. Because the biomechanics of the hip are improved by displacing the hip nearer the midline, a Trendelenburg limp often is eliminated.

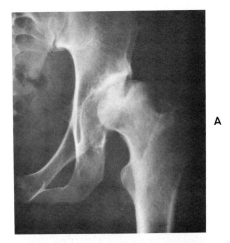

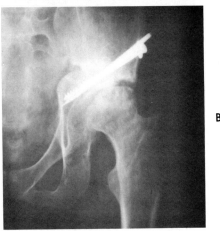

Fig. 2-96 **A,** Young adult with painful acetabular dysplasia before Chiari osteotomy. **B,** After surgery. Note that optional internal fixation has been used in this patient. (Courtesy Dr. R. Betz.)

▲ *Technique (Chiari).* Place the patient supine on a fracture table with the feet fastened to the traction plate. Now slightly abduct and externally rotate the affected hip. Make an anterolateral approach about 10 cm long. Develop the interval between the tensor fasciae latae and the sartorius muscles, and retract the former laterally. Now incise the iliac epiphysis in line with the iliac crest. With a periosteal elevator detach the lateral half of the epiphysis along with the tensor fasciae latae and the anterior part of the gluteus medius.

Now dissect these muscles subperiosteally and retract them posteriorly. Insert a periosteal elevator between the capsule of the hip and the gluteus minimus. Dissect subperiosteally posteriorly to the point where the pelvis curves inferiorly. Now with a curved periosteal elevator dissect subperiosteally farther posteriorly until the sciatic notch is reached. Replace this elevator with a flexible metal ribbon retractor 3 cm wide. This completes the dissection posteriorly. Now

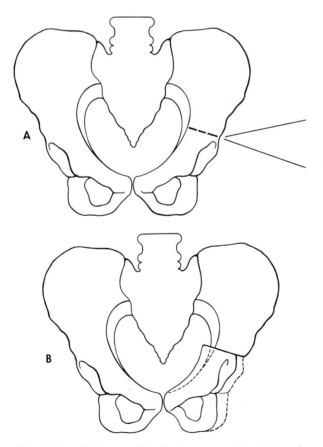

Fig. 2-97 Chiari medial displacement osteotomy. **A,** Line of osteotomy extending from immediately superior to lip of acetabulum into sciatic notch. Osteotomy may be curved to facilitate femoral head coverage. **B,** Completed osteotomy with medial displacement of distal fragment for interpositional capsular arthroplasty.

return anteriorly to the medial aspect of the ilium. With a periosteal elevator strip the iliacus muscle and the underlying periosteum posteriorly to the sciatic notch.

Once the sciatic notch is reached, replace the elevator with a flexible metal ribbon retractor that touches and overlaps the ribbon retractor already in the notch. With curved scissors separate the rectus muscle and its reflected head from the capsule of the hip joint. Now divide the reflected head. The osteotomy should be made precisely between the insertion of the capsule and the reflected head of the rectus muscle, following the capsular insertion in a curved line and ending distal to the anteroinferior iliac spine anteriorly and in the sciatic notch posteriorly. Do not open or damage the capsule of the joint. After the line of the osteotomy has been determined, start the osteotomy with a straight, narrow osteotome, opening the lateral table of the ilium along this line.

At the beginning determine the exact position of the osteotome by image intensification or by roentgenograms. Direct the osteotomy superiorly approximately 20 degrees toward the inner table of the ilium (Fig. 2-97). Change the position of the osteotome as necessary to make the osteotomy curve superiorly. Do not direct the osteotomy more than 20 degrees superiorly because it then might enter the sacroiliac joint. Furthermore, do not splinter the inner cortex of the ilium.

When the osteotomy has been completed, displace the hip medially by releasing the traction on the extremity and by forcing the limb into abduction. The distal fragment then displaces medially, hinging at the symphysis pubis. If, however, the adductor muscles are extremely relaxed, it may be necessary to manipulate the head manually or displace the distal fragment with an instrument. Be sure the distal fragment is displaced far enough medially so that the proximal fragment covers the femoral head completely. Optional internal fixation may be inserted to secure and maintain adequate displacement.

After the displacement has been completed, decrease the abduction of the limb to about 30 degrees. If the capsule is loose, perform a capsulorrhaphy. Now check the position of the hip and the osteotomy by image intensification or by roentgenograms. Replace and suture the iliac apophysis, and close the wound. Apply a spica cast with the hip in 20 to 30 degrees of abduction, neutral rotation, and neutral extension.

▲ *Postoperative management.* In children and adults the cast is removed at 6 to 8 weeks, and active and passive exercises of the hip are started. Partial weight bearing on crutches is allowed and progressed as tolerated.

Congenital Hip Dislocation in the Adolescent and Young Adult

In children older than 8 to 10 years of age or in young adults in whom the femoral head cannot be pulled distally to the level of the acetabulum, only palliative salvaging operations are possible. Rarely a femoral shortening combined with a pelvic osteotomy could be considered, but the chances of creating a hip to last a lifetime are minimal. After a few years degenerative arthritic changes develop in the hip joint. When these changes cause enough pain or limitation of motion to require additional surgery, a reconstructive operation such as a total hip arthroplasty may be indicated at the appropriate age. Arthrodesis now is rarely indicated for an old unreduced dislocation and is contraindicated in bilateral dislocations. In bilateral dislocations in this age-group the hips should be left unreduced, and total hip arthroplasties may be carried out during adulthood (Fig. 2-98). Patients with a reduced femoral head but painful acetabular dysplasia may be treated with an appropriately selected pelvic osteotomy.

CONGENITAL AND DEVELOPMENTAL COXA VARA

The term *congenital coxa vara* has been applied to two types of coxa vara seen in infancy and childhood. The first type is present at birth, is rare, and is associated with other congenital anomalies such as proximal femoral focal deficiency or anomalies in other parts of the body such as cleidocranial dysostosis. The second type, usually not discovered until walking is begun, is more common than the first and is associated with no other abnormality except possibly a congenitally short femur.

Coxa vara, often bilateral, is characterized by a progressive decrease in the angle between the femoral neck and shaft, a progressive shortening of the limb,

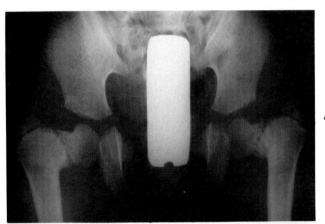

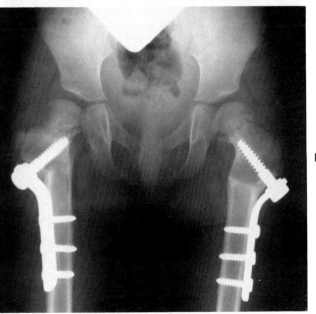

Fig. 2-99 Congenital coxa vara. **A,** Preoperative roentgenogram shows neck-shaft angle of less than 90 degrees. **B,** After bilateral subtrochanteric osteotomies and internal fixation with Campbell hip screws.

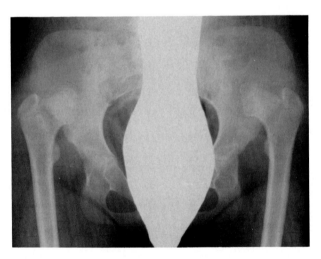

Fig. 2-98 Bilateral untreated congenital dislocation of hip in 12-year-old girl.

and the presence of a defect in the medial part of the neck. Microscopic examination reveals that the tissue in this defect consists of cartilage that, because the columnar arrangement of its cells is irregular and ossification within it is atypical, resembles an abnormal physis. The adjacent metaphyseal bone is osteoporotic, its trabeculae being atrophic, and occasionally it contains large groups of cartilage cells. When walking is begun, the forces that the femoral neck must withstand are of course increased, and because the neck is weak, varus deformity gradually develops.

As the patient becomes older and heavier, the deformity increases until the greater trochanter eventually lies superior to the femoral head; furthermore, pseudarthrosis of the femoral neck may develop. In adults the trochanter may come to lie several inches superior to the head, and when pseudarthrosis is present, the head may be widely separated from the neck. After the age of 8 years the likelihood of obtaining a hip whose function approaches normal diminishes rapidly.

The treatment of choice for correction of developmental coxa vara is subtrochanteric osteotomy to place the femoral neck and head in an appropriate valgus position with the shaft of the femur. Surgery is indicated when the neck-shaft angle is 110 degrees or less. The subtrochanteric osteotomy is fixed internally with either a blade-plate or screw-plate combination (see Fig. 2-99). Although biomechanically this may provide enough rigid internal fixation to eliminate the need for postoperative immobilization, a spica cast should be worn until union is complete.

Regardless of the method of osteotomy, the deformity can recur, and children should be examined periodically after surgery until their growth is complete. In addition, a significant number of children with coxa vara have associated femoral hypoplasia or limb length discrepancy, which ultimately may require limb length equalization.

▲ *Technique (valgus osteotomy for developmental coxa vara).* Perform an adductor tenotomy through a small medial incision. Expose the trochanter and proximal shaft of the femur through a lateral, longitudinal incision. If a screw and side plate device is used for internal fixation, insert the screw in the midline of the femoral neck as determined by image intensification or both anteroposterior and lateral roentgenograms. Insert the screw as close as possible to the trochanteric apophysis without entering it. If possible, center the screw in the femoral neck distal to the abnormal physis. If this is technically impossible, center the screw in the femoral head. Then make a transverse osteotomy slightly distal to the screw at about the level of the lesser trochanter. If necessary, take a small lateral wedge of bone to correct the neck-shaft angle (approximately 135 to 150 degrees). Then fix the side plate to the shaft of the femur in the usual manner. Irrigate the wound and close it in layers, inserting irrigation-suction drainage if desired. Apply a 1½ cast.

▲ *Postoperative management.* The cast is removed 8 to 12 weeks after surgery when roentgenographic union of the osteotomy has occurred. Regular follow-up includes the assessment of possible recurrence of the deformity and the development of progressive limb length discrepancy that requires treatment.

EXSTROPHY OF BLADDER

Exstrophy of the bladder occurs as a result of a congenital failure of fusion of the tissues of the midline of the body. The major anomaly is a maldevelopment of the lower part of the abdominal wall and the anterior wall of the bladder so that the anterior surface of the posterior wall of the bladder is exposed to the exterior. Hernias and other defects of the anterior abdominal wall also may be present more proximally. As noted by O'Phelan, however, the orthopaedic surgeon becomes involved in treatment because of the diastasis of the symphysis pubis, the lateral flare of the innominate bones, and the resultant lateral displacement and external rotation of the acetabula that, if left uncorrected, would result in a wide-based, waddling, externally rotated gait. Other orthopaedic anomalies may be associated with exstrophy of the bladder, including congenital dislocation or dysplasia of the hip and myelomeningocele.

Because most of the urologic structures are present or bifid, reconstruction is possible. Unless the symphysis pubis is approximated, however, urologic reconstruction is followed by complications such as the formation of fistulae or recurrences. These complications seem to be caused by tension placed on the soft tissues during closure, and this tension can be relieved by repair of the symphysis pubis. O'Phelan described the results of bilateral posterior iliac osteotomies and approximation of the symphysis. First osteotomies of the iliac bones near the sacroiliac joints are made. Then 1 week later the symphysis pubis is approximated by sutures. The procedure may be done in one stage instead of two. O'Phelan has altered his wiring technique because in his earlier patients the wire tended to break or cut through the pubic rami. After the symphysis pubis has been reduced and fixed, the urologic structures can be reconstructed without undue tension, and the gait is improved (Fig. 2-100).

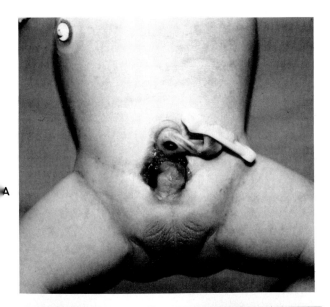
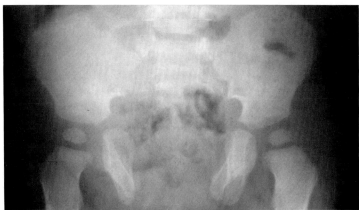
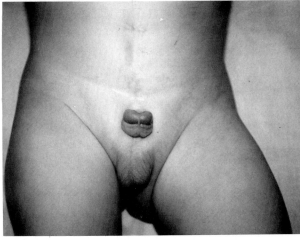
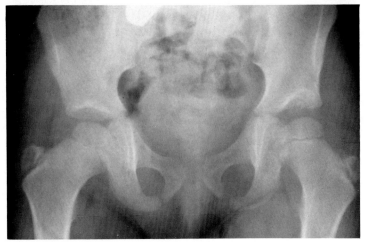

Fig. 2-100 **A,** Congenital exstrophy of bladder in newborn male. **B,** Note pubic diastasis on roentgenogram. **C,** After bilateral posterior iliac osteotomies and anterior reconstruction. **D,** At 5 years of age.

After posterior iliac osteotomy and approximation of the symphysis pubis, the most common complication is cutting of the wire through the symphysis pubis and into the neck of the reconstructed urethra. Because of this possibility, a generous posterior iliac osteotomy is needed to allow the wings of the ilium to be rotated without tension on the symphysis pubis anteriorly. Preoperative CT scans will outline the three-dimensional anatomy of the pelvis and help determine how much rotation of the iliac wings will be required to allow adequate apposition of the symphysis pubis.

This technique has been modified with acceptable results. The procedure is performed in one stage, first the posterior iliac osteotomies, then repair of the anterior structures by a urologic surgeon, and finally repair of the symphysis pubis. A heavy, nonabsorbable suture may be substituted for wire fixation.

◤ *Technique (O'Phelan).* Place the patient prone on the operating table. On one side make a curved incision starting along the lateral part of the posterior iliac crest, extending inferiorly toward the posterosuperior iliac spine, and turning caudally for a short

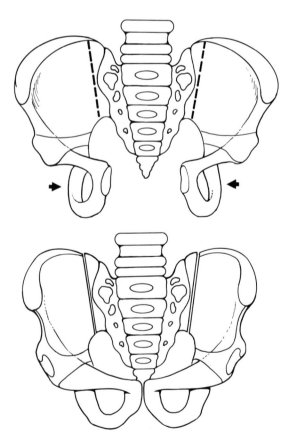

Fig. 2-101 Technique for reconstruction in exstrophy of bladder (see text). (Redrawn from Furnas DW, Haq MA, and Somers G: Plast Reconstr Surg 56:61, 1975.)

distance along the sacroiliac joint. Identify the fascial plane between the sacrospinalis, the quadratus lumborum, and the oblique abdominal muscles medially and superiorly and the gluteal muscles inferiorly. Then detach the gluteal muscles from the ilium by subperiosteal dissection, and retract them laterally to expose the posterior surface of the ilium and the greater sciatic notch. Release the soft tissue attachments on the iliac crest and the cartilaginous epiphysis to expose the anteroposterior thickness of the ilium. Then clear the medial surface of the pelvis down to the sciatic notch. Identify the sciatic notch and carefully insert a blunt retractor into it to provide counterpressure during the osteotomy and to prevent injury to the neurovascular structures. Now with a small osteotome make a vertical osteotomy about 2.5 cm lateral to the sacroiliac joint from the crest of the ilium to the sciatic notch (Fig. 2-101). Divide the bone completely, including both cortices, and use a bone or a laminar spreader to separate the fragments. Unless both cortices are divided, the deformity will recur. Now perform the same procedure on the opposite side. After osteotomies have been performed on both sides, manipulate the pelvis by applying pressure in a medial and anterior direction on both sides to bring the pubic rami together.

If the posterior iliac osteotomies allow easy apposition of the pubic symphysis anteriorly, the anterior reconstruction may be done in the same operative procedure. Place the patient supine, and have the urologic surgeon suitably prepare the operative field and carefully identify the abnormal bladder and urethral structures. When these structures are ready for reconstruction, expose the symphysis pubis and the pubic rami by subperiosteal and subperichondral dissection. Then approximate the symphysis pubis by pushing the pelvis medially on both sides. Circle each superior pubic ramus with a heavy wire loop and tighten each; then place a third wire through each of the first two loops, and with the symphysis approximated tighten this wire appropriately. A heavy, nonabsorbable suture may be used instead of wire loops. After the urologic surgeon has repaired the genitourinary tissues and the abdominal wall, place the patient in a well-molded bilateral spica cast with the hips in neutral rotation to keep the bone and soft structures anteriorly approximated as well as possible.

◤ *Postoperative management.* The cast is worn until there is conclusive roentgenographic evidence that the osteotomies have healed with solid mature bone. This generally will require 4 to 12 weeks, depending on the age of the child. Follow-up evaluation should include careful assessment of hip dysplasia or neurologic impairment in the lower extremities that requires treatment.

Trunk and Upper Extremity

CONGENITAL ELEVATION OF SCAPULA (SPRENGEL DEFORMITY)

In Sprengel deformity the scapula lies more superiorly than it should in relation to the thoracic cage and usually is hypoplastic and misshapen. Other congenital anomalies may be present such as cervical ribs, malformations of ribs, and anomalies of the cervical vertebrae (Klippel-Feil syndrome); rarely one or more scapular muscles are partly or completely absent. Impairment never is severe unless the deformity too is severe. When the deformity is mild, the scapula is only slightly elevated and is a bit smaller than normal, and its motion is only mildly limited, but when it is severe, the scapula is very small and may be so elevated that it almost touches the occiput. The patient's head often is deviated toward the affected side. In about one third of the patients an extra ossicle, the omovertebral bone, is present: this is a rhomboidal plaque of cartilage and bone, lying in a strong fascial sheath, that extends from the superior angle of the scapula to the spinous process, lamina, or transverse process of one or more lower cervical vertebrae.

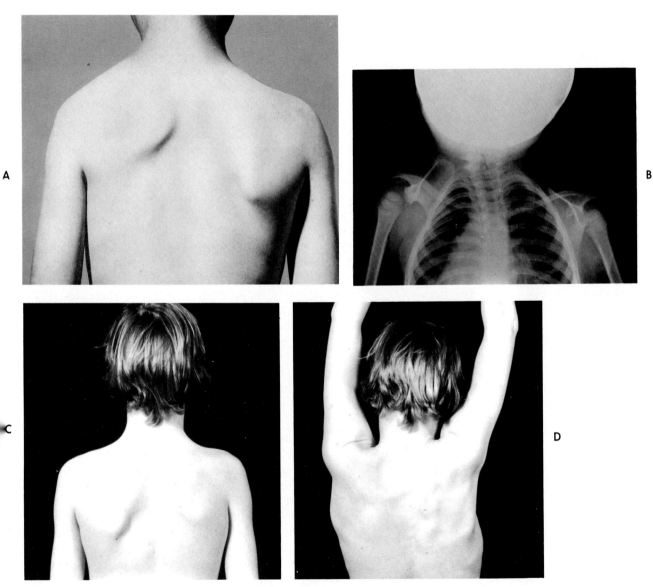

Fig. 2-102　**A,** Sprengel deformity *(left)* in 5-year-old boy. **B,** Posteroanterior roentgenogram shows congenital elevation of left scapula. **C,** Sixteen-year-old boy after Woodward procedure (note midline scar). **D,** Active abduction of shoulders and scapulae.

Sometimes a well-developed joint is found between it and the scapula; sometimes it is attached to the scapula by fibrous tissue only; rarely it makes a solid osseous ridge between the spinal column and the scapula.

When deformity and impairment are mild, no treatment is indicated; when they are more severe, surgery may be indicated, depending on the age of the patient and the severity of any associated deformities. The results of surgery occasionally are disappointing because the deformity is never simply elevation of the scapula alone; it always is complicated by malformations and contractures of the soft structures of the region.

An operation to bring the scapula inferiorly to near its normal position may be attempted after the child is about 3 years of age. However, the earlier surgery is performed after 3 years of age, the better are the results because as the child grows, the operation becomes more difficult and ultimately impossible. In older children an attempt to bring the scapula inferiorly to its normal level may injure the brachial plexus.

Numerous operations have been described to correct Sprengel deformity. Two surgical techniques are commonly used. Green described surgical release of muscles from the scapula along with excision of the supraspinatus portion of the scapula and any omovertebral bone. The scapula then is moved inferiorly to a more normal position and the muscles are reattached. Woodward described transfer of the origin of the trapezius muscle to a more inferior position on the spinous processes. This procedure is generally preferred and is described here (Fig. 2-102).

Brachial plexus palsy is the most severe complication of surgery for Sprengel deformity. The scapula in this deformity is hypoplastic compared with the normal scapula. At surgery attention should be directed at placing the spine of the scapula at the same level as that on the opposite side rather than effecting exact alignment of the inferior angle of the scapulae. Several authors have recommended morcellation of the clavicle on the ipsilateral side as a first step in the surgical treatment of Sprengel deformity to avoid brachial plexus palsy. This is not a routine part of surgical treatment but is recommended in severe deformity or in children who show signs of brachial plexus palsy after surgical correction.

◣ *Technique (Woodward).* Place the patient prone on the operating table, and prepare and drape the shoulder so that both the involved shoulder girdle and the arm can be manipulated. Make a midline incision from the spinous process of the first cervical vertebra distally to that of the ninth thoracic vertebra (Fig. 2-103, *A*). Undermine the skin and subcutaneous tissues laterally to the medial border of the scapula. Next identify the lateral border of the trapezius muscle in the distal end of the incision, and by blunt dissection separate it from the underlying latissimus dorsi muscle. By sharp dissection free the fascial sheath of origin of the trapezius from the spinous processes. Identify the origins of the rhomboideus major and minor muscles, and by sharp dissection free them from the spinous processes. Now free the rhomboids and the superior part of the trapezius from the muscles of the chest wall anterior to them. Retract the freed sheet of muscles laterally to expose any omovertebral bone or fibrous bands attached to the superior angle of the scapula. By extraperiosteal dissection excise any omovertebral bone, or if the bone is absent, excise any fibrous band or contracted levator scapulae muscle; avoid injuring the spinal accessory nerve, the nerves to the rhomboids, or the transverse cervical artery. If the supraspinous part of the scapula is deformed, resect it along with its periosteum; this releases the levator scapulae muscle (if not already excised), allowing the shoulder girdle to move more freely (Fig. 2-103, *B*). Divide transversely the remaining narrow attachment of the trapezius muscle at the level of the fourth cervical vertebra. Now displace the scapula along with the attached sheet of muscles distally until its spine lies at the same level as that of the opposite scapula (Fig. 2-103, *C*). While holding the scapula in this position, reattach the aponeuroses of the trapezius and rhomboid muscles to the spinous processes at a more inferior level. In the distal part of the incision create a fold in the origin of the trapezius muscle, and either excise the excess tissue or incise the fold and overlap and suture in place the resultant free edges (Fig. 2-103, *D*).

◣ *Postoperative management.* A Velpeau bandage is applied and is worn for about 2 weeks. Active and passive range-of-motion exercises are begun.

◣ *Technique for morcellation of clavicle (Robinson et al).* Make a straight incision over the clavicle extending from 1.5 cm lateral to the sternoclavicular joint to 1.5 cm medial to the acromioclavicular joint. Expose the clavicle subperiosteally. Now divide the bone 2 cm from each end, remove it, and cut it into small pieces (morcellate). Then replace the pieces in the periosteal sleeve and close with interrupted sutures. Close the subcutaneous tissues and skin in a routine manner.

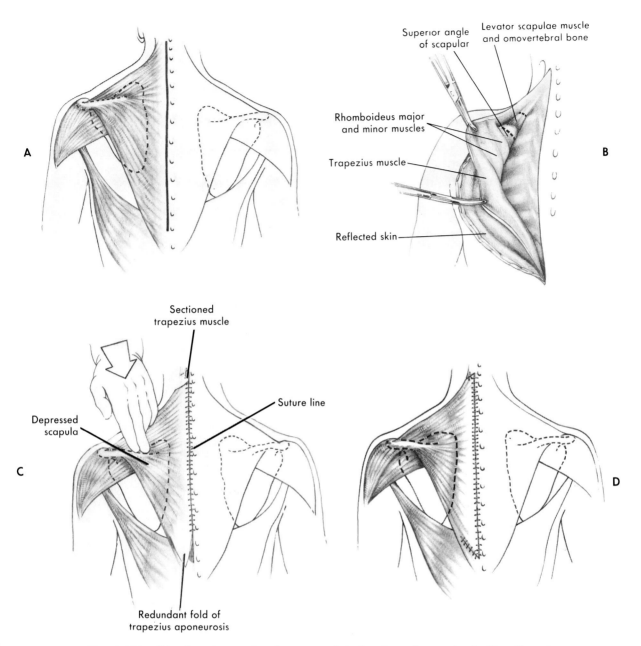

Fig. 2-103 Woodward operation for congenital elevation of scapula. **A,** Elevation of scapula and extensive origin of trapezius; skin incision. **B,** Skin has been incised in midline. Origins of trapezius and of rhomboideus major and minor have been freed from spinous processes, and these muscles have been retracted laterally. Levator scapulae, any omovertebral bone, and any deformed superior angle of scapula are to be excised. **C,** Remaining narrow attachment of trapezius superiorly has been divided at level of C4. Scapula and attached sheet of muscles have been displaced inferiorly, and aponeuroses of trapezius and rhomboids have been reattached to spinous processes at more inferior level. Thus a redundant fold of trapezius aponeurosis in formed inferiorly. **D,** Fold of trapezius aponeurosis has been incised, and resultant free edges have been overlapped and sutured in place. Free superior edge of trapezius also has been sutured. (Modified from Woodward JW: J Bone Joint Surg 43A:219, 1961.)

CONGENITAL TORTICOLLIS

Congenital torticollis, or wryneck, is caused by fibromatosis within the sternocleidomastoid muscle. Its cause is unknown. A mass either is palpable at birth or becomes so, usually during the first 2 weeks. It is more common on the right than on the left side. It may involve the muscle diffusely, but more often it is localized near the clavicular attachment of the muscle. It attains maximum size within 1 or 2 months and then may remain the same size or become smaller; usually it diminishes and disappears within a year. If it fails to disappear, then the muscle becomes permanently fibrotic and contracted and causes torticollis that also is permanent unless treated (Fig. 2-104).

There is a reported incidence of congenital dislocation of the hip or dysplasia of the acetabulum ranging from 7% to 20% in children with torticollis. Careful screening and, if necessary, roentgenographic examination are indicated.

When congenital torticollis is seen in early infancy, it is impossible to tell whether the mass causing it will disappear spontaneously. Consequently during infancy only conservative treatment is indicated. The parents should be instructed to stretch the sternocleidomastoid muscle by manipulating the head manually. Excising the lesion during infancy is unjustified; surgery should be delayed until evolution of the fibromatosis is complete, and then, if necessary, the muscle may be released at one or both ends. Coventry and Harris, in a study of 35 infants with congenital torticollis seen at the Mayo Clinic, found that conservative treatment at home by the family produced excellent results in 30. In only five patients was surgical release of the muscle necessary. The authors believe that if the muscle is still contracted after the child is 1 year old, it should be released, but they also believe that surgery at any age up to 12 years would produce as good a result as operation earlier because asymmetry of the face and skull still could correct itself during the remaining period of growth.

Canale et al evaluated 57 patients with congenital torticollis who were treated between 1941 and 1977. They found that if congenital torticollis persisted beyond the age of 1 year, it did not resolve spontaneously. Children with torticollis who were treated during the first year of life had better results than those treated later, and an exercise program was more likely to be successful when the restriction of motion was less than 30 degrees and there was no facial asymmetry or the facial asymmetry was noted only by the examiner. Nonoperative therapy after the age of 1 year rarely was successful. Regardless of the type of treatment, established facial asymmetry and limitation of motion of more than 30 degrees at the beginning of treatment usually precluded a good result.

Any permanent torticollis slowly becomes worse during growth. The head becomes inclined toward the affected side and the face toward the opposite side. When the deformity is severe, the ipsilateral shoulder becomes elevated, and the frontooccipital diameter of the skull may become shorter than normal. Such severe deformity could and should be prevented by surgery during childhood. Unfortunately many patients are first seen only after the deformities have become fixed and the remaining growth potential is insufficient to correct them.

Several operations have been devised to release the sternocleidomastoid muscle at the clavicle. Unipolar release of the muscle distally is appropriate for mild or moderate deformity. Bipolar release proximally and distally may be indicated for severe torticollis.

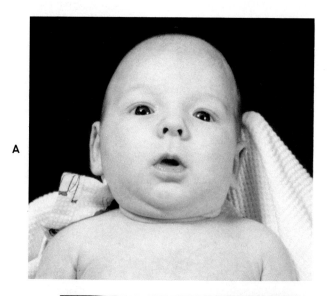

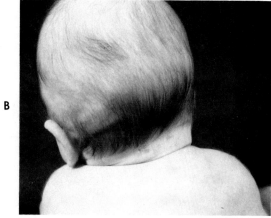

Fig. 2-104 Congenital torticollis *(left)* in 3-month-old female infant. **A,** Anterior view. **B,** Posterior view.

Unipolar release. Ling, in a review of 103 patients treated for torticollis, found that open tenotomy of the sternocleidomastoid muscle could be followed by tethering of the scar to the deep structures, reattachment of the clavicular head or the sternal head of the sternocleidomastoid muscle, loss of contour of the muscle, failure to correct the tilt of the head, or failure of facial asymmetry to correct. Because tethering of the scar to the deep structures is common before the age of 1 year, Ling recommends that the operation be delayed until later, when the child is between the ages of 1 and 4 years.

▶ *Technique.* Make an incision 5 cm long just superior to and parallel to the medial end of the clavicle (Fig. 2-105), and deepen it to the tendons of the sternal and clavicular attachments of the sternocleidomastoid muscle. Incise the tendon sheath longitudinally, and pass a hemostat or other blunt instrument posterior to the tendons. Then by traction on the hemostat draw the tendons outside the wound, and then superior and inferior to the hemostat clamp them and resect 2.5 cm of their inferior ends. If contracted, divide the platysma muscle and adjacent fascia. Then with the head turned toward the affected side and the chin depressed, explore the wound digitally for any remaining bands of contracted muscle or fascia, and if any are found, divide them under direct vision until the deformity can, if possible, be overcorrected. If after this procedure overcorrection is not possible, then make a small transverse incision inferior to the mastoid process and carefully divide the muscle near the bone. Take care to avoid damaging the spinal accessory nerve. Close the wound or wounds, and apply a bulky dressing that holds the head in the overcorrected position.

▶ *Postoperative management.* At 1 week physical therapy, including manual stretching of the neck to maintain the overcorrected position, is begun. Manual stretching should be continued three times daily for 3 to 6 months. During this time the patient may sleep with halter traction on the head. The use of plaster casts or braces usually is unnecessary (Fig. 2-106).

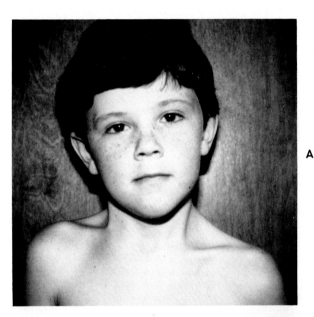

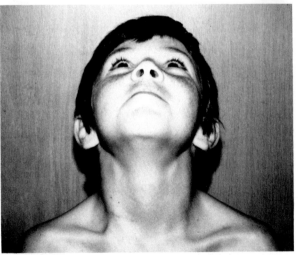

Fig. 2-106 Seven-year-old boy with right torticollis. **A,** Before unipolar supraclavicular release. **B,** Note scar superior to clavicle in transverse line of skin crease.

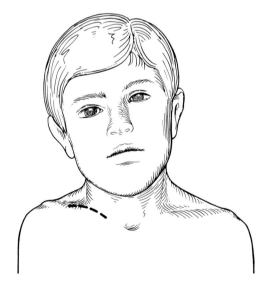

Fig. 2-105 Unipolar release for torticollis. Note line of skin incision.

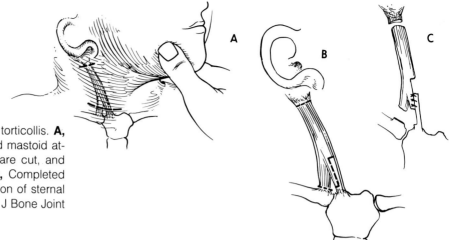

Fig. 2-107 Bipolar Z-plasty operation for torticollis. **A,** Location of skin incisions. **B,** Clavicular and mastoid attachments of sternocleidomastoid muscle are cut, and Z-plasty is performed on sternal origin. **C,** Completed operation; note preservation of medial portion of sternal attachment. (Redrawn from Ferkel RD et al: J Bone Joint Surg 65A:894, 1983.)

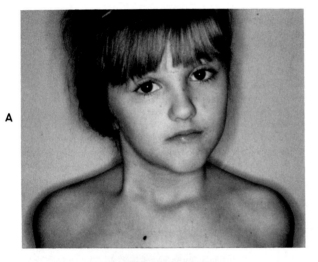

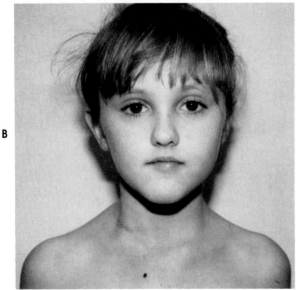

Fig. 2-108 Bipolar release for congenital torticollis. **A,** Severe congenital right torticollis in 8-year-old girl. **B,** After bipolar release.

Bipolar release. Surgical correction in older children with severe deformity or after failed operation usually requires a bipolar release of the sternocleidomastoid muscle. Ferkel et al described a modified bipolar release and Z-plasty of the muscle for use in these circumstances.

▲ *Technique (Ferkel et al).* Make a short transverse proximal incision behind the ear, and divide the sternocleidomastoid muscle insertion transversely just distal to the tip of the mastoid process (Fig. 2-107). With this limited incision the spinal accessory nerve is avoided, although the possibility that the nerve may take an anomalous route is always borne in mind. Then make a distal incision, 4 to 5 cm long in line with the cervical skin creases one fingerbreadth proximal to the medial end of the clavicle and the sternal notch. Divide the subcutaneous tissue and platysma muscle, exposing the clavicular and sternal attachments of the sternocleidomastoid muscle. Carefully avoid the anterior and external jugular veins and the carotid vessels and sheath during the dissection. Then cut the clavicular portion of the muscle transversely, and perform a Z-plasty on the sternal attachment so as to preserve the normal V-contour of the sternocleidomastoid muscle in the neckline. Obtain the desired degree of correction by manipulating the head and neck during the release. Occasionally, release of additional contracted bands of fascia or muscle is necessary before closure. Close both wounds with subcuticular sutures.

▲ *Postoperative management.* Physical therapy, consisting of stretching, muscle strengthening, and active range-of-motion exercises, is instituted in the early postoperative period. Head halter traction or a cervical collar also may be used during the initial 6 to 12 weeks after surgery (Fig. 2-108).

CONGENITAL PSEUDARTHROSIS OF CLAVICLE

Congenital pseudarthrosis of the clavicle is a rare anomaly. Several theories concerning its cause have been proposed. One is that the clavicle develops in two separate masses by medial and lateral ossification centers; thus pseudarthrosis could be explained by failure of ossification of the precartilaginous bridge that normally would connect the two ossification centers. Another is that the lesion may be caused by direct pressure from the subclavian artery on the immature clavicle on the right. In one review, congenital pseudarthrosis of the clavicle was found to occur almost invariably on the right side. In a series of 60 unilateral lesions, 59 were on the right, and in the one patient with a pseudarthrosis on the left, dextrocardia was found.

Pseudarthrosis of the clavicle is present at birth and usually is in the middle third of the clavicle (Fig. 2-109).

Congenital pseudarthrosis of the clavicle requires treatment, not because of hypermobility of the shoulder girdle but usually because it is unsightly. Spontaneous union is unknown, and consequently any desired union requires open reduction and bone grafting. Most surgeons agree that the ideal time for grafting is between the ages of 3 and 5 years. Although it can be performed at any age, the older the patient is, the more difficult is the grafting. Simple resection of the prominent ends of the bone has resulted in pain, prominence of the ends during movements of the shoulder, and asymmetry of the shoulder girdles.

Union is easier to obtain in congenital pseudarthrosis of the clavicle than in that of the tibia. Almost any type of bone grafting suitable for traumatic nonunion of the clavicle has been satisfactory in pseudarthrosis, but open reduction and internal fixation with plate and screws and autogenous iliac bone grafting have produced the best results (Fig. 2-110).

▶ *Technique.* Make a transverse 3-inch (7.5 cm) incision centered over the body of the clavicle, approximately a fingerbreadth above the superior border of the bone. Carry sharp dissection through the subcutaneous tissue to expose the clavicle, both medially and laterally and in the central third in the area of the pseudarthrosis. Expose the bone subperiosteally, taking care to protect the underlying neurovascular structures. Debride the site of the pseudarthrosis of all fibrous and cartilaginous tissue down to normal bone both medially and laterally. Bend a four-hole plate (either semitubular or dynamic compression) to fit the contours of the bone. Then fix the plate to the clavicle in the usual manner. Obtain autogenous iliac grafts, and place them on the superior, inferior, and posterior aspects of the pseudarthrosis. Close the

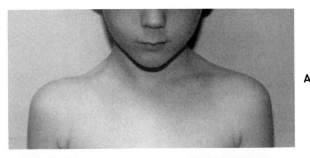
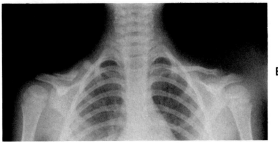

Fig. 2-109   Congenital pseudarthrosis of clavicle. **A,** Subcutaneous prominence in middle third of right clavicle in 4-year-old child. **B,** Pseudarthrosis of right clavicle on roentgenogram.

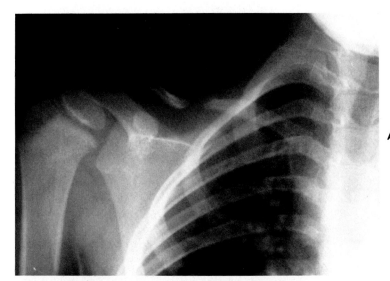
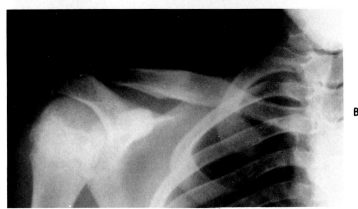

Fig. 2-110   **A,** Congenital pseudarthrosis of right clavicle before plating and bone grafting. **B,** At 7 years of age after plate removal.

wound in layers and the skin with subcuticular sutures.

▶*Postoperative management.* A collar and cuff are worn for 3 to 6 weeks. The plate may be removed at 12 to 24 months when roentgenographic union is present.

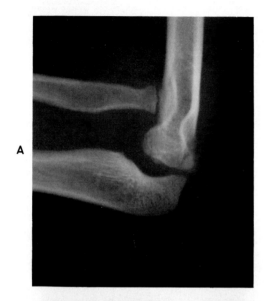
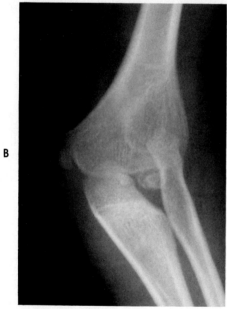

Fig. 2-111   Congenital dislocation of radial head. **A,** Lateral view. **B,** Anteroposterior view.

CONGENITAL DISLOCATION OF RADIAL HEAD

Congenital dislocation of the radial head is rare but should be suspected when the head has been dislocated for a long time but there is no evidence that the ulna has been fractured. The roentgenographic findings are fairly characteristic. The radial shaft is abnormally long, and the ulna is usually abnormally bowed. The radial head is dislocated, frequently posteriorly but sometimes anteriorly, is rounded, showing little if any depression for articulation with the capitellum, and is usually smaller than normal; occasionally there is an area of ossification in the tissues about it. The capitellum also may be small, and the radial notch of the ulna that should articulate with the radial head may be small or absent (Fig. 2-111).

Congenital dislocation of the radial head may be familial, especially on the paternal side. It sometimes is associated with chondroosteodystrophy.

A congenitally dislocated radial head usually is irreducible either manually or surgically because of adaptive changes in the soft tissues and the absence of normal surfaces for articulation with the ulna and humerus. Consequently open reduction of the dislocation and reconstruction of the annular ligament in childhood are inadvisable. Any impairment usually is caused by restriction of rotation of the forearm, and in children physical therapy to improve this motion is the only treatment indicated. If pain persists into adulthood, the radial head and neck may be excised. Any resection of the radial head should be postponed until growth is complete, but even then it may not improve motion because of the contractures of the soft tissues.

CONGENITAL PSEUDARTHROSIS OF RADIUS

Congenital pseudarthrosis of the radius is extremely rare. In patients with neurofibromatosis the pseudarthrosis develops from a cyst in the radius, and patients usually have skin manifestations of neurofibromatosis or a strong family history of the disease.

In each case reported, pseudarthrosis of the radius occurred in the distal third of the bone, and the distal fragment was quite short. Because the lesion is near the distal radial physis, the ends of the bone are attenuated, and the ulna is relatively long, the treatment of choice is dual onlay bone grafting as recommended by Boyd for congenital pseudarthrosis of the tibia (p. 122). This operation restores length, provides a viselike grip on the osteoporotic distal fragment, increases the size of the distal end of the proximal fragment, and usually results in satisfactory union (Fig. 2-112).

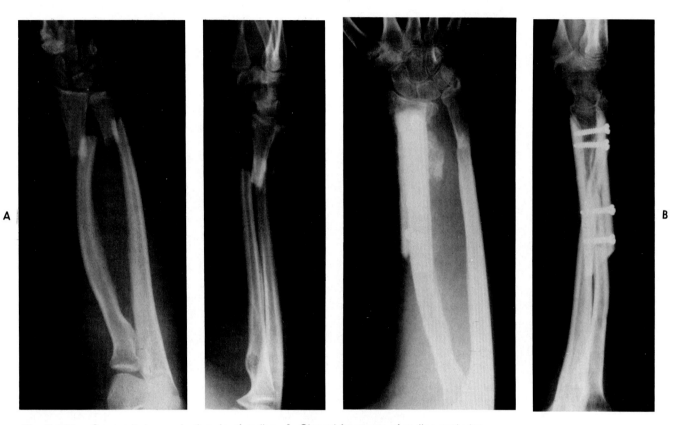

A **B**

Fig. 2-112 Congenital pseudarthrosis of radius. **A,** Closed fractures of radius and ulna in child with manifestations of neurofibromatosis. **B,** Union of radius after treatment by dual onlay bone grafting.

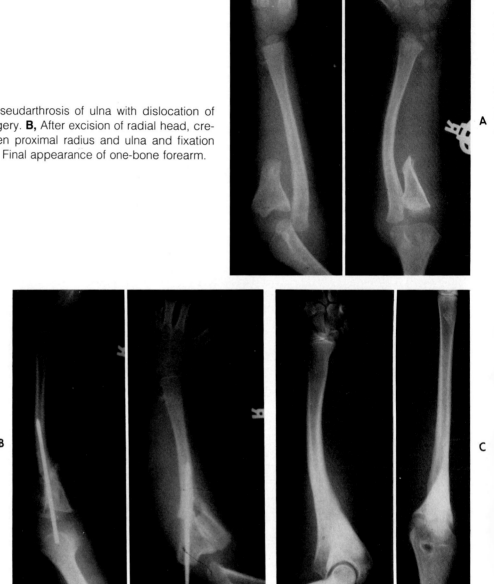

Fig. 2-113   Congenital pseudarthrosis of ulna with dislocation of radial head. **A,** Before surgery. **B,** After excision of radial head, creation of synostosis between proximal radius and ulna and fixation with intramedullary nail. **C,** Final appearance of one-bone forearm.

CONGENITAL PSEUDARTHROSIS OF ULNA

Congenital pseudarthrosis of the ulna in neurofibromatosis is extremely rare. Five patients with solitary ulnar pseudarthroses have been reported, and one patient had involvement of both bones of the distal forearm. One pseudarthrosis of the ulna occurred through a localized lytic lesion similar to type 2 congenital pseudarthrosis of the tibia, and all the others showed sclerotic tapering of the ends of the bones. The ununited ulna produces angulation of the radius, shortening of the forearm, and dislocation of the radial head (Fig. 2-113).

Bone grafting of congenital pseudarthrosis of the ulna usually has failed, but because significant bowing of the radius develops in the very young child, early surgery is indicated. When the pseudarthrosis has developed through a cystic lesion, early curettage of the cyst, internal fixation of the bone, and bone grafting usually are successful. In established pseudarthrosis with tapering of the ends of the bone, the distal ulna should be excised early to relieve its tethering effect on the radius; then the forearm is fitted with a suitable brace. If the radial head dislocates, it should be excised and a synostosis (one-bone forearm) produced between the radius and ulna (Fig. 2-112). Osteotomy of the distal radius to correct bowing also may be indicated.

CONGENITAL RADIOULNAR SYNOSTOSIS

Congenital radioulnar synostosis usually involves the proximal ends of the bones, fixing the forearm in pronation. It more often is bilateral than unilateral. Often there is a familial predisposition, and the deformity seems to be transmitted on the paternal side of the family. Wilkie has noted two types. In the first the medullary canals of the radius and ulna are joined. The proximal end of the radius is malformed and is fused to the ulna for a distance of several centimeters (Fig. 2-114). The radius is longer and larger than the ulna, and its shaft arches anteriorly more than is normal. In the second type the radius is fairly normal, but its proximal end is dislocated either anteriorly or posteriorly and is fused to the proximal ulnar shaft; the fusion is neither as extensive nor as intimate as in the first type. Wilkie states that the second type often is unilateral and that sometimes other deformity, such as a supernumerary thumb, absence of the thumb, or syndactyly, also is present.

Congenital radioulnar synostosis is for several important reasons difficult to treat. The fascial tissues are short and their fibers are abnormally directed, the interosseous membrane is narrow, and the supinator muscles may be abnormal or absent. The anomalies in the forearm may be so widespread that sometimes no rotation is possible, even after the radius and ulna have been separated and the interosseous membrane has been split throughout its length. Simply excising the fused part of the radius never improves function. It is inadvisable to perform any operation with the hope of obtaining pronation and supination. Fortunately most patients are not disabled enough to justify an extensive operation. Any disabling pronation deformity should be corrected by rotational osteotomy; then motion of the shoulder, especially when the elbow is extended, compensates well for the deformity.

A
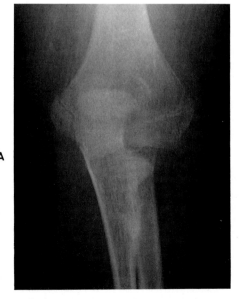

B
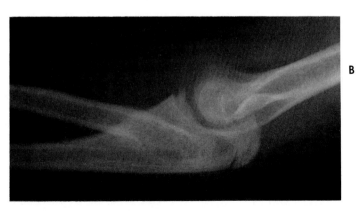

Fig. 2-114   Congenital radioulnar synostosis. **A,** Anteroposterior view. **B,** Lateral view.

REFERENCES
Anomalies of foot
Congenital metatarsus adductus

Berman A and Gartland JJ: Metatarsal osteotomy for the correction of adduction of the fore part of the foot in children, J Bone Joint Surg 53A:498, 1971.

Bleck E: Metatasus adductus: classification and relationship to outcomes of treatment, J Pediatr Orthop 1983.

Heyman CH: The surgical release of fibrous tissue structures resisting correction of congenital clubfoot and metatarsus varus. In American Academy of Orthopaedic Surgeons: Instructional course lectures, vol 16, St Louis, 1959, The CV Mosby Co.

Heyman CH, Herndon CH, and Strong JM: Mobilization of the tarsometatarsal and intermetatarsal joints for the correction of resistant adduction of the fore part of the foot in congenital clubfoot or congenital metatarsus varus, J Bone Joint Surg 40A:299, 1958.

Kendrick RE et al: Tarsometatarsal mobilization for resistant adduction of the fore part of the foot: a follow-up study, J Bone Joint Surg 52A:61, 1970.

Lichtblau S: Section of the abductor hallucis tendon for correction of metatarsus varus deformity, Clin Orthop 110:227, 1975.

Lloyd-Roberts GC and Clark RC: Ball and socket ankle joint in metatarsus adductus varus (S-shaped or serpentine foot), J Bone Joint Surg 55B:193, 1973.

McCormick DW and Blount WP: Metatarsus adductovarus: "skewfoot," JAMA 141:449, 1949.

Ponseti IV and Becker JR: Congenital metatarsus adductus: the results of treatment, J Bone Joint Surg 48A:702, 1966.

Stark JG, Johanson JE, and Winter RB: The Heyman-Herndon tarsometatarsal capsulotomy for metatarsus adductus: result in 48 feet, J Pediatr Orthop 7:305, 1987.

Clubfoot

Abrams RC: Relapsed club foot. The early results of an evaluation of Dillwyn Evans' operation, J Bone Joint Surg 51A:270, 1969.

Addison A, Fixsen JA, and Lloyd-Roberts GC: A review of the Dillwyn Evans type collateral operation in severe clubfeet, J Bone Joint Surg 65B:12, 1983.

Anderson AF and Fowler SB: Anterior calcaneal osteotomy for symptomatic juvenile pes planus, Foot Ankle 4:274, 1984.

Ashby ME: Roentgenographic assessment of soft tissue medial release operations in club foot deformity, Clin Orthop 90:146, 1973.

Bényi P: A modified Lambrinudi operation for drop foot, J Bone Joint Surg 42B:333, 1960.

Björnness T: Congenital clubfoot: a follow-up of 95 persons treated in Sweden from 1940-1945 with special reference to their social adaption and subjective symptoms from the foot, Acta Orthop Scand 46:848, 1975.

Carpenter EB and Huff SH: Selective tendon transfers for recurrent club foot, South Med J 46:220, 1953.

Carroll NC: Congenital clubfoot: pathoanatomy and treatment. In The American Academy of Orthopaedic Surgeons: Instructional course lectures, vol 36, St Louis, 1987, The CV Mosby Co.

Crawford AH, Marxen JL, and Osterfeld DL: The Cincinnati incision: a comprehensive approach for surgical procedures of the foot and ankle in childhood, J Bone Joint Surg 64A:1355, 1982.

Cummings J and Lovell W: Current concepts: operative treatment of congenital idiopathic clubfoot, J Bone Joint Surg 70A:1108, 1988.

Dekel S and Weissman SL: Osteotomy of the calcaneus and concomitant plantar stripping in children with talipes cavo-varus, J Bone Joint Surg 55B:802, 1973.

De Langh R et al.: Treatment of clubfoot by posterior capsulectomy, Clin Orthop 106:248, 1975.

Dillwyn-Evans D: Relapsed club foot, J Bone Joint Surg 43B:722, 1961.

Duckworth T and Smith TWD: The treatment of paralytic convex pes valgus, J Bone Joint Surg 56B:305, 1974.

Dwyer FC: Osteotomy of the calcaneum for pes cavus, J Bone Joint Surg 41B:80, 1959.

Dwyer FC: The treatment of relapsed club foot by the insertion of a wedge into the calcaneum, J Bone Joint Surg 45B:67, 1963.

Dwyer FC: The present status of the problem of pes cavus, Clin Orthop 106:254, 1975.

Fisher RL and Shaffer SR: An evaluation of calcaneal osteotomy in congenital clubfoot and other disorders, Clin Orthop 70:141, 1970.

Galdino MJ Jr et al: Triple arthrodesis in young children: a salvage procedure after failed releases in severely affected feet, Foot Ankle 7:319, 1987.

Garceau GJ: Talipes equino-varus. In American Academy of Orthopaedic Surgeons: Instructional course lectures, vol 7, Ann Arbor, Mich, 1950, JW Edwards Co.

Garceau GJ and Palmer RM: Transfer of the anterior tibial tendon for recurrent club foot: a long-term follow-up, J Bone Joint Surg 49A:207, 1967.

Ghali NN et al: The results of pantalar reduction in the management of congenital talipes equinovarus, J Bone Joint Surg 65B:1, 1983.

Gordon SL and Dunn EJ: Peroneal nerve palsy as a complication of clubfoot treatment, Clin Orthop 101:229, 1974.

Grill F and Franke J: The Ilizarov distractor for the correction of relapsed or neglected clubfoot, J Bone Joint Surg 69B:593, 1987.

Herndon CH and Heyman CH: Problems in the recognition and treatment of congenital convex pes valgus, J Bone Joint Surg 45A:413, 1963.

Hersh A and Fuchs LA: Treatment of the uncorrected clubfoot by triple arthrodesis, Orthop Clin North Am 4:103, 1973.

Herzenberg JE et al: Clubfoot analysis with three-dimensional computer modeling, J Pediatr Orthop 8:257, 1988.

Irani RN and Sherman MS: The pathological anatomy of club foot, J Bone Joint Surg 45A:45, 1963.

Kite JH: Principles involved in treatment of club foot, J Bone Joint Surg 21:595, 1939.

Kite JH: Congenital metatarsus varus (a study based on four hundred cases). In The American Academy of Orthopaedic Surgeons: Instructional course lectures, vol 7, Ann Arbor, Mich, 1950, JW Edwards Co.

Kite JH: Conservative treatment of the resistant recurrent clubfoot, Clin Orthop 70:93, 1970.

Kuhlmann RF: A survey and clinical evaluation of the operative treatment for congenital talipes equinovarus, Clin Orthop 84:88, 1972.

Lambrinudi C: New operation on drop-foot, Br J Surg 15:193, 1927.

Lambrinudi C: A method of correcting equinus and calcaneus deformities at the sub-astragaloid joint, Proc R Soc Med 26:788, 1933.

LaReaux RL and Hosey T: Results of surgical treatment of talipes equino valgus by means of navicular-cuneiform arthrodesis with midcuboid osteotomy, J Foot Surg 26:412, 1987.

Lichtblau S: A medial and lateral release operation for club foot: a preliminary report, J Bone Joint Surg 55A:1377, 1973.

Lloyds-Roberts GC, Swann M, and Catterall A: Medial rotational osteotomy for severe residual deformity in club foot: a preliminary report on a new method of treatment, J Bone Joint Surg 56B:37, 1974.

Lovell WW and Hancock CI: Treatment of congenital talipes equinovarus, Clin Orthop 70:79, 1970.

McKay DW: New concept of and approach to clubfoot treatment. Section I. Principles and morbid anatomy, J Pediatr Orthop 2:347, 1982.

McKay DW: New concept of and approach to clubfoot treatment. Section II. Correction of clubfoot, J Pediatr Orthop 3:10, 1983.

McKay DW: New concept of and approach to clubfoot treatment. Section III. Evaluation and results, J Pediatr Orthop 3:141, 1983.

Ponseti IV and Smoley EN: Congenital club foot: the results of treatment, J Bone Joint Surg 45A:261, 1963.

Porter RW: Congenital talipes equinovarus. I. Resolving and resistant deformities, J Bone Joint Surg 69B:822, 1987.

Reimann I and Becker-Anderson H: Early surgical treatment of congenital clubfoot, Clin Orthop 102:200, 1974.

Reimann I and Werner HH: Congenital metatarsus varus: on the advantages of early treatment, Acta Orthop Scand 46:857, 1975.

Roberts JM: Bone procedures for treatment of persistent clubfoot, Personal communication, 1988.

Sell LS: Tibial torsion accompanying congenital club-foot, J Bone Joint Surg 23:561, 1941.

Silver CM, Simon SD, and Litchman HM: Long-term follow-up observations on calcaneal osteotomy, Clin Orthop 99:181, 1974.

Simons GW: Complete subtalar release in club feet. I. A preliminary report, J Bone Joint Surg 67A:1044, 1985.

Simons GW: Complete subtalar release in club feet. II. Comparison with less extensive procedures, J Bone Joint Surg 67A:1056, 1985.

Tachdjian MO: Congenital convex pes valgus, Orthop Clin North Am 3:131, 1972.

Tayton K and Thompson P: Relapsing club feet: late results of delayed operation, J Bone Joint Surg 61B:474, 1979.

Thompson TC: Astragalectomy and the treatment of calcaneovalgus, J Bone Joint Surg 21:627, 1939.

Toohey JS and Campbell P: Distal calcaneal osteotomy in resistant talipes equinovarus, Clin Orthop 197:224, 1985.

Turco VJ: Surgical correction of the resistant club foot: one-stage posteromedial release with internal fixation: a preliminary report, J Bone Joint Surg 53A:477, 1971.

Turco VJ: Resistant congenital clubfoot. In The American Academy of Orthopaedic Surgeons: Instructional course lectures, vol 24, St Louis, 1975, The CV Mosby Co.

Victoria-Diaz A and Victoria-Diaz J: Pathogenesis of idiopathic clubfoot, Clin Orthop 185:14, 1984.

Weseley MS and Barenfeld PA: Mechanism of the Dwyer calcaneal osteotomy, Clin Orthop 70:137, 1970.

Weseley MS, Barenfeld PA, and Barrett N: Complications of the treatment of clubfoot, Clin Orthop 84:93, 1972.

Wilcox PG and Weiner DS: The Akron midtarsal dome osteotomy in the treatment of rigid pes cavus: a preliminary review, J Pediatr Orthop 5:333, 1985.

Wynne-Davies R: Talipes equinovarus: a review of eighty-four cases after completion of treatment, J Bone Joint Surg 46B:464, 1964.

Zimny ML et al: An electron microscopic study of the fascia from the medial and lateral sides of clubfoot, J Pediatr Orthop 5:577, 1985.

Congenital vertical talus

Becker-Andersen H and Reimann I: Congenital vertical talus: re-evaluation of early manipulative treatment, Acta Orthop Scand 45:130, 1974.

Colton CL: The surgical management of congenital vertical talus, J Bone Joint Surg 55B:566, 1973.

Dunn HK and Samuelson KM: Flat-top talus: a long-term report of twenty club feet, J Bone Joint Surg 56A:57, 1974.

Green NA: One stage release for congenital vertical talus. Paper presented at the meeting of the Pediatric Orthopaedic Society, Hilton Head, SC, May 17-20, 1989.

Grice DS: An extra-articular arthrodesis of the subastragalar joint for correction of paralytic flat feet in children, J Bone Joint Surg 34A:927, 1952.

Grice DS: Further experience with extra-articular arthrodesis of the subtalar joint, J Bone Joint Surg 37A:246, 1955.

Grice DS: The role of subtalar fusion in the treatment of valgus deformities of the feet. In The American Academy of Orthopaedic Surgeons: Instructional course lectures, vol 16, St Louis, 1959, The CV Mosby Co.

Guttman G: Modification of the Grice-Green subtalar arthrodesis in children, J Pediatr Orthop 1:219, 1981.

Harrold AJ: Congenital vertical talus in infancy, J Bone Joint Surg 49B:634, 1967.

Harrold AJ: The problem of congenital verticle talus, Clin Orthop 97:133, 1973.

Jacobsen ST and Crawford AH: Congenital vertical talus, J Pediatr Orthop 3:306, 1983.

Jayakumar S and Cowell HR: Rigid flatfoot, Clin Orthop 122:77, 1977.

Kumar SJ, Cowell HR, and Ramsey PL: Foot problems in children. I. Vertical and oblique talus. In American Academy of Orthopaedic Surgeons: Instructional course lectures, vol 31, St Louis, 1982, The CV Mosby Co.

McCall RE et al: The Grice extraarticular subtalar arthrodesis: a clinical review, J Pediatr Orthop 5:442, 1985.

Scott SM, Janes PC, and Stevens PM: Grice subtalar arthrodesis followed to skeletal maturity, J Pediatr Orthop 8:176, 1988.

Tarsal coalition

Conway JJ and Cowell HR: Tarsal coalition: clinical significance and roentgenographic demonstration, Radiology 92:799, 1969.

Cowell HR: Tarsal coalition: review and update. In American Academy of Orthopaedic Surgeons: Instructional course lectures, vol 31, St Louis, 1982, The CV Mosby Co.

Cowell HR and Elener V: Rigid painful flatfoot secondary to tarsal coalition, Clin Orthop 177:54, 1983.

Danielson LG: Talo-calcaneal coalition treated with resection, J Pediatr Orthop 7:513, 1987.

Harris RI: Rigid valgus foot due to talocalcaneal bridge, J Bone Joint Surg 37A:169, 1955.

Harris RI and Beath T: Etiology of peroneal spastic flatfoot, J Bone Joint Surg 30B:624, 1948.

Herzenberg JE et al: Computerized tomography of talocalcaneal tarsal coalition: a clinical and anatomic study, Foot Ankle 6:273, 1986.

Kumar SJ, Cowell HR, and Ramsey PL: Foot problems in children. I. Vertical and oblique talus. In American Academy of Orthopaedic Surgeons: Instructional course lectures, vol 31, St Louis, 1982, The CV Mosby Co.

Swiotkowski MF, Scranton PE, and Hansen S: Tarsal coalitions: long-term results of surgical treatment, J Pediatr Orthop 3:287, 1983.

Accessory navicular, adolescent hallux valgus, and cleft foot

Cedell CA and Åström M: Proximal metatarsal osteotomy in hallux valgus, Acta Orthop Scand 53:1013, 1982.

Das De S: Distal metatarsal osteotomy for adolescent hallux valgus, J Pediatr Orthop 4:32, 1984.

Gardner RC: Improving operative technique and post-operative course of McBride bunionectomy, Orthop Rev 11(4):35, 1973.

Goldner J and Gaines R: Adult and juvenile hallux valgus: analysis and treatment, Orthop Clin North Am 7:863, 1976.

Hansen C: Hallux valgus treated by the McBride operation, Acta Orthop Scand 45:778, 1974.

Houghton G and Dickson R: Hallux valgus in the younger patient, J Bone Joint Surg 61B:176, 1979.

Kidner FC: The prehallux (accessory scaphoid) in its relation to flatfoot, J Bone Joint Surg 11:831, 1929.

Luba R and Rosman M: Bunions in children: treatment with a modified Mitchell osteotomy, J Pediatr Orthop 4:44, 1984.

McBride E: Hallux valgus bunion deformity. In The American Academy of Orthopaedic Surgeons: Instructional course lectures, vol 9, St Louis, 1952, The CV Mosby Co.

McBride E: Hallux valgus, bunion deformity: its treatment in mild, moderate and severe stage, J Int Coll Surg 21:99, 1954.

McBride E: Surgical treatment of hallux valgus bunions, Am J Orthop Surg 5:44, 1963.

McKeever DC: Arthrodesis of the first metatarsophalangeal joint for hallux valgus, halux rigidus, and metatarsal primus varus, J Bone Joint Surg 34A:129, 1952.

Meyerding HW and Upshaw JE: Heredofamilial cleft foot deformity (lobster-claw or splitfoot), Am J Surg 74:889, 1947.

Schofield S: A modification of McBride's operation for adolescent hallux valgus, J Bone Joint Surg 64B:119, 1982 (abstract).

Scranton PE and Zuckerman JD: Bunion surgery in adolescents: results of surgical treatment, J Pediatr Orthop 4:39, 1984.

Simmonds F and Menelaus M: Hallux valgus in adolescents, J Bone Joint Surg 42B:761, 1960.

Anomalies of toes

Dennyson WG, Bear JN, and Bhoola KD: Macrodactyly in the foot, J Bone Joint Surg [BR] 59B(3):355, 1977.

Diamond LS and Gould VE: Macrodactyl of the foot: surgical syndactyly after wedge resection, South Med J 67:645, 1974.

Farmer AW: Congenital hallux varus, Am J Surg 95:274, 1958.

Kelikian H, Clayton L, and Loseff H: Surgical syndactylia of the toes, Clin Orthop 19:209, 1961.

Lapidus PW: Transplantation of the extensor tendon for correction of the overlapping fifth toe, J Bone Joint Surg 24:555, 1942.

Leonard MH and Rising EE: Syndactylization to maintain correction of overlapping fifth toe, Clin Orthop 43:241, 1965.

Ruiz-Mora, J: Plastic correction of overriding fifth toe, vol 6, Orthopaedic Letters Club, 1954.

Scrase WH: The treatment of dorsal adduction deformities of the fifth toe, J Bone Joint Surg 36B:146, 1954.

Thompson TC: Surgical treatment of disorders of the fore part of the foot, J Bone Joint Surg 46A:1117, 1964.

Venn-Watson EA: Problems in polydactyly of the foot, Orthop Clin North Am 7:909, 1976.

Congenital angular deformities of leg and congenital pseudarthrosis

Aegerter EE: The possible relationship of neurofibromatosis, congenital pseudarthrosis, and fibrous dysplasia. J Bone Joint Surg 32A:618, 1950.

Andersen KS: Congenital pseudarthrosis of the tibia and neurofibromatosis, Acta Orthop Scand 47:108, 1976.

Badgley CE, O'Connor SJ, and Kudner DF: Congenital kyphosocoliotic tibia, J Bone Joint Surg 34A:349, 1952.

Baw S: The transarticular graft for infantile pseudarthrosis of the tibia: a new technique, J Bone Joint Surg 57B:63, 1975.

Boyd HB: Congenital pseudarthrosis: treatment by dual bone grafts, J Bone Joint Surg 23:497, 1941.

Boyd HB: Pathology and natural history of congenital pseudarthrosis of the tibia, Clin Orthop 166:5, 1982.

Boyd HB and Fox KW: Congenital pseudarthrosis: follow-up study after massive bone-grafting, J Bone Joint Surg 30A:274, 1948.

Boyd HB and Sage FP: Congenital pseudarthrosis of the tibia, J Bone Joint Surg 40A:1245, 1958.

Charnley J: Congenital pseudarthrosis of the tibia treated by the intramedullary nail, J Bone Joint Surg 38A:283, 1956.

Crossett LS et al: Congenital pseudarthrosis of the tibia: long-term follow-up, Orthop Trans 10(3):499, 1986, and Clin Orthop August 1989.

Dooley BJ, Menelaus MB, and Paterson DC: Congenital pseudarthrosis and bowing of the fibula, J Bone Joint Surg 56B:739, 1974.

Gordon L, Weulker N, and Jergensen H: Vascularized fibular grafting for the treatment of congenital pseudarthrosis of the tibia, Orthopedics 9:825, 1986.

Grogan DP, Love SM, and Ogden JA: Congenital malformations of the lower extremities, Orthop Clin North Am 18:537, 1987.

Heyman CH, Herndon CH, and Heiple KG: Congenital posterior angulation of the tibia with talipes calcaneus: a long-term report of eleven patients, J Bone Joint Surg 41A:476, 1959.

Hsu LCS et al: Valgus deformity of the ankle in children with fibular pseudarthrosis: results of treatment by bone-grafting of the fibula, J Bone Joint Surg 56A:503, 1974.

Ilizarov GA: The principles of the Ilizarov method, Bull Hosp Jt Dis Orthop Inst 48:1, 1988.

Krida A: Congenital posterior angulation of the tibia: a clinical entity unrelated to congenital pseudarthrosis, Am J Surg 28:98, 1951.

Langenskiöld A: Pseudarthrosis of the fibula and progressive valgus deformity of the ankle in children: treatment by fusion of the distal tibial and fibular metaphyses: review of three cases, J Bone Joint Surg 49A:463, 1967.

Lawsing JF III et al: Congenital pseudarthrosis of the tibia: successful one stage transposition of the fibula into the distal tibia: a case report, Clin Orthop 110:201, 1975.

Leung PC: Congenital pseudarthrosis of the tibia. Three cases treated by free vascularized iliac crest graft, Clin Orthop 175:45, 1983.

Masserman RL, Peterson HA, and Bianco AJ Jr: Congenital pseudarthrosis of the tibia: a review of the literature and 52 cases from the Mayo Clinic, Clin Orthop 99:140, 1974.

McFarland B: Pseudarthrosis of the tibia in childhood, J Bone Joint Surg 33B:36, 1951.

Morrissy RT: Congenital pseudarthrosis of the tibia: factors that affect results, Clin Orthop 166:21, 1982.

Morrissy RT, Riseborough EJ, and Hall JE: Congenital pseudarthrosis of the tibia, J Bone Joint Surg 63B:367, 1981.

Murray HH and Lovell WW: Congenital pseudarthrosis of the tibia: a long-time follow-up study, Clin Orthop 166:14, 1982.

Nimami A et al: Free vascularized fibular grafts in the treatment of congenital pseudarthrosis of the tibia, Microsurgery 8:111, 1987.

Mullay HH and Lovell WW: Congenital pseudarthrosis of the tibia: a long-term follow-up study, Clin Orthop 166:14, 1982.

Paterson D: Treatment of nonunion with a constant direct current: a totally implantable system, Orthop Clin North Am 15:47, 1984.

Paterson DC and Simonis RB: Electrical stimulation in the treatment of congenital pseudarthrosis of the tibia, J Bone Joint Surg 67B:454, 1985.

Pho RWH et al: Free vascularized fibular graft in the treatment of congenital pseudarthrosis of the tibia, J Bone Joint Surg 67B:64, 1985.

Purvis GD and Holder JE: Dual bone graft for congenital pseudarthrosis of the tibia: variations of technic, South Med J 53:926, 1960.

Rathgeb JM, Ramsey PL, and Cowell HR: Congenital kyphoscoliosis of the tibia, Clin Orthop 103:178, 1974.

Sharrard WJW: Treatment of congenital and infantile pseudarthrosis of the tibia with pulsing electromagnetic fields, Orthop Clin North Am 15:143, 1984.

Sofield HA: Congenital psuedarthrosis of the tibia, Clin Orthop 76:33, 1971.

Sofield HA and Millar EA: Fragmentation realignment, and intramedullary rod fixation of deformities of the long bones in children: a ten-year appraisal, J Bone Joint Surg 41A:1371, 1959.

Umber JS and Coleman SS: Congenital pseudoarthrosis of the tibia (abstract), Orthop Trans 2:212, Nov 1978.

Umber JS, Moss SW, and Coleman SS: Surgical treatment of congenital pseudarthrosis of the tibia, Clin Orthop 166:28, 1982.

Weiland AJ: Elective microsurgery for orthopaedic reconstruction. III. Vascularized bone transfers. In The American Academy of Orthopaedic Surgeons: Instructional course lectures, vol 33, St Louis, 1984, The CV Mosby Co.

Constrictures of leg

Cozen L and Brockway A: Z-plasty procedure for release of constriction rings. In Operative orthopedic clinics, Philadelphia, 1955, JB Lippincott Co.

Peet EW: Congenital constriction bands. In Rob C and Smith R, editors: Operative surgery, part 10, Philadelphia, 1959, FA Davis Co.

Sarnat BG and Kagan BM: Prenatal constricting band and pseudoarthrosis of the lower leg, Plast Reconstr Surg 47:547, 1971.

Congenital hyperextension and dislocation of knee

Bell MJ, Atkins RM, and Sharrard WJW: Irreducible congenital dislocation of the knee: aetiology and management, J Bone Joint Surg 69B:403, 1987.

Curtis BH and Fisher RL: Congenital hyperextension with anterior subluxation of the knee: surgical treatment and long-term observations, J Bone Joint Surg 51A:255, 1969.

Ferris B and Aichroth P: The treatment of congenital knee dislocation: a review of nineteen knees, Clin Orthop 216:136, 1987.

Johnson E, Audell R, and Oppenheim WL: Congenital dislocation of the knee, J Pediatr Orthop 7:194, 1987.

Katz MP, Grogono BJ, and Soper KC: The etiology and treatment of congenital dislocation of the knee, J Bone Joint Surg 49B:112, 1967.

Niebauer JJ and King DE: Congenital dislocation of the knee, J Bone Joint Surg 42A:207, 1960.

Nogi J and MacEwen GD: Congenital dislocation of the knee, J Pediatr Orthop 2:509, 1982.

Roach JW and Richards BS: Instructional case: congenital dislocation of the knee, J Pediatr Orthop 8:226, 1988.

Congenital dislocation of patella

Green JP and Waugh W: Congenital lateral dislocation of the patella, J Bone Joint Surg 50B:285, 1968.

McCall RE and Lessenberry HB: Case report: bilateral congenital dislocation of the patella, J Pediatr Orthop 7:100, 1987.

Stanisavljevic S, Zemenick G, and Miller D: Congenital, irreducible, permanent lateral dislocation of the patella, Clin Orthop 116:190, 1975.

Støren H: Congenital complete dislocation of patella causing serious disability in childhood: the operative treatment, Acta Orthop Scand 36:301, 1965.

Congenital and developmental dislocation of hip

Artz TD et al: Neonatal diagnosis, treatment and related factors of congenital dislocation of the hip, Clin Orthop 110:112, 1975.

Ashley KR, Larsen LJ, and James PM: Reduction of dislocation of the hip in older children: a preliminary report, J Bone Joint Surg 54A:545, 1972.

Barlow TG: Early diagnosis and treatment of congenital dislocation of the hip, J Bone Joint Surg 44B:292, 1962.

Berman L, Catterall A, and Meire HB: Ultrasound of the hip: a review of the applications of a new technique, Br J Radiol 59:13, 1986.

Betz RR et al: Long-term follow-up of Chiari pelvic osteotomies for dysplastic hips, Orthop Trans 8:394, 1984 (abstract).

Bos CFA et al: Magnetic resonance imaging in congenital dislocation of the hip, J Bone Joint Surg 70B:174, 1988.

Bowen J and Kasser J: The pelvic harness, Wilmington, Del, 1982, AI duPont Institute (pamphlet).

Browning WH, Rosenkrantz H, and Tarquinio T: Computed tomography in congenital hip dislocation. The role of acetabular anteversion, J Bone Joint Surg 64A:27, 1982.

Bucholz RW and Ogden JA: Patterns of ischemic necrosis of the proximal femur in nonoperatively treated congenital hip disease. In The Hip: Proceedings of the sixth open scientific meeting of The Hip Society, St Louis, 1978, The CV Mosby Co.

Canale ST et al: Pelvic displacement osteotomy for chronic hip dislocation in myelodysplasia, J Bone Joint Surg 57A:177, 1975.

Castelein RM and Sauter AJM: Ultrasound screening for congenital dysplasia of the hip in newborns: its value, J Pediatr Orthop 8:666, 1988.

Chiari K: Pelvic osteotomy as shelf operation. Paper presented at the meeting of the Neuvième Congrès Internationale de Chirurgia Orthopédique, Wien (Hofburg), 1963.

Chiari K: Medial displacement osteotomy of the pelvis, Clin Orthop 98:55, 1974.

Chuinard EG: Femoral osteotomy in the treatment of congenital dysplasia of the hip, Orthop Clin North Am 3:157, 1972.

Coleman SS: The incomplete pericapsular (Pemberton) and innominate (Salter) osteotomies: a complete analysis, Clin Orthop 98:116, 1974.

Coleman SS: Treatment of congenital dislocation of the hip in the older child. In Ahstrom JP, editor: Current practice in orthopaedic surgery, vol 6, St Louis, 1975, The CV Mosby Co.

Coleman SS: Congenital dysplasia and dislocation of the hip. St Louis, 1978, The CV Mosby Co.

Coleman SS: Classics in orthopaedics. Diagnosis and treatment of congenital hip dislocation. Paper presented at the sixth annual meeting of the Mid-America Orthopaedic Association, Tucson, March 16-20, 1988.

Coleman SS and MacEwen GD: Congenital dislocation of the hip in infancy, In The American Academy of Orthopaedic Surgeons: Instructional course lectures, vol 21, St Louis, 1972, The CV Mosby Co.

Colton CL: Chiari osteotomy for acetabular dysplasia in young subjects, J Bone Joint Surg 54B:578, 1972.

Dega W, Król J, and Polakowski L: Surgical treatment of congenital dislocation of the hip in children: a one-stage procedure, J Bone Joint Surg 41A:920, 1959.

Denton JR and Ryder CT: Radiographic follow-up of Salter innominate osteotomy for congenital dysplasia of the hip, Clin Orthop 98:210, 1974.

Edelson JG et al: Congenital dislocation of the hip and computerized axial tomography, J Bone Joint Surg 66B:472, 1984.

Eppright RH: Dial osteotomy of the acetabulum, J Bone Joint Surg 58A:283, 1976.

Exner GU: Ultrasound screnning for hip dysplasia in neonates, J Pediatr Orthop 8:656, 1988.

Eyre-Brook AL, Jones DA, and Harris FC: Pemberton's acetabuloplasty for congenital dislocation or subluxation of the hip, J Bone Joint Surg 60B:18, 1978.

Ferguson AB Jr: Primary open reduction of congenital dislocation of the hip using a median adductor approach, J Bone Joint Surg 55A:671, 1973.

Fletcher RR and Johnson CE II: Greater trochanteric advancement for the treatment of coxa brevis associated with congenital dislocation of the hip, Orthopedics 8:519, 1985.

Frank GR and Michael HR: Treatment of congenital dislocation of the hip: results obtained with the Pemberton and Salter osteotomies, South Med J 60:975, 1967.

Frankel CJ: Results of treatment of irreducible congenital dislocation of the hip by arthrodesis, J Bone Joint Surg 30A:422, 1948.

Gage JR and Winter RB: Avascular necrosis of the capital femoral epiphysis as a complication of closed reduction of congenital dislocation of the hip: a critical review of twenty years' experience at Gillette Children's Hospital, J Bone Joint Surg 54A:373, 1972.

Galeazzi R: Uber die Torsion des verrenkten oberen Femurendes und ihre Beseitigung, Verh Dtsch Ges Orthop Chir, p. 334, 1910.

Galpin RD et al: One-stage treatment of congenital dislocation of the hip, including femoral shortening, J Bone Joint Surg 71A:734, 1989.

Graf R: Sonographie der Sauglinshufte Bucherei des Orthopaden, Stuttgart, FRG, 1985, Ferdinand Enke Verlag.

Gregosiewicz A and Wośko I: Risk factors of avascular necrosis in the treatment of congenital dislocation of the hip, J Pediatr Orthop 8:17, 1988.

Grill F et al: The Pavlik harness in the treatment of congenital dislocating hip: report on a multicenter study of the European Paediatric Orthopaedic Society, J Pediatr Orthop 8:1, 1988.

Gruel CR et al: Teratologic dislocation of the hip, J Pediatr Orthop 6:693, 1986.

Harris NH, Lloyd-Roberts GC, and Gallien R: Acetabular development in congenital dislocation of the hip: with special reference to the indications for acetabuloplasty and pelvic or femoral realignment osteotomy, J Bone Joint Surg 57B:46, 1975.

Henard DC and Calandruccio RA: Experimental production of roentgenographic and histological changes in the capital femoral epiphysis following abduction, extension and internal rotation of the hip, J Bone Joint Surg 52A:601, 1970 (abstract).

Hilgenreiner H: Zur Fruhdiagnose und Fruhbehandlung der angeborenen Huftgelenkverrenkung, Med Clin 21:1385, 1925.

Hoffman DV, Simmons EH, and Barrington TW: The results of the Chiari osteotomy, Clin Orthop 98:162, 1974.

Ilfeld FW et al: Postnatal developmental dislocation of the hip. Poster exhibit, presented at the annual meeting of The American Academy of Orthopaedic Surgeons, Las Vegas, Feb 1989.

Jones DA: Sub-capital coxa valga after varus osteotomy for congenital dislocation of the hip: a report of six cases with a minimum follow-up of nine years, J Bone Joint Surg 59B:152, 1977.

Kalamchi A and MacEwen GD: Avascular necrosis following treatment of congenital dislocation of the hip, J Bone Joint Surg 62A:876, 1980.

Kalamchi A and MacFarlane R III: The Pavlik harness: results in patients over three months of age, J Pediatr Orthop 2:3, 1982.

Kasser JR, Bowen JR, and MacEwen GD: Varus derotation osteotomy in the treatment of persistent dysplasia in congenital dislocation of the hip, J Bone Joint Surg 67A:195, 1985.

Klisić P and Jankovic L: Combined procedure of open reduction and shortening of the femur in treatment of congenital dislocation of the hips in older children, Clin Orthop 119:60, 1976.

Klisić P, Jankovic L, and Basara V: Long-term results of combined operative reduction of the hip in older children, J Pediatr Orthop 8:532, 1988.

Kumar SJ: Hip spica application for the treatment of congenital dislocation of the hip, J Pediatr Orthop 1:97, 1981.

Lang P et al: Three-dimensional CT and MR imaging in congenital dislocation of the hip: clinical and technical considerations, J Comput Assist Tomogr 12:459, 1988.

Magilligan DJ: Calculation of the angle of anteversion by means of horizontal lateral roentgenography, J Bone Joint Surg 38A:1231, 1956.

Mau H et al: Open reduction of congenital dislocation of the hip by Ludloff's method, J Bone Joint Surg 53A:1281, 1971.

McKay DW: A comparison of the innominate and the pericapsular osteotomy in the treatment of congenital dislocation of the hip, Clin Orthop 98:124, 1974.

Mitchell GP: Arthrography in congenital displacement of the hip, J Bone Joint Surg 45B:88, 1963.

Mitchell GP: Chiari medial displacement osteotomy, Clin Orthop 98:146, 1974.

Moen C and Lindsey RW: Computerized tomography with routine arthrography in early evaluation of congenital hip dysplasia, Orthop Rev 15:71, 1986.

Monticelli G: Intertrochanteric femoral osteotomy with concentric reduction of the femoral head in treatment of residual congenital acetabular dysplasia, Clin Orthop 119:48, 1976.

Mubarak SJ, Leach J, and Wenger DR: Management of congenital dislocation of the hip in the infant, Contemp Orthop 15:29, 1987.

O'Hara JN, Bernard AA, and Dwyer N St JP: Early results of medial approach open reduction in congenital dislocation of the hip: use before walking age, J Pediatr Orthop 8:288, 1988.

Ortolani M: Congenital hip dysplasia in the light of early and very early diagnosis, Clin Orthop 119:6, 1976.

Paterson DC: Innominate osteotomy: its role in the treatment of congenital dislocation and subluxation of the hip joint, Clin Orthop 98:198, 1974.

Pemberton PA: Pericapsular osteotomy of the ilium for treatment of congenital subluxation and dislocation of the hip, J Bone Joint Surg 47A:65, 1965.

Pemberton PA: Pericapsular osteotomy of the ilium for the treatment of congenitally dislocated hips, Clin Orthop 98:41, 1974.

Pérez A and Noguera JG: Experience with innominate osteotomy (Salter) and medial displacement osteotomy (Chiari) in the treatment of acetabular dysplasia: preliminary report of 82 operations, Clin Orthop 98:133, 1974.

Perkins G: Signs by which to diagnose congenital dislocation of the hip, Lancet 1:648, 1928.

Peterson HA et al: The use of computerized tomography in dislocation of the hip and femoral neck anteversion in children, J Bone Joint Surg 63B:198, 1981.

Ponseti I: Non-surgical treatment of congenital dislocation of the hip, J Bone Joint Surg 48A:1392, 1966.

Race C and Herring JA: Congenital dislocation of the hip: evaluation of closed reduction, J Pediatr Orthop 3:166, 1983.

Ramsey PL, Lasser S, and MacEwen GD: Congenital dislocation of the hip: use of the Pavlik harness in the child during the first six months of life, J Bone Joint Surg 58A:1000, 1976.

Ring PA: The treatment of unreduced congenital dislocation of the hip in adults, J Bone Joint Surg 41B:299, 1959.

Roth A, Gibson DA, and Hall JE: The experience of five orthopedic surgeons with innominate osteotomy in the treatment of congenital dislocation and subluxation of the hip, Clin Orthop 98:178, 1974.

Saies AD, Foster BK, and Lequesne GW: The value of a new ultrasound stress test in assessment and treatment of clinically detected hip instability, J Pediatr 8:436, 1988.

Salter RB: Innominate osteotomy in the treatment of congenital dislocation and subluxation of the hip, J Bone Joint Surg 43B:518, 1961.

Salter RB: Role of innominate osteotomy in the treatment of congenital dislocation and subluxation of the hip in the older child, J Bone Joint Surg 48A:1413, 1966.

Salter RB: Specific guidelines in the application of the principle of innominate osteotomy, Orthop Clin North Am 3:149, 1972.

Salter RB: Editorial comment: osteotomy of the pelvis, Clin Orthop 98:2, 1974.

Salter RB and Dubos JP: The first fifteen years' personal experience with innominate osteotomy in the treatment of congenital dislocation and subluxation of the hip, Clin Orthop 98:72, 1974.

Salter RB, Hansson G, and Thompson GH: Innominate osteotomy in the management of residual congenital subluxation of the hip in young adults, Clin Orthop 182:53, 1984.

Salvati EA and Wilson PD: Treatment of irreducible hip subluxation by Chiari's iliac osteotomy: a report of results in 19 cases, Clin Orthop 98:151, 1974.

Schoenecker PL and Strecker WB: Congenital dislocation of the hip in children: comparison of the effects of femoral shortening and of skeletal traction in treatment, J Bone Joint Surg 66A:21, 1984.

Schwartz DR: Acetabular development after reduction of congenital dislocation of the hip: a follow-up study of fifty hips, J Bone Joint Surg 47A:705, 1965.

Serafinov L: Biomechanical influence of the innominate osteotomy on the growth of the upper part of the femur, Clin Orthop 98:39, 1974.

Severin E: Congenital dislocation of the hip: development of the joint after closed reduction, J Bone Joint Surg 32A:507, 1950.

Shih C-H and Shih H-N: One-stage combined operation of congenital dislocation of the hips in older children, J Pediatr Orthop 8:535, 1988.

Smith WS et al: Correlation of postreduction roentgenograms and thirty-one-year follow-up in congenital dislocation of the hip, J Bone Joint Surg 50A:1081, 1968.

Somerville EW: Development of congenital dislocation of the hip, J Bone Joint Surg 35B:568, 1953.

Somerville EW: Open reduction in congenital dislocation of hip, J Bone Joint Surg 35B:363, 1953.

Somerville EW: Results of treatment of 100 congenitally dislocated hips, J Bone Joint Surg 49B:258, 1967.

Somerville EW: A long-term follow-up of congenital dislocation of the hip, J Bone Joint Surg 60B:25, 1978.

Somerville EW and Scott JC: The direct approach to congenital dislocation of the hip, J Bone Joint Surg 39B:623, 1957.

Staheli LT: Technique: slotted acetabular augmentation, J Pediatr Orthop 1:321, 1981.

Steel HH: Triple osteotomy of the innominate bone, J Bone Joint Surg 55A:343, 1973.

Szöke N, Kühll L, and Heinrichs J: Ultrasound examination in the diagnosis of congenital hip dysplasia of newborns, J Pediatr Orthop 8:12, 1988.

Toby EB et al: Postoperative computed tomographic evaluation of congenital hip dislocation, J Pediatr Orthop 7:667, 1987.

Trevor D, Johns DL, and Fixsen JA: Acetabuloplasty in the treatment of congenital dislocation of the hip, J Bone Joint Surg 57B:167, 1975.

Utterback TD and MacEwen GD: Comparison of pelvic osteotomies for the surgical correction of the congenital hip, Clin Orthop 98:104, 1974.

Viere R et al: Use of the Pavlik harness in the treatment of CDH: an analysis of treatment failures. Paper presented at the annual meeting of the Pediatric Orthopaedic Society of North America, Colorado Springs, Colo, May 5-8, 1988.

von Rosen S: Further experience with congenital dislocation of the hip in the newborn, J Bone Joint Surg 50B:538, 1968.

Wagner H: Osteotomies for congenital hip dislocation. In The Hip Society: Proceedings of the fourth open scientific meeting of The Hip Society, 1976, St Louis, 1976, The CV Mosby Co.

Wagner H: Femoral osteotomies for congenital hip dislocation. In Weil VH, editor: Progress in orthopaedic surgery, vol 2, Berlin, 1978, Springer-Verlag.

Waters P et al: Salter innominate osteotomies in congenital dislocation of the hip, J Pediatr Orthop 8:650, 1988.

Weinstein SL and Ponseti IV: Congenital dislocation of the hip: open reduction through a medial approach, J Bone Joint Surg 61A:119, 1979.

Wenger DR: Congenital hip dislocation: techniques for primary open reduction including femoral shortening. In AADS Instr Course Lect 38:343, 1989.

Wynne-Davies R: Acetabular dysplasia and familial joint laxity: two etiological factors in congenital dislocation of the hip. A review of 589 patients and their families, J Bone Joint Surg 52B:704, 1970.

Congenital and developmental coxa vara

Amstutz HC and Wilson PD Jr: Dysgenesis of the proximal femur (coxa vara) and its surgical management, J Bone Joint Surg 44A:1, 1962.

Fisher RL and Waskowitz WJ: Familial developmental coxa vara, Clin Orthop 86:2, 1972.

Kalamchi A, Cowell HR, and Kim KI: Congenital deficiency of the femur, J Pediatr Orthop 5(2):129, 1985.

Ogden JA et al: Proximal femoral epiphysiolysis in the neonate, J Pediatr Orthop 4(3):285, 1984.

Pappas AM: Congenital abnormalities of the femur and related lower extremity malformations: classification and treatment, J Pediatr Orthop 3(1):45, 1983.

Richie MF and Johnston CE II: Management of developmental coxa vara in cleidocranial dysostosis, Orthopedics 12(7):1001, 1989.

Weinstein JN, Kuo KN, and Millar EA: Congenital coxa vara: a retrospective review: J Pediatr Orthop 4(1):70, 1984.

Exstrophy of bladder

Aadalen RJ et al: Exstrophy of the bladder: long-term results of bilateral posterior iliac osteotomies and two stage anterior repair, Orthop Trans 1:93, May 1977 (abstract).

Aadlen RJ et al: Exstrophy of the bladder: long-term results of bilateral posterior iliac osteotomies and two-stage anatomic repair, Clin Orthop 151:193, 1980.

Cracciolo A III and Hall CB: Bilateral iliac osteotomy: the first stage in repair of exstrophy of the bladder, Clin Orthop 68:156, 1970.

Furnas DW, Haq MA, and Somers G: One-stage reconstruction for exstrophy of the bladder in girls, Plast Reconstr Surg 56:61, 1975.

Grotte G and Sevastikoglou JA: A modified technique for pelvic reconstruction in the treatment of exstrophy of the bladder, Acta Orthop Scand 37:197, 1966.

O'Phelan EH: Iliac osteotomy in exstrophy of the bladder, J Bone Joint Surg 45A:1409, 1963.

Congenital elevation of scapula (Sprengel deformity)

Cavendish ME: Congenital elevation of the scapula, J Bone Joint Surg 54B:395, 1972.

Chung SMK and Farahvar H: Surgery of the clavicle in Sprengel's deformity, Clin Orthop 116:138, 1976.

Chung SMK and Nissenbaum MM: Congenital and developmental defects of the shoulder, Orthop Clin North Am 6:381, 1975.

Halley DK and Eyring EJ: Congenital elevation of the scapula in a family, Clin Orthop 97:31, 1973.

Galpin RD and Birch JG: Congenital elevation of the scapula (Sprengel's deformity), Orthopedics 10(6):965, 1987.

McClure JG and Raney RB: Anomalies of the scapula, Clin Orthop 110:22, 1975.

Robinson RA et al: The surgical importance of the clavicular component of Sprengel's deformity, J Bone Joint Surg 49A1481, 1967 (abstract).

Woodward JW: Congenital elevation of the scapula: correction by release and transplantation of muscle origins: a preliminary report, J Bone Joint Surg 43A:219, 1961.

Congenital torticollis

Canale ST, Griffin DW, and Hubbard CN: Congenital muscular torticollis: a long-term follow-up, J Bone Joint Surg 64A:810, 1982.

Coventry MB and Harris L: Congenital muscular torticollis in infancy: some observations regarding treatment, J Bone Joint Surg 41A:815, 1959.

Ferkel RD et al: Muscular torticollis: a modified surgical approach, J Bone Joint Surg 65A:894, 1983.

Hummer CD Jr and MacEwen GD: The coexistence of torticollis and congenital dysplasia of the hip, J Bone Joint Surg 54A:1255, 1972.

Ling CM: The influence of age on the results of open sternomastoid tenotomy in muscular torticollis, Clin Orthop 116:142, 1976.

Congenital pseudarthrosis of clavicle, radius, and ulna

Ali MS and Hooper G: Congenital pseudarthrosis of the ulna due to neurofibromatosis, J Bone Joint Surg [Br] 64(5):600, 1982

Aegerter EE: The possible relationship of neurofibromatosis, congenital pseudarthrosis, and fibrous dysplasia, J Bone Joint Surg 32A:618, 1950.

Alldred AJ: Congenital pseudarthrosis of the clavicle, J Bone Joint Surg 45B:312, 1963.

Baldwin DM and Weiner DS: Congenital bowing and intraosseous neurofibroma of the ulna: a case report, J Bone Joint Surg 56A:803, 1974.

Bargar WL, Marcus RE, and Ittleman FP: Late thoracic outlet syndrome secondary to pseudarthrosis of the clavicle, J Trauma 24(9):857, 1984.

Bayne LG: Congenital pseudarthrosis of the forearm, Hand Clin 1(3):457, 1985.

Bell DF: Congenital forearm pseudarthrosis: report of six cases and review of the literature, J Pediatr Orthop 9(4):438, 1989.

Boyd HB: Congenital pseudarthrosis: treatment by dual bone grafts, J Bone Joint Surg 23:497, 1941.

Boyd HB and Fox KW: Congenital pseudarthrosis: follow-up study after massive bone-grafting, J Bone Joint Surg 30A:274, 1948.

Brooks S: Bilateral congenital pseudarthrosis of the clavicles: case report and review of the literature, Br J Clin Pract 38(11-12):432, 1984.

Burge P and Benson M: Bilateral congenital pseudarthrosis of the olecranon, J Bone Joint Surg [Br] 69(3):460, 1987.

Fabry G et al: Treatment of congenital pseudarthrosis with the Ilizarov technique, J Pediatr Orthop 8(1):67, 1988.

Gallien R: Accessory bone at the insertion of the levator scapulae muscle in a Sprengel deformity, J Pediatr Orthop 5(3):352, 1985.

Gibson DA and Carroll N: Congenital pseudarthrosis of the clavicle, J Bone Joint Surg 52B:629, 1970.

Greenberg LA and Schwartz A: Congenital pseudarthrosis of the distal radius, South Med J 68:1053, 1975.

Herman S: Congenital bilateral pseudarthrosis of the clavicles, Clin Orthop 91:162, 1973.

Herring JA and Roach JW: Congenital pseudarthrosis of the radius (clinical conference), J Pediatr Orthop 5(3):367, 1985.

Lloyd-Roberts GC, Apley AG, and Owen R: Reflections upon the aetiology of congenital pseudarthrosis of the clavicle: with a note on cranio-cleido dysostosis, J Bone Joint Surg 57B:24, 1975.

Lombard JJ: Pseudarthrosis of the clavicle: a case report, S Afr Med J 66(4):151, 1984.

Ostrowski DM: Congenital pseudarthrosis of the forearm [letter], J Hand Surg [Am] 14(2 Pt 1):318, 1989.

Ostrowski DM, Eilert RE, and Waldstein G: Congenital pseudarthrosis of the ulna: a report of two cases and a review of the literature, J Pediatr Orthop 5(4):463, 1985.

Owen R: Congenital pseudarthrosis of the clavicle, J Bone Joint Surg 52B:644, 1970.

Richin PF et al: Congenital pseudarthrosis of both bones of the forearm: a case report, J Bone Joint Surg 58A:1032, 1976.

Schnall SB, King JD, and Marrero G: Congenital pseudarthrosis of the clavicle: a review of the literature and surgical results of six cases, J Pediatr Orthop 8(3):316, 1988.

Sellers DS et al: Congenital pseudarthrosis of the forearm, J Hand Surg [Am] 13(1):89, 1988.

Sofield HA and Millar EA: Fragmentation, realignment, and intramedullary rod fixation of deformities of the long bones in children: a ten-year appraisal, J Bone Joint Surg 41A:1371, 1959.

Sprague BL and Brown GA: Congenital pseudarthrosis of the radius, J Bone Joint Surg 56A:191, 1974.

Wall JJ: Congenital pseudarthrosis of the clavicle, J Bone Joint Surg 52A:1003, 1970.

Zaman M: Pseudoarthrosis of the radius associated with neurofibromatosis: a case report, J Bone Joint Surg 59A:977, 1977.

Congenital radioulnar synostosis

Bauer M and Jonsson K: Congenital radioulnar synostosis: radiological characteristics and hand function—case reports, Scand J Plast Reconstr Surg—Hand Surg 22(3):251, 1988.

Griffet J et al: Congenital superior radioulnar synostoses: a study of 43 cases, Int Orthop 10(4):265, 1986.

Hankin FM et al: Ulnar nerve palsy following rotational osteotomy of congenital radioulnar synostosis, J Pediatr Orthop 7(1):103, 1987.

Hansen OH and Andersen NO: Congenital radio-ulnar synostosis: report of 37 cases, Acta Orthop Scand 41:225, 1970.

Okrent DH and McFadden JC: Radiologic case study: congenital radioulnar synostosis, Orthopedics 9(10):1452, 1986.

Simmons BP, Southmayd WW, and Riseborough EJ: Congenital radioulnar synostosis, J Hand Surg [Am] 8(6):829, 1983.

Wilkie DPD: Congenital radio-ulnar synostosis, Br J Surg 1:366, 1913-1914.

Congenital dislocation of radial head

Almquist EE, Gordon LH, and Blue AI: Congenital dislocation of the head of the radius, J Bone Joint Surg 51A:1118, 1969.

Exarhou EI and Antoniou NK: Congenital dislocation of the head of the radius, Acta Orthop Scand 41:551, 1970.

Gattey PH and Wedge JH: Unilateral posterior dislocation of the radial head in identical twins, J Pediatr Orthop 6(2):220, 1986.

Gleason TF and Goldstein WM: Traumatic recurrent posterior dislocation of the radial head: a case report, Clin Orthop 184:186, 1984.

Keats S: Congenital bilateral dislocation of head of the radius in a seven-year-old child, Orthop Rev 3:33, Aug 1974.

Lancaster S and Horowitz M: Lateral idiopathic subluxation of the radial head: case report, Clin Orthop 214:170, 1987.

Luke DL, Schoenecker PL, and Gilula LA: Imaging rounds #100: congenital dislocation of the radial head, Orthop Rev 18(8):911, 1989.

Woo CC: Traumatic radial head subluxation in young children: a case report and literature review, J Manipulative Physiol Ther 10(4):191, 1987.

3 Congenital Limb Deficiency and Limb Length Discrepancy

JOHN E. HERZENBERG

CONGENITAL DEFICIENCIES OF LONG BONES

The first scientific approach to the problem of congenital long-bone deficiencies was devised by Frantz and O'Rahilly in 1961. Their widely used classification describes deficiencies as terminal or intercalary. In terminal deficiencies, there is an amputation with no body parts distal to the site (Fig. 3-1, *A*). In intercalary deficits, a middle segment is missing, but the distal segments are present (Fig. 3-1, *B*). Terminal and intercalary deficiencies are further defined as transverse or longitudinal. For example, complete absence of a hand at the wrist is a terminal transverse deficiency (Fig. 3-2). A complete hand without a radius or ulna is an intercalary transverse deficiency. An example of terminal longitudinal deficiency is fibular hemimelia in which the lateral two rays are also missing. Fibular hemimelia in which the foot is normal is an intercalary longitudinal deficiency.

In 1964, Swanson, in conjunction with the American Society for Surgery of the Hand and the International Federation of Societies for Surgery of the Hand, devised a more specific classification scheme. Although this system was devised originally for upper extremity deficiencies, it is applicable to the lower extremity. Like its predecessor, the Swanson classification scheme aids in taxonomy but not in treatment planning. Day modified the Frantz and O'Rahilly system to expand the scope of classification (Fig. 3-3). The Terminology Committee of the Pediatric Orthopaedic Society of North America is currently devising a further modification to help simplify classification of congenital limb deficiencies.

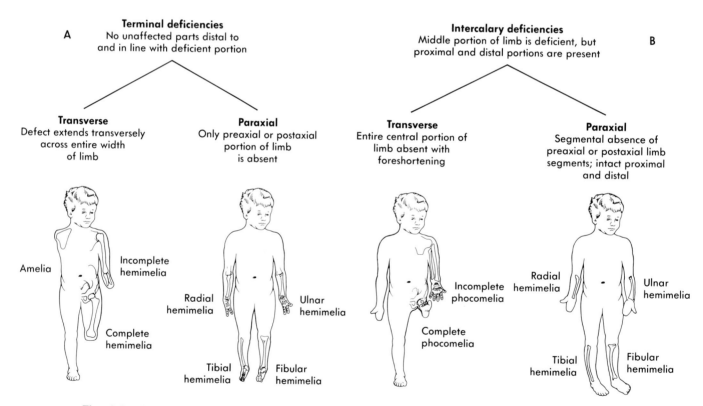

Fig. 3-1 Frantz-O'Rahilly classification of congenital limb deficiencies. (Modified from Hall CB, Brooks MB, and Dennis JF: JAMA 181:590, 1962.)

Tibial Hemimelia

Since the first description by Otto in 1841, tibial hemimelia has been described under a variety of names, including congenital longitudinal deficiency of the tibia, congenital dysplasia of the tibia, paraxial tibial hemimelia, tibial dysplasia, and congenital deficiency or absence of the tibia. This condition actually represents a spectrum of deformities, ranging from total absence of the tibia (the most severe form) to mild hypoplasia of the tibia (the least severe form). The incidence of this condition has been estimated at 1 per million live births and may be bilateral in as many as 30% of patients. It usually occurs sporadically, although familial cases with either autosomal dominant or recessive transmission patterns have been reported. At least four distinct syndromes have tibial hemimelia as a component: polydactyly–triphalangeal thumb syndrome (Werner syndrome), tibial hemimelia diplopodia, tibial hemimelia–split hand/foot syndrome, and tibial hemimelial-micromelia-trigonal brachycephaly syndrome. Although the exact cause is unknown, Sweet and Lane described a murine model for tibial hemimelia in which the dominant mutation was shown to reside on the X chromosome.

Clinical Presentation

The involved leg is short, and the fibular head is palpable if it is proximally displaced. The foot is held in severe equinovarus and the hindfoot is stiff. In older children, the proximal tibial anlage may be palpable, even if it is not roentgenographically visible. The knee is generally flexed and, in more severe deformities, quadriceps insufficiency causes a lack of knee extension. Careful clinical evaluation of the quadriceps extensor mechanism is important, since this has significant prognostic value regarding potential for reconstruction of the knee. The femur may be mildly shortened, and rotational malalignment is frequent.

Associated anomalies are common, including hip dysplasia, proximal femoral focal deficiency, partial absence of the fibula, partial absence of the medial rays of the foot, popliteal webbing, knee flexion contractures, syndactyly, duplication of the femur, polydactyly, tarsal coalition, cleft hand, clubfoot, radial dysplasia, coxa valga, lumbosacral defects, hemivertebrae, hypoplastic thumb, scoliosis, and Sprengel deformity. Congenital heart disease, genitourinary abnormalities, and hernias have also been reported.

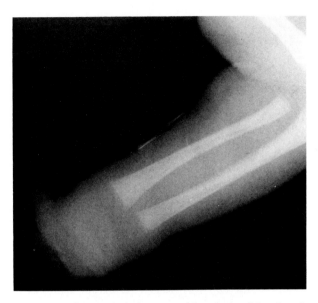

Fig. 3-2 Congenital absence of hand at wrist, a terminal transverse deficiency.

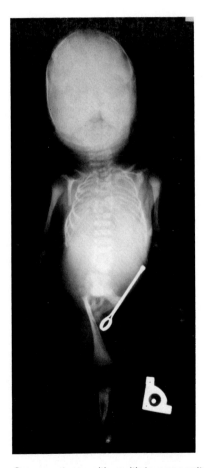

Fig. 3-3 Some patients with multiple congenital anomalies defy description. This child has a single femur with double distal epiphyses, duplication of the tibia, malformed pelvis, and multiple hemivertebrae.

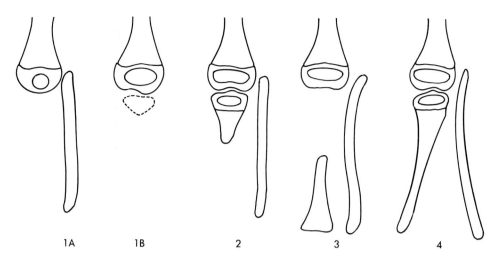

1A   1B   2   3   4

Fig. 3-4 Classification of tibial hemimelia. In type 1A fibula is dislocated proximally, there is no roentgenographic evidence of tibia, and distal femoral epiphysis is smaller than normal side. In type 1B, fibula is dislocated proximally, and there is proximal tibial anlage that may be visible on ultrasound or magnetic resonance imaging studies but cannot be seen with plain roentgenograms at birth. Type 2 deformity has proximal dislocation of fibula and roentgenographically visible proximal tibia with normal appearing knee joint. In type 3, fibula is dislocated proximally, distal tibia is roentgenographically visible, but proximal tibia is not seen. In type 4, fibula is migrated proximally and there is diastasis of distal tibiofibular joint. (Modified from Jones E, Barnes J, and Lloyd-Roberts GC: J Bone Joint Surg 60B:31, 1978.)

Classification

The most widely used classification of tibial hemimelia is that of Jones, Barnes, and Lloyd-Roberts, based on the early roentgenographic presentation; treatment recommendations are given for each type (Fig. 3-4).

In type 1A deformity there is a complete roentgenographic absence of the tibia and a hypoplastic distal femoral epiphysis (compared to the normal side). In type 1B deformity there is also no roentgenographic evidence of a tibia, but the distal femoral epiphysis appears more normal in size and shape. This difference is critical, since the type 1B deformity has a proximal tibial cartilaginous anlage that can be expected to ossify with time. Modern imaging techniques, such as arthrography, ultrasound, and magnetic resonance imaging, have shown this cartilaginous anlage in type 1B deformity (Fig. 3-5, *A* and *B*). Type 2 deformity has a roentgenographically visible proximal tibia of varying size from birth. The fibula is usually normal in size, but the head is proximally dislocated (Fig. 3-5, *A*). Type 3 deformity, in which the proximal tibia is not roentgenographically visible, is rare. The distal tibial epiphysis is sometimes visible, along with a mature distal metaphysis; however, there may be only a diffuse calcified density within the distal tibial anlage. The distal femoral epiphysis is usually well formed, but the upper end of the fibula is proximally dislocated. Although the distal femoral epiphysis is usually of normal size, the knee is generally unstable. In type 4 deformity, the tibia is shortened and there is a proximal migration of the fibula with distal tibial fibular diastasis (Fig. 3-6). This has also been called congenital diastasis of the ankle joint and congenital tibiofibular diastasis. Very few type 4 deformities have been reported.

Pathologic Anatomy

Several authors have described the pathologic findings in tibial hemimelia. The superficial peroneal nerve may terminate at the level of the ankle. Leg muscles that normally insert on the plantar surface of the foot tend to blend into a common tendon sheet. The talus and calcaneus are frequently congenitally fused. The anterior tibial artery is absent and the plantar arterial arch is incomplete. Similar vascular findings in clubfoot and fibular hemimelia suggest etiologic theories of reduced vascular flow as a cause. Associated anomalies are generally most severe when the tibia is least developed.

Treatment

As with all congenital lower limb deficiencies, the goal of treatment is a functional limb equal in length to the normal limb. The type of surgical treatment is dependent on the roentgenographic classification and clinical appearance. For severe deficiencies, amputation and prosthetic rehabilitation are the most practical means of treatment. Type 1A lesions are most frequently treated with knee disarticulation; however, type 1B deformities can often be reconstructed to yield a functional knee joint.

The two options for treatment of type 1A deformity are knee disarticulation or knee reconstruction (with or without foot amputation). The easiest and frequently most effective option is knee disarticulation followed by above-knee prosthetic fitting. This provides a definitive solution with one operation. Knee disarticulation is preferred over above-knee amputa-

tion, since above-knee amputation for type 1A deformity may result in skin problems from bony stump overgrowth. Because the expected femoral growth is often diminished, the end result of a knee disarticulation may be a functional above-knee amputation level. Children treated in this manner are almost uniformly active, functional prosthetic users. Attempts to correct the equinovarus and absent knee joint frequently result in repeated operations and eventual failure. It may be reasonable to preserve the foot in bilateral deformities, since limb length discrepancy is not a problem, but attempts to reconstruct the knee in conjunction with foot amputation have produced mixed results.

Brown described reconstruction of type 1A tibial hemimelia in two patients in whom the fibula was surgically transferred into the intercondylar notch to create a tibia (Fig. 3-9). In 1972, Brown and Pohnert reported 40 patients treated with this procedure, of whom 22 were functioning satisfactorily and 18 required secondary revision procedures for flexion deformities of the knee. Brown redefined his indica-

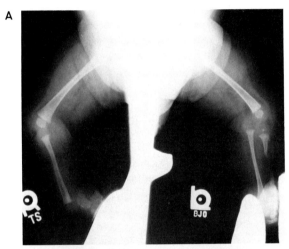

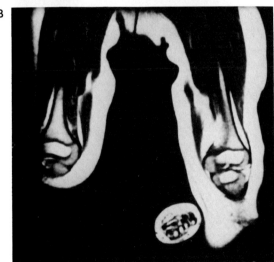

Fig. 3-5 **A,** Newborn with bilateral tibial hemimelia. Note proximal tibial remnant on left and none on right. Distal femoral epiphyses are equally well developed. Therefore left side is type 2 deformity and right side is type 1B deformity. **B,** Magnetic resonance imaging of same patient shows proximal tibial anlage on both sides. Left side, however, has bony epiphysis, whereas right side is purely cartilaginous. Flexion contracture of both knees in these coronal images obscures lower legs.

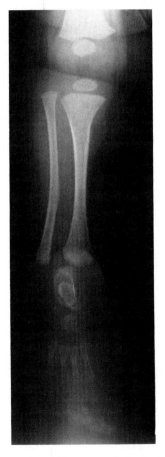

Fig. 3-6 Newborn with congenital diastasis of ankle representing type 4 tibial hemimelia. Notice absence of first ray.

tions as a child under 1 year of age (preferably under 6 months) with the physical potential to walk, functioning quadriceps, and full passive extension of the knee. Subsequent authors have reported failure of the procedure to reliably obtain good results. In reports by Jayakumar and Eilert, Schoenecker et al, and Loder and Herring, poor results ranged from 50% to 100%, with the majority of patients requiring further surgery because of knee joint instability or stiffness. The success of the Brown procedure probably depends on the presence of a functioning quadriceps mechanism, the absence of flexion contracture, and a proximal tibial anlage.

In types 1B and 2 deformities a functional knee joint exists, and knee disarticulation generally is not required if the quadriceps mechanism is functional. A proximal tibial fibular synostosis combined with a Syme amputation is the treatment of choice (Fig. 3-7). Making a synostosis between the fibula and tibia creates a more uniform, in-line, weight-bearing mechan-

ical axis. When the fibula is not transferred to the tibia, a peculiar curved hypertrophied fibula develops, causing a secondary deformity. Fusing the fibula underneath the tibia encourages its transformation into a more tibia-like bone. The Syme amputation is preferred to a through-bone amputation to prevent transdiaphyseal problems of bony stump overgrowth and to preserve maximum length of the stump.

Attempts have been made to treat tibial hemimelia with surgical equalization of leg length, production of a plantigrade foot, and creation of a stable knee, but traditional leg lengthening procedures, soft tissue reconstruction, and casting have not reliably achieved these goals in patients with tibial hemimelia. For this reason, the treatment pendulum has swung toward early amputation and prosthetic rehabilitation. With the recent introduction to North America of the Ilizarov method of extremity reconstruction, the pendu-

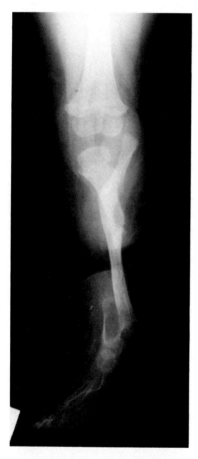

Fig. 3-7 Child 1½ years old with type 2 tibial hemimelia underwent transfer of fibula to tibia. Because periosteal sleeve was left intact, connection between transferred distal fibula and original proximal fibula reformed. Syme amputation may be considered as a second stage.

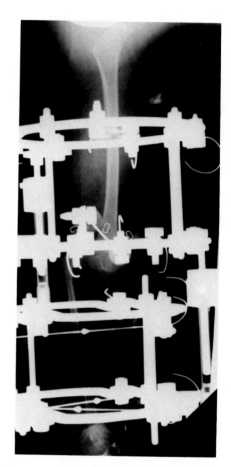

Fig. 3-8 Roentgenogram of 18-month-old child with type 1B tibial hemimelia undergoing reconstruction with Ilizarov apparatus. Fibula is pulled distally to level of cartilage anlage of proximal tibial epiphysis. Bent Kirschner wire had been inserted at distal tip of proximal tibial anlage at time of an open procedure to release soft tissue between fibula and distal femur and proximal tibia.

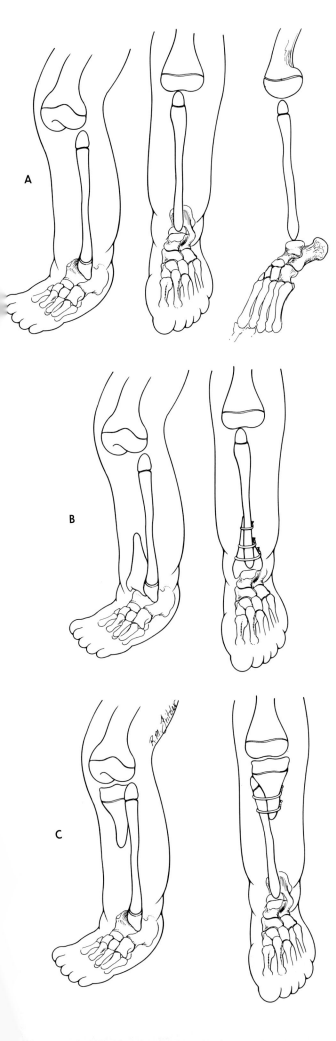

lum may eventually swing back toward restoration of leg length, production of a plantigrade foot, and achievement of a stable knee with a functional range of motion (Fig. 3-8), but at present the primary treatment remains early amputation and prosthetic rehabilitation.

Other ingenious procedures have been used for reconstruction in children with tibial hemimelia. In ipsilateral femoral deficiency, arthrodesis of the fibula may be performed, or, in younger children, chondrodesis, aligning the fibula directly with the femur and the intercondylar notch. Combining this with a Syme amputation significantly lengthens the effective lever arm of the femur. Although Syme and Boyd amputations have been the accepted treatments to make prosthetic rehabilitation easier, other alternatives have been described. If a family is absolutely opposed to amputation of the foot, an acceptable alternative is to reconstruct the foot and ankle complex by implanting the distal fibula into the talus in an extreme equinus position to increase the length of the limb (Fig. 3-9, A). Elaborate prostheses can be constructed to take advantage of this extra length while accommodating the foot.

In type 1B deficiency, a knee joint exists even if it cannot be seen on roentgenograms, and functional reconstruction may be possible, as in a type 2 deficiency. In both of these types, a proximal tibial segment is present. The recommended treatment is transection of the proximal fibula at the level of the distal tip of the proximal tibial remnant and transfer of the distal fibula to fuse with the tibial remnant. Putti used a side-to-side configuration (Fig. 3-9, B and C), but most authors now prefer end-to-end fusions between the tibial remnant and the fibula. Although it would seem preferable to wait until the proximal tibial anlage ossifies, Jones et al reported that stability can be achieved even when the proximal tibia is purely cartilaginous. At a second stage, amputation of the foot is performed to facilitate prosthetic rehabilitation. Retention of the foot during the proximal tibial reconstruction is helpful because it serves as a fixation point for a long-leg cast.

Fig. 3-9 Variations on Putti procedure for reconstruction of congenital absence of tibia. **A,** Fibula is inserted into hindfoot with foot in severe equinus to lengthen it. Fibula has also been transferred to intercondylar notch. **B,** Fibula has been transferred to intercondylar notch and distal tibiofibular synostosis has been created. **C,** Type 2 deficiency. Fibula has been synostosed to proximal tibia and inserted into hindfoot with foot positioned in equinus to achieve additional length.

Newer techniques of limb reconstruction, such as those described by Ilizarov, may allow equalization of limb lengths in severe tibial hemimelia, even when associated with severe equinovarus deformity, but currently the best results are obtained with foot amputation and prosthetic limb equalization in types 1B or 2 deficiency. Some authors recommend knee disarticulation even in type 2 deficiencies, if there are severe knee flexion contractures preoperatively. Proximal tibial or fibular synostosis is not absolutely indicated for all type 2 deformities; the literature is replete with reports of satisfactory prosthetic rehabilitation after the Syme amputation alone; however, if the fibula is transferred under the tibial remnant, it can be expected to reliably remodel and eventually form into a large tibia-like bone.

Type 3 deficiencies are extremely rare and, in the limited reports available, have been treated with amputations of the foot at either the Syme or Chopart level. In these patients the knee joint is generally stable, with the fibula proximally displaced. These patients function well as below-knee amputees. In some patients tibiofibular synostosis may be possible.

For patients with type 4 deficiency, treatment must be individualized. The Syme amputation provides excellent function. Customized reconstruction of the ankle joint to retain the foot and ankle has also been described; however, most patients require subsequent limb lengthening.

Fibular transfer

▶ *Technique (Brown)* (Fig. 3-10). Make an anterior semicircular incision starting at the knee laterally just proximal to the fibular head, extending inferiorly to the level of the distal femoral epiphysis, then extending proximally and medially to allow access to the entire distal femur (Fig. 3-10, *A*). Develop the skin flaps just above the deep fascia, and incise the lateral retinacular ligaments longitudinally parallel to the patella and quadriceps mechanism (Fig. 3-10, *B*). Dissect the patellar tendon free for later transplantation into the proximal fibula. Dissect the deep ligamentous tissues and fibrous tissues between the proximal end of the fibula and the lateral femoral condyle, incising them sufficiently to mobilize the proximal fibula for distal medial transfer (Fig. 3-10, *C*). Excise all attachments to the proximal fibula, including the biceps tendon. Section the pointed proximal fibular head trans-

versely to produce a flatter surface (Fig. 3-10, *D*). Free any dense adhesions underneath the medial femoral condyle to make room for the transferred fibula, which is held with crossed Kirschner wires. Align the fibula in the axial, coronal, and sagittal planes with the longitudinal axis of the femur. Reef the soft tissues to form a tight knee capsule and maintain patellar alignment. Attach the distal end of the patellar tendon to the proximal fibula to provide an extensor mechanism.

If the fibula is too long, perform a segmental resection distally to allow satisfactory alignment and use intramedullary Steinmann pin fixation (Fig. 3-10, *E*). Drive a wire from proximal to distal down the medullary canal of the fibula and out through the ankle joint. After reducing the fibula under the femur, drive the wire back up into the femur for fixation across the new knee (Fig. 3-10, *F*). Close the wounds and apply a cast extending from the toes to the groin, with the knee joint in maximal extension and neutral varus-valgus alignment. A Syme amputation can be done either simultaneously or as a secondary reconstructive operation.

▶ *Postoperative management.* The crossed Kirschner wires are removed 4 to 6 weeks after surgery. Intramedullary Kirschner wires are backed out to allow knee motion at 4 to 6 weeks. If the fibular osteotomy has healed, the knee wire may be removed completely. Vigorous physical therapy and splinting programs are necessary to promote formation of a neoarthrosis.

Distal fibulotalar arthrodesis

▶ *Technique.* Place the patient supine on the operating table. Approach the distal fibulotalar articulation anterolaterally to expose both bones. Dissect soft tissue to allow central placement of the body of the talus onto the distal end of the fibula. Create a trough through the dome of the talus into which the distal fibula is placed plantigrade and in neutral alignment with the foot. If necessary, fix the fibulotalar articulation with longitudinal and crossed Kirschner wires. Remove the cartilage from the distal fibular epiphysis and from the dome of the talus to allow bone-to-bone contact. Close the wound and apply a long-leg, bent-knee cast.

▶ *Postoperative management.* The cast is worn until the arthrodesis has united, usually 12 to 16 weeks.

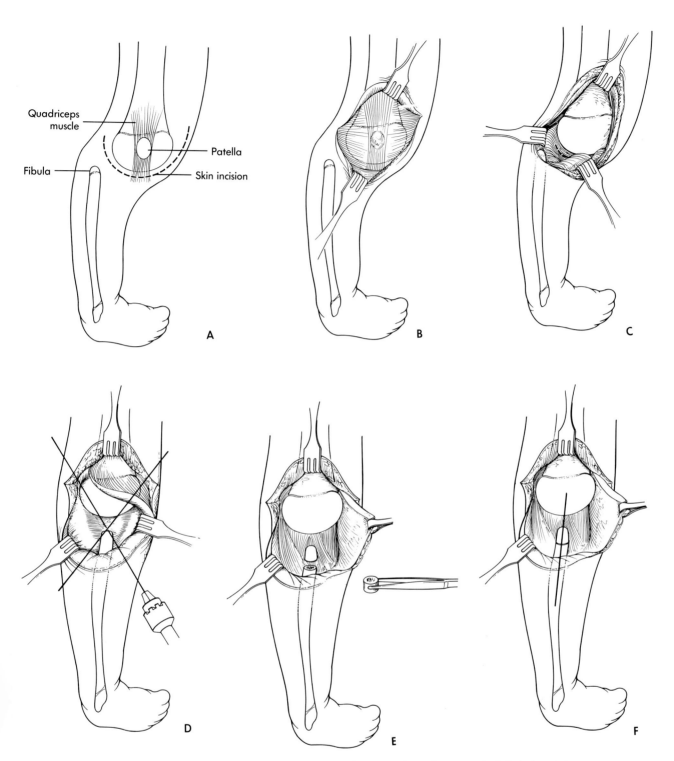

Fig. 3-10 Brown procedure. **A,** Incision begins anterolaterally, extends inferiorly, and ends anteromedially. **B** and **C,** Interposed tissues between the displaced proximal fibula and distal femur must be completely sectioned. **D,** Fibula is then brought down underneath femur and held with crossed Kirschner wires or with intramedullary Kirschner wire. **E** and **F,** If fibula cannot be brought down to level of intercondylar notch, segmental resection of fibula can be performed and fixed with intramedullary Kirschner wire. (Modified from Brown FW: J Bone Joint Surgery 47A:695, 1965.)

Proximal tibiofibular synostosis

▶ *Technique* (Fig. 3-7). Make an anterolateral incision beginning at the proximal fibula and extending distally and anteriorly to the junction of the proximal and middle thirds of the tibia. Protect the peroneal nerve. Dissect a sufficient portion of the anterior compartment musculature from the proximal medial tibia to expose the proximal tibial cartilaginous anlage (in type 1B deficiency) or the bony proximal tibia (in type 2 deficiency). Leave the proximal attachments of the fibula intact, but perform a subperiosteal dissection of the fibula. At an appropriate point opposite the distal end of the proximal tibial anlage, perform an osteotomy of the fibula. Drill an appropriate-size Steinmann pin distally through the medullary canal out the plantar aspect of the foot. Reduce the fibula on the proximal tibia, and drive the intramedullary pin retrograde into the proximal tibial remnant. If necessary, pass the pin into the distal femur for stability. Distally, bend the pin 90 degrees and cut it off below the level of the skin to be removed 6 to 8 weeks later. Immobilize the leg in a long-leg cast.

At a later date, the foot is amputated. The tip of the proximal tibial remnant should be sectioned sufficiently to create a wide surface for either chondrodesis or synostosis with the fibula. The periosteum of the fibula should be sutured to the proximal tibial remnant if possible to prevent reformation of the fibula.

Fibular Hemimelia

Fibular hemimelia, also known as congenital absence of the fibula, congenital deficiency of the fibula, paraxial fibular hemimelia, and aplasia or hypoplasia of the fibula, is the most common long bone deficiency (followed by aplasia of the radius, femur, tibia, ulna, and humerus). Whether or not vascular dysgenesis and relative ischemia affects the developing mesenchyme and causes the skeletal dysplasia seen in fibular hemimelia is still conjectural. There are no clear genetic or toxic pathogenetic mechanisms. Fibular hemimelia consists of a spectrum of anomalies, the least severe of which is mild fibular shortening and the most severe, total absence of the fibula associated with defects in the femur, tibia, and foot.

Clinical Presentation

The clinical presentation depends on the specific classification and associated anomalies. Generally, there is leg length discrepancy with equinovalgus deformity of the foot, flexion contracture of the knee, femoral shortening, instability of the knee and ankle, and a stiff hindfoot with absent lateral rays (Fig. 3-11). Although equinovalgus is by far the most common foot deformity, equinovarus and calcaneovalgus have also been reported. Clinical problems are leg length inequality and foot and ankle instability. In bilateral involvement the leg length discrepancy is generally manifested as disproportionate dwarfism, since both sides are usually affected to a similar degree.

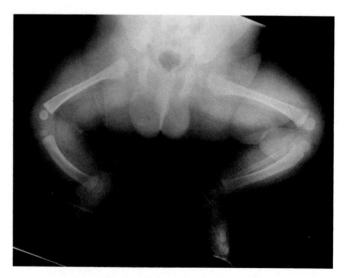

Fig. 3-11 Roentgenogram of infant with classical fibular hemimelia. Femur and tibia are both short, and foot is in valgus with absent lateral rays.

Classification

A modified classification scheme has been proposed by Achterman and Kalamchi (Fig. 3-12), who distinguished a type 1 deformity (hypoplasia of the fibula) from a type 2 deformity (complete absence of the fibula). Type 1 deformity is further subdivided into types 1A and 1B. In type 1A, the proximal fibular epiphysis is distal to the proximal tibial physis and the distal fibular physis is proximal to the talar dome. In type 1B, deficiency of the fibula is more severe, with 30% to 50% of the length of the fibula missing and no distal support for the ankle joint (Fig. 3-13). Achterman and Kalamchi described abnormalities of

the femur with hypoplasia of the patella and lateral femoral condyle. The cruciate ligaments were also clinically unstable. Bowing of the tibia was found most often in patients with type 2 deficiencies. Ball and socket ankle joints were present in most patients with type 1A deficiencies, and more severe foot and ankle problems were found in those with type 2 deformities. However, some patients with type 2 deformities had a relatively stable ankle joint despite the absence of a fibula, and others had complete instability of the tibiotalar articulation. Tarsal coalitions and absence of the lateral rays were frequent.

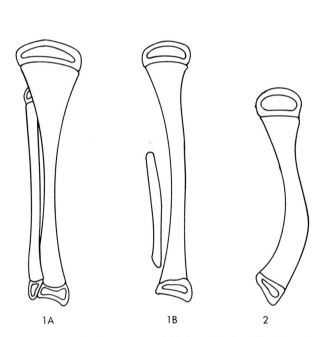

1A   1B   2

Fig. 3-12 Achterman and Kalamchi classification of fibular hemimelia. Type 1A: proximal fibular epiphysis is more distal and distal fibular epiphysis is more proximal than normal. Type 1B: more severe deficiency of fibula with at least 30% to 50% of fibula missing and no distal support to ankle joint. Type 2: completely absent fibula with bowing and shortening of tibia. (Modified from Achterman C and Kalamchi A: J Bone Joint Surg 61B:133, 1979.)

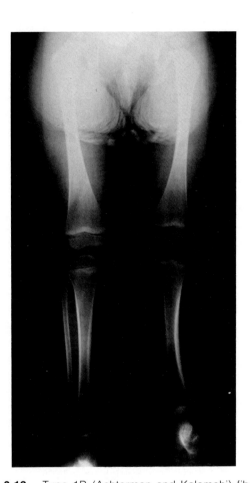

Fig. 3-13 Type 1B (Achterman and Kalamchi) fibular hemimelia with very hypotrophic, faintly visible fibula, mild shortening of femur, and moderate shortening of tibia. Overall alignment of limb is valgus.

Treatment

Reasonably accurate growth predictions for treatment and prognosis can be made for the newborn with congenital fibular hemimelia and should be discussed with the parents before treatment is begun.

For an anticipated mild leg length discrepancy, the goals of treatment are equalization of limb length and correction of the foot deformity. Shoe lifts are prescribed during the growth period and epiphysiodesis of the normal leg is performed at the appropriate time so that leg lengths are equal at the end of skeletal growth. If contralateral epiphysiodesis or shortening would result in unacceptable overall diminution of height, then the physician is faced with a difficult decision: either the short leg is lengthened, or the foot is amputated and length is equalized with a prosthesis. Several studies have examined the validity of predicting leg length inequality. Kruger and Talbott found that more severe shortening was associated with more normal feet; other series have found just the opposite. Generally, the percentage of shortening seen in an infant remains relatively constant throughout childhood, so reasonable predictions of final leg length discrepancy can be made based on very early roentgenograms. If the predicted discrepancy is more than can be corrected with limb equalization procedures, then a Syme amputation and prosthetic rehabilitation are recommended. Early amputation aids psychologic acceptance of amputation for both the parents and the child. Some authors recommend reconstruction of the ankle joint with soft tissue procedures or bony reconstruction of a stable ankle mortice. Thomas and Williams recommend Gruca's operation to reconstruct the ankle joint even when eventual amputation is recommended, since this allows the child to spend the major portion of the growing and developmental years without having to rely on prostheses. Other authors, however, have found that children undergoing amputation in late childhood or early adolescence frequently stated that they wished they had had definitive amputation much earlier. Therefore, the Gruca procedure is rarely indicated—only when the foot is to be salvaged and the ankle requires stabilization.

For more severe deformities of the foot, multiple soft tissue releases have not reliably obtained a plantigrade foot. More severe foot deformities also may be accompanied by more severe degrees of limb shortening. Faced with the prospect of multiple and unpredictable surgeries to correct both limb length and foot deformities, early amputation and prosthetic reconstruction are usually considered the best option.

The maximum amount of limb length discrepancy that can be corrected with a lengthening procedure has been variously described. Kowamura stated that lengthening greater than 10% of the length of the involved bone is inadvisable, but greater lengthenings are now routinely being performed, in particular with the Ilizarov technique. Currently, the Syme amputation and prosthetic fitting are recommended when limb length discrepancy is predicted to be significant and the foot is deformed. Another advantage of early amputation is the decreased number of hospitalizations and surgical procedures required. Children who undergo amputation at an early age have an excellent emotional adaptation to their disability, with good functional and cosmetic results.

Various reconstructive procedures have been described. For equinovalgus deformity, both posterior and lateral releases are required. The tendo Achilles as well as the fibrocartilaginous anlage of the absent fibula must be released. In older children, ankle valgus can be corrected with a dome or varus supramalleolar osteotomy. Varus osteotomy shortens the limb somewhat but also eliminates the medial prominence associated with a simple closing wedge osteotomy (Figs. 3-14 and 3-17).

At the time of the Syme amputation, any residual bowing of the tibia may be corrected with an osteotomy. Although a Boyd amputation offers greater length than a Syme, it should be used cautiously in very young children, for the Boyd amputation leaves a remnant of calcaneus that can migrate posteriorly (Fig. 3-15). Prophylactic sectioning of the tendo Achilles should be considered when amputation is performed for congenital limb deficiencies.

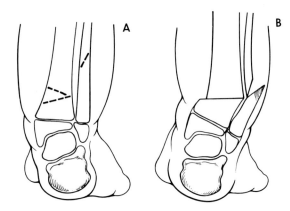

Fig. 3-14   Closing wedge technique **(A)** can result in a translation deformity with a very prominent medial malleolus **(B).**

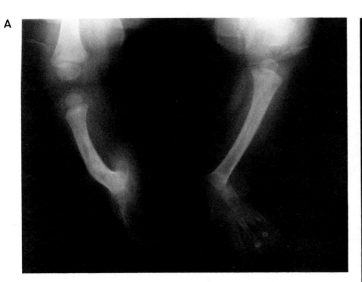

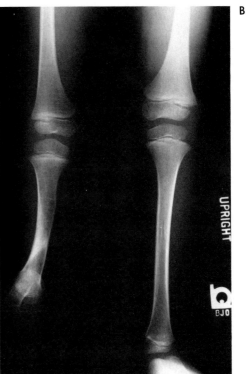

Fig. 3-15   A, Bilateral type 2 deficiencies affecting right side more severely than left side. There are four rays on left foot and only three on right. **B,** Follow-up after Boyd amputation on right and foot centralization on left. (Courtesy RN Hensinger, MD.)

Stabilization of the ankle

▲ *Technique (Gruca)* (Fig. 3-16). Make an anterior incision to obtain exposure of the distal tibia. Fashion an oblique osteotomy from a point between the lateral and middle thirds of the distal tibial articular surface, through the epiphysis, and extending proximally and medially (Fig. 3-16, *A*). Displace this osteotomy medially and proximally for about 1.5 cm. Make the approach in such a way as to ensure the periosteum of the lateral and posterolateral surface of the tibia is undisturbed. Leave the deltoid ligament intact and free the talus enough so that it can shift into the new mortice created by the osteotomy. Place a cortical graft between the two fragments of the distal tibia, and fix the osteotomy and graft with lag screws or Kirschner wires (Fig. 3-16, *B*). As the anatomic axis of the talus and calcaneus is shifted toward the midline, the valgus deformity is corrected. Soft tissue releases are performed as necessary at the time of the reconstruction.

▲ *Postoperative management.* A short leg, nonwalking cast is worn for 8 to 12 weeks until the osteotomy has healed.

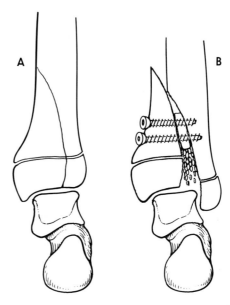

Fig. 3-16   Gruca procedure as modified by Serafin. This osteotomy splits distal tibia and moves medial portion proximally to create mortice for talus. Distal lateral tibia, in effect, becomes fibula, stabilizing talus. (Modified from Serafin J: J Bone Joint Surg 49B:59, 1967.)

Varus supramalleolar osteotomy of the ankle

▶ *Technique (Wiltse)* (Fig. 3-17). Make an anterior approach to the distal tibia and a lateral approach to the distal fibula. Create a triangular osteotomy, removing a segment of bone that can be used for bone graft (Fig. 3-17, *A*). The base of the triangle is parallel to the ground, but not parallel to the ankle joint. Make an oblique osteotomy of the distal fibula. Displace the distal segments proximally and laterally to avoid excessive prominence of the medial malleolus (Fig. 3-17, *B*). Fix the osteotomy with Steinmann pins and apply a long-leg cast.

▶ *Postoperative management.* Weight bearing is prohibited until there is adequate healing of the osteotomy.

Proximal Femoral Focal Deficiency

Like many other congenital longitudinal and transverse deficiencies, proximal femoral focal deficiency (PFFD) includes a broad spectrum of defects. Mild forms result in minor hypoplasia of the femur, whereas severe involvement may result in complete agenesis of the femur (Fig. 3-18). Most commonly, PFFD consists of a partial skeletal defect in the proximal femur with a variably unstable hip joint, shorten-

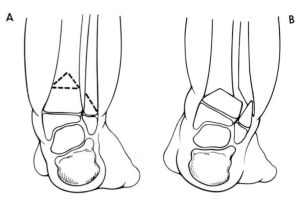

Fig. 3-17 Wiltse's varus osteotomy for valgus ankle joint. This osteotomy corrects translation that occurs during closing wedge osteotomy **(A).** Translatory shift occurs because deformity is present in ankle joint and yet osteotomy is done more proximally in metaphysis. **B,** Translating distal fragment laterally results in more natural contour of ankle.

Fig. 3-18 **A,** Infant with severe proximal femoral focal deficiency. In addition to absent femur, tibia is short and lateral ray is absent. **B,** At age 5, after Boyd amputation. Note that distal femoral epiphysis is seen but there is no femoral shaft or head. Acetabulum shows no sign of development. Cartilage anlage of distal femoral epiphysis was present at birth but not yet roentgenographically evident.

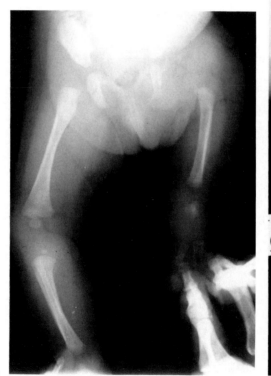

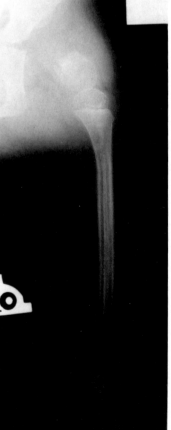

A

B

ing, and associated other anomalies. Most patients with PFFD, especially those with bilateral involvement, have associated anomalies, the most common of which are fibular hemimelia and agenesis of the cruciate ligaments of the knee. A variety of other congenital anomalies have been reported in association with PFFD, including clubfoot, congenital heart anomalies, spinal dysplasia, and facial dysplasias.

The incidence of PFFD has been reported to be 1 per 50,000 live births. Maternal diabetes has been implicated in femoral hypoplasia.

Classification

Aitken's four-part (A, B, C, D) classification is one of the earliest attempts to provide a systematic taxonomy of this condition (Fig. 3-19). In class A there is a normal acetabulum and femoral head, with shortening of the femur and absence of the femoral neck on early roentgenograms. With age, the cartilaginous neck ossifies, although this is frequently associated with a pseudarthrosis. This may heal, but the usual roentgenographic picture shows severe proximal femoral varus with significant shortening of the limb.

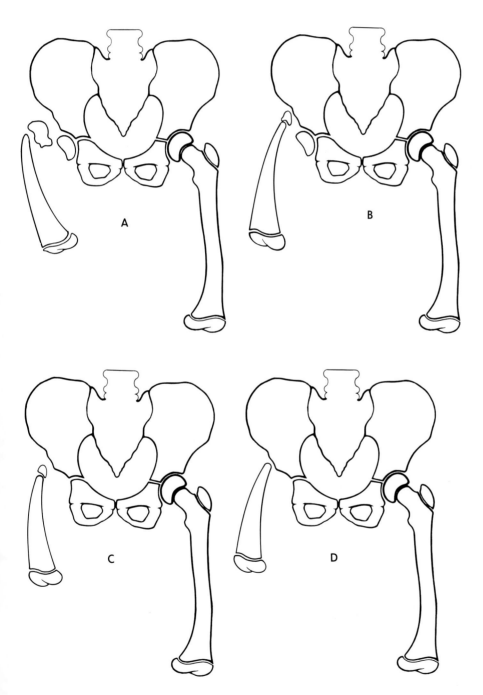

Fig. 3-19 Aitken classification of proximal femoral focal deficiency. **A,** In class A, hip joint appears formed but there is absence of femoral neck on early roentgenograms and shortening of femur. Pseudarthrosis of femoral shaft to head is usually present. **B,** In class B, femoral head is more rudimentary and there is more significant deficiency of proximal shaft of femur. Pseudarthrosis between femoral shaft and head is always present. **C,** In class C there is no femoral head, acetabulum is shallow, and proximal femur is represented only by small tuft. **D,** In class D deficiencies, there is no femoral head or acetabulum, and more significant deficiency of femoral shaft is present.

Table 3-1   Nine Pappas classes of congenital abnormalities of the femur

	Class I	Class II (Aitken D)	Class III (Aitken B)	Class IV (Aitken A)
Femoral shortening (%)	—	70-90	45-80	40-67
Femoral-pelvic abnormalities	Femur absent Ischiopubic bone structures underdeveloped and deficient Lack of acetabular development	Femoral head absent Ischiopubic bone structures delayed in ossification	No osseous connection between femoral shaft and head Femoral head ossification delayed Acetabulum may be absent Femoral condyles maldeveloped Infrequent irregular tuft on proximal end of femur	Femoral head and shaft joined by irregular calcification in a fibrocartilaginous matrix
Associated abnormalities	Fibula absent	Tibia shortened Fibula, foot, knee joint, and ankle joint abnormal	Tibia shortened 0%-40% Fibula shortened 5%-100% Patella absent or small and high riding Knee-joint instability frequent Foot malformed	Tibia shortened 0%-20% Fibula shortened 4%-60% Knee-joint instability frequent Foot small with infrequent malformations
Treatment objectives	Prosthetic management	Pelvic-femoral stability through prosthetic management	Union between femoral shaft and hip for hip stability Prosthetic management	Union between femoral head, neck, and shaft Prosthetic management

From Pappas AM: J Pediatr Orthop 3:45, 1983.

Class V (Aitken A)	Class VI	Class VII	Class VIII	Class IX
48-85	30-60	10-50	10-41	6-20
Femur incompletely ossified, hypoplastic, and irregular Midshaft of femur abnormal	Distal femur short, irregular, and hypoplastic Irregular distal femoral diaphysis	Coxa vara Hypoplastic femur Proximal femoral diaphysis irregular with thickened cortex Lateral femoral condyle deficiency frequent Valgus distal femur	Coxa valga Hypoplastic femur Femoral head and neck smaller Proximal femoral physis horizontal Abnormality of femoral condyles frequent with associated bowing of shaft and valgus of distal femur	Hypoplastic femur
Tibia shortened 4%-27% Fibula shortened 10%-100% Knee-joint instability frequent Severe malformations of the foot frequent	Single bone lower leg Patella absent Foot malformed	Tibia shortened <10%-24% Fibula shortened <10%-100% Lateral and high riding patella frequent	Tibia shortened 0%-36% Fibula shortened 0%-100% Lateral and high riding patella frequent Foot malformed	Tibia shortened 0%-15% Fibula shortened 3%-30% Additional ipsilateral and contralateral malformations frequent
Prosthetic management	Prosthetic management	Extremity length equality Improved alignment of (a) proximal and (b) distal femur	Extremity length equality Improved alignment of (a) proximal and (b) distal femur	Extremity length equality

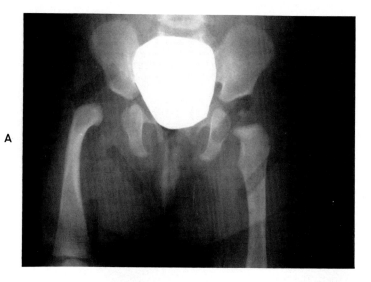

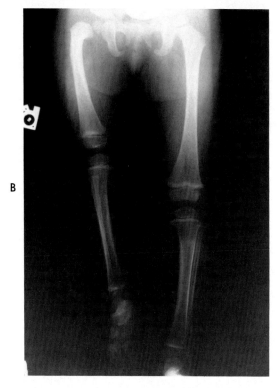

Fig. 3-20 **A,** A 4-month-old infant with PFFD on right. Although proximal capital epiphysis is not yet ossified, well-developed acetabulum indicates that femoral head is present. **B,** At age 11 years, varus angulation of proximal femur and mild shortening in tibia.

Class B is similar to class A in that an acetabulum and femoral head are present (see Fig. 3-20); however, there is no bony connection between the proximal femur and the femoral head, and a pseudarthrosis is present. In class C there is further degradation in the formation of the hip, characterized by a dysplastic acetabulum, absent femoral head, and short femur. A small, separate ossific tuft can be seen at the proximal end of the femur. In class D the acetabulum, femoral head, and proximal femur are totally absent. Unlike class C, there is no ossified tuft capping the proximal femur in class D. Class D patients often have bilateral anomalies.

Other authors have expanded the definition of PFFD to include lesser expressions of femoral malformation. Pappas, in his evaluation of 125 patients with PFFD, described nine classes that range from a complete absence of the proximal femur (class I) to mild femoral aplasia (class IX). The Pappas class II corresponds to an Aitken class D, the Pappas class III corresponds to an Aitken class B, and the Pappas class IV and V may be correlated with an Aitken class A (Table 3-1). Kalamchi and co-workers developed a simplified classification scheme for congenital deficiency of the femur that included five groups: group I, short femur and intact hip joint; group II, short femur and coxa vara of the hip; group III, short femur but well-developed acetabulum and femoral head; group IV, absent hip joint and dysplastic femoral segment; and group V, total absence of the femur.

In their review of 69 patients Gillespie and Torode found that two major groups could be identified for treatment purposes. Group I patients had a hypoplastic femur in which both the hip and knee were reconstructable and leg equalization was sometimes possible. Group II patients exhibited a "true" PFFD, where the hip joint was markedly abnormal. Although some of these patients had tenuous connections between the femoral head and the proximal femur, the alignment and surrounding musculature were markedly abnormal. Additionally, these legs were too shortened, rotated, and marred by flexion contractures of the hip and knee to be reconstructable. These patients required only the reconstructive procedures that facilitate prosthetic fitting.

Treatment

The major problems facing these children are limb length inequality and variable inadequacy of the proximal femoral musculature and hip joint. Treatment is highly individualized and ranges from amputation and prosthetic rehabilitation to limb salvage, lengthening, and hip reconstruction. The natural history of the particular variant and the limitations of surgical reconstruction must be considered.

Often surgical reconstruction of any kind is not indicated. Most authors agree that bilateral PFFD is best treated without surgery (Fig. 3-21). These patients can walk well without prostheses, but for social or cosmetic reasons, extension prostheses may be provided. The patients learn to accept their short stature

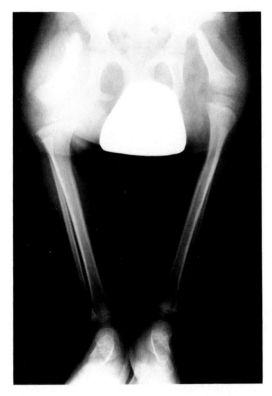

Fig. 3-21 Severe (class D) bilateral PFFD in 3-year-old boy. Note total lack of formation of acetabulum.

and are quite functional. Foot surgery may be required to correct other associated anomalies. Limb lengthening is not indicated in these patients, since extreme lengthening would be necessary and the hips are unstable. Knee fusion is not indicated, because the knee functions in conjunction with the hip pseudarthrosis to provide useful motion.

Stability of the hip is important in determining treatment. In patients with both a femoral head and acetabulum (Aitken classes A and B), many authors have recommended surgery to establish continuity between the femoral head and the femur, but this may be technically difficult if there is little bone stock to work with in the proximal femur. For this reason, surgery is best delayed until there is adequate ossification of the femoral head and proximal metaphysis. In some patients the femur is so short that a simultaneous knee fusion is performed, creating a one-bone leg (Fig. 3-22). With limited bone stock for proximal fixation, autogenous bone graft should be added to the pseudarthrosis site. Although the roentgenographic picture may be improved with correction of the proximal pseudarthrosis, it remains to be shown that function is improved. In fact, many patients treated nonoperatively have good motion and reasonably good function. Stabilizing the proximal pseudarthrosis may diminish the overall range of motion of the hip. For less severe proximal femoral dysplasia (Pappas classes VII, VIII, and IX), hip reconstruction is limited to osteotomies that improve biomechanical alignment. Care must be taken not to damage the proximal femoral physis in these children who already have problems with diminished growth of the femur.

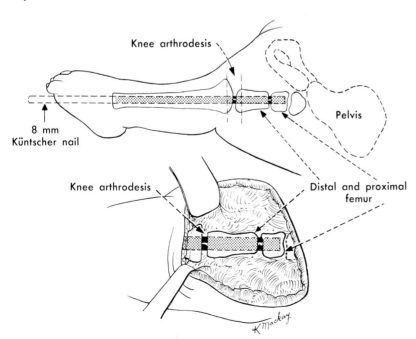

Knee arthrodesis

8 mm
Küntscher nail

Knee arthrodesis

Pelvis

Distal and proximal
femur

Fig. 3-22 When proximal femur is small and has pseudarthrosis between femoral neck and shaft, it can be stabilized to create better lever arm. Simultaneously knee arthrodesis can be performed to create one-bone leg. If possible, intramedullary fixation should stop just short of proximal femoral physis. (Courtesy RE King.)

For more severe deficiencies in which there is no femoral head or acetabulum (Aitken classes C and D or Pappas classes II and III), most authors recommend that no attempts be made at hip reconstruction, although there are notable exceptions. King recommends iliofemoral fusion, which requires a simultaneous Chiari osteotomy to create a suitable bony bed to receive the small femoral remnant, allowing the knee joint to assume the function of the hip joint (Fig. 3-23). Fixson and Lloyd-Roberts also use this technique, with additional bone graft to ensure fusion. Although this technique eliminates the hip instability, it may severely limit mobility of the thigh. Even with a certain amount of instability, the knee generally functions as a hinge joint providing flexion and extension only. Rotation and abduction are lost after iliofemoral arthrodesis. Steel et al reported four patients with iliofemoral fusion for Aitken class C or D deficiencies and argued that untreated patients have progressive instability and proximal migration of the femur that interfere with prosthetic fitting and function. Steel's technique includes closing wedge osteotomies to eliminate the anterior bowing and to fuse the femur to the ilium so that the shaft is pointed as anteriorly as possible. This allows the knee joint to extend fully to simulate the 90 degrees of hip flexion required for sitting and to flex 90 degrees to simulate the neutral position of the hip required for walking.

Surgical limb lengthening, with or without contralateral shortening, should be considered only if the femur is intact. In 1982, Herring and Coleman suggested 10 to 12 cm as the maximum amount of lengthening possible in a single long bone with congenital deficiency and, combined with contralateral shortening, 17 cm as the maximum amount of inequality that could be corrected. They recommended limb lengthening only in femurs with over 60% of predicted femoral length or less than 17 cm of pro-

jected shortening; other prerequisites for lengthening were hip stability and a stable plantigrade foot. Gillespie and Torode, using Wagner's technique of leg lengthening (Fig. 3-24), suggested that lengthening be considered for femurs that are at least 60% of the normal length. The Ilizarov method of lengthening, using thin-wire circular external fixators, may extend these limits. The Ilizarov device allows extension proximally or distally with hinges to prevent knee and hip subluxation. Regardless of technique, limb lengthening in patients with PFFD is difficult, with the ever-present danger of knee and hip subluxation. For predicted discrepancies greater than 12 to 14 cm, lengthening may be performed in two stages: one at age 8 or 9 years and a second during the early teens. Depending on predictions of the patient's overall height based on the normal leg, a contralateral epiphysiodesis may be indicated.

If limb lengthening is not feasible, various approaches are available to facilitate prosthetic rehabilitation. Most children with PFFD can learn to walk without a prosthesis, but a prosthesis helps equalize leg lengths. An extension prosthesis is acceptable for a small child, but when the child becomes a teenager, a more cosmetically pleasing prosthesis is facilitated by amputation of the foot. Amputation of the foot should be performed between the ages of 1 and 2 years, before the parents and child become psychologically attached to the concept of having a foot and an extension prosthesis. An alternative approach is to use the prosthesis to mold the foot into equinus so that it fits into an above-knee amputation prosthetic socket. The socket is fashioned to include the entire femur. Later an arthrodesis can be performed, if necessary, to facilitate prosthetic fitting. It is possible, however, that some knee motion within the stump of the prosthesis may serve as a protective mechanism for the abnormal proximal hip. If a knee arthrodesis is performed, the potential benefits in gait and prosthetic fitting may be outweighed by the increased stress placed on the proximal femur and proximal hip articulation and pseudarthrosis, if present.

Currently knee arthrodesis and foot amputation are the preferred treatment in significant deformities, rather than limb lengthening (Fig. 3-25, *A* and *B*). Either ankle disarticulation, Syme amputation, or Boyd amputation may be used. The heel pad is stabilized by either the Syme or Boyd amputation, an advantage over a simple ankle disarticulation. The Boyd amputation saves the entire calcaneus and provides a slightly more bulbous stump and additional length. If the combined length of the tibia, femoral remnant, and foot is greater than the femur on the opposite side, taking into account potential growth, then there is no advantage in the small increase and additional

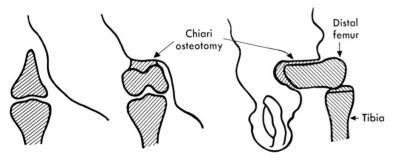

Fig. 3-23   King's reconstruction for type D proximal femoral focal deficiency. Distal femur is fused directly to pelvis and knee joint functions as hip joint. To allow patient to flex "hip" to sit in chair and extend "hip" to stand, femoral segment is fused to pelvis at 90-degree angle. (Courtesy RE King.)

length provided with the Boyd amputation. It is possible to fuse the knee over an intramedullary nail and still allow longitudinal growth of the distal femoral and proximal tibial physes.

Prosthetic reconstruction can be facilitated in severe cases with an early Syme amputation. The child is followed with serial scanograms until sufficient data have been collected to construct a working Moseley straight-line graph; then further surgery can be planned. If knee arthrodesis is elected to improve prosthetic fitting and gait, the physes around the knee can be epiphysiodesed if necessary to ensure that the prosthetic knee will be at the same level as the contralateral normal knee when the child achieves skeletal maturity. Precise predictions are not necessary, since small amounts of additional shortening in the involved leg can be readily accommodated by the prosthesis. If, however, the involved femorotibial unit is longer than the contralateral normal femur, the prosthetic knee must be placed in a distal position, which is less cosmetically desirable. While this can be treated with a leg-shortening procedure at skeletal maturity, a simpler preventative procedure, such as an epiphysiodesis during the growing years, is preferable.

• • •

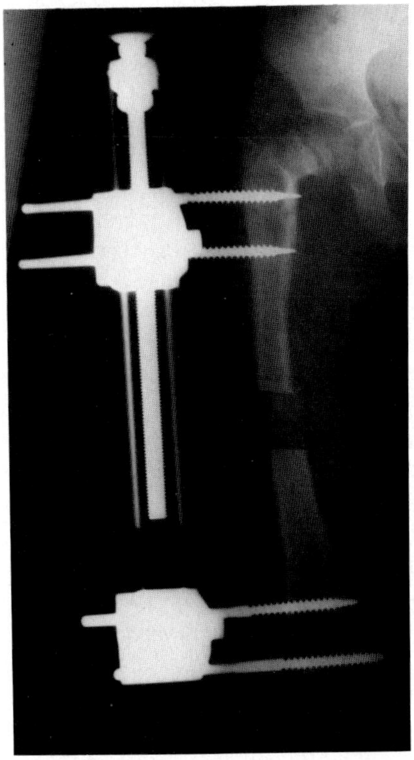

Van Nes described his below-knee rotation plasty in 1950, although it was originally performed by Borggreve some 20 years before. The operation has been modified by Hall, and later by Gillespie and Torode, to make it more suitable for reconstruction in PFFD. This reconstruction should be considered in patients who, because of significant femoral shortening, are not candidates for a femoral lengthening. This procedure combines arthrodesis of the knee with rotation of the distal tibia 180 degrees externally so that the ankle joint becomes a functional knee joint: ankle plantar flexion becomes "knee" extension and ankle dorsiflexion becomes "knee" flexion. A reasonably stable hip joint and a well-functioning ankle are required for this technique. Unfortunately, many patients with PFFD also have fibular hemimelia, with a poorly functioning ankle joint. An arc of ankle motion of at least 90 degrees is required for rotation plasty reconstruction to be beneficial. The femur, knee, and tibia should equal the length of the oppo-

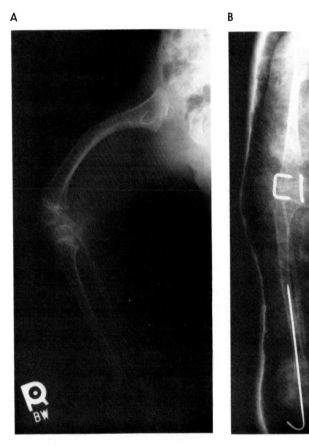

Fig. 3-25 **A,** A 7-year-old child with PFFD. Femur is severely shortened and tibia is relatively hypoplastic. **B,** Surgical management consisted of Boyd ankle amputation, stabilization with intramedullary Steinmann pin, and arthrodesis of knee joint with staples. Functionally, this patient can be rehabilitated as knee disarticulation amputee.

Fig. 3-24 Wagner lengthening in mild proximal femoral focal deficiency. There is strong tendency for osteotomy to drift into varus alignment with monolateral fixator.

site femur, but this is usually not the case, so ipsilateral knee epiphysiodesis is done to equalize the reconstructed "femoral unit" and the contralateral normal femur. There are some problems that must be discussed with the patient and parents before this type of reconstruction. First, the appearance of the leg, with the foot rotated backwards, can be psychologically disturbing; great care should be taken in preoperative consultation to make this clear. It is helpful to have another patient who has already undergone the procedure demonstrate how the prosthesis functions. If this is not possible, then the family should be shown photographs and drawings of a rotation plasty. Another problem, particularly in young children, is derotation of the surgically rotated foot. Of 20 patients with Van Nes rotation plasty reported by Kostuik et al, 12 patients required a subsequent derotation, and half of those required a second derotation operation. They recommend that this reconstruction be deferred until the age of 12 years. Torode and Gillespie modified the procedure to limit the amount of derotation.

Rotation plasty

▶ *Technique (modified Van Nes)* (Fig. 3-26). Position the patient prone and drape the entire limb free so that the skin is exposed from the toes to the iliac crest. Place a small towel under the sacrum. Begin the incision proximal and lateral to the knee and extend it across the knee distally along the subcutaneous crest of the tibia. Elevate the flaps medially and laterally to expose the knee capsule and patellar tendon. Divide the patellar tendon and open the knee capsule transversely. Apply traction on the capsule proximally and distally to expose the knee joint fully by dividing the collateral ligaments and anterior, medial, and lateral capsule. On the medial side, carefully dissect out the insertion of the adductor magnus up to the level of the femoral artery. Divide the adductor magnus to enable the artery to derotate anteriorly and to limit postoperative derotation. Trace the femoral artery distally and posteriorly as it becomes the popliteal artery. Divide the medial hamstring muscles at their insertion. On the lateral side, carefully dissect out the peroneal nerve. If the fibula is deficient, the anatomic relationship between the peroneal nerve and the proximal fibular head may be abnormal. To prevent damage to the peroneal nerve, trace the nerve proximally to its point of origin on the sciatic nerve. Release any fascial attachments distally over the peroneal nerve.

After the major neurovascular structures have been completely identified and protected, divide the posterior knee capsule and section the origins of the gastrocnemius heads. The only remaining attachments from the femur to the tibia are the skin, subcutaneous tissues, and neurovascular structures. Release the lateral hamstrings. With an osteotome or oscillating saw, remove the articular cartilage of the proximal tibia down to the level of the proximal tibial epiphysis. Do not dissect into the proximal tibial physis.

If the leg needs to be shortened, shorten the femur by removing both the distal femoral epiphysis and physis. Next, insert an intramedullary Rush rod through the distal femur proximally, exiting through the piriformis fossa into the buttock. If necessary, ream the femur with a drill to prevent comminution of the femur during the nail insertion. Make a small incision in the buttock where the nail exits. Then remove the nail and reinsert it from proximal to distal through the femur and into the tibia, stopping short of the distal tibial physis. While the nail is being inserted, rotate the tibia externally to relax the peroneal nerve. Gently transfer the femoral popliteal artery anteriorly through the adductor hiatus. If the leg cannot be comfortably rotated through the knee arthrodesis, obtain additional rotation through a separate osteotomy in the midshaft of the tibia, which will also be stabilized by the intramedullary nail. Additional shortening can be performed through the tibia if necessary. In such cases a fibular osteotomy is also performed. Attempt to rotate the extremity 180 degrees. If the rotation places too much torque on the vascular structures and the distal pulses are lost, derotate the leg through the knee until the pressure on the vessels is relieved. Close and apply a plaster cast, maintaining rotation.

▶ *Postoperative management.* If derotation of the foot was required to achieve vascular pressure, then the foot is rotated serially using successive hip spica casts to turn the foot on the axis of the intramedullary nail. When the osteotomies are healed, the child is fitted with a modified below-knee prosthesis. Although it is possible to amputate the toes to make the foot look more like a below-knee stump and less like a backwards foot, most patients decline this option.

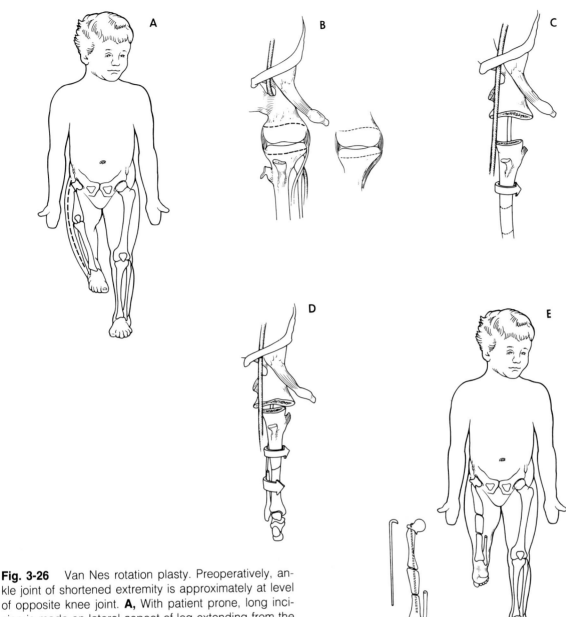

Fig. 3-26 Van Nes rotation plasty. Preoperatively, ankle joint of shortened extremity is approximately at level of opposite knee joint. **A,** With patient prone, long incision is made on lateral aspect of leg extending from the hip to midshaft of tibia. **B,** Quadriceps and sartorious tendons are taken down distally to expose adductor hiatus and femoral artery, and peroneal nerve is dissected free. Lines of resection are indicated. Preoperatively it is important to determine predicted length of extremity to decide whether to preserve distal femoral epiphysis or proximal tibial epiphysis. **C,** After resection of knee joint and freeing up femoral-popliteal artery, tibia is rotated externally 140 degrees. **D,** Further rotation of additional 40 degrees may be obtained by osteotomizing tibia. In this way, total amount of stretch on soft tissues is spread over longer distance. External rotation is preferred to internal rotation to prevent stretch of peroneal nerve. **E,** Fixation with intramedullary Rush rod should be augmented by spica cast. (Modified from Torode IP and Gillespie R: J Bone Joint Surg 65B:569, 1983.)

AMPUTATIONS

Although most of the basic surgical principles of amputation in adults apply to children, there are important differences. Most amputations in children are performed for congenital conditions. Either the child is born without a portion of the limb, or an amputation is performed to facilitate reconstruction and prosthetic rehabilitation in a deficient limb. Trauma accounts for most acquired amputations in children. Unlike typical adult dysvascular patients, children may tolerate skin grafts over stumps and, to a certain extent, tension at the suture line. Most revision surgery in children with congenital amputations involves the lower extremity. Revision amputation surgery in upper extremity limb deficiency is rarely required. Prosthetic fitting after amputation in children should begin after complete wound healing and standard stump preparation. A rigid postoperative plaster dressing that is bivalved to allow for swelling is preferred. When the wounds are sufficiently healed, stump wrapping with elastic bandages is begun to prepare the stump for a prosthesis. Phantom pain and phantom sensations are problems in child amputees, especially after tumor surgery. Neuroma formation is rare, but gentle handling of the nerves and sectioning with a sharp knife without applying excessive traction on the nerves should be a routine part of amputation surgery in children.

In planning amputation surgery, maximal length should be preserved to provide maximal lever arm strength for powering a prosthesis. Physes should be preserved whenever possible to ensure continued growth of the limb. This is particularly true for the physes around the knee, which provide the majority of growth in the lower extremity, and the physes around the shoulder and wrist, which provide the majority of longitudinal growth in the upper extremity. Although amputation through a long bone in a growing child can result in appositional terminal overgrowth, this is not adequate reason for sacrificing length. In below-knee amputation in a young child, it is highly likely that the fibula, and to a lesser extent the tibia, will overgrow, but this can be satisfactorily remedied by revision surgery. Although knee disarticulation would prevent overgrowth, it is far more important to preserve the knee joint to power a below-knee prosthesis than to prevent overgrowth of the stump. Even short below-knee segments should be preserved if possible in growing children. Loder and Herring found that the gait characteristics of children with knee disarticulations were not a problem for moderate activities, but the inability to run well with a knee disarticulation placed significant limitations on sports activities. Since the proximal tibial physis contributes the majority of the growth of the tibia, an initially short stump has the potential to become a longer, more functional stump. Furthermore, in older children, it is possible to lengthen a short below-knee stump using the Ilizarov technique to provide a more functional below-knee stump.

Terminal overgrowth has been reported most frequently in the humerus, followed by the fibula, tibia,

Fig. 3-27 A, Newborn with congenital amputation through proximal tibia. **B,** At 5 years of age, continued growth of distal stump and penciling resulted in protrusion of bone from skin.

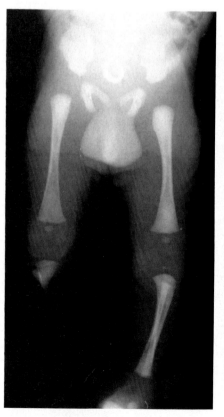

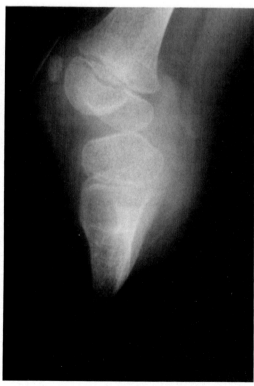

A

B

and femur. Because it appears to be caused by appositional periosteal bone formation distally and not by epiphyseal growth proximally (Fig. 3-27), epiphysiodesis does not prevent stump overgrowth. A variety of techniques have been devised to prevent stump overgrowth, but none has been completely successful. Small bone spurs that form at the edge of the transected bone do not constitute true overgrowth and rarely require surgical removal. Stump overgrowth occurs in both congenital and traumatic amputations. Another unusual problem, unique to the growing child with a below-knee amputation, was recently described by Mowery, Herring, and Jackson. They found patellar dislocations to be a common problem in adolescents, and in all patients they found patella alta, presumably caused by the force of the patellar tendon–bearing prosthesis against the lower surface of the patella. They postulated that this elongation of the patellar tendon might be prevented by earlier modifications of the prosthesis to distribute the force around a greater area rather than concentrating it on the patellar tendon.

Although the standard amputation techniques are described in Chapter 19, important variations of amputations around the ankle exist for reconstruction in a congenitally limb-deficient child. The two most common reconstructive amputations performed for congenitally limb-deficient children are the Syme and Boyd procedures. Syme amputation is a modified ankle disarticulation. The Boyd procedure amputates all of the foot bones, except the calcaneus, and fuses the calcaneus to the distal tibia.

Many studies have documented excellent results with both the Syme and Boyd amputations, yet the literature seems to favor a well-performed Boyd amputation over a Syme amputation. The problems encountered in Syme amputations in children have been overgrowth of retained calcaneus apophyses, heel pad migration, and exostosis formation. Advantages of the Boyd operation are the additional length gained and the prevention of the posterior displacement of the heel pad, which occurs in many patients with a Syme amputation. However, it is important to position the calcaneus in proper alignment for the Boyd amputation. If the calcaneus is not aligned correctly, it angulates into equinus and interferes with weight bearing.

A problem common to both the Syme and Boyd amputations is the flare of the distal tibial metaphysis, causing a bulbous shape to the distal stump and necessitating a special prosthesis with a removable medial window. However, in children with congenital limb deficiencies such as tibial hemimelia and fibula hemimelia the distal ankle is relatively hypoplastic, so a bulbous stump is usually not a problem. A common problem in the Syme amputation is posterior migration of the heel pad, despite attempts to anchor the heel pad distally. The Boyd amputation obviates this problem by producing an arthrodesis of the calcaneus to the distal tibia, although this may be difficult to achieve in very young children whose calcaneus is largely cartilaginous.

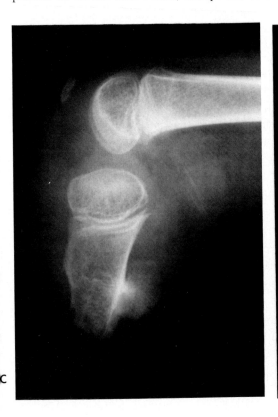

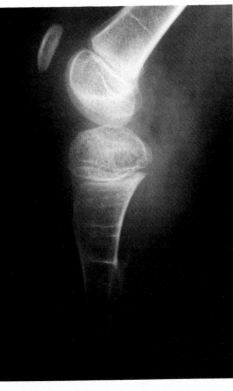

Fig. 3-27, cont'd C, After resection, distal stump is squared off, but bone spur is formed posteriorly. **D,** At 9 years of age further growth and penciling of stump necessitated repeat revision of distal tip of tibia. (Courtesy RN Hensinger, MD.)

C

D

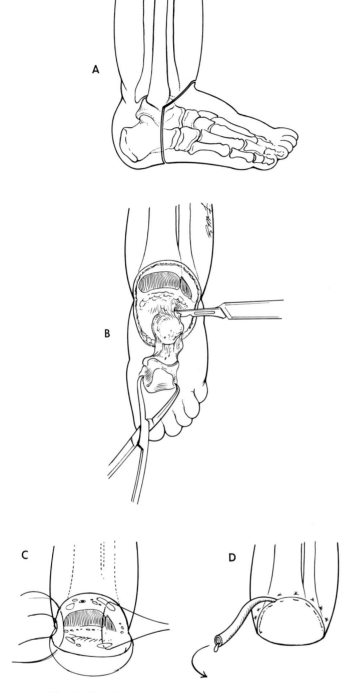

Ankle Disarticulation

▶ *Technique (Syme amputation)* (Fig. 3-28). Make a fishmouth incision beginning at the lateral malleolus, extending over the dorsum of the foot, and ending 1 cm distal to the medial malleolus. The plantar portion should extend distally enough to allow adequate skin closure anteriorly. Place the foot in as much equinus as possible to expose the anterior ankle capsule and divide it. Next, divide the deltoid ligament between the talus and the medial malleolus, but do not damage the nearby posterior tibial vessels. Section the lateral ligaments between the calcaneus and fibula. Grasp the talus with a large clamp and further force it into equinus to permit dissection of the posterior ankle capsule. Make a subperiosteal dissection of the calcaneus in its posterior aspect through the ankle joint. Cut the tendo Achilles at its point of insertion into the calcaneus, but do not "button hole" through the skin. Place further traction on the hindfoot and further hyperflexion into equinus, and dissect the soft tissues with a periosteal elevator and a knife, being certain to stay in the subperiosteal plane to avoid damaging the heel pad. Continue the dissection until the entire calcaneus is excised. To anchor the heel pad, drill holes in the anterior aspect of the distal tibia and use stout sutures from the distal aspect of the heel pad, anchoring it in the aponeurosis of the distal tibia. In children, it is not necessary to remove the cartilage of the distal tibia, but if desired the flare of the medial malleolus and distal fibula may be trimmed to create a more even weight-bearing surface. Pull the flexor tendons distally, transect them, and allow them to retract. Ligate the posterior tibial artery and anterior tibial artery as distally as possible to prevent ischemic necrosis of the flaps. Insert suction drains in the wound and close the skin in layers. Apply a rigid plaster dressing to decrease pain after surgery; bivalve the cast to allow for swelling.

▶ *Postoperative management.* Weight bearing on the stump in a cast is delayed until there is adequate healing of the wound.

Fig. 3-28 Syme amputation. **A,** Fishmouth incision. **B,** Enucleation of talus and calcaneus. **C,** Plantar flap sutured to distal tibia. **D,** Completed closure with drain.

Hindfoot Amputation

▶ *Technique (Boyd amputation)* (Fig. 3-29). Make a fishmouth incision in the manner described for the Syme amputation. Elevate the skin flaps proximally and amputate the forefoot through the midtarsal joints. Excise the entire talus, using sharp dissection. With an oscillating saw or osteotome, transect the distal end of the calcaneus. In a similar manner remove the articular surface of the subtalar joint on the calcaneus perpendicular to the long axis of the tibia. Resect an adequate amount of the distal tibial articular cartilage so that the bony epiphysis of the distal tibia is exposed. Shape the calcaneus to fit accurately against the surface of the distal tibial epiphysis. Stabilize this with a smooth Steinmann pin that enters the heel pad and provides fixation to the tibia by crossing the distal tibial physis into the metaphysis. Occasionally, the tendo Achilles must be severed to allow accurate positioning of the calcaneus. It is important to shift the calcaneus anteriorly before fixing it with the Steinmann pin. Section the medial and lateral plantar nerves and allow them to retract. Section the posterior tibial artery and anterior tibial artery as distally as possible to prevent wound necrosis. Close the wound over drains and apply a plaster cast. For young children, a hip spica cast may be necessary.

▶ *Postoperative management.* The intramedullary pin usually can be removed at 6 weeks and a new cast applied for an additional 6 weeks. Following this, the stump usually is healed sufficiently for prosthetic rehabilitation.

Fig. 3-29 Boyd amputation. **A,** Fishmouth incision is fashioned for ease of closure. Resected areas of bone are shaded. **B,** Cartilage of distal tibia should be removed, shaving it down gradually until bony epiphysis of distal tibia is reached. Calcaneus should be shifted anteriorly and tendo Achilles sectioned to prevent its proximal migration. **C,** Intramedullary fixation with a smooth pin facilitates fusion of calcaneus to epiphysis of distal tibia.

LIMB LENGTH DISCREPANCY

Limb length equality is not simply a cosmetic concern, it is also a functional concern. The short leg gait is awkward, increases energy expenditure because of the excessive vertical rise and fall of the pelvis, and may result in scoliosis and back pain from longstanding significant discrepancies. In a study of 23 young adults with untreated limb length inequality of 1.2 to 5.2 cm, Papaioannou, Stokes, and Kenright found compensatory scoliosis and decreased spinal mobility, but no back pain. Giles and Taylor, and Friberg studied much larger groups of patients and concluded that significant limb length inequality is associated with low back pain and that the pain is helped by limb equalization.

Limb length inequality may result from trauma or infection that damages the physis, from asymmetric paralytic conditions (such as polio or cerebral palsy), or from tumors or tumorlike conditions that affect bone growth (such as juvenile rheumatoid arthritis or postfracture hypervascularity) by stimulating asymmetric growth. Idiopathic unilateral hypoplasia or hyperplasia are other common causes of limb length inequality.

The treatment of limb length inequality must be tailored to the specific condition and needs of the individual patient. Treatment plans can be formulated only after a careful evaluation that includes assessment of the chronologic and skeletal ages of the patient, the current and predicted discrepancy in limb lengths, the predicted adult height, the cause of the disorder, the functional status of the joints, and the social and psychologic background of the patient and family.

Clinical Assessment

The simplest means of measuring limb length discrepancy is to place wooden blocks of known heights under the short leg until the pelvis is level, but asymmetric pelvic development or pelvic obliquity may cause miscalculation. Measurement may also be made from the anterosuperior iliac spine to the medial malleolus. Clinical evaluation should also include as-

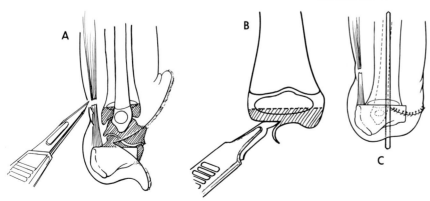

sessment of any rotational and angular deformities, foot height differences, scoliosis, pelvic obliquity, and joint mobility and function. In certain paralytic conditions, particularly spastic diplegia, mild shortness of the paralytic side can actually improve gait by allowing the paralytic foot to clear the floor easier during the swing phase of gait. Flexion contractures of the knee and hip make the limb appear shorter than it really is, both on clinical and roentgenographic examination. The goals of treatment are balanced spine and pelvis, equal limb lengths, and a correct mechanical weight-bearing axis. In patients with rigid scoliosis and an oblique lumbosacral take-off, some degree of limb length discrepancy may be desirable to preserve a balanced spine.

Roentgenographic measurements are important for accuracy, since clinically palpable landmarks may be inaccurate. Two commonly used roentgenographic techniques for measuring limb length discrepancy are the orthoroentgenogram and the scanogram. Both techniques involve placing a radiopaque ruler under the limbs. The orthoroentgenogram is made on a long cassette that includes the hip, knee, and ankle on a single exposure, which results in a magnification error and makes it unacceptably inaccurate ex-

cept in small children. The scanogram uses separate exposures of the hip, knee, and ankle, so there is little parallax error. It does, however, require that the child remain still for all three exposures. For this reason, orthoroentgenograms are preferred in small children and scanograms in older, more cooperative children. A view of the left wrist is obtained to estimate skeletal age from the Gruelich and Pyle atlas. For children under the age of 5, this is not necessary, since the skeletal and chronologic ages are not significantly different.

CT scanograms have been proposed as an improvement over standard scanograms. The radiation exposure is less and accuracy is not compromised. On lateral CT scanograms, accurate measurement can be made of even the limb with a flexion deformity, as shown by Huurman et al. On biplanar CT scanograms, as proposed by Carey et al, foot height can also be measured. Further advances and availability of digital imaging technology may result in further decreases in radiation exposures.

Two widely used techniques exist for predicting growth and helping decide the timing of growth arrest procedures. The first technique is the Green-Anderson growth remaining chart (Fig. 3-30). Proper

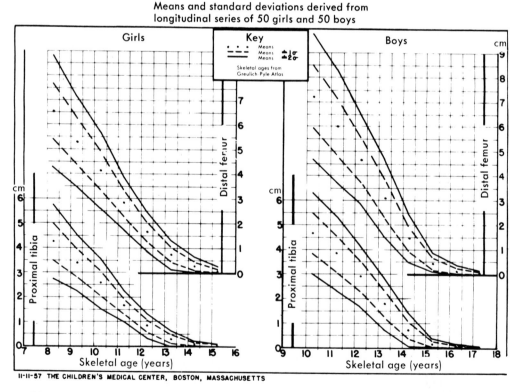

Fig. 3-30 Green-Anderson growth prediction chart shows amount of growth remaining in distal femur and proximal tibia (see text). (From Anderson M, Green WT, and Messner MB: J Bone Joint Surg 45A:1, 1963.)

use of this chart requires the clinician to estimate the percentage of growth inhibition for the individual patient by taking two interval measurements separated by at least 3 months. The growth difference between the involved limb and the normal limb is multiplied by 100, and that result is divided by the growth of the normal limb. Moseley simplified the Green-Anderson growth remaining chart by mathematically manipulating the original data to allow it to fit on a straight line graph that is both visually graphic and easier to apply (Fig. 3-31). It obviates the need for mathematical calculations of growth inhibition and provides a ready prediction of the results of epiphysiodesis, lengthening, and shortening (Fig. 3-32). Reference slopes are provided for predicting future limb growth after epiphysiodesis of the distal femur, the proximal tibia, or both. The difference between the slopes of the normal leg and the short leg is the growth inhibition. Lengthening the short leg in a growing child can be depicted by a sharp vertical rise, followed by a continued gradual slope equivalent to the slope of growth before lengthening.

One criticism of the Green-Anderson tables and Moseley straight line graph for leg length inequality is that they do not include an estimation for foot height. For example, a discrepancy of 4 cm by roentgenographic scanograms may be 5 cm by the clinical block technique, if the short leg also has a smaller foot and ankle unit.

There are some fundamental problems with both the Green-Anderson and the Moseley methods. The original data may not be applicable to modern children. The skeletal age according to Greulich and Pyle's atlas is at best an approximation. Human growth is not always mathematically predictable, for it is influenced by nutritional, metabolic, hormonal, and socioeconomic factors. Shapiro identified five distinct patterns of limb length discrepancy in a review of over 800 children, implying that growth inhibition may differ in certain etiologies of limb length discrepancy, making standard growth prediction charts inaccurate. For example, limb length discrepancy in some children with juvenile rheumatoid arthritis and Perthes' disease may follow an upward slope–downward slope pattern in which the discrepancy corrects itself. In overgrowth after a femoral fracture, the pattern of growth may level off and, after a short period, the discrepancy remains constant. Despite these atypical patterns, most leg length discrepancies follow the traditional growth prediction curves.

Simpler methods of predicting growth are available. The Menelaus method is convenient, because it requires no special charts or graphs and relies on chronologic age rather than skeletal age. Menelaus assumes that in adolescents over 9 years of age the distal femur grows ⅜ in/yr, the proximal tibia grows ¼ in/yr, and growth ceases at age 14 years in girls and age 16 years in boys. Using this technique, Menelaus achieved a final limb length discrepancy of less than ¾ inch in 94% of patients who underwent epiphysiodesis. In summary, all the methods are, at best, approximations. A final discrepancy after treatment of 1 to 1.5 cm clinically should be considered a successful outcome.

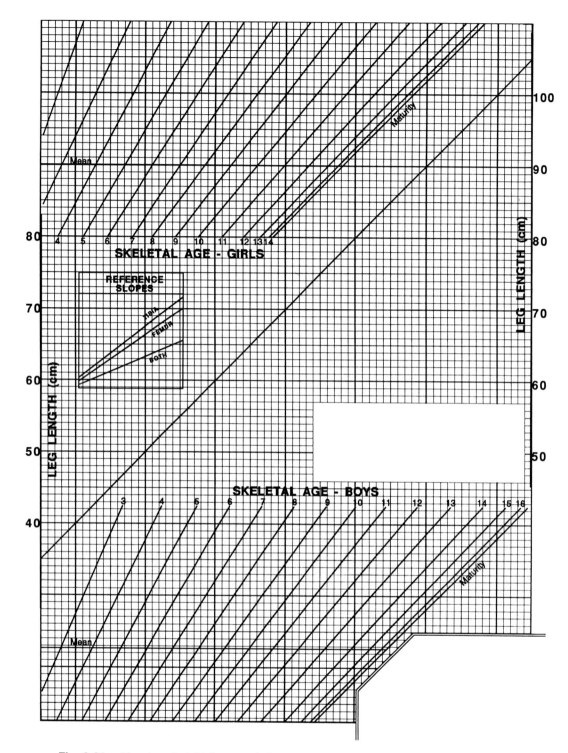

Fig. 3-31 Moseley straight line graph for predicting future growth. (From Moseley CF: J Bone Joint Surg 59A:174, 1977.)

A THE DEPICTION OF PAST GROWTH

At each visit to the hospital obtain these three values:

1. The length of the normal leg measured by orthoroentgenogram from the most superior part of the femoral head to the middle of the articular surface of the tibia at the ankle,
2. The length of the short leg, and
3. The radiologic estimate of skeletal age.

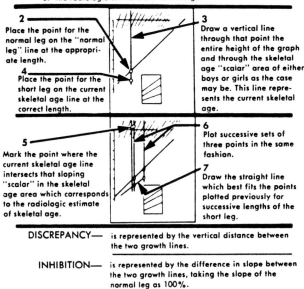

2
Place the point for the normal leg on the "normal leg" line at the appropriate length.

4
Place the point for the short leg on the current skeletal age line at the correct length.

3
Draw a vertical line through that point the entire height of the graph and through the skeletal age "scalar" area of either boys or girls as the case may be. This line represents the current skeletal age.

5
Mark the point where the current skeletal age line intersects that sloping "scalar" in the skeletal age area which corresponds to the radiologic estimate of skeletal age.

6
Plot successive sets of three points in the same fashion.

7
Draw the straight line which best fits the points plotted previously for successive lengths of the short leg.

DISCREPANCY— is represented by the vertical distance between the two growth lines.

INHIBITION— is represented by the difference in slope between the two growth lines, taking the slope of the normal leg as 100%.

B THE PREDICTION OF FUTURE GROWTH

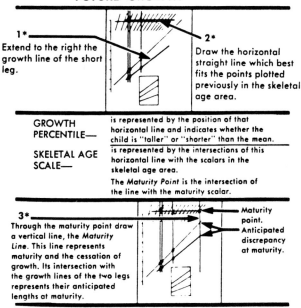

1*
Extend to the right the growth line of the short leg.

2*
Draw the horizontal straight line which best fits the points plotted previously in the skeletal age area.

GROWTH PERCENTILE— is represented by the position of that horizontal line and indicates whether the child is "taller" or "shorter" than the mean.

SKELETAL AGE SCALE— is represented by the intersections of this horizontal line with the scalars in the skeletal age area.

The *Maturity Point* is the intersection of the line with the maturity scalar.

3*
Through the maturity point draw a vertical line, the *Maturity Line*. This line represents maturity and the cessation of growth. Its intersection with the growth lines of the two legs represents their anticipated lengths at maturity.

→ Maturity point.
→ Anticipated discrepancy at maturity.

*In keeping a child's graph up to date it is recommended that these lines be drawn in pencil. The addition of further data makes this method more accurate and may require slight changes in the positions of these lines.

C THE EFFECT OF SURGERY

EPIPHYSEODESIS

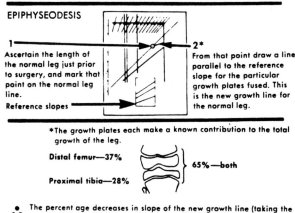

1
Ascertain the length of the normal leg just prior to surgery, and mark that point on the normal leg line.

Reference slopes

2*
From that point draw a line parallel to the reference slope for the particular growth plates fused. This is the new growth line for the normal leg.

*The growth plates each make a known contribution to the total growth of the leg.

Distal femur—37%
Proximal tibia—28%
} 65%—both

• The percent age decreases in slope of the new growth line (taking the
•• previous slope as 100%) exactly represents the loss of the contribution of the fused growth plate(s).

LENGTHENING

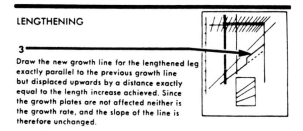

3
Draw the new growth line for the lengthened leg exactly parallel to the previous growth line but displaced upwards by a distance exactly equal to the length increase achieved. Since the growth plates are not affected neither is the growth rate, and the slope of the line is therefore unchanged.

D THE TIMING OF SURGERY

EPIPHYSEODESIS

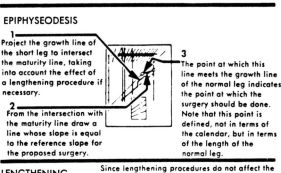

1
Project the growth line of the short leg to intersect the maturity line, taking into account the effect of a lengthening procedure if necessary.

2
From the intersection with the maturity line draw a line whose slope is equal to the reference slope for the proposed surgery.

3
The point at which this line meets the growth line of the normal leg indicates the point at which the surgery should be done. Note that this point is defined, not in terms of the calendar, but in terms of the length of the normal leg.

LENGTHENING
Since lengthening procedures do not affect the rate of growth, the timing of this procedure is not critical and will be governed by clinical considerations.

E POST-SURGICAL FOLLOW-UP

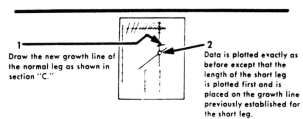

1
Draw the new growth line of the normal leg as shown in section "C."

2
Data is plotted exactly as before except that the length of the short leg is plotted first and is placed on the growth line previously established for the short leg.

Fig. 3-32 Instructions for using Moseley straight line graph for leg length discrepancy. (From Moseley CF: J Bone Joint Surg 59A:174, 1977.)

Treatment

Four types of treatment are available for limb length equalization: shoe lift or prosthetic conversion, epiphysiodesis of the long leg, shortening of the long leg (in patients too old for epiphysiodesis), and lengthening of the short leg.

Nonsurgical Treatment

For small discrepancies of 2 cm or less, no treatment is necessary. If a patient desires, a 1-cm shoe lift can be provided to wear inside the shoe. The entire discrepancy need not be compensated, since people rarely stand erect with both knees and hips straight and many people have small (1-cm) differences that are functionally insignificant. The degree of discrepancy that can be made up with an internal shoe lift is limited, however, and for differences of 2 to 4 cm, a lift on the outside of the shoe is necessary, although it can taper towards the front of the shoe. For small discrepancies a heel lift can be used, and for larger differences, a full sole lift. To limit the amount of external lift, the shoemaker can shave down the heel on the long-leg shoe by 1 cm. A shoe lift can be used for larger discrepancies if the patient declines shortening or lengthening. However, lifts of 5 to 10 cm are unsightly, unstable, and may need additional uprights on an ankle-foot orthosis (AFO) to help support the ankle. Extension prostheses are "modified shoe lifts" in that the foot is not amputated. Instead, the foot is forced into an equinus position and fit into a custom prosthesis that has a prosthetic foot distal to the natural foot (Fig. 3-33). Conversion with a Syme or Boyd amputation is preferred, however, since prosthetic fitting is easier.

Surgical Treatment

Theoretically, lengthening of the short limb is optimal treatment, but technical difficulty and frequent complications of lengthening procedures have made them an infrequent choice. For the growing child, epiphysiodesis is a relatively simple procedure with reasonably low morbidity and fast recovery. In the adolescent too old for effective epiphysiodesis, limb shortening is an accurate, safe, and simple procedure, with a complication rate only slightly higher than epiphysiodesis. Joint stiffness after shortening is rare, since the muscles are made somewhat slack by shortening the limb, unlike lengthening, which frequently results in permanent joint stiffness and subluxation.

There are several disadvantages of shortening: (1) the normal limb is operated on rather than the pathologic limb, and if there is a deformity in the short limb, a second operation may be needed to correct that deformity; (2) the resultant body proportions may be cosmetically unpleasing after shortening, as shown by Wagner (Fig. 3-34); (3) the degree of shortening possible is limited because of the inability of the muscles to adapt to shortenings of greater than 5 cm; (4) the final height after shortening or epiphysiodesis may be unacceptably low.

Based on skeletal age, an estimation of predicted adult height can be made with the Bayley-Pinneau tables using the Green-Anderson assumption that skeletal age correlates with the percent of mature height. These tables take into account the child's current height, chronologic age, and skeletal age. An estimation of the adult height is helpful in determining if lengthening is appropriate. For example, in an adolescent boy with a predicted height of 5 feet 11 inches, shortening by 2 inches is not as unpalatable as it would be if the predicted height were 5 feet.

Recent advancements in technology, including Russian and Italian systems of distraction osteogenesis, represent improvements over the Wagner method and have promising initial results, but long-term results are still forthcoming.

Fig. 3-33 Special (leg-lengthening) extension prosthesis can be used to treat 18 cm of shortening secondary to PFFD. Equinus position of foot is necessary to ensure good fit. (From Meyer E and Petersen D. In Hungerford DS, editor: Progress in orthopaedic surgery, 1977, Berlin, Springer-Verlag.)

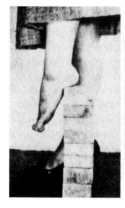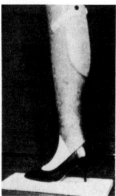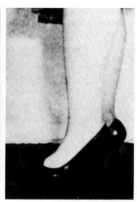

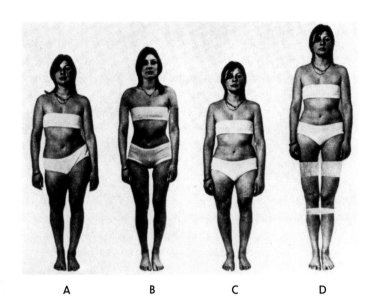

Fig. 3-34 Composite photography to illustrate results of various treatment maneuvers. **A,** A 24-year-old female with 8½ cm of leg-length discrepancy. Right hip was destroyed by infection during infancy and left knee underwent epiphysiodesis to limit resultant discrepancy. **B,** After 8½-cm femoral lengthening with Wagner technique. **C,** Composite picture showing appearance if 8½ cm of left femoral shortening had been performed. **D,** Composite picture showing result if epiphysiodesis had not been performed and if total discrepancy was corrected with femoral lengthening. (From Wagner H. In Hungerford DS, editor: Progress in orthopaedic surgery, Berlin, 1977, Springer-Verlag.)

Epiphysiodesis. Phemister described epiphysiodesis in 1933, and his original technique, with minor modifications, has been valuable for limb length equalization. Most authors recommend epiphysiodesis when 2 to 5 cm of shortening is required; however, Menelaus and others recommend epiphysiodesis for discrepancies of up to 8 to 10 cm to prevent the complications of limb lengthening.

Phemister removed a rectangular piece of the lateral cortex on either side of the epiphysis and reinserted it in a reversed position (Fig. 3-35). White developed special hollow chisels to remove a square block of bone and curetted the physeal cartilage deep in the hole before replacing the bone block in a reversed position.

A newer technique of epiphysiodesis involves the use of percutaneous instrumentation to obliterate the physis through small, cosmetically pleasing incisions. Experimental evidence reported by Canale, Russell, and Holcomb and by Ogilvie indicates that the physis can be effectively obliterated by this technique. Early clinical results from Canale et al and from Bowen and Johnson support these findings. Angled curets may be used instead of high-speed burrs to scrape the physeal cartilage.

Regardless of technique, careful preoperative timing and consideration of the final height of the knee are important. For discrepancies involving the femur and tibia, epiphysiodesis of both may be required to ensure that the knees and pelvis will be level. Operative complications are uncommon, yet reported complications include cutaneous nerve entrapment, infection, asymmetric arrest, undercorrection, and overcorrection.

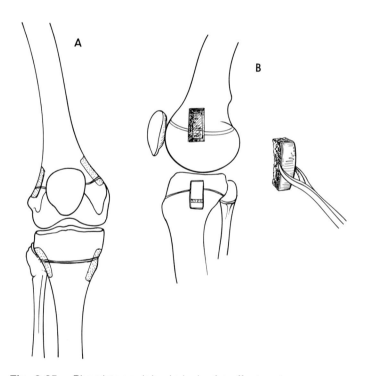

Fig. 3-35 Phemister epiphysiodesis. An offset rectangular section of bone including growth plate is removed **(A)** and reinserted upside down to act as bony bridge **(B).** (Modified from Phemister DB: J Bone Joint Surg 15:1, 1933.)

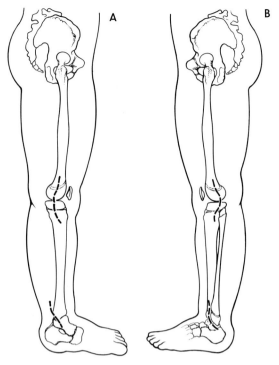

Fig. 3-36 **A,** Medial and, **B,** lateral surgical approaches to physes around knee. (Modified from Abbott LC and Gill GG: Arch Surg 46:591, 1943.)

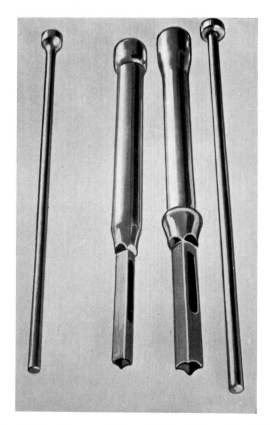

Fig. 3-37 Square hollow chisels designed by J. Warren White for epiphysiodesis. Obturators aid in removal of bone block from chisel.

Physeal exposure around the knee

▶ *Technique (Abbott and Gill)* (Fig. 3-36). Flex the knee 30 degrees to relax the hamstring muscles, and make a lateral incision 6.5 cm proximal to the lateral femoral condyle, continuing distally between the biceps tendon and iliotibial band to the fibular head, then extending anteriorly over the lateral aspect of the tibia. Enter the interval between the lateral intermuscular septum and the vastus lateralis. Ligate the superior geniculate arteries. Make a vertical incision in the periosteum over the physeal plate, and identify the thin "white line" of the physeal cartilage. Protect the peroneal nerve behind the fibular head, and incise the periosteum over the anterior aspect of the fibular head. Reflect the anterior compartment muscles of the tibia distally to expose the proximal tibial physis. On the medial side, make a curved incision starting at the adductor tubercle, and continuing first posteriorly and then anteriorly along the sartorius tendon. Ligate the geniculate arteries. Open the periosteum of the distal femur between the vastus medialis and the vastus intermedius muscles. Keep the dissection subperiosteal to avoid entering the knee joint. Over the proximal tibia, retract the pes anserinus tendon posteriorly, ligate the geniculate arteries, and make a vertical incision to facilitate a subperiosteal exposure to locate the physis.

Four short (2.5 cm) incisions may be used rather than two long ones to improve cosmesis. Dissection of the peroneal nerve is not mandatory. Fluoroscopy or image intensification, using needles to locate the physes, is helpful in placing the incisions. Preoperative roentgenograms showing the relation of the distal femoral physis to the patella also aid placement of the incision.

Open epiphysiodesis

▶ *Technique (White)* (Fig. 3-37). Expose the medial and lateral physis as described. With a ½-inch square mortising chisel, remove a square of bone that contains the physis, approximately ½ to ¾ of an inch deep. Place the chisel diagonally so that two opposite points of the square are on the physis. Gently work the chisel side to side, and loosen the bone plug, removing it in one piece if possible. Curet the physis toward the midline anteriorly and posteriorly, but leave the curettings in place. Reinsert the bone plug, turning it 90 degrees so that the physeal cartilage of the bone plug is now vertical. Tamp the bone plug to prevent displacement. For the fibular physis, simply scoop out the physis from anterior to posterior cortex with a curet through a small incision. Close the incisions and apply a long-leg splint.

▲ *Postoperative management.* Active range of motion exercises are begun within a week of surgery, and partial weight bearing with crutches is allowed. The splint is removed at 3 weeks. Fusion is usually evident on roentgenograms in 3 to 6 months.

Percutaneous epiphysiodesis

▲ *Technique (Canale).* After administration of general anesthesia place the patient supine on the operating table. Prepare the limb in the standard fashion and drape it free. A tourniquet may be used if desired. Place a hemostat on the lateral aspect of the leg to locate the lateral portion of the distal femoral physis. After the physis is located with image intensification, make a small, vertical, or horizontal stab wound approximately 1.5 cm in length medially and laterally. Place a smooth Steinmann pin or Kirschner wire into the physis and drill it into the lateral side of the distal femoral physis (Fig. 3-38, *A*). Confirm correct positioning of the pin on both anteroposterior and lateral image intensification views. Rotate the image intensifier rather than the leg, because rotation of the leg causes the iliotibial band and medial musculature to become extremely taut and interfere with placement of instruments. Place a cannulated reamer over the guide pin (Fig. 3-38, *B*) and drill into the physis approximately halfway across; verify this with image intensification (Fig. 3-38, *C*). After removal of the reamer, introduce a high-speed pneumatic drill (such as the Hall drill) with a dental burr. Take care to protect the skin during drilling to prevent heat necrosis of the skin; using a guard for the dental burr is helpful. Alternatively, use straight and curved curets to remove the physis. Ream the physis proximally and distally, anteriorly and posteriorly, especially at the periphery, to create a "bulls-eye" effect in the center of the physis at the lateral periphery.

It is not necessary to remove the entire physis. A lucent area or blackout effect will be noted on image intensification where the physis and surrounding bone have been removed. If the bulls-eye effect is not achieved, use a curet or larger reamer (such as from an adult compression hip screw set) and repeat the procedure on the medial side with frequent image intensification evaluation. Often the medial and lateral defects can be connected. Thoroughly irrigate to remove all loose pieces of cartilage and cancellous bone. Close the wounds with subcutaneous sutures and apply a sterile dressing.

▲ *Postoperative management.* Immediate weight bearing in a soft knee immobilizer is allowed. The immobilizer is worn for approximately 2 to 3 weeks.

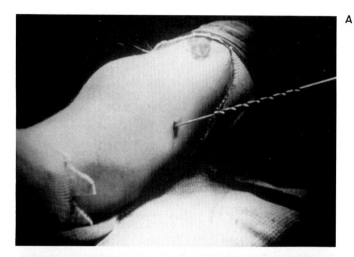
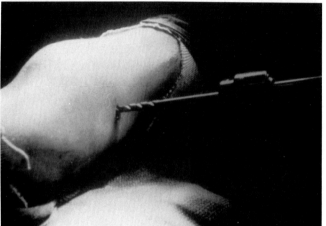
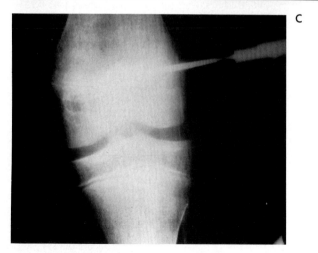

Fig. 3-38 Percutaneous epiphysiodesis. **A,** Insertion of guide pin. **B,** Cannulated reamer. **C,** Obliteration of peripheral physis.

The same technique is used in the proximal tibial physis, except that the tibial physis is more undulating than the femoral, requiring more careful drilling.

Epiphysiodesis of the proximal fibular physis may not be necessary, especially if the desired growth arrest in the proximal tibia is less than 2.5 cm. Proximal fibular epiphysiodesis can be accomplished using a small Steinmann pin, a small cannulated reamer, and a hand drill or hand curet under direct vision through a small separate incision. Because of the possibility of mechanical or thermal damage to the peroneal nerve, power instruments should not be used in this area.

As a modification of this technique, a radiolucent imaging table may be used instead of a fracture table. Use a tourniquet, and make the stab wound large enough to insert a ¼-inch drill bit to broach the cortex. Curet the physis with angled and straight curets, using the image intensifier as needed (Fig. 3-39).

A knee immobilizer is worn for 10 to 14 days; then active range of motion exercises are begun. Crutches are used for guarded weight bearing for the first 4 weeks.

Bowen and Johnson described a similar technique for use in the distal femur, but discouraged its use in the proximal tibia because of the danger of injury to the peroneal nerve. If used in the proximal tibia, it is important to palpate the fibular head, make the incision over the physis under image control, and stay anterolateral. A drill is not required to broach the proximal fibular cortex; a small straight curet works well and does not risk injury to the peroneal nerve.

Limb shortening. Shortening is usually reserved for the skeletally mature patient who can accept the loss of stature necessary to equalize limb lengths. When planning surgery, both ultimate length and alignment should be considered. Wagner outlined the standard approach to limb shortening, but improvements have been made in femoral shortening techniques, such as a closed technique for diaphyseal shortening in the femur developed by Winquist and Hansen. In the femur, 5 to 6 cm is the maximum length that can be removed without seriously affecting muscle function; in the tibia, the maximum is probably 2 to 4 cm, although Menelaus reported resection of 5.1 cm of the tibia in one patient.

In general, femoral shortenings are tolerated better than tibial shortenings because the soft tissue muscular envelope is much larger, making skin closure easier, offering a better cosmetic result, and ensuring prompt union of the osteotomy. However, if the discrepancy is largely confined to the tibia, a tibial shortening is preferred to make the knee heights level.

Wagner recommends metaphyseal osteotomy if angular or rotational correction is required and diaphyseal osteotomy if shortening alone is necessary. Proximal metaphyseal osteotomy in the femur has fewer complications than distal osteotomy, which may compromise knee motion. Distal femoral metaphyseal osteotomy should be avoided unless necessary for correction of angular deformity. The development of interlocking intramedullary fixation has made diaphyseal shortening preferable to metaphyseal osteotomy in the femur, even if rotational correction is neces-

• • •

Fig. 3-39 A, Percutaneous epiphysiodesis using small curets introduced through drill holes in medial and lateral cortices. **B,** After vigorous curettage under fluoroscopic control, contrast dye can be introduced to produce "physigram" to document completeness of curettage.

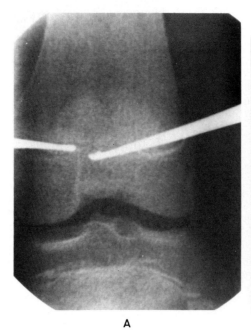

A

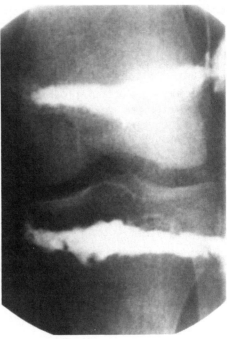

B

sary. Preferably, shortening with an intramedullary saw by closed means may be delayed in children until they approach skeletal maturity to allow fixation with an interlocking intramedullary nail.

Proximal femoral metaphyseal shortening

▲ *Technique (Wagner)* (Fig. 3-40, *A*). Preoperatively, plan the osteotomy to provide the needed angular correction, using tracing paper to outline the osteotomy cuts. Through a proximal lateral incision, split the fascia lata and elevate the vastus lateralis and the periosteum. Fashion an insertion site for the right angle blade plate or hip screw according to the preoperative plan. Mark the bone to control rotation, and remove the proscribed segment with an oscillating saw. Leave a spike of medial cortex and lesser trochanter intact to act as a buttress. Remove the segment, and bring the distal fragment into direct apposition with the proximal segment. Apply the osteosynthesis plate, and insert the screws to create compression across the osteotomy.

Distal femoral metaphyseal shortening

▲ *Technique (Wagner)* (Fig. 3-40, *B*). Make a careful preoperative plan on tracing paper, outlining the planned resection and angular correction. Make a lateral incision through the fascia lata, and elevate the vastus lateralis anteriorly, avoiding the knee joint. Use the blade plate seating device to prepare the entrance for the blade plate. With an oscillating saw, make the proximal osteotomy and then the distal osteotomy. For added stability, try to preserve a medial spike of bone with the distal fragment. Impact the two fragments, apply the blade under compression, and insert a distal femoral sliding screw and fixation plate device.

Proximal tibial metaphyseal shortening

▲ *Technique (Wagner)* (Fig. 3-41). Through a lateral incision, resect a portion of the fibula at the junction of the proximal and middle thirds. Make a separate anterior incision to expose the proximal tibia subperiosteally. Resect the desired amount of bone (not to exceed 4 cm, except in unusual circumstances) below the tibial tubercle with an oscillating saw. Hold the two bone ends under compression with a T-plate. Perform a prophylactic fasciotomy. Wound closure may be difficult because of the nature of the skin about the proximal tibia.

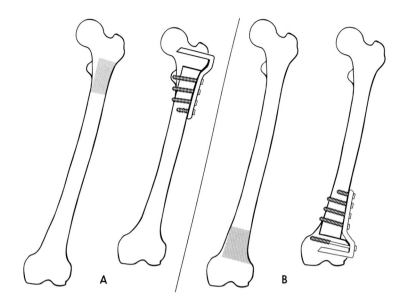

Fig. 3-40　**A,** Wagner technique for proximal femoral metaphyseal shortening. **B,** Wagner technique for distal femoral metaphyseal shortening. (Modified from Wagner H. In Hungerford DS, editor: Progress in orthopaedic surgery, Berlin, 1977, Springer-Verlag.)

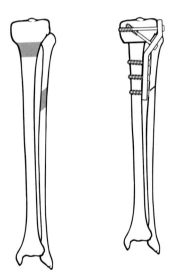

Fig. 3-41　Wagner technique for proximal tibial metaphyseal shortening. (Modified from Wagner H. In Hungerford DS, editor: Progress in Orthopaedic Surgery, Berlin, 1977, Springer-Verlag.)

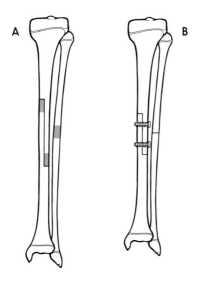

Fig. 3-42 Technique for tibial diaphyseal shortening in skeletally immature patients. (Modified from Broughton NS, Olney BW, and Menelaus NB: J Bone Joint Surg 71B:242, 1989.)

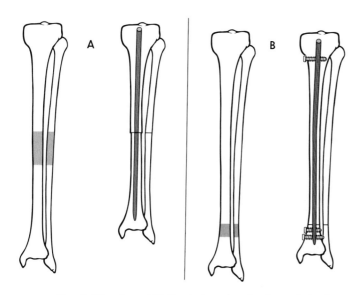

Fig. 3-43 **A** and **B,** Technique for diaphyseal shortening with intramedullary fixation. **B,** Distal tibial shortening with locked intramedullary nail. (Modified from Wagner H. In Hungerford DS, editor: Progress in orthopaedic surgery, Berlin, 1977, Springer-Verlag.)

Tibial diaphyseal shortening

▲ *Technique (Broughton, Olney, and Menelaus)* (Fig. 3-42, *A* and *B*). Make a longitudinal incision over the anteromedial surface of the tibia. Perform a subperiosteal dissection, and make a step-cut osteotomy, removing the desired amount of bone and allowing for 5 to 7.5 cm of overlap after shortening. Through a separate incision remove an equivalent amount of bone from the midshaft of the fibula. Shorten the leg and fix the step-cut with two lag screws or, for mature patients, an intramedullary nail (Fig. 3-43).

Femoral diaphyseal shortening

▲ *Technique (Winquist and Hansen)* (Fig. 3-44, *A* and *B*). Position the patient on a fracture table in the lateral position. Use the standard techniques for closed intramedullary nailing (p. 52) and ream to the desired width in 0.5-mm increments. Adjust the saw for the appropriate depth according to the preoperative plan and insert the saw until, with the blade fully retracted, the measuring device is seated firmly against the greater trochanter. While an assistant applies pressure to hold the measuring device in place for both the proximal and distal saw cuts, deploy the saw blade in increments, making complete revolutions. If necessary, back up one index notch to repeat the cuts if the blade is getting stuck. Slowly continue cutting until the final index mark is reached, at which point the blade is fully deployed. The most difficult area to cut is posteriorly in the linea aspera. If necessary, complete the cut percutaneously with a thin osteotome. The next larger size blade and cam can be inserted to get a larger cutting diameter, but this can be difficult if the canal is not reamed widely enough.

After completing the first cut, retract the blade fully, and withdraw it slightly to allow manipulation of the leg. Remove the leg from traction, manipulate the osteotomy to complete it, and sever the periosteum. Remove the foot or traction bale from the fracture table and angulate the distal femur 60 to 70 degrees in all directions to tear the periosteum, then replace the traction. Advance the measuring device handle distally while holding the locking nut in place. The amount of distance that develops between these two components should equal the amount of femur to be resected. Spin the locking nut distally to lock the measuring device handle. With the assistant holding the measuring device firmly against the greater trochanter, make the second (proximal) osteotomy in the same fashion as the first. After completing the second osteotomy, retract the blade fully and remove the saw.

A

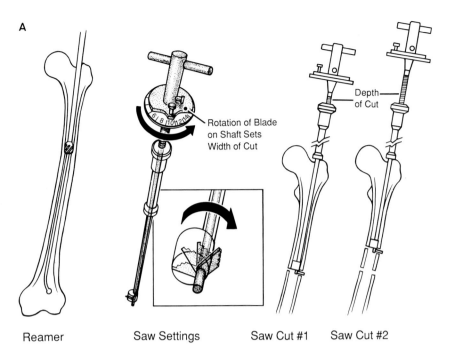

Reamer Saw Settings Saw Cut #1 Saw Cut #2

Fig. 3-44 **A,** Closed femoral diaphyseal shortening as described by Winquist and Hansen (see text). Intramedullary canal is reamed with standard cannulated reamer. Special intramedullary saw is inserted into reamed canal. One or two rotations are made with saw at each setting and saw is progressively opened until blade is completely exposed. **B,** After making both saw cuts, intercalary segment is split using back-cutting chisel. Rotational alignment and distraction can be controlled with locked intramedullary nail. **C,** A 16-year-old girl underwent 4 cm closed femoral shortening. Shortly after surgery, intercalary fragment is seen around site of osteotomy acting as bone graft. **D,** Osteotomy is healed 8 weeks later. Note 4 mm of distraction occurred postoperatively after osteotomy. Locking the nail is recommended to preserve alignment and length if necessary.

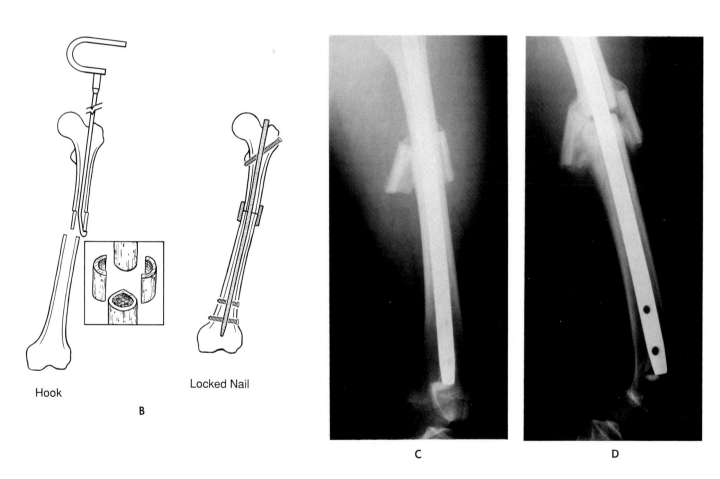

Hook Locked Nail

B

C D

Insert an appropriate size internal chisel, hook the medial aspect of the intercalary segment, and pound on the handle backward to split the bone. Repeat this maneuver at least one more time on the lateral segment. Use the hook of the chisel to push the fragments out away from the canal. Have the unscrubbed surgeon again remove the foot or traction bale from the fracture table and impact the osteotomy, displacing the segmental fragments to either side, using the chisel to manipulate the osteotomized fragments if necessary. Pass a nail-driving guide wire across the osteotomy, and insert an appropriate size nail for fixation, while the unscrubbed surgeon maintains rotational alignment. If a locked nail is used, be certain that the rotational alignment is absolutely correct. Steinmann pins may be inserted into the lateral aspect of the distal femoral condyle and the greater trochanter just before the first osteotomy to serve as references for rotational alignment control.

▲ *Postoperative management.* A knee splint is used to stabilize the shortened quadriceps mechanism, and a vigorous strengthening program is instituted. Rehabilitation is faster if the patient has undergone a preoperative quadriceps strengthening program. Derotation or distraction at the osteotomy site may occur if a locked nail is not used.

Limb lengthening. A limb lengthening program requires a patient and family fully committed to maximal participation in an extended project. The success of a limb lengthening procedure is largely dependent on patient effort in physiotherapy and care of the external fixator. Although recent technical improvements have reduced the frequency of serious complications associated with limb lengthening, the process remains difficult and should be performed by surgeons with appropriate experience.

Shortening procedures are preferable for many patients who are candidates for a limb lengthening. Patients who are unable to participate in frequent follow-up, or who do not have the support to care for the fixator properly and to undergo vigorous physiotherapy, are best treated by means other than lengthening. Limb lengthening candidates and their parents should meet other patients in various stages of the lengthening process.

Salter described acute distraction and interposition grafting through the innominate bone. Millis and Hall reported a modification of this technique: they achieved an average lengthening of 2.3 cm in 20 patients with acetabular dysplasia with femoral shortening, pure limb length inequality, decompensated scoliosis, and primary intrapelvic asymmetry. This technique may be useful in patients who also require acetabular reconstruction, but epiphysiodesis or gradual distraction lengthening techniques are more reliable alternatives for isolated limb length discrepancy.

Transiliac lengthening

▲ *Technique (Millis and Hall)* (Figs. 3-45, *A* and *B,* and 3-46). Use the same approach to the pelvis as for the Salter innominate osteotomy (see Chapter 2). Use a Gigli saw to make the osteotomy from the sciatic notch to the anteroinferior iliac spine. Introduce a lamina spreader into the anterior aspect of the osteotomy. Have an assistant apply caudally directed pressure on the iliac crest to prevent displacement of the proximal fragment by shear force through the sacroiliac joint, while another assistant applies traction to the femur, keeping the knee flexed to relax the sciatic nerve. Fashion a full-thickness block of iliac crest bone graft into a trapezoidal shape. The height of the graft directly superior to the acetabulum will determine the amount of lengthening. Wedge the iliac graft into the distraction site and hold it with two large threaded Steinmann pins that transfix the proximal fragment, the graft, and the distal fragment. Postoperative traction is applied for 5 days. Begin range of motion exercises on the third day and touch down weight bearing on the seventh day. Full weight bearing is delayed until there is roentgenographic evidence of graft incorporation (at 3 to 6 months).

Fig. 3-45 A, Acute transiliac lengthening accomplished by modification of Salter technique. Instead of triangular graft, square or trapezoidal graft is employed. The larger the graft, the more lengthening is achieved. **B,** Acetabular dysplasia and mild limb length inequality. Pelvic obliquity results in compensatory scoliosis. In middle figure, block has been placed underneath short leg. While this balances pelvis and straightens spine, it causes acetabulum to be even more vertical. On right, transiliac lengthening is performed to simultaneously improve femoral acetabular coverage and regain length. (Modified from Millis MB and Hall JE: J Bone Joint Surg 61A:1182, 1979.)

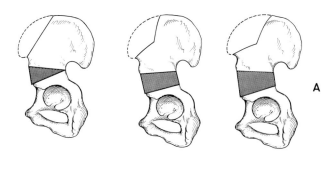

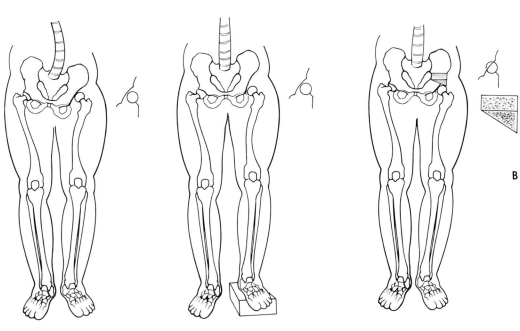

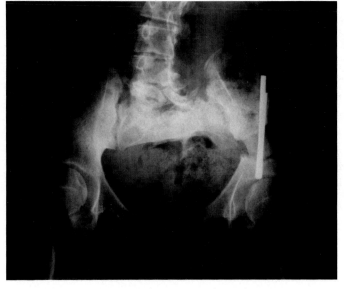

Fig. 3-46 Transiliac lengthening with trapezoidal graft.

Lengthening by slow distraction. Osteotomy followed by gradual distraction of the bone fragments with a mechanical apparatus has been the basic procedure for limb lengthening since Putti's report of the technique in 1921. Methods of both osteotomy and fixation have been modified by several authors, including Abbott, Barr and Ober, Bost and Larsen, White, Anderson, and Sofield. However, disturbingly high complication rates (Fig. 3-47) were reported with all methods, including deep infection, nonunion, fracture after plate removal, malunion, and nerve palsy. Wagner introduced a low-profile, mobile, monolateral fixator which improved results, and DeBastiani designed a similar but more versatile fixator. In the early 1950s, Ilizarov devised a thin-wire, circular external fixator for fracture fixation and found that slow distraction with the device caused regeneration of bone in the distraction gap. For lengthening procedures, he used a percutaneous "corticotomy" in which the accessible cortices of a long bone

are cut with a 5-mm osteotome through a 10-mm skin incision (Fig. 3-48) without penetrating the medullary canal. After 5 to 7 days, distraction is begun at the rate of 0.25 mm four times a day. The thin wires (1.8 mm or 1.5 mm) are tensioned up to 130 kg to provide adequate stiffness for bone segment stability. Simultaneous or sequential correction of axial, translational, and rotational deformities is possible. In children, the fixator is worn approximately 1 month for each centimeter of lengthening, and in adults, about 1.5 months for each centimeter. This lengthy period of fixator wear is one of the major disadvantages of Ilizarov's technique. The Ilizarov apparatus has been modified by Catagni et al, who replaced the semicircular rings with 90-degree and 120-degree arches, which attach to bone with standard 5-mm half-pins, and by Monticelli and Spinelli who combined heavy transfixation pins with thin-tensioned wires.

Paley classified complications of limb lengthening as *problems, obstacles,* and *complications.* A problem,

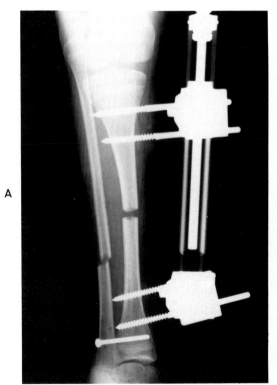 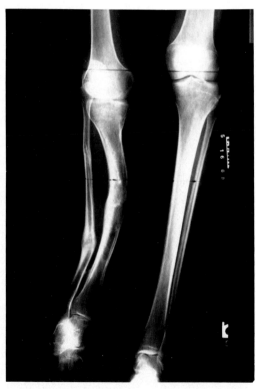

Fig. 3-47   A, Wagner lengthening in an adolescent with tibial hemimelia. **B,** Follow-up 4 years later shows results of several complications encountered during and after lengthening. Fibula remains elevated; tibia, which fractured after plate removal, has healed in valgus alignment; foot is in severe equinus, and leg length discrepancy persists.

such a minor pin tract infection, can be dealt with in an outpatient setting. An obstacle requires a secondary procedure, such as repeat corticotomy for premature consolidation of the lengthening gap. Neither problems nor obstacles necessarily prevent a good result. A complication is an unexpected sequela that compromises the final result. A minor complication, such as residual equinus contracture, can be treated surgically to improve the result. A major complication, such as permanent nerve palsy, might not be improved by surgery.

Methods of lengthening

Of the multiple techniques for limb lengthening, the Wagner method using open osteotomy has been the most widely used, but newer techniques of percutaneous corticotomy are becoming more popular. Two basic types of external fixators are available for limb lengthening after percutaneous corticotomy: large half-pin monolateral devices and thin-wire circular devices. The large half-pin devices are relatively simple to apply but are limited in correcting angular and rotational deformities and do not effect simultaneous correction of complex deformities. The original Wagner device is adjustable in only two planes, and the Hoffman modification in one additional plane. DeBastiani's device (Orthofix) can be converted from a lengthening to a correction device. Circular devices use transfixion wires that limit muscle and joint motion more than monolateral fixators. The Ilizarov device is modular and can be adapted with extensions and hinges to lengthen and correct angular and translational deformities simultaneously. Rotational deformities can be corrected either at the time of fixator application or later by applying outriggers to the rings. The circular devices are more difficult to apply than monolateral fixators, and extensive training and experience are recommended before using them.

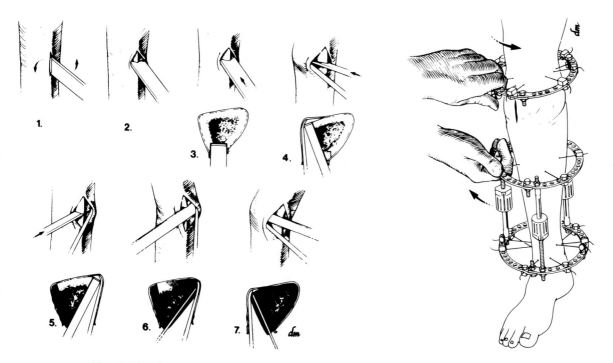

Fig. 3-48 Percutaneous tibial corticotomy modified from Ilizarov. Entire tibia is cut through 1.5-cm incision centered over anterior crest. Small elevator lifts periosteum on medial and lateral cortices. A 5-mm osteotome is used to first cut medial cortex then lateral cortex. Osteotome is reinserted in medial cortex and twisted 90 degrees to help fracture posterior cortex. This maneuver is repeated along lateral cortex. If necessary, Ilizarov rings can be used to complete posterior aspect of corticotomy by externally rotating distal segment. (From Paley D et al: Clin Orthop 241:146, 1989.)

Tibial lengthening

▲ *Technique (Wagner)* (Fig. 3-49). Position the patient supine on a radiolucent table. Expose the distal lateral fibula, and insert two cortical screws 1.5 cm apart to transfix the fibula to the tibia to prevent proximal migration of the fibula during lengthening. Transect the fibula just proximal to the upper screw. Next insert the proximal and distal four parallel Schanz screws anteromedially through stab incisions in the subcutaneous border of the tibia, parallel to the plane of the knee joint. Make an anterior incision and dissect subperiosteally to expose the midshaft of the tibia. Make a transverse osteotomy with an oscillating saw and incise the periosteum. Close the wounds over drains and attach the distraction device. Lengthen the tendo Achilles if the lengthening is to be substantial.

▲ *Postoperative management.* Distraction is continued 1.5 mm daily (about 1 cm/wk). Partial weight bearing with forearm crutches and vigorous physiotherapy are instituted as soon as possible. Dry bandages are used to protect the pin sites, and antibiotic powder or spray is used as necessary. After the length has been achieved, an osteosynthesis plate is applied over the anterolateral surface of the tibia. If insufficient callus is present, autologous corticocancellous bone graft is added. Protected weight bearing is continued and the plate is removed when the tibia appears normal and the medullary canal is reconstituted.

• • •

Dick recommends cleaning the pin sites with alcohol three to four times daily and does not permit weight bearing. Coleman modified Wagner's procedure by making an oblique osteotomy of the fibula and fixing the distal tibia and fibula with only one screw, by routinely performing an anterior compartment fasciotomy, and by decompressing the peroneal nerve prophylactically in congenital deformities.

▲ *Technique (DeBastiani—Orthofix).* Place the patient supine on a radiolucent table. Resect 2 cm of the distal fibula through a lateral approach. Use the mated drills, drill guides, and screw guides to insert the conical self-tapping cortical and cancellous screws. Insert a cancellous screw 2 cm distal to the medial aspect of the knee, parallel to the knee joint. Place the appropriate rigid template parallel to the diaphysis of the tibia and insert the distal-most screw. Next go to the proximal part of the template and insert the next screw in the fourth template hole distal to the upper screw. The last screw to be placed is in the distal template, in the hole farthest away from the distal-most screw. Remove the template and perform a corticotomy just distal to the tibial tubercle. Incise the skin and periosteum anteriorly, longitudinally. Under direct vision, drill a series of unicortical holes in the tibia. Set the drill stop at 1 cm to prevent penetration of the marrow. Use a thin osteotome to connect the drill holes, and to divide along the posteromedial cortex and posterolateral cortex, as much as can be done safely. Flex the tibia at the corticotomy to crack the posterior aspect of the tibia. Apply the Orthofix lengthener. If the Orthofix fracture fixation device is used, fix the ball joint rigidly with a small amount of methyl methacrylate. Suture the periosteum and close the skin over drains.

▲ *Postoperative management.* Partial weight bearing and physiotherapy are begun immediately. Distraction is delayed until callus is roentgenographically visible, usually by day 10 to 15. Distraction is begun at 0.25 mm every 6 hours but may be reduced if pain or muscle contraction occurs. Roentgenographs are made 1 week after distraction to ensure a complete corticotomy, and at 4-week intervals thereafter. If the regenerated callus is of poor quality, distraction is stopped for 7 days. Recompression is indicated for gaps in the callus and for evidence of excessive neurovascular distraction. At the end of the desired lengthening, the body-locking screw mechanism is tightened and the distraction mechanism is removed from the fixator. Full weight bearing is allowed until good callus consolidation is seen and then the body-locking screw is unlocked to allow dynamic axial compression. The fixator is removed when corticalization is complete. If stability is confirmed, screws are removed. If there is any doubt about the stability of the bone, the fixator is replaced for an additional period.

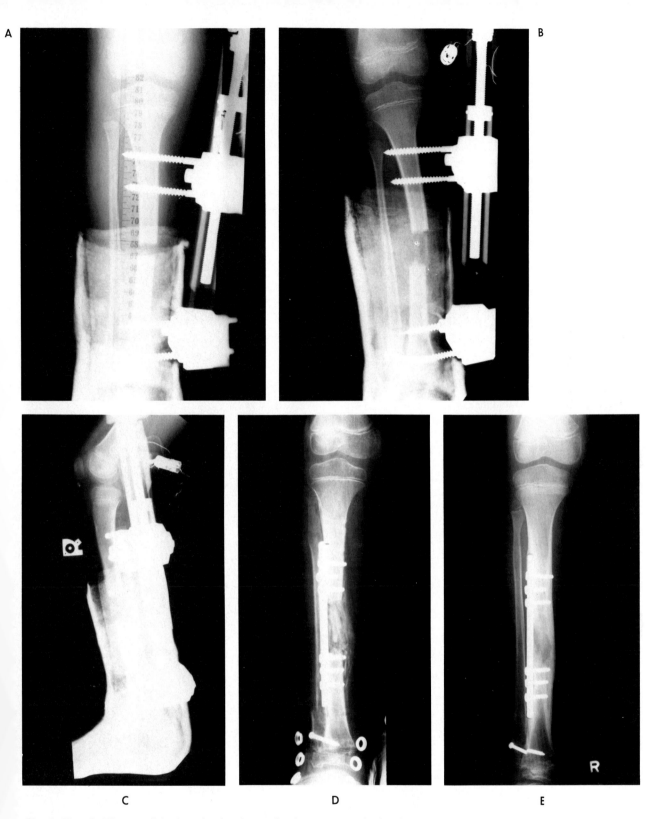

Fig. 3-49 A, Wagner tibial lengthening immediately postoperatively, showing a 1.2-cm initial diastasis. **B,** After gradual lengthening, note the valgus deformation beginning to occur. The fibula underwent a spontaneous epiphysiolysis in response to lengthening. **C,** Lateral roentgenogram during tibial lengthening. Note short-leg cast applied around fixator to keep foot from developing equinus. **D,** At the end of lengthening, after application of Wagner plate, bone grafting, and removal of fixator. Note regenerate bone formation formed in proximal fibula after epiphysiolysis. **E,** Six months later, previous roentgenogram shows incorporation of bone graft and neocorticalization. Proximal fibular physis appears intact despite having undergone epiphysiolysis. (Courtesy Dr. TF Kling.)

▲ *Technique (modified Ilizarov)* (Fig. 3-50). *Preconstruction:* Assemble a frame consisting of four equal Ilizarov rings sized to the particular patient; use the smallest diameter rings that leave sufficient space for swelling after surgery. There should be one fingerbreadth of space between the proximal ring and the tibial tubercle, and two fingerbreadths posteriorly at the largest diameter of the posterior calf muscles. The proximal-most ring may be a ⅝-inch ring to allow more knee flexion after surgery, particularly if the ipsilateral femur is to be lengthened at the same time, since full rings would touch each other after relatively little knee flexion, limiting knee mobility. Connect the upper two rings with 20- or 40-mm threaded hexagonal sockets for better stability. In small patients, there may be room proximally for only one ring and a drop wire (Fig. 3-51). The distal

two rings may be spaced farther apart than the top two rings for better stability of the distal ring construct, but for significant lengthenings, it is better to have the distal two-ring construct relatively farther away from the intended proximal metaphyseal corticotomy site. Such an arrangement maximizes the amount of soft tissue that is available to stretch to contribute to the overall lengthening. For the initial preconstruction, use only two connections between

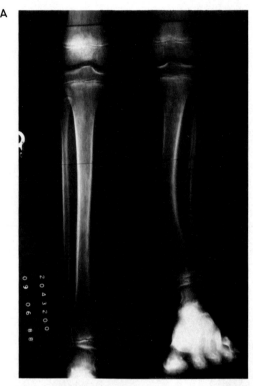
A,

Fig. 3-50   A, Congenital posteromedial bow in 11-year-old girl. Although deformity largely corrected spontaneously, child is left with 6 cm of shortening and valgus angulation in midshaft of tibia. **B,** Double-level tibial lengthening. Lower corticotomy is made at apex of angular deformity in midshaft and upper corticotomy could have been made more proximally in metaphyseal region. After distraction with appropriately placed hinge, more distal corticotomy not only opens up for elongation, but also corrects valgus deformity. Final result after removal of fixator shows excellent regenerate bone formation in gaps. This 6 cm lengthening required 4½ months in fixator. Premature consolidation of proximal fibular osteotomy resulted in spontaneous proximal fibular epiphysiolysis.

B,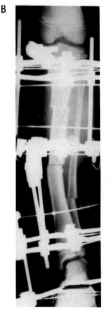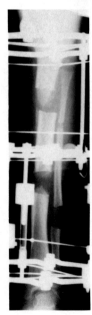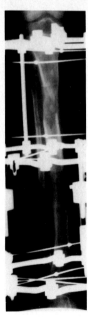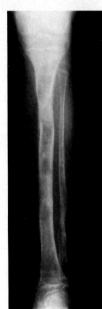

each pair of rings, one anteriorly and one directly posteriorly. Plan the frame so that the central connection bolts are centered directly over the tibial tubercle and the anterior crest of the tibia. Assemble all the rings symmetrically. To compensate for the inevitable anterior and valgus angulation that occurs during routine tibial lengthening, some surgeons connect the upper two-ring set to the lower two-ring set with anterior and posterior threaded rods attached to the lower of the proximal two rings with conical washer couples. These allow a tilt of up to 7 degrees to be built into the system. Adjust the frame so that the proximal rings are higher anteriorly and medially. The frame is applied in this "cockeyed" position, but after the corticotomy is made, the conical washer bolts are removed and all four rings are brought into parallel alignment, placing the tibia into about 5 degrees of prophylactic recurvatum and varus.

Application: Position the patient on a radiolucent table, and apply a tourniquet to the upper thigh. Through a lateral incision, expose the midfibula with subperiosteal dissection and transect it with an oscil-

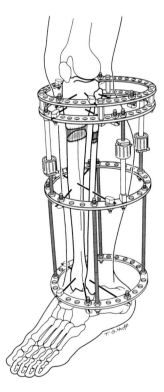

Fig. 3-51 Typical Ilizarov frame for moderate tibial lengthening. In skeletally immature child with intact physes, there would not be room in proximal segment for two rings. Single ring distal to proximal tibial physis is used with drop-wire for additional segmental stabilization of proximal segment. For significant amounts of lengthening, third ring may be placed more distal to allow greater mass of soft tissue for recruitment into lengthening process.

lating saw. Release the tourniquet and close the fibular wound in layers. If desired, perform a subcutaneous fasciotomy at the time of the fibular osteotomy. Under fluoroscopic control, insert a reference wire from medial to lateral, parallel to the knee joint, just below the proximal tibial physis. Use 1.8-mm wires in large children and adolescents and 1.5-mm wires in smaller children. Place another reference wire from medial to lateral parallel to the ankle joint just proximal to the distal tibial physis, parallel with the first wire, and perpendicular to the mechanical axis of the leg. Attach the preassembled frame to these two reference wires. Use the standard Ilizarov principles of wire insertion and fixation at all times: wires should be pushed or gently tapped through the soft tissues, rather than drilled, especially when exiting close to neurovascular structures. When passing wires through the anterior compartment muscles, hold the foot dorsiflexed for the same reason. Incise the skin to allow for passage of olive wires. Never pull or bend a wire to the ring. Instead, build up to the wire with washers or posts as necessary to avoid undue torque and undesirable moments on the bone. Tension the wires to 130 kg, unless the wire is suspended off of a ring, in which case 50 to 90 kg is used to prevent warping of the ring. It is best to use two wire tensioners to tension two wires simultaneously on the same ring, if possible, to prevent warping of the ring. After tensioning and securing the wires, cut the ends long (about 4 cm) and curl the ends of the wire directly over the wire-fixation bolt to allow later retensioning, if necessary. Once the two reference wires are attached to the frame and tensioned, the frame can act as a drill guide for the remaining wires. The wires in the first ring are the initial transverse reference wire and a medial face wire that is parallel to the medial surface of the tibia. Place a third wire from the fibular head into the tibia to prevent dissociation of the proximal tibiofibular joint during lengthening. This wire does not put the peroneal nerve at risk if the fibular head is readily palpable. Do not use an olive wire because it would compress the proximal tibiofibular joint. Ideally, this wire should be proximal to the proximal fibular physis. In the second ring, place a transverse wire and another medial face wire, avoiding the pes anserinus tendons, if possible. Since there is a strong tendency to valgus during proximal tibial lengthenings, place olive wires on the top and bottom rings laterally and on the middle two rings medially to function as handles or fulcrum points for bending the tibia into varus.

Corticotomy: Remove the two threaded rods connecting the proximal fixation block with the distal fixation block. Make a 2-cm incision over the crest of the tibia, just below the tibial tubercle. Incise the periosteum longitudinally, and insert a small periosteal elevator into the wound. Elevate a narrow portion of periosteum the width of the small periosteal elevator along the medial and lateral surfaces of the tibia. Insert a ½-inch osteotome transversely into the thick anterior cortex but do not violate the medullary canal. Use a ¼-inch or 5-mm osteotome to score the medial side, then the lateral side. The periosteal elevator can be placed flush along the bone to act as a directional guide for the osteotome. The corticotomy is guided both by feel and by hearing the sound change when the osteotome exits the back cortex. On the medial side, there are no important structures at risk; on the lateral cortex, the tibialis posterior muscle belly is between the bone and the deep neurovascular structures. After cutting the medial then lateral cortices, withdraw the ¼-inch osteotome, and reinsert it along the medial cortex. Turn the osteotome 90 degrees to spread the cortices apart, thus cracking the posterior cortex. Repeat this maneuver at the lateral cortex, if needed. The corticotomy can also be completed by externally rotating the distal tibia, but do not internally rotate the tibia for fear of stretching the peroneal nerve.

Assembly: Reduce the fracture and insert four distraction rods or graduated telescopic rods, approximately 90 degrees apart, between the middle two rings. Close the corticotomy site, over a drain if necessary, and apply compressive dressings. Dress the wire sites with foam sponges held in place by plastic clips or rubber stoppers. If rubber stoppers are used, put them on before fixing the wires to the rings. Using a different color stopper to identify the olive side of an olive wire is helpful when the device is removed.

▶ *Postoperative management.* Physical therapy and crutch walking with partial weight bearing are begun immediately. Distraction is delayed for 5 to 7 days. In children, the distraction rate is 0.25 mm four times daily. The patient is taught to care for the pins before discharge from the hospital, usually 5 to 7 days after surgery. Roentgenograms are made 7 to 10 days after distraction begins to document separation at the corticotomy site. Regenerated bone should be seen in the gap by 4 to 6 weeks, although linear streaks of regenerated bone are usually visible before then, particularly in younger children. If the regenerated bone formation is insufficient, the rate of distraction should be slowed, stopped, or in some cases, temporarily reversed. Weight bearing and functional activity of the limb aid in maturation of the regenerated bone. During distraction, knee flexion contractures and ankle equinus contractures can be prevented with prophylactic splints and orthoses. The fixator is removed when there is evidence of corticalization of the re-

generated bone and the patient is able to walk without aids.

Modifications: For significant lengthenings, especially when ankle mobility is not normal before the surgery, the foot may be fixed into the lengthening device by inserting an olive wire from each side of the calcaneus, approximately at right angles to one another. These are attached to an appropriate size half ring. This half ring must be within 2 cm of the back of the heel to capture the obliquely placed wires anteriorly. The heel ring is connected to the lower-most ring of the lengthening frame with short plates and threaded rods. The connections may be removed periodically to exercise the ankle, and the heel ring and wires may be removed after lengthening is complete, to prevent subtalar stiffness. A custom orthosis can be constructed to accommodate the foot construct.

For lengthenings over 6 cm, double-level lengthening speeds up the process and reduces the time in the fixator by about 40%. In this modification, three rings are used, with a drop wire off each ring to give "bilevel" fixation at each segment. The frame is preconstructed with prophylactic varus and recurvatum built into the construct between the top and middle rings. The fibula should have one wire transfixing it at each of the three rings. Two fibular osteotomies and two corticotomies are required, one of each just below the proximal ring and one of each just above the distal ring. A heel ring and wires are added to prevent equinus of the ankle. The bottom two rings can be connected to provide a stable handle on the distal segments to complete the proximal corticotomy, and the top two rings can be connected to complete the distal corticotomy.

If a fixed knee contracture develops during lengthening, the frequency of physical therapy treatments should be increased. If the knee contracture does not respond to physical therapy and splinting, the frame may be extended proximally to the femur and a hinge incorporated at the approximate axis of rotation of the knee. The device can then be used to slowly distract and correct the knee contracture.

To correct other deformities of the tibia while lengthening, the Ilizarov frame may be modified with hinges to effect angular and translational correction simultaneously. Internal rotation may be corrected distally by osteotomy at the time of fixator application. Proximally, internal rotation should be corrected gradually after the lengthening is completed, but before the regenerated bone is solid. The use of the Ilizarov device for multiplane corrections and for simultaneous distal fibular transport (for fibular hemimelia) should be attempted only by surgeons with experience in these techniques.

Femoral lengthening

▲ *Technique (Wagner)* (Fig. 3-52). Place the patient supine on a radiolucent table with a bolster under the ipsilateral buttock. Insert the two most proximal pins with an image intensifier at the level of the lesser trochanter, and the two most distal pins at the level of the superior pole of the patella. Predrill the 6.5-mm self-tapping Schanz pins with a 3.2-mm drill bit, and insert them in a plane perpendicular to the long axis of the femur with a drill guide. The two-pin groupings should be made in the same plane. Expose the midshaft of the femur subperiosteally through a posterolateral approach in the interval between the vastus lateralis and the biceps femoris. Make a transverse osteotomy of the femur with an oscillating saw, and close the wound over drains. Attach the distraction device to the Schanz pins, leaving 1 to 2 cm of clearance to allow for swelling of the lateral thigh. Apply 5 to 6 mm of acute distraction to prevent painful contact between the bone fragments.

▲ *Postoperative management.* Distraction is continued by turning the knob of the device one complete turn daily. This lengthens the femur by 1.5 mm. The distraction may be divided if one complete turn is too painful. Partial weight bearing with forearm crutches is encouraged, and vigorous physiotherapy of the hip and knee is mandatory. Varus and anterior angulation may be corrected by adjusting the linkage between the Schanz pins and the lengthener. Daily pin care is necessary to prevent pin sepsis. If the skin becomes very tented over the pins, it should be incised under local anesthesia. The hamstrings and adductors may be lengthened if necessary. After the desired length has been achieved, a plate and, if necessary, autologous bone graft are applied. After the plate and bone graft are applied and the skin is closed over a drain, the fixator is removed. Weight bearing is gradually increased. The plate is removed when there is normal reconstitution of the femur and medullary canal.

• • •

A   B   C

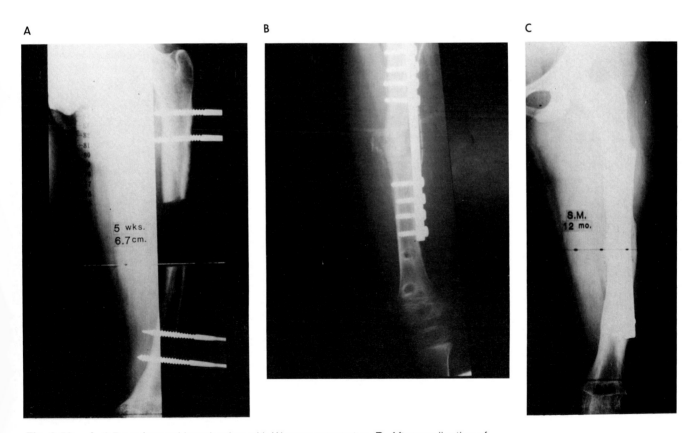

Fig. 3-52   **A,** 6.7 cm femoral lengthening with Wagner apparatus. **B,** After application of Wagner plate and bone graft and immediately after removal of the external fixator. **C,** Follow-up at 12 months shows hypertrophy of the callus.

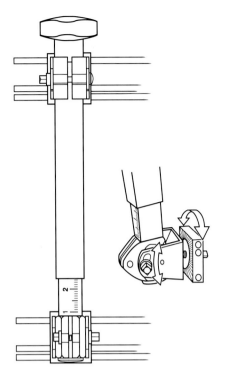

Fig. 3-53 Hoffman modification of Wagner device allows rotation in three planes.

The Hoffman modification of the Wagner device allows rotation in three planes and is somewhat easier to apply (Fig. 3-53). A 4.5-mm drill bit is used to predrill the holes for a 6-mm half pin. Dick recommends transection of the periosteum and acute distraction of 10 mm, followed by daily distraction of 1 to 2 mm. He also excises a tract of iliotibial band and intermuscular septum. Tenotomy of the adductors may decrease varus deviation during lengthening. Special plates, without screw holes in the area of the lengthening gap, have been designed to prevent plate breakage.

Coleman recommends plate removal in two stages to prevent fracture through the stress-shielded bone or screw holes. At the first stage, half the screws are removed completely, and the remaining half are loosened by one or two turns and removed with the plate 6 to 12 months later.

◣ *Technique (DeBastiani—Orthofix)* (Figs. 3-54 and 3-55). Place the patient supine on a radiolucent table. Use the mated drills, drill guides, and screw guides to insert the conical self-tapping cortical and cancellous screws. Insert a cortical screw at the level of the lesser trochanter, perpendicular to the shaft of the femur. Attach the rigid template; insert the distal-most screw next, being careful to line the template up parallel to the shaft of the femur. Return to the proximal end of the template and insert the next screw in the fourth template hole distal to the upper screw. The last screw to be placed is in the distal template, in the hole farthest away from the distal-most screw. Remove the template and perform a corticotomy 1 cm distal to the proximal two screws (just distal to the iliopsoas insertion). Incise the anterior thigh skin longitudinally, and dissect bluntly between the sartorius muscle and the tensor fasciae latae muscle, and through the substance of the vastus intermedius and rectus femoris muscles. Incise the periosteum longitudinally, and elevate it laterally and medially. Under direct vision, drill a series of 4.8-mm unicortical holes in the visible aspect of the anterior two thirds of the circumference of the femur. Set the drill stop at 1 cm to prevent penetration of the marrow. Use a thin osteotome to connect the drill holes without violating the marrow. Flex the femur at the corticotomy to crack the posterior cortex, completing the corticotomy. Do not use the Orthofix pins as a handle to complete the corticotomy, or they may loosen. Reduce the fracture, and apply the Orthofix lengthener. If the Orthofix fracture-fixation device is used, fix the ball joint rigidly with a small amount of methyl methacrylate. Suture the periosteum and close the skin over drains. The use of six pins has recently been recommended for femoral lengthening to gain stability and to resist a tendency for varus deviation.

▲*Postoperative management.* Same as for tibial lengthening.

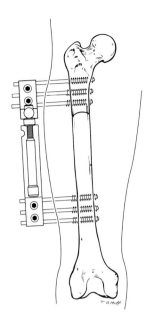

Fig. 3-54 Orthofix device for femoral lengthening. To control varus deviation, three screws are used proximally and three screws distally, or frame may be applied with prophylactic valgus built into construct.

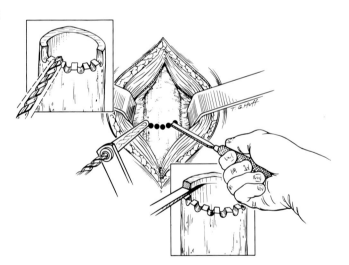

Fig. 3-55 DeBastiani technique for corticotomy. Using limited open exposure, Orthofix drill is used to make multiple drill holes in anterior half of bone. These holes are connected with 5-mm osteotome. Osteotome is used to complete corticotomy posteriorly without drill holes. (Modified from Aldegheri R, Renzi-Brivio L, and Agostini S: Clin Orthop 241:137, 1989.)

▲ *Technique (modified Ilizarov)* (Fig. 3-56, *A, B,* and *C*).
Preconstruction: The standard femoral lengthening frame consists of a proximal fixation block made of two arcs, a distal fixation block made of two identical-size rings, and an "empty" middle ring (usually one size larger than the distal femoral rings) to link the two fixation blocks. Preconstruct the frame before surgery to decrease the time spent in the operating room. Use the smallest-diameter rings that leave sufficient space for swelling after surgery, because smaller rings give a more mechanically stable construct. There should be one fingerbreadth of space between the distal ring and the anterior thigh and two fingerbreadths posteriorly at the largest diameter of the posterior calf muscles. The distal-most ring may be a ⅝-inch ring to allow more knee flexion after surgery. This is particularly important if there is to be a simultaneous lengthening of the ipsilateral tibia with proximal tibial rings. (Full rings would touch each other after relatively little knee flexion, limiting knee mobility.) Connect the bottom two rings initially with two 20- or 40-mm threaded hexagonal sockets for better stability, one positioned directly anteriorly and one directly posteriorly. In small patients, there may be room distally for only one ring and a drop

wire. Plan the frame so that the central connection bolts are centered directly over the anterior and posterior midlines. Choose two parallel arcs to match the contour of the proximal lateral thigh, usually a 90-degree arc most proximally and a 120-degree arc below it. This causes less impingement of the proximal end of the fixator against the lower abdomen and pelvis during hip flexion. Connect the two arcs with two 40-mm hexagonal sockets. The reach of the 120-degree arc can be extended by attaching two oblique supports off the first and last holes on the arc. Attach the oblique support to the empty middle ring, which will not hold any wires but will allow a more even 360-degree push-off between the distal fixation block and the proximal fixation block. Connect the empty middle ring to the distal fixation block with two threaded rods, one anteriorly and one medially, to align the empty ring with the distal ring block anteriorly and medially where the soft tissue sleeve of the thigh is minimal and the larger, empty ring laterally and posteriorly where extra skin clearance is required. Later, it will be necessary to build out from the distal block laterally and posteriorly with short connection plates to have additional threaded rods or graduated telescopic rods in these locations.

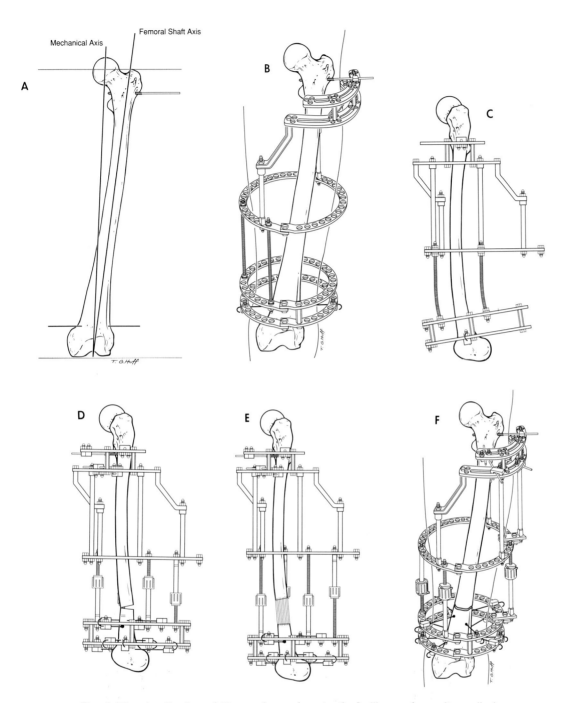

Fig. 3-56   Application of Ilizarov frame (see text). **A,** Ilizarov frame is applied perpendicular to mechanical axis, not femoral shaft axis. Distally, reference wire is placed parallel to femoral condyles. Proximally, reference pin is drilled perpendicular to mechanical axis. **B,** Ilizarov femoral-lengthening frame is constructed on proximal and distal reference pins. Middle ring is larger in diameter than distal two rings to accommodate conical shape of thigh. **C,** Lateral view of frame after lengthening of anterior threaded rod to tilt distal ring block as shown. Remainder of wires and pins will be inserted with frame in this position. **D,** Lateral view of frame after corticotomy, when upper and lower segments have been brought into alignment. Notice how this places femur into slight recurvatum at corticotomy. **E,** After lengthening, prophylactic recurvatum is now diminished. **F,** Completed femoral frame. Graduated telescopic distractors are placed in alternating up-down position for greater stability. Olive wires add greater stability to construct. "Empty" middle ring serves as even push-off point.

Reference wires: Position the patient supine with a folded sheet under the ipsilateral buttock. A radiolucent table that splits at the lower extremities, allowing removal of the part of the table under the involved leg, is helpful. Place the foot on a Mayo stand or other small table to permit flexion and extension of the knee and hip to allow assessment of acceptable placement of the wires in the soft tissues around the knee. Use fluoroscopy to insert the proximal reference pin and the distal reference wire. In the distal femur, use 1.8-mm wires and in the proximal femur, use the Ilizarov 5-mm conical self-drilling, self-tapping screws. If preferred, other heavy-gauge half pins, particularly those designed to be predrilled, may be substituted. When using conical pins, be careful not to back them out once they are inserted, or they will loosen. Under fluoroscopic control, insert an olive wire from lateral to medial, parallel to the

knee joint as the distal reference wire, parallel to the femoral condyles at the level of the adductor tubercle. For the proximal reference pin, insert a half pin just distal to the level of greater trochanter, parallel to an imaginary line drawn from the tip of the greater trochanter to the center of the femoral head, normally within 3 degrees of being parallel to the axis of the knee joint. The proximal and distal reference wires should be parallel to one another and perpendicular to the mechanical axis (Fig. 3-57); however, they are not perpendicular to the anatomic axis of the femur. This is important because lengthening should take place along the mechanical axis of the femur rather than the femoral shaft axis. Failure to adhere to this principle disrupts the normal mechanical axis and causes medialization of the knee.

Secure the preassembled frame to the top reference pin and bottom reference wire, and check to make sure there is adequate clearance between the skin and the frame and that all the connections are tight. Tension the wires to 130 kg of force after fixing the olive end of the wire to the distal ring. Secure the proximal half pin with either a monopin fixation clamp or a buckle clamp. Now loosen the anterior and medial connections between the distal fixation block and the empty ring. Distract slightly to tilt the frame into about 5 degrees of recurvatum, then tighten the connections. From this point on, the frame can be used as a drill guide for insertion of the remaining wires and pins. The frame is fixed in this apex anterior position, because, after corticotomy, the proximal and distal blocks are tilted back into parallel alignment, causing the femur to be in slight recurvatum at the corticotomy site. This will spontaneously correct as the normal recurvatum forces occur during lengthening.

Fixation: Insert two oblique smooth wires on the distal ring and one medial olive wire and an oblique smooth wire on the ring above. Some important technical points must be remembered while inserting the wires. When inserting a wire from the anterior thigh to the posterior thigh, first flex the knee 45 degrees as the wire penetrates the anterior skin. Next flex the knee 90 degrees as the wire penetrates the quadriceps muscle. Now drill the wire through the bone just to the opposite cortex. Tap the wire through the soft tissue, keeping the knee fully extended as the wire traverses the hamstrings; flex the knee to 45 degrees as the wire exits the skin. After each wire is inserted, move the knee from full extension to 90 degrees of flexion. The wire should "float" in the soft tissue and should not be pulled by the muscle or cause tenting of the skin. This technique of wire placement helps minimize skin irritation and joint contractures. If a wire does not exit directly in the

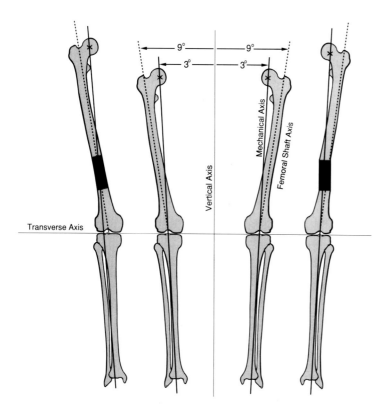

Fig. 3-57 Difference between lengthening of femoral shaft axis and lengthening of mechanical axis of femur. On left, femur has been lengthened along its femoral shaft axis. Knee is moved medially so that line drawn from center of femoral head to center of ankle passes lateral to intercondylar notch. On right, lengthening has been done parallel to mechanical axis, allowing mechanical axis to remain aligned properly. It does, however, give slight zig-zag appearance to femur.

plane of the ring, build the ring up to the level of the wire with either washers or posts. Do not bend the wire in any plane to get it to lie more closely to the ring. In the proximal arc, add one more pin anteriorly, on the opposite side of the arc, to avoid the reference pin. This pin should not be inserted any more medially than the anterosuperior iliac spine, or the femoral nerve will be at risk. On the second arc, place two additional pins, one on each side of the arc, in the oblique plane between the two top pins. The ideal mechanical placement of wires and pins should approach 90 degrees when viewed axially, within anatomic limits. A 90-degree fixation spread within a given ring or a given fixation block resists bending moments in a more uniform manner. Olive wires add mechanical strength to the construct, but should not be overused. The olive wires function as fulcrums, acting on the bone to resist or correct axial deviation. Lengthenings around the knee tend to angulate into valgus, whereas lengthenings near the ankle and hip tend to angulate into varus. All sites are prone to anterior angulation. The olive wires in the femoral construct are strategically placed to resist valgus angulation. An additional olive wire may be placed opposite to the lateral olive wire of the distal ring to lock the distal ring into place, if desired.

Corticotomy: Remove the anterior and medial connecting rods from between the empty ring and the distal fixation block. Make a ½-inch incision in the lateral skin just proximal to the distal fixation block. Incising the fascia lata transversely makes the lengthening process easier and diminishes the tendency for valgus angulation. Dissect bluntly down to the bone with Mayo scissors, and insert a small, sharp periosteal elevator down to the lateral cortex of the femur. With a knife, make a longitudinal incision through the periosteum, and then use the elevator to strip a thin, 1-cm wide section of periosteum anterior and posterior, as much as can be reached. Transect the lateral cortex with a ½-inch osteotome, then cut the anterior and posterior cortex with a ¼-inch osteotome, including the linea aspera. Do not violate the medullary canal. Fracture the medial-most cortex by bending the femur. Be sure the fragments demonstrate enough motion to indicate that the corticotomy is complete, but do not widely displace the two segments. Reduce the fracture and align the proximal and distal fixation blocks so they are parallel. This will create a small amount (5 degrees) of prophylactic recurvatum in the femur, which will spontaneously correct as the natural tendency for procurvatum appears during lengthening (Fig. 3-56, *C, D,* and *E*). Use four upright threaded rods or short graduated telescopic tubes to connect the distal fixation block with the empty ring. Complete the frame by adding components until there are four connectors between every arc or ring in the frame. Close the skin over a drain and apply a pressure dressing to the lateral wound. Dress the wire and pin sites with sponges. Apply rubber stoppers to each wire and pin site before attaching them to the frame. The stoppers help to maintain slight pressure on the pin dressings and to minimize pin-skin interface motion, which is a prelude to pin infections. Wrap the proximal four pins tightly with stretch gauze to minimize skin motion over these pins.

▲ *Postoperative management.* Physical therapy and protected weight bearing with crutches are begun immediately. Knee flexion of at least 45 to 75 degrees is encouraged, but the knee is splinted in extension at night. Lengthening is begun on the fourth to sixth day after surgery, depending on the age of the patient, and progresses at 0.25 mm four times daily. The patient should be taught how to lengthen before discharge from the hospital, and a record of lengthening should be maintained. Although lengthening at precisely every 6 hours is desirable, it is far more practical to lengthen at breakfast, lunch, dinner, and bedtime. A preoperative lateral view of the knee is essential to help judge early signs of subluxation, especially during large lengthenings in patients with congenital deficiencies of the femur. Roentgenograms should be made 7 to 10 days after lengthening is begun to ensure distraction of the corticotomy. If there is insufficient regenerate bone after 4 to 6 weeks, the rate of distraction may be adjusted. Once the desired length has been achieved, the fixator is kept in place until there is corticalization of the regenerated bone. Some surgeons "train" the regenerated bone before fixator removal by placing it under slight compression or by retensioning the wires. Weight bearing and fixator stability are critical factors in producing healthy regenerate bone. At the time of fixator removal, the knee may be manipulated if necessary, but only before removal of the device. Protected weight bearing and vigorous physical therapy are continued and activity is gradually increased.

• • •

If deviation of the mechanical axis or deformity of the proximal femur requires treatment, the Ilizarov frame and application are modified to accommodate these needs. Hinges may be placed at the lengthening corticotomy site to effect angular correction. Immediate correction of proximal deformities may be achieved by percutaneous osteotomy between the proximal two arcs. The arcs are initially angulated relative to one another, the osteotomy is performed, and the arcs are brought immediately into parallel alignment to effect the desired correction.

Humeral lengthening

▶ *Technique (Modified Ilizarov)* (Fig. 3-58). *Preconstruction and fixation:* The humeral frame is analogous to the femoral frame. Proximally, use two half pins on an arc and a third drop pin on a multiple-pin fixation clamp. Distally, use three 1.5-mm wires in the distal humerus, attached with posts as necessary to a ⅝-inch ring. The ⅝-inch ring allows flexion of the elbow during treatment. Use the oblique supports to extend the reach of the proximal arc to the ends of the ⅝-inch ring distally. Insert the proximal reference pin perpendicular to the humerus through the deltoid muscle. Insert the distal reference wire from the medial epicondyle to the lateral epicondyle. Insert the remaining two distal wires medially in the interval between the median and ulnar nerves. They may be oriented in the coronal plane rather than the axial plane to make placement easier. Take care not to injure the neurovascular structures. Ideally, an olive wire should be placed both medially and laterally to lock the distal ring and prevent side-to-side sliding on the wires. When inserting a wire from the lateral side, be sure to stop drilling when the medial cortex is broached. Proceed by tapping the pin out through the medial soft tissue to prevent injury to the medial neurovascular structures.

Corticotomy: The ideal location for humeral

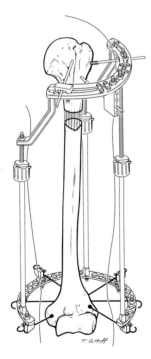

Fig. 3-58 Typical configuration of humeral lengthening ring (see text). Three half-pins are placed proximally in metaphyseal region. Corticotomy is made distal to insertion of deltoid and pectoralis major.

lengthening corticotomy is just distal to the pectoralis major. Approach this through an anterolateral 2-cm incision. Identify the radial nerve and sharply incise the periosteum. Elevate a narrow transverse strip of the periosteum, and score the anterolateral cortex with a ½-inch osteotome. Complete the medial and lateral corticotomies with a ¼-inch osteotome. To complete the posterior corticotomy, turn the elevator 90 degrees to act like a lamina spreader and manipulate the humerus if necessary. Reduce the fracture and apply the frame with three or four distraction rods. Close the corticotomy. Distraction is begun 5 to 7 days after surgery. If a radial palsy develops during lengthening, the rate of distraction is slowed or temporarily halted. The fixator is removed after the regenerated bone has sufficiently healed.

Complications

All types of limb lengthening devices and techniques have some complications in common, but certain complications are more or less likely to occur with a given device. The most common problem is pin tract infection, which can be minimized by careful pin insertion technique. For thin wires, the pin should be inserted through the skin directly at the level the wire is to enter bone to prevent tenting of the skin. At the end of the procedure, moving the nearby joints through a full range of motion will identify skin tenting over wires, and the sites can be released with a scalpel. The thin transfixion wires seem to cause fewer problems than the large half pins, but skin and muscle motion over any wire or pin can cause irritation and eventually infection. The motion of skin over pins and wires should be minimized by special dressing techniques. For thin-wire fixators, commercially available 1-inch foam cubes with a slit are placed around the pin site. The slit is then stapled or sutured to prevent the cube from falling off. Finally, a clip or previously applied rubber stopper is lowered on to the foam to apply mild pressure on the skin. Excessive pressure should be avoided, particularly over bony prominences, or an ulceration may occur. For large pins, particularly in the thigh, surgical gauze can be wrapped snugly around two or more neighboring pins to apply pressure to the skin around the pins. All wire and pin care should include daily sterilization with an antiseptic such as Betadine or Hibistat, but only a small amount (1 ml per pin, daily) should be used so as not to irritate the skin. The solution can be diluted if the alcohol content irritates the patient's skin, or a nonirritating antibiotic ointment such as Neosporin can be used.

At the first sign of a pin tract infection, broad-spectrum oral antibiotics should be given, local pin care should be intensified, and if necessary, the pin site should be incised to promote drainage. If the infection does not improve with these measures, the pin may have to be removed. If pin removal jeopardizes the stability of the construct, a replacement pin should be inserted. With the Ilizarov apparatus, this is relatively simple: a wire can be placed in a nearby hole or dropped off the ring on a post to avoid the previously infected pin site. With monolateral fixators, it is more difficult to reinsert a replacement pin away from the infected area. For severe infections, the pin tract and bone should be curetted.

The most difficult complications that occur during lengthening are related to the muscles. In theory, the bones can be lengthened by virtually any amount, but the muscles have a limited ability to stretch. Typically, the muscles that cause the most problems are the triceps surae during tibial lengthening and the quadriceps during femoral lengthening. Knee flexion contracture is common during tibial lengthening and can be prevented with prophylactic splinting, especially at night. Custom orthoses or commercially available Dynasplints are helpful. Vigorous and frequent physical therapy is also critical. Prophylactic treatment should be begun within 1 week of the original surgery. For tibial lengthenings greater than 4 to 5 cm, the foot should be fixed in neutral position by applying a posterior plaster splint for monolateral fixators or by placing two wires in the heel and connecting them to a ring attached to the main frame of a thin-wire circular fixator. The heel pins should be removed as soon as possible after lengthening is completed (provided the knee is not contracted), to allow the subtalar joint and ankle to regain motion. If there is residual contracture of the tendo Achilles at the end of treatment, lengthening should be considered. Any preoperative tendo Achilles contracture should be corrected before or during tibial lengthening.

Joint subluxation or dislocation has been reported during femoral lengthenings, especially if either the hip or knee joint is unstable before the surgery (as is frequently the case in PFFD). For hips with varus deformities, corrective valgus osteotomy should be delayed until after lengthening. The cruciate ligaments are generally deficient in PFFD, making knee subluxation more likely, and prophylactic fixation of the knee joint with a mobile hinge is possible with the Ilizarov apparatus. A posteriorly dislocated tibia can be slowly pulled back anteriorly with a mobile Ilizarov hinge on a rail, to reduce the dislocation and allow simultaneous knee motion. With the monolateral fixators, these options are not available. For hip subluxation, traction and bed rest are usually sufficient to reduce the subluxation.

Neurovascular complications are usually related to faulty pin placement, but may result from stretching during lengthening. If the rate of distraction is 1 mm/day, then the neurovascular tissues are almost always able to stretch to accommodate the lengthening. Decreasing or temporarily stopping the distraction is usually sufficient. If a cutaneous nerve is tented over a wire or pin, the problem can be solved by removing the pin. Hypertension rarely is seen with slow gradual distraction.

Bony complications of distraction osteogenesis include premature consolidation and delayed consolidation. In Wagner lengthenings, common problems were deep infection, pseudarthrosis, plate breakage, and malunion. With distraction osteogenesis, by either the Ilizarov or DeBastiani techniques, the problems of delayed and premature consolidation can usually be solved without compromising a satisfactory end result. Premature consolidation results from an excessive latency period. For femoral lengthenings in children, a latency period of 5 days is recommended, and for tibial lengthenings, 7 days. For older patients, and in cases of compromised vascularity to the limb, longer latency periods may be appropriate. To prevent premature consolidation of the fibula in tibial lengthenings, a standard open osteotomy of the fibula may be performed instead of the corticotomy. In some cases of premature consolidation, the patient reports that it became successively more difficult to lengthen, until finally a loud "pop" was felt, followed by short but intense pain. This scenario describes spontaneous rupture through the consolidated regenerate bone. The ends should be brought back to the level of apposition seen before the fracture; after a brief latency period, lengthening is begun again.

Delayed consolidation is more common with diaphyseal lengthening than with metaphyseal corticotomy. Contributing factors include frame instability, overvigorous initial corticotomy with excessive stripping of the periosteum, and overly fast distraction, especially after too brief a latency period. Underlying medical or nutritional problems and lack of exercise are other contributing factors. In addition to correcting these mitigating factors, the surgeon can slow or cease distraction, or compress the bone and alternatively compress and lengthen. Walking and normal use of the limb should always be encouraged. In adult patients and older children the best regenerate bone is made by patients who are active and who take only sparing amounts of analgesics. Bone grafting with autologous cancellous graft of the gap is a final resort. Extra precautions should be made during the preparing and draping of the fixator, since the pin sites may harbor bacteria. With Wagner lengthening, bone grafting of the gap is expected, but it is easier to drape the monolateral fixators out of the sterile operative site. The problem of malunion and axial deviations during lengthening has been discussed in the previous sections describing technique.

REFERENCES
Congenital long bone deficiencies

Aitken GT: Congenital lower limb deficiencies. In The American Academy of Orthopaedic Surgeons: instructional course lectures, vol 24, St Louis, 1975, The CV Mosby Co.

Burtch RL, Fishman S, and Kay HW: Nomenclature for congenital skeletal limb deficiencies, a revision of the Frantz and O'Rahilly classification, Artif Limbs 10:24, 1966.

Day HJB: Nomenclature and classification in congenital limb deficiency. In Murdoch G and Donovan RG, editors: Amputation surgery and lower limb prosthesis. Oxford, 1988, Blackwell Scientific Publications, Ltd.

Frantz CH and O'Rahilly R: Congenital skeletal limb deficiencies, J Bone Joint Surg 43A:1202, 1961.

Kay HW: A proposed international terminology for the classification of congenital limb deficiencies, Inter-Clin Info Bull 13(7):1, 1974.

Lenz W: Genetics and limb deficiencies, Clin Orthop 148:9, 1980.

O'Rahilly R: Morphological patterns in limb deficiencies and duplications, Am J Anat 89:135, 1951.

Rogala ET, Wynne-Davies R, and Little-John, A: Congenital limb anomalies: frequency and aetiological factors, J Med Genet 11:221, 1974.

Swanson AB: A classification for congenital limb malformations, J Hand Surg 1A:8, 1976.

Swinyard CA: Limb development and deformity: problems of evaluation and rehabilitation, Springfield, Ill, 1969, Charles C Thomas, Publisher.

Tibial hemimelia

Aitken GT: Amputation as a treatment for certain lower-extremity congenital anomalies, J Bone Joint Surg 41A:1267, 1959.

Aitken GT: Tibial hemimelia. In A symposium on selected lower limb anomalies: surgical and prosthetic management, Washington, DC, 1971, National Academy of Sciences.

Aitken GT: The child amputee: an overview, Orthop Clin North Am 3(2):447, 1972.

Aitken GT: Congenital lower limb deficiencies. In American academy of orthopaedic surgeons: instructional course lectures, vol 24, St Louis, 1975, The CV Mosby Co.

Bose K: Congenital diastasis of the inferior tibiofibula joint: report of a case, J Bone Joint Surg 58A:886, 1976.

Brown FW: Construction of a knee joint in congenital total absence of the tibia (paraxial hemimelia tibia): a preliminary report, J Bone Joint Surg 47A:695, 1965.

Brown FW: The Brown operation for total hemimelia tibia. In Aitken GT, editor: Selected lower-limb anomalies: surgical and prosthetics management, Washington, DC, 1971, National Academy of Sciences.

Brown FW and Pohnert WH: Construction of a knee joint in meromelia tibia (congenital absence of the tibia): a fifteen-year follow-up study, J Bone Joint Surg 54A:1333, 1972.

Clark MW: Autosomal dominant inheritance of tibial meromelia: report of a kindred, J Bone Joint Surg 57A:262, 1975.

der Kaloustian VM and Mnaymneh WA: Bilateral tibia aplasia with lobster-claw hands: a rare genetic entity, Acta Pediatr Scand 62:77, 1973.

Exner G: The treatment of congenital tibial defect by means of Hahn's plastic surgery (translocation of the fibula), Z Orthop 103(2):193, 1967.

Frantz CH and O'Rahilly R: Congenital skeletal limb deficiencies, J Bone Joint Surg 43A:1202, 1961.

Garbarino JL et al: Congenital diastasis of the inferior tibiofibular joint: a review of the literature and report of two cases, J Pediatr Orthop 5:225, 1985.

Gilsanz V, Teitelbaum G, and Condon VR: Clubfoot deformity and tibiofibular diastasis, AJR 140(4):759, 1983.

Hall CB, Brooks MB, and Dennis JF: Congenital skeletal deficiencies of the extremities: classification and fundamentals of treatment, JAMA 181:590, 1962.

Hancock CI and King RE: The one-bone leg, Inter-Clin Info Bull 7(3):11, 1967.

Henkel L and Willert HG: Dysmelia: a classification and a pattern of malformation in a group of congenital defects of the limbs, J Bone Joint Surg 51B:399, 1969.

Herring JA and Lloyd-Roberts G: Instructional case: management of tibial dysplasia, J Pediatr Orthop 1:339, 1981.

Hootnick DR, Packard DS, and Levinsohn EM: Congenital tibia aplasia with preaxial polydactyly: soft tissue anatomy as a clue to teratogenesis, Teratology 27:169, 1983b.

Hootnick D et al: The natural history and management of congenital short tibia with dysplasia or absence of the fibula, J Bone Joint Surg 59B(3):267, 1977.

Hootnick DR et al: Soft tissue anomalies in a patient with congenital tibial aplasia and talocalcaneal synchrondrosis, Teratology 36(2):153, 1987.

Jayakumar SS and Eilert RE: Fibular transfer for congenital absence of the tibia, Clin Orthop 139:97, 1979.

Jones E, Barnes J, and Lloyd-Roberts GC: Congenital aplasia and dysplasia of the tibia with intact fibula: classification and management, J Bone Joint Surg 60B:31, 1978.

Kalamchi A and Dawe RV: Congenital deficiency of the tibia, J Bone Joint Surg 67B:581, 1985.

Karchinov K: Congenital diplopodia with hypoplasia or aplasia of the tibia: a report of six cases, J Bone Joint Surg 55B:604, 1973.

Lamb DW, Wynne-Davies R, and Whitmore JM: Five-fingered hand associated with partial or complete tibial absence and pre-axial polydactyly: a kindred of 15 affected individuals in five generations, J Bone Joint Surg 65B:60, 1983.

Loder RT and Herring JA: Fibular transfer for congenital absence of the tibia, a reassessment, J Pediatr Orthop 7(1):8, 1987.

Narang IC, Mysorekar VR, and Mathur BP: Diplopodia with double fibula and agenesis of tibia: a case report, J Bone Joint Surg 64B:206, 1982.

Ogden JA: Ipsilateral femoral bifurcation and tibial hemimelia: a case report, J Bone Joint Surg 58A:712, 1976.

Ono N et al: A case of congenital tibial deficiency with other severe limb anomalies, Hokkaido J Orthop Trauma Surg 26(1-2):127, 1982.

Pappas AM, Hanawalt BJ, and Anderson M: Congenital defects of the fibula, Orthop Clin North Am 3:187, 1972.

Pashayan H et al: Bilateral aplasia of the tibia, polydactyly, and absent thumb in father and daughter, J Bone Joint Surg 53B:495, 1971.

Schoenecker PL et al: Congenital tibial dysplasia with intact fibula, J Pediatr Orthop 5:751, 1985.

Sturz H and Witt AN: Aplasia of the tibia: a case report with observation for 38 years (author's transl), Z Orthop 118:862, 1980.

Tuli SM and Varma BP: Congenital diastasis of tibio-fibular mortise, J Bone Joint Surg 54B:346, 1972.

Williams L et al: Tibial dysplasia: a study of the anatomy, J Bone Joint Surg 65B:157, 1983.

Fibular hemimelia

Achterman C and Kalamchi A: Congenital deficiency of the fibula, J Bone Joint Surg 61B:133, 1979.

Aitken GT: Congenital short femur with fibular hemimelia, J Bone Joint Surg 56A:1306, 1974.

Aitken GT: Congenital lower limb deficiencies. In The American Academy of Orthopaedic Surgeons: instructional course lectures, vol 24, St Louis, 1975, The CV Mosby Co.

Amstutz HC: Natural history and treatment of congenital absence of the fibula, J Bone Joint Surg 54A:1349, 1972.

Anderson L, Westin GW, and Oppenheim WL: Syme amputation in children: indications, results, and long-term follow-up, J Pediatr Orthop 4(5):550, 1984.

Arnold WD: Congenital absence of the fibula, Clin Orthop 14:20, 1959.

Bohne WHO and Root L: Hypoplasia of the fibula, Clin Orthop 125:107, 1977.

Coventry MB and Johnson EW Jr: Congenital absence of the fibula, J Bone Joint Surg 34A:941, 1952.

Duraiswami PK: Experimental causation of congenital skeletal defects and its significance in orthopaedic surgery, J Bone Joint Surg 34B:646, 1952.

Epps EH and Schneider PL: Treatment of hemimelias of the lower extremity, J Bone Joint Surg 71A:2, 1989.

Farmer AW and Laurin CA: Congenital absence of the fibula, J Bone Joint Surg 42A:1, 1960.

Frantz CH and O'Rahilly R: Congenital skeletal limb deficiencies, J Bone Joint Surg 43A:1202, 1961.

Grogan DP, Love SM, and Ogden JA: Congenital malformations of the lower extremities, Orthop Clin North Am 18:537, 1987.

Hootnick DR, Levinsohn EM, and Packard DS Jr: Midline metatarsal dysplasia associated with absent fibula, Clin Orthop 150:1123, 1980.

Hootnick D et al: The natural history and management of congenital short tibia with dysplasia or absence of the fibula, J Bone Joint Surg 59B:267, 1977.

Hootnick DR et al: Vascular dysgenesis associated with skeletal dysplasia of the lower limb, J Bone Joint Surg 62A:1123, 1980.

Jansen K and Anderson KS: Congenital absence of the fibula, Acta Orthop Scand 45:446, 1974.

Kawamura B et al: Limb lengthening by means of subcutaneous osteotomy: experimental and clinical studies, J Bone Joint Surg 50A:851, 1968.

Kruger LM: Recent advances in surgery of lower limb deficiencies, Clin Orthop 148:97, 1980.

Kruger LM and Talbott RD: Amputation and prosthesis as definitive treatment in congenital absence of the fibula, J Bone Joint Surg 43A:625, 1961.

Lenz W: Genetics and limb deficiencies, Clin Orthop 148:9, 1980.

Pappas AM, Hanawalt BJ, and Anderson M: Congenital defects of the fibula, Orthop Clin North Am 3:187, 1972.

Serafin J: A new operation for congenital absence of the fibula: preliminary report, J Bone Joint Surg 49B:59, 1967.

Thomas IH and Williams PF: The Gruca operation for congenital absence of the fibula, J Bone Joint Surg 69B:587, 1987.

Thompson TC, Straub LR, and Arnold WD: Congenital absence of the fibula, J Bone Joint Surg 39A:1229, 1957.

Weiner DS, Greenberg B, and Shamp N: Congenital re-duplication of the femur associated with paraxial fibular hemimelia, J Bone Joint Surg 60A:554, 1978.

Westin GW, Sakai DN, and Wood WL: Congenital longitudinal deficiencies of the fibula: follow-up treatment by Syme amputation, J Bone Joint Surg 58A:492, 1976.

Wiltse LL: Valgus deformity of the ankle: a sequel to acquired or congenital abnormalities of the fibula, J Bone Joint Surg 54A:595, 1972.

Wood WL, Zlotsky N, and Westin GW: Congenital absence of the fibula: treatment by Syme amputation—indications and technique, J Bone Joint Surg 47A:1159, 1965.

Proximal femoral focal deficiency

Acker RB: Congenital absence of femur and fibula: report of two patients, Clin Orthop 15:203, 1959.

Aitken GT: Amputation as a treatment for certain lower-extremity congenital abnormalities, J Bone Joint Surg 41A:1267, 1959.

Aitken GT: Proximal femoral focal deficiency: definition, classification, and management. In Aitken GT, editor: Proximal femoral focal deficiency: a congenital anomaly, Washington, DC, 1969, National Academy of Sciences.

Aitken GT: Congenital short femur with fibular hemimelia, J Bone Joint Surg 56A:1306, 1974.

Amstutz HC and Wilson PD Jr: Dysgenesis of the proximal femur (coxa vara) and its surgical management, J Bone Joint Surg 44A:1, 1962.

Bevan-Thomas WH and Millar EA: A review of proximal focal femoral deficiency, J Bone Joint Surg 49A:1376, 1967.

Bochmann D: Prosthetic devices for the management of proximal femoral focal deficiency, Ortho-Pros 4, 1980.

Borggreve J: Arch Orthop Chir 28:175, 1930. (Cited in Van Nes, CP: Rotation-plasty for congenital defects of the femur, making use of the ankle of the shortened limb to control the knee joint of a prosthesis, J Bone Joint Surg 32B:12, 1950).

Cristini JA: Surgical management of the proximal femoral focal deficient extremity, J Bone Joint Surg 55A:424, 1973.

Emery SF and Yngve DA: Congenital short femur, Orthopedics 10:1094, 1987.

Epps HE: Current concepts review: proximal femoral focal deficiency, J Bone Joint Surg 65A:867, 1983.

Fixsen JA and Lloyd-Roberts GC: The natural history and early treatment of proximal femoral dysplasia, J Bone Joint Surg 56B:86, 1974.

Fock G and Sulaman M: Congenital short femur, Acta Orthop Scand 37:294, 1965.

Frantz CH and O'Rahilly R: Congenital skeletal limb deficiencies, J Bone Joint Surg 43A:1202, 1961.

Gillespie R and Torode IP: Classification and management of congenital abnormalities of the femur, J Bone Joint Surg 65B:557, 1983.

Gilsanz V: Distal focal femoral deficiency, Radiology 147:105, 1983.

Grogan DP, Love SM, and Ogden JA: Congenital malformations of the lower extremities. Orthop Clin North Am 18(4):537, 1987.

Gupta DK and Gupta SK: Familial bilateral proximal femoral focal deficiency, J Bone Joint Surg 66A:1470, 1984.

Hall JE and Bochman D: The surgical and prosthetic management of proximal femoral focal deficiency. In Aitken GT, editor: Proximal femoral focal deficiency: a congenital anomaly. Washington, DC, 1969, National Academy of Sciences.

Hamanishi C: Congenital short femur: clinical, genetic and epidemiological comparison of the naturally occurring condition with that caused by thalidomide, J Bone Joint Surg 62B:307, 1980.

Hootnick D et al: The natural history and management of congenital short tibia with dysplasia or absence of the fibula: a preliminary report, J Bone Joint Surg 59B:267, 1977.

Johansson E and Aparisi T: Missing cruciate ligament in congenital short femur, J Bone Joint Surg 65A:1109, 1983.

Johnston CE: Congenital short femur with coxa vara, Orthopedics 6:892, 1983.

Kalamchi A, Lowell HE, and Kim KI: Congenital deficiency of the femur, J Pediatr Orthop 5:129, 1985.

King RE: Some concepts of proximal femoral focal deficiency. In Aitken GT, editor: Proximal femoral focal deficiency: a symposium, Washington, DC, 1969, National Academy of Sciences.

Koman LA, Meyer LC, and Warren FH: Proximal femoral focal deficiency: a 50-year experience, Dev Med Child Neurol 24:344, 1982.

Koman LA, Meyer LC, and Warren FH: Proximal femoral deficiency: natural history and treatment, Clin Orthop 162:135, 1982.

Kostuik JP et al: Van Nes rotational osteotomy for treatment of proximal femoral focal deficiency and congenital short femur, J Bone Joint Surg 57A:1039, 1975.

Kritter AE: Tibial rotation-plasty for proximal femoral focal deficiency, J Bone Joint Surg 59A:927, 1977.

Lange DR, Schoenecker PL, and Baker CL: Proximal femoral focal deficiency: treatment and classification in forty-two cases, Clin Orthop 135:15, 1978.

Lloyd-Roberts GC and Stone KH: Congenital hypoplasia of the upper femur, J Bone Joint Surg 45B:557, 1963.

Mital MA, Masalawalla KS, and Desai MG: Bilateral congenital aplasia of the femur, J Bone Joint Surg 45B:561, 1963.

Morgan JD and Somerville EW: Normal and abnormal growth at the upper end of the femur, J Bone Joint Surg 42B:264, 1960.

Panting AL and Williams PF: Proximal femoral focal deficiency, J Bone Joint Surg 60B:46, 1978.

Pappas AM: Congenital abnormalities of the femur and related lower extremity malformations: classifications and treatment, J Pediatr Orthop 3:45, 1983.

Richardson EG and Ramback BE: Proximal femoral focal deficiency: a clinical appraisal, South Med J 72:166, 1979.

Riedel F and Froster-Iskenius Ursula: Caudal dysplasia and femoral hypoplasia-unusual facies syndrome: different manifestations of the same disorder? Eur J Pediatr 144:80, 1985.

Ring PA: Congenital short femur: simple femoral hypoplasia, J Bone Joint Surg 41B:73, 1959.

Shands AR Jr and MacEwen GD: Congenital abnormalities of the femur, Acta Orthop Scand 32:307, 1962.

Steel HH et al: Iliofemoral fusion for proximal femoral focal deficiency, J Bone Joint Surg 69A:837, 1987.

Torode IP and Gillespie R: Rotationplasty of the lower limb for congenital defects of the femur, J Bone Joint Surg 65B:569, 1983.

Tsou PM: Congenital distal femoral focal deficiency: report of a unique case, Clin Orthop 162:99, 1982.

Van Nes CP: Rotationplasty for congenital defects of the femur, J Bone Joint Surg 32B:12, 1950.

Westin GW: Congenital absence of the femur: a rational approach, J Bone Joint Surg 46A:1380, 1964.

Westin GW and Gunderson FO: Proximal femoral focal deficiency: a review of treatment experiences. In Aitken GT, editor: Proximal femoral focal deficiency: a congenital anomaly, Washington DC, 1969, National Academy of Sciences.

Amputations and congenital deficiency of upper extremities

Abraham E et al: Stump overgrowth in juvenile amputees, J Pediatr Orthop 6:66, 1986.

Aitken GT: Amputation as a treatment for certain lower-extremity congenital abnormalities, J Bone Joint Surg 41A:1267, 1959.

Aitken GT: Surgical amputation in children, J Bone Joint Surg 45A:1735, 1963.

Aitken GT: Management of severe bilateral upper limb deficiencies, Clin Orthop 37:53, 1964.

Aitken GT: The child amputee: an overview, Orthop Clin North Am 3:2, 447, 1972.

Aitken GT and Frantz CH: The juvenile amputee, J Bone Joint Surg 35A:659, 1953.

Anderson L, Westin GW, and Oppenheim WL: Syme amputation in children: indications, results, and long-term follow-up, J Pediatr Orthop 4(5):550, 1984.

Blum CE and Kalamchi A: Boyd amputations in children, Clin Orthop 165:138, 1982.

Brooks MB and Mazet R: Prosthetics in child amputees, Clin Orthop 9:190, 1957.

Buttomley AH: Myoelectric control of powered prostheses, J Bone Joint Surg 47B:411, 1965.

Christie J et al: A study of stump growth for children with below-knee amputations, J Bone Joint Surg 61B:464, 1979.

Davidson WH and Bohne WHO: The Syme amputation in children, J Bone Joint Surg 57A:905, 1975.

Day HJB: Prosthetic management of congenital lower limb deficiency. In Murdoch G and Donovan RG, editors: Amputation surgery and lower limb prosthetics, Oxford, 1988, Blackwell Scientific Publications, Ltd.

Day HJB: Prosthetic treatment of congenital upper limb deficiency. In Murdoch G and Donovan RG, editors: Amputation surgery and lower Limb Prosthetics, Oxford, 1988, Blackwell Scientific Publications, Ltd.

Dresher CS and Macdonell JA: Total amelia, J Bone Joint Surg 47A:511, 1965.

Eilert RE and Jayakumar SS: Boyd and Syme ankle amputations in children, J Bone Joint Surg 58A(8):1138, 1976.

Fergusson CM, Morrison JD, and Kenwright J: Leg-length inequality in children treated by Syme's amputation, J Bone Joint Surg 69B:433, 1987.

Fletcher I: Review of the treatment of thalidomide children with limb deficiencies in Great Britain, Clin Orthop 148:12, 1980.

Frantz C.H and Aitken GT: Management of the juvenile amputee, Clin Orthop 9:30, 1959.

Glynn MK et al: Management of the upper-limb-deficient child with a powered prosthetic device, Clin Orthop 209:202, 1986.

Greene WB and Cary JM: Partial foot amputations in children: a comparison of the several types with the Syme amputation, J Bone Joint Surg 64A:438, 1982.

Hall CB: Recent concepts in the treatment of the limb-deficient child, Artif Limbs 10:36, 1966.

Harris RI: Syme's amputation: the technical details essential for success, J Bone Joint Surg 38B:614, 1956.

Keier AN, Rozhkov AV, and Shatilov OY: Management of short stumps. In Murdoch G and Donovan RG, editors: Amputation surgery and lower limb prosthetics, Oxford, 1988, Blackwell Scientific Publications.

Kruger LM and Talbott RD: Amputation and prosthesis as definitive treatment in congenital absence of the fibula, J Bone Joint Surg 43A:625, 1961.

Lamb DW and Law HT: Upper-limb deficiencies in children. In Prosthetic orthotic and surgical management, Boston, 1987, Little, Brown & Co, Inc.

Lamb DW and Scott H: Management of congenital and acquired amputations in children, Orthop Clin North Am 12:973, 1981.

Lamb DW, Simpson DC, and Pirie RB: The management of lower limb phocomelia, J Bone Joint Surg 52B:688, 1970.

Lambert CN, Hamilton RC, and Pellicore RH: The juvenile amputee program: its social and economic value, J Bone Joint Surg 51A:1135, 1969.

Loder RT and Herring JA: Disarticulation of the knee in children: a functional assessment, J Bone Joint Surg 69A:1155, 1987.

Marquardt E: The Heidleberg pneumatic arm prosthesis, J Bone Joint Surg 47B:425, 1965.

Marquardt E: The multiple limb-deficient child, In American academy of orthopaedic surgeons: Atlas of limb prosthetics, St Louis, 1981, The CV Mosby.

Marquardt EG and Buff HU: Total management of the limb-deficient child. In Murdoch G and Donovan RG, editors: Amputation surgery and lower limb prosthetics, Oxford, 1988, Blackwell Scientific Publications.

Mazet R Jr: Syme's amputation: a follow-up study of 51 adults and 32 children, J Bone Joint Surg 50A:1549, 1968.

Mowery CA, Herring JA, and Jackson D: Dislocated patella associated with below-knee amputation in adolescent patients, J Pediatr Orthop 6:299, 1986.

Peacock K and Tsai TM: Comparison of functional results of replantation versus prosthesis in a patient with bilateral arm amputation, Clin Orthop 214:153, 1987.

Popov B: The bioelectrically controlled prosthesis, J Bone Joint Surg 47B:421, 1965.

Rosenfelder R: Infant amputees: early growth and care, Clin Orthop 148:41, 1980.

Scotland TR and Galway HR: A long-term review of children with congenital and acquired upper limb deficiency, J Bone Joint Surg 65B:346, 1983.

Scott RN: Surgical implications of myoelectric control, Clin Orthop 61:248, 1968.

Shaperman J and Sumida CT: Recent advances in research in prostheses for children, Clin Orthop 148:26, 1980.

Shaperman J and Sumida CT: Recent advances in research in prosthetics for children, Clin Orthop 148:26, 1980.

Simpson DC and Lamb DW: A system of powered prostheses for severe bilateral upper limb deficiency, J Bone Joint Surg 47B:442, 1965.

Sorbye R: Myoelectric prosthetic fitting in young children, Clin Orthop 148:34, 1980.

Speer DP: The pathogenesis of amputation stump overgrowth, Clin Orthop 159:294, 1981.

Swanson AB: The Krukenberg procedure in the juvenile amputee, J Bone Joint Surg 46A:1540, 1964.

Tooms RE: The amputee. In Lovell WW and Winter RB, editors: Pediatric orthopaedics, 2 ed, Philadelphia, 1978, JB Lippincott Co.

Tubiana R: Krukenberg's operation, Orthop clin north am 12:819, 1981.

Von Saal G: Epiphysiodesis combined with amputation, J Bone Joint Surg 21:442, 1939.

Limb length discrepancy

Abbott LC: The operative lengthening of the tibia and fibula, J Bone Joint Surg 9:123, 1927.

Aldegheri R, Giampaolo T, and Lavini F: Epiphyseal distraction: chondrodiatasis, Clin Orthop 241:117, 1989.

Aldegheri R, Giampaolo T, and Lavini F: Epiphyseal distraction: hemichondrodiatasis, Clin Orthop 241:128, 1989.

Aldegheri R, Renzi-Brivio L, and Agostini S: The callotasis method of limb lengthening, Clin Orthop 241:137, 1989.

Aldegheri R et al: Lengthening of the lower limbs in achondroplastic patients: a comparative study of four techniques, J Bone Joint Surg 70B:1, 69, 1988.

Alho A et al: Filling of a bone defect during experimental osteotaxis distraction, Acta Orthop Scand 53:29, 1982.

Allan FG: Bone lengthening, J Bone Joint Surg 30B:490, 1948.

Allan PG: Simultaneous femoral and tibial lengthening, J Bone Joint Surg 45B:206, 1963.

Amstutz HC and Sakai DN ed: Symposium: equalization of leg lengths, Clin Orthop 136:2, 1978.

Anderson M and Green WT: Length of the femur and the tibia: norms derived from orthoroentgenograms of children from five years of age until epiphyseal closure, Am J Dis Child 75:279, 1948.

Anderson M, Green WT, and Messner MB: Growth and predictions of growth in the lower extremities, J Bone Joint Surg 45A:1, 1963.

Anderson MT, Messner MB, and Green WT: Distribution of lengths of the normal femur and tibia in children from one to eighteen years of age, J Bone Joint Surg 46A:1197, 1964.

Anderson WV: Leg lengthening, J Bone Joint Surg 35B:150, 1952.

Armour PC and Scott JHS: Equalisation of leg length, J Bone Joint Surg 63B:4,587, 1981.

Armstrong PF: Attempts to accelerate longitudinal bone growth. In Uhthoff HK and Wiley JJ, editors: Behavior of the growth plate, New York, 1988, Raven Press.

Aronson J et al: Mechanical induction of osteogenesis: the importance of pin rigidity, J Pediatr Orthop 8:396, 1988.

Aronson J et al: The histology of distraction osteogenesis using different external fixators, Clin Orthop 241:106, 1989.

Aston JW and Henley MB: Physeal growth arrest of the distal radius treated by the Ilizarov technique, Orthop Rev 18:813, 1989.

Axer A, Elkon A, and Eliahu HE: Hypertension as a complication of limb lengthening, J Bone Joint Surg 48(A):520, 1966.

Baker GCW: Periosteal division in the management of the short leg in childhood, J Bone Joint Surg 66B:276, 1984.

Barr JS and Ober FR: Leg lengthening in adults, J Bone Joint Surg 15:674, 1933.

Bayley N: Growth curves of height and weight by age for boys and girls scaled according to physical maturity, J Pediat 45:187, 1956.

Bayley N and Pinneau SR: Tables for predicting adult height from skeletal age: revised for use with the Greulich-Pyle hand standards, J Pediatr 49:423, 1952.

Beals RK: Hemihypertrophy and hemihypotrophy, Clin Orthop 166:199, 1982.

Bjerkreim I: Limb lengthening by physeal distraction, Acta Orthop Scand 60:140, 1989.

Bjerkreim I and Hellum C: Femur lengthening using the Wagner technique, Acta Orthop Scand 54:263, 1983.

Blachier D, Trevous L, and Carlioz H: Progressive femoral lengthening by the Wagner technique: a report of 48 cases, Rev Chir Orthop 72:495, 1986.

Blair VP III et al: Epiphysiodesis: a problem of timing, J Pediatr Orthop 2:281, 1982.

Blount WP: Unequal leg length in children, Surg Clin North Am 38:1107, 1958.

Blount WP: A mature look at epiphyseal stapling, Clin Orthop 77:158, 1971.

Blount WP and Clarke GR: Control of bone growth by epiphyseal stapling: a preliminary report, J Bone Joint Surg 31A:464, 1949.

Bohlman HR: Experiments with foreign materials in the region of the epiphyseal cartilage plate of growing bones to increase their longitudinal growth, J Bone Joint Surg 11:365, 1929.

Bost FC and Larsen LJ: Experiences with lengthening of the femur over an intramedullary rod, J Bone Joint Surg 38A:567, 1956.

Bosworth DM: Skeletal distraction of the tibia, Surg Gynecol Obstet 66:912, 1938.

Bowen RJ and Johnson WJ: Percutaneous epiphysiodesis, Clin Orthop 190:170, 1984.

Brockway A and Fowler SB: Experience with 105 leg lengthening operations, Surg Gynecol Obstet 75:252, 1942.

Brockway A, Craig WA, and Cockrell BR: End-result study of sixty-two stapling operations, J Bone Joint Surg 36A(1):63, 1954.

Broughton NS, Olney BW, and Menelaus MB: Tibial shortening for leg length discrepancy, J Bone Joint Surg 71B(2):242, 1989.

Brown K et al: Epiphyseal growth after free fibular transfer with and without microvascular anastomosis: an experiment study in the dog, J Bone Joint Surg 65B:493, 1983.

Bylander B, et al: A roentgen stereophotogrammetric analysis of growth arrest by stapling, J Pediatr Orthop 1(1):81, 1981.

Cameron BM: A technique for femoral shaft shortening: a preliminary report, J Bone Joint Surg 39A:1309, 1957.

Cambras RA et al: Limb lengthening in children, Orthopedics 7:468, 1984.

Canale ST, Russell TA, and Holcomb RL: Percutaneous epiphysiodesis: experimental study and preliminary clinical results, J Pediatr Orthop 6:150, 1986.

Carpenter EB and Dalton JB Jr: A critical evaluation of a method of epiphyseal stimulation: follow-up notes on article previously published, J Bone Joint Surg 45A:642, 1963.

Carroll NC et al: Experimental observations on the effects of leg lengthening by the Wagner method, Clin Orthop 160:251, 1981.

Castle E: Epiphyseal stimulation, J Bone Joint Surg 53A:326, 1971.

Caton J: Leg lengthening with the Ilizarov technique: analysis and results of a multicenter study, Rev Chir Orthop 73(suppl 2):23, 1987.

Cattaneo R et al: Limb lengthening in achondroplasia by Ilizarov's method, Int Orthop 12:173, 1988.

Cauchoix J and Morel G: One stage femoral lengthening, Clin Orthop 136:66, 1978.

Chandler D et al: Results of 21 Wagner limb lengthenings in 20 patients, Clin Orthop 230:217, 1988.

Chacha PB and Chong KC: Experience with tibial lengthening in Singapore, Clin Orthop 125:100, 1977.

Chan KP and Hodgson AR: Physiologic leg lengthening: a preliminary report, Clin Orthop 68:55, 1970.

Christensen NO: Growth arrest by stapling: an experimental study of longitudinal bone growth and morphology of the growth region, Acta Orthop Scand Suppl 151:3, 1973.

Cleveland RH et al: Determination of leg length discrepancy: a comparison of weight-bearing and supine imaging, Invest Radiol 23(4):301, 1988.

Codivilla A: On the means of lengthening in the lower limbs, the muscles and tissues which are shortened through deformity, Am J Orthop Surg 2:353, 1905.

Coleman SS: Current concepts of tibial lengthening, Orthop Clin North Am 3:201, 1972.

Coleman SS and Noonan TD: Anderson's method of tibial lengthening by percutaneous osteotomy and gradual distraction: experiences with 31 cases, J Bone Joint Surg 49A:263, 1967.

Coleman SS and Stevens PM: Tibial lengthening, Clin Orthop 136:92, 1978.

Compere EL: Indications for and against the leg-lengthening operation: use of the tibial bone graft as a factor in preventing delayed union, non-union, or late fracture, J Bone Joint Surg 18:692, 1936.

Connolly JF et al: Epiphyseal traction to correct acquired growth deformities: an animal and clinical investigation, Clin Orthop 202:258, 1986.

Cundy P et al: Skeletal age estimation in leg length discrepancy, J Pediatr Orthop 8:513, 1988.

Dale GG and Harris WR: Prognosis of epiphyseal separation: an experimental study, J Bone Joint Surg 40B:116, 1958.

Dal Monte A and Donzeccio O: Tibial lengthening according to Ilizarov in congenital hypoplasia of the leg, J Pediatr Orthop 76:135, 1987.

Dal Monte A and Donzelli O: Comparison of different methods of leg lengthening, J Pediatr Orthop 8:62, 1988.

Dal Monte A et al: Humeral lengthening in hypoplasia of the upper limb, J Pediatr Orthop 5:202, 1985.

dePablos J, Villas C, and Canadell J: Bone lengthening by physial distraction: an experimental study, Int Orthop 10:163, 1986.

DeBastiani G: Chrondal diastasis-controlled symmetrical distraction of the epiphyseal plate and limb lengthening in children, J Bone Joint Surg 68B:550, 1986.

DeBastiani G et al: Limb lengthening by distraction of the epiphyseal plate, J Bone Joint Surg 68B:545, 1986.

DeBastiani G et al: Limb lengthening by callus distraction (callotasis), J Pediatr Orthop 7:1299 1987.

DeBastiani G et al: Epiphyseal distraction: chondrodiastasis and hemichondrodiatasis, In Uhthoff HJK and Wiley JJ, editors: Behavior of the growth plate, New York, 1988, Raven Press.

Dick HM and Petzokdt RI: Lengthening of the ulna in radial agenesis: a preliminary report, J Hand Surg 2:175, 1977.

Dick HM and Tietjen R: Humeral lengthening for septic neonatal growth arrest, J Bone Joint Surg 60A:1138, 1978.

Eichler J: Methodological errors in documenting leg length and leg length discrepancies. In Hungerford DS, editor: Progress in or-

thopaedic surgery, vol 1, Leg length discrepancy: the injured knee. New York, 1977, Springer-Verlag.

Elo JO: The effect of subperiosteally implanted autogenous whole-thickness skin graft on growing bone: an experimental study, Acta Orthop Scand Suppl 45, 1960.

Eyring EJ: Staged femoral lengthening, Clin Orthop 136:83, 1978.

Fishbane BM and Riley LH: Continuous transphyseal traction: experimental observation, Clin Orthop 136:120, 1978.

Fjeld TO and Steen H: Limb lengthening by low rate epiphyseal distraction: an experimental study in the caprine tibia, J Orthop Res 6:360, 1988.

Fleming B et al: A biomechanical analysis of the Ilizarov external fixator, Clin Orthop 241:95, 1989.

Frankel VH, Gold S, and Golyakhovsky V: The Ilizarov technique, Bull Hosp J Dis 48(1):17, 1988.

Freiberg AH: Codivilla's method of lengthening the lower extremity, Surg Gynecol and Obstet 14:614, 1912.

Friberg O: Clinical symptoms and biomechanics of lumbar spine and hip joint in leg length inequality, Spine 8:643, 1983.

Friberg O, Koivisto E, and Wegelius C: A radiographic method for measurement of leg length inequality, Diagn Imag Clin Med 54:78, 1985.

Ganel A, Israeli A, and Horoszowski H: Fatal complications of femoral elongation in an achondroplastic dwarf, Clin Orthop 185:69, 1984.

Ganel A et al: Leg lengthening in achondroplastic children, Clin Orthop 144:194, 1979.

Giles LGF and Taylor JR: Low back pain associated with leg length inequality, Spine 6:510, 1981.

Glass RBJ and Poznanski AK: Leg length determination with biplanar CT scanograms, Radiology 156:833, 1985.

Granberry WM and James JM: The lack of effect of microwave diathermy on rate of growth of bone of the growing dog, J Bone Joint Surg 45A:773, 1963.

Green SA: Ilizarov external fixation, technical and anatomical considerations. Bull Hosp Joint Dis 48(1):28, 1988.

Green WT and Anderson M: Experiences with epiphyseal arrest in correcting discrepancies in length of the lower extremities in infantile paralysis: a method of predicting the effect, J Bone Joint Surg 29:659, 1947.

Green WT and Anderson M: Epiphyseal arrest for the correction of discrepancies in length of the lower extremities, J Bone Joint Surg 39A:853, 1957.

Greulich WW and Pyle SI: Radiographic atlas of skeletal development of the hand and wrist, ed 2, Stanford, Calif, 1959, Stanford University Press.

Grill F: Distraction of the epiphyseal cartilage as a method of limb lengthening, J Pediatr Orthop 4:105, 1984.

Grill F: Correction of complicated extremity deformities by external fixation, Clin Orthop 241:166, 1989.

Grill F and Franke J: The Ilizarov distractor for the correction of relapsed or neglected clubfoot, J Bone Joint Surg 69B:593, 1987.

Gross R: Leg length discrepancy: how much is too much? Orthopedics 1:305, 1978.

Gross RH: An evaluation of tibial lengthening procedures, J Bone Joint Surg 53A:693, 1971.

Grundy PF and Roberts CJ: Does unequal leg length cause back pain? a case-control study, Lancet 256, 1984.

Haas SL: Mechanical retardation of bone growth, J Bone Joint Surg 30A:506, 1948.

Haas SL: Stimulation of bone growth, Am J Surg 95:125, 1958.

Hang Y and Shih JD: Tibial lengthening, Clin Orthop 125:94, 1977.

Heims CA and McCarthy S: CT scanograms for measuring leg-length discrepancy, Radiology 151:802, 1984.

Herring JA and Coleman SS: Femoral lengthening, J Pediatr Orthop 2:432, 1982.

Herron LD, Amstutz HC, and Pakal DN: One stage femoral lengthening in the adult, Clin Orthop 136:74, 1978.

Hogberg N and Lindstrom A: Aspects of epiphyseodesis, Acta Orthop Scand 27:69, 1957.

Hood RW and Riseborough EJ: Lengthening of the lower extremity by the Wagner method: a review of the Boston Children's Hospital experience, J Bone Joint Surg 63A:1122, 1981.

Houghton GR and Rooker GD: The role of the periosteum in the growth of long bones: an experimental study in the rabbit, J Bone Joint Surg 61B:218, 1979.

Huurman WW et al: Limb-length discrepancy measured with computerized axial tomographic equipment, J Bone Joint Surg 69A:699, 1987.

Ilizarov GA: The principles of the Ilizarov method, Bull Hosp Joint Dis 48:1, 1988.

Ilizarov GA: Experimental studies of bone elongation. In Coombs R, Green S, and Sarmiento A, editors: External fixation and functional bracing, London, 1989, Orthotext.

Ilizarov GA: Angular deformities with shortening. In Coombs R, Green S, and Sarmiento A, editors: External fixation and functional bracing, London, 1989, Orthotext.

Ilizarov GA: The tension-stress effect on the genesis and growth of tissues. II. The influence of the rate and frequency of distraction, Clin Orthop 239:263, 1989.

Ilizarov GA: The tension-stress effect on the genesis and growth of tissues. I. The influence of stability of fixation and soft tissue preservation, Clin Orthop 238:249, 1989.

Janes JM and Jennings WK: Effect of induced arteriovenous fistula on leg length: ten-year observations, Proc Mayo Clinic 36:1, 1961.

Jenkins DHR, Cheng DHF, and Hodgson AR: Stimulation of bone growth by periosteal stripping: a clinical study, J Bone Joint Surg 57B:482, 1975.

Johansson JE and Barrington TW: Femoral shortening by a step-cut osteotomy for leg-length discrepancy in adults, Clin Orthop 181:132, 1983.

Johnson JTH and Southwick WO: Growth following transepiphyseal bone grafts: an experimental study to explain continued growth following certain fusion operations, J Bone Joint Surg 42A:1381, 1960.

Jones DC and Moseley CF: Subluxation of the knee as a complication of femoral lengthening by the Wagner technique, J Bone Joint Surg 67:33, 1985.

Kaplan EG and Kaplan GS: Metatarsal lengthening by use of autogenous bone graft and internal wire compression fixation: a preliminary report, J Hand Surg 2:394, 1977.

Kawamura B, Hosono S, and Takahashi T: The principles and technique of limb lengthening, Int Orthop 5:69, 1981.

Kawamura B, et al: Limb lengthening by means of subcutaneous osteotomy: experimental and clinical studies, J Bone Joint Surg 50A:851, 1968.

Kawamura B: Limb lengthening, Orthop Clin North Am 9:155, 1978.

Kempf I, Grosse A, and Abalo C: Locked intramedullary nailing: its application to femoral and tibial axial, rotational, lengthening, and shortening osteotomies, Clin Orthop 212:165, 1986.

Kenwright J, Bentley G, and Morgan JD: Leg lengthening, Acta Orthop Scand 41:454, 1970.

Kenwright J et al: Effect of controlled axial micromotion on healing of tibial fractures, Lancet 2:8517, 1986.

Kogutt MS: Computed radiographic imaging: use in low-dose leg length radiography, AJR 148:1205, 1987.

Korkala O, et al: Experimental lengthening of tibial diaphysis: gap healing with or without gradual distraction, Arch Orthop Trauma Surg 107:172, 1988.

Kuntscher G: Intramedullary surgical technique and its place in orthopaedic surgery: my present concept, J Bone Joint Surg 47A:809, 1965.

Lamoureux J and Verstreken L: Progressive upper limb lengthening in children: a report of two cases, J Orthop Pediatr 6:481, 1986.

Letts RM and Meadows L: Epiphysiolysis as a method of limb lengthening, Clin Orthop 133:230, 1978.

Leung JCY et al: Viscoelastic behaviour of tissue in leg lengthening by distraction, Clin Orthop 139:102, 1979.

Liedberg E and Persson BM: Technical aspects of midshaft femoral shortening with Kuntscher nailing, Clin Orthop 136:62, 1978

Lynch MC and Taylor JF: Periosteal division and longitudinal growth in the tibia of the rat, J Bone Joint Surg 69B(5):812, 1987.

MacEwen DG and Case JL: Congenital hemihypertrophy, Clin Orthop 50:147, 1967.

MacNicol MF and Catto AM: Twenty-year review of tibial lengthening for poliomyelitis, J Bone Joint Surg 64B:607, 1982.

Malhis TM and Bowen JR: Tibial and femoral lengthening: a report of 54 cases, J Pediatr Orthop 2:487, 1982.

Manning C: Leg lengthening, Clin Orthop 136:105, 1978.

Matev IB: Thumb reconstruction through metacarpal bone lengthening, J Hand Surg 5:482, 1980.

Matev IB: The bone lengthening method in hand reconstruction: twenty years' experience, J Hand Surg 14:376, 1989.

Mayhall WST: Leg length discrepancy treated by epiphysiodesis, Orthop Rev 7(4):41, 1978.

McCarroll HR: Trials and tribulations in attempted femoral lengthening, J Bone Joint Surg 32A:132, 1950.

McCullough J and Kenwright J: The prognosis in congenital lower limb hypertrophy, Acta Orthop Scand 50:307, 1979.

McGibbons KC, Deacon AE, and Raisbeck CC: Experiences in growth retardation with heavy vitallum staples, J Bone Joint Surg 44:36, 1962.

Menelaus MB: Correction of leg length discrepancy by epiphyseal arrest, J Bone Joint Surg 48B:336, 1966.

Merle D'Aubigne R and Dubousset J: Surgical correction of large length discrepancies in the lower extremities of children and adults, J Bone Joint Surg 53A:411, 1971.

Mezhenina EP et al: Methods of limb elongation with congenital inequality in children, J Pediatr Orthop 4:201, 1984.

Millis MB and Hall JE: Transiliac lengthening of the lower extremity: a modified innominate osteotomy for the treatment of postural imbalance, J Bone Joint Surg 61A:1182, 1979.

Monticelli G and Spinelli R: Distraction epiphysiolysis as a method of limb lengthening. I. Experimental study, Clin Orthop 154:254, 1981.

Monticelli G and Spinelli R: Distraction epiphysiolysis as a method of limb lengthening. III. Clinical applications, Clin Orthop 154:274, 1981.

Monticelli G and Spinelli R: Leg lengthening by closed metaphyseal corticotomy, Ital J Orthop Traumatol 4:139, 1983.

Monticelli G, Spinelli R, and Bonucci EL: Distraction epiphysiolysis as a method of limb lengthening. II. Morphologic investigations, Clin Orthop 154:262, 1981.

Morscher E and Figner G: Measurement of leg length. In Hungeford, DS, editor: Progress in orthopaedic surgery, vol 1, Leg length discrepancy: the injured knee. New York, 1977, Springer-Verlag.

Moseley CF: A straight-line graph for leg length discrepancies, J Bone Joint Surg 59A:174, 1977.

Moseley CF: A straight line graph for leg length discrepancies, Clin Orthop 136:33, 1978.

Moseley CF: Leg length discrepancy, Orthop Clin North Am 18(4):529, 1987.

Moseley C and Mosca V: Complications of Wagner leg lengthening. In Uhthoff HK and Wiley JJ, editors: Behavior of the growth plate, New York, 1988, Raven Press.

Newschwander GE and Gunst RM: Limb lengthening with the Ilizarov external fixator, Orthop Nurs 8:15, 1989.

Noble J et al: Limb lengthening by epiphysial distraction, J Bone Joint Surg 60B:139, 1978.

Noble J et al: Breaking force of the rabbit growth plate and its application to epiphyseal distraction, Acta Orthop Scand 53:13, 1982.

Ogilvie JW: Epiphysiodesis: evaluation of a new technique, J Pediatr Orthop 6:147, 1986.

Olerud C, Danckwardt-Lilliestrom G, Olerud S: Genu recurvatum caused by partial growth arrest of the proximal tibial physis: simultaneous correction and lengthening with physeal distraction, Arch Orthop Trauma Surg 106:64, 1986.

Paley D: Current techniques of limb lengthening, J Pediatr Orthop 8:73, 1988.

Paley D: The principles of deformity correction by the Ilizarov technique: technical aspects, Techniques in Orthop 4:15, 1989.

Paley D: Problems, obstacles and complications of limb lengthening by the Ilizarov technique, Clin Orthop 250:81, 1990.

Paley D et al: The biology and biomechanics of the Ilizarov external fixator, Clin Orthop 241:95, 1989.

Paley D et al: Ilizarov treatment of tibial nonunions with bone loss, Clin Orthop 241:146, 1989.

Papaioannou T, Stokes I, and Kenwright J: Scoliosis associated with limb-length inequality, J Bone Joint Surg 64A(1):59, 1982.

Paterson JMH, Waller CS, and Catterall A: Lower limb lengthening by a modified Wagner technique, J Pediatr Orthop 9:129, 1989.

Peltonen J: Bone formation and remodeling after symmetric and asymmetric physeal distraction, J Pediatr Orthop 9:191, 1989.

Petty W, Winter RB, and Felder D: Arteriovenous fistula for treatment of discrepancy in leg length, J Bone Joint Surg 56A:582, 1974.

Phemister DB: Operative arrestment of longitudinal growth of bones in the treatment of deformities, J Bone Joint Surg 15:1, 1933.

Pilcher MF: Epiphysial stapling: thirty-five cases followed to maturity, J Bone Joint Surg 44B:82, 1962.

Poirier H: Epiphyseal stapling and leg equalization, J Bone Joint Surg 50B:61, 1968.

Price CT: Metaphyseal and physeal lengthening, In The American Academy of Orthopaedic Surgeons: Instructional course lectures, vol 38, St. Louis, 1989, CV Mosby Co.

Price CT and Mills W: Radial lengthening for septic growth arrest: case report, J Pediatr Orthop 3(1):88, 1983.

Pritchett JW: Lengthening the ulna in patients with hereditary multiple exostoses, J Bone Joint Surg 68A:561, 1986.

Putti V: Operative lengthening of the femur, Surg Gynecol Obstet 58:318, 1934.

Pyka WR and Nagel DA: Use of the Ilizarov external fixator for tibial lengthening: case report, Contemp Orthop 17:15, 1988.

Rainey RK: Operative femoral shortening by closed intramedullary technique, Orthop Rev 8(1):36, 1984.

Ratliff AHC: The short leg in poliomyelitis, J Bone Joint Surg 41B:56, 1959.

Regan JM and Chatterton C: Deformities following surgical epiphyseal arrest, J Bone Joint Surg 28:165, 1946.

Rezaian SM: Tibial lengthening using a new extension device, J Bone Joint Surg 58A:239, 1976.

Rezaian SM and Abtahi M: A simple and safe technique for tibial lengthening, Clin Orthop 207:216, 1986.

Salai M et al: Subluxation of the hip joint during femoral lengthening, J Pediatr Orthop 5:642, 1985.

Schopler SA, Lawrence JF, and Johnson MK: Lengthening of the humerus for upper extremity limb length discrepancy, J Pediatr Orthop 4:477, 1986.

Shapiro F: Fractures of the femoral shaft in children: the overgrowth phenomenon, Acta Orthop Scand 52:649, 1981.

Shapiro F: Ollier's disease: an assessment of angular deformity, shortening, and pathological fracture in twenty-one patients, J Bone Joint Surg 64A:95, 1982.

Shapiro F: Developmental patterns in lower extremity length discrepancies, J Bone Joint Surg 69A:684, 1987.

Shapiro F: Longitudinal growth of the femur and tibia after diaphyseal lengthening, J Bone Joint Surg 69A:684, 1987.

Shapiro F, Simon S, and Glincher MJ: Hereditary multiple exostosis: anthropometric roentgenographic and clinical aspects, J Bone Joint Surg 61A:815, 1979.

Siffert RS: Lower limb-length discrepancy, J Bone Joint Surg 68A(7):1101, 1987.

Simon S, Whippen J, and Shapiro F: Leg-length discrepancies in monoarticular and pauciarticular juvenilerheumatoid arthritis, J Bone Joint Surg 63A:209, 1981.

Skirving AP and Newman JH: Elongation of the first metatarsal, J Pediatr Orthop 1:508, 1981.

Sledge CB and Noble J: Experimental limb lengthening by epiphyseal distraction, Clin Orthop 136:111, 1978.

Smith DJ: Assessment of the accuracy of three techniques to predict leg length discrepancy, Orthopedics 5:737, 1982.

Sofield HA, Blair SJ, and Millar EA: Leg-lengthening: a personal follow-up of forty patients some twenty years after the operation, J Bone Joint Surg 40A:311, 1958.

Spinelli R: Bone lengthening through physeal distraction-separation, In Uhthoff HK and Wiley JJ, editors: Behavior of the growth plate, New York, 1988, Raven Press.

Stephens DC: Femoral and tibial lengthening, J Pediatr Orthop 3:424, 1983.

Stephens DC, Herrick W, and MacEwen GD: Epiphysiodesis for limb length inequality: results and indications, Clin Orthop 136:41, 1978.

Stephens DC et al: Epiphysiodesis for limb length inequality: results and indications, Clin Orthop 136:41, 1978.

Straub LR, Thompson TC, and Wilson PD: The results of epiphyseodesis and femoral shortening in relation to equalization of limb length, J Bone Joint Surg 27:254, 1945.

Tajana GF, Morandi M, and Zembo MM: The structure and development of osteogenetic repair tissue according to Ilizarov technique in man, Orthopedics 12:515, 1989.

Talab Y, Hamdan J, and Ahmed M: Orthopaedic causes of hypertension in pediatric patients, J Bone Joint Surg 64A:291, 1982.

Taylor JF and Warrell E: The effect of local trauma on tibial growth, J Bone Joint Surg 59B:503, 1977.

Thompson TC, Straub LR, and Campbell RD: An evaluation of femoral shortening with intramedullary nailing, J Bone Joint Surg 36A:43, 1954.

Thornton L: A method of subtrochanteric limb shortening, J Bone Joint Surg 31A:81, 1949.

Tupman GS and Bath E: Treatment of inequality of the lower limbs, J Bone Joint Surg 42B(3):489, 1960.

Urano Y and Kobayashi A: Bone lengthening for shortness of the fourth toes, J Bone Joint Surg 60A:91, 1979.

Wagner H: Surgical lengthening or shortening of femur and tibia: technique and indications. In Hungerford DS, editor: Progress in orthopaedic surgery, vol 1, Leg length discrepancy: the injured knee, New York, 1977, Springer-Verlag.

Wagner H: Operative lengthening of the femur, Clin Orthop 136:125, 1978.

Westh RN and Menelaus MB: A simple calculation for the timing of epiphyseal arrest, J Bone Joint Surg 63B:117, 1981.

Westin GW: Femoral lengthening using a periosteal sleeve: report on twenty-six cases, J Bone Joint Surg 48A(8):836, 1987.

Wilde GP and Baker GC: Circumferential periosteal release in the treatment of children with leg-length inequality, J Bone Joint Surg 69B(5):817, 1987.

Wilk LH and Badgley CE: Hypertension: another complication of the leg-lengthening procedure, J Bone Joint Surg 45A:1262, 1963.

Wilson AJ and Ramsby GR: Skeletal measurements using a flying spot digital imaging device, AJR 149:339, 1987.

Winquist RA: Closed intramedullary osteotomies of the femur, Clin Orthop 212:157, 1986.

Winquist RA, Hansen ST Jr, and Pearson RE: Closed femoral shortening, J Bone Joint Surg 57A:135, 1975.

Yabsley RH and Harris WR: The effect of shaft fractures and periosteal stripping on the vascular supply to epiphyseal plates, J Bone Joint Surg 47A:551, 1965.

Yosipovitch Z and Palti Y: Alterations in blood pressure during leg lengthening, J Bone Joint Surg 49:1352, 1967.

Zimbler S et al: Correction of leg length discrepancy: use of epiphyseodesis (Tufts experience). In Uhthoff HK and Wiley JJ, editors: Behavior of the growth plate, New York, 1988, Raven Press.

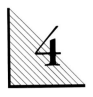

4 Congenital Anomalies of the Hand

PHILLIP E. WRIGHT
MARK T. JOBE

PRINCIPLES OF MANAGEMENT

The difficulties in treating congenital anomalies of the hand have long been recognized. Flatt cautioned that "congenital malformations are some of the most difficult problems confronting the hand surgeon." Milford observed that "a single surgical procedure cannot be standardized to suit even similar anomalies." Space precludes discussion of every treatment of each anomaly. Included here are those procedures that have been shown to be safe and effective in most situations.

Treatment for the child with a congenital hand deformity may be sought at birth or later in development. Involvement may be unilateral or bilateral; the anomaly may be an isolated condition, or it may be a single manifestation of a malformation syndrome or skeletal dysplasia. Early evaluation by the hand surgeon usually is desirable, not because of urgency to begin treatment but to help with the concerns of the parents. Parents usually have considerable anxiety because of personal guilt feelings, the appearance of the hand, the future function of the hand, and the possibility of subsequent siblings being similarly affected. To adequately inform the parents and to dispel as much anxiety as possible, it is helpful for the surgeon to be familiar with the modes of inheritance, as well as the preferred treatment and prognosis, of each condition. Although specific considerations and indications for surgical and nonsurgical treatment are discussed with each individual condition, the amazing ability of children to compensate functionally for deformity should be remembered.

Table 4-1 Distribution of primary diagnoses: in descending order of incidence

Type of anomaly	No. of cases		Percent
Syndactyly		443	17.5
Polydactyly—all		361	14.3
Polydactyly, radial	162		6.4
Polydactyly, ulnar	130		5.2
Polydactyly, central	69		2.7
Amputation—all		179	7.1
Amputation, hand/ digits	77		3.0
Amputation, arm/ forearm	75		3.0
Amputation, wrist	27		1.1
Camptodactyly		173	6.9
Clinodactyly		142	5.6
Brachydactyly		131	5.2
Radial clubhand		119	4.7
Central defects		99	3.9
Thumb, hypoplastic		90	3.6
Acrosyndactyly		83	3.3
Trigger digit		59	2.3
Poland syndrome		56	2.2
Apert syndrome		52	2.1
Constriction bands		51	2.0
Musculotendinous de- fects		49	1.9
Madelung deformity		43	1.7
Thumb, absent		34	1.4
Ulnar finger/metacarpal absent		31	1.2
Ulnar hypoplasia		31	1.2
Synostosis, radioulnar		29	1.2
Ulnar clubhand		25	1.0
Thumb, triphalangeal		21	0.8
Hypoplasia, whole hand		21	0.8
Macrodactyly		21	0.8
Phocomelia		19	0.8
Thumb, adducted		18	0.7
Radial hypoplasia		17	0.7
Symphalangism		13	0.5
Other		115	4.6
		2525	100.0

From Flatt A: The care of congenital hand anomalies, St Louis, 1977, The CV Mosby Co.

INCIDENCE AND CLASSIFICATION

Congenital malformations of the hand encompass a myriad of deformities, all of which carry different functional and cosmetic implications for the patient and parents. Unfortunately, they occur with relative frequency. In 1982 the Congenital Malformations Committee of the International Federation of Societies for Surgery of the Hand reported an incidence of approximately 11 anomalies per 10,000 population. These data were accumulated in seven centers located in the United Kingdom, Japan, and the United States. A similar incidence was reported earlier by Conway and Bowe (1:626 live births). The most commonly encountered anomalies of the hand are syndactyly, polydactyly, congenital amputations, camptodactyly, clinodactyly, and radial clubhand. The most common anomaly reported in the Iowa study (Flatt) was syndactyly, as opposed to polydactyly in the Asian series (Tables 4-1 and 4-2).

The classification system devised by Swanson et al, which currently is accepted by the American Society for Surgery of the Hand and the International Federation of Societies for Surgery of the Hand, separates

Table 4-2 Diagnoses in Yokohama patients

Type of anomaly	No. of cases	Percent
Syndactyly	23	10.1
Polydactyly	65	28.6
Brachydactyly	19	8.4
Brachysyndactyly	10	4.4
Symphalangism	1	0.5
Annular grooves	3	1.3
Ectrodactyly		
Cleft hand	12	5.3
Ectrosyndactyly	17	7.5
Amputation	16	7.0
Microdactyly	5	2.2
Floating thumb	5	2.2
Hypoplasia of the thumb	3	1.3
Five finger	2	0.9
Monodactyly	1	0.5
Floating small finger	1	0.5
Defect of fifth meta- carpus	1	0.5
Macrodactyly	3	1.3
Clinodactyly	3	1.3
Clubhand	14	6.1
Phocomelia	2	0.9
Others	21	9.3
	227	

Modified from Yamaguchi S et al: Incidence of various congenital anomalies of the hand from 1961 to 1972. In Proceedings of the sixteenth annual meeting of the Japanese Society for Surgery of the Hand, Fukuoka, 1973.

congenital anomalies of the hand into seven categories (see box). This classification is based on specific embryologic failures and has eliminated confusing Greek and Latin terms and eponyms. It is based in part on the system outlined by Frantz and O'Rahilly in which four patterns of deficiencies were identified on the basis of certain skeletal deficiencies: terminal transverse, terminal longitudinal, intercalary transverse, and intercalary longitudinal. After extensive clinical application and testing, Flatt found that this system permitted full categorization of complex deformities. It does not delineate etiologic factors, treatment, or prognosis.

CLASSIFICATION OF CONGENITAL ANOMALIES OF THE HAND

  I. Failure of formation of parts (arrest of development)
 II. Failure of differentiation (separation) of parts
III. Duplication
 IV. Overgrowth (gigantism)
  V. Undergrowth (hypoplasia)
 VI. Congenital constriction band syndrome
VII. Generalized skeletal abnormalities

Isolated deformities that commonly are nongenetic include unilateral transverse failure of formation, deficiencies as a result of constriction bands, longitudinal radial and ulnar dysplasias, macrodactyly, and preaxial polydactyly. Isolated deformities that usually are autosomal dominant include lobster claw deformity, symphalangism, brachydactyly, triphalangeal thumb, camptodactyly, and postaxial polydactyly. Syndactyly may occur sporadically or as a dominant trait. The malformation syndromes and skeletal dysplasias have different patterns of inheritance.

FAILURE OF FORMATION (ARREST OF DEVELOPMENT)
Transverse Deficiencies

Transverse deficiencies include those deformities in which there is complete absence of parts distal to some point on the upper extremity, producing amputation-like stumps that allow further classification by naming the level at which the remaining stump terminates. Wynne-Davies reported the incidence of transverse deficiencies to be 6.8 per 10,000. Most transverse deficiencies (98%) are unilateral, and the most common level is the upper third of the forearm. There is no particular sex predilection. Except

for thalidomide, no particular cause has been established, and in the usual unilateral transverse deficiency there is no genetic basis, although the rare bilateral or multiple transverse deficiencies may be inherited as an autosomal recessive trait. Transverse deficiencies usually do not occur in association with malformation syndromes, but anomalies reported to occur in association with transverse deficiencies include hydrocephalus, spina bifida, myelomeningocele, clubfoot, radial head dislocation, and radioulnar synostosis.

The newborn with a transverse deficiency usually has a slightly bulbous, well-padded stump. In the more distal deficiencies, rudimentary, vestigal digital "nubbins" are common (Fig. 4-1). Hypoplasia of the more proximal muscles helps differentiate these deficiencies from those associated with congenital bands. In the more common upper forearm amputation, the forearm usually is no more than 7 cm long at birth and can be expected to measure no more than 10 cm by skeletal maturity. In midcarpal amputations, the second most frequent level of deficiency, the rudimentary digital remnants usually are nonfunctional. Although the affected forearm may be relatively shorter than the normal side, pronation and supination usually are possible. These children generally are of normal intelligence.

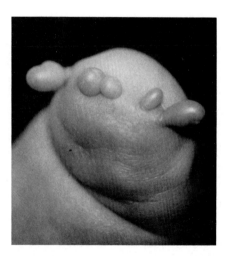

Fig. 4-1 Failure of formation (digital nubbins). Wrist motion allows use as assisting hand.

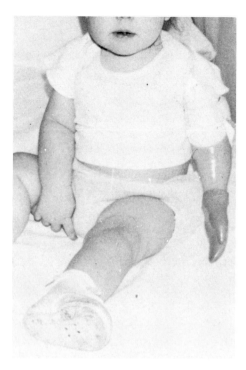

Fig. 4-2 Passive plastic mitten prosthesis. (From Pellicore RJ and Tooms RE: The juvenile amputee: prosthetic management. Section I. Upper limb prosthetic management. In AAOS: Atlas of limb prosthetics: surgical and prosthetic principles, St Louis, 1981, The CV Mosby Co.)

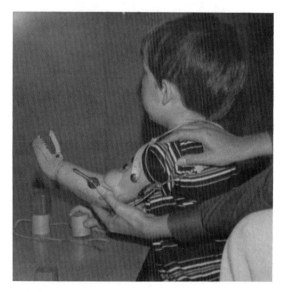

Fig. 4-3 CAPP terminal device, actively opened by patient.

Prosthetic Management

For those patients who do not require surgery, treatment usually has consisted of early prosthetic fitting of the deficient limb, preferably by the time the child is crawling and certainly by the time of independent ambulation. The child's development of manual and bimanual skills progresses in an orderly and predictable pattern. Until the age of 9 months, prehension is achieved primarily by bilateral palmar grasp. Single-hand grasp develops next, and by the age of 12 to 18 months, thumb-to-finger pinch is possible. The ability to grasp an object is believed to precede the ability to release. By the age of 24 months the child should have developed coordinated shoulder positioning, grasp, and release. The fitting of the upper limb prosthesis should complement and enhance these developmental milestones. The choice of prosthetic design is based on the level of amputation, the age and mental capacity of the child, and occasionally certain socioeconomic conditions that may determine availability and practicality of more complicated prostheses.

For the rare child with complete arm amputation, especially if bilateral, conventional body-powered prostheses that include an elbow are unlikely to be of functional benefit. For most children with congenital above-elbow amputations, a rigid elbow is used initially. When the passive mitten initially used as a terminal device is exchanged for an actively opened split hook, usually at age 18 months, the rigid elbow is replaced by a friction elbow. At about 3 years of age, dual terminal devices and elbow controls may be tried. For bilateral above-elbow amputations, only the preferred or dominant side is fitted with a dual-control, articulated prosthesis.

For the child with an amputation at the upper third of the forearm, a passive plastic mitten prosthesis (Fig. 4-2) is introduced between the ages of 3 and 6 months, followed by the addition of an actively opened, Plastisol-covered, split hook at 12 to 18 months of age. A Child Amputee Prosthetic Program (CAPP) terminal device (Fig. 4-3) may be substituted if preferred. Training with a functional device is begun at 18 months of age. The CAPP device can be used until the child is about 6 years old. The prosthesis also is of some benefit in providing stability during sitting and may assist the child in pulling to a standing position. Although standard prosthetic fitting usually is satisfactory, a myoelectric prosthesis (Fig. 4-4) has been shown to be useful and appropriate for the preschool-aged child and may be considered between the ages of 2 and 4 years.

Prosthetic treatment for the child with a midcarpal amputation is somewhat more controversial. Although the carpal bones cannot be seen roentgenographically until about the age of 6 to 8 months, their presence improves the prognosis because minimal shortening of the forearm can be expected. Delay in carpal bone maturation rarely is encountered. The long, below-elbow stump is so useful for stabilizing objects and assisting in bimanual functions for which sensibility is required that the benefits of a prosthesis are debatable. Options include use of an open-ended volar plate secured to the forearm, which permits simple grip between stump and plate, an open-ended volar plate with a terminal hook, and an artificial hand driven by the radiocarpal motion. Terminal sensibility is sacrificed with the last option, but a good cosmetic effect is achieved. Regardless of the prosthesis chosen, therapist-supervised training sessions are essential. These sessions should be scheduled at regular intervals, particularly when a new prosthesis is introduced, and coordinated follow-up should be maintained among patient, family, therapist, orthotist, and physician. Most children do well with prostheses, although it is common for adolescents, particularly boys, to reject the prosthesis for a time before resuming its use.

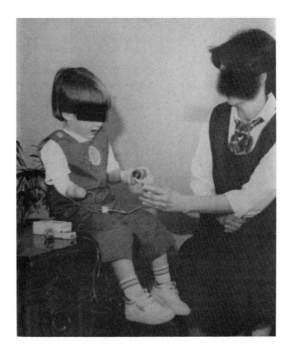

Fig. 4-4　Myoelectric prosthesis. Practice sessions are essential for child to learn to use this prosthesis effectively.

Surgical Treatment

There are few indications for surgical intervention in children with transverse deficiencies of the upper extremity. Epps et al in 1980 reported only 85 operations performed on 1077 children with upper extremity congenital amputations.

Amputation of nonfunctional digital remnants often is performed for psychologic and cosmetic benefits. Complete amputation of all digits often gives the hand the bizarre appearance of a little paw with small nubbins attached. As stated by Littler and emphasized by Flatt, it often is wise to alter the "stigma of congenitalism" and make the deformity appear acquired. Simple elliptic excision is appropriate.

Krukenberg reconstruction and Nathan and Nguyen modification. Krukenberg in 1917 described a procedure consisting of separation of the radius and ulna to allow a sensate, "chopstick"-like forearm. The Krukenberg reconstruction (Fig. 4-5) is best for the child with bilateral below-elbow amputation who is visually impaired and for the child with unilateral amputation in an underdeveloped country with limited prosthetic resources. Swanson and Swanson reported that persons with bilateral amputations found this adaptation much more useful than mechanical prostheses and that they transferred dominance to this limb when a prosthesis was used on the other limb. Chan et al also emphasized that younger children adapt more quickly and that parents readily accept the procedure as they see their children advance from a one-handed pattern to a two-handed activity pattern. This reconstruction does not preclude the use of a prosthesis for cosmesis when desired. Surgical prerequisites include a stump length of at least 8 cm from the insertion of the biceps, relatively normal forearm musculature, and a patient and family who are willing to undergo a somewhat disfiguring operation to improve function. Nathan and Nguyen described a modification of this procedure that requires extensive excision of muscle and allows closure of skin flaps without the use of skin grafts.

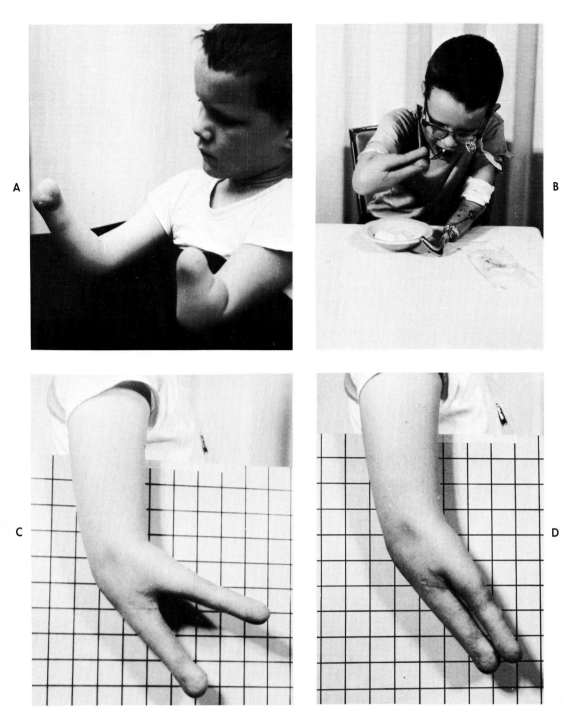

Fig. 4-5   Krukenberg reconstruction. This procedure is usually best for visually impaired children with bilateral below-elbow amputations, **A,** especially in regions with limited prosthetic resources. **B,** After reconstruction, child uses reconstructed limb as dominant hand. **C** and **D,** Tips of rays can be separated about 7.5 cm, and pinch and grasp are excellent. (From Swanson AB: J Bone Joint Surg 46A:1540, 1964.)

▶ *Technique (Krukenberg; Swanson and Swanson)* **(Fig. 4-6).** Make a longitudinal incision on the flexor surface of the forearm slightly toward the radial side (Fig. 4-6, *A*); make a similar one on the dorsal surface slightly toward the ulnar side, but on this surface elevate a V-shaped flap to form a web at the junction of the rays (Fig. 4-6, *B*). Now separate the forearm muscles into two groups (Fig. 4-6, *C* and *D*): on the radial side carry the radial wrist flexors and extensors, the radial half of the flexor digitorum sublimis, the radial half of the extensor digitorum communis, the brachioradialis, the palmaris longus, and the pronator teres; on the ulnar side carry the ulnar wrist flexors and extensors, the ulnar half of the flexor digitorum sublimis, and the ulnar half of the extensor digitorum communis. If they make the stump too bulky or the wound hard to close, resect as necessary the pronator quadratus, the flexor digitorum profundus, the flexor pollicis longus, the abductor pollicis longus, and the extensor pollicis brevis; take care here not to disturb the pronator teres. Next incise the interosseous membrane throughout its length along its ulnar attachment, taking care not to damage the interosseous vessel and nerve. The radial and ulnar rays now can be separated 6 to 12 cm at their tips depending on the size of the forearm; motion at their proximal ends occurs at the radiohumeral and proximal radioulnar joints. The opposing ends of the rays should touch; if not, perform an osteotomy of the radius or ulna as necessary. Now the adductors of the radial ray are the pronator teres, the supinator, the flexor carpi radialis, the radial half of the flexor digitorum sublimis, and the palmaris longus; the abductors of the radial ray are the brachioradialis, the extensor carpi radialis longus, the extensor carpi radialis brevis, the radial half of the extensor digitorum communis, and the biceps. The adductors of the ulnar ray are the flexor carpi ulnaris, the ulnar half of the flexor digitorum sublimis, the brachialis, and the anconeus; the abductors of the ulnar ray are the extensor carpi ulnaris, the ulnar half of the extensor digitorum communis, and the triceps.

Remove the tourniquet, obtain hemostasis, and observe the circulation in the flaps. Now excise any excess fat, rotate the skin around each ray, and close the skin over each so that the suture line is not on the opposing surface of either (Fig. 4-6, *E* and *F*). Excise any scarred skin at the ends of the rays and, if necessary to permit closure, shorten the bones; in children the skin usually is sufficient for closure and the bones must not be shortened because growth at the distal physes will still be incomplete. Preserve any remaining rudimentary digit. Next suture the flap in place at the junction of the rays and apply any needed split-thickness graft. Insert small rubber drains and, with the tips of the rays separated 6 cm or more, apply a compression dressing.

▶ *Postoperative management.* The limb is constantly elevated for 3 to 4 days. The sutures are removed at about 2 weeks. At 2 to 3 weeks rehabilitation to develop abduction and adduction of the rays is begun.

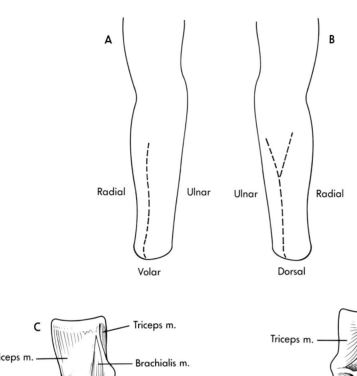

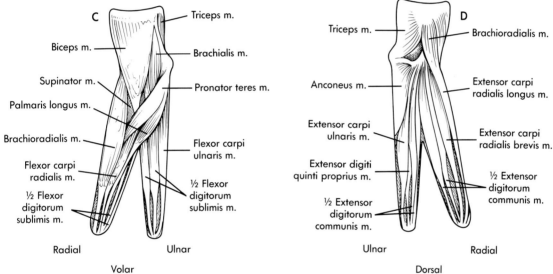

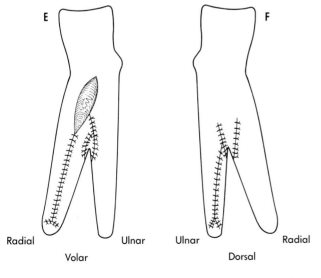

Fig. 4-6 Krukenberg reconstruction (see text). **A,** Incision on flexor surface of forearm. **B,** Incision on dorsal surface. **C** and **D,** Forearm muscles have been separated into two groups. **E,** Skin closure on flexor surface of forearm; elliptical area indicates location of any needed split-thickness skin graft. **F,** Skin closure on dorsal surface. (Modified from Swanson AB: J Bone Joint Surg 46A:1540, 1964.)

▶ *Technique (Nathan and Trung)* (Fig. 4-7). Under tourniquet control, make an incision beginning on the dorsoulnar aspect of the forearm at the junction of the proximal and middle thirds. Continue this incision distally in an S-shaped fashion to create proximal ulnar and distal radial-based flaps. Continue this incision palmarward and proximally to create opposing distal ulnar and proximal radial-based flaps, again in an S-shaped fashion. Sharply incise the underlying fascia in line with the skin incision, taking care to preserve the cutaneous nerves. Excise the palmaris longus, the flexor carpi radialis, and the entire flexor superficialis muscles. Be careful to preserve the blood supply to the flexor digitorum profundus. Divide the flexor digitorum profundus into radial and ulnar halves with blunt dissection. Excise the pronator quadratus, carefully preserving the anterior interosseous artery and nerve. Dorsally, identify and preserve the brachioradialis. The extensor carpi radialis longus and brevis, abductor pollicis longus, and extensor pollicis brevis may be excised to allow for primary skin closure. Next make an opening between the radial and ulnar halves of the extensor digitorum communis. Gently divide the interosseous membrane by pulling apart the stumps of the radius and ulna, thus splitting the fibers. Close the wound over rubber drains, beginning distally and closing the radial stump first. A flap or graft should not be necessary for closure. Release the tourniquet after closure, and check that the skin blanches and fills. Apply a compressive dressing, separating the tips of the rays 6 cm or more.

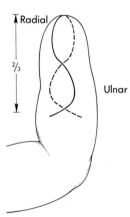

Fig. 4-7 Modified S-shaped incisions for Krukenberg reconstruction (see text). *Solid line,* Volar incision; *dotted line,* dorsal incision. (From Nathan PA and Trung NB: J Hand Surg 2:127, 1977.)

▶ *Postoperative management.* The limb is elevated continuously for 48 hours. The drains are removed in routine fashion, and sutures are removed at 2 weeks. Two to three weeks after surgery, rehabilitation is begun to develop abduction and adduction of the rays.

Metacarpal lengthening. Metacarpal lengthening usually is reserved for transverse deficiencies at the level of the metacarpophalangeal joints in the child with at least one remaining digit. Osteotomy of a digital ray with gradual distraction and subsequent bone grafting was first described by Matev in 1967 for a deficient thumb, and there have been few reports advocating this procedure for congenital absence of fingers. The procedure requires judgment and experience and should be performed by surgeons knowledgeable in the special needs and expectations of these patients and the techniques and realistic results of the procedure. According to Kessler et al and Cowen and Loftus, metacarpal lengthening is best performed between the ages of 5 and 11 years. An average of 4 to 5 cm of length may be gained, but improved function and cosmesis may not be achieved. Complications include pin tract infection, neurovascular compromise, and distal ulcerations. Ilizarov of Russia has reported gains in length and improved function with his distraction/fixation apparatus, but reports in the English literature are presently insufficient for definitive conclusions.

▶ *Technique (Kessler et al).* Under tourniquet control, make longitudinal dorsal incisions over or between the metacarpals to be lengthened. Perform an osteotomy of the appropriate metacarpals, and insert two wires transversely through the skin and metacarpals, both proximal and distal to the osteotomy (Fig. 4-8). Close the incisions in a routine manner, and apply the distraction apparatus.

▶ *Postoperative management.* The hand is elevated continuously for 48 hours. Distraction is done at a rate of 1 mm per day and should be painless. Distraction is terminated at any signs of vascular or neurologic impairment. Bone grafting is performed after maximum safe lengthening has been accomplished.

Fig. 4-8 Metacarpal lengthening with distraction. **A,** Distraction apparatus. *Left,* Older design; *right,* currently used design, consisting of two separate and independently acting parts. **B,** Aplasia of all digits and hypoplastic thumb. **C,** Thumb metacarpal is fully developed, but all other digits have only remnants of bases. **D** and **E,** Appearance and function after reconstruction. (From Kessler I, Baruch A, and Hecht O: J Hand Surg 2:394, 1977.)

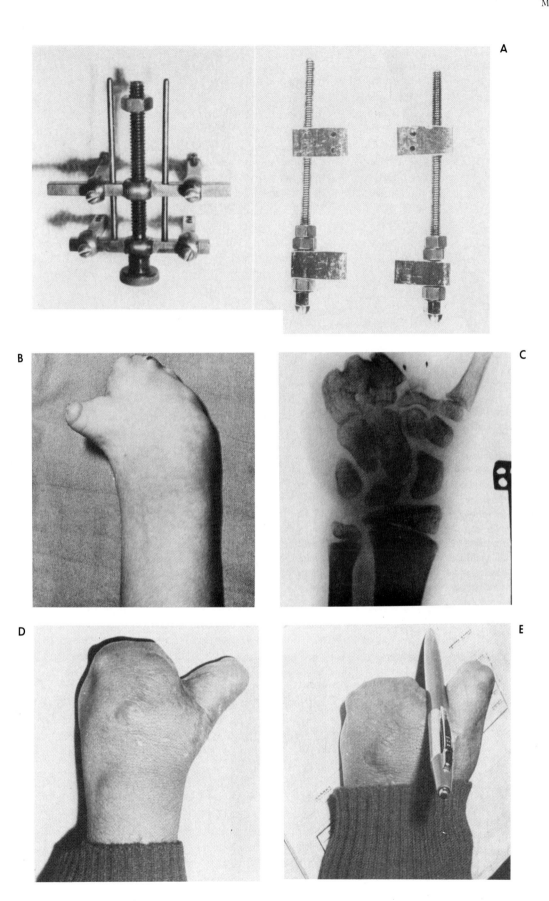

Longitudinal Deficiencies

Longitudinal deficiencies include all failure-of-formation anomalies that are not considered transverse deficiencies. In this category are phocomelia, radial ray dysplasia, ulnar ray dysplasia, and central dysplasia. To further identify these malformations, all absent or deficient bones are named. Any bone not named is assumed to be present. In the Iowa study these deformities comprised 9.3% of reported malformation, compared with the 7.1% incidence of transverse deficiencies.

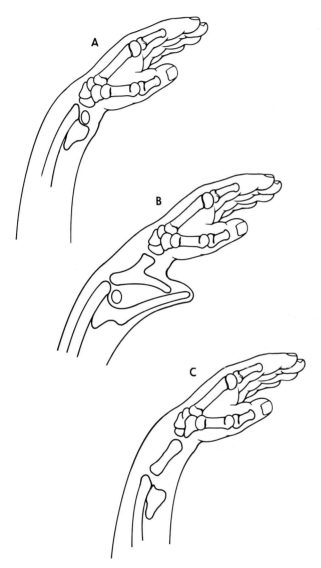

Fig. 4-9 Three types of phocomelia described by Frantz and O'Rahilly. **A,** Hand attached to shoulder with no intermediate humeral or forearm segment. **B,** Hand attached to shoulder with abnormal humeral, radial, and ulnar segment intervening. **C,** Hand attached to shoulder with intervening humeral segment without forearm segment. (Redrawn from Frantz CH and O'Rahilly R: J Bone Joint Surg 43A:1202, 1961.)

Phocomelia

Phocomelia is derived from the Greek words meaning *seal limb* or *flipper*. It represents the most profound expression of longitudinal reduction of a limb because an intercalated segment is absent. The term is used to describe a condition in which the hand is suspended from the body near the shoulder; the hand usually is deformed and contains only three or four digits. No definite inheritance pattern has been established; the anomaly was extremely rare until the appearance of thalidomide-related deformities in the 1950s. In 1977 Flatt reported an incidence of phocomelia of 0.8% in 2525 congenital hand malformations. In 1962 Taussig reported an incidence of 60% in infants born to mothers taking thalidomide between days 38 and 54 after conception.

Frantz and O'Rahilly described three anatomic types of phocomelia: (1) complete phocomelia with absence of all limb bones proximal to the hand, (2) absence or extreme hypoplasia of proximal limb bones with forearm and hand attached to the trunk, and (3) hand attached directly to the humerus (Fig. 4-9). Associated deformities include radial ray deficiencies in thalidomide-related phocomelia, cleft lip, and cleft palate (Robert's syndrome). Scoliosis and cardiac, skin, chromosomal, and calcification aberrations also have been reported.

Although children with phocomelia show slight differences in the overall length and appearance of the limb and different degrees of humeral, forearm, and hand deficiencies, the clavicle and scapula always are present. The scapula often is deficient laterally, and active abduction of the extremity is difficult, usually achieved by a sudden, jerking type of motion. The abducted position usually can be maintained only by the patient gripping his ear. There is no true elbow joint. The hand usually has only three or four digits, and the thumb usually is absent. Active and passive motion at the metacarpophalangeal and proximal interphalangeal joints varies considerably. Marked difficulty in moving the hand to the midline progresses as the patient grows and the chest widens. By maturity the patient usually is unable to reach the mouth, face, and genitalia and is unable to clasp the hands together, creating considerable functional and psychologic impairment.

Treatment. Treatment of these patients generally is conservative. Various ingenious devices have been developed to assist in hygiene, feeding, and dressing, and these play a major role in the child's achieving independence. Conventional prostheses designed to increase length usually are rejected. Surgery plays a minor role in treatment of phocomelia and generally is indicated only for shoulder instability, limb shortening, or inadequate thumb opposition. The clavicular turn-down operation described by Sulamaa and Ryoppy to gain length and shoulder stability has had disappointing results and has not been shown to improve the overall function of the limb. Rotational osteotomy of one of the digits with web space deepening may improve thumb opposition, but the specific technique for phocomelia has not been well-described or tested.

Radial Clubhand–Radial Deficiencies

Radial ray deficiencies include all malformations with longitudinal failure of formation of parts along the preaxial or radial border of the upper extremity: deficient or absent thenar muscles; a shortened, unstable, or absent thumb; and a shortened or absent radius, commonly referred to as *radial clubhand*. These conditions may occur as isolated deficiencies, but more commonly they occur to some degree in association with each other. Radial clubhand occurs in an estimated 1:100,000 live births. It comprised 4.7% of congenital anomalies in the Iowa series and 6.1% in the Yokohama series. Bilateral deformities occur in approximately 50% of patients; when unilateral, the right side is more commonly affected. Both sexes are equally affected. Complete radial absence is more common than partial absence.

In most cases of radial clubhand the cause is unknown and the deformities are believed to occur sporadically. Of 35 patients with radial clubhand Lamb (1977) found no blood relatives to at least the third degree with similar deficiencies; 12 of 35 had mothers who were known to have taken thalidomide. In a later study Wynne-Davies and Lamb found a higher proportion of a first-degree relative with minor congenital anomalies than would be expected from a random survey, which suggests a genetic contribution. They also found that twice as many of their patients were born during the summer quarter than during the winter quarter, and they presumed some environmental factor. Radial deficiencies in association with Fanconi's anemia and thrombocytopenia are inherited as an autosomal recessive trait; in association with Holt-Oram syndrome, in an autosomal dominant pattern.

The currently accepted and most useful classification of congenital radial dysplasias is a modification of that proposed by Heikel, in which four types are described (Fig. 4-10). In type I (short distal radius) the distal radial physis is present but is delayed in appearance, the proximal radial physis is normal, the radius is only slightly shortened, and the ulna is not bowed. In type II (hypoplastic radius), both distal and proximal radial physes are present but delayed in appearance, which results in moderate shortening of the radius and thickening and bowing of the ulna.

Type III deformity (partial absence of the radius) may be proximal, middle, or distal, with absence of the distal third most common; the carpus usually is radially deviated and unsupported and the ulna is thickened and bowed. The type IV pattern (total absence of the radius) is the most common, with radial deviation of the carpus, palmar and proximal subluxation, frequent pseudoarticulation with the radial border of the distal ulna, and a shortened and bowed ulna.

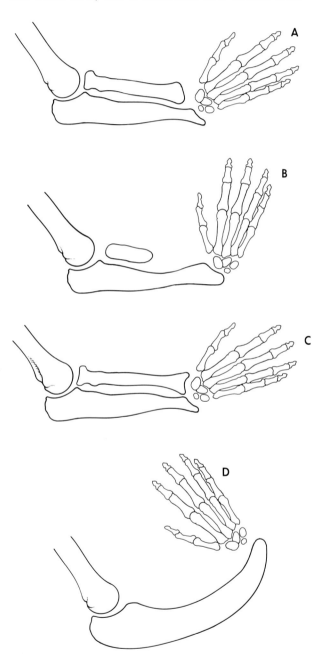

Fig. 4-10 Heikel classification of radial dysplasia. **A,** Type I—short distal radius. **B,** Type II—hypoplastic radius. **C,** Type III—partial absence of radius. **D,** Type IV—total absence of radius. (Redrawn from Heikel HV: Acta Orthop Scand Suppl 39:1, 1959.)

Variable degrees of thumb deficiencies are frequent with all patterns.

Associated cardiac, hemopoietic, gastrointestinal, and renal abnormalities occur in approximately 25% of patients with radial clubhand and may pose significant morbidity and mortality risks. The most frequently associated syndromes are Holt-Oram syndrome, Fanconi's anemia, thrombocytopenia–absent radius (TAR) syndrome, and the VATER syndrome, which consists of vertebral segmentation deficiencies, anal atresia, tracheoesophageal fistula, esophageal atresia, renal abnormalities, and radial ray deficiencies. In the Holt-Oram syndrome the cardiac abnormality, most commonly atrial septal defect, requires surgical correction before any upper limb reconstruction. Children with Fanconi anemia, a pancytopenia of early childhood, have a very poor prognosis, and death usually occurs 2 to 3 years after onset of the disease. In the TAR syndrome the thrombocytopenia usually resolves by the age of 4 to 5 years and, although it may delay reconstruction, is not a contraindication to surgical treatment. Approximately half these patients also have cardiac defects. Successful treatment of the associated abnormalities usually is possible, and upper extremity reconstruction may be appropriate in selected patients. Radial deficiency also is associated with trisomy 13 and trisomy 18; these children have multiple congenital defects and mental deficiency that may make reconstruction inappropriate despite significant deformity.

The anatomic pathology of congenital absence of the radius has been extensively reviewed by Kato, Heikel, and Flatt. The scapula, clavicle, and humerus often are reduced in size, and the ulna is characteristically short, thick, and curved, with an occasional synostosis with any radial remnant. Total absence of the radius is most frequent, but in partial deficiencies the proximal end of the radius is present most often. The scaphoid and trapezium are absent in more than half these patients; the lunate, trapezoid, and pisiform are deficient in 10%; and the thumb, including the metacarpal and its phalanges, is absent in more than 80%, although a rudimentary thumb is not uncommon. The capitate, hamate, triquetrum, and the ulnar four metacarpals and phalanges are the only bones of the upper extremity that are present and free from deficiencies in nearly all patients. The muscular anatomy, although highly variable, always is deficient. Muscles that frequently are normal are the triceps, extensor carpi ulnaris, extensor digiti quinti proprius, lumbricals, interossei (except for the first dorsal interossei), and hypothenar muscles. The long head of the biceps is almost always absent and the short head is hypoplastic. The brachialis often is deficient or absent as well. The brachioradialis is absent in nearly 50% of patients. Both the extensors carpi radialis longus and brevis frequently are absent or may be fused with the extensor digitorum communis. The pronator teres often is absent or rudimentary, inserting into the intermuscular septum. The palmaris longus often is defective. The flexor digitorum superficialis usually is present and is abnormal more frequently than is the flexor digitorum profundus. The pronator quadratus, extensor pollicis longus, abductor pollicis longus, and flexor pollicis longus muscles usually are absent. The peripheral nerves generally have an anomalous pattern with the median nerve the most clinically significant. The nerve is thicker than normal and runs along the preaxial border of the forearm just beneath the fascia. In 25% of patients it bifurcates distally with a dorsal branch running a course similar to the dorsal cutaneous branch of the superficial radial nerve, which frequently is absent. This nerve is at considerable risk during radial dissections because it is quite superficial and, as stated by Flatt, "represents a strong and unyielding bowstring of the radially bowed forearm and hand." The radial nerve frequently terminates at the level of the lateral epicondyle just after innervating the triceps. The ulnar nerve characteristically is normal according to most authors, and the musculocutaneous nerve usually is absent. The vascular anatomy usually is represented by a normal brachial artery, a normal ulnar artery, a well-developed common interosseous artery, and an absent radial artery.

The obvious deformity of a short forearm and radially deviated hand is almost invariably present at birth. A prominent knob at the wrist usually represents the distal end of the ulna. The forearm is between 50% and 75% of the length of the contralateral forearm, a ratio that usually remains the same throughout periods of growth. The thumb characteristically is absent or severely deficient; the contralateral thumb is deficient in unilateral as well as bilateral cases. Duplication of the thumb has been reported by Kummel. The hand often is relatively small. The metacarpophalangeal joints usually have limited flexion and some hyperextensibility. Flexion contractures often occur in the proximal interphalangeal joints. Stiffness of the elbow in extension, probably the result of weak elbow flexors, frequently is associated with radial clubhand. Most authors emphasize the elbow extension contracture as an extremely important consideration in evaluating these patients for reconstruction. Because of the radial deviation of the hand, the child usually can reach the mouth without the need of elbow flexion. If untreated, the deformity does not appear to worsen over time, but prehension is limited and the hand is used primarily to trap objects between it and the forearm. Lamb found that unilateral involvement did not significantly affect the activities of daily living, but bilateral involvement reduced activities by one third. Associated cardiac or hematologic problems may worsen the overall prognosis.

Nonsurgical management. Immediately after birth the radial clubhand often can be corrected passively, and early casting and splinting generally are recommended. A light, molded plastic, short-arm splint is applied along the radial side of the forearm and is removed only for bathing until the infant begins to use the hands; then it is worn only during sleep. Riordan recommends applying a long-arm corrective cast as soon after birth as possible. The cast is applied in three stages by means of a technique similar to that used for clubfoot casting. The hand and wrist are corrected first, then the elbow is corrected as much as possible. Although correction usually is achieved in the infant, Milford concluded that casting and splinting in a child younger than 3 months of age often is impractical. Lamb reported that elbow extension contracture can be improved by splinting with the hand and wrist in neutral position; 20 of his 27 patients improved to 90 degrees. He also cautioned that elbow flexion never improves after centralization procedures. As the child matures and ulnar growth continues, splinting is inadequate to maintain correction. There is no satisfactory conservative therapy for the significant thumb deformities associated with radial clubhand.

Surgical treatment. Although surgery may be postponed for 2 to 3 years with adequate splinting, there is general agreement favoring surgical correction at 3 to 6 months of age in children with inadequate radial support of the carpus. Pollicization, when indicated, follows at 9 to 12 months of age if possible. Specific contraindications to surgical treatment include severe associated anomalies not compatible with long life, inadequate elbow flexion, mild deformity with adequate radial support (type I and some type II deformities), and older patients who have accepted the deformities and have adjusted accordingly. Reconstruction of these limbs requires familiarity with the concepts and surgical details of three types of procedures: centralization of the carpus on the forearm, thumb reconstruction, and occasionally transfer of the triceps to restore elbow flexion.

Centralization of hand

Centralization of the hand over the distal ulna was first reported in 1893 by Sayre, who suggested sharpening the distal end of the ulna to fit into a surgically created carpal notch. Lidge modified this method by leaving the ulnar physis intact, providing the forerunner of modern centralization techniques. Other procedures have been performed in an attempt to stabilize the hand on the forearm. Hoffa in 1890 performed a distal transverse osteotomy of the ulna to simply realign the ulna. Bardenheuer (1894) suggested splitting the distal ulna longitudinally to allow the carpus to become wedged between the two halves. Albee (1919) attempted to create a radius with a free tibial graft. Starr (1949) and Riordan (1955) used a nonvascularized fibular graft to support the carpus, but fibular growth did not continue and the deformity recurred. Delorme (1969) suggested intramedullary fixation of the carpus on the ulna. Incisions and surgical approaches also have varied. Manske and McCarroll prefer transverse ulnar incisions, removing an ellipse of skin. Watson et al prefer ulnar and radial Z-plasty incisions to allow removal of the distal radial anlage, which they believe essential. The creation of a carpal notch to stabilize the carpus on the ulna also is controversial. Lamb believes this essential and recommends that the depth of the notch equal the transverse diameter of the distal ulna, which usually requires removal of all the lunate and most of the capitate. Watson et al do not excise any of the carpus because of the possibility of affecting growth of the forearm. In 12 patients with centralization procedures, about 30 degrees of radial deviation had recurred at an average follow-up of 10 years, a result comparable to procedures that create a carpal notch. Buck-Gramcko (1985) also does not remove any of the carpus. When the carpal notch is not created, the distal ulna is reported to broaden and take on the roentgenographic appearance of a normal distal radius. Bora et al recommend adjunctive tendon transfers in which the flexor digitorum superficialis from the central digits is transferred around the postaxial side of the forearm into the dorsal aspect of the metacarpal shafts, the hypothenar muscles are transferred proximally along the ulnar shaft, and the extensor carpi ulnaris is transferred distally along the shaft of the metacarpal of the little finger; however, in their report this failed to prevent the 25 to 35 degrees of recurrent radial deviation. Most authors agree that it is beneficial to use a Kirschner wire to secure alignment of the long or index metacarpal with the ulna for at least 6 weeks. Ulnar osteotomy is required if the ulna is so bowed that the Kirschner wire cannot be passed along its medullary canal.

Centralization has been shown to improve function, particularly in bilateral involvement. Bora et al reported total active digital motion of 54% of normal after surgery, compared with 27% in untreated patients. Forearm length was functionally doubled, and the metacarpal-ulnar angle averaged 35 degrees after surgery, compared with 100 degrees in untreated patients. Tsuyuguchi et al, however, reported that only 6 of their 12 patients were satisfied with the results despite obvious functional gains.

Complications reported in association with centralization include growth arrest of the distal ulna, ankylosis of the wrist, recurrent instability of the wrist, damage to neural structures (particularly the anomalous median nerve), vascular insufficiency of the hand, wound infection, necrosis of wound margins, fracture of the ulna, and pin migration and breakage. Major neurovascular complications are rare.

▶ *Technique (Manske et al)*. Begin the incision just radial to the midline on the dorsum of the wrist at the level of the distal ulna, and proceed ulnarward in a transverse direction to a point radial to the pisiform at the volar wrist crease. Pass the incision through the bulbous soft tissue mass on the ulnar side of the wrist, incising considerable fat and subcutaneous tissue (Fig. 4-11, *A*).

Identify and preserve the dorsal sensory branch of the ulnar nerve, which is deep in the subcutaneous tissue and lies near the extensor retinaculum. Expose the extensor retinaculum and the base of the hypothenar muscles. It is not necessary to identify the ulnar artery or nerve on the volar aspect of the wrist (Fig. 4-11, *B*).

Identify and dissect free the extensor carpi ulnaris tendon at its insertion on the base of the fifth metacarpal, and detach and retract it proximally. Next identify and retract radially the extensor digitorum communis tendons. This exposes the dorsal and ulnar aspects of the wrist capsule. Incise the capsule transversely, thus exposing the distal ulna (Fig. 4-11, *C*).

The carpal bones are a cartilaginous mass deep in the wound on the radial side of the ulna. The carpoulnar junction is most easily identified by dissecting from proximal to distal along the radial side of the distal ulna. Take care not to mistake one of the intercarpal articulations for the carpoulnar junction.

Now define the cartilaginous mass of carpal bones, and excise a square segment of its midportion (measuring approximately 1 × 1 cm) to accommodate the distal ulna. Dissect free the distal ulnar epiphysis from the adjacent soft tissue, and square it off by shaving perpendicular to the shaft (Fig. 4-11, *D*). Take care not to injure the physis or the attached soft tissue.

Place the distal ulna in the carpal defect, and stabilize it with a smooth Kirschner wire (Fig. 4-11, *E*). In practice, this usually is accomplished by passing the Kirschner wire proximally down the shaft of the distal ulna to emerge at the olecranon (or at the midshaft if the ulna is bowed.) Then pass the wire distally across the carpal notch into the third metacarpal. Cut off the proximal end of the wire beneath the skin.

Stabilize the ulnar side of the wrist by imbricating the capsule or by suturing the distal capsule to the periosteum of the shaft of the distal ulna. (If there is insufficient distal capsule, suture the cartilaginous carpal bones to the periosteum.) Obtain additional stabilization by advancing the extensor carpi ulnaris tendon distally and reattaching it to the base of the fourth or fifth metacarpal (Fig. 4-11, *F*). Also advance the origin of the hypothenar musculature proximally, and suture it to the ulnar shaft to provide additional stability to the wrist. Excise the bulbous excess of the skin and soft tissue, and suture the skin. This results in a pleasing cosmetic closure and helps stabilize the hand in the ulnar position.

▶ *Postoperative management.* The wrist is immobilized in a plaster cast for 6 weeks and then is placed in a removable orthoplast splint. The Kirschner wire is removed at 6 to 12 weeks. Children are encouraged to wear the splint until skeletal maturity.

Fig. 4-11 Centralization arthroplasty technique, transverse ulnar approach (see text). **A,** Incision. **B,** Exposure of muscle, tendon, and nerve. **C,** Capsular incision. **D,** Exposure of carpoulnar junction and excision of segment of carpal bones. **E,** Insertion of Kirschner wire. **F,** Reattachment of extensor carpi ulnaris tendon. (Redrawn from Manske PR et al: J Hand Surg 6:423, 1981.)

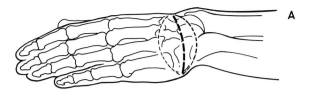

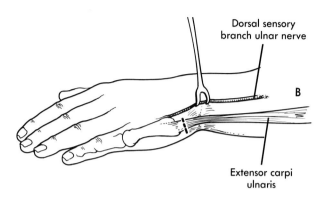

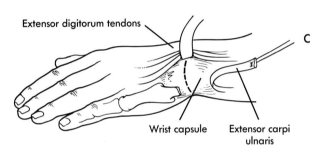

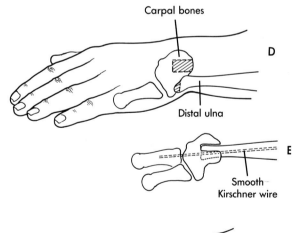

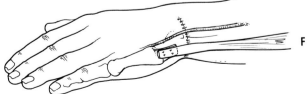

▶ *Technique (Watson et al).* Under pneumatic tourniquet control, make two skin incisions (Fig. 4-12, *A*). On the radial aspect perform a standard 60-degree Z-plasty with a longitudinal central limb to obtain lengthening along the longitudinal axis of the forearm. On the ulnar aspect perform a similar Z-plasty but with a transverse central limb to take up skin redundancy in this area, transposing the excess tissue to the deficient radial wrist area (Fig. 4-12, *B*). Once the skin incisions are completed, carry the dissection along the radial side, identifying the median nerve (Fig. 4-12, *C*). The median nerve is more radially located than usual and may be the most superficial structure encountered after the radial skin incision is made. Identification and preservation of the "radial-median" nerve are vital to the resulting functional capacity of the hand. Continue the dissection ulnarward, resecting the fibrotic distal radial anlage, which may act as a restricting band, to maintain the hand in radial deviation (Fig. 4-12, *D*). Next identify and protect the ulnar nerve and artery through the ulnar incision to allow complete dissection around the distal ulna without damage to critical structures (Fig. 4-12, *E*). Perform a complete capsular release of the ulnocarpal joint, taking care to avoid injury to the ulnar physis. At this point the hand should be fully movable, attached to the forearm only by the skin, the dorsal and palmar tendons, and the preserved neurovascular structures.

Take care to remove all the fibrotic material in the "center" of the wrist and forearm area. The ulna and ulnar incision should be clearly visible through the radial incision, and the reverse also should be true. It should not be necessary to remove any carpal bones or to remodel the distal ulna to maintain the hand in a centralized position. Pass a 0.045 inch Kirschner wire through the lunate, capitate, and long finger metacarpal, exiting through the metacarpophalangeal joint (Fig. 4-12, *F*). Centralize the hand in the desired position, and pass the Kirschner wire in a retrograde fashion into the ulna to maintain the position of the hand (Fig. 4-12, *G*). Deflate the tourniquet, and obtain hemostasis before skin closure or deflate the tourniquet immediately after the application of the dressing and splint. Apply a bulky hand dressing with a dorsal plaster splint extending above the elbow. Before discontinuing anesthesia, ensure that circulation in the hand is satisfactory.

▶ *Postoperative management.* The hand is elevated for 24 to 48 hours. The dressing is changed and sutures are removed 2 weeks after surgery. A long-arm cast is applied and worn for an additional 4 weeks. The Kirschner wire is removed at 6 weeks, and a short-arm cast is applied to be worn an additional 3 weeks. Night splinting is continued until physeal closure to avoid recurrence of radial deviation.

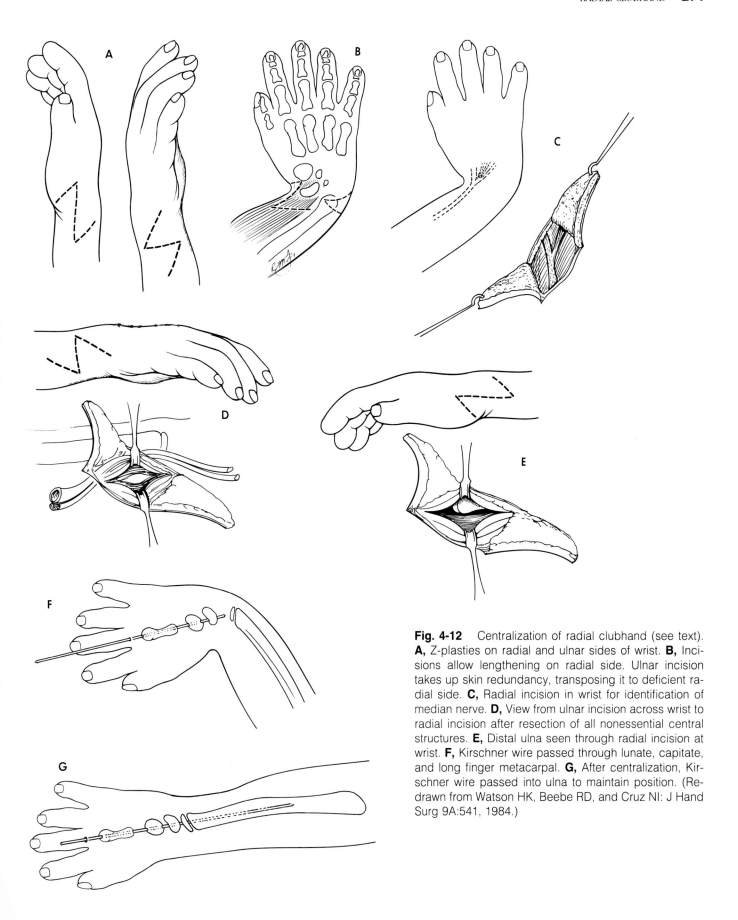

Fig. 4-12 Centralization of radial clubhand (see text). **A,** Z-plasties on radial and ulnar sides of wrist. **B,** Incisions allow lengthening on radial side. Ulnar incision takes up skin redundancy, transposing it to deficient radial side. **C,** Radial incision in wrist for identification of median nerve. **D,** View from ulnar incision across wrist to radial incision after resection of all nonessential central structures. **E,** Distal ulna seen through radial incision at wrist. **F,** Kirschner wire passed through lunate, capitate, and long finger metacarpal. **G,** After centralization, Kirschner wire passed into ulna to maintain position. (Redrawn from Watson HK, Beebe RD, and Cruz NI: J Hand Surg 9A:541, 1984.)

Centralization of hand and tendon transfers

▲ *Technique (Bora et al)* (Fig. 4-13, *A* and *B*). Bora et al suggest that treatment be started immediately after birth with corrective casts to stretch the radial side of the wrist. At the age of 6 to 12 months the hand is centralized surgically over the distal end of the ulna and tendon transfers are carried out 6 to 12 months later.

Stage I: Make a radial S-shaped incision, and excise the radiocarpal ligament. Isolate and excise the lunate and capitate. Then make a longitudinal incision over the distal ulnar epiphysis, free it from the surrounding tissue, and preserve the tendons of the extensor carpi ulnaris and extensor digitorum quinti minimus. Transpose the distal end of the ulna through the plane between the flexor and extensor tendons and into a slot formed by the removal of the lunate and capitate. With the distal end of the ulna at the base of the long finger metacarpal transfix it with a smooth Kirschner wire. Check the position of the ulna and carpus by roentgenograms in the operating room to ensure that the ulna is aligned with the long axis of the long finger metacarpal. Now suture the dorsal radiocarpal ligament over the neck of the ulna, close the skin, and apply a long-arm cast with the elbow at 90 degrees. When the deformity is unilateral, the wrist and hand should be placed in neutral, and when it is bilateral, they should be placed in 45 degrees of pronation on one side and 45 degrees of supination on the other. The cast is removed at 6 weeks, and a splint is applied for night wear.

Stage II (Fig. 4-13, *B*): Three tendon transfers are performed 6 to 12 months after the centralization procedure. Before attempting to transfer the flexor digitorum sublimis tendons, test for function because in some instances the sublimis tendon is nonfunctioning in one or more of the three ulnar digits. Passively maintain the metacarpophalangeal joints and the wrist joint in hyperextension and the interphalangeal joints in extension, and release one finger at a time. An intact sublimis tendon will flex the proximal interphalangeal joint of the released finger.

Make a midlateral incision on the ulnar side of the long finger at the level of the proximal interphalangeal joint. Divide the sublimis tendon at the level of the middle phalanx, and divide also the chiasm of the decussating fibers. Perform a similar procedure on the ring finger. Next make a short transverse incision on the volar aspect of the forearm and pull the two tendons into it. At the site of previous dorsal incision reenter the wrist and transfer the sublimis tendons subcutaneously around the ulnar side of the ulna to the dorsum of the hand. Loop the tendon from the long finger around the shaft of the index finger metacarpal and the tendon from the ring finger around the shaft of the long finger metacarpal (Fig. 4-13). Transpose the tendons extraperiostally, and suture them back to themselves with the wrist in 15 degrees of dorsiflexion and maximum ulnar deviation. Now transfer the extensor carpi ulnaris tendon distally along the shaft of the little finger metacarpal and transfer the origin of the hypothenar muscles proximally along the ulnar shaft. Thus an effort is made to maintain balance and prevent recurrence of the deformity.

▲ *Postoperative management.* A cast is applied after the procedure and is worn for 1 month; after this a night splint is worn for at least 3 months. Careful follow-up should be made to observe for possible recurrence of deformity. A night splint may be used for several years.

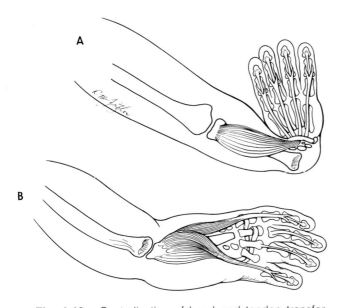

Fig. 4-13 Centralization of hand and tendon transfer (see text). **A,** Volar aspect of radial clubhand deformity showing right-angle relationship of hand and forearm and acute angulation of extrinsic flexor tendons. **B,** Volar aspect after centralization and transfer of superficialis tendons of ring and long fingers. (Redrawn from Bora FW Jr: J Bone Joint Surg 52A:966, 1970.)

Pollicization for reconstruction of the thumb with radial clubhand

Although the thumb frequently is absent or severely deficient in radial dysplasia, children usually are able to adapt to the thumbless hand with ulnar-side-of-index to radial-side-of-middle finger prehension and finger-to-palm prehension after centralization. Despite this adaptability, overall function and self-care activities are impaired and can be improved with successful pollicization. Because normal, as well as compensatory, prehensile patterns are firmly established within the first year of life, it is desirable that surgical reconstruction be performed early. Pollicization is recommended for both unilateral and bilateral cases. If a "floating" thumb deformity is present, with inadequate musculotendinous and bony elements, the remnant should be amputated before pollicization to allow reconstruction of a stable thumb. The parents must be clearly informed that the floating thumb is of no functional use and will be discarded after the operation.

Gossett was the first to report replacement of the thumb with the index finger, and the index finger continues to be the preferred donor digit if it is not too deficient. Despite reports of successful single-stage toe-to-hand transfers, in the congenitally deficient thumb the index is preferred because the appearance is more acceptable and there is less donor site morbidity (Fig. 14-14). Buck-Gramcko (1971) reported that results were better when pollicization was performed in the first year of life; his youngest patient was 11 weeks old. Side-to-side grip between index and middle fingers, particularly for smaller objects, persisted in children whose reconstruction was performed later in life. He emphasized the importance of removing the entire index metacarpal except for the head, which acts as the new trapezium. The index finger must be rotated 160 degrees and placed in 40 degrees of palmar abduction for optimal function and appearance. Hyperextension instability at the index metacarpophalangeal joint is prevented by positioning the metacarpal head in 70 to 80 degrees of hyperextension before fixation. The reattached intrinsic muscles are important in the function of the thumb and in the formation of a new thenar eminence for cosmesis as well. Milford stressed the importance of suturing the intrinsic tendons into the lateral bands to enhance extension.

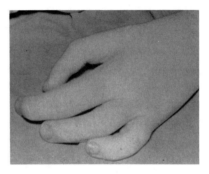

Fig. 4-14   Appearance of hand after pollicization.

▲ *Technique (Buck-Gramcko).* Make an S-shaped incision down the radial side of the hand just onto the palmar surface. Begin the incision near the base of the index finger on the palmar aspect, and end it just proximal to the wrist. Make a slightly curved transverse incision across the base of the index finger on the palmar surface, connecting at right angles to the distal end of the first incision (Fig. 4-15, *A*). Make a third incision on the dorsum of the proximal phalanx of the index finger from the proximal interphalangeal joint extending proximally to end at the incision around the base of the index finger (Fig. 4-15, *B*). Through the palmar incision, free the neurovascular bundle between the index and middle fingers by ligating the artery to the radial side of the middle finger. Then separate the common digital nerve carefully into its component parts for the two adjacent fingers so that no tension will be present after the index finger is rotated. Sometimes an anomalous neural ring is found around the artery; split this ring carefully so that angulation of the artery after transposition of the finger will not occur. When the radial digital artery to the index finger is absent, it is possible to perform the pollicization on a vascular pedicle of only one artery. On the dorsal side, preserve at least one of the great veins.

Now, on the dorsum of the hand, sever the tendon of the extensor digitorum communis at the metacarpophalangeal level. Detach the interosseus muscles of the index finger from the proximal phalanx and the lateral bands of the dorsal aponeurosis. Partially strip subperiosteally the origins of the interosseus muscles from the second metacarpal, being careful to preserve the neurovascular structures.

Now, perform an osteotomy and resect the second metacarpal as follows. If the phalanges of the index finger are of normal length, resect the whole metacarpal with the exception of the base of the metacarpal, which must be retained to obtain the proper length of the new thumb. When the entire metacarpal is resected except for the head, rotate the head as shown in Fig. 4-15, *E,* and attach it by sutures to the joint capsule of the carpus and to the carpal bones, which in young children can be pierced with a sharp needle. Rotate the digit 160 degrees to allow apposition (Fig. 4-15, *F*). Bony union is not essential, and fibrous fixation of the head is sufficient for good function. When the base of the metacarpal is retained, fix the metacarpal head to its base with one or two Kirschner wires, again in the previously described position. In attaching the metacarpal head, bring the proximal phalanx into complete hyperextension in relation to the metacarpal head for maximum stability of the joint. Unless this is done, hyperextension is likely at the new "carpometacarpal" joint (Fig. 4-15, *G*). Suture the proximal end of the detached extensor digitorum communis tendon to the base of the former proximal phalanx (now acting as the first metacarpal) to become the new "abductor pollicis longus." Section the extensor indicis proprius tendon, shorten it appropriately, and then suture it by end-to-end anastomosis.

Suture the tendinous insertions of the two interosseus muscles to the lateral bands of the dorsal aponeurosis by weaving the lateral bands through the distal part of the interosseus muscle and turning them back distally to form a loop that is sutured to itself. In this way, the first palmar interosseus will become an "adductor pollicis" and the first dorsal interosseus an "abductor brevis" (Fig. 4-15, *H*).

Close the wound by fashioning a dorsal skin flap to close the defect over the proximal phalanx, and fashion the rest of the flaps as necessary for skin closure as in Fig. 4-15, *C* and *D*.

▲ *Postoperative management.* The hand is immobilized for 3 weeks, and then careful active motion is begun.

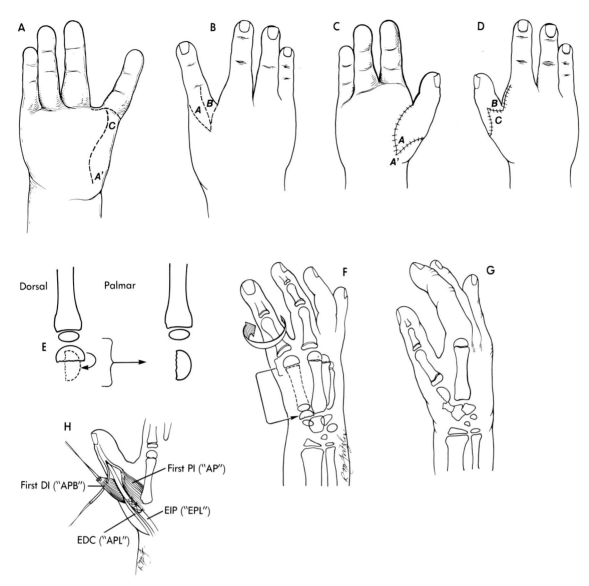

Fig. 4-15 Pollicization of index finger. **A** and **B,** Palmar and dorsal skin incisions. **C** and **D,** Appearance after wound closure. **E,** Rotation of metacarpal head into flexion to prevent postoperative hyperextension. **F,** Index finger rotated about 160 degrees along long axis to place finger pulp into position of opposition. **G,** Final position of skeleton in about 40 degrees of palmar abduction with metacarpal head secured to metacarpal base or carpus. **H,** Reattachment of tendons to provide control of new thumb. First palmar interosseous *(PI)* functions as adductor pollicis *(AP);* first dorsal interosseous *(DI),* as the abductor pollicis brevis *(APB);* extensor digitorum communis *(EDC),* as abductor pollicis longus *(APL);* and extensor indicis proprius *(EIP),* as extensor pollicis longus *(EPL).* (Redrawn from Buck-Gramcko D: J Bone Joint Surg 53A:1605, 1971.)

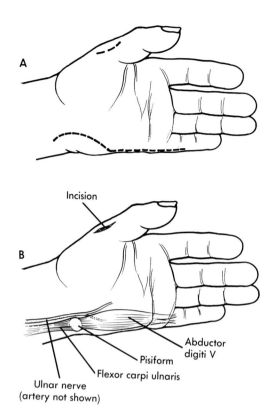

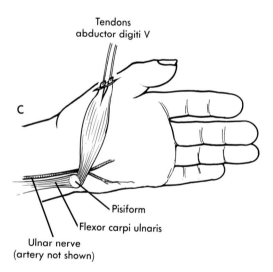

Fig. 4-16 Abductor digiti minimi opponensplasty (see text). **A,** Incision. **B,** Detachment of tendinous insertions. **C,** Abductor digiti minimi passed through subcutaneous tunnel. (Redrawn from Manske PR and McCarroll HR Jr: J Hand Surg 3:552, 1978.)

Opponensplasty

Abductor digiti minimi opponensplasty, as described by Huber, may be appropriate for the rare patient with only isolated thenar asplasia in association with the radial clubhand or for patients with weakness in apposition after pollicization. Manske and McCarroll reported improvement in appearance, dexterity, strength, and usefulness of the thumb in 20 of 21 patients with an average age at operation of 4 years, 9 months.

▶ *Technique (Manske and McCarroll).* Make an incision beginning over the ulnar border of the proximal phalanx of the little finger and palm, curving radialward proximal to the metacarpophalangeal joint, and crossing the wrist crease on the radial side of the pisiform (Fig. 4-16, *A*). Detach the tendinous insertions into the extensor hood and the proximal phalanx of the little finger, retaining as much tendon length as possible (Fig. 4-16, *B*). Starting distally, dissect the abductor digiti minimi muscle out of its fascial sheath to its origin at the pisiform, taking care to avoid dissection on the proximal and radial sides of the muscle where the neurovascular structures enter. Make a second incision over the dorsoradial aspect of the metacarpophalangeal joint of the thumb, and pass the muscle through a large subcutaneous tunnel between the thumb incision and the proximal ulnar incision (Fig. 4-16, *C*). Be certain that the muscle glides freely in the tunnel and is not restricted by soft tissue.

The method of insertion of the transferred tendon at the metacarpophalangeal joint (Fig. 4-17, *A*) depends on the patient's deformity. In patients with thenar aplasia with other radial anomalies, suture one of the transferred slips to the soft tissue at the radial aspect of the base of the proximal phalanx and the other to the extensor pollicis longus muscle at the level of the metacarpophalangeal joint, as recommended by Riordan, Powers, and Hurd (1975) (Fig. 4-17, *B*). In patients with isolated thenar aplasia, stabilize the metacarpophalangeal joint by imbricating the ulnar capsule in a pants-over-vest fashion (Fig. 4-17, *C*). Then suture one of the tendinous insertions to the radial capsule and the other to the imbricated ulnar capsule and to the extensor pollicis longus tendon. If the opponensplasty is performed after pollicization, suture one slip to the radial lateral band and the other to the central slip at the proximal interphalangeal joint of the pollicized finger (Fig. 4-17, *D*). Close the incisions in routine fashion, and apply a bulky dressing and splint, holding the thumb in opposition.

▶ *Postoperative management.* Three weeks after surgery the bulky dressing is removed and the thumb is taped into opposition for an additional 3 weeks; the child is encouraged to use the hand. Six weeks after surgery, all dressings are discontinued. Formal retraining of the transfer usually is not necessary.

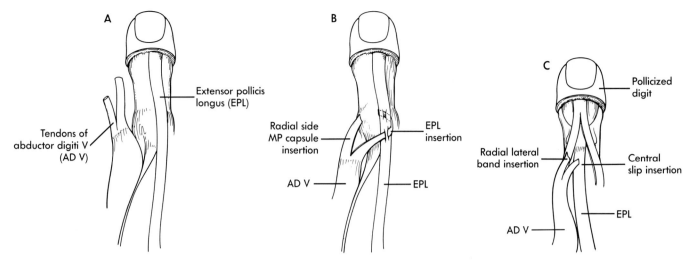

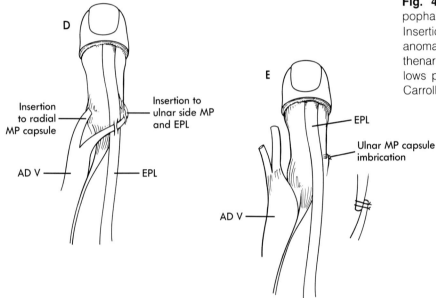

Fig. 4-17 **A,** Tendon insertion at thumb metacarpophalangeal joint depends on patient's deformity. **B,** Insertion in patients with thenar aplasia and other radial anomalies. **C** and **D,** Insertion in patients with isolated thenar aplasia. **E,** Insertion when opponensplasty follows pollicization. (Redrawn from Manske PR and Mc-Carroll HR Jr: J Hand Surg 3:552, 1978.)

Triceps transfer to restore elbow flexion

An elbow stiff in extension is a contraindication for centralization; rarely, however, a child may have passive elbow flexion but minimal or no active flexion because of complete absence of elbow flexors. Menelaus reported that triceps transfer restored elbow flexion in two patients when performed 2 to 3 months after centralization; both improved from a preoperative passive range of motion of 0 to 45 degrees to a postoperative active range of motion of 0 to 90 degrees.

▲ *Technique (Menelaus).* Make a lateral incision to expose the lower end of the triceps muscle and the anterior, lateral, and posterior aspects of the proximal end of the ulna. Identify the triceps insertion, and dissect a tongue of periosteum from the proximal end of the ulna in continuity with the triceps tendon. Dissect the triceps proximally to the midarm level. Identify and mobilize the ulnar nerve; then perform a posterior capsulotomy of the elbow. Roll the periosteal tongue and the triceps tendon, and pass this through a tunnel created in the coronoid process of the ulna. Secure the transfer with a nonabsorbable suture. Close the wound, and apply a splint or cast with the elbow in 120 degrees of flexion.

▲ *Postoperative management.* The transfer is protected in a long-arm cast for 4 to 6 weeks. The sutures are removed at 2 weeks. After cast removal, gentle active exercises are begun, supporting the limb in a 90-degree, long-arm, posterior splint that is worn between exercise periods and during sleep.

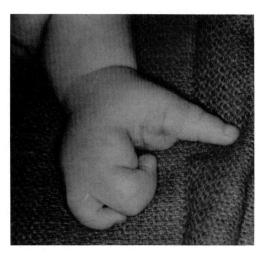

Fig. 4-18 Typical pattern of central deficiency with central V-shaped cleft.

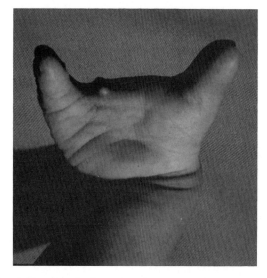

Fig. 4-19 Atypical pattern of central deficiency with U-shaped deficiency involving index, middle, and ring fingers.

Cleft Hand–Central Deficiencies

Central deficiencies of the hand include those malformations in which there is a longitudinal failure of formation of the second, third, or fourth ray. Also included in this category are those deformities in which there is severe suppression of the radial four rays, leaving a one-digit (fifth ray) hand. Further suppression that results in the digitless hand is considered a transverse deficiency. Common names for this deformity include ectrodactyly, crab claw, lobster claw, and cleft hand. It is exceedingly rare, with an incidence of approximately 1:90,000 live births. This group of malformations constituted 3.9% of the Iowa series. The first description of central deficiencies was published in 1770 by Hartsinck, who reported certain blacks called *Touwingas* or "two-fingered Negroes" in Dutch Guiana who had similar bilateral hand and foot deformities.

Central deficiencies are commonly classified into two main patterns of deformity: typical and atypical. The typical pattern is a central V-shaped cleft with variable degrees of deficiency of the middle ray (Fig. 4-18). Syndactyly between the ulnar and radial two digits is common. The deformity typically is bilateral with similar bilateral foot deformities. The atypical pattern, initially described by Lange, is a severe U-shaped deficiency that involves the index, middle, and ring ray, leaving only a thumb and little finger attached to the hand (Fig. 4-19). This deformity usually is unilateral without associated foot deformities. Flatt suggested that the typical and atypical forms are distinctly different not only in appearance but also in cause and that the term *cleft hand* should refer only to typical patterns and the term *lobster claw* should refer to the fully developed atypical pattern. Flatt's classification of these malformations includes four groups: group 0, all bones present; group 1, one ray involved; group 2, two rays involved; and group 3, three rays involved. These groups are further divided into three subgroups based on the degree of finger involvement (Fig. 4-20). This classification is more complicated but helps eliminate some confusion.

EXAMPLES OF CLASSIFICATION GROUPS

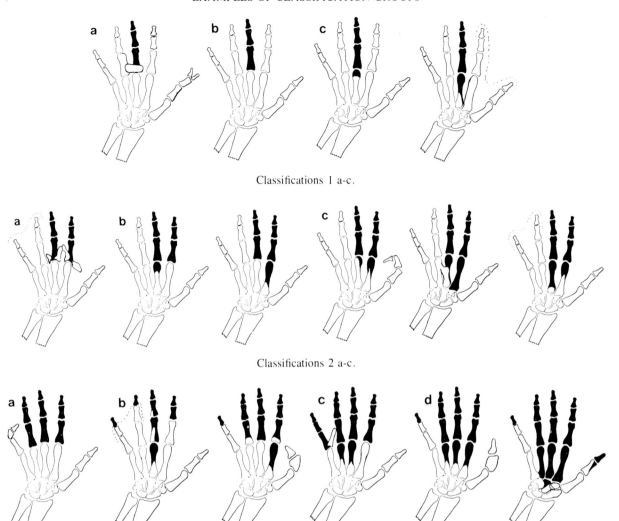

Classifications 1 a-c.

Classifications 2 a-c.

Classifications 3 a-d.

Fig. 4-20 Flatt classification of central deficiencies. Group 0—all bones present; group 1—one ray involved; group 2—two rays involved; and group 3—three rays involved. (From Nutt JN and Flatt AE: J Hand Surg 6:48, 1981.)

The cause of central deficiencies is unknown, and most of cases occur sporadically. An autosomal dominant mode of inheritance frequently is seen in the typical pattern, but penetrance often is incomplete. Maisels suggested a centripetal suppression theory according to which milder deformities have only a simple cleft without significant tissue loss, but as the severity of suppression increases, absence of the central ray is seen first, followed by loss of the radial rays and eventually loss of all rays (Fig. 4-21). Müller emphasized the etiologic differences between cleft hand and symbrachydactyly, noting that cleft hand seems to result from primary insufficiency of the central ectodermal ridge, whereas symbrachydactyly may result from primary failure of formation of the underlying bone. This would explain the absence of terminal digital remnants in pure central longitudinal deficiencies. The association of cleft hand and central polydactyly also has been established, emphasizing the complexity of these deformities.

Anomalies that occur most often in association with central hand deficiencies include cleft foot, cleft lip, and cleft palate; congenital heart disease, imperforate anus, anonychia, cataracts, and deafness also have been reported. Barsky reported that five of nine patients had cleft foot and three of nine had cleft lip and palate. In Flatt's series major musculoskeletal anomalies in addition to hand deformities included hypoplasia or pseudarthrosis of the clavicle, absent pectoralis major muscle, short humerus, synostosis of the elbow, short forearm, absent ulna, radioulnar synostosis, bilateral absence of the tibia, bilateral dislocation of the hip, short femur, hypoplastic patella, clubfoot, calcaneovalgus foot, cavovarus foot, deviated nasal septum, and congenital ptosis. Five patients had associated genitourinary system anomalies.

The typical cleft hand pattern of a central V-shaped defect in the palm is present at birth. The middle finger usually is entirely missing, and frequently the two remaining digits on each side of the cleft have vary-

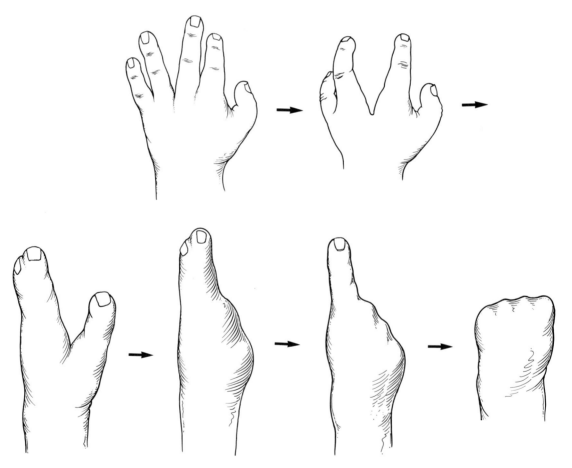

Fig. 4-21   Maisels' suppression theory. Milder deformities have only simple cleft without significant tissue loss, but as severity of suppression increases, absence of central first ray is followed by loss of radial rays and eventually loss of all rays. (Redrawn from Maisels DO: Br J Plast Surg 23:269, 1970.)

ing degrees of webbing, often causing a thumb adduction contracture. Similar foot deformities are frequent. Occasionally, the index finger may be missing as well, but rarely are the ring and middle fingers absent. In the atypical pattern, only two fingers are present, one along the radial border and one along the ulnar border. A shallow U-shaped defect intervenes along the distal palm. The most lateral (radial) ray often lies in the same plane as the most medial (ulnar) ray. The deformity usually is unilateral, without associated foot deformity. In the most severe forms all digits except for the small finger may be absent.

Roentgenographic findings are highly variable. Transversely oriented bones and occasionally a delta phalanx may be seen. There may appear to be two metacarpals supporting one digit or a split metacarpal supporting two digits. Carpal coalition is present in older children.

Children with these deformities develop amazing dexterity but frequently hide their hand in a pocket to avoid drawing attention to its clawlike appearance. This is particularly true in grade school and in new surroundings but seems to diminish as the patient matures. Even patients with the atypical pattern may develop adequate pinch and grasp.

Treatment. There is no appropriate nonsurgical treatment for these deformities, and the use of prostheses, as recommended in the early writing of Fort, has been essentially abandoned except on rare occasions when requested for cosmesis. The surgical management must be individualized according to the deformity and available anatomy. General principles of hand surgery are applicable, in that good pinch and grasp are the primary goals, followed by acceptable cosmesis if possible. Surgical reconstruction includes closure of the cleft, release of syndactyly, correction of thumb adduction contracture, removal of transverse or other deforming bony elements, and correction of delta phalanx. In the atypical pattern, deepening of the palm for grasp, osteotomies of the ulnar or radial metacarpals to allow better opposition, tendon transfers in the hypoplastic hand to restore digital motion, and possibly single-stage toe-to-hand transfer for the one-digit hand occasionally are needed.

In planning the sequence and timing of surgery, the recommendations of Flatt should be carefully reviewed. Syndactyly should be released in the normal time sequence: the border digits by 6 months of age and the central digits by 18 months of age. After a recovery period of 6 months, closure of the cleft alone

or closure of the cleft with correction of thumb adduction contracture may be performed. Often it is difficult to determine the extent of thumb mobility required by the patient. A minor adduction contracture usually does not require correction. To close the cleft, bony elements that block closure should be removed sparingly because central metacarpal loss may weaken the palm and lead to cleft recurrence. If cleft closure is performed simultaneously with first web space deepening, the index metacarpal may be transferred to the long metacarpal position by means of the Snow and Littler or Miura and Komada technique. The technique described by Miura and Komada is less demanding technically and produces comparable results with less risk of complications. Ueba also described a technique helpful for palmar cleft with absence of the long finger, especially when the cleft hand is combined with a narrow thumb web. All functioning digits with any proximal phalanx should be spared because these usually significantly improve grasp. A delta phalanx should be corrected at about 3 years of age, especially if it is causing radial deviation of the thumb or ulnar deviation of the little finger.

In the atypical pattern the thumb or little finger, or both, usually are hypoplastic to some extent, making pinch impossible; deepening of the palm and possibly metacarpal osteotomies performed between the ages of 2 and 3 years should improve grasp. In hands of nearly normal size, tendon transfers usually are unnecessary; however, in severely hypoplastic hands (less than 50% of normal), tendon transfers may be needed to supplement the available motors. These transfers should be delayed until the age of 3 years.

If only one digit exists, a single-stage toe-to-hand transfer may be performed around the age of 18 months. The strongest indications for this procedure in a child are complete adactyly, complete absence of a thumb, or a nonfunctional thumb with two or fewer fingers on the same hand. Although Gilbert has reported success with this technique, there are a number of problems associated with the procedure. Incorporation of the transferred digit into a functional pattern may be difficult for a child who has never had a thumb, tendon transfers may be required because of deficient donor tendons, anomalous vascular patterns may be present, identification of a recipient branch of the median nerve may be difficult, and a branch of the superficial radial nerve or an adjacent digital nerve may be required to reinnervate the transferred toe.

Cleft closure

▶ *Technique (Barsky).* Under tourniquet control, sharply elevate a distally based diamond-shaped flap from one side of the opposing sides of the involved fingers (Fig. 4-22, *A*). Place the flap slightly dorsally to allow for a gentle slope of the commissure. Make the flap approximately 1 cm at the base and 1.5 times longer than wide. Defat the flap down to the subdermal vascular plexus. Make an incision from the free end of the flap along the opposing surfaces of the cleft. Expose the metacarpals extraperiosteally. Excise excess soft tissue and bony elements that will prevent apposing of the metacarpals. Drill two holes in each metacarpal just proximal to the heads, and place a heavy suture through the holes (Fig. 4-22, *B*). Approximate the metacarpals, and tie the suture to secure the correction. Close the dorsal and palmar skin incisions from proximal to distal. Excise excess skin to create interdigitating flaps along the dorsal and palmar surfaces. Place the finger flap into the commissure, and before suturing the flap, excise excess skin from the dorsum of the hand rather than from the flap (Fig. 4-22, *C*). Apply a well-molded, long-arm cast to the level of the metacarpal heads over a minimum amount of bandages.

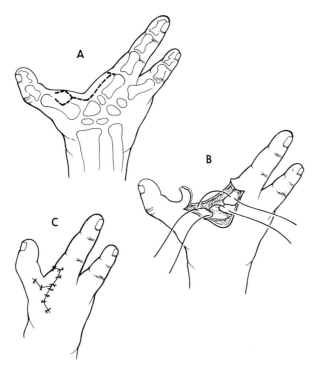

Fig. 4-22 Barsky technique of cleft closure (see text). **A**, Skin incision. **B**, Approximation of metacarpals with heavy sutures passed through holes drilled in bone. **C**, Flap used to create new web and skin on dorsal and palmar surfaces. (Redrawn from Barsky AJ: J Bone Joint Surg 46A:1707, 1964.)

▶ *Postoperative management.* The cast is worn for 3 to 4 weeks. If there is a tendency for the thumb to separate excessively, apply another cast for an additional 2 to 3 weeks; then allow regular use of the hand. Special therapy usually is not required.

Combined cleft closure and release of thumb adduction contracture

▶ *Technique (Snow and Littler).* First make incisions that outline the sides of the cleft on the dorsal surfaces of the index and ring fingers, joining the incisions where the V-shaped apex extends proximal to the level of the metacarpal head. Then make a small, straight incision on the ulnar side of the index finger to accommodate a small flap that will be used to make a commissure (Fig. 4-23, *A*). Raise this flap on the radial side of the ring finger. As the incisions pass the metacarpal heads, curve them back proximally onto the palm, almost parallel to each other and lying to the cleft side of the midline of the two fingers (Fig. 4-23, *B*). Do not extend the incisions any further into the palm than a point opposite the V-shaped apex of the dorsal incision. This is the palmar flap that will create the new thumb web.

To release the thumb adduction contracture, make another incision beginning on the dorsum of the thumb web at the same level as the V-shaped cleft incision. Extend the incision distally, parallel with the index split incision until it reaches the distal edge of the thumb-index web. This creates a strip of dorsal skin that is left connected to the index finger and the dorsum of the hand and that will cover the dorsal veins and extensor tendons of the index finger.

Develop the split flap from the dorsum, carefully tying the dorsal veins in the incision; do not dissect them off the flap. The flap will be compromised unless venous drainage is good. Also carefully protect and preserve the branches of the median nerve.

Next develop the thumb-index incision and release the fibrous bands between the two metacarpals. Detach the origins of the first dorsal interosseous from these bones. The adductor muscle and the radial belly of the flexor pollicis brevis muscle may have to be elevated from their origins; the radial artery must be protected during this step. Occasionally, the dissection will have to be carried down to the capsule of the carpometacarpal joint, and sometimes the capsule must be incised to permit full thumb abduction.

Now perform an osteotomy of the index ray at its base and transfer it to the third metacarpal (Fig. 4-23, *C*). If the third metacarpal is small, shape the index ray into a peg and impale it into the base of the third metacarpal. If enough bone is present, fix the index metacarpal to the base of the third metacarpal with Kirschner wire (Fig. 4-23, *D*). Carefully align the

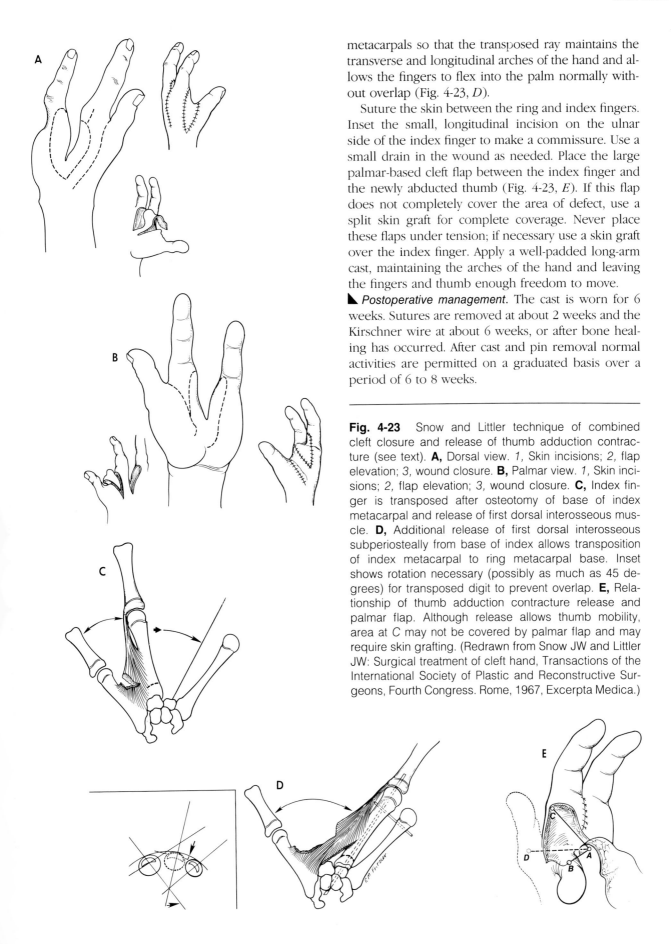

metacarpals so that the transposed ray maintains the transverse and longitudinal arches of the hand and allows the fingers to flex into the palm normally without overlap (Fig. 4-23, *D*).

Suture the skin between the ring and index fingers. Inset the small, longitudinal incision on the ulnar side of the index finger to make a commissure. Use a small drain in the wound as needed. Place the large palmar-based cleft flap between the index finger and the newly abducted thumb (Fig. 4-23, *E*). If this flap does not completely cover the area of defect, use a split skin graft for complete coverage. Never place these flaps under tension; if necessary use a skin graft over the index finger. Apply a well-padded long-arm cast, maintaining the arches of the hand and leaving the fingers and thumb enough freedom to move.

▶ *Postoperative management.* The cast is worn for 6 weeks. Sutures are removed at about 2 weeks and the Kirschner wire at about 6 weeks, or after bone healing has occurred. After cast and pin removal normal activities are permitted on a graduated basis over a period of 6 to 8 weeks.

Fig. 4-23 Snow and Littler technique of combined cleft closure and release of thumb adduction contracture (see text). **A,** Dorsal view. *1,* Skin incisions; *2,* flap elevation; *3,* wound closure. **B,** Palmar view. *1,* Skin incisions; *2,* flap elevation; *3,* wound closure. **C,** Index finger is transposed after osteotomy of base of index metacarpal and release of first dorsal interosseous muscle. **D,** Additional release of first dorsal interosseous subperiosteally from base of index allows transposition of index metacarpal to ring metacarpal base. Inset shows rotation necessary (possibly as much as 45 degrees) for transposed digit to prevent overlap. **E,** Relationship of thumb adduction contracture release and palmar flap. Although release allows thumb mobility, area at *C* may not be covered by palmar flap and may require skin grafting. (Redrawn from Snow JW and Littler JW: Surgical treatment of cleft hand, Transactions of the International Society of Plastic and Reconstructive Surgeons, Fourth Congress. Rome, 1967, Excerpta Medica.)

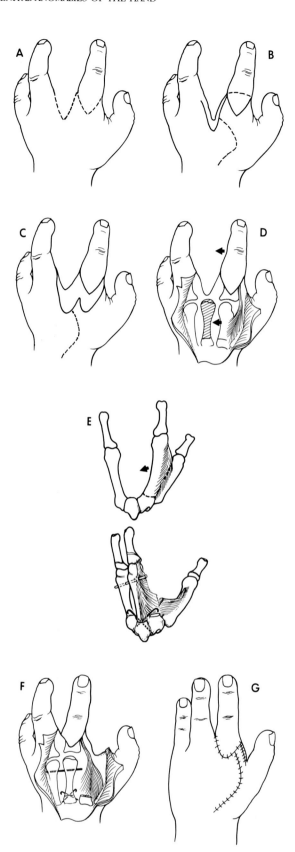

▲ *Technique (Miura and Komada)* (Fig. 4-24). Make a linear incision beginning on the radial side of the base of the ring finger and continuing to the ulnar side of the base of the index finger and crossing the cleft space. Make a curved incision around the base of the index finger at the level desired for the new thumb web space. Then detach the index metacarpal at its base along with the first dorsal interosseous muscle. If exposure is not adequate, make another dorsal skin incision to expose just the bases of the index and long metacarpals. Release the fascia of the adductor pollicis and the first dorsal interosseous. If the base of the third metacarpal is present, impale the index ray on the base of the third metacarpal and fix it with Kirschner wires. Reconstruct the transverse metacarpal ligament with two or three soft tissue sutures between the index and ring fingers. Fashion the flap for the thumb web from the skin radial to the curved incision along the original cleft. Close the skin. Apply a long-arm cast molded over the metacarpals to prevent separation of the cleft.

▲ *Postoperative management.* The cast and skin sutures are removed at 3 weeks. Additional casting may be required if there is any laxity in the cleft. After final cast removal gradual resumption of normal activities is permitted over a period of 6 to 8 weeks.

Fig. 4-24 Reconstruction of cleft hand with adducted thumb. **A,** Initial skin incision on dorsum of hand. **B,** Additional incisions *(broken line)* to expose metacarpal dorsally and finger on palmar surface. **C,** Index finger skin flaps. **D,** Scheme for transposing index metacarpal to middle metacarpal position. **E,** Bone transposition: fasciae of first dorsal interosseous and adductor pollicis are released and muscle may require release. **F,** Transposition of index and release of thumb completed. **G,** After wound closure. (Redrawn from Miura T and Komada T: Plast Reconstr Surg 64:65, 1979.)

▶ *Technique (Ueba)* (Fig. 4-25). Make a V-shaped skin incision, in the form of a triangular skin flap, on the radial side of the ring finger (Fig 4-25, *A*). This flap is used to form the commissure. Make a second skin incision, beginning from the palmar end of the previous skin incision and extending to the ulnar side of the palm (Fig.4-25, *B*). Make a third skin incision around the base of the index finger; then place an incision at the bottom of the cleft to connect the previous incisions (Fig. 4-25, *C*). Elevate the interdigital palmar and dorsal skin flaps, and sever the fibrous bands between the thumb and index finger to widen the thumb web as much as possible (Fig. 4-25, *D*). Elevate the periosteum around the second metacarpal, and transfer the metacarpal ulnarward, taking care not to injure the ulnar nerve. Shift the second metacarpal slightly ulnarward, and supinate it so that the index finger flexes without overlapping the ring finger. Fix the second metacarpal to the fourth metacarpal with one or two Kirschner wires and a nonabsorbable suture or long-lasting absorbable suture around the metacarpal necks.

Then connect the common extensor tendons to the index and ring fingers with a free tendon graft taken from the palmaris longus muscle. Pass this tendon graft through the extensor tendons at the level of the metacarpophalangeal joints, reflect its ends, and suture them to the extensor aponeurosis (Fig. 4-25, *E*). After rotating the flaps (Fig. 4-25, *F*), make suture lines transversely to conceal the original cleft and deepen the thumb web (Fig. 4-25, *G*). Close the skin with absorbable sutures. Apply a long-arm cast, molded to avoid recurrence of the cleft.

▶ *Postoperative management.* The cast and any remaining sutures are removed at 3 weeks when a second cast is applied. The cast and Kirschner wires are removed at about 6 weeks or when bone healing is complete. Resumption of normal activities is allowed during the next 4 to 6 weeks.

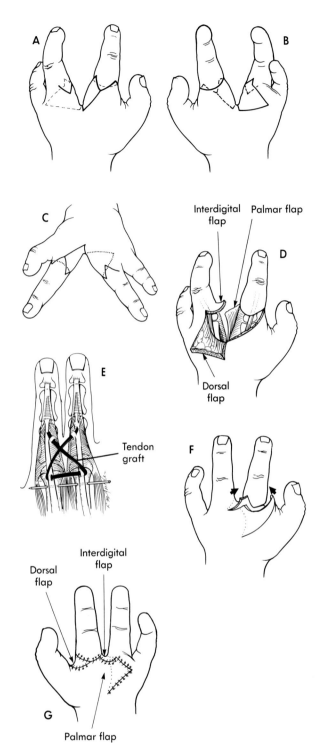

Fig. 4-25 Ueba technique for cleft hand. **A,** Dorsal view of incisions. *Solid line,* Dorsal incisions; *broken line,* palmar incisions. **B,** Palmar view of incisions. *Solid line,* Palmar incision; *broken line,* dorsal incisions. **C,** Incisions from web space. *Solid line,* Dorsal incisions; *broken line,* palmar incisions. **D,** Flaps developed and elevated. **E,** Flaps rotated. **F,** Reconstruction of extensor tendon with graft; Kirschner wire stabilizes index to ring metacarpal. **G,** Appearance of palm after wound closure. (Redrawn from Ueba Y: J Hand Surg 6:557, 1981.)

Deepening of web and metacarpal osteotomy

▶ *Technique*. It usually is safer to undertake correction in two stages. First deepen the web by Z-plasty and remove any redundant bone segments or rudimentary digits. Later, shorten a metacarpal if needed or rotate one or both to provide appositional pinch between the digits. Apply a long-arm cast.

▶ *Postoperative management*. The sutures are removed at 2 weeks and the cast at 4 to 6 weeks. Normal activities are resumed during the next 4 to 6 weeks.

Tendon transfer for type II deformities

▶ *Technique (Flatt)*. This procedure requires a good, stable, passive range of motion in the border digits. Identify the donor tendons, either wrist flexors or extensors, through appropriate incisions. Harvest the palmaris longus tendon to be used as a graft for the transfers. Secure the graft to the donor tendons with a Pulver-Taft weave, and secure the distal ends into the terminal phalanges of the border digits with pull-out wire.

▶ *Postoperative management*. The wrist is splinted in mild flexion for 3 weeks; then the pull-out wire and skin sutures are removed. Normal activities are gradually resumed during the next 4 to 6 weeks.

Ulnar Clubhand–Ulnar Deficiencies

Ulnar deficiencies are those malformations in which there is longitudinal failure of formation along the postaxial border of the upper extremity. The most common form is a partial deficiency of the ulna and the ulnar two digits, commonly referred to as *ulnar clubhand*. Other terms for this deformity include ulnar dysmelia, paraxial ulnar hemimelia, and congenital absence of the ulna. Ulnar deficiencies are among the rarest of congenital hand anomalies, with a relative incidence one tenth to one third that of radial deficiencies.

The cause of this rare anomaly is unknown, and its occurrence is sporadic. The only report that suggests a familial pattern is that of Roberts in 1886 in which he reported the deformity in three successive generations.

Swanson recognizes four types of ulnar deficiency (Fig. 4-26): type 1, hypoplasia or partial defect of the ulna; type 2, total defect of the ulna; type 3, total or partial defect of the ulna with humeroradial synostosis; and type 4, total or partial defect of the ulna associated with congenital amputation at the wrist. Partial absence of the ulna is more common than total absence, the reverse of radial deficiencies. In Swanson's series 53.4% of patients had humeroradial synostosis and 5.7% had congenital amputations at the wrist.

Anomalies associated with ulnar deficiencies, unlike radial deficiencies, are almost solely limited to the musculoskeletal system and include clubfoot, fibular deficiencies, spina bifida, femoral agenesis, mandibular defects, and absence of the patella. Carpal

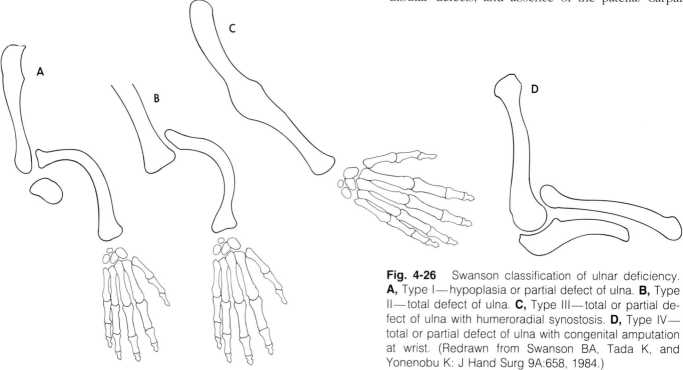

Fig. 4-26 *Swanson classification of ulnar deficiency.* **A,** Type I—hypoplasia or partial defect of ulna. **B,** Type II—total defect of ulna. **C,** Type III—total or partial defect of ulna with humeroradial synostosis. **D,** Type IV—total or partial defect of ulna with congenital amputation at wrist. *(Redrawn from Swanson BA, Tada K, and Yonenobu K: J Hand Surg 9A:658, 1984.)*

bone deformities are common because of severe deformity and coalition. Digital malformation occurs in 89% of patients, and radial head dislocation is frequent.

Varying degrees of deficiency along the ulnar side of the hand are present at birth. The forearm usually is shortened and frequently bowed. The small and ring fingers usually are absent. Syndactyly of the remaining digits is common. The middle and index finger, as well as the thumb, are absent in about two thirds of patients. Forearm bowing with radial convexity is caused by the tethering effect of the ulnar anlage. Ulnar deviation of the hand usually correlates with the degree of radial bowing and increased ulnar slope to the distal radius, as does supination deformity of the forearm. The elbow usually is restricted in motion and may be fused. The deformity is more commonly unilateral.

Roentgenograms usually show a typical pattern (Fig. 4-27) of an absent distal ulna and a bowed radius with an increased ulnar slope along its distal articular surface. The pisiform and hamate usually are absent, and frequently there are coalitions of the other carpal bones. It often is difficult to determine the presence or absence of the proximal ulna because mineralization may not occur until the child is 1 year of age.

Nonsurgical management. Initial management of ulnar clubhand in the infant consists of corrective casting and splinting. A long-arm cast is applied in the method of Riordan, applying the hand section first, then joining the hand to the forearm in the corrected position, and finally joining the forearm to the arm in 90 degrees of elbow flexion. Frequent cast changes are necessary and should be continued until correction is achieved. Removable splints may be used to maintain correction. This should be continued until the child is 6 months of age, at which time exploration and excision of the ulnar anlage should be considered if significant radial bowing is present.

Surgical treatment. Indications for surgical intervention are syndactyly, radial bowing and presence of an ulnar anlage, dislocation of the radial head with limited elbow extension and forearm pronation and supination, and internal rotation deformity of the humerus. Surgical separation of the syndactyly should be performed in accordance with standard syndactyly protocol: separation of the thumb and index finger by 6 months of age and of central syndactyly by 18 months of age. Malrotation, as well as syndactyly, of the thumb may require first metacarpal derotational osteotomy to correct the supination deformity. This procedure usually requires a local rotational flap to create the web and should be performed 6 months after syndactyly release.

Most authors agree that an ulnar anlage should be excised to prevent further radial bowing and shortening. Straub first called attention to the fibrocartilage anlage that spans the gap between proximal ulna and distal radius and ulnar carpus. This anlage does not appear to grow and acts as a tether to deform the radius and carpus with subsequent bowing of the radial shaft and dislocation of the radial head. Ogden et al recommend routine resection of the distal end of the fibrocartilaginous mass before the age of 2 to 3 years. Riordan recommends resection before 6 months of age. Broudy and Smith recommend removal of the distal ulnar anlage when there is progressive or severe ulnar deviation of the hand at the radiocarpal joint, increased radial bowing, or gradual dislocation of the radial head. If bowing is severe, wedge osteotomy of the radius may be necessary at the time of anlage excision.

If radial head dislocation blocks extension of the elbow, creation of a one-bone forearm should be considered. If the block in extension is acceptable and functional pronation and supination are preserved, then surgical treatment probably will not improve function. If there is marked shortening and bowing of the radius with considerable forearm instability and restriction of elbow motion, then creation of a one-bone forearm probably will improve function. For this procedure to be successful, some proximal ulna must be present. The proximal radius usually is excised several months before the creation of the one-bone forearm because simultaneous performance of the two procedures might be too extensive.

Internal rotation deformity of the humerus may be present with humeroradial synostosis and requires correction if it impairs function.

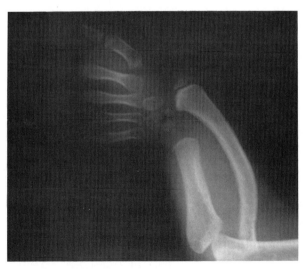

Fig. 4-27 Roentgenographic appearance of type I ulnar clubhand.

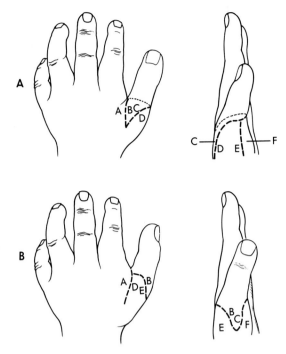

Fig. 4-28   Rotational osteotomy of first metacarpal. **A,** Incision. **B,** After osteotomy, dorsal V-flap is rotated volarly. (Redrawn from Broudy AS and Smith RJ: J Hand Surg 4:304, 1979.)

Rotational osteotomy of the first metacarpal

▶ *Technique (Broudy and Smith).* Under tourniquet control, make a transverse, racquet-shaped skin incision on the volar aspect and extend it to a V-shaped tongue at the middorsum of the first metacarpal. The apex of the V lies at the level of the first metacarpal (Fig. 4-28, *A*) base to allow adequate exposure for osteotomy. Make a proximal longitudinal incision on the radiovolar side of the first metacarpal, 120 degrees from the apex of the V (Fig. 4-28, *B*). Perform an osteotomy of the base of the first metacarpal, and position the metacarpal in the desired amount of pronation. Fix the metacarpal in position with Kirschner wires, suture the V flap into the opened linear incision, and close the V defect in a side-to-side manner. Apply a long-arm cast.

▶ *Postoperative management.* The cast is removed 6 weeks after surgery, and progressive activity is begun. Kirschner wires are removed 6 weeks after surgery or when bone healing is complete. A removable, short-arm, thumb spica splint is worn during sleep for another 6 weeks.

Excision of the ulnar anlage

▶ *Technique (Flatt).* Under tourniquet control, make a lazy S–shaped incision along the postaxial border, carrying it across the wrist crease to the midcarpal level. Because of the absence of the extrinsic flexor muscles, the ulnar neurovascular bundle and the anlage lie close together in the subcutaneous tissues. Free and protect the neurovascular bundle before dissecting the anlage off its carpal attachment. Remove at least one third of the forearm length. Incise the soft tissues on the ulnar side of the wrist joint sufficiently to allow full correction of the hand on the distal radial articular surface. The hand should flop over into neutral or even slight radial deviation; if it must be pushed into neutral, release more of the soft tissue. Close the wound with nonabsorbable sutures, and apply a well-molded, long-arm cast.

▶ *Postoperative management.* Remaining sutures are removed 3 weeks after surgery, and the cast is changed. The cast is removed 6 weeks after surgery, and normal activities are resumed gradually during next 4 to 6 weeks.

Creation of one-bone forearm

▲ *Technique (Straub).* Make a curved longitudinal dorsoradial incision beginning just proximal to the elbow and ending at the middle or distal third of the forearm. Expose and excise the fibrocartilaginous band that extends distally from the ulnar fragment; in excising this band, free its proximal end by performing an osteotomy on the distal end of the fragment. Next expose the radial nerve at the elbow, and trace it distally to its interosseous branch; this branch and its enclosing supinator muscle may be grossly displaced by the dislocation of the proximal radius. Develop the cleavage between the dorsal and volar muscles of the forearm while carefully protecting the important neurovascular structures in the antecubital area. Then at the level of the distal end of the ulnar fragment, divide the radial shaft and excise its proximal part, including the radial head (Fig. 4-29, *A*). Place the proximal end of the distal radial fragment against the distal end of the ulnar fragment (Fig. 4-29, *B*), and fix them together with a Kirschner wire passed distally through the olecranon (Fig. 4-29, *C*). Close the skin with absorbable or nonabsorbable sutures. Apply a long-arm cast with the elbow flexed about 90 degrees.

▲ *Postoperative management.* The cast is changed 2 weeks after surgery, and any remaining sutures are removed. A long-arm cast is worn for a total of 8 weeks after surgery. The cast and Kirschner wire or Steinmann pin fixation are removed at 8 weeks or when bone healing is complete. Normal activities are resumed after another 6 to 8 weeks.

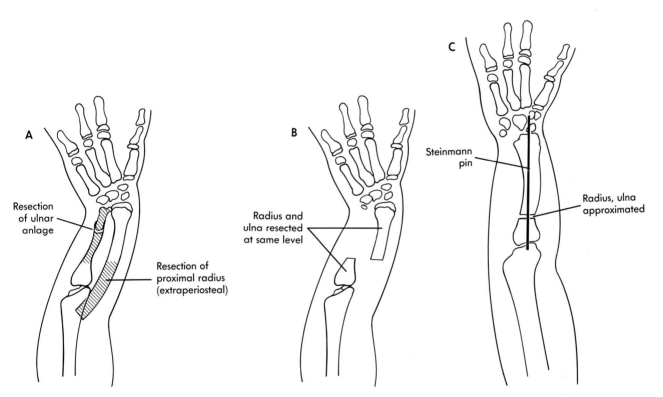

Fig. 4-29 Creation of one-bone forearm. **A,** Resection of distal ulnar anlage and proximal radius *(shaded areas).* **B,** Alignment of distal radius and proximal ulna. **C,** Kirschner wire extending into carpals used to stabilize radial and ulnar segments.

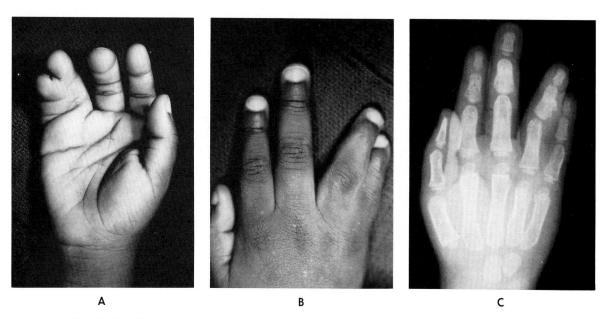

A   B   C

Fig. 4-30   Simple syndactyly in a 5-year-old child. Fingers are bridged only by skin and other soft tissues. **A,** Palmar view. **B,** Dorsal view. **C,** Roentgenogram. Note angular deformity of ring finger.

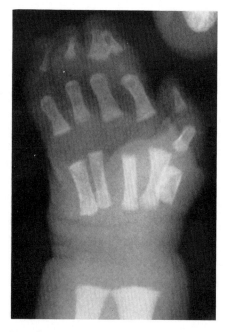

Fig. 4-31   Complex syndactyly. Common bony elements are shared by involved fingers.

FAILURE OF DIFFERENTIATION
Syndactyly

Syndactyly, or "webbed fingers," is due to the failure of the fingers to separate during embryologic development. It is the most common congenital anomaly of the hand, occurring in 1:2000 births. The specific cause is unknown, but it is believed to result from an abnormal slowing of growth and development of the finger buds during the seventh and eighth weeks of gestation. Although most are sporadic occurrences, Flatt found a family history of syndactyly in 40% of his patients, which suggests heredity as one factor. Several pedigrees have shown an autosomal dominant trait for long-ring finger syndactyly, but penetrance has been incomplete.

Syndactylies are classified as complete or incomplete and as simple or complex. Complete syndactyly is present when the fingers are joined from the web to the finger tip; incomplete syndactyly indicates that the fingers are joined from the web to a point proximal to the finger tips. Simple syndactyly exists when only skin or other soft tissue bridges the fingers (Fig.

4-30); complex syndactyly occurs when there are common bony elements shared by involved fingers (Fig. 4-31). Acrosyndactyly refers to lateral fusion of adjacent digits at their distal ends with proximal fenestrations between the joined digits. Brachysyndactyly denotes associated shortening of the syndactyl digits. Anomalies that may be found in association with syndactyly include webbing of the toes, polydactyly, constriction rings, brachydactyly, cleft feet, hemangioma, absence of muscles, spinal deformities, funnel chest, and heart disorders. Apert syndrome and Poland syndrome characteristically include multiple syndactylies.

Syndactyly occurs between the long and ring fingers in more than 50% of patients (Fig. 4-32); the fourth web, second web, and first web are affected in diminishing frequencies. The syndactyly is bilateral in about half the patients, and boys are more frequently affected than are girls. The intervening skin usually is normal although deficient compared with the normal hand, a fact that is important in the consideration of surgical correction. The two nails may be completely separate, or the digits may share a common nail without intervening eponychium. If the fingers are of relatively similar length, flexion and extension usually are normal. Abnormally tight fascial bands usually are present within the web, minimizing any lateral movement between the involved digits. Frequently there are anomalous sharings of musculotendinous units, nerves, and vessels between joined digits. The phalanges usually are normal in the simple pattern; in the complex pattern, however, various interosseous connections range from duplication patterns, to branching patterns, to shared patterns. Differentiation of the joints also may be incomplete. Rarely is there any angular deformity of the digits at birth unless a delta phalanx is present. If a central syndactyly involves the middle and ring or middle and index fingers, angular deformities develop slowly. If, however, the syndactyly involves the ring and little fingers or index finger and thumb, then a gradual flexion contracture, lateral deviation, and rotation deformity usually develop in the longer of the two digits within the first year of life. In Poland syndactyly or syndrome, the sternocostal portion of the ipsilateral pectoralis major muscle is absent. The hand deformity includes unilateral shortening of the index, long, and ring fingers, multiple simple incomplete syndactylies, and hypoplasia of the hand (Fig. 4-33).

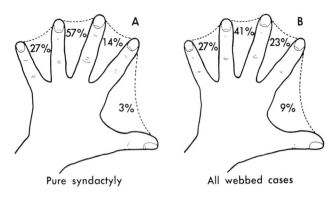

Fig. 4-32 Site of syndactyly. **A,** Percentage incidence when only true syndactyly of simple or complex type is considered. **B,** Total count incidence in which associated conditions (all webbed digits) are included. (From Flatt AE: Practical factors in the treatment of syndactylism. In Littler JW et al: Symposium of reconstructive hand surgery, vol 9, St. Louis, 1974, The CV Mosby Co.)

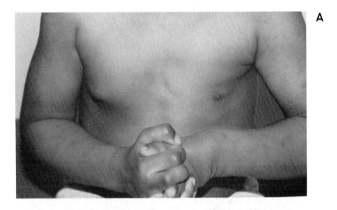

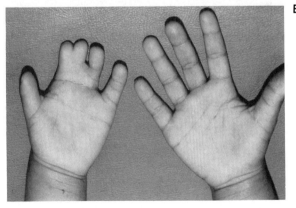

Fig. 4-33 Poland syndrome in 9-year old child. **A,** Hypoplasia of pectoralis muscle. **B,** Brachysyndactyly. (Courtesy Dr. George L. Burruss, Memphis.)

Treatment

Surgical intervention is not urgent. While awaiting the appropriate age for reconstruction, parents should be encouraged to massage the web in an attempt to stretch the intervening skin to facilitate later surgery. Surgical reconstruction is best done before the child is of school age. Kettlekamp and Flatt found results better in children older than 18 months at the time of correction, especially in the final appearance of the commissure. There is a tendency for the web to migrate distally and the commissure to contract if surgery is performed at an earlier age. If the syndactyly involves the second or third web space and there are no other deformities of the involved fingers, surgery should be delayed until the child is at least 18 months of age. When digits of different sizes are completely involved, whether the syndactyly is simple or complex, early separation, between the ages of 6 and 12 months, is best because of the likelihood of angular, rotational, and flexion deformities. These deformities are difficult to correct, and preventing them takes precedence over the possibility of distal web migration and commissure contracture. When multiple digits are involved, the border digits should be released early, followed by subsequent releases after a 6-month waiting period. Simultaneous releases of the radial and ulnar sides of a finger are contraindicated and may jeopardize the viability of the finger.

The surgical procedure includes three technical steps: separation of the digits, commissure reconstruction, and resurfacing of the intervening borders of the digits. Early attempts at separation incorporated such techniques as passage of setons, use of ligatures, and straight linear incisions. Pieri in 1949 condemned the use of straight incisions and favored a zig-zag incision to prevent linear contracture along the long axis of the finger; all currently accepted methods incorporate this principle. Shared digital nerves are carefully split longitudinally to preserve innervation to both digits. Common digital arteries may extend into the web and require ligation of one of more branches. Care should be taken to avoid devascularizing the digit. When the nail is shared, an additional longitudinal strip of nail and underlying matrix usually must be removed to match the normal nail width. Osseous structures usually are divided longitudinally with a scalpel if the procedure is performed at an early age.

Special attention must be given to the reconstruction of the web commissure. The normal commissure has a sloping configuration from proximal dorsal to distal palmar. Dorsally, it begins at about the level of the transverse metacarpal ligament and extends distally and palmarward to about the level of the proxi-mal digital flexion crease, usually at about the midpoint of the bony proximal phalanx. Distally, the commissure forms a rectangle between the small and ring and index and middle fingers. In some hands the commissure between the middle and ring fingers forms a V or U shape. Distal web span must be greater than proximal web span to allow abduction of the fingers about the axis of the metacarpophalangeal joint. In recreating a commissure with normal appearance and function, a properly designed local flap generally is preferable to a skin graft to minimize commissure contracture. Numerous local flaps have been designed, but the most commonly used are the dorsal "pantaloon" flap described by Bauer et al, the matching volar and dorsal proximally based V-shaped flaps conceived by Zeller and popularized by Cronin and by Skoog, and the "butterfly" flap devised by Shaw et al. Woolf and Broadbent described the butterfly flap as useful for partial simple syndactyly that ends proximal to the proximal interphalangeal joint (Fig. 4-34).

Regardless of flap design, in resurfacing the intervening borders of the digits, there never is enough skin for primary closure of each digit. This phenomenon can be clearly demonstrated to the parents by comparing the sum of the circumferences of two individual fingers with that of the circumference of two fingers held together; the latter is always less. The zig-zag incision is designed to create interdigitating volar and dorsal flaps for one finger; the other finger requires either full- or split-thickness skin grafting (full-thickness grafting usually is preferred). Grafts should be avoided at the base of the ring finger where wearing of a ring may be bothersome. The

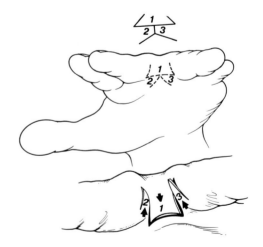

Fig. 4-34 Butterfly flap technique for release of syndactyly. Flaps are designed in web space to form dorsal rectangle; then flaps are rotated to deepen web. (Redrawn from Woolf RM and Broadbent TR: Plast Reconstr Surg 49:48, 1972.)

parents should be informed that recurrence and angular deformity are possible despite a well-designed and well-executed reconstruction and that future revision may be necessary. Toledo and Ger found reoperation necessary in 59% of patients with major associated anomalies and in 30% of patients with syndactyly as the primary abnormality.

The most common complication of syndactyly reconstruction is scar deformity of the digit or web. Distal migration of the web may occur, particularly if surgery is performed before the child is 18 months old. The most catastrophic complication is circulatory insufficiency to the finger, resulting in loss of the digit. This rarely has been reported and should not occur if the syndactyly on each side of the finger is released in stages.

▲ *Technique (Bauer et al).* Outline all incisions carefully with a skin-marking pen (Fig. 4-35, *A* and *B*). First cut a single rectangular skin flap from the dorsal surface of the two webbed fingers for the new web between these fingers. Base it proximally at the level of an adjacent normal web; make it wide enough to form a normal web and long enough to reach the palmar edge of the new web. Now separate the fingers with longitudinal dorsal and palmar incisions on the ring finger along the ulnar side of the abnormal web (toward the radial side of the ring finger); locate and curve these incisions so that they outline the flaps that will cover the ulnar side of the middle finger. Take care not to injure the digital nerve of the ring finger. Raise these flaps, and remove from them any excess subcutaneous fat to give the middle finger a more normal shape. Suture them together on the ulnar side of the middle finger; then suture the web flap in place (Fig. 4-35, *C*). Cover the defect on the ring finger with a full-thickness free graft taken from the groin. If the fingernails are confluent, they should be separated, and the matrix at their margins should be removed so that the grafts can be brought around to the edge of each nail. When a finger is webbed on both sides, it is safer to separate only one side at a time.

Place Xeroform gauze over the grafts, and then carefully insert a wet contour dressing between the fingers; begin at the web space and pack distally so that the fingers are held in wide abduction and extension. Then apply a dry dressing and a plaster splint to immobilize the fingers and wrist.

▲ *Postoperative management.* The hand is elevated for a week or more before redressing.

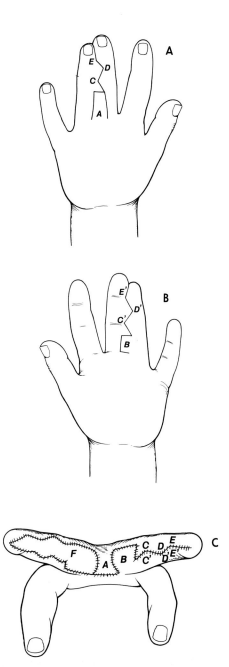

Fig. 4-35 Syndactyly release. **A,** Dorsal skin incisions. Rectangular dorsal flap *(A)* is designed for web; alternating flaps *(C, D,* and *E)* are arranged to interdigitate with volar flaps. **B,** Palmar skin incisions. Rectangular flap *(B)* is arranged to cover radial side of ring finger; remaining flaps *(C', D', E')* are arranged to interdigitate with dorsal flaps. **C,** Separation is completed, flaps have been sutured into place covering radial side of ring finger and web. Skin graft is required for ulnar side of middle finger. (Redrawn from Bauer TB, Tondra JM, and Trusler HM: Plast Reconstr Surg 17:385, 1956.)

▲ *Technique (Skoog).* With a skin pencil outline the incisions to be made on the fingers. Design dorsal and volar flaps so that when mobilized they will cover most of the denuded side of one finger without tension (Fig. 4-36, *A* and *B*). Make the free borders of the flaps irregular by designing small triangular points at the level of the interphalangeal joints. In planning the flaps so that they fit each other, first out-

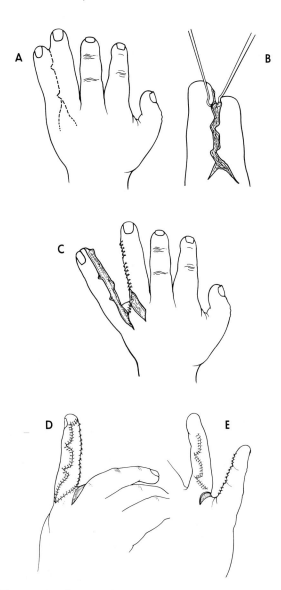

Fig. 4-36 Skoog technique for syndactyly. **A** and **B**, Dorsal and volar skin incisions. **C,** Web space reconstruction, closure ring finger. **D** and **E**, Dorsal and volar views, skin graft in place on little finger and graft in web space.

line the incision on one side and then establish the key points for the incision on the opposite side by pushing straight needles vertically through the web. Then elevate the tourniquet and raise the flaps consisting mainly of the skin that forms the abnormal web. In raising the flaps preserve all subcutaneous tissue and be careful not to sever digital nerves and arteries. Then release the tourniquet and control all bleeding. Using the triangular flaps, reconstruct the web space (Fig 4-36, *C*). On one finger close the flaps as planned and cover the small remaining defect at the dorsomedial aspect of the base of this finger (Fig. 4-36, *D*) by a full-thickness skin graft obtained from the inguinal region. Then make a pattern of the denuded area on the adjacent finger and on the new web and obtain a matching full-thickness graft again from the inguinal region. Carefully suture the graft in place (Fig. 4-36, *E*), and close the donor area. Then apply a pressure dressing: place Xeroform gauze over the grafts and suture lines, spread the fingers widely and place between them wet cotton pressed to fit the contours of the fingers and web, and then wrap on dry gauze and Webril. Next apply a plaster splint; extend it proximal to the elbow if necessary to ensure sufficient immobilization.

When more than two fingers are involved in the syndactyly, it is safer to separate only one side of a single finger at a time.

▲ *Postoperative management.* The hand is elevated for at least 3 days after surgery. At 10 to 14 days the dressing is changed, if necessary with the patient under general anesthesia. Sutures may be removed at this time. Another bandage is maintained for an additional 10 to 14 days, and gradual resumption of normal activities is allowed.

Apert Syndrome

In 1906 Apert described a patient with a group of deformities that included atypical facies and multiple complex syndactylies of the hand, which he called *acrocephalosyndactyly.* Despite its rarity (1:200,00 births), much has been written about the management of the complex hand deformities in this syndrome. The condition is believed to result from a single gene mutation in one of the parents and can be passed in dominant and recessive forms; sporadic occurrences also are possible. Apert syndrome was classified into two main categories by Blank: true or typical, characterized by multiple complex syndactylies, and atypical, with only partial syndactylies.

At birth these patients have a high, broad forehead and a flattened occiput. The eyes are widely set with the outer canthus lower than the inner canthus. The lower jaw is prominent, and the maxilla is shortened (Fig. 4-37, *A*). Mental retardation is common but not universal. There may be associated visceral abnormalities. These patients usually can be expected to live well into adulthood. The hand deformities are typically symmetric. The hand is spoon-shaped with a tapering terminal end and complex syndactyly of the index, middle, and ring fingers (Fig. 4-37, *B*). The little finger usually shows complete simple syndactyly with the ring finger. Often a nail is shared between the index, long, and ring fingers. Syndactyly also may occur between the thumb and index finger. The fingers have limited motion because of incomplete joint development, and they usually are shortened. Five digits usually are present, distinguishing Apert syndrome from Carpenter syndrome (acrocephalopolysyndactyly) in which polydactyly also is present. The arm and forearm frequently are shortened with limited elbow motion. The untreated hand functions in a spoonlike fashion with either a two-handed or a thumb-to-side-of-index-finger prehensile pattern.

Treatment

Reconstructive surgery usually improves hand function in these patients by creating a three-fingered hand with an opposable thumb. The surgical management should follow the protocol outlined by Flatt. In the child younger than 2 years, bilateral simultaneous reconstructive procedures may be carried out because the child is not dependent on self-care. In the older child only one hand at a time should be reconstructed. The border digits should be released before the child is 1 year old. If the thumb is not included in the syndactyly, a simple four-part Z-plasty is used to deepen the first web. Six to 9 months later, release of the central syndactylies and deletion of the middle finger at the metacarpophalangeal joint are performed. This deletion provides the necessary skin coverage and good sensibility to the remaining digits. Flatt found more deformity in patients with a ray amputation of the middle finger and ulnar transposition of the index finger, and this procedure is not recommended.

◣ *Technique (Flatt)*. Stage I, release of the border digits, is performed before the age of 1 year. After application and inflation of a tourniquet, incise the border syndactylies as described by Bauer et al to release the small, ring, and index fingers and the thumb. If the thumb is not included in the syndactyly, deepen the web with a four-part Z-plasty (p. 309). Close the skin flaps with interrupted sutures, and cover the remaining defects with a full-thickness skin graft.

Stage II is performed 6 to 9 months later to allow for revascularization and softening of the tissues. Make the incisions on the long finger to create flaps as described by Bauer et al, using all the skin overlying the middle digit. After the flaps are elevated, ampute the middle digit at the metacarpophalangeal joint. Use the overlying skin to reconstruct the remaining commissure between the index and ring fingers and to cover the fingers. Close the flaps in routine fashion and use a full-thickness skin graft if necessary to cover the remaining defects. Apply sterile dressings of moistened cotton batting between the webs and apply a plaster splint to maintain positioning. The splint is worn 4 weeks, and then active motion of the hand is encouraged.

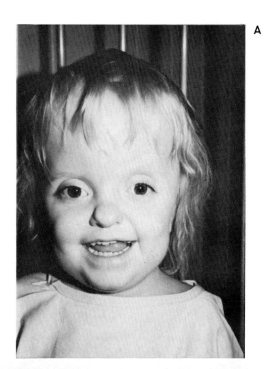

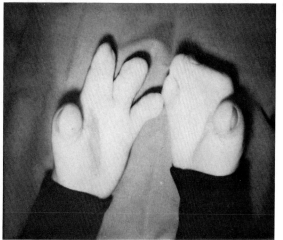

Fig. 4-37 Apert syndrome. **A,** Characteristic facial features of high forehead and wide-set eyes. **B,** Complex syndactyly involving all fingers of both hands; left hand has syndactyly release.

DUPLICATION (POLYDACTYLY)

Duplication of digits, or polydactyly, is a common and conspicuous hand anomaly. It was recorded in biblical literature as long ago as 3000 years, and approximately 9000 to 10,000 new cases are recorded each year. Polydactyly is classified into three main categories: preaxial, duplication of the thumb (bifid thumb); central, duplication of the index, middle, or ring fingers; and postaxial, duplication of the small finger. Also included in the general category of duplication is ulnar dimelia or mirror hand, an exceedingly rare anomaly.

Preaxial Polydactyly (Bifid Thumb)

The bifid thumb represents a complete or partial duplication of the thumb (Fig. 4-38). It is the most common duplication pattern in white and oriental populations, occurring in 1:3000 births. It usually is unilateral; only 9 of 70 patients in Wassel's series had bilateral involvement. The cause of the bifid thumb is unknown. Most occur sporadically, which suggests environmental factors rather than genetic predisposi-

tion. Preaxial polydactyly has been produced in the offspring of rats by the administration of cytosine arabinoside during pregnancy. When the thumb duplication is associated with a triphalangeal thumb, an autosomal dominant pattern and sporadic occurrence have been identified. Bifid thumb typically occurs as an isolated deformity unassociated with other malformation syndromes, but visceral anomalies have been rarely reported, particularly hand-heart or Holt-Oram syndrome.

Wassel described a group of 70 patients with bifid thumbs and suggested a now widely used classification (Fig. 4-39): type I, partial duplication of the distal phalanx and a common epiphysis; type II, complete duplication, including the epiphysis of the distal phalanx; type III, duplication of the distal phalanx and bifurcation of the proximal phalanx; type IV, complete duplication of distal and proximal phalanges; type V, complete duplication of distal and proximal phalanges with bifurcation of the metacarpal; type VI, complete duplication of the distal and proximal phalanx and the metacarpal; and type VII, variable degrees of

Fig. 4-38 Varied manifestations of bifid thumb ranging from partial **(A)** to complete **(D)** duplication of thumb. Wassel's type IV **(B)** is the most common.

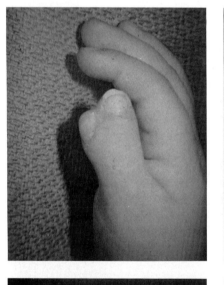
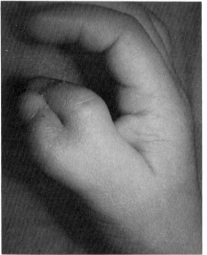
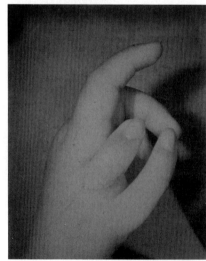
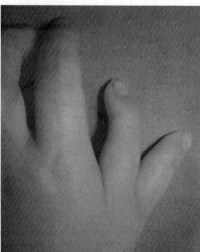

duplication associated with a triphalangeal thumb. In Wassel's series type IV was the most common pattern (47%), followed by type VII (20%) and type II (15%). Wood found that type 4 and type 7 deformities could be further subdivided depending on the extent of duplication and triphalangism.

The deformity usually is unilateral, and clinical appearance varies from mild widening of the thumb tip to complete duplication of the entire thumb. Typically there is some degree of hypoplasia of both duplicates, and more commonly the radial duplicate is the more hypoplastic. There may be convergence or divergence of the duplications. Occasionally the thumb has decreased pronation, placing it in the same plane as the other digits. Anatomic dissections have revealed fibrous interconnections between the two thumbs. The nail may be one large, conjoined nail with a central longitudinal groove, or it may be completely duplicated. The ulnar-innervated intrinsic muscles to the thumb (adductor pollicis and deep head of the flexor pollicis brevis) typically insert on the ulnarmost thumb duplicate, and the median-innervated intrinsic muscles to the thumb (abductor pollicis, superficial head of the flexor pollicis brevis, and opponens pollicis) typically insert on the radial-most thumb duplicate. Extrinsic flexor and extensor tendons may be duplicated and usually are eccentrically placed along each thumb. The phalanges may be angulated, and there may be an associated delta phalanx. The joints usually are stiff, with a widened joint surface. The collateral ligaments of the duplicated joints often are shared, with insufficiency in the space along the adjacent sides. Wide variations may occur in the neurovascular anatomy. Both radial and ulnar neurovascular bundles to the digits may be completely duplicated or may be shared with small separate branches that supply the individual digits.

Treatment

Surgical correction of the bifid thumb almost always is indicated, not only for the obvious cosmetic improvement but also for better function. Occasionally, if the thumb appears only slightly broader than expected, with underlying roentgenographic evidence of duplication, then surgery might not improve the condition. Surgical reconstruction generally is performed when the child is about 18 months of age but no later than 5 years of age if possible. Later revisions may be required, and fusions needed for late angular deformities and instability may be performed at around 8 to 10 years of age. Simple excision of the more hypoplastic digit rarely results in a satisfactory thumb because of progressive angulation and instability. For types I and II bifid thumbs a combination procedure (Bilhaut-Cloquet) is recommended. More proximal duplication requires excision of the most hypoplastic thumb, narrowing of the widened proximal articular surface, ligament reconstruction, intrinsic transfer, and centralization of the extrinsic flexor and extensor tendons.

Late angular deformity and instability are the most frequent complications, and these may require further ligament reconstruction, corrective closing wedge osteotomy, or perhaps arthrodesis. Miura has successfully treated this Z-collapse at the thumb interphalangeal joint with a rotation skin flap on the concave side of the deformity, combined with excision of the radial half of the extensor tendon and transfer of the flexor tendon into the ulnar side of the distal phalanx. Other reported complications include infection, scar contracture, joint stiffness, inadequate tendon excursion, residual prominence at the previous site of duplication, and a narrowed first web space. Loss of sensibility or viability of the digit rarely is encountered if surgical details are carefully observed.

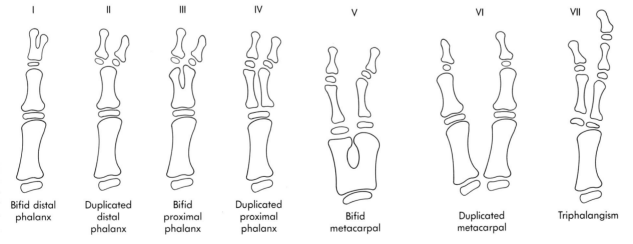

I	II	III	IV	V	VI	VII
Bifid distal phalanx	Duplicated distal phalanx	Bifid proximal phalanx	Duplicated proximal phalanx	Bifid metacarpal	Duplicated metacarpal	Triphalangism

Fig. 4-39 Wassel classification of thumb polydactyly. (Redrawn from Wassel HD: Clin Orthop 64:175, 1969.)

Types I and II bifid thumbs

▶ *Technique (Bilhaut-Cloquet)* (Fig. 4-40). Under tourniquet control, make a central wedge-shaped incision from dorsal to palmar over the involved thumb tip, extending proximally to the level of bifurcation. The dorsal component of the incision will pass through the nail and nail bed. Incise the central component of the underlying tendon and bone of the duplicated structures in line with the skin incision. Carefully approximate the articular surface and physis of the remaining parts of the distal phalanx, and secure them with a transverse Kirschner wire. This may be difficult because of tightening of the collateral ligaments. Carefully suture the nail bed with 6-0 absorbable suture, and close the skin with interrupted sutures. Apply a short- or long-arm thumb spica cast, depending on the patient's age. Younger children require the long-arm cast.

▶ *Postoperative management.* The cast is removed 4 to 6 weeks after surgery, and the Kirschner wire may be removed 6 weeks after surgery. Progressively increased use is allowed after removal of the cast and wire.

Types III through VI bifid thumbs

▶ *Technique (Lamb; Marks and Bayne).* Under tourniquet control, make a racquet-shaped incision over the most hypoplastic thumb (usually the radialmost digit). If the ulnar thumb is the more affected, it should be removed instead. Through the incision expose the abductor pollicis brevis tendon as it inserts into the proximal phalanx of the radialmost thumb and carefully preserve this tendon. If the ulnar thumb is to be excised, then identify the adductor pollicis and carefully preserve it. Detach the collateral ligament distally from the phalanx that is to be excised. Strip the collateral ligament proximally off the metacarpal or phalanx with a strip of periosteum to allow adequate exposure of the joint. Excise the supernu-

merary digit with the part of the metacarpal or phalanx with which it articulates (Fig. 4-41, *A*). Centralize the remaining digit over the remaining articular surface (Fig. 4-41, *B*), and suture the collateral ligament and intrinsic tendon securely to the phalanx (Fig. 4-41, *C*). Secure this alignment with a longitudinal Kirschner wire placed across the joint (Fig. 4-41, *D*). Check the alignment of the extensor and flexor tendons to ensure that they track centrally along the digit. Partial resection or transfer of the tendons may be required to achieve a central line of pull. Close the skin with simple interrupted sutures. A Z-plasty also may be required if there is inadequate skin along the ulnar border for a tension-free closure.

▶ *Postoperative management.* The thumb is immobilized for about 4 weeks, at which time the wire may be removed and the hand mobilized. A protective splint may be required for another 3 to 4 weeks.

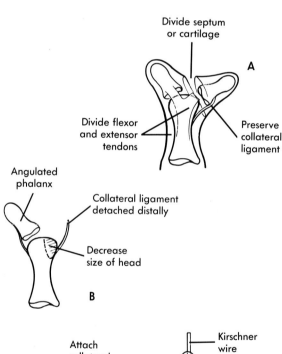

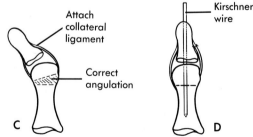

Fig. 4-41 Technique for asymmetric duplication (see text). **A,** Removal of less functional component. **B,** Transfer of collateral ligament. **C,** Osteotomy of proximal phalanx. **D,** Kirschner wire fixation. (Redrawn from Marks TW and Bayne LG: J Hand Surg 3:107, 1978.)

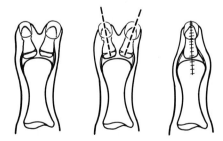

Fig. 4-40 Bilhaut-Cloquet technique for symmetric thumb duplication in which duplicate digits are joined at midline after excision of excess central soft and osseous tissue (see text). (Redrawn from Marks TW and Bayne LG: J Hand Surg 3:107, 1978.)

Triphalangeal Thumb

As the name implies, the triphalangeal thumb has three phalanges instead of the normal two. This uncommon anomaly, which can be inherited as an autosomal dominant trait, has been associated with maternal use of thalidomide. Two major types of triphalangeal thumbs are most common: one has a small, wedge-shaped extra ossicle (delta phalanx, p. 323) that causes an angular deformity without significantly increasing thumb length; the other has an extra phalanx that is normal or nearly normal and creates the appearance of a five-finger hand (Fig. 4-42). Buck-Gramcko described a transitional type in which a trapezoidal extra phalanx causes both increased length and angular deformity (Fig. 4-43). The triphalangeal thumb also has been classified as opposable or nonopposable. The most common hand anomaly associated with triphalangeal thumb is a bifid thumb; other associated conditions include cleft foot, tibial defects, congenital heart disease, Fanconi anemia, anomalies of the gastrointestinal tract, and chromosomal anomalies.

In type I deformities (delta phalanx) the thumb is deviated ulnarward in the area of the interphalangeal joint. Roentgenograms show either a delta phalanx or a trapezoidal extra phalanx. In type II deformities (five-fingered hand), the thumb is longer than normal and lies in the same plane as the other fingers. Extra skin creases overlie the additional interphalangeal joint. Patients with type II deformities are unable to oppose the thumb to the other digits and tend to use side-to-side prehension. Hypoplasia of the thenar muscles often is associated with type II deformities and further hinders opposition. Polydactyly usually is present, and 60% of patients have significant web space contractures. Roentgenograms show a complete extra, rectangular phalanx; the duplicated phalanx typically is the middle phalanx.

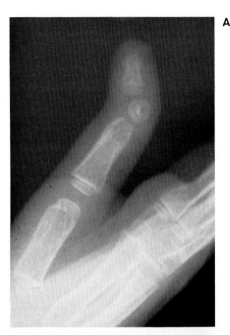

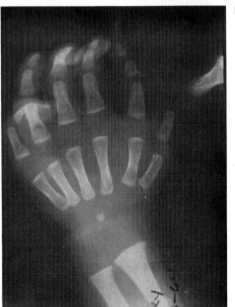

Fig. 4-43 Roentgenographic appearance of triphalangeal thumb. **A,** Type I. **B,** Type II with associated duplication.

Fig. 4-42 Clinical appearance of triphalangeal thumb associated with duplication (Wassel type VII).

Treatment

Although nonsurgical treatment does not correct the condition, surgical intervention is not required for all children with triphalangeal thumbs, especially those with type I deformities. The goals of surgical treatment are correction of angular deformity, restoration of normal length, correction of web contracture, and improvement of opposition. Removal of the abnormal phalanx along with reconstruction of the collateral ligament allows remodeling of the joint surfaces and usually provides adequate stability, especially if performed during the first year of life; however, Wood reported late instability and angular deformity in 10 of 29 patients after ligamentous reconstruction. Reduction osteotomy, as described by Peimer, will correct the angulation deformity with less chance of ligamentous instability. This osteotomy is best performed when the child is between 24 and 30 months of age and the physis is clearly visible on roentgenogram. Late instability can be treated with arthrodesis. Contracture of the first web space may be released with a four-part Z-plasty as described by Woolf and Broadbent (p. 309). Severe contracture

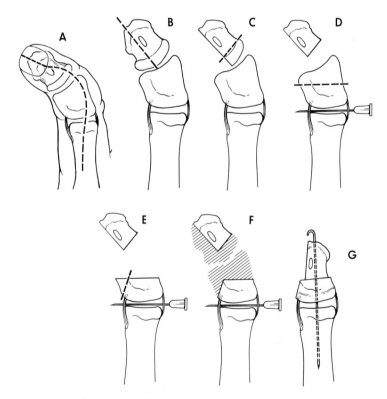

Fig. 4-44 Reduction osteotomy (see text). **A,** Dorsal incision. **B,** Narrowing of distal phalanx. **C,** Excision of distal physis. **D,** Needle placed across PIP joint to orient transverse osteotomy. **E,** Completion of osteotomy. **F,** Combined osteotomies form closing wedge to shorten and realign thumb. **G,** Bone ends are fixed with smooth wires. (Redrawn from Peimer CA: J Hand Surg 10A:376, 1985.)

may require a dorsal rotation flap as described by Strauch and Spinner. Thenar hypoplasia may require opponensplasty with the use of the abductor digiti minimi (p. 311) or ring sublimis (p. 310). For type II deformity (five-fingered hand), pollicization of the radialmost digit, as described by Buck-Gramcko (p. 274), is recommended.

Surgical correction also may be required for associated anomalies such as polydactyly. Wood outlined treatment guidelines for duplication associated with triphalangism of the thumb. If the duplication is a Wassell type IV (p. 297), the radialmost digit should be excised when the child is about 6 months old. In Wassell type VII duplication (complete duplication), the triphalangeal thumb should be removed. The remaining thumb may require web reconstruction and metacarpal osteotomy to complete the pollicization.

Reduction osteotomy

▲ *Technique (Peimer).* Mark the preoperative roentgenograms, or make a sketch of the phalangeal and physeal deformities, to plan the location of the osteotomies and the amount to be resected. Use a skin marking pen to mark the curved dorsal incision, including the nail and matrix that must be removed (Fig. 4-44, *A*). Make a curved incision through the nail, matrix, and skin down to the level of the paratenon. Elevate skin flaps, and expose the middle and distal phalanges by dividing and reflecting the extensor pollicis longus tendon just proximal to its insertion on the distal phalanx. Use a scalpel or fine bone-cutting forceps to narrow the distal phalanx to the desired width, taking care to avoid fragmenting the phalanx. Expose the distal phalangeal physis with the first longitudinal cut (Fig. 4-44, *B*). With a scalpel perform a transverse osteotomy, completely excising the physis (Fig. 4-44, *C*). Perform a second transverse osteotomy in the middle of the middle phalanx distal to the normal horizontal portion of the physis. Confirm that the second osteotomy is parallel to the proximal interphalangeal joint by inserting a thin hypodermic needle into the joint to determine the joint line (Fig. 4-44, *D*). With the second transverse osteotomy, expose the abnormal longitudinal portion of the C-shaped middle phalangeal physis and completely excise the distal portion of the middle phalanx and the abnormal physis without cutting the collateral ligament (Fig. 4-44, *E*). After removing the bone fragments, place the remaining bone in a closing-wedge position to realign and shorten the thumb (Figs. 4-44, *F* and *G*). If necessary, use bone-cutting forceps or a small rasp to contour the bony surfaces. Align the bone ends, and fix them with one or two smooth 0.028-inch or 0.035-inch Kirschner wires. Transfix the retained interphalangeal joint if additional stability is needed. Check the adequacy of resection and realignment, and confirm the Kirschner wire placement and phalangeal position with roentgenograms. Shorten and repair the extensor pollicis longus tendon with fine sutures. Release the tourniquet, excise redundant skin, and close the wound. Cut and bend the Kirschner wires, leaving them protruding through the skin. Apply a long plaster, opponens gauntlet splint that extends above the elbow.

▶ *Postoperative management.* If necessary the splint can be removed for wound inspection during the first 2 to 3 weeks after surgery, but the hand is kept well-splinted for 6 to 8 weeks. The Kirschner wires are removed after 6 to 8 weeks or when bone healing is evident on roentgenograms. Splinting usually is not required after pin removal. Physical therapy may be helpful in regaining motion in older patients.

Postaxial Polydactyly

Duplication of the small finger is the most common pattern of duplication in the black population. It occurs in approximately 1:300 black births, with a relative frequency of 8:1 compared with duplication of other digits. The true incidence is impossible to determine because many of these children have the extra digit removed in the nursery, although this probably is done less frequently than in the past. Stelling and Turek classified postaxial polydactyly into three types based on the degree of duplication: type 1, duplication of soft parts only; type 2, partial duplication of the digit, including the osseous structures (Fig. 4-45); and type 3, complete duplication of the ray, including the metacarpal. Type 3 duplication is rare.

Duplication of the small finger is believed to be genetically determined. Types 2 and 3 duplications are believed to be inherited as dominant traits with marked penetrance. The type 1 pattern is multifactorial, involving two genes with incomplete penetrance. Persons with type 2 or 3 deformities may produce offspring with any of the three types, whereas those with type 1 deformities produce only children with type 1 patterns. Autosomal recessive inheritance also has been identified in association with multiple abnormalities.

The typical black child with a supernumerary digit likely inherited it as an autosomal dominant trait and has no other abnormalities; postaxial polydactyly in the white child frequently is associated with more serious abnormalities. The most common local associated anomaly is syndactyly, but there may be multiple deformities, as well as chromosomal abnormalities.

Infants with postaxial polydactyly may have a well-formed extra digit along the ulnar border of the small finger (type 2) or may have only a rudimentary soft tissue tag (type 1). Both digits usually are hypoplastic to some degree. Angular deformity may be present at birth or may occur later during growth.

Treatment

The use of ligatures around the base of type 1 postaxial duplication is not recommended because of reports of fatal hemorrhage. In type 2 duplications the extra digit should be excised through an elliptic incision, usually when the child is about 1 year old. A frequent complication is an unsightly bump caused by a retained segment of duplicated metacarpal head.

▶ *Technique.* Under tourniquet control make an elliptic incision around the base of the extra digit. Leave excess skin at the time of initial incision, and excise this as appropriate at the time of closure. Identify, ligate, and divide the neurovascular bundle to the extra digit. For a type I duplication, complete the excision at this point and close the skin with simple closure. For type II duplication, identify and preserve the abductor digiti quinti minimi tendon. Expose the area of bone bifurcation subperiosteally. Identify and preserve the ulnar collateral ligament if the bifurcation is in the area of the joint. Amputate the extra digit, and trim any excess bone in the area of the bifurcation. Reconstruct the collateral ligament and abductor insertion if violated. Close the skin with simple interrupted sutures. Apply a soft bandage.

▶ *Postoperative management.* A very young child may require a cast for a short time (10 days), but generally no immobilization is necessary. Sutures are removed at 2 weeks, and unlimited activity is allowed.

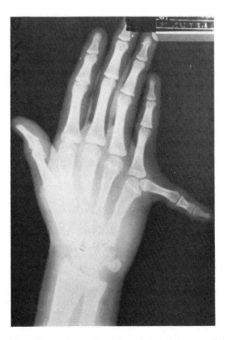

Fig. 4-45 Type 2 postaxial polydactyly: partial duplication of digit including osseous structures.

Central Polydactyly

Central polydactyly refers to duplication of the index, middle, or ring finger. It rarely occurs as a solitary deformity and usually is associated with complex syndactyly. The most typical pattern is type 2 central polydactyly concealed within a syndactyly between the middle and ring fingers. Polydactyly of the index finger and polysyndactyly of the middle and ring fingers probably are inherited as autosomal dominant traits. Associated anomalies include polydactyly and syndactyly of the toes.

Treatment

In isolated central polydactyly, excision of the most hypoplastic digit is performed in keeping with surgical principles of polydactyly reconstruction. In the central polysyndactyly pattern, surgical options include syndactyly reconstruction with excision of the extra digit or creation of a three-fingered hand, which Flatt believes gives better results. The complexity of these deformities requires astute surgical judgment and an individualized approach. Surgical reconstruction should be performed by the time the child is 6 months old to prevent further angular deformity. As many normal-appearing fingers as possible should be reconstructed. Amputation of a functionless digit may be performed later.

Ulnar Dimelia

Ulnar dimelia, commonly called *mirror hand,* occurs as radial and ulnar clusters of fingers in the same hand that are near mirror images of each other. It is considered a duplication phenomenon of the ulnar half of the forearm, wrist, and hand, but because there is complete substitution of the radial components as well, this anomaly is not so easily classified as pure duplication. It is an exceedingly rare anomaly, with few reports in the literature. The largest reported series is that of Harrison et al in which they describe the deformity in three patients. The cause is unknown, but its occurrence usually is sporadic. It is believed to result from an aberration in the control process of the apical ectodermal ridge of the limb bud. When associated with fibular dimelia, it may be explained as a single gene mutation transmitted as an autosomal dominant trait. Ulnar dimelia usually is associated with some degree of hypoplasia of the arm and scapula. The only distant associated anomaly is fibular dimelia with absence of the tibia.

The deformity usually is unilateral and grotesque, with multiple fingers dangling from a somewhat normal palm. The hand usually has six to eight well-formed fingers that may all lie in nearly the same plane or with slight opposition between the two halves. The postaxial digits appear slightly more normal than the preaxial digits. There is no thumb. Syndactyly may be present. The digits may be somewhat flexed because of deficient extensors, and the hand usually is radially deviated at the wrist and extension of wrist may not be possible. The wrist and elbow appear thick, elbow motion is decreased, and the arm is shortened. The ulna and ulnar carpal bones are completely duplicated, the scaphoid and trapezium are replaced, and the distal ulnar epiphysis is broadened. At the elbow each of the duplicated ulnae articulates with the distal humerus separately, and they tend to face each other somewhat. There is no capitellum on the distal humerus.

Treatment

Parents should be encouraged to maintain passive range of motion in the fingers, wrist, elbow, and shoulder by gentle stretching exercises until the child reaches an appropriate age for reconstruction, usually by the age of 2 years. During this period the child should be carefully observed during play to determine which radial digit may function best as the thumb. Surgical intervention should be performed early to prevent the inevitable psychologic trauma to the parents, which also may be sensed by the child. No single surgeon has accumulated enough experience to clearly delineate the best method of treating the many complex problems involved with this deformity. Problems that require correction include limited movement of the elbow, limited pronation and supination, limited movement of the wrist, excessive number of fingers, inadequate finger extension, absence of the thumb, and inadequate first web space.

To improve elbow flexion, Harrison et al excised the upper 1-inch portion of the lateral ulna in a 1-year-old patient and achieved 40 degrees of elbow flexion; by the time the child was 12 years old, however, the elbow again had stiffened into extension. Most authors recommend this treatment method for limited elbow flexion but emphasize postoperative muscle strengthening. Pronation and supination also may be improved, but rotation osteotomy may be required to place the forearm in a more functional position. Limitation of wrist extension by palmar and radial contractures may require Z-plasty and lengthening of the contracted tendons and capsule. The flexor carpi radialis muscle may be transferred to the dorsum to aid extension, and Gorriz recommends transferring the flexor digitorum superficialis of the pollicized finger to the dorsum of the index metacarpal. Wrist arthrodesis may be necessary for recurrent wrist instability; this procedure can be performed when the child is about 12 years of age. Pollicization may be performed in one stage as based on the principles of Buck-Gramcko (p. 274), using the most functional of the radial digits. The excess radial digits are deleted, including the metacarpal and carpal bones. The excess skin is used as a filleted flap to recreate a first web space. Tendon transfers may be necessary to improve finger extension with the use of donor tendons from the amputated digits or the flexor carpi ulnaris if duplicated.

Excision of proximal ulna

▶ *Technique.* Under tourniquet control if possible, place a longitudinal incision over the proximal aspect of the preaxial ulnar bone. Expose the proximal ulna extraperiosteally, preserving a sufficient periosteal and ligamentous strip to reconstruct a collateral ligament. Excise a sufficient amount of the ulna, along with its remaining periosteum, to allow adequate extension and flexion, usually approximately 1 inch of bone. Check the stability of the elbow, close the incision in layers, and apply a long-arm cast with the elbow in 90 degrees of flexion.

▶ *Postoperative management.* The cast is worn for 3 to 6 weeks depending on the stability of the elbow. Neurovascular status must be carefully monitored. After the cast is removed, active assisted flexion and extension exercises are begun. A night splint is recommended to hold the elbow in 90 degrees of flexion until the child can actively flex the elbow against resistance. Emphasis should be placed on strengthening the elbow flexors and extensors to maintain motion achieved at surgery.

Reconstruction of hand and wrist

▶ *Technique.* Before inflation of the tourniquet, carefully plan the incision to allow pollicization of the most functional digit, as well as fillet-type amputations of the excessive digits and exposure of the neurovascular bundles to the digit chosen for pollicization. After the incisions and skin flaps have been designed, exsanguinate the limb and inflate the tourniquet. Make the incisions and carefully dissect the common neurovascular bundles to the middle digit in each web space. Ligate the bifurcation to each adjacent digit. Carefully dissect the common digital nerves to the thenar level before division. Carefully preserve the digital nerves and dorsal veins to the pollicized digit. Next dissect out the tendons to the pollicized digit; if there are bifurcations of these tendons, divide the abnormal insertions to the neighboring tendons. Amputate the extra digits, including the metacarpal and articulating carpal bones. Preserve the extensor tendons to the excised digits, if present, to use later to reinforce finger extension or thumb abduction. Shorten the metacarpal of the pollicized digit by performing an osteotomy just proximal to the metacarpal neck and scarring the remaining shaft. Rotate the head of the metacarpal into 120 degrees of flexion and 90 degrees of pronation, and secure it in this position with two sutures or a Kirschner wire, which allows appropriate shortening and opposition of the pollicized digit. Then suture the intrinsic muscles to the lateral bands of the extensor mechanism of the pollicized digit to augment adduction and abduction. Now use the fillet flaps from the deleted digits to reconstruct a first web space. Remove any excess skin to allow appropriate closure of the shortened, pollicized digit. If increased extension of the wrist is needed, divide the flexor digitorum sublimis muscle at the level of the A-1 pulley into the pollicized digit and transfer it to the dorsal base of the second metacarpal. Deflate the tourniquet, check the viability of the remaining digits and flaps, and apply a bulky dressing with a long-arm posterior splint supporting the elbow at 90 degrees, the wrist at neutral or in slight extension, and the thumb in the abducted position.

▶ *Postoperative management.* The splint is worn for 3 weeks but may be changed for suture removal and wound inspection. After splint removal an exercise program is begun and a removable night splint is used to hold the thumb in the opposed position for an additional 3 months.

OVERGROWTH (MACRODACTYLY)

Macrodactyly is a rare congenital anomaly in which there is enlargement of the finger. Flatt found macrodactyly in only 19 of 1476 patients with congenital hand anomalies, an incidence of 0.9%. The index finger is involved most frequently. Macrodactyly does not appear to be an inherited condition. Although its cause is uncertain, three possible factors are strongly suspected: abnormal nerve supply, abnormal blood supply, and abnormal humoral mechanism. Some have postulated that macrodactyly is an aborted type of neurofibromatosis; however, other manifestations of this disease usually are not seen in these patients. Barsky described two types of true macrodactyly: static enlargement of the digit without progression as the child grows and progressive enlargement out of proportion to normal growth. The latter form may not enlarge during infancy but begins to enlarge rapidly during early childhood; this form frequently is associated with angular deformity. Macrodactyly most commonly exists without other conditions, but syndactyly is associated with macrodactyly in about 10% of patients. Some patients with neurofibromatosis will develop macrodactyly.

In static macrodactyly the deformity is present in infancy. There usually is diffuse enlargement of the digit; however, the distal and palmar tissues usually appear more enlarged than the dorsal and proximal tissues. The finger grows but in proportion to normal digital growth. Progressive macrodactyly occurs in early childhood as a rapidly enlarging digit, frequently with an angular deformity that makes the finger banana shaped (Fig. 4-46). The skin may be thickened and the nails hypertrophied. The phalanges always are involved, and the metacarpals may be enlarged as well. With maturity the enlarged digit begins to lose motion. Later in life symptoms of carpal tunnel syndrome may develop, with complaints of paresthesias and hypesthesias. Trophic ulcers also may develop over the involved digit. Involvement usually is unilateral, and multiple digits are affected two to three times as often as single digits. If the thumb is involved, a characteristic abduction and hyperextension deformity results. It generally is believed that all the tissues of the involved finger are enlarged; however, some have noted sparing of the tendons and vessels. The nerves that innervate the involved territory are characteristically enlarged. In a rare type of macrodactyly, which Kelikian called *hyperostotic variety,* there may be osteocartilaginous deposits around the joints.

Treatment

There are no satisfactory nonsurgical methods of controlling macrodactyly. Attempts to compress the digit with elastic wrapping have been unsuccessful. Indications for surgery include enlargement, angulation, carpal tunnel syndrome, and causalgia. For the progressively enlarging digit, a debulking procedure usually is needed. With this procedure as much excess tissue as possible is excised from one half the digit; 3 months later the other half is debulked. This procedure may be required several times during the growth period. Tsuge proposed that the disproportionate growth is a result of excessive neural input and recommended that the digital nerves be stripped

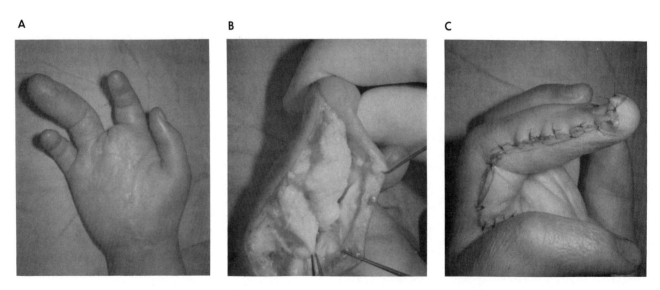

Fig. 4-46   **A,** Recurrent macrodactyly in 6-year-old child 2 years after debulking procedure of ring finger and amputation of middle finger. **B,** Intraoperative photograph shows enlargement of digital nerve. **C,** Wound closure after debulking.

of one half their fascicles at the time of debulking. He also recommended complete excision of the enlarged digital nerves during debulking as the most effective way of controlling progressive macrodactyly, believing that this causes only minimal neural impairment in children. Kelikian recommended segmental resection of the tortuous digital nerves with end-to-end repair.

Physeal arrest after the digit has reached estimated adult length also is frequently recommended. Clifford recommends drill holes through the physes, Jones recommends resection of the epiphyses, and Wood uses a high-speed drill for epiphysiodesis of all phalanges. Various methods of digital shortening also have been described, including simple amputation of the distal phalanx and filleting of the distal phalanx, with transfer of the nail and matrix onto the end of the middle phalanx, with or without some of the underlying distal phalanx. In the angulated finger, closing wedge osteotomies through either the proximal or middle phalanx are necessary for correction. Millesi described a complicated technique for shortening the enlarged thumb, in which parts of the distal and proximal phalanges are removed and the distal interphalangeal joint is preserved. Amputation is used only as a last resort in the adult with a severe and bothersome deformity, but it may be the only choice to provide relief.

The most common complication is recurrence, which is expected after debulking. Flap necrosis is a major surgical complication, and some have recommended excision of the overlying skin and replacement with a full-thickness skin graft to avoid this problem. Careful attention to flap design may help prevent skin necrosis. Operating on only one side of the finger at a time minimizes the risk of circulatory disturbance.

Debulking

▸ *Technique (Tsuge).* Under tourniquet control, make a midlateral incision the length of the involved digit. Identify and dissect out the digital nerve. Excise all excessive adipose tissue. If the digital nerve is grossly enlarged, half the fascicles may be stripped and excised as recommended by Tsuge. If the digital nerve is excessively tortuous, then a section may be resected and an end-to-end repair performed as described by Kelikian. Resect matching sections of the

volar half of the distal phalanx and the dorsal half of the middle phalanx (Fig. 4-47, *A*), and reduce the fragments (Fig. 4-47, *B*). Remove excessive skin, close the incision (Fig. 4-47, *C*), and apply a bulky hand dressing. No particular postoperative protection is required. Debulking of the opposite side of the digit can be performed 3 months after the first procedure.

Epiphysiodesis

▸ *Technique.* Under tourniquet control, make a midlateral incision the length of the entire finger. Identify the physes of the proximal, middle, and distal phalanges, and perform epiphysiodesis of these with a high-speed burr or curet and cautery. Close the incision, and apply a finger splint, which is worn for 3 weeks.

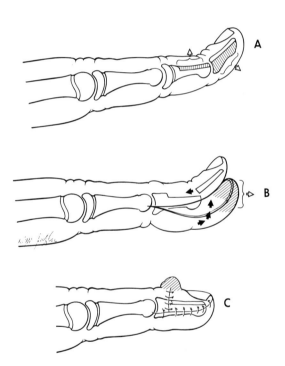

Fig. 4-47 Digital shortening for macrodactyly (Tsuge). **A,** Matching sections *(shaded areas)* of volar half of distal phalanx and dorsal half of middle phalanx are removed. **B,** Distal phalanx is reduced on middle phalanx, with preservation of dorsal skin bridge but removal of excess soft tissue. **C,** Soft tissue closure is completed, accepting some excess dorsal soft tissue. (Redrawn from Tsuge K: J Hand Surg 10A:968, 1985.)

Digital shortening

▶ *Technique.* Under tourniquet control, make an L-shaped incision beginning at the midlateral aspect of the proximal phalangeal joint and extending distally to a level just proximal to the germinal matrix (Fig. 4-48, *A*). Carry the incision transversely across the dorsum of the finger. Remove the distal half of the middle phalanx and the proximal part of the distal phalanx. Using a rongeur, sharpen the distal end of the remaining middle phalanx to a point to fit into the intramedullary canal of the distal phalanx (Fig. 4-48, *B*). Place the distal phalanx onto the middle phalanx, and fix it with a Kirschner wire to recess the finger (Fig. 4-48, *C*). Excess volar soft tissue can be removed at a later stage. Close the incision, and apply a finger splint to be worn for 3 weeks.

Thumb shortening

▶ *Technique (Millesi).* Under tourniquet control, excise the distal half of the nail and nail matrix, as well as the underlying distal phalangeal tuft (Fig. 4-49, *A*). Through a dorsal longitudinal incision overlying the middle and distal phalanx, remove the middle third of the distal phalanx and the middle third of the overlying nail and matrix. Next remove the middle third of the middle phalanx by performing parallel oblique osteotomies (Fig. 4-49, *B*). Reduce the two remaining longitudinal components of the distal phalanx, and pin them with a transverse Kirschner wire. Reduce the distal and proximal fragments of the middle phalanx in a shortened fashion, and pin them with an oblique Kirschner wire (Fig. 4-49, *C*). Close the wound by carefully approximating the skin edges as well as the nail matrix, leaving the Kirschner wires protruding through the skin. Apply a thumb splint.

▶ *Postoperative management.* The splint is worn for 3 weeks. The Kirschner wires are removed when the osteotomies are healed, usually by 4 to 6 weeks.

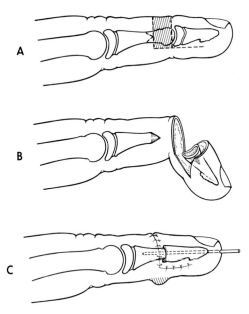

Fig. 4-48 Digital shortening for macrodactyly (Barsky). **A,** L-shaped midlateral and dorsal incisions allow removal of excess dorsal tissue and distal half of middle phalanx and proximal portion of distal phalanx *(shaded area).* **B,** Bone ends are prepared for pencil-cone reduction. **C,** Distal phalanx is reduced on middle phalanx and secured with Kirschner wire. (Redrawn from Barsky AJ: J Bone Joint Surg 49A:1255, 1967.)

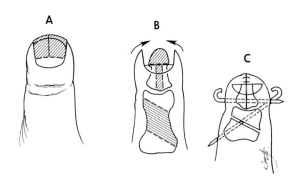

Fig. 4-49 Thumb reduction for macrodactyly (Millesi). **A,** Removal of distal half of nail and distal phalanx preserving eponychial tissue. **B,** Reduction osteotomies performed through dorsal incision. **C,** Remaining bone reduced and pinned. (Redrawn from Millesi H: Macrodactyly: a case study. In Littler JW et al: Symposium on reconstructive hand surgery, St Louis, 1974, The CV Mosby Co.)

UNDERGROWTH

Congenital hand anomalies classified as *undergrowth* deformities are those in which there is incomplete development, making the entire upper extremity or any of its parts smaller or deficient. Hypoplasia of digital parts often occurs with other deformities of the hand such as radial clubhand, syndactyly, and even macrodactyly. Its use as a separate category is best limited to those deformities that present a formed but deficient part without other anomalies.

Hypoplastic Thumb

The designation *hypoplastic thumb* generally applies to any thumb with some degree of deficiency in any of its anatomic parts—osseous, musculotendinous, or ectodermal. The thumb may be functional but simply shorter than normal or, in the most severe manifestation, totally absent. The hypoplastic thumb constituted 3.6% of anomalies in Flatt's series and 1.3% of the Yokohama series; hypoplasia of the whole hand represented 0.8% in Flatt's series and absence of the thumb, 1.4%. Because of the wide variety of deformities produced by hypoplasia of the thumb, etiologic factors also are varied. Many of these deformities are sporadic occurrences, but some are transmitted genetically or are associated with specific syndromes. The six types of hypoplastic thumb are based on the appearance of the deformity and the deficient structures. They include short thumb, adducted thumb, abducted thumb, floating thumb, absent thumb, and clasped thumb.

Short Thumb

The normal thumb extends to about the level of the proximal interphalangeal joint of the index finger; a thumb is considered "short" if its length is less than this. Hypoplasia of any or all osseous components produces a thumb that is significantly shorter than normal. The short thumb frequently is associated with other anomalies and syndromes. When the metacarpal is short and slender, it may be a manifestation of a syndrome such as Fanconi, Holt-Oram, or Juberg-Hayward; it also may be associated with other malformations of the spine and cardiovascular and gastrointestinal systems. When the metacarpal is short and broad, it may be associated with Cornelia de Lange syndrome, hand-foot-uterus syndrome, diastrophic dwarfism, or myositis ossificans progressiva. Shortening of the proximal phalanx of the thumb may be associated with brachydactyly. The distal phalanx may be broad and short in association with Rubinstein-Taybi, Apert, Carpenter, or hand-foot-uterus syndrome. The thumb may be radially deviated ("hitchhiker's thumb") or very short and stubby ("potter's thumb" or "murderer's thumb"). A slender distal phalanx may be associated with Fanconi or Holt-Oram syndrome.

Treatment. If the hypoplastic thumb is only short, surgical correction rarely is indicated. If prehension is significantly limited, deepening of the web space may be sufficient to create a relative lengthening of the thumb in relation to objects that are grasped. This may be achieved with a two- or four-limb Z-plasty.

Adducted Thumb

The adducted thumb usually is caused by absence or partial absence of the thenar muscles, which results in deficient opposition. Strauch and Spinner noted that these thumbs often lack a functional flexor pollicis longus muscle. The radial collateral ligament of the thumb metacarpophalangeal joint also may be deficient. The thumb usually is shortened and tapered, with a flattened thenar eminence and a deficient first web space. The deformity usually is transmitted as an autosomal dominant trait and usually is unilateral.

Treatment. The goals of surgical reconstruction of the adducted thumb are correction of the adduction contracture and restoration of opposition. The adduction contracture may be corrected by a two- or four-limb Z-plasty or a sliding dorsal flap raised from the radial side of the index finger. The two-limb Z-plasty rarely attains adequate correction. The two most popular techniques for restoration of opposition are the ring flexor superficialis tendon opponensplasty and the abductor digiti quinti opponensplasty, as described by Huber and popularized by Littler and Cooley. The Huber procedure allows creation of a more nearly normal-appearing thenar eminence. Littler also described the use of an abdominal flap (Fig. 4-50) for reconstruction of the adducted thumb.

Simple Z-plasty of the thumb web

▸ *Technique.* Before inflating the tourniquet, diagram the appropriate skin incision, designing the flap with its longitudinal axis along the distal ridge of the first web space and extending from the proximal thumb crease to approximately 1 cm proximal to the proximal digital crease of the index finger at a point that corresponds to the radial confluence of the proximal and middle palmar creases. Draw an oblique proximal palmar limb, as well as a distal dorsal limb, at an approximately 60-degree angle, with the lengths of both limbs corresponding to the longitudinal incision (Fig. 4-51, *A*). In designing these flaps, keep in mind the basic principle of all Z-plasty procedures: all flap sides must be of equal lengths. Now inflate the tourniquet, and make the appropriate incisions as outlined. Elevate the flaps sharply, carefully undermining to avoid vascular compromise. If additional depth is needed, sharply dissect the distal edge of the web space musculature to obtain a partial recession. Reverse the flaps and carefully suture them with interrupted 6-0 nylon sutures or absorbable skin sutures (Fig. 4-51, *B*). Mattress sutures may be used to help prevent tip necrosis. Deflate the tourniquet, check for adequate blood supply to the flaps, and apply a sterile dressing with the thumb splinted in the abducted, opposed position.

▸ *Postoperative management.* The splint and sutures are removed 2 weeks after surgery, and free use of the hand is allowed if healing has progressed adequately.

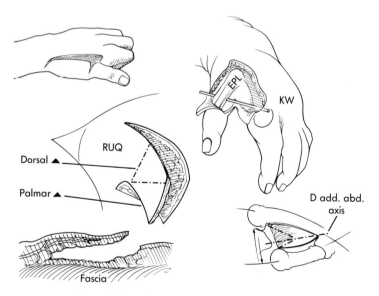

Fig. 4-50 Correction of adduction contracture of thumb using abdominal flap based on thoracoepigastric vessels. (Redrawn from Littler JW: Clin Orthop 13:182, 1959.)

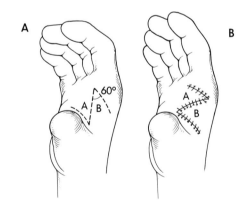

Fig. 4-51 Simple Z-plasty of thumb web. **A,** Incisions. **B,** Closure after reversal of flaps.

Four-limb Z-plasty

◣*Technique (modified from Broadbent and Woolf).* Before inflating the tourniquet, outline the flaps. Make the longitudinal axis of the Z-plasty along the distal edge of the thumb web ridge, extending from the ulnar margin of the proximal thumb crease to an area approximately 1 cm proximal to the proximal digital crease of the index finger. Draw proximal palmar and distal dorsal limbs at 90-degree angles to the longitudinal axis; the lengths of these limbs should equal that of the longitudinal incision (Fig. 4-52, *A*). Bisect each angle with an additional oblique limb, again with the length corresponding to the length of the other flap margins (Fig. 4-52, *B*). Then inflate the tourniquet and make the appropriate incisions. Sharply elevate the flaps, elevating the skin as well as a small amount of subcutaneous tissue. For further deepening, perform a small recession of the thumb web musculature in its midsubstance. Do not perform a complete myotomy. Interdigitate the appropriate flaps, and suture them with 6-0 monofilament nylon. It is helpful to label the flaps before incision; if labeled *1, 2, 3,* and *4,* beginning from the radialmost flap and ending at the ulnarmost flap, the sequence after interdigitation should be *3, 1, 4, 2,* (Fig. 4-52, *C*). Then deflate the tourniquet, inspect the flaps for viability, and apply a bulky dressing with the thumb splinted in the abducted position.

◣*Postoperative management.* The sutures and splint are removed 14 days after surgery. If desired, a small web-spacer splint may be used for an additional 2 weeks.

Web deepening with sliding flap

◣*Technique (Brand)* (Fig. 4-53). Before inflating the tourniquet, design the flaps by drawing a line dorsally from the apex of the first and second metacarpals and extending it distally to the radial side of the proximal phalanx of the index finger. Then curve the line back across the web space into the palm proximally to the apex of the first and second metacarpals. Exsanguinate the arm, inflate the tourniquet, and make the skin incisions as outlined. Sharply elevate the skin flaps with a small amount of subcutaneous tissue. Release any thickened dorsal and volar fascia carefully to avoid injury to the neurovascular structures. If severe contracture is present, incise the capsule of the carpometacarpal joint of the thumb. Pull the thumb away from the palm, and hold it with a Kirschner wire. Allow the flap to slide with the thumb, and use it to cover the thumb and palmar web. Cover the dorsal defect with a split-thickness skin graft. Suture the flaps in place with interrupted 6-0 nylon sutures, and secure and bolster the skin graft. Deflate the tourniquet, inspect the flaps for via-

bility, and apply a sterile dressing with the thumb splinted in the abducted position.

◣*Postoperative management.* Sutures are removed at 2 weeks and the Kirschner wire at 4 weeks, after which unrestricted motion of the thumb is allowed.

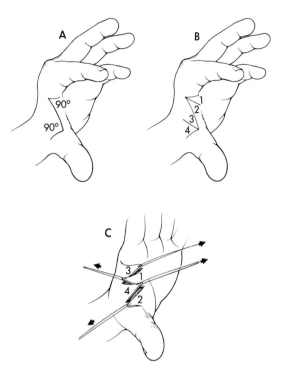

Fig. 4-52   Four-flap Z-plasty for lengthening first web in adducted thumb. **A,** Ninety-degree dorsal and volar flaps are marked in first web. **B,** These are then bisected to create four flaps. **C,** Flaps are elevated, transposed, and interdigitated to complete lengthening. (Redrawn from Woolf RM and Broadbent TR: Plast Reconstr Surg 49:48, 1972.)

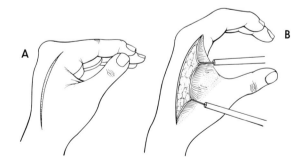

Fig. 4-53   Dorsal sliding flap for correction of adduction deformity of first web. **A,** Incision. **B,** Radial flap is undermined and dorsal defect is covered with split-thickness skin graft.

Ring sublimis opponensplasty

▶ *Technique (Riordan).* Expose the sublimis tendon of the ring finger through an ulnar midlateral incision over the proximal interphalangeal joint, and divide the tendon at the level of the joint or just proximal to it. Divide the chiasm, thus separating the two slips of tendon at the level of the joint so that they will pass around the profundus and can be easily withdrawn at the wrist. Now expose the flexor carpi ulnaris tendon through an L-shaped incision that extends proximally along the flexor carpi ulnaris tendon and distally turns radialward parallel to the flexor creases of the wrist. To make a pulley, cut halfway through the flexor carpi ulnaris tendon at a point approximately 6.3 cm proximal to the pisiform (Fig. 4-54). Then strip the radial half of the tendon distally almost to the pisiform and create a loop large enough for the sublimis tendon to pass through easily; carry the end of the radial segment of the flexor carpi ulnaris through a split in the remaining half of the tendon, loop it back, and suture it to the remaining half. Now make a wide C-shaped incision on the thumb as follows. Begin on the dorsum of the thumb just proximal to the interphalangeal joint, and proceed proximally and volarward around to the radial aspect of the thumb. At a point just proximal to the metacarpophalangeal joint curve the incision dorsalward in line with the major skin creases of the thenar eminence. Preserve on the dorsoradial aspect of the thumb the fine sensory nerve from the superficial branch of the radial nerve. Expose and define the extensor pollicis longus tendon over the proximal phalanx, the extensor aponeurosis over the metacarpophalangeal joint, and the tendon of the abductor pollicis brevis. Now at the wrist identify the sublimis tendon to the ring finger and withdraw it into the forearm incision. Pass the tendon through the loop fashioned from the flexor carpi ulnaris. Then, with a small hemostat or a tendon carrier, pass the tendon subcutaneously across the thenar eminence in line with the fibers of the abductor pollicis brevis.

Now make a small tunnel for insertion of the transfer by burrowing between two small parallel incisions in the abductor pollicis brevis tendon. Split the end of the sublimis tendon for approximately 2.5 cm, or more if necessary, and pass one half of it through the tunnel. Now separate the extensor aponeurosis from the periosteum of the proximal phalanx of the thumb, make a small incision in it 6 mm distal to the first tunnel, and pass the same strip of sublimis through it. Bring the slip out from beneath the aponeurosis through a small longitudinal slit in the long extensor tendon about 3 mm proximal to the interphalangeal joint.

Now determine the proper tension for the transfer. Grasp the two slips of sublimis with small hemostats and cross them. With the thumb in full opposition and the wrist in a straight line, place the two overlapping slips of sublimis under some tension. Releasing the thumb and passively flexing the wrist should completely relax the transfer so that the thumb can be brought into full extension and abduction; extending the wrist 45 degrees should place enough tension on the transfer to bring the thumb into complete opposition and the tip of the thumb into complete extension. If the tension is insufficient, increase it and repeat the test. When the correct tension has been determined, suture the slips of sublimis together with the cut ends buried (Fig. 4-54, *inset*). Now anchor the transfer and the tendon of the abductor pollicis brevis to the joint capsule with a single nylon or wire suture so that the transfer passes over the exact middle of the metacarpal head; this prevents later displacement of the tendon toward the palmar aspect of the joint during opposition. Close the wound with nonabsorbable sutures, and immobilize the hand in a pressure dressing and a dorsal plaster splint as follows. Place the wrist in 30 degrees flexion, the fingers in the functional position, and the thumb in full opposition with the distal phalanx extended; place a few layers of gauze between the individual fingers to prevent maceration of the skin.

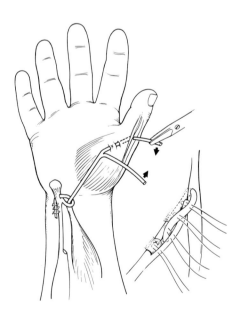

Fig. 4-54 Opponensplasty of ring sublimis for adduction contracture of thumb (see text).

◣ *Postoperative management.* At 3 weeks the dressing and splint are removed and active motion is begun, but the thumb is supported with an opponens splint for an additional 6 weeks. Many patients can oppose the thumb as soon as the splint is removed. When the sublimis of the ring finger has been used for the transfer, as in the Riordan technique, training in its use may be facilitated by asking the patient to place the tip of the thumb against the ring finger; this maneuver produces flexion of the ring finger and an automatic attempt to oppose the thumb with the transferred sublimis. In patients with weak quadriceps muscles who habitually rise from a sitting position by pushing up with the flattened hands or in patients who use crutches, the transfer must be protected for 3 months or longer, or it will be overstretched and cease to function.

Abductor digiti quinti opponensplasty

◣ *Technique (Huber; Littler and Cooley).* Make a curved palmar incision along the radial border of the abductor digiti quinti muscle belly extending from the proximal side of the pisiform proximally to the ulnar border of the little finger distally. Free both tendinous insertions of the muscle, one from the extensor expansion and the other from the base of the proximal phalanx. Lift the muscle from its fascial compartment, and carefully expose its neurovascular bundle. Isolate the bundle, taking care not to damage the veins. Next free the origin of the muscle from the pisiform, but retain the origin on the flexor carpi ulnaris tendon; now the muscle can be mobilized enough for its insertion to reach the thumb. Make a curved incision on the radial border of the thenar eminence, and create across the palm a subcutaneous pocket to receive the transfer. Now fold the abductor digiti quinti muscle over about 170 degrees (like a page of a book) and pass it subcutaneously to the thumb. Suture its tendons of insertion to the insertion of the abductor pollicis brevis. Throughout the procedure avoid compression of and undue tension on the muscle and its neurovascular pedicle. Apply a carefully formed light compression dressing and then a volar plaster splint to hold the thumb in abduction and the wrist in slight flexion.

Abducted Thumb

The abducted thumb deformity was described in 1919 by Tupper who reported four patients with mildly hypoplastic thumbs and associated abduction deformities. He called this *pollex abductus* and believed it resulted from an abnormal insertion of the flexor pollicis longus muscle into an otherwise normal extensor pollicis longus muscle, causing marked abduction of the proximal phalanx of the thumb. This

was verified at the time of reconstruction, when he also noted deficiencies in the thenar musculature, adduction contracture of the first metacarpal with web space deficiency, marked laxity of the ulnar collateral ligament, radial and superficial displacement of the flexor pollicis longus, and inability to flex the interphalangeal joint of the thumb. This is an extremely rare deformity, and since the first report only five more cases have been reported.

Treatment. There have been almost as many surgical procedures described for the abducted thumb as there have been cases reported: release of the bifurcated tendon insertion and reattachment to the metacarpal neck; release of the tendon distally, withdrawal at the wrist, and reattachment to the distal phalanx; and release of the anomalous slip to the extensor pollicis longus muscle, with an ulnarward shift of the extensor pollicis longus at the metacarpophalangeal joint. All procedures have been combined with release of the radial collateral ligament and reefing of the ulnar collateral ligament of the metacarpophalangeal joint, and some have required a secondary opponensplasty. Blair and Omer described a technique in which the flexor pollicis longus is released from its abnormal tendinous insertion and centralized by moving it ulnarward. To complete the transfer the abductor pollicis brevis musculotendinous junction is divided, the flexor pollicis longus tendon is transferred under the intrinsic muscle, and the intrinsic muscle is reattached. They did not find it necessary to reconstruct the ulnar collateral ligament. For severe web space contracture Bayne recommends a staged procedure in which the web space is first released and maintained with a Kirschner wire (Fig. 4-55) followed in 6 weeks by a Riordan opponensplasty that uses the ring sublimis and by reconstruction of the ulnar collateral ligament that uses one slip of the sublimis.

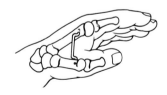

Fig. 4-55 Staged reconstruction for abducted thumb in which adduction contracture is released and maintained with interposed Kirschner wire; this may be followed in 6 weeks by reconstruction of ulnar collateral ligament and ring sublimis opponensplasty. (Redrawn from Dobyns JH, Wood VE, and Bayne LG: Congenital hand deformities. In Green DP, editor: Operative hand surgery, ed 2, New York, 1988, Churchill Livingstone.)

▶ *Technique (Blair and Omer).* Under tourniquet control, make a zig-zag palmar incision along the thumb to allow exploration of the flexor pollicis longus, the ulnar collateral ligament, and the extensor pollicis longus. Develop the flaps, and identify and protect the digital nerves. Identify the abnormal tendinous slip of the flexor pollicis longus that passes over the radial border of the thumb and into the extensor pollicis longus, usually between the metacarpophalangeal joint and the interphalangeal joint. Release this abnormal insertion sharply. Release the insertion of the abductor pollicis brevis (Fig. 4-56, *A*). Transfer the flexor pollicis longus tendon ulnarly under the abductor pollicis brevis tendon (Fig. 4-56, *B*). If the abduction deformity of the thumb metacarpophalangeal joint cannot be corrected, release the radial collateral ligament. Suture the abductor pollicis

brevis tendon into its normal insertion (Fig. 4-56, *C*). This technique centralizes the flexor pollicis longus and constructs a sling at the metacarpophalangeal joint. If there is continued laxity of the ulnar collateral ligament of the thumb metacarpophalangeal joint, use the abnormal tendon slip to reinforce the ligament. Suture the skin with simple interrupted sutures, and apply a modified thumb spica cast that extends beyond the interphalangeal joint dorsally and stops proximal to the metacarpophalangeal joint on the volar side. This prevents hyperextension and abduction of the thumb but allows metacarpophalangeal flexion and flexor tendon excursion.

▶ *Postoperative management.* The cast is removed at 6 weeks, and unlimited motion of the hand is allowed.

Floating Thumb (Pouce Flottant)

Floating thumb refers to a small, slender thumb that appears to dangle from the radial border of the hand. Typically there are two phalanges, a fingernail, no metacarpophalangeal joint, and no first metacarpal (Fig. 4-57). The trapezium and scaphoid also often are absent. The thumb takes origin somewhat more distally than usual, and there is neither extrinsic nor intrinsic muscle function.

Treatment. Amputation is the treatment of choice, followed by index finger pollicization. Despite gallant attempts to restore stability and function to these severely deficient and useless thumbs, the results have not been as rewarding as with pollicization. In bilateral cases, pollicization of one side should be performed early; the parents then may decide concerning the other side.

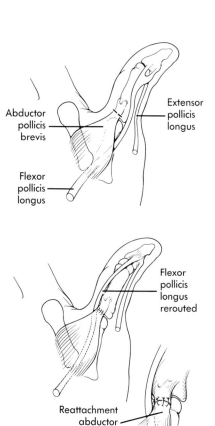

Fig. 4-56 Rerouting of flexor pollicis longus for abducted thumb (see text). Flexor pollicis is centralized after tenotomy and reattachment of abductor pollicis brevis. (Redrawn from Blair W and Omer G: J Hand Surg 6:241, 1981.)

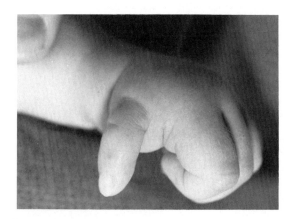

Fig. 4-57 Floating thumb (pouce flottant) deformity.

Absent Thumb

This is the most severe manifestation of the hypoplastic thumb and may be associated with radial ray deficiencies, ring D chromosome abnormalities, Holt-Oram syndrome, trisomy 18 syndrome, Rothmund-Thomson syndrome, and thalidomide use. Radial clubhand also is associated with an absent thumb except in the thrombocytopenia–absent radius (TAR) syndrome. Absence of the thumb creates an extreme functional impairment, particularly if bilateral. The development of a strong lateral pinch between the index and long fingers compensates for the absence of the thumb, and a fairly strong grip may be developed. Rotational deformity of the fingers allows limited opposition.

Treatment. Function and appearance can be improved with satisfactory pollicization of the index finger. The timing of pollicization is based on the child's natural development of prehensile activities. Because this develops early, beginning at the age of 3 months, the best time for pollicization is between the ages of 6 and 12 months to allow some growth of the hand before surgery. The choice of procedure usually is between recession or pollicization of the index finger. Recession is preferable in the older child with a strong lateral pinch between index and long fingers because this pattern may persist despite pollicization. This operation recesses the index finger to make it more resemble a thumb and provides a wider gap between the index and long fingers.

Recession of the index finger

▶ *Technique (Flatt).* Under tourniquet control, make a dorsal longitudinal 1-cm incision in the first web space. Divide the deep transverse metacarpal ligament, palmar and dorsal fascia, and intertendinous connections between the index and middle finger metacarpals. Take care to avoid injury to the neurovascular structures. Make a second short, curved dorsoradial incision at the base of the index metacarpal. Expose the base of the index metacarpal, and perform an osteotomy (Fig. 4-58, *A*). The metacarpal now may be easily grasped and maneuvered. Reposition the metacarpal into 20 degrees of radial abduction, 35 degrees of palmar abduction, and 100 to 110 degrees of axial rotation (Fig. 4-58, *B*). Recess the metacarpal by removing 1.5 to 2 cm of the metacarpal shaft. When the desired position and recession are achieved, pass a Kirschner wire into adjacent metacarpals to fix the index metacarpal in this position. Close the incision routinely (Fig. 4-58, *C*), and apply a well-padded, long-arm cast that holds the repositioned index finger in abduction.

▶ *Postoperative management.* The cast is changed 2 weeks after the operation, and the skin sutures are removed. A long-arm cast that supports the pollicized index finger is applied and worn for 4 more weeks. The Kirschner wire is removed when bone healing is complete, usually 4 to 6 weeks after the operation, and progressively increasing activities are allowed. The thumb is splinted in a resting position for another 4 to 6 weeks.

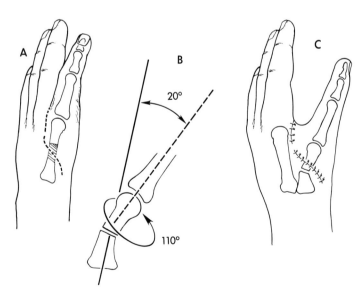

Fig. 4-58 Recession of index finger. **A,** Two incisions are required: intermetacarpal ligament is cut through distal incision, and osteotomy of index metacarpal is performed through proximal incision. **B,** Distal portion of index is rotated 110 degrees and abducted 20 degrees palmarward. **C,** Skin closure. (Redrawn from Flatt AE: The care of congenital hand anomalies, St Louis, 1977, The CV Mosby Co.)

Congenital Clasped Thumb

Congenital clasped thumb is an unusual condition in which the thumb is positioned in adduction and extreme flexion at the metacarpophalangeal joint. Underlying hypoplasia or absence of the extensor pollicis brevis muscle is usual, and the extensor pollicis brevis or extensor pollicis longus may be absent. Some degree of total thumb hypoplasia may be present. This may be an isolated deformity, or it may be associated with clubfoot deformities and several well-defined syndromes. There is no single cause, but the deformity results from an imbalance between the flexors and extensors of the thumb. Weckesser et al called this deformity a syndrome and classified it into four distinct types on the basis of etiologic factors: group 1, deficient extension only; group 2, flexion contracture combined with deficient extension; group 3, hypoplasia of the thumb, including tendon and muscle deficiencies; and group 4, those deformities that do not easily fit any of the other three categories. Group 1 syndrome appears to be transmitted as a sex-linked recessive gene because it is more common in boys and frequently is bilateral.

At birth the thumb usually is flexed into the palm, with the deformity typically located at the metacarpophalangeal joint, unlike trigger thumb deformity. During the first few weeks of life it is typical for an infant to clutch the thumb, but normally the thumb is released intermittently. If no active extension at the metacarpophalangeal joint is demonstrated after prolonged observation and particularly by the age of 3 months, the diagnosis of congenital clasped thumb is established.

Nonsurgical management. Most clasped thumb deformities are deficiencies of extension only (group 1) and usually respond to early splinting in extension and abduction. Weckesser et al recommend the use of a plaster splint, which is changed every 6 weeks and continued for 3 to 6 months. The long-term results of this protocol appear satisfactory if the initial response to splinting is good. If at the end of 3 to 6 months of splinting there is no evidence of active extension of the metacarpophalangeal joint, further splinting will probably not be beneficial. This lack of response to splinting usually indicates that the extrinsic extensors are extremely deficient (the usual case) or totally absent and that a tendon transfer is required to restore function.

Surgical treatment. Useful donor tendons for an inadequate extensor pollicis longus muscle are the palmaris longus, brachioradialis, extensor carpi radialis longus, extensor indicis proprius, and flexor superficialis muscles. The extensor pollicis longus is an ideal motor muscle, but it may be absent as well. Flatt prefers to use the brachioradialis with a tendon graft.

The extensor pollicis brevis muscle may be replaced with the extensor indicis proprius muscle. Significant web space contracture also may require reconstruction.

For group 3 deformities with significant hypoplasia of the thenar muscles and abductor pollicis longus and instability of the metacarpophalangeal joint, Neviaser recommends a single-stage operation involving chondrodesis of the metacarpophalangeal joint, replacement of the extensor pollicis longus with the extensor indicis proprius, replacement of the abductor pollicis longus with the palmaris longus, and a Huber opponensplasty (p. 311). Web space reconstruction usually is necessary in these patients. With this protocol Neviaser obtained useful grasp and pinch in eight patients with no complications, despite the magnitude of the surgery. These procedures should be performed after the first year of life and before the child reaches school age.

Group 2 clasped thumb deformity

▶ ***Technique.*** Stage 1 is release of web space contracture, which is performed as described on p. 308. Stage II is restoration of thumb extension (Fig. 4-59) with the use of the extensor indicis proprius.

Under tourniquet control, make a short transverse incision at the base of the index metacarpal and locate the extensor indicis proprius tendon. Divide the tendon at its confluence with the extensor hood. Next make a short transverse incision over the dorsum of the wrist in line with the extensor indicis proprius

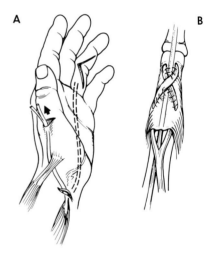

Fig. 4-59 Littler's technique for correction of congenital clasped thumb. **A,** Path of transferred tendon. **B,** Suture of transferred tendon. (Redrawn from Crawford HH, Horton CE, and Adamson JE: J Bone Joint Surg 48A:82, 1966.)

tendon and withdraw the tendon into this wound. Make a bayonet-shaped incision over the dorsoulnar aspect of the thumb centered over the metacarpophalangeal joint. Identify the extensor pollicis longus tendon if present, and retract it to one side. Create a tunnel through the base of the proximal phalanx from the ulnar aspect to the radial aspect distal to the physis. Reroute the tendon of the extensor indicis proprius subcutaneously from the wrist to the base of the thumb, passing it through the osseous tunnel and suturing it back on itself. If the extensor pollicis longus is absent or severely deficient, choose either the flexor digitorum sublimis to the ring finger or the brachioradialis, with a palmaris longus tendon graft for the donor muscle. If the flexor digitorum sublimis is selected, make a transverse incision at the base of the ring finger on the palmar aspect and release the sublimis tendon just proximal to Camper's chiasm. Make a short longitudinal incision over the palmar aspect of the wrist proximal to the flexion crease, and identify the ring sublimis tendon (Fig. 4-59, *A*). Deliver the sublimis tendon into this wound, reroute it subcutaneously around the radial border of the wrist deep to the abductor pollicis longus tendon, and suture it into the remnants of the extensor pollicis longus at the distal phalanx (Fig. 4-59, *B*). If there is no distal tendon in which to suture the donor, create a periosteal flap to anchor the distal insertion of the tendon. Fix the thumb in extension with Kirschner wire, close the incision in routine fashion, and apply a splint with the thumb in extension and abduction.

▶ *Postoperative management.* Six weeks after surgery the Kirschner wire is removed. The hand is held in a plaster splint for an additional 2 months. Some type of thumb support, such as a removable splint, should be continued for about 4 months before unrestricted activity is allowed.

Group 3 clasped thumb deformity

▶ *Technique (modified from Neviaser).* Under tourniquet control, make a dorsal incision over the thumb metacarpophalangeal and interphalangeal joints (Fig. 4-60, *A*). If the metacarpophalangeal joints are unstable to both radial and ulnar stresses, perform a dorsal capsulotomy and identify the articular surfaces of the metacarpal and proximal phalanx. Shave the articular cartilage with a scalpel to expose the epiphyseal bone, and pin the joint with a Kirschner wire. Next make a short transverse dorsal incision at the base of the index finger to expose the extensor indicis proprius tendon. Make a transverse dorsal incision over the wrist in line with the tendon, divide the tendon distally, and deliver it into the wound (Fig. 4-60, *B*). Reroute the tendon subcutaneously, and suture it into

the soft tissue around the base of the distal phalanx or beneath a periosteal flap. Now make a short transverse palmar incision at the wrist over the palmaris longus tendon. Divide this tendon at its insertion into the palmar fascia, and route it subcutaneously, passing it through an osseous tunnel created at the base of the thumb proximal phalanx just distal to the physis; suture the tendon back on itself (Fig. 4-60, *C*). Next perform an opponensplasty as described on p. 311, perform a Z-plasty reconstruction of the web space contracture (p. 309), and derotate the thumb metacarpal if necessary by sharply incising the capsule of the trapeziometacarpal joint and pronating the thumb 90 degrees. Fix this with a Kirschner wire. Close the incisions in routine fashion, and apply a splint with the thumb in the corrected position.

▶ *Postoperative management.* The Kirschner wires are removed 6 weeks after surgery, and progressive motion is allowed. The thumb is protected in a night splint for another 3 to 4 weeks.

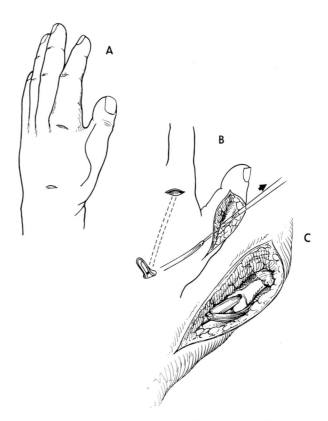

Fig. 4-60   Transfer of extensor indicis proprius for absent extensor pollicis brevis. **A,** Incisions. **B,** Extensor indicis proprius is passed through bony tunnel in proximal phalanx of thumb and, **C,** sutured to itself. (Redrawn from Dobyns JH, Wood VE, and Bayne LG: Congenital hand deformities. In Green DP, editor: Operative hand surgery, ed 2, New York, 1988, Churchill Livingstone.)

Hypoplastic Hands and Digits

Hypoplastic hands or digits are those in which there is defective or incomplete development of the part. Like syndactyly, elements of hypoplasia are seen in almost all hand deformities, and this term is best limited to those fingers and hands in which there is relatively symmetric deficiency of the part without associated deformity. Hypoplasia of the entire hand accounted for 0.8% of the deformities in the Iowa series and brachydactyly ("short fingers"), 5.2%. The single most commonly hypoplastic bony segment is the middle phalanx (brachyphalangia or brachymesophalangia). Brachymetacarpia ("short metacarpal") also is included with the hypoplastic deformities if present early, but this is extremely rare and usually is not noted until after the adolescent growth spurt.

Brachydactyly has played an important role in the genetic literature as the first example of mendelian inheritance demonstrated in human beings. Shortening of the fingers usually is considered a dominant trait, but further genetic variations also have been described. If a person with brachydactyly marries a normal individual, about half their offspring will have brachydactyly. Sporadic cases do occur, but no specific etiologic factor has been identified.

Brachyphalangia usually occurs alone, but it may occur in association with similar toe deformities. Shortening of the middle phalanges is common in malformation syndromes such as Treacher Collins, Bloom, Cornelia de Lange, Holt-Oram, Silver, and Poland syndromes. In Poland syndrome the shortening usually is unilateral. Brachydactyly E, as defined by Bell, consists of brachymetacarpia of the long, ring, and little fingers in association with pseudohypoparathyroidism. Other conditions associated with brachymetacarpia include the syndromes of Turner, Biemond, and Silver.

There is no useful classification for the hypoplastic hand or digits. Geneticists have devised several detailed groupings of this disorder in an attempt to better record patterns of inheritance, but for the most part these serve no useful purpose in determining management of the deformities.

Hypoplasia of the digits may range from simple shortening (most common) to a small hand with nothing more than nubbins for fingers. In some patients this may represent an intermediate entity between congenital amputation and hypoplastic digits. There usually is some degree of hypoplasia of all tissues, not just the osseous structures. Except for the nubbinlike fingers, function usually is near normal. Brachymetacarpia usually is noted during the teenage growth spurt as a depression of one or more metacarpal heads with the fist clenched. The ulnar two fingers are most commonly affected.

Nonsurgical Management

Single-digit shortening, particularly of the little finger, requires no surgical correction. Although a single short digit surrounded by digits of normal length may be cosmetically unsatisfactory, functional limitation usually is minimal and digital lengthening will not improve function and may result in stiffness.

Surgical Treatment

Lengthening procedures have been recommended for brachymetacarpia to improve appearance of the metacarpal row and increase grip strength. Wood found that more than 1 cm of shortening may disrupt the metacarpal arch and cause decreased grip strength. Tajima described a single-stage lengthening using a V-shaped metacarpal osteotomy with an interpositional bone graft. Buck-Gramcko detaches the interossei and intermetacarpal ligaments at the time of osteotomy (Fig. 4-61). Despite success with lengthening procedures, these should be discouraged for the adult patient whose only concern is the appearance of the hand.

For the hypoplastic hand with no functioning digits or preservation of only one digit, consideration may be given to more complex and less predictable procedures, but this is a controversial area of reconstructive hand surgery. It generally is accepted that, with

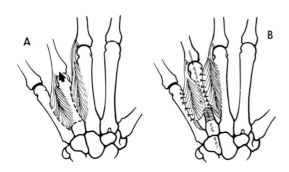

Fig. 4-61 Buck-Gramcko technique for lengthening brachymetacarpia in the hypoplastic hand. **A,** Detachment of interossei and intermetacarpal ligaments and metacarpal osteotomy. **B,** Interposition bone graft fixed with Kirschner wire. (Redrawn from Dobyns JH, Wood VE, and Bayne LG: Congenital hand deformities. In Green DP, editor: Operative hand surgery, ed 2, New York, 1988, Churchill Livingstone.)

the exception of the soft tissue nubbin, any digit regardless of size will be of some use to the patient. The musculotendinous structures in these fingers usually are extremely deficient, with little if any excursion. Added length created by distraction techniques or web deepening may produce a sense of improved function. A one-stage, nonvascularized, toe-phalanx transplantation as an interpositional or terminal graft may be beneficial for the extremely hypoplastic digit. Even if the periosteum and physis are preserved, growth of the transferred phalanx does not continue. The 1970 report of Matev of an average 3.3 cm lengthening of the thumb metacarpal in three adult patients with traumatic amputations sparked interest in the use of similar techniques for lengthening the severely hypoplastic digit. The usual technique includes division of the metacarpal bone and periosteum, application of external fixation, and gradual distraction of approximately 1 mm/day until the desired length is achieved or neurovascular or cutaneous limits are reached. Cowen and Loftus reported lengthening of the entire palm through the carpometacarpal joints with the use of distal metacarpal and proximal carpal pins. Although the usual length achieved is from 25 to 50 mm, Cowen and Loftus reported gaining as much as 7 cm. Ilizarov also has reported lengthening of hand and forearm bones with his distraction apparatus. Lengthening within a digit should be avoided; the shortest bone to which the device can be applied is about 3 cm.

Metacarpal lengthening

◣ *Technique (Tajima)* (Fig. 4-62). Under tourniquet control, make a dorsal longitudinal incision over the shortened metacarpal. Retract the extensor tendon to one side, and expose the metacarpal shaft subperiosteally. Perform two V-shaped osteotomies at the junction of the proximal and middle thirds of the bone. Expose the deep transverse metacarpal ligament distally and incise it. Sharply detach the interosseous muscle on both sides of the metacarpal. Now manually distract the metacarpal to ensure that the osteotomies are adequate. Harvest the iliac crest bone graft, and fashion it to fill the gap in the lengthened bone. Insert the graft, and secure it with a longitudinal Kirschner wire. Reattach the interosseous muscle to the periosteum through separate drill holes into either the bone graft or the metacarpal, depending on where the interosseous muscle falls into place after lengthening. Suture the skin in routine fashion, and apply a cast or splint.

◣ *Postoperative management.* The osteotomy is protected with a cast or splint until union occurs, but motion of the finger is begun 3 weeks after surgery. The Kirschner wire may be removed at 6 weeks.

Toe-phalanx transplantation

◣ *Technique.* Under tourniquet control, make a dorsal longitudinal incision over the second toe, which usually is excessively long and is the donor of choice; similar grafts may be harvested from the third or fourth toes if desired. Carry the incision through the skin, subcutaneous tissue, and extensor mechanism. Harvest the proximal phalanx, including the periosteum, as described by Goldberg and Watson, in an attempt to retain physeal growth. Close the donor site with simple sutures. The cartilage over each end of the donor phalanx may or may not be retained, depending on whether some pseudojoint function is desirable. Make a dorsal longitudinal incision over the hypoplastic digit, which may be represented only by an empty skin tube. Place the toe phalanx within the hypoplastic digit in axial alignment with the adjacent bone, and secure it with a longitudinal Kirschner wire. This may be used as an interpositional graft or terminal graft. Close the skin with interrupted sutures, and apply a supportive dressing. After the digit viability is certain, apply a cast of appropriate length.

◣ *Postoperative management.* The cast is maintained for approximately 6 weeks. Kirschner wires are removed, and activities are gradually increased.

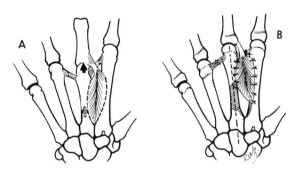

Fig. 4-62 Tajima technique for metacarpal lengthening in hypoplastic hand. **A,** Chevron osteotomy is made in shortened metacarpal; interosseous muscle and transverse metacarpal ligaments are released. **B,** Bone graft is interposed and secured with axial Kirschner wire; transverse metacarpal ligaments are repaired if possible. (Redrawn from Dobyns JH, Wood VE, and Bayne LG: Congenital hand deformities. In Green DP, editor: Operative hand surgery, ed 2, New York, 1988, Churchill Livingstone.)

Lengthening with distraction

▲ *Technique (Cowen and Loftus; stage I).* Under tourniquet control, make a Z-type incision on the dorsum of the hand and perform an osteotomy of the involved metacarpal or metacarpals. Manually distract the bone to ensure complete release of the soft tissues. Insert a transverse 0.062-inch Kirschner wire through the metacarpal distal to the osteotomy site. Insert this wire into the rectangular blocks of the distraction device. Using the device as a drill guide, place two additional Kirschner wires transversely through the metacarpal if possible. Use the same technique to insert the proximal wires. Release the tourniquet, and observe circulation. Make a few turns of the distraction device. Close the incision in routine fashion. If complete closure is not possible after distraction, the open portion of the incision may be allowed to granulate or may be covered with a split-thickness graft.

▲ *Postoperative management.* The patient is kept in the hospital for a few days after the procedure for careful observation. The patient or parents are instructed to increase the distraction by one third of a turn three times daily or one half turn twice daily. This amounts to approximately 1 mm of lengthening per day. This process is continued until the desired length is achieved and may require as much as 3 months. Close observation by the surgeon and the family during this process is mandatory to recognize any neurovascular compromise. When desired lengthening is obtained or neurovascular or cutaneous limits have been reached, the second stage of the procedure is performed.

▲ *Technique (stage II).* Make a dorsal incision over the metacarpal or metacarpals that are to be grafted. Harvest donor bone graft from the iliac crest, ulna, fibula, or toe phalanx, and insert this into the bony defect created by distraction. Stabilize the graft with a longitudinal Kirschner wire or leave the external fixator in place. Close the incision, deflate the tourniquet, and apply a short-arm cast with a protective plaster bow in older children or a long-arm cast in infants.

▲ *Postoperative management.* After 1 to 2 weeks the cast is replaced by a sling or wrap that covers the entire hand and distraction device. The apparatus and Kirschner wires are removed when sufficient time has passed to allow bone healing, usually after 8 or more weeks. The hand is protected with a cast or splint as needed, depending on the roentgenographic and clinical progress.

CONGENITAL RING SYNDROME

Congenital ring syndrome or congenital constriction band syndrome occurs when deep cutaneous creases encircle a limb as if a string were tightly tied around the part (Fig. 4-63). Its frequent association with congenital amputations and acrosyndactyly led to this malformation's designation as a syndrome. Other terms used to describe this condition include Streeter bands or dysplasia, annular grooves or defects, and intrauterine amputation. Patterson reported an incidence of 1:15,000 births. Constriction bands represented 2.0% of anomalies in Flatt's series. The more distal rings are more common, as is involvement of the central digits.

There is no evidence that congenital ring syndrome is an inherited condition. Kino believes the cause to be an external effect of amniotic adhesions formed in utero after hemorrhages in the distal rays. Patterson and Streeter theorize failure of development of subcutaneous tissue in the same manner that normal skin creases are formed. There is general agreement that these malformations occur somewhat later than 5 to 7 weeks' gestation when the majority of hand anomalies occur. The youngest fetus described by Potter was at 10 weeks of gestation.

Patterson includes four types of deformity in constriction ring syndrome: (1) a simple ring usually occurring transversely, but occasionally obliquely, around the limb or digit, (2) a deeper ring often associated with abnormality of the part distally, usually lymphedema, (3) fenestrated syndactyly (acrosyndactyly) or lateral fusion of adjacent digits at their distal ends with proximal fenestrations between the in-

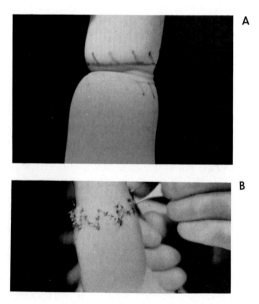

Fig. 4-63   A, Congenital ring syndrome in 3-month-old child. **B,** Z-plasty's release of constrictures.

tervening skin and soft tissue, and (4) intrauterine amputation in which the soft tissues are more affected than the bone, which may protrude as in a guillotine amputation; there are no rudimentary parts distally and the proximal limb parts are normally developed. These four types may be present in any combination in a single child, but they do not occur constantly with any other type of anomaly of the limbs. Syndactyly, hypoplasia, brachydactyly, symphalangism, symbrachydactyly, and camptodactyly have been reported in up to 80% of patients with congenital ring syndrome, and clubfoot, cleft lip, cleft palate, and cranial defects in 40% to 50%. Generally, there are no associated visceral malformations, but one of Flatt's patients had a patent ductus arteriosus.

These malformations usually are asymmetric. The grooves or rings vary in circumferential extent and depth and at times appear as normal but misplaced skin creases. Lymphedema distal to the crease is frequent. With shallow rings the skin often is normal but subcutaneous tissue usually is deficient. With deeper rings the superficial blood vessels that run across the ring are absent although deep vessels are intact. Digits distal to the rings may be shortened or completely amputated. Terminal simple syndactyly with small fenestrations through the proximal web is frequent; Miura reported acrosyndactyly in 26 of 55 patients with congenital constriction band syndrome. The rings are not static in their effect. If the ring is deep and unrelenting, there may be progressive necrosis beneath the ring, with increased scarring, constriction, and vascular impairment. In 58% of Flatt's patients distal lymphedema, cyanosis, and worsening at the site of constriction occurred before surgical intervention. Rarely does the ring progress to cause frank necrosis of the distal part.

Treatment

For very shallow, incomplete creases with no distal lymphedema, surgical intervention usually is unnecessary except to improve appearance. The creases should be observed for gradual improvement in appearance, which may occur as "baby fat" is lost. If creases are deep enough to cause lymphedema or impairment of circulation, they should be excised down to normal tissue and the defect should be closed with multiple Z-plasty procedures. If the ring completely encircles the part, the safer approach is staged excision of one half of the groove with Z-plasty closure, followed by a second operation 2 to 3 months later. Lymphedema and cyanosis usually gradually improve after release. Simple excision of the groove with simple everting closure generally is inadequate because circumferential scar contracture may occur.

Acrosyndactyly is a frequent component of this syndrome. Because all finger tips frequently are bound together, permanent deformity will result unless early syndactyly reconstruction is performed. Release of the border digits should be done within the first 6 months of life, followed by release of the central digits when the child is about 18 months of age. Finger stiffness at the proximal interphalangeal joints is common after syndactyly release. Short digits may require lengthening by osteotomy and distraction. The shortened thumb may require deepening of the web space or lengthening by the method of Søiland in which an extremely shortened index finger is added to the top of the thumb. Amputations in this syndrome usually have adequate or abundant soft tissue coverage and rarely require surgical reconstruction.

Multiple Z-plasty release of congenital ring

▲ *Technique.* If the congenital ring is deep and completely encircles the limb or finger, plan to correct only half of the ring in the initial procedure. Before inflating the tourniquet, mark out the multiple Z-plasty sites along the constricting ring (Fig. 4-64, *A*). Exsanguinate the limb, and inflate the tourniquet. Excise half the constricting ring, and then sharply incise the Z-plasty sites to elevate the flaps. Suture the flaps in an appropriate interdigitating fashion to allow for lengthening of the constricting ring (Fig. 4-64, *B*). Deflate the tourniquet, and apply a bulky dressing with a short-arm or long-arm splint.

▲ *Postoperative management.* The splinting is maintained for 2 to 3 weeks. Sutures are removed after 10 to 14 days. The other half of the constricting ring can be similarly reconstructed after 2 to 3 months.

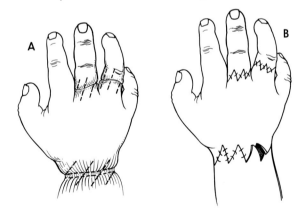

Fig. 4-64 Multiple Z-plasties for severe congenital ring syndrome. **A,** Band is completely excised after it is ascertained that no deep fascial constriction remains. Only volar half of ring should be corrected at initial procedure. **B,** Z-plasty closure. (Redrawn from Dobyns JH, Wood VE, and Bayne LG: Congenital hand deformities. In Green DP, editor: Operative hand surgery, ed 2, New York, 1988, Churchill Livingstone.)

MISCELLANEOUS ANOMALIES
Congenital Trigger Digits

Congenital trigger digit occurs when the normal gliding movement of the flexor tendon is impeded within the digital flexor sheath. Unlike adults with stenosing tenovaginitis the congenitally involved finger usually shows a persistent flexion deformity rather than actual "triggering" (Fig. 4-65, *A*). This is a relatively rare condition, found in only 2.3% of Flatt's patients. It occurs far more commonly in the thumb and is bilateral in about 25% of patients. The condition occurs sporadically and is not believed to be an inherited trait. Trigger digits typically occur without other anomalies, but an association with trisomy 13 has been reported.

Approximately 25% of trigger digits are noted at birth; frequently the condition is not noted until the age of 1 or 2 years at which time the child has a relatively fixed flexion posture of the interphalangeal joint of the thumb. Even with some force it may not be possible to fully extend the interphalangeal joint of the thumb. Dellon and Hansen reported an occasional extension posture of the thumb and involvement of multiple digits. The abnormal clicking or snapping usually is not the presenting complaint commonly seen in adults. This condition must be differentiated from the clasped thumb deformity in which there is primarily metacarpophalangeal flexion.

The pathologic anatomy responsible for trigger digits includes narrowing and thickening of the sheath, with occasional formation of a ganglion cyst. An intratendinous nodule may be present proximal to the first annular pulley. Chronic inflammation also is frequent. Fixed contractures are unlikely if the condition resolves or is corrected before the child is 3 years old. Spontaneous resolution occurs in about 30% of children whose condition appears within the first year of life and in about 12% of those in whom it occurs between the ages of 6 months and 2 years.

Treatment

Because spontaneous resolution can be expected in about 30% of children whose condition becomes apparent within the first year of life, observation and gentle manipulation are appropriate. Splinting may be attempted, but this has not been shown to be of benefit. If the condition does not resolve spontaneously, surgical intervention should not be delayed beyond the age of 3 years. Surgical release of the first annular pulley should be performed at about the age of 2 years if spontaneous resolution has not occurred. In the rare instance in which multiple trigger digits fixed in extension prevent the child from making a fist, surgical intervention should be earlier (around the age of 1 year). Accidental nerve injury may be avoided by first making a shallow incision and identifying the digital nerves. Lacerated digital nerves and tendons should be repaired. Recurrence is unlikely if release is adequate.

Release of congenital trigger thumb

▶ *Technique.* Under tourniquet control, make a transverse incision at the volar crease of the metacarpophalangeal joint of the thumb. Carefully protect the two digital nerves. The flexor sheath usually is quite prominent just beneath the subcutaneous fat. Identify the proximal edge of the first annular pulley, and completely incise it longitudinally under direct vision. Shaving the nodule and excising a segment of the A-1 pulley usually are unnecessary. Close the wound (Fig. 4-65, *B*), and apply a soft dressing. No particular immobilization is required. This procedure may be performed in a similar fashion in other involved digits.

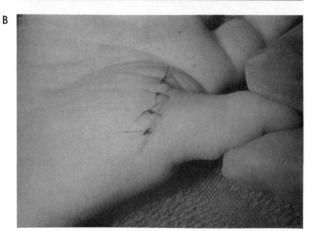

A

B

Fig. 4-65   **A,** Trigger thumb in 2-year-old child. **B,** After release.

Camptodactyly

Camptodactyly is a flexion deformity of the proximal interphalangeal joint that usually involves only the little finger (Fig. 4-66). This type of bent-finger deformity should be distinguished from clinodactyly in which the finger is bent either radialward or ulnarward. Camptodactyly occurs in fewer than 1% of the population and was found in 6.9% of the anomalies in Flatt's series. There is a strong hereditary predisposition in many patients in whom the deformity is transmitted as an autosomal dominant trait. Sporadic cases also occur. All structures that could possibly cause flexion deformity at the proximal interphalangeal joint have been considered as possible etiologic factors. Kilgore found a stout band of tissue in association with Landsmeer's ligament. McFarlane et al found an abnormal insertion of the lumbrical tendon into the flexor superficialis tendon, the capsule of the metacarpophalangeal joint, or the extensor expansion of the adjacent finger in all 21 of their patients. This appears to support the view of Millesi that camptodactyly is due to relative imbalance between the flexors and extensors. Smith and Kaplan suggested relative shortening in the flexor superficialis muscle/tendon unit because the deformity usually could be corrected with simultaneous flexion of the wrist. Other theories include contractures of the collateral ligaments or volar plate, insufficient palmar skin, and congenital fibrous substrata in the subcutaneous tissues.

There appear to be two types of camptodactyly, based on the age at which the deformity occurs. The first type occurs in infancy and affects both sexes equally. This is the more common type, occurring in about 80% of patients. The second type occurs during adolescence and affects mostly girls. Camptodactyly commonly is associated with many syndromes including trisomy 13, oculodentodigital, orofaciodigital, Aarskog, and cerebrohepatorenal syndromes.

Most patients are seen with a flexion deformity of the proximal interphalangeal joint during the first year of life. About two thirds have bilateral deformities, which are not necessarily symmetric in severity. The metacarpophalangeal joint usually is held in hyperextension to compensate for the flexed posture. Rotational deformity may cause mild overlapping of fingers. In young children the deformity disappears when the wrist is flexed, but in older children the flexion deformity usually is fixed. If left untreated, 80% will worsen, especially during the period of growth acceleration. The deformity usually does not progress after the age of 18 to 20 years. Rarely, pain and swelling are present.

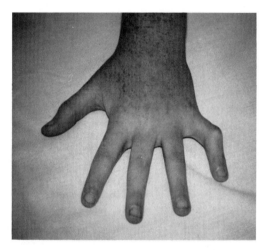

Fig. 4-66 Campodactyly (flexion deformity of proximal interphalangeal joint) involving only little finger.

Treatment

Neither nonsurgical nor surgical treatment of camptodactyly has been particularly predictable or satisfying. Engber and Flatt reported that 20% of patients improved with nonsurgical treatment and only 35% improved with surgical treatment. Miura reported full-time dynamic splinting in 24 patients until full extension was achieved, followed by splinting for 8 hours a day. Good results were obtained as long as splinting was continued, but some flexion deformity recurred when splinting was discontinued. It is reasonable to advise patients with mild deformities to live with their deformities. For young children in whom the deformity disappears with wrist flexion and for whom the parents desire surgical correction, release of the sublimis tendon may correct the deformity and prevent worsening during growth. This usually should be performed by the age of 4 years. In older children and young adults in whom the deformity can be corrected with splinting but who continue to have weak extension at the proximal inter-phalangeal joint, release of the flexor digitorum sublimis muscle and transfer into the extensor apparatus, as advocated by Millesi and by Lankford, is advised. A volar release, including local skin flap and volar plate release, has been used before tendon transfer to allow passive correction of the flexion deformity.

▲ *Technique (McFarlane et al)* (Fig. 4-67). Under tourniquet control, make a straight midline incision over the finger so that a Z-plasty closure can be achieved as necessary. Divide the flexor digitorum sublimis tendon just proximal to the vinculum longum, and transfer it through the lumbrical canal to the dorsal surface of the finger. Suture the sublimis tendon to the extensor apparatus with nonabsorbable sutures. Tension the transferred tendon so that normal stance of the digit is achieved in all wrist positions. If correction of the deformity is not complete, consideration can be given to a proximal release of the volar plate; however, it is best to accept a flexion deformity of approximately 20 degrees. Insert a Kirschner wire through the proximal interphalangeal joint to maintain extension. Close the skin with single or multiple Z-plasty procedures. Apply a short-arm cast with the metacarpophalangeal joints in 90 degrees of flexion and the digits fully extended.

▲ *Postoperative management.* The cast and Kirschner wire are removed 4 weeks after surgery. A dorsal splint with a metacarpal stop to prevent overstretching of the transferred tendon is worn for another 4 weeks.

Kirner Deformity

This anomaly, originally described by Kirner in 1927, consists of palmar and radial curving of the distal phalanx of the little finger. It is an unsightly deformity that occurs only infrequently; David and Burwood determined an incidence of 1:410 live births in their survey of 3000 patients. The deformity occurs more frequently in girls and may rarely affect several fingers. Sporadic, as well as familial, occurrences have been reported, and there is no known specific etiologic factor. A similar deformity may result from frostbite, physeal fracture, and infection. Kirner deformity has been associated with Cornelia de Lange, Silver, and Turner syndromes.

The deformity typically is seen when the child is around the age of 8 to 10 years and appears as a beaked little finger tip with increased convexity of the fingernail. The finger tip curves radially and toward the palm. The deformity usually is bilateral and symmetric. Although it may be progressive, usually it is not painful. Roentgenograms reveal a broadened physis with irregularities of the metaphysis. The typical curvature can be seen within the distal phalanx (Fig. 4-68, *A*).

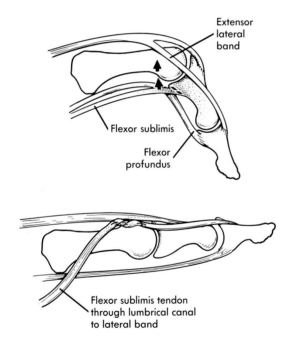

Fig. 4-67 Technique for correction of campodactyly. Flexor superficialis tendon is transferred to extensor apparatus. (Redrawn from Dobyns JH, Wood VE, and Bayne LG: Congenital hand deformities. In Green DP, editor: Operative hand surgery, ed 2, New York, 1988, Churchill Livingstone.)

Treatment

For mild deformities either splinting or no treatment may be appropriate. More severe deformities in skeletally mature patients require one or more osteotomies of the terminal phalanx, as described by Carstam and Eiken. No effective treatment has been described for correction of the nail deformity.

▲ *Technique (Carstam and Eiken)* (Fig. 4-68, *B*). Under tourniquet control, make a radial midlateral incision over the distal phalanx of the involved finger. Expose the distal phalanx subperiosteally, and make two osteotomies through the volar three fourths of the diaphysis. Using a periosteal hinge left intact on the dorsum of the phalanx, correct the deformity. This periosteal hinge also helps control rotation of the fragments. Complete correction of the deformity may be blocked by a curved nail deformity. Place a longitudinal Kirschner wire through the phalanx and the distal interphalangeal joint to hold the correction. If the phalanx is extremely small, insert a Kirschner wire extraperiosteally along the volar aspect of the phalanx to act as an internal splint. Close the incisions in routine fashion, and apply a long-arm or short-arm splint.

▲ *Postoperative management.* The splint and Kirschner wire are removed 4 to 6 weeks after surgery. Usually no specific postoperative therapy is necessary. Activities are permitted depending on the clinical and roentgenographic signs of healing.

Delta Phalanx

The delta phalanx is an abnormal, trapezoidal-shaped phalanx that appears triangular on roentgenogram (Fig. 4-69) and derives its name from the Greek *delta*. The abnormal physis is C- or J-shaped and tends to bracket one side of the phalanx. The incidence of this deformity in the general population has not been established. The specific cause is not known, but in as many as 44% of patients there is a strong family history and autosomal dominant transmission. Delta phalanx rarely is an isolated anomaly and usually occurs in association with such entities as polydactyly, syndactyly, symphalangism, cleft foot, triphalangeal thumb, central hand deficiency, ulnar clubhand, Apert syndrome, Poland syndrome, diastrophic dwarfism, and Holt-Oram syndrome.

The delta phalanx causes an angular deformity of the digit in the frontal plane. When in the border digits, the finger tends to deviate toward the hand. The angulation frequently is mild but, when severe, may cause an unacceptable appearance. According to Flatt this anomaly most commonly occurs in the proximal phalanx of the thumb in association with triphalangeal thumb and in the middle phalanx of the small finger. The next most frequent location is the proximal phalanx of the ring finger. Progressive angulation is inevitable.

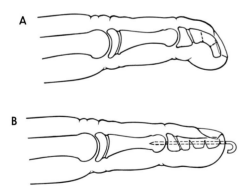

Fig. 4-68   Correction of Kirner deformity. **A,** Deformity. **B,** Multiple opening wedge osoteomies in distal phalanx fixed with Kirschner wire. (Redrawn from Carstam N and Eiken O: J Bone Joint Surg 52A:1663, 1970.)

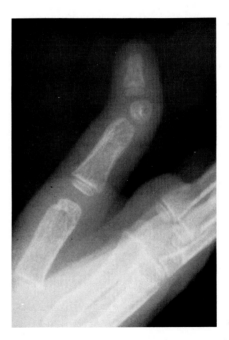

Fig. 4-69   Roentgenographic appearance of delta phalanx.

Treatment

Moderate angulation of the finger produced by the delta phalanx is awkward and unsightly. Nonsurgical treatment will not alter progression, and surgical intervention should be aimed at narrowing the digit, straightening the phalanx, and destroying the abnormal portion of the physis. If associated with central polydactyly, the delta phalanx should be excised along with the extra digit with a syndactyly-type reconstruction. If associated with a triphalangeal thumb, the delta phalanx should be excised and the joint ligaments reconstructed. The deformity may recur after osteotomy. Reverse wedge osteotomy, as described by Carstam and Theander, is preferable to simple opening wedge osteotomy. Carstam and Theander reported elimination or marked reduction of clinodactyly in all their patients. Vickers described a procedure in which he resected the isthmus of the continuous epiphysis and inserted an interpositional fat graft. He reported spontaneous angular correction and growth of the phalanx in 11 patients. Smith described a technique in which he performed an opening wedge osteotomy of the delta phalanx and inserted a bone graft obtained from the distal phalanx (Fig. 4-70).

Reverse wedge osteotomy

▲ *Technique (Carstam and Theander)* (Fig. 4-71). Under tourniquet control, make a curved dorsal incision over the involved phalanx, extending from the distal portion of the proximal phalanx, over the entire length of the middle phalanx, and onto the proximal portion of the distal phalanx. Carefully mobilize the edges of the extensor tendon so that both borders of the delta phalanx in the middle phalanx can be seen. Identify and protect the insertion of the central extensor slip. Remove a wedge-shaped piece of bone from the central portion of the delta phalanx, either by using a scalpel if it is mostly cartilaginous or by carefully picking away at it with sharp bone cutters, as described by Flatt. Reverse this wedge-shaped piece of bone, and insert it into the defect after correcting the angular deformity. Place a longitudinal Kirschner wire through the distal phalanx and into the proximal phalanx to hold the corrected position; leave the wire protruding through the distal end of the finger. Close

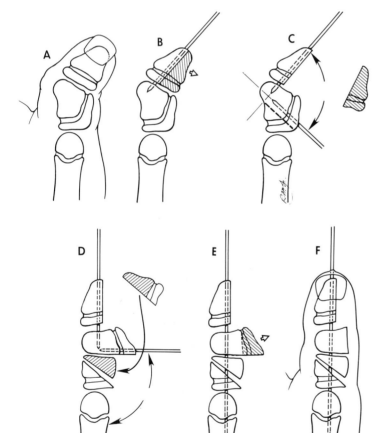

Fig. 4-70 Modified opening wedge technique for correction of delta phalanx as described by Smith. (Redrawn from Dobyns JH, Wood VE, and Bayne LG: Congenital hand deformities. In Green DP, editor: Operative hand surgery, ed 2, New York, 1988, Churchill Livingstone.)

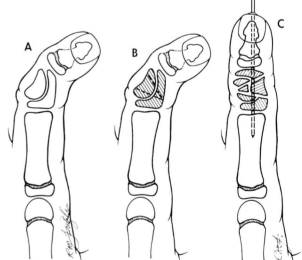

Fig. 4-71 Reverse wedge osteotomy for correction of delta phalanx. **A,** Delta phalanx involving middle phalanx. **B,** Wedge-shaped piece of bone is removed from central portion. **C,** Wedge is reversed and reinserted after correction of angular deformity; Kirschner wire is used for fixation. (Redrawn from Carstam N and Theander G: Scand J Plast Reconstr Surg 9:199, 1975.)

the incision in routine fashion, and apply a long- or short-arm splint.

▲ *Postoperative management.* The splint and Kirschner wire are removed 4 to 6 weeks after surgery. Gradually increased activity is permitted depending on clinical and roentgenographic healing.

Madelung Deformity

Madelung deformity is an abnormality of the palmar ulnar part of the distal radial epiphysis in which progressive ulnar and volar tilt develops at the distal radial articular surface, with dorsal subluxation of the distal ulna. The deformity probably was first described by Malgaigne in 1855 and later by Madelung in 1878. It is believed to be a congenital disorder although it seldom is obvious until late childhood or adolescence. It is a rare anomaly, accounting for only 1.7% of hand anomalies in Flatt's series. The cause of Madelung deformity is uncertain; however, it has been shown to be transmitted in an autosomal dominant pattern. Other Madelung-like deformities have occurred after trauma, as reported by Vender and Watson in a gymnast, and after infection and neoplasm. There is no definitive method of distinguishing these from idiopathic Madelung deformity. Vender and Watson classified Madelung and Madelung-like deformities into four groups: posttraumatic, dysplastic (dyschondrosteosis or diaphyseal aclasis), genetic (e.g., Turner syndrome), and idiopathic. They believe that acquired deformities usually can be distinguished by a lack of appropriate physical findings, unilaterality, less severe carpal deformities, and the appropriate history of repetitive injury or stress.

A deformity of the wrist similar to Madelung deformity frequently is associated with dyschondrosteosis, the most common form of mesomelic dwarfism. This disorder consists of mild shortness of stature, shortness of the middle segment of the upper and lower extremities, and Madelung deformity. Other associated conditions include mucopolysaccharidosis, Turner syndrome, achondroplasia, multiple exostoses, multiple epiphyseal dysplasia, and dyschondroplasia (Ollier disease).

The typical Madelung deformity consists of volar subluxation of the hand, with prominence of the distal ulna and volar and ulnar angulation of the distal radius. It is more commonly bilateral and affects girls more frequently than boys. A family history of the deformity often is present. The deformity usually manifests in late childhood or early adolescence, with decreased motion and minimal pain. As growth occurs the deformity worsens in appearance. Roentgenographic abnormalities are seen in the radius, ulna, and carpal bones (Fig. 4-72). The radius is curved,

with its convexity dorsal and radial and a similar angulation of the distal radial articular surface. The forearm is relatively short. The distal radial epiphysis is triangular in shape because of the failure of growth in the ulnar and volar aspects of the physis; early closure of these aspects of the physis also is frequent. Osteophyte formation may be visible at the volar ulnar border of the radius. The ulna is subluxated dorsally, the ulnar head is enlarged, and overall length of the ulna is decreased. The carpus appears to have subluxated ulnarward and palmarward into the distal radioulnar joint, which usually is spread apart. The carpus appears wedge-shaped with its apex proximal within the lunate.

Treatment

Because children with Madelung deformity usually have minimal pain and excellent function, a conservative approach is warranted initially. Surgery should be considered for severe deformity or persistent pain, usually from ulnocarpal impingement of the carpus. Distal radial osteotomy with ulnar shortening (Milch recession) is a preferred treatment in skeletally immature patients. The radial osteotomy may be a closing or opening wedge as needed for alignment. Osteotomy combined with a judicious Darrach excision of the distal ulnar head may be used in skeletally mature patients. The deformity may recur after either procedure, and range of motion of the forearm usually does not improve after surgery.

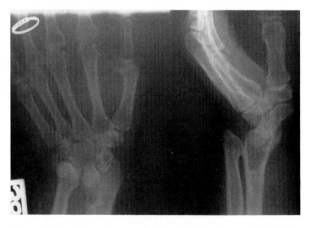

Fig. 4-72 Roentgenographic appearance of Madelung deformity. Note abnormalities of radius, ulna, and carpal bones.

Correction of Madelung deformity

▶ *Technique (Ranawat et al)* (Fig. 4-73). Make a dorsal longitudinal incision over the distal forearm, detach the extensor retinaculum from the radius over the extensor digitorum communis tendons, and reflect the retinaculum and the tendon of the extensor digiti minimi ulnarward. If the patient is skeletally mature, expose the distal radioulnar joint and excise about 1 cm of the distal ulna. If the patient is skeletally immature, expose the ulnar shaft and perform an appropriate cuff recession as described by Milch. Next perform an osteotomy parallel to the distal articular surface of the radius. Resect an appropriate wedge of bone based radially and dorsally from the distal end of the proximal fragment of the radius and appose the raw surfaces. Stabilize the osteotomy with Kirschner wires so that the distal articular surface of the radius is facing volarward 0 to 15 degrees to the long axis of the radius and ulnarward 60 to 70 degrees. Close the incision in routine fashion, and apply a long-arm cast.

▶ *Postoperative management.* The cast and pins are removed 4 weeks after surgery, and active exercises of the wrist are begun. The osteotomy is protected with a cast or splint until there are sufficient roentgenographic and clinical signs of bone healing. Normal activities are progressively resumed. After the final cast is removed, protective splinting may be necessary for 8 to 10 weeks after surgery.

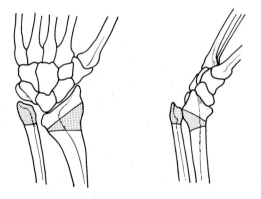

Fig. 4-73 Reconstruction of Madelung deformity. Dorsal and radial based closing wedge osteotomy of radius is performed in conjunction with Darrach excision. Correct alignment is obtained, and plate and screws are used for fixation. (Redrawn from Ranawat CS, DeFiore J, and Straub LR: J Bone Joint Surg 57A:772, 1975.)

REFERENCES
General

Beals RK and Crawford A: Congenital absence of the pectoral muscles, Clin Orthop 119:166, 1976.

Birch-Jensen A: Congenital deformities of the upper extremities, Odense, Denmark, 1949, Ejnar Muntsgaads Forleg.

Cheng JCY, Chow SK, and Leung PC: Classification of 578 cases of congenital upper limb anomalies with the IFSSH system—a 10 years' experience. J Hand Surg 12A:1055, 1987.

Conway H and Bowe J: Congenital deformities of the hands, Plast Reconstr Surg 18:286, 1956.

Dobyns JH, Wood VE, and Bayne LG: Congenital hand deformities. In Green DP, editor: Operative hand surgery, ed 2, New York, 1988, Churchill-Livingstone.

Flatt AE: The care of congenital hand anomalies, St Louis, 1977, The CV Mosby Co.

Frantz CH and O'Rahilly R: Congenital skeletal limb deficiencies, J Bone Joint Surg 43A:1202, 1961.

Huber E: Hilfsoperation bei Medianuslahmung, Dtsch Z Chir 162:271, 1921.

Imamura T and Miura T: The carpal bones in congenital hand anomalies: a radiographic study in patients older than ten years, J Hand Surg 13A:650, 1988.

Lamb DW: The practice of hand surgery, ed 2, Oxford, 1989, Blackwell Scientific Publications.

Lamb DW and Scott H: Management of congenital and acquired amputation in children, Orthop Clin North Am 12:997, 1981.

Littler JW: Introduction to surgery of the hand, Reconstr Plast Surg 4:1543, 1964.

MacDonnell JA: Age of fitting upper extremity prostheses in children, J Bone Joint Surg 40A:655, 1958.

Marcer E: Intervento per correggere la clinodattilia metacarpofalangia, Clin Ortop 1:111, 1949.

Matev IB: Thumb reconstruction in children through metacarpal lengthening, Plast Reconstr Surg 64:665, 1979.

Milford L: The hand: congenital anomalies. In Crenshaw AH, editor: Campbell's operative orthopaedics, ed 7, St Louis, 1987, The CV Mosby Co.

Ogino T: A clinical and experimental study of teratogenic mechanism of cleft hand, polydactyly and syndactyly, Nippon Seikeigeka Gakkai Zasshi 53:535, 1979.

O'Rahilly R: Morphologic patterns in limb deficiencies and duplications, Am J Anat 89:135, 1956.

Silverman ME, Copeland AJ Jr, and Hurst JW: The Holt-Oram syndrome: the long and short of it, Am J Cardiol 25:11, 1970.

Stelling F: The upper extremity. In Ferguson AB, editor: Orthopedic surgery in infancy and childhood, Baltimore, 1963, The Williams & Wilkins Co.

Stetten DW: Idiopathic progressive curvature of the radius, or so-called Madelung's deformity of the wrist (carpus varus and carpus valgus), Surg Gyn Obstet 8:4, 1909.

Swanson AB: A classification for congenital limb malformations, J Hand Surg 1:8, 1976.

Swanson AB, Barsky AJ, and Entin M: Classification of limb malformations on the basis of embryological failures, Surg Clin North Am 48:1169, 1968.

Temtamy SA and McKusick VA: Absence deformities as isolated malformations, Birth Defects 14:36, 1978.

Temtamy SA and McKusick VA: Absence deformities as part of syndromes, Birth Defects 14:73, 1978.

Turek SI: Orthopaedic principles and their application, Philadelphia, 1967, JB Lippincott Co.

Watson-Jones R: Fractures and joint injuries, ed 3, vol 2, Baltimore, 1943, Williams & Wilkins.

Wynne-Davies R and Lamb DW: Congenital upper limb anomalies: an etiologic grouping of clinical, genetic, and epidemiologic data from 382 patients with "absence" defects, constriction bands, polydactylies, and syndactylies, J Hand Surg 10A (6 pt 2):958, 1985.

Wynne-Davies R et al: Congenital abnormalities of the hand. In Lamb DW, Hooper G, and Kuczynski K, editors: The practice of hand surgery, ed 2, Oxford, 1989, Blackwell Scientific Publications.

Yamaguchi S et al: Restoration of function to congenitally deformed hands. Proceedings of the sixteenth annual meeting of the Japanese Society for Surgery of the Hand, Fukuoka, 1973.

Transverse deficiencies

Chan KM et al: The Krukenberg procedure: a method of unilateral anomalies of upper limb in Chinese children, J Hand Surg 9A:548, 1984.

Cowen NJ and Loftus JM: Distraction augmentation manoplasty; technique for lengthening digits for the entire hand, Orthop Rev 7:45, 1978.

Epps C, Burkhalter W, and McCollough NC III: Modern amputation surgery and prosthetic techniques. In The American Academy of Orthopaedic Surgeons Instructional course lectures, Presented in Atlanta, 1980.

Ilizarov GA: Clinical application of the tension-stress effect of limb-lengthening, Clin Orthop 250:8, 1990.

Kessler I, Baruch A, and Hecht O: Experience with distraction lengthening of digital rays in congenital anomalies, J Hand Surg 2:394, 1977.

Krukenberg H: Uber Platiches Unwertung von Amputationstumpen, Stuttgart, 1917, Ferdinand Enk.

Matev I: A new method of thumb reconstruction. Paper presented at the Anglo-Scandinavian Symposium of Hand Surgery, Lausanne, Switzerland, May 26-27, 1967.

Nathan PA and Trung NB: The Krukenberg operation: a modified technique avoiding skin grafts, J Hand Surg 2:127, 1977.

Swanson AB and Swanson G deG: The Krukenberg procedure in the juvenile amputee, Clin Orthop 148:55, 1980.

Phocomelia

Lamb DW, MacNaughtan AK, and Fragiadakis EG: Phocomelia of the upper limb, Hand 3:200, 1971.

Sulamaa M and Ryoppy S: Early treatment of congenital bone defects of the extremities: aftermath of thalidomide disaster, Lancet 1:130, 1964.

Taussig HB: A study of the German outbreak of phocomelia: the thalidomide syndrome, JAMA 180:1106, 1962.

Radial deficiencies

Albee FH: Formation of radius congenitally absent: condition seven years after implantation of bone graft, Ann Surg 87:105, 1928.

Bora FW et al: Radial clubhand deformity: long-term follow-up, J Bone Joint Surg 63A:741, 1981.

Buck-Gramcko D: Radialization as a new treatment for radial club hand, J Hand Surg 10A (pt2):964, 1985.

Buck-Gramcko D: Pollicization of the index finger: method and results in aplasia and hypoplasia of the thumb, J Bone Joint Surg 53A:1605, 1971.

DeLorme TL: Treatment of congenital absence of radius by transepiphyseal fixation, J Bone Joint Surg 51A:117, 1969.

Goldberg MJ and Meyn M: The radial clubhand, Orthop Clin North Am 7:341, 1976.

Gosset J: La pollicisation de l'index, J Chir (Paris) 65:403, 1949.

Harrison SH: Pollicization in cases of radial club hand, Br J Plast Surg 23:192, 1970.

Heikel HVA: Aplasia and hypoplasia of the radius, Acta Orthop Scand (suppl) 39:1, 1959.

Kato K: Congenital absence of the radius, with review of the literature and report of three cases, J Bone Joint Surg 6:589, 1924.

Kummel W: Die Missbildungen der Extremitäten durch Defekt, Verwachsung und Ueberzahl, Heft 3, Kassel, Germany, 1895, Bibliotheca Medica.

Lamb DW: The treatment of radial club hand: absent radius, aplasia of the radius, hypoplasis of the radius, radial paraxial hemimelia, Hand 4:22, 1972.

Lamb DW: Radial club hand, a continuing study of sixty-eight patients with one hundred and seventeen club hands, J Bone Joint Surg 59A:1, 1977.

Lamb DW, Wynne-Davies R, and Soto L: An estimate of the population frequency of congenital malformations of the upper limb, J Hand Surg 7:557, 1982.

Lidge RT: Congenital radial deficient club hand, J Bone Joint Surg 51A:1041, 1969.

Manske PR and McCarroll HR Jr: Abductor digiti minimi opponensplasty in congenital radial aplasia, J Hand Surg 3:522, 1978.

Manske RP, McCarroll HR Jr, and Swanson K: Centralization of the radial club hand: ulnar surgical approach, J Hand Surg 6:423, 1981.

Menelaus MB: Radial club hand with absence of the biceps muscle treated by centralization of the ulna and triceps transfer: report of two cases, J Bone Joint Surg 58B:488, 1976.

Riordan DC: Congenital absence of the radius, J Bone Joint Surg 37A:1129, 1955.

Riordan DC: Congenital absence of the radius, a 15-year follow-up, J Bone Joint Surg 45A:1783, 1963.

Riordan DC, Powers RC, and Hurd RA: The Huber procedure for congenital absence of thenar muscle. Presented to the Annual Meeting of the American Society for Surgery of the Hand, San Francisco, Feb 27, 1975.

Sayre RH: A contribution to the study of club-hand, Trans Am Orthop Assoc 6:208, 1893.

Skerik SK and Flatt AE: The anatomy of congenital radial dysplasia: its surgical and functional implications, Clin Orthop 66:125, 1969.

Starr DE: Congenital absence of the radius: a method of surgical correction, J Bone Joint Surg 27:752, 1945.

Tsuyuguchi Y et al: Radial ray deficiency, J Pediatr Orthop 7:699, 1987.

Watson HK, Beebe RD, and Cruz NI: Centralization procedure for radial clubhand, J Hand Surg 9A:541, 1984.

Wynne-Davies R and Lamb DW: Congenital upper limb anomalies, J Hand Surg 10A (6 pt 2):958, 1985.

Central deficiencies

Barsky AJ: Cleft hand: classification, incidence, and treatment, J Bone Joint Surg 46A:1707, 1964.

Flatt AE and Wood VE: Multiple dorsal rotation flaps from the hand for thumb web contractures, Plast Reconstr Surg 45:258, 1970.

Fort AJA: Des difformities congenitales et acquises des doigts, et des moyens d'y remedier, Paris, 1869, Adrien Delahaye.

Gilbert A: Toe transfers for congenital hand defects, J Hand Surg 7A:118, 1982.

Hartsinck JJ: Beschryving van Guiana, of de wilde Kust in Zuid-America, vol 2, Amsterdam, 1770, Gerrit Tielenburg.

Lange M: Grundsatzliches uber die Beurteilung der Enstehung und Bewertung atypischer Handund Fussmissbildungen, Verh Dtsch Orthop Ges 31, Kongress Konigsberg/Pr Z Orthop (suppl) 31:80, 1936.

Maisels DO: Lobster-claw deformities of the hands and feet, Br J Plast Surg 23:269, 1970.

Manske PR: Cleft hand and central polydactyly in identical twins: a case report, J Hand Surg 8:906, 1983.

Milford L: The split (cleft) hand. Paper presented at Symposium on Congenital Hand Deformities, American Society for Surgery of the Hand, Atlanta, 1978.

Miura T and Komada T: Simple method for reconstruction of the cleft hand with an adducted thumb, Plast Reconstr Surg 64:65, 1979.

Müller W: Die angeborenen Fehlbildugen der menschlichen Hand, Leipzig, Germany, 1937, Thieme.

Nutt JN III and Flatt AE: Congenital central hand deficit, J Hand Surg 6:48, 1981.

Snow JW and Littler JW: Surgical treatment of cleft hand. Transactions of the International Society for Plastic Reconstructive Surgery, Fourth Congress, Rome, 1967, Excerpta Medical Foundation.

Tada K, Yonenobu K, and Swanson AB: Congenital central ray deficiency in the hand—a survey of 59 cases and subclassification, J Hand Surg 6:434, 1981.

Ueba Y: Plastic surgery for cleft hand, J Hand Surg 6:557, 1981.

Watari S and Tsuge K: A classification of cleft hands, based on clinical findings, Plast Reconstr Surg 64:381, 1979.

Ulnar deficiencies

Broudy AS and Smith RJ: Deformities of the hand and wrist with ulnar deficiency, J Hand Surg 4:304, 1979.

Ogden JA, Watson HK, and Bohne W: Ulnar dysmelia, J Bone Joint Surg 58A:467, 1976.

Roberts AS: A case of deformity of the forearm and hands with an unusual history of hereditary congenital deficiency, Ann Surg 3:135, 1886.

Straub LR: Congenital absence of ulna, Am J Surg 109:300, 1965.

Swanson AB, Tada K, and Yonenobu K: Ulna ray deficiency: its various manifestations, J Hand Surg 9A:658, 1984.

Syndactyly

Bauer TB, Tondra JM, and Trusler HM: Technical modification in repair of syndactylism, Plast Reconstr Surg 17:385, 1956.

Cronin TD: Syndactylism: results of zig-zag incision to prevent postoperative contracture, Plast Reconstr Surg 18:460, 1956.

Kettlekamp DB and Flatt AE: An evaluation of syndactyly repair, Surg Gynecol Obstet 133:471, 1961.

Miura T: Syndactyly and split hand, Hand 8:125, 1976.

Pieri G: Processo operatorio per la cura sindattilia grave, Chir Ital 3-4:258, 1949.

Shaw DT et al: Interdigital butterfly flap in the hand (the double-opposing Z-plasty), J Bone Joint Surg 55A:1677, 1973.

Skoog T: Syndactyly: a clinical report on repair, Acta Chir Scand 130:537, 1965.

Sugiura Y: Poland's syndrome: clincoroentgenographic study on 45 cases, Cong Anom 16:17, 1976.

Toledo LC and Ger E: Evaluation of the operative treatment of syndactyly, J Hand Surg 4:556, 1979.

Woolf RM and Broadbent TR: The four-flap Z-plasty, Plast Reconstr Surg 49:48, 1972.

Zeller S: Abhandlung uber die ersten Erscheinungen venerischer Lokal-Krankheits-Formen, und deren Behandlung, sammt einer kurzen Anzeige zweier neuen Operazions-Methoden, nahmlich: die angebornen verwachsenen Finger, und die Kastrazion betreffend, Wien, 1810, JG Binz.

Apert syndrome

Apert E: De l'acrocephalosyndactylie, Bull Mem Soc Med Hop Paris 23:1310, 1906.

Blank CE: Apert's syndrome: a type of acrocephalosyndactyly: observations on a British series of thirty-nine cases, Ann Hum Genet 24:151, 1960.

Hoover GH, Flatt AE, and Weiss MW: The hand in Apert's syndrome, J Bone Joint Surg 52A:877, 1970.

Preaxial polydactyly

Bilhaut M: Guerison d'un pouce bifide per un nouveau procede operatoire, Cong Fren Chir 4:576, 1890.

Marks TW and Bayne LG: Polydactyly of the thumb: abnormal anatomy and treatment, J Hand Surg 3:107, 1978.

Mirua T: Non-traumatic flexion deformity of the proximal interphalangeal joint—its pathogenesis and treatment, Hand 15:25, 1983.

Wassel HD: The results of surgery for polydactyly of the thumb: a review, Clin Orthop 64:175, 1969.

Wood VE: Polydactyly and the triphalangeal thumb, J Hand Surg 3:436, 1978.

Central polydactyly

Manske PR: Cleft hand and central polydactyly in identical twins: a case report, J Hand Surg 8:906, 1983.

Tada K et al: Central polydactyly—a review of 12 cases and their surgical treatment, J Hand Surg 7:460, 1982.

Ulnar dimelia

Buck-Gramcko D: Operative Behandlung einer Spiegelbild-Deformität der hand (mirror hand—doppelte ulna mit polydaktylie). Traitement operatoire d'une difformite en miroir de l'avant-bras (deboublement du cutitus et des doigts cubitaux), Ann Chir Plast 9:180, 1964.

Gorriz G: Ulnar dimelia—a limb without anteroposterior differentiation, J Hand Surg 7A:466, 1982.

Harrison RG, Pearson MA, and Roaf R: Ulnar dimelia, J Bone Joint Surg 42B:549, 1960.

Perini G: Dimelia ulnare e suo trattamento chirurgico, Arch Putti Chir Organi Mov 6:363, 1965.

Stalling F: The upper extremity. In Ferguson AB, editor: Orthopedic surgery in infancy and childhood, Baltimore, 1963, Williams & Wilkins.

Turek SL: Orthopaedic principles and their application, Philadelphia, 1967, JB Lippincott Co.

Macrodactyly

Barsky AJ: Macrodactyly, J Bone Joint Surg 49A:1255, 1967.

Clifford RH: Treatment of macrodactylism: case report, Plast Reconstr Surg 23:245, 1959.

Jones KG: Megalodactylism: case report of a child treated by epiphyseal resection, J Bone Joint Surg 45A:1704, 1963.

Kelikian H: Congenital deformities of the hand and forearm, Philadelphia, 1974, WB Saunders Co.

Millesi H: Macrodactyly: a case study. In Littler JW, Cramer LM, and Smith JW, editors: Symposium on reconstructive hand surgery, St Louis, 1974, The CV Mosby Co.

Tsuge K: Treatment of macrodactyly, J Hand Surg 10A:968, 1985.

Wood VE: Macrodactyly, J Iowa Med Soc 59:922, 1969.

Hypoplastic thumb

Bayne LG: Abducted thumb (congenital hand deformities). In Green DP, editor: Operative hand surgery, New York, 1988, Churchill-Livingstone.

Blair WF and Omer GE Jr: Anomalous insertion of the flexor pollicis longus, J Hand Surg 6:241, 1981.

Brand PW and Milford LW: Web deepening with sliding flap for adducted thumb in the hand. In Crenshaw AH, editor: Campbell's operative orthopaedics, ed 4, St Louis, 1963, The CV Mosby Co.

Broadbent TR and Woolf RM: Flexion-abduction deformity of the thumb—congenital clasped thumb, Plast Reconstr Surg 34:612, 1964.

Egloff DV and Verdan Cl: Pollicization of the index finger for reconstruction of the congenitally hypoplastic or absent thumb, J Hand Surg 8:839, 1983.

Fitch RD, Urbaniak JR, and Ruderman RJ: Conjoined flexor and extensor pollicis longus tendons in hypoplastic thumb, J Hand Surg 9A:417, 1984.

Littler JW and Cooley SGE: Opposition of the thumb and its restoration by abductor digiti quinti transfer, J Bone Joint Surg 45A:1389, 1963.

Manske PR: Redirection of the extensor pollicis longus in the treatment of spastic thumb-in-palm deformity, J Hand Surg 10A:533, 1985.

Neviaser RJ: Congenital hypoplasis of the thumb with absence of the extrinsic extensors, abductor pollicis longus, and thenar muscles, J Hand Surg 4:301, 1979.

Riordan DC: Tendon transfers in hand surgery, J Hand Surg 8 (5 pt 2):748, 1983.

Strauch B and Spinner M: Congenital anomaly of the thumb: absent intrinsics and flexor pollicis longus, J Bone Joint Surg 58A:115, 1976.

Tsuyuguchi Y et al: Congenital clasped thumb: a review of forty-three cases, J Hand Surg 10A:613, 1985.

Tupper JW: Pollex abductus due to congenital malposition of the flexor pollicis longus, J Bone Joint Surg 51A:1285, 1969.

Weckesser EC, Reed JR, and Heiple KG: Congenital clasped thumb (congenital flexion-adduction deformity of the thumb), J Bone Joint Surg 50A:1417, 1968.

Hypoplastic hands and digits

Bell J: On brachydactyly and symphalangism. In Penrose LS, editor: The treasury of human inheritance, vol 5, Cambridge, 1951, Cambridge University Press.

Buck-Gramcko D: Pollicization of the index finger: method and results in aplasia and hypoplasia of the thumb, J Bone Joint Surg 53A:1605, 1971.

Carroll RE and Green DP: Reconstruction of hypoplastic digits using two phalanges, J Bone Joint Surg 57A:727, 1975.

Cowen NJ: Surgical management of the hypoplastic hand, In Cowen NJ, editor: Practical hand surgery, Miami, 1980, Symposia Specialties, Inc.

Cowen NJ and Loftus JM: Distraction augmentation manoplasty: technique for lengthening digits for the entire hand, Orthop Rev 7:45, 1978.

Goldberg NH and Watson HK: Composite toe (phalanx with epiphysis) transplants in the reconstruction of the aphalangic hand, Orthop Trans 5:98, 1981.

Huber E: Hilfsoperation bei onedianuslahmung, Dtsch Z Chir 162:271, 1921.

Ilizarov GA, Shtin VP, and Ledyaev VI: The course of reparative regeneration of cortical bone in distraction osteosynthesis under various conditions of fragment fixation, Eksp Khr Anesteziol 14:3, 1969.

Matev IB: Thumb reconstruction after amputation at the metacarpophalangeal joint by bone lengthening, J Bone Joint Surg 52A:957, 1970.

Peimer CA: Combined reduction osteotomy for triphalangeal thumb, J Hand Surg 10A:376, 1985.

Tajima T: Operative treatment of congenital hand anomalies, Clin Orthop Surg 11:475, 1976.

Tupper JW: Pollex abductus due to congenital malposition of the flexor pollicis longus, J Bone Joint Surg 51A:1285, 1969.

Wood VE: Polydactyly and the triphalangeal thumb, J Hand Surg 3:436, 1978.

Congenital ring syndrome

Kino Y: Clinical and experimental studies of the congenital constriction band syndrome with emphasis on its etiology, J Bone Joint Surg 57A:636, 1975.

Miura T: Congenital constriction band syndrome, J Hand Surg 9A:82, 1984.

Patterson TJS: Congenital ring-constrictions, Br J Plast Surg 14:1, 1961.

Potter EL: Pathology of the foetus and the newborn, Chicago, 1953, Year Book Medical Publishers, Inc.

Salama R and Weisman SL: Congenital bilateral anomalous band between flexor and extensor pollicis longus tendons, Hand 7:25, 1975.

Søiland H: Lengthening a finger with the "on the top" method, Acta Chir Scand 122:184, 1961.

Streeter GL: Focal deficiencies in fetal tissues and their relation to intra-uterine amputation. In Contributions to embryology, No 126, vol 22, Washington, DC, 1930, Carnegie Institute of Washington.

Temtamy SA and McKusick VA: Digital and other malformations associated with congenital ring constrictions, Birth Defects 14:547, 1978.

Congenital trigger digits

Dellon AL and Hansen FC: Bilateral inability to grasp due to multiple (ten) congenital trigger fingers, J Hand Surg 5:470, 1980.

Dinham JM and Meggitt DF: Trigger thumbs in children, J Bone Joint Surg 56B:153, 1974.

Camptodactyly

Engber WM and Flatt AE: Camptodactyly: an analysis of sixty-six patients and twenty-four operations, J Hand Surg 2:216, 1977.

Kilgore ES Jr and Graham WP III: Camptodactyly. In The hand, Philadelphia, 1977, Lea & Febiger.

Lankford LL: Correspondence club letter, No 1975-1, Dallas, May, 1975.

McFarlane RM, Curry GJ, and Evans HB: Anomalies of the intrinsic muscles in camptodactyly, J Hand Surg 8:531, 1983.

Millesi H: Camptodactyly. In Littler JW, Cramer LM, and Smith JW, editors: Symposium on reconstructive hand surgery, St Louis, 1974, The CV Mosby Co.

Miura T: Non-traumatic flexion deformity of the proximal interphalangeal joint—its pathogenesis and treatment, Hand 15:25, 1983.

Oldfield MC: Campdactodactyly: flexor contractures of the fingers in young girls, Br J Plast Surg 8:312, 1956.

Smith RJ and Kaplan EB: Camptodactyly and similar atraumatic flexion deformities of the proximal interphalangeal joints of the fingers, J Bone Joint Surg 50A:1187, 1968.

Kirner deformity

Carstam N and Eiken O: Kirner's deformity of the little finger, J Bone Joint Surg 52A:1663, 1970.

David TJ and Burwood RL: The nature and inheritance of Kirner's deformity, J Med Genet 9:430, 1972.

Dykes RG: Kirner's deformity of the little finger, J Bone Joint Surg 60B:58, 1978.

Kirner J: Doppelseitige Verkrummung des Kleinfingergrundgliedes als selbstandiges Krankheitsbild, Fortschr Rontgenstr 36:804, 1927.

Todd AH: Case of hereditary contracture of the little fingers, Lancet 2:1088, 1929.

Delta phalanx

Carstam N and Theander G: Surgical treatment of clinicodactyly caused by longitudinally bracketed diaphysis (delta phalanx), Scand J Plast Reconstr Surg 9:199, 1975.

Smith RJ: Osteotomy for "delta-phalanx" deformity, Clin Orthop 123:91, 1977.

Madelung deformity

Darrach W: Habitual forward dislocation of the head of the ulna, Ann Surg 57:928, 1913.

Gelberman RH and Bauman T: Madelung's deformity and dyschondrosteosis, J Hand Surg 5:338, 1980.

Madelung V: Die spontane Subluxation der Hand nach vome, Verh Dtsch Ges Chir 7:259, 1878.

Malgaigne JF: Traité des fractures et des luxations, 2:711, 1855.

Milch H: Cuff resection of the ulna for malunited Colles' fracture, J Bone Joint Surg 23:311, 1941.

Ranawat CS, DeFiore J, and Straub LR: Madelung's deformity: an end-result study of surgical treatment, J Bone Joint Surg 57A:722, 1975.

Vender MI and Watson HK: Acquired Madelung-like deformity in a gymnast, J Hand Surg 13A:19, 1988.

Vickers DW: Langenskiöld's operation (physiolysis) for congenital malformations of bone producing Madelung's deformity and clinicodactyly, J Bone Joint Surg 66B:778, 1984.

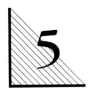

5 Skeletal and Genetic Dysplasias

JAMES H. BEATY

The skeletal dysplasias (osteochondrodysplasias) and genetic dysplasias include a wide variety of disorders characterized by intrinsic bone disturbance, generalized metabolic disorders, and ectodermal deformity. The overall size and shape of the limbs and trunk are affected, and a generalized disturbance in the development of the skull, spine and extremities occurs to varying degrees. Disproportionate short stature (dwarfism) is frequent, and the standing height for patients with many of the skeletal dysplasias falls below the fifth percentile for age.

Although the most commonly accepted nomenclature is based on the International Nomenclature of Constitutional Diseases of Bone (1983), terminology for skeletal dysplasias typically is derived from several different sources. Regardless of the designation of any particular dysplasia, a descriptive term to indicate the portion of the limb with the greatest involvement is helpful, such as rhizomelic (proximal), mesomelic (middle), and acromelic (distal). Diagnosis of the specific dysplasia is important to determine the appropriate treatment and accurate genetic counseling for the family.

Included in this chapter are some of the more common skeletal and genetic dysplasias affecting infants and children and the surgical procedures sometimes recommended for these patients.

ACHONDROPLASIA

Achondroplasia (chondrodysplasia fetalis, chondrodystrophic dwarfism) is the most common form of dwarfism; 80% to 90% of children with achondroplasia are born to families with normal parents and siblings, most likely as the result of a dominant gene mutation. For these families the possibility of giving birth to another achondroplastic child is equal to that of the rest of the population. Because achondroplasia is an autosomal dominant disorder, the possibility of having an achondroplastic child is 50% if one parent is achondroplastic and the other is not; if both parents are achondroplastic, the likelihood of having an achondroplastic child is 75%.

The primary defect in achondroplasia is abnormal endochondral bone formation with normal periosteal and intramembranous ossification. Interstitial cartilage production is affected, and the cartilage of the physis fails to proliferate. Since ossification remains unaffected, the long bones increase in length—but growth is very slow, producing rhizomelic extremities with greater shortening of the proximal segment than the distal segment. This is most obvious in long bones with a rapid rate of growth, particularly the humerus and femur. The remaining portions of the physis and articular cartilage are normal, producing short, wide bones with normal articular surfaces.

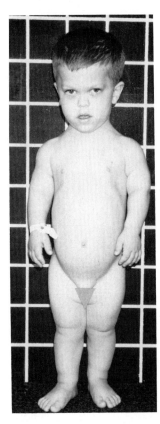

Fig. 5-1   Achondroplasia in 6-year-old boy. Note characteristic rhizomelia with short humerus and femur, disproportionate trunk-to-extremities length, frontal bossing, and short, broad hands.

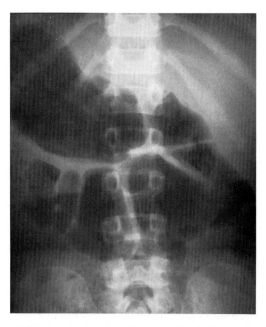

Fig. 5-2   Lumbar spine in achondroplasia. Note decrease in interpedicular distance from upper lumbar spine to sacrum.

Clinical features. The distinctive characteristics of achondroplasia are easily recognized at birth: dwarfism secondary to overall reduction in height from shortness of the lower limbs; disproportion between the height of the trunk and extremities, with the greatest amount of shortening in the proximal segments of the limbs; enlarged skull with prominent frontal region and depression of the bridge of the nose; and short, broad hands with the characteristic "trident" hand unable to adduct the middle and ring fingers in extension (Fig. 5-1). Children younger than 12 months of age may have a kyphotic deformity at the thoracolumbar junction and lordosis in the upper thoracic region. Once ambulation begins, lumbar lordosis gradually becomes exaggerated and hip flexion contractures develop. Bowing of the lower extremities, most commonly a genu varum deformity, may occur, and occasionally a valgus deformity develops at the knee.

Roentgenographic features. A mild kyphotic deformity at the thoracolumbar junction and hyperlordosis in the lumbar region may exist during infancy. With growth, the interpedicular distance from the upper lumbar spine to the sacrum decreases, in contrast to normal individuals in whom this distance remains the same or slightly increases (Fig. 5-2). The pelvis is wide with a general reduction in the size of the sciatic notch, the iliac crests are square, and the acetabulum is broad and flat. The increased width of the pelvis compared with its depth gives it the characteristic "champagne glass" appearance (Fig. 5-3). The diaphyses of long bones appear normal in diameter, with flaring in the metaphyseal area. The physes are notched with an inverted V centrally, particularly in the distal femur. The fibula appears longer than the tibia, and the head of the fibula may be at the level of the knee joint (Fig. 5-4).

Orthopaedic treatment. Spinal deformity, with occasional neurologic dysfunction, most often requires treatment in adults with achondroplasia, who have a relatively high incidence of lumbar disk disease or spinal stenosis. MRI and CT are helpful before surgical decompression of the stenotic lumbar spine in patients with neurologic symptoms.

Genu varum occurs in more than half of all patients with achondroplasia. Severe deformity may require surgical correction, most commonly proximal tibial and fibular osteotomies (Fig. 5-5). For the occasional child with severe genu valgum, osteotomy of the distal femur may be required. Limb lengthening procedures in these children have recently been reported, but the total social, psychologic, and orthopaedic benefits are inconclusive.

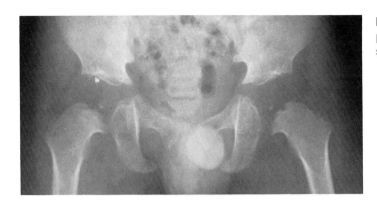

Fig. 5-3 Pelvis in achondroplasia. "Champagne glass" pelvis, small sciatic notch, squared iliac crests, and flat acetabulum.

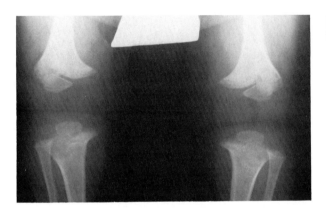

Fig. 5-4 Knee in achondroplasia. Notched, inverted V in distal femoral physis and proximal fibular overgrowth.

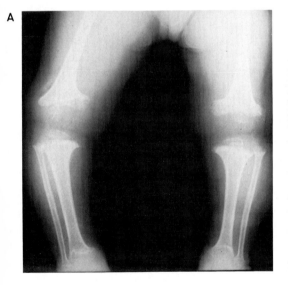

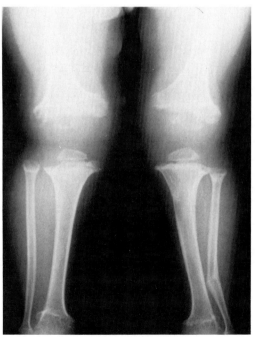

Fig. 5-5 Achondroplasia: bilateral genu varum in 5-year-old boy, greater in right leg than in left. **A,** Preoperative standing anteroposterior roentgenogram. **B,** After bilateral tibial and fibular osteotomies.

MULTIPLE EPIPHYSEAL DYSPLASIA

Multiple epiphyseal dysplasia (MED) is one of the more common osteochondrodysplasias. The milder form of this disorder is known as Ribbing disease to distinguish it from the more severe form described by Fairbank. Multiple epiphyseal dysplasia is usually transmitted as an autosomal dominant disorder, although autosomal recessive transmission has been reported. The primary defect is endochondral ossification not only in the epiphyses but also in the region of the physes.

Clinical features. Multiple epiphyseal dysplasia is characterized by short-limbed disproportionate dwarfing of varying degrees, and symptoms usually do not appear until after walking age. The disorder is diagnosed in most children between the ages of 5 and 15 years. The joints, primarily the hips, knees and ankles, are symmetrically affected. Angular deformities, particularly coxa vara and genu varum or valgum, are usually associated with flexion contractures of the hips and knees. The spine is usually not involved, and the face and head are normal.

Roentgenographic features. The primary roentgenographic changes are irregular ossification in the epiphyses of the long bones, particularly the femur and humerus. Epiphyseal ossification is usually delayed, and once ossification begins it is irregular and mottled in appearance.

Joint deformities in multiple epiphyseal dysplasia are caused by mechanical factors and by growth. Malalignment of the extremities may alter mechanical forces across the joints in the lower extremities and cause deformity and early osteoarthritis. The hips are the most severely deformed. The proximal femoral epiphyses appear late and when ossified are small and fragmented, leading to progressive deformity, including coxa vara, with subsequent hip joint subluxation and premature osteoarthritis (Fig. 5-6).

Multiple epiphyseal dysplasia must be differentiated from the rare incidence of bilateral, symmetric Perthes disease. The delayed bone age typical of Perthes disease is not seen in multiple epiphyseal dysplasia, and a skeletal survey may be helpful in children with suspected bilateral Perthes disease to rule out an osteochondrodysplasia. Anteroposterior roentgenograms of the knees and the ankles are the most useful views (Fig. 5-7). The lack of ossification in the lateral aspect of the distal tibial epiphysis, or the so-called slant sign, is occasionally seen but is not a universal finding.

Some recent reports have indicated that Perthes-like changes may be superimposed on the irregular ossification of multiple epiphyseal dysplasia. Current imaging techniques such as bone scans and MRI are being used to evaluate the association of avascular necrosis with multiple epiphyseal dysplasia.

Orthopaedic treatment. Osteoarthritis of the hip is the most common problem requiring surgery in patients with multiple epiphyseal dysplasia. Subluxation of the femoral head with hinged abduction occasionally occurs in adolescent patients, and valgus subtrochanteric osteotomy may be performed to prevent further instability and deformity; varus derotational osteotomy is contraindicated because of preexisting coxa vara. Any realignment osteotomy of the hip must be performed with the realization that early osteoarthritis is almost inevitable.

Severe, symptomatic valgus deformity of the knee or ankle may be corrected by osteotomy, but when supracondylar femoral osteotomy is used for correction of severe genu valgum, the coxa vara deformity may also require correction to ensure physiologic joint alignment after any osteotomy about the knee. Realignment osteotomies should be performed on patients close to skeletal maturity unless symptoms require earlier surgery. Occasionally severe limb length discrepancy may require epiphysiodesis for limb equalization.

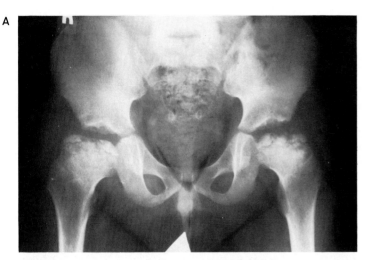

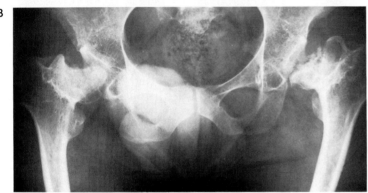

Fig. 5-6 Multiple epiphyseal dysplasia (MED). **A,** Coxa vara and fragmented, Perthes-like appearance of proximal femoral epiphyses in 7-year-old boy. **B,** Severe deformity and subluxation in 26-year-old man.

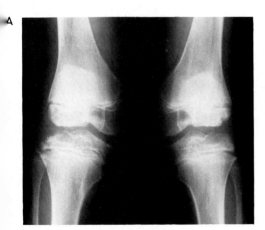

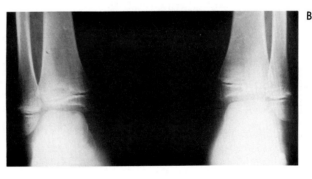

Fig. 5-7 Multiple epiphyseal dysplasia (MED). **A,** Anteroposterior roentgenogram of knees shows irregular articular surfaces of femoral condyle and tibial plateau. **B,** Anteroposterior roentgenogram of ankles. Note epiphyseal irregularity ("slant sign") of distal tibial epiphysis.

SPONDYLOEPIPHYSEAL DYSPLASIA CONGENITA

Spondyloepiphyseal dysplasia congenita affects the vertebrae and physes, causing short-trunk disproportionate dwarfism. It is transmitted as an autosomal dominant disorder, although most occurrences are sporadic—the results of new mutation. The primary abnormality is in the proliferative zone of the physis.

Clinical features. Spondyloepiphyseal dysplasia congenita may be diagnosed at birth because of the characteristic roentgenographic appearance of the vertebrae and epiphyses of long bones. Cleft palate and clubfoot are commonly associated anomalies. The hands and feet are usually normal in length, in contrast to the extreme shortness of the proximal and middle segments of the extremities. Severe genu valgum usually develops with growth, but genu varum may occur.

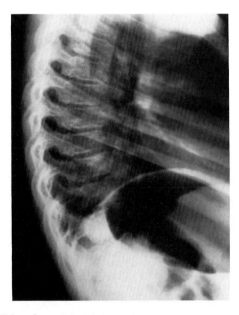

Fig. 5-8 Spondyloepiphyseal dysplasia. Platyspondyly of thoracic spine with wedging of vertebral bodies.

Myopia or retinal detachment has been reported in more than half of children with spondyloepiphyseal dysplasia congenita in some series, and ophthalmology consultation is recommended at appropriate intervals.

Roentgenographic features. Ossification of the epiphyses is delayed in children with spondyloepiphyseal dysplasia congenita, especially of the proximal femoral epiphyses. Roentgenograms of the spine show varying degrees of platyspondyly and posterior wedging of the vertebral bodies (Fig. 5-8). Progressive kyphoscoliosis may develop in late adolescence. Odontoid hypoplasia or os odontoideum may lead to atlantoaxial instability. Delayed ossification of the proximal femoral epiphyses causes coxa vara deformity in almost all patients, and the distal femoral and tibial epiphyses are flattened with irregular articular surfaces. Genu valgum is commonly associated with overgrowth of the medial femoral condyle.

Orthopaedic treatment. Odontoid hypoplasia or os odontoideum in children with spondyloepiphyseal dysplasia congenita should be thoroughly evaluated and aggressively treated. Posterior atlantoaxial fusion is indicated for signs and symptoms of myelopathy and for instability of more than 5 mm. Scoliosis develops in most children with spondyloepiphyseal dysplasia congenita. Curves of less than 40 degrees in skeletally immature patients may be treated initially with bracing. Posterior spinal fusion is recommended for curves that progress despite brace treatment or which initially measure more than 50 degrees.

Subtrochanteric valgus osteotomy may be indicated for severe coxa vara deformity in which the femoral neck-shaft angle is less than 110 degrees. The neck-shaft angle should be corrected to 140 degrees or more to help prevent recurrence of the deformity. Extension of the distal femur in conjunction with the valgus osteotomy decreases the flexion deformity of the hip and may improve excessive lumbar lordosis.

Before any osteotomy about the hip or knee, the alignment of the entire extremity must be considered. Severe genu valgum may require varus supracondylar femoral osteotomy, but the alignment of the hip, knee, and ankle should be evaluated before osteotomy of the knee alone.

SPONDYLOEPIPHYSEAL DYSPLASIA TARDA

Spondyloepiphyseal dysplasia tarda primarily affects the spine and the epiphyses of the larger, more proximally located joints, particularly the hip. Spondyloepiphyseal dysplasia tarda may be transmitted as an X-linked recessive disorder, autosomal dominant, or autosomal recessive trait. The X-linked type affecting males only is most common. Hip or spine involvement is usually not apparent until after 4 years of age and typically may not be diagnosed until the age of 10. Symptomatic scoliosis is frequent, but the most common problem is deformity of the hip or knee, with progressive osteoarthritis becoming symptomatic by early adolescence in many patients.

Roentgenographic features. The most common roentgenographic finding is symmetric involvement of the shoulders, hips, and knees. Delayed ossification predisposes these joints to deformation and early osteoarthritis. Because atlantoaxial instability may be caused by odontoid hypoplasia or os odontoideum, roentgenographic assessment should include lateral flexion and extension views of the cervical spine. Platyspondyly affects the remainder of the spine to a varying degree, and scoliosis is common.

Orthopaedic treatment. The treatment for scoliosis in spondyloepiphyseal dysplasia tarda is similar to that for adolescent idiopathic scoliosis. Orthotic treatment is recommended for curves approaching 30 degrees in the skeletally immature patient. In patients with atlantoaxial instability, neurologic symptoms, or excessive laxity, posterior C1-C2 spinal fusion should be considered.

The typical early symptomatic osteoarthritis of the hip in spondyloepiphyseal dysplasia tarda usually requires total hip arthroplasty during early adulthood; reconstructive osteotomy of the hip is rarely performed (Fig. 5-9). Occasionally realignment osteotomies of the knee and ankle are also required.

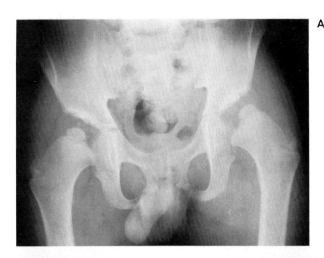

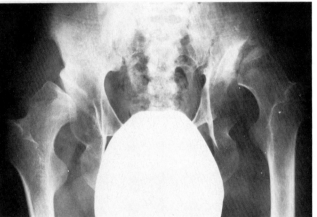

Fig. 5-9 Spondyloepiphyseal dysplasia tarda. **A,** Early femoral head changes in 8-year-old boy. **B,** Subluxation and osteoarthritis of hips in 33-year-old man.

METAPHYSEAL CHONDRODYSPLASIA

Metaphyseal chondrodysplasia includes a group of dysplasias characterized by roentgenographic changes in the metaphyses of long bones with normal epiphyses. These rare disorders are caused primarily by abnormal mineralization in the metaphyseal region of the long bones and defects in the proliferative and hypertrophic zones of the physes. The two most common types of metaphyseal chondrodysplasia are those described by Schmid and McKusick; Jansen described a rare third type.

Clinical features. The Schmid type of metaphyseal chondrodysplasia is most common. It causes short stature, bowing of the lower extremities, increased

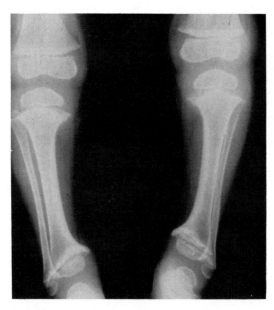

Fig. 5-10 Metaphyseal chondrodysplasia, Schmid type. **A,** Varus deformity of knee and ankle with distal fibular overgrowth.

lordosis, and a waddling gait. This type of metaphyseal chondrodysplasia is often misdiagnosed as vitamin D–resistant rickets. It is transmitted as an autosomal dominant disorder. The lower extremities are more severely involved than the upper extremities with typical varus deformities of the knees and ankles.

The McKusick type of metaphyseal chondrodysplasia is a distinct entity originally called "cartilage-hair hypoplasia," partly because of the sparse, light-colored hair of children with this disorder. It is a common cause of dwarfing among the Amish population of North America, with an incidence of 2 per 1000 live births, but is less frequent in the general population than the Schmid type. The McKusick type of metaphyseal chondrodysplasia is an autosomal recessive disorder. Genu varum in the McKusick type is mild compared with that in the Schmid type. Distal fibular overgrowth causes varus deformity of the ankle.

Roentgenographic features. Atlantoaxial instability and thoracic scoliosis have been reported in the Schmid type of metaphyseal chondrodysplasia. Varus deformities of the knee and ankle may worsen with growth and weight-bearing (Fig. 5-10). In the McKusick type, a greater degree of shortening exists in the long bones, particularly in the lower extremities. Coxa vara and genu varum are less common and less severe than in the Schmid type.

Orthopaedic treatment. Lateral flexion and extension roentgenograms should be carefully evaluated for evidence of atlantoaxial instability in patients with the McKusick type of metaphyseal chondrodysplasia. Coxa vara in the McKusick type rarely requires subtrochanteric valgus osteotomy. Genu varum seen in early infancy tends to improve spontaneously with growth, but corrective osteotomy is required, rarely, if the deformity does not improve.

LARSEN SYNDROME

Larsen syndrome is a rare skeletal dysplasia affecting the extremities, the face, and the spine. Its primary manifestations are multiple, fixed joint dislocations. It is inherited as an autosomal dominant disorder, but autosomal recessive transmission has been reported.

Clinical features. Common facial findings include a prominent forehead, ocular hypertelorism, and depression of the nasal bridge. Bilateral radial head dislocations with associated cubitus varus are common. Thoracic or lumbar scoliosis may be present, and lumbar lordosis may be increased by bilateral hip dislocations. Anterior dislocations of the knees and severe equinovarus or equinovalgus deformities of the feet are also common.

Roentgenographic features. The most frequent problems are dislocations of the radial head, knee, and hip, but dislocations have been reported in numerous other joints in the upper and lower extremities (Fig. 5-11). Screening roentgenograms of the cervical, thoracic, and lumbar parts of the spine should be obtained to detect other congenital anomalies.

Orthopaedic treatment. Because Larsen syndrome is a rare dysplasia, the diagnosis should not be made unless the characteristic facial features and other bony anomalies exist in addition to the classic multiple joint dislocations. The dislocations of the hip and knee and the foot deformity do not usually respond to conservative treatment and typically require surgical correction. The surgical treatment of dislocations of the knee and hip is similar to that of teratologic dislocation of the hip and congenital dislocation of the knee (see Chapter 2). The knee dislocation should be corrected before treatment of the hip.

The frequency of cervical spine anomalies associated with Larsen syndrome mandates thorough evaluation of the cervical spine with routine screening roentgenograms and, if necessary, flexion and extension lateral views before the administration of general anesthesia. Surgical stabilization occasionally is required for severe cervical kyphosis or C1-C2 instability. Posterior spinal fusion alone may not be sufficient for children with severe kyphosis or large multilevel segmental loss of posterior elements. In rare circumstances, staged anterior and posterior fusions are required.

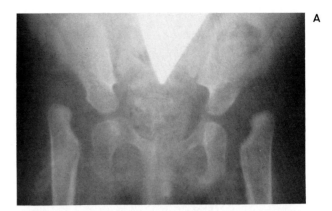

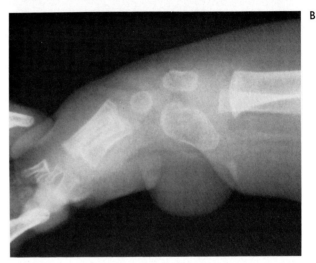

Fig. 5-11 Larsen syndrome. **A,** Bilateral teratologic hip dislocations. **B,** Severe, fixed teratologic clubfoot.

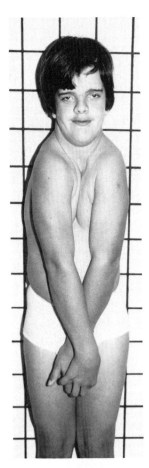

Fig. 5-12   Cleidocranial dysplasia in 15-year-old boy with bilateral absence of middle third of clavicle and nearly complete shoulder apposition.

CLEIDOCRANIAL DYSPLASIA

Cleidocranial dysplasia (cleidocranial dysostosis) involves that part of the skeleton formed by intramembranous ossification—particularly the facial bones, the cranium, the clavicle, and the pelvis. It is an autosomal dominant disorder causing generalized disturbance of bone growth and development in the bones formed by intramembranous ossification. Approximately 30% of these cases are spontaneous mutations; the patients have no family history of the disorder.

Clinical features. Common facial features include frontal bossing, hypertelorism, and dental abnormalities such as delayed or absent eruption of permanent teeth and defective tooth formation. Palpable defects of the clavicle are common. Patients missing all or significant portions of the clavicle have excessive mobility and may be able to appose their shoulders completely (Fig. 5-12).

Roentgenographic features. The clavicle may be completely absent or hypoplastic; more frequently, though, the central third of the clavicle is absent and the medial and lateral portions remain. The most common finding on pelvic roentgenogram is partial or total absence of the pubis with failure of closure of the pubic symphysis; the iliac crest may also be hypoplastic. Scoliosis may be caused by hemivertebrae formation.

Orthopaedic treatment. Surgical treatment for the defect in the clavicle is generally not required. Occasionally recurrent dislocation of the elbow or shoulder requires surgical correction. Even more rarely, symptoms from the brachial plexus in the distal upper extremity may require surgical removal of the remaining fragment of the clavicle. Attempts at reconstruction of the defect in the clavicle are not recommended. In the rare patients with associated coxa vara, a subtrochanteric valgus osteotomy may be performed if the femoral neck-shaft angle is 110 degrees or less.

DIASTROPHIC DYSPLASIA

Diastrophic dysplasia is a rare skeletal dysplasia causing abnormalities of the hands, feet, and ears and characteristic extreme short-limbed dwarfism. Initially described by Lamy and Maroteaux, who suggested the name "diastrophic dwarfism," it is transmitted as an autosomal recessive disorder; the parents of a child with diastrophic dysplasia have a 25% chance of giving birth to another affected child. The etiology is unknown, but diastrophic dysplasia is believed to be a neuromesodermal defect secondary to failure of normal collagen to form.

Clinical features. Diastrophic dysplasia is usually obvious at birth because of the extremely short stature and micromelia. Some children die during infancy from respiratory failure. Severe scoliosis with kyphosis and severe bilateral clubfoot deformities usually exist at birth. Specific abnormalities of the hand include the so-called hitchhiker thumb with radial subluxation of the metacarpophalangeal joint and excessive shortening of the first metacarpal. The rigid bilateral clubfoot deformities usually resist nonoperative treatment. The spinal deformities are also severe, and progressive thoracic kyphoscoliosis or cervical kyphosis is frequent.

Roentgenographic features. Congenital anomalies of the spine have been reported in large series and are associated with progressive spinal deformity, which typically requires early surgery. The long tubular bones are short and broad and have marked flaring in the metaphyses. A rhizomelic pattern of shortening exists in the upper and lower extremities. The proximal femoral epiphyses are delayed in appearance and ossification pattern. Early osteoarthritis and bilateral hip dislocations are common.

Orthopaedic treatment. Because of the multiple skeletal deformities in children with diastrophic dysplasia, including spinal deformity, deficient joint motion and contractures, severe bilateral clubfeet, and early onset of osteoarthritis, treatment should be directed to the specific problems that are responsive to appropriate orthopaedic treatment.

Cervical kyphosis is the most critical consideration because of the risk of quadriparesis from progressive kyphosis. Lateral flexion and extension cervical spine roentgenograms should be obtained to assess the stability at the apex of the kyphosis. MRI may be helpful in assessing spinal cord compression when neurologic symptoms exist. Surgical intervention is recommended for neurologic involvement; usually both anterior and posterior surgical approaches are required because of kyphosis in association with spina bifida.

Thoracolumbar spinal deformity is frequent in patients with diastrophic dysplasia. Bracing may be used initially in an attempt to control spinal deformity, but surgical treatment is recommended, even in the very young patient, if the deformity progresses. For kyphosis of greater than 50 degrees, anterior fusion should be followed by posterior fusion.

The bilateral clubfoot deformity in diastrophic dysplasia is extremely rigid and resistant to manipulation and casting. Surgical release is technically difficult because of the small size and rigidity of the foot and probably should be delayed until the child is 12 to 18 months of age. The commonly associated dislocation of the hip is also difficult to correct because of other skeletal deformities, primarily of the spine and foot, which require aggressive treatment. Treatment of the hip with soft tissue release and osteotomies is not recommended. If possible, severe contractures about the hip and knee should be corrected to allow weight bearing. Occasionally in the adult with severely symptomatic osteoarthritis of the hip, total hip arthroplasty is recommended.

CHONDROECTODERMAL DYSPLASIA

Chondroectodermal dysplasia (Ellis–van Creveld syndrome) is a rare syndrome characterized by short-limbed disproportionate dwarfism, dysplasia of fingernails and toenails, and polydactyly. It is transmitted as an autosomal recessive trait and is most common among the Amish of Pennsylvania. The incidence in this group is approximately 5 per 1000 live births.

Clinical features. Most children with chondroectodermal dysplasia have congenital heart disease, and approximately one third of infants are stillborn or die of cardiopulmonary causes.

Postaxial polydactyly of the hands is extremely common, occasionally involving the feet as well. Syndactyly of digits may also occur. The nails of the hands and feet are dysplastic. Generally acromesomelic shortening in the lower extremities occurs with valgus deformity of the knee, which tends to progress with growth.

Roentgenographic features. The middle phalanges of the hands and feet typically have cone-shaped epiphyses. The radial head may be dislocated, and the proximal radius and distal ulna may be hypoplastic. Early ossification of the femoral head is frequent and may be apparent in utero, making the diagnosis possible before birth. The fibulae are disproportionately shorter than the tibiae. Epiphyseal growth disturbance of the proximal tibia may cause a progressive valgus deformity at the knee.

Orthopaedic treatment. Correction of the polydactyly and syndactyly is recommended before 12 to 18 months of age. The progressive genu valgum usually requires surgical correction, and a supracondylar femoral osteotomy is indicated for genu valgum exceeding 20 degrees to correct the angular deformity and the externally rotated knee.

Preoperative roentgenograms should be studied carefully before a plan is made for surgical correction. Realignment may require a femoral varus derotational osteotomy of the hip combined with supracondylar varus femoral osteotomy and, if necessary, a proximal tibial and fibular osteotomy. The valgus deformity of the knee may recur because of growth disturbance of the lateral portion of the proximal tibial epiphysis. Close observation is recommended throughout skeletal growth, and a second osteotomy may be required.

DYSPLASIA EPIPHYSEALIS HEMIMELIA

Dysplasia epiphysealis hemimelia (Trevor disease) is a rare disorder in which osteocartilaginous growths involve the tarsal bones and the epiphyses of the long bones in the lower extremities. The medial or lateral half of long bones is most frequently involved, especially the distal femur, distal tibia, and talus. The medial aspect of a single extremity is more frequently affected than the lateral aspect.

Clinical features. Dysplasia epiphysealis hemimelia may become evident at any age, although the diagnosis is most commonly made during adolescence. Frequent clinical findings include loss of motion in the extremities, asymmetric joint enlargement, and symptoms of locking and pain (Fig. 5-13). Angular deformity, particularly varus or valgus deformity of the knee or ankle, may occur. Limb length inequality may progress with growth. The pathologic process is similar to that of an intraarticular osteochondroma.

Roentgenographic features. Dysplasia epiphysealis hemimelia may appear as an irregular, lobulated

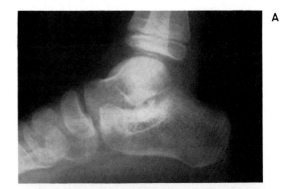

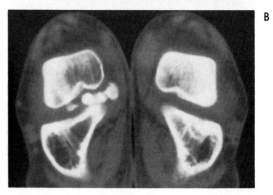

Fig. 5-13 Dysplasia epiphysealis hemimelia in 9-year-old referred for treatment of peroneal spastic flatfoot. **A,** Lateral view of ankle and foot showing sclerosis of middle facet and subtalar joint. **B,** CT scan demonstrates deformity of talus medially into medial facet of subtalar joint.

mass or as a sessile-based lesion similar to an osteochondroma protruding from the medial or lateral half of an epiphysis or a carpal or tarsal bone, most commonly in the knee, ankle, talus, and tarsal navicular (Fig. 5-14). More than one bone in the same extremity may be involved, but bilateral involvement has not been reported.

Orthopaedic treatment. There have been no reports of malignant transformation of this lesion, so treatment should be directed toward functional symptoms. If the mass interferes with joint range of motion, then excision is recommended. If an associated angular deformity beyond physiologically acceptable limits exists, then osteotomy may be required. If limb length discrepancy progresses, appropriate treatment is recommended to obtain limb length equalization by adulthood. Sometimes joint deformity is so severe that fusion is required during adolescence or arthroplasty of the hip or knee is required during adulthood.

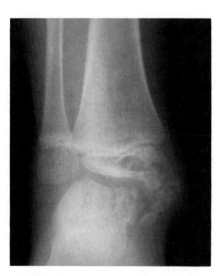

Fig. 5-14 Dysplasia epiphysealis hemimelia. Anteroposterior roentgenogram of ankle reveals deformity of medial half of talus beneath medial malleolus.

DIAPHYSEAL DYSPLASIA

Diaphyseal dysplasia (progressive diaphyseal dysplasia, Engelmann disease) is a rare disorder characterized by wide diaphyses and excessive periosteal and endosteal bone formation with sclerosis. It is believed to be transmitted as an autosomal dominant disorder.

Clinical features. Patients with mild forms of diaphyseal dysplasia may have apparently normal limbs and only occasional pain. More severely involved patients have chronic vague pain and muscle-wasting in the lower extremities. Walking may be delayed, or the older child may be unable to run.

Roentgenographic features. Skeletal involvement is usually bilateral and symmetric. The tibia and femur are most commonly affected, but the fibula or upper extremity long bones are occasionally involved. Roentgenograms show uniform enlargement of the bone's diaphyseal aspect with thickened cortices. With progression of the disease the medullary canal becomes narrow and may be obliterated. Hematopoietic dysfunction occasionally occurs in the severely involved patient.

Ribbing disease (hereditary multiple dyphyseal sclerosis) is a variant of Engelmann disease occurring in young patients in whom fewer bones are involved. The progressive nature of this disorder is not evident.

Orthopaedic treatment. There is no specific treatment for diaphyseal dysplasia. Occasionally a biopsy is recommended to confirm the diagnosis.

NEUROFIBROMATOSIS

Neurofibromatosis (von Recklinghausen disease) is a multisystemic hereditary disorder characterized by abnormalities of the supportive tissue of the central and peripheral nervous systems and associated with various anomalies of the skeleton, skin, and soft tissues. It is transmitted as an autosomal dominant trait, but mutations do occur. Its etiology is not completely understood, but the disease is considered to be a hamartomatous disorder, probably of neural crest origin, involving the neurectoderm, mesoderm, and endoderm, with the potential of appearing in almost all organ systems. The incidence of neurofibromatosis has been estimated as 1 in 2500 to 3000 live births.

Historically, three clinical forms were recognized: peripheral, central, and mixed. Currently a two-part classification is used: neurofibromatosis 1, or NF 1 (peripheral), and neurofibromatosis 2, or NF 2 (central). Multiple hyperpigmented areas and neurofibromas are characteristic of NF 1; acoustic nerve tumors, with or without other intercranial and interspinal tumors, are characteristic of NF 2. NF 1 is most common.

Clinical features. Soft tissue findings include café-au-lait spots, nodules (dermal neurofibromas), nevi (hyperpigmentation), hypertrophic villi (elephantiasis), plexiform neurofibromas, verrucous hyperplasia, and axillary freckles. These manifestations occur in widely varying degrees and in patients of different ages. The café-au-lait spots usually appear by the age of 9 years. The cutaneous nodules appear only after puberty and are manifestations of long-standing disease. Nevi are present in only about 6% of children with neurofibromatosis. Elephantiasis occurs more frequently in adults, but 10% of patients with these large soft tissue masses are children. In as many as 25% of patients with neurofibromatosis, café-au-lait spots are the only manifestations of the disease throughout their lifetimes. In 1987 the National Institutes of Health established diagnostic criteria for neurofibromatosis (see box at left), two or more of which should be met for the diagnosis to be made.

Roentgenographic features. Scoliosis is the most common skeletal defect associated with neurofibromatosis, occurring in as many as 60% of patients. The scoliosis is usually in the thoracic area and tends to produce a short-segmented, sharply angulated curve involving four to six vertebrae; it is usually progressive (Fig. 5-15). Severe kyphosis is frequently associated with the scoliosis, and anomalies of the cervical spine are common. Disorders of bone growth are frequently associated with changes in the soft tissues overlying the bony deformity.

The association of pseudarthrosis with neurofibromatosis has long been recognized. The single bone most commonly affected is the tibia. Bowing of the tibia is typically anterolateral and is usually evident within the first 2 years of life (Fig. 5-16). Pseudarthrosis may be congenital or may develop after a fracture or after osteotomy. Most patients with congenital pseudarthrosis of the tibia ultimately meet the diagnostic criteria for neurofibromatosis.

Other bony manifestations of neurofibromatosis include erosive defects from contiguous tumors and subperiosteal bone proliferation (calcifying hematoma).

Soft tissue neoplasms are also frequent, and the discovery of a mass by the parents is the single most common criterion leading to a diagnosis of neurofibromatosis. Malignancy is a significant risk in patients with neurofibromatosis; chances for it increase with age, from about 7% in children to 20% in adults. The list of malignant tumors associated with neurofibromatosis has greatly expanded within the last decade and includes neurofibrosarcoma, nonlymphocytic leukemia, Wilms' tumor, and urogenital rhabdomyosarcoma.

DIAGNOSTIC CRITERIA FOR NEUROFIBROMATOSIS

1. Six or more cafe au lait macules with their greatest diameters more than 5 mm in prepubertal children and more than 15 mm in postpubertal persons
2. Two or more neurofibromas of any type of one plexiform neurofibroma
3. Freckling in the axillary or inguinal region
4. Optical glioma
5. Two or more Lisch nodules (iris hamartomas)
6. A distinctive osseous lesion, such as sphenoid dysplasia or thinning of long bone cortex without pseudarthrosis
7. A first-degree relative (parent, sibling, or offspring) with neurofibromatosis identified by criteria *1* through *6*

From National Institutes of Health: Neurofibromatosis, Consensus Development Conference Statement 6(12):13, 1987.

Orthopaedic treatment. Spinal deformities, limb length discrepancy, and pseudarthrosis of the tibia most frequently require orthopaedic treatment in patients with neurofibromatosis. The scoliotic deformity can be either nondysplastic or dysplastic. The nondysplastic curvature resembles idiopathic scoliosis in location and progression and can generally be treated in a similar manner (see Chapter 10). Most scoliosis in patients with neurofibromatosis, however, is dysplastic with changes such as rib pencilling, spindling of the transverse processes, vertebral scalloping, severe apical vertebral rotation, foraminal enlargement, and adjacent soft tissue neurofibroma. Posterior fusion, with or without instrumentation, usually achieves stability for scoliosis alone; dysplastic kyphoscoliosis may require both anterior and posterior fusion. Because of the frequency of cervical spine deformities in these patients, the cervical spine should be carefully evaluated on roentgenograms before either skull traction or general anesthesia is administered.

Limb length discrepancy in children with neurofibromatosis may vary from mild hemihypertrophy to two to three times normal size in both length and circumference. Standard limb equalization procedures may be successful in mild and moderate deformities, but amputation is occasionally required for severe, untreated deformities.

The treatment and prognosis of pseudarthrosis of the tibia is dependent on the type of congenital anterolateral bowing (p. 119). The mainstay of treatment of pseudarthrosis of the tibia has been bone grafting, with reported success rates ranging from 31% to 56%. Newer techniques, including electrical stimulation, vascularized bone grafting, intramedullary rodding, and the Ilizarov procedure, show promising results, with reported success rates of 70% to 100%; there are, however, no long-term studies for evaluation of these modalities.

Large neurofibromas should be followed with periodic roentgenographic evaluation. Lesions in areas not clearly defined on roentgenogram or by physical examination may be regularly evaluated with MRI or CT scanning. Increasing size and pain suggest malignant transformation, for which appropriate treatment should be undertaken.

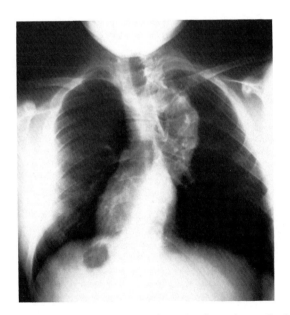

Fig. 5-15 Sharply angulated cervicothoracic scoliosis in 14-year-old boy with neurofibromatosis.

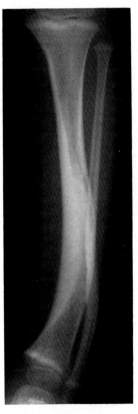

Fig. 5-16 Neurofibromatosis. Congenital pseudarthrosis of left tibia (type II) with anterolateral angulation.

DOWN SYNDROME

Down syndrome is a genetic disorder characterized by trisomy for all or a large portion of chromosome 21. The overall incidence is 1 in 600 live births, but the incidence increases progressively with maternal age.

Clinical features. Down syndrome is usually obvious at birth because of the characteristic facial features of hypoplastic maxilla and nasal bones, flattening of the nasal bridge, ocular hypertelorism, and a protuding, hypertrophied, fissured tongue. Children with Down syndrome have varying degrees of intellectual impairment, and many have congenital heart or gastrointestinal anomalies.

Roentgenographic features. The most common roentgenographic finding is the characteristic appearance of the pelvis with wide iliac wings and an acetabulum more horizontal than normal. Roentgenograms of the skull may show microcephaly, flattening of the occiput, abnormal convexity of the frontal region, and persistent widening of the sutures.

Orthopaedic treatment. The majority of orthopaedic problems in children with Down syndrome are secondary to hypotonia, ligamentous laxity, and hyperflexibility. Common problems include pes planus, genu valgum, recurrent dislocation of the patella, scoliosis, recurrent dislocation of the hip, and instability of the cervical spine.

Atlantoaxial instability is reported to occur in approximately 15% of children with Down syndrome. A small percentage of these children have excessive laxity or neurologic symptoms that require posterior spinal fusion. Screening for atlantoaxial instability should be performed before the child begins an educational program or participates in any activities that involve flexion and extension of the cervical spine. Scoliosis in children with Down syndrome rarely requires surgical correction. Deformities of the foot or lower extremity should be corrected only if they prohibit ambulation. Sometimes recurrent dislocation of the hip requires surgical correction, but initial treatment of hip dislocation should be reduction and immobilization in a spica cast. For recurrent dislocation of the hip the recommended treatment is capsular plication, either anteriorly or posteriorly depending on the direction of dislocation, and associated femoral or pelvic osteotomy (Fig. 5-17). Capsular plication may be effective in very young children (younger than 5 years of age), but the older the child with recurrent dislocation is, the more likely it is that a femoral osteotomy, pelvic osteotomy, or both will be required in combination with the capsular plication. Most often, femoral derotational osteotomy is performed for posterior dislocation and Salter osteotomy is performed for recurrent anterior dislocation.

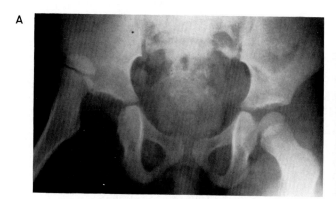
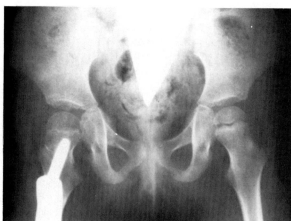

A
B

Fig. 5-17 Down syndrome. **A,** Recurrent posterior dislocation of right hip in 3-year-old girl. **B,** After posterior capsular plication and femoral derotation osteotomy.

MUCOPOLYSACCHARIDOSIS

Mucopolysaccharidosis is a group of widely varying skeletal disorders characterized by an inability to metabolize one or more mucopolysaccharides normally. These substances thus accumulate in tissues such as the brain, viscera, eyes, heart, lungs, and joints. Five different types of mucopolysaccharidosis are generally distinguished, depending on the mode of inheritance, the specific mucopolysaccharide involved, and the clinical and roentgenographic features. With the exception of Morquio syndrome, the mucopolysaccharidosis share a clinical-roentgenographic pattern of varying severity known as dysostosis multiplex. Although no specific therapy is available for treatment of the mucopolysaccharidoses, some recent reports indicate that bone marrow transplantation may be beneficial for some patients with these disorders.

Clinical features. The clinical presentation of the disorder depends on which mucopolysaccharides are involved, since some have a greater toxic effect on the central nervous system, others on the eye, and others on the skeleton.

Roentgenographic features. Characteristic roentgenographic deformities include wide metacarpals with tapered ends, distal radius and ulna pointing toward one another, varus of the humerus, valgus of the hips, flared iliac wings, dysplastic acetabula, inferoanterior beak in one or more upper lumbar vertebral bodies, J-shaped sella turcica, and flattened mandibular condyle. Myelography may show a thickened dura with narrowing of the contrast media space but without narrowing of the bony canal. These findings must be correlated with clinical findings and biochemical findings for definitive diagnosis of a specific type of mucopolysaccharidosis.

Orthopaedic treatment. Orthopaedic treatment of children with mucopolysaccharidosis is generally aimed at prolonging ambulation and improving hygiene and caretaking. Release of flexion contractures or correction of lower extremity angular deformities may be indicated, and some patients require spinal fusion for cervical spine instability. The specific musculoskeletal problems must be evaluated for each child and treated appropriately.

Morquio syndrome is transmitted as an autosomal recessive trait and is usually diagnosed in children between the ages of 18 months and 2 years because of a waddling gait, genu valgum, thoracic kyphosis, and pectus carinatum. Dwarfism is mainly of the short-trunk type, but as the child grows the lower limbs become shorter because of increasing genu valgum and deformity about the hip joints. Joint laxity and pes planus are common. Fine corneal opacities may be seen on careful slit-lamp examination. Repeated urinalysis is often necessary to detect keratosulfate in the urine.

Roentgenographic findings in infants are primarily in the spine, the pelvis, and the hands. Flattened vertebrae (platyspondyly) are seen in the thoracolumbar area, with the "tongue" deformity visible on the lateral view. Hypoplasia of the odontoid process or hypermobility of the upper cervical spine is frequent and is best seen on flexion-extension views. The acetabula are apparently oversized, and there is a valgus deformity of the hips. Some reports indicate acetabular dysplasia and an increased tendency toward subluxation or dislocation of the hip. The cervical instability may require fusion to the occiput, and multiple osteotomies may be needed for correction of genu valgum.

Hurler syndrome is an autosomal recessive disorder, usually manifested by the age of 2 to 3 years by progressive mental retardation or stunting of growth. The characteristic "gargoyle face" begins to appear, with thickened lips, wide nostrils, and large ears (Fig. 5-18). Hair becomes coarser. Progressive flexion contractures of the elbows, knees, and hips cause progressive disability in walking. Occasionally, blindness and deafness occur. The liver and spleen are enlarged, and joint motion is limited. Corneal opacities may exist. Kyphosis is frequent. Urinalysis shows increased excretion of heparitin sulfate and dermatan sulfate.

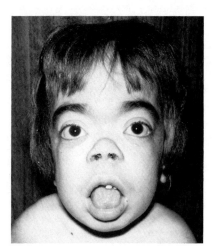

Fig. 5-18   Hurler syndrome. Characteristic "gargoyle" face: thickened lips, wide nostrils, and coarse hair.

The most characteristic roentgenographic finding is anteroinferior "beaking" of the vertebrae in the thoracolumbar area (Fig. 5-19). Orthopaedic treatment should be directed at symptomatic relief of low back or joint pain, and the short life span of these patients (few survive beyond adolescence) should be kept in mind before any orthopaedic treatment is considered.

Hunter syndrome is a sex-linked recessive trait affecting only males. It has clinical features similar to those of Hurler syndrome, but is milder and more slowly progressive. The mental retardation is not as severe as in Hurler syndrome, and onset is slightly later in life. Joint contractures most frequently affect the shoulders, with mild clawing of the fingers and occasional flexion contractures of the knees. Dwarfism and deafness are frequent, as are heart defects. Urinalysis shows increased excretion of dermatan sulfate and heparitin sulfate. Roentgenographic findings are similar to those in Hurler syndrome, but much less severe (Fig. 5-20). Vertebral beaking is marked,

even in infants, but the epiphyses of the long bones show no or only mild changes. Because this a sex-linked disorder, genetic counseling is imperative.

Sanfilippo syndrome is an autosomal recessive disease that usually does not become manifest until early childhood, usually as a behavioral problem or a "spastic" gait; mental retardation also begins in early childhood. Reflexes in the lower extremities may be hyperactive, with or without clonus. There are generally no marked joint contractures and no clawing of the fingers. Deafness is frequent, but there are no corneal opacities. Urinalysis shows increased heparitin sulfate. This form of mucopolysaccharidosis is often misdiagnosed as cerebral palsy; the key to differentiation is the increase in behavioral problems in conjunction with the increasing lower extremity spasticity. Most of these children are bedridden by adolescence and frequently die in early adulthood from respiratory distress. Orthopaedic treatment is indicated only for improvements in hygiene or caretaking.

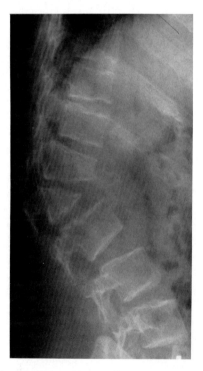

Fig. 5-19   Hurler syndrome. Severe wedging of vertebrae can be seen at thoracolumbar spine junction.

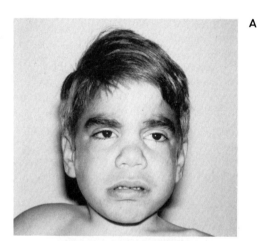

A

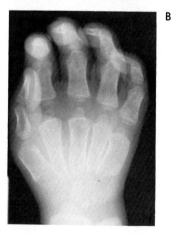

B

Fig. 5-20   Hunter syndrome. **A,** Characteristic facial features in 9-year-old boy. **B,** Anteroposterior roentgenogram of hand showing short, wide, dysplastic metacarpals and phalanges.

APERT SYNDROME

Apert syndrome is a rare condition primarily affecting the skull, feet, and hands. It is believed to be caused by a primary germ plasm defect causing premature fusion of the bones of the skull and syndactyly of the hands and feet.

Characteristic facial features include elongation, wide-spaced eyes, and strabismus (Fig. 5-21). The extremity manifestations include syndactyly of the hands or feet, which may be simple or complex but more frequently involves severe fusions of multiple digits.

Syndactyly of the hands generally requires surgical correction between the ages of 6 and 18 months (see Chapter 4). If syndactyly of the feet causes functional problems or difficulty in shoe fitting, then surgical correction is recommended.

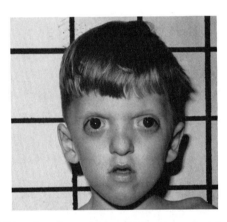

Fig. 5-21 Apert syndrome. Note characteristic facial elongation and wide-spaced eyes.

MULTIPLE HEREDITARY OSTEOCHONDROMATOSIS

Multiple hereditary osteochondromatosis (diaphyseal aclasis, hereditary multiple exostoses, multiple cartilaginous exostosis) is one of the most common skeletal dysplasias, with an incidence of approximately 10 per 1 million in the general population. It is transmitted as an autosomal dominant trait, and men and women are equally affected. The osteochondromas may be found throughout the skeleton, but the most common sites are the tubular long bones, iliac crests, scapulae, and ribs. The ends of the long bones, responsible for most of the longitudinal growth of the diaphysis, are often the most severely affected, as are the bones with the smallest cross-sectional area at the physes. For example, the radius and ulna are generally affected at their distal ends where most of the physeal growth in the forearm occurs, but the ulna is affected more severely because of its smaller cross-sectional area.

The osteochondromas may be large, sessile masses or pedunculated exostoses arising from the metaphyseal regions of long bones in close proximity to the physes.

Clinical features. Most patients with multiple hereditary osteochondromatosis are identified during the first decade of life. Pain or a palpable mass may be the initial presenting complaint. Pain is most common in the region of musculotendinous structures near adjacent lesions. Unusual complications have been reported, particularly with lesions in the pelvis that affect the visceral structures. Occasionally a painful nonunion results from fracture of an osteochondroma. The most serious complication is the risk of transformation to chondrosarcoma, reported to occur in from 0.5% or less to 1.5% of patients well into adulthood.

Roentgenographic features. In the upper extremity the most common deformity is shortening and bowing of the forearm. The ulna is usually more severely affected, with a pseudo-Madelung deformity distally, subluxation or dislocation of the radial head, and progressive shortening of the ulna.

Coxa valga is common in patients with multiple osteochondroma about the hip. Valgus deformity of the knee may be associated with valgus deformity of the ankle caused by shortening of the fibulae, valgus tibiae, and wedge-shaped distal tibial epiphyses (Fig. 5-22).

Orthopaedic treatment. Surgical excision of the exostoses is recommended if pain is associated with specific lesions. It should include extracapsular dissection and excision of the entire cartilaginous cap and adjacent periosteum. The adjacent physes should be avoided during the surgical dissection. Transformation to a malignant chondrosarcoma should be considered if a lesion increases in size and causes pain after skeletal maturity.

Current recommendations for treatment of progressive forearm and wrist deformity include lengthening of the ulna and either distal radial osteotomy or distal radial lateral hemiepiphysiodesis. These procedures may be performed in addition to excision of the distal exostoses (Fig. 5-23). Rarely, for severe shortening of the ulna a one-bone forearm procedure (p. 179) is preferable to ulnar lengthening. If the dislocated radial head is painful at skeletal maturity, it should be removed.

Progressive angular deformity of the ankle may be treated with supramalleolar osteotomy or a well-timed hemiepiphysiodesis. Occasionally tibial or distal femoral osteotomy may be required for severe genu valgum. Lesions in the region of the fibular head and neck may require excision and peroneal nerve decompression. Progressive limb length discrepancy in patients with asymmetric limb involvement may require limb equalization by epiphysiodesis or, rarely, limb-lengthening procedures.

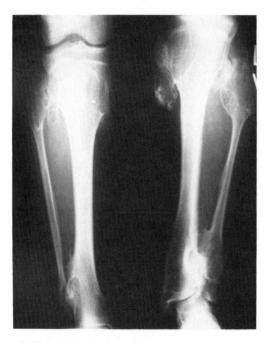

Fig. 5-22 Multiple hereditary osteochondromatosis. Note numerous sessile lesions of tibiae and fibulae and valgus deformity of left ankle.

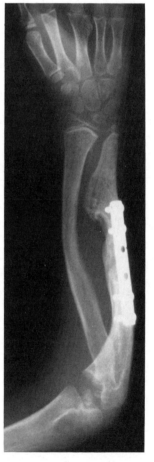

Fig. 5-23 Multiple hereditary osteochondromatosis. Progressive shortening of ulna has been treated by ulnar lengthening.

ENCHONDROMATOSIS

Enchondromatosis, or Ollier disease, is characterized by multiple cartilaginous lesions within the metaphyseal regions of tubular bones. The lesions appear to arise from the physes and result from the failure of normal endochondral ossification. No pattern of heredity to this disorder is known.

Clinical features. Enchondromatosis is usually evidenced in early childhood by the development of palpable masses on the extremities or trunk. Unilateral angular deformity or shortening of an extremity is common, and significant bowing and shortening of the forearm may occur in addition to a valgus or varus deformity in the lower extremity, which causes limb length discrepancy.

Patients with enchondromatosis are at risk for the development of a secondary chondrosarcoma, especially those with multiple soft tissue hemangiomas (Maffucci syndrome). A pattern of rapid growth of the lesion or increasing pain should prompt thorough evaluation, including biopsy if appropriate.

Roentgenographic features. The most common roentgenographic finding is a radiolucent area of cartilage in the metaphysis with irregular areas of calcification in a longitudinal or streaking pattern. In addition to the characteristic expansile lesions, shortening with associated angular deformity and limb length discrepancy may occur in an asymmetric pattern (Fig. 5-24).

Orthopaedic treatment. Osteotomy may be required for correction of severe angular deformity in the lower extremities. Osteotomies may be performed through areas of enchondromatosis, which appear to heal easily, as do pathologic fractures. Limb length discrepancy may require observation throughout adolescence and limb equalization by standard techniques of epiphysiodesis or limb lengthening. Individual lesions in the digits of the hand should be curetted and grafted if they become large enough to interfere with function.

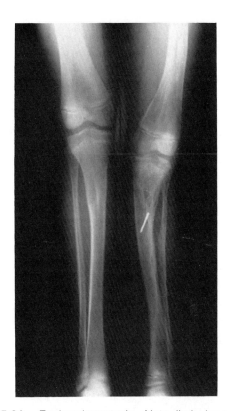

Fig. 5-24 Enchondromatosis. Note limb length discrepancy with involvement of distal femur and proximal tibia.

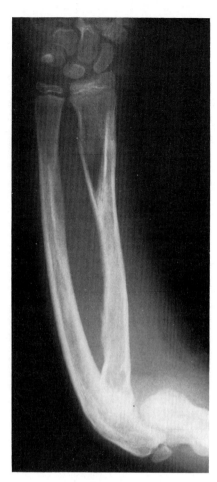

Fig. 5-25 Melorheostosis. Note flowing candle wax appearance of distal radius, angulation of proximal ulna, and dislocation of radial head.

MELORHEOSTOSIS

Melorheostosis, also known as "flowing wax bone," is a rare disorder in which calcified streaks extend longitudinally along the axis of long bones.

Clinical features. Clinical manifestations vary from mild to severe. In mild involvement this disorder may be an incidental finding on roentgenograms obtained for another problem. In the more severely involved patients there may be limitation of joint motion and soft tissue and bony contractures, especially about the hip and knee. With severe involvement the skin appears shiny and tense with edema and induration of the soft tissues. Occasionally underlying muscle atrophy and weakness exist in addition to compression of neurovascular structures. Limb length discrepancy, with or without angular deformity, may be the primary manifestation (Fig. 5-25).

Roentgenographic features. The characteristic roentgenographic appearance is melting wax along the side of a candle, which is caused by the longitudinal densities along the long axis of the tubular bones. The lesions are generally diaphyseal but may extend into metaphyseal and epiphyseal regions.

Orthopaedic treatment. Severe contractures about joints sometimes require surgical release. Rarely, severe limb length discrepancy and angular deformity may require osteotomy and either epiphysiodesis or limb lengthening as indicated.

CHONDRODYSPLASIA PUNCTATA

Chondrodysplasia congenita punctata (Conradi disease, chondrodysplasia faetalis hypoplastica, dysplasia epiphysealis punctata) is characterized by multiple punctate calcifications appearing in infancy and during skeletal maturation. The disorder is transmitted as an autosomal dominant trait, although the majority of cases are the result of spontaneous mutation.

Clinical features. Cataracts and alopecia exist in a significant number of patients, and severe delays in motor development and microcephaly are common in the rhizomelic form. Orthopaedic abnormalities include limb length discrepancy, coxa vara, flexion contractures of joints in the lower extremities, clubfoot, and significant spinal deformities including atlantoaxial instability and congenital scoliosis and kyphosis.

Roentgenographic features. The characteristic punctate calcifications are apparent at birth and usually resolve by the time the child is 12 to 24 months of age (Fig. 5-26). Secondary centers of ossification, especially the proximal femoral epiphyses, are delayed in appearance. Congenital hemivertebrae or congenital unilateral bars and odontoid hypoplasia may be seen in the spine.

Orthopaedic treatment. The most difficult problems in chondrodysplasia punctata are the spinal deformities. Atlantoaxial instability should be carefully evaluated. Scoliosis or kyphosis associated with congenital anomalies may be rapidly progressive and require early surgical correction. Lower extremity deformities include coxa vara, limb length discrepancy, and flexion contractures of the knee or hip; these contractures rarely require surgical release. Coxa vara with a femoral neck-shaft angle of less than 110 degrees should be treated with valgus subtrochanteric osteotomy. Occasionally limb length discrepancy requires equalization by appropriately timed epiphysiodesis or limb lengthening. Although epiphysiodesis is not recommended because of the already short stature, limb lengthening should be undertaken only if appropriate principles of limb lengthening are followed (see Chapter 3).

Clinical photographs in this chapter are courtesy of Dr. Sid Wilroy.

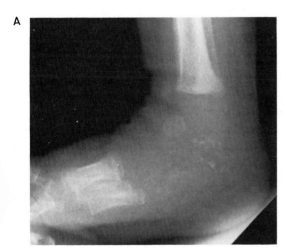
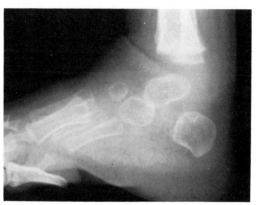

Fig. 5-26 Chondrodysplasia punctata. **A,** Newborn with clubfoot. Note characteristic punctate calcification in calcaneus. **B,** Progression of ossification 18 months later.

REFERENCES

General

Bailey JA II: Disproportionate short stature, Philadelphia, 1973, WB Saunders Co.

Bassett GS and Scott CI Jr: The osteochondrodysplasias. In Morrissy RT (ed): Lovell and Winter's pediatric orthopaedics, ed 3, Philadelphia, 1990, JB Lippincott Co.

Diamond LS: Management of inherited disorders of the skeleton. In Instructional Course Lectures. The American Academy of Orthopaedic Surgeons, vol 25, St Louis, 1976, The CV Mosby Co.

Dutton RV: A practical radiologic approach to skeletal dysplasias in infancy, Radiol Clin North Am 25:1211, 1987.

Fairbank T: An atlas of general affectations of the skeleton, Edinburgh, 1959, Churchill Livingstone.

Lenzi L and Capilupi B: International nomenclature of constitutional diseases of bone: revision 1983, Ital J Orthop Traumatol 11:249, 1985.

Kaitila II, Leisti JT, and Rimoin DL: Mesomelic skeletal dysplasias, Clin Orthop 114:94, 1976.

Kaufman HJ: Classification of the skeletal dysplasias and the radiologic approach to their differentiation, Clin Orthop 114:12, 1976.

McKusick VA: Heritable disorders of connective tissues, St Louis, 1972, The CV Mosby Co.

Orioli IM, Castilla EE, and Barbosa-Neto JG: The birth prevalence rates for the skeletal dysplasias, J Med Genet 23:328, 1986.

Rimoin DL, Silberberg R, and Hollister DW: Chondro-osseous pathology in the chondrodystrophies, Clin Orthop 114:137, 1976.

Spranger JW, Langer LO, and Wiedermann HR: Bone dysplasias, Philadelphia, 1974, WB Saunders Co.

Stelling FH III: The hip in heritable conditions of connective tissue, Clin Orthop 90:33, 1973.

Wynne-Davies R, Hall CM, and Apley AG: Atlas of skeletal dysplasias, New York, 1985, Churchill Livingstone.

Achondroplasia

Bailey JA: Orthopaedic aspects of achondroplasia, J Bone Joint Surg 52A:1285, 1970.

Boden SD et al: Metatrophic dwarfism: uncoupling of endochondral and perichondral growth, J Bone Joint Surg 69A:174, 1987.

Herring JA: Kyphosis in an achondroplastic dwarf, J Pediatr Orthop 3:250, 1983.

Kopits SE: Orthopedic complications of dwarfism, Clin Orthop 114:153, 1976.

Rimoin DL et al: Metatropic dwarfism, the Kniest syndrome, and the pseudoachondroplastic dysplasias, Clin Orthop 114:70, 1976.

Multiple epiphyseal dysplasia

Anderson PE Jr et al: Bilateral femoral head dysplasia and osteochondritis: multiple epiphyseal dysplasia tarda, spondyloepiphyseal dysplasia tarda, and bilateral Legg-Perthes disease, Acta Radiol 29:705, 1988.

Crossan JF, Wynne-Davies R, and Fulford GE: Bilateral failure of the capital femoral epiphysis: bilateral Perthes disease, multiple epiphyseal dysplasia, pseudoachondroplasia, and spondyloepiphyseal dysplasia congenita and tarda, J Pediatr Orthop 3:297, 1983.

Herring JA and Hotchkiss BL: Legg-Perthes disease versus metaphyseal epiphyseal dysplasia, J Pediatr Orthop 7:341, 1987.

MacKenzie WG et al: Avascular necrosis of the hip in multiple epiphyseal dysplasia, J Pediatr Orthop 9:666, 1989.

Spranger J: The epiphyseal dysplasias, Clin Orthop 114:46, 1976.

Versteylen RJ et al: multiple epiphyseal dysplasia complicated by severe osteochondritis dissecans of the knee: incidence in two families, Skeletal Radiol 17:407, 1988.

Spondyloepiphyseal dysplasia

Bannerman RM, Ingall GB, and Mohn JF: X-linked spondyloepiphyseal dysplasia tarda: clinical and linkage data, J Med Genet 8:291, 1971.

Carter C and Sutcliffe J: Genetic varieties of spondyloepiphyseal dysplasia. In Symposium ossium, Edinburgh, 1970, Churchill Livingstone.

Crossan JF, Wynne-Davies R, and Fulford GE: Bilateral failure of the capital femoral epiphysis: bilateral Perthes disease, multiple epiphyseal dysplasia, pseudoachondroplasia, and spondyloepiphyseal dysplasia congenita and tarda, J Pediatr Orthop 3:297, 1983.

Diamond LS: A family study of spondyloepiphyseal dysplasia, J Bone Joint Surg 52A:1587, 1970.

Fisher RL: Unusual spondyloepiphyseal and spondylometaphyseal dysplasias of childhood, Clin Orthop 100:78, 1974.

Kaibara N et al: Spondyloepiphyseal dysplasia tarda with progressive arthropathy, Skeletal Radiol 10:13, 1983.

Kozlowski K: Metaphyseal and spondylometaphyseal chondrodysplasias, Clin Orthop 114:83, 1976.

Schantz K, Andersen PE Jr, and Justesen P: Spondyloepiphyseal dysplasia tarda: report of a family with autosomal dominant transmission, Acta Orthop Scand 59:716, 1988.

Wynne-Davies R and Hall C: Two clinical variants of spondyloepiphyseal dysplasia congenita (with and without severe coxa vara), J Bone Joint Surg 64B:435, 1982.

Metaphyseal chondrodysplasia

Cooper RR and Ponseti IV: Metaphyseal dysostosis: description of an ultrastructural defect in the epiphyseal plate chondrocytes; case report, J Bone Joint Surg 55A:485, 1973.

Evans R and Caffey J: Metaphyseal dysostosis resembling vitamin D–refractory rickets, Am J Dis Child 95:640, 1958.

Fisher RL: Unusual spondyloepiphyseal and spondylometaphyseal dysplasias of childhood, Clin Orthop 100:78, 1974.

Jansen M: Über atypische Chondrodystrophie (Achondroplasie) und über eine noch nicht beschriebene angeborene Wachstumsstörung des Knochensystems: Metaphysäre Dysostosis, Z Orthop Chir 61:2255, 1934.

Kozlowski K: Metaphyseal and spondylometaphyseal chondrodysplasias, Clin Orthop 114:83, 1976.

McKusick VA: Heritable disorders of connective tissue, ed 4, St Louis, 1972, The CV Mosby Co.

Schmid F: Beitrag zur Dysostosis enchondrolic Metaphysaria, Monatsschr Kinderheilkd 97:393, 1949.

Wasylenko MJ, Wedge JH, and Houston CS: Metaphyseal chondrodysplasia, Schmid type: a defect of ultrastructural metabolism; case report, J Bone Joint Surg 62A:660, 1980.

Larsen syndrome

Bowen JR, Ortega K, Ray S, et al: Spinal deformities in Larsen syndrome, Clin Orthop 197:159, 1985.

Habermann ET, Sterling A, and Dennis RI: Larsen's syndrome: a heritable disorder, J Bone Joint Surg 58A:558, 1976.

Larsen LJ, Schottstaedt ER, and Bost FC: Multiple congenital dislocations associated with characteristic facial abnormality, J Pediatr 37:574, 1950.

Oki T, Terashima Y, Murachi S, et al: Clinical features and treatment of joint dislocations in Larsen's syndrome: report of three cases in one family, Clin Orthop 119:206, 1976.

Cleidocranial dysplasia

Dore DD, MacEwen GD, and Boulos MI: Cleidocranial dysostosis and syringomyelia: review of the literature and case report, Clin Orthop 214:229, 1987.

Kerr HD: Cleidocranial dysplasia, J Rheumatol 15:359, 1988.

Richie MF and Johnston CE II: Management of developmental coxa vara in cleidocranial dysostosis, Orthopedics 12:1001, 1989.

Diastrophic dysplasia

Bethem D, Winter RB, and Lutter L: Disorders of the spine in diastrophic dwarfism, J Bone Joint Surg 62A:529, 1980.

Herring J: The spinal disorders in diastrophic dwarfism, J Bone Joint Surg 60A:177, 1978.

Hollister DW and Lackman RS: Diastrophic dwarfism, Clin Orthop 114:61, 1976.

Horton WA et al: Growth curves for height for diastrophic dysplasia, spondyloepiphyseal dysplasia congenita, and pseudoachondroplasia, Am J Dis Child 136:316, 1982.

Lamy M and Maroteaux P: Le nanisme diastrophique, Presse Med 68:1977, 1960.

Chondroectodermal dysplasia

Ellis RWB and van Creveld S: A syndrome characterized by ectodermal dysplasia, polydactyly, chondrodysplasia, and congenital morbus cordia, Arch Dis Child 16:65, 1940.

Kaitila II, Leisti JT, and Rimoin DL: Mesomelic skeletal dysplasias, Clin Orthop 114:94, 1976.

Dysplasia epiphysealis hemimelia

Fairbank HAT: Dysplasia epiphysialis multiplex, Br J Surg 34:225, 1947.

Greenspan A et al: Mixed sclerosing bone dysplasia coexisting with dysplasia epiphysealis hemimelica (Trevor-Fairbank disease), Skeletal Radiol 15:452, 1982.

Hensinger RN et al: Familial dysplasia epiphysealis hemimelia, associated with chondromas and osteochondromas: report of a kindred with variable presentations, J Bone Joint Surg 56A:1513, 1974.

Kettelkamp DB, Campbell CJ, and Bonfiglio M: Dysplasia epiphysealis hemimelia: a report of fifteen cases and a review of the literature, J Bone Joint Surg 48A:746, 1966.

Schier CK et al: Ribbing's disease: radiographic-scintigraphic correlation and comparative analysis with Englemann's disease, J Nucl Med 28:244, 1987.

Trevor D: Tarso-epiphyseal aclasis: a congenital error of epiphyseal development, J Bone Joint Surg 32B:204, 1950.

Diaphyseal dysplasia

Hundley JD and Wilson FC: Progressive diaphyseal dysplasia: review of the literature and report of seven cases in one family, J Bone Joint Surg 55A:461, 1973.

Kaftori JK, Kleinhaus U, and Naveh Y: Progressive diaphyseal dysplasia (Camurati-Englemann): radiographic follow-up and CT findings, Radiology 164:777, 1987.

Haveh Y et al: Progressive diaphyseal dysplasia: evaluation of corticosteroid therapy, Pediatrics 75:321, 1985.

Ribbing S: Hereditary multiple diaphyseal sclerosis, Acta Radiol 31:522, 1949.

Schier CK et al: Ribbing's disease: radiographic-scintigraphic correlation and comparative analysis with Englemann's disease, J Nucl Med 28:244, 1987.

Stenzler S et al: Progressive diaphyseal dysplasia presenting as neuromuscular disease, J Pediatr Orthop 9:463, 1989.

Wirth CR, Kay J, and Bourke R: Diaphyseal dysplasia (Engelmann's syndrome): a case report demonstrating a deficiency in cortical haversian system formation, Clin Orthop 171:186, 1982.

Neurofibromatosis

Chaglassian JH, Riseborough EJ, and Hall JL: Neurofibromatosis scoliosis: natural history and results of treatment in 37 cases, J Bone Joint Surg 58A:695, 1976.

Crawford AH: Neurofibromatosis in the pediatric patient, Orthop Clin North Am 9(1):11, 1978.

Crawford AH: Neurofibromatosis. In Morrissy RT (ed): Lovell and Winter's pediatric orthopaedics, ed 3, Philadelphia, 1990, JB Lippincott Co.

Crawford AH and Bagemary N: Osseous manifestations in neurofibromatosis in childhood, J Pediatr Orthop 6:72, 1986.

Curtis BH et al: Neurofibromatosis with paraplegia: report of eight cases, J Bone Joint Surg 51A:843, 1969.

Ducatman BS, Scheithaur BW, and Dahlin DC: Malignant bone tumors associated with neurofibromatosis, Mayo Clin Proc 58:578, 1983.

Gregg PJ et al: Pseudarthrosis of the radius associated with neurofibromatosis, Clin Orthop 171:175, 1982.

Kullmann L and Wouters HW: Neurofibromatosis, gigantism and subperiosteal hematoma: report of two children with extensive subperiosteal bone formation, J Bone Joint Surg 54B:130, 1977.

McKeen EA et al: Rhabdomyosarcoma complicating multiple neurofibromatosis, J Pediatr 93:992, 1978.

National Institute of Health: Neurofibromatosis, Consensus Development Conference Statement 6(12):13, 1987.

Veliskakis KP, Wilson PD Jr, and Levine DB: Neurofibromatosis and scoliosis: significance of the short angular spine curvature, J Bone Joint Surg 52A:833, 1970.

von Recklinghausen F: Ueber die multiplen Fibrome der haut und ihre Beziehung zur den multiplen Neuromen, Berlin, 1882, Hirschwald.

Wellwood JM, Bulmer JA, and Graff DJC: Congenital defects of the tibia in siblings with neurofibromatosis, J Bone Joint Surg 53B:314, 1971.

Whitehouse D: Diagnostic value of the café-au-lait spots in children, Arch Dis Child 41:316, 1966.

Winter RB, Lonstein JE, and Anderson M: Neurofibromatosis and hyperkyphosis: a review of 33 patients with kyphosis of 80 degrees or greater, J Spine Disorders 1:39, 1988.

Winter RB et al: Spine deformity in neurofibromatosis: a review of one hundred and two patients, J Bone Joint Surg 61A:677, 1979.

Yong-Hing K, Kalamchi A, and MacEwen GD: Cervical spine abnormalities in neurofibromatosis, J Bone Joint Surg 61A:695, 1979.

Down syndrome

Aprin H, Zink WP, and Hall JE: Management of dislocation of the hip in Down syndrome, J Pediatr Orthop 5:428, 1985.

Beaty JH: Cervical spine (atlantoaxial) instability in children with Down syndrome, Down Syndrome News 12:117, 1988.

Bennet GC et al: Dislocation of the hip in trisomy 21, J Bone Joint Surg 64B:289, 1982.

Diamond LS, Lynne D, and Sigman B: Orthopedic disorders in patients with Down's syndrome, Orthop Clin North Am 12:57, 1981.

Dugdale TW and Renshaw TS: Instability of the patellofemoral joint in Down syndrome, J Bone Joint Surg 68A:405, 1986.

Gore DR: Recurrent dislocation of the hip in a child with Down's syndrome, J Bone Joint Surg 63A:823, 1981.

Pueschel SM et al: Symptomatic atlantoaxial subluxation in persons with Down syndrome, J Pediatr Orthop 4:682, 1984.

Semine AA et al: Cervical-spine instability in children with Down syndrome (trisomy 21), J Bone Joint Surg 60A:649, 1978.

Mucopolysaccharidoses

Kelly TE: The mucopolysaccharidoses and mucolipidoses, Clin Orthop 114:116, 1976.

Wakai S et al: Skeletal muscle involvement in mucopolysaccharidosis type IIA: severe type of Hunter syndrome, Pediatr Neurol 4:178, 1988.

Apert syndrome

Beligere N, Harris V, and Pruzansky S: Progressive bony dysplasia in Apert syndrome, Radiology 139:593, 1981.

Sherk HH, Whitaker LA, and Pasquariello PS: Facial malformations and spinal deformities: a predictable relationship, Spine 7:526, 1982.

Multiple hereditary osteochondromatosis

Fogel GR et al: Management of deformities of the forearm in multiple hereditary osteochondromas, J Bone Joint Surg 66A:670, 1984.

Pritchett JW: Lengthening of the ulna in patients with hereditary multiple exostoses, J Bone Joint Surg 68B:561, 1986.

Peterson HA: Multiple hereditary osteochondromata, Clin Orthop 329:222, 1989.

Snearly WN and Peterson HA: Management of ankle deformities in multiple hereditary osteochondromata, J Pediatr Orthop 9:427, 1989.

Shapiro F, Simon S, and Glimcher MJ: Hereditary multiple exostoses: anthropometric, roentgenographic, and clinical aspects, J Bone Joint Surg 61A:815, 1979.

Enchondromatosis

Ben-Itzhak I et al: The Maffucci syndrome, J Pediatr Orthop 8:345, 1988.

Fogel GR et al: Management of deformities of the forearm in multiple hereditary osteochondromas, J Bone Joint Surg 66A:670, 1984.

Lucas D, Tupler R, and Enneking WF: Multicentric chondrosarcomas associated with Ollier's disease: review and case report, J Fla Med Assoc 77:24, 1990.

Paterson DC et al: Generalized enchondromatosis: a case report, J Bone Joint Surg 71:133, 1989.

Swartz HS et al: The malignant potential of enchondromatosis, J Bone Joint Surg 69A:269, 1987.

Urist MR: A 37-year follow-up evaluation of multiple-stage femur and tibia lengthening in dyschondroplasia (enchondromatosis) with a net gain of 23.3 centimeters, Clin Orthop 242:137, 1989.

Melorheostosis

Abdul KFW et al: Intramedullary osteosclerosis: a report of the clinicopathologic features of five cases, Orthopedics 11:1667, 1988.

Khurana JS et al: Case report 510: melorheostosis of ilium, femur, and adjacent soft tissues, Skeletal Radiol 17:539, 1988.

Lee SH and Sanderson J: Hypophosphataemic rickets and melorheostosis, Clin Radiol 40:209, 1989.

Chondrodysplasia punctata

Bethem D: Os odontoideum in chondrodystrophia calcificans congenita: a case report, J Bone Joint Surg 64A:1385, 1982.

Crossan JF, Wynne-Davies R, and Fulford GE: Bilateral failure of the capital femoral epiphysis: bilateral Perthes disease, multiple epiphyseal dysplasia, pseudoachondroplasia, and spondyloepiphyseal dysplasia congenita and tarda, J Pediatr Orthop 3:297, 1983.

6 Developmental Problems in the Lower Extremity

JAMES H. BEATY

Although the complex process of growth and development involves the entire musculoskeletal system of the child, the orthopaedist is concerned primarily with the patterns and rates of growth of the spine and extremities. The proximal and distal physes of each long bone are responsible for most of the growth of the extremities, with additional contributions from the epiphyses. The spine and skull also contribute to the child's overall skeletal height. In the upper extremity the majority of growth of the limb is provided by the physes of the proximal humerus and the distal radius and ulna. In the lower extremity the distal femoral and proximal tibial physes provide 65% of the growth of the limb.

This information has practical clinical application because any serious injury, such as from trauma or infection, to the physes of the proximal humerus or distal radius causes numerous clinical problems, and injury to the physes around the knee can cause significant limb length discrepancy and angular deformity. Injury to physes that contribute less growth to the extremities is less likely to cause significant clinical problems. Evaluation of the overall growth and development may be aided by determining the relationship of chronologic age to skeletal age, using a standard roentgenographic atlas of skeletal age. This comparison is important not only in the treatment of common conditions such as limb length discrepancy and scoliosis, but also in the choice and timing of many surgical procedures.

Another aspect of growth and development is the variety of physiologic conditions seen in the growing child. Most physiologic conditions improve or correct with growth, but in some adolescents and young adults, severe physiologic conditions have neither corrected with growth nor responded to conservative treatment.

Because the lower extremities are the most commonly affected, this chapter discusses only those conditions of the lower extremities related to growth and development that occasionally require surgical correction, including pes planus, skewfoot, torsional problems, genu varum, and genu valgum.

FLEXIBLE FLATFOOT

The treatment of flexible flatfoot (pes planus) is one of the more controversial areas in pediatric orthopaedics. Few studies have attempted to assess the natural history and long-term results of untreated flexible flatfoot. Staheli found that flatfeet are the rule in infants, common in children, and within a large range of normal in adults. Wenger et al found no correlation between the use of corrective footwear and the correction of flatfoot with growth.

Although the cause is not completely understood, flexible flatfoot is thought to result from an abnormality in the bone-ligament complex of the foot that causes loss of the longitudinal arch and mild to moderate abduction of the forefoot with associated heel valgus. During weight bearing, longitudinal forces are directed medially, accentuating the heel valgus and forefoot pronation. Occasionally a mild to moderate contracture of the tendo Achilles is associated with a more severe flexible flatfoot.

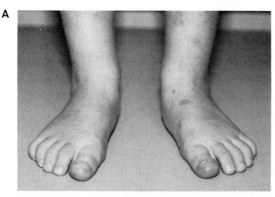

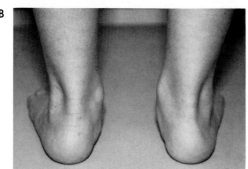

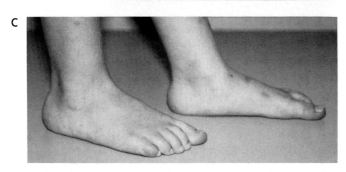

Fig. 6-1 Flexible flatfoot in 4-year-old child. **A,** Forefoot abduction, pronation. **B,** Heel valgus, mild tendo Achilles contracture. **C,** Loss of longitudinal arch.

Clinical Findings

The appearance of flexible flatfoot in children is related to their age and weight-bearing status, with extreme variability in the appearance of the longitudinal arch. The infant may have a large fat pad overlying the longitudinal arch that completely obliterates the normal contour of the midfoot ("fat foot"). In contrast, the condition is more easily detected in the older child who is weight-bearing during examination (Fig. 6-1).

The range of motion of the subtalar joint should be evaluated by gentle inversion and eversion of the calcaneus. Since the differential diagnosis of flexible flatfoot in young adolescents includes tarsal coalition, any limitation in subtalar motion should be evaluated with appropriate roentgenographic studies.

In severe, symptomatic flexible flatfoot a callus may develop along the longitudinal arch of the foot. Pain along the medial aspect of the midfoot and hindfoot and excessive shoe wear are not uncommon.

Roentgenographic Findings

Roentgenographic examination usually is not recommended for asymptomatic flatfoot. If a possibility of tarsal coalition or congenital vertical talus exists, or if surgery is being considered, appropriate roentgenograms for the differential diagnosis or standing anteroposterior and lateral views should be obtained.

Roentgenographic features of severe flexible flatfoot include an increase in the talocalcaneal angle (measured on the anteroposterior roentgenogram) to greater than 40 degrees (the normal angle is 20 to 35 degrees). On the lateral view the talonavicular joint may appear to "sag." The most reliable roentgenographic measurement is the talo–first metatarsal angle on the lateral view. In normal feet this is 0 degrees; in the mild flexible flatfoot, up to 15 degrees; in the moderate flexible flatfoot, between 15 and 40 degrees; and in the severe flexible flatfoot, greater than 40 degrees (Fig. 6-2).

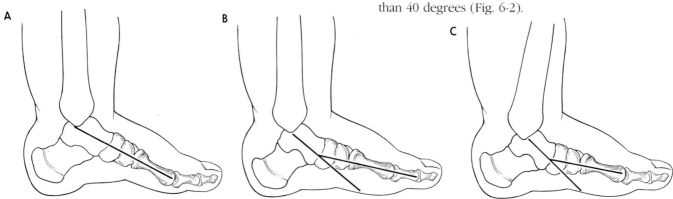

Fig. 6-2 Flexible flatfoot evaluated by lateral talo–first metatarsal angle. **A,** Normal (0 degrees). **B,** Mild (15 degrees). **C,** Severe (40 degrees). (Redrawn from Bordelon RL: Clin Orthop 181:7, 1983.)

Treatment

Children with asymptomatic flexible flatfeet require little treatment. Three common clinical situations include parental concern about the appearance of the flexible flatfoot, foot or leg pain, and excessive shoe wear. Occasionally the latter may require a trial of shoe modification.

Rarely, a child with significant pain or grossly excessive shoe wear may require a custom-molded orthosis that can be shifted to various types of shoes. The family should be aware that an orthosis is designed to relieve pain and improve shoe wear but does not correct the flatfoot.

Few children or young adults with flexible flatfeet develop pain or impairment severe enough to warrant surgical correction. The rare patient with significant pain and more-than-normal shoe wear may require operative intervention, but conservative treatment should be continued until the need for surgery is clearly indicated; careful patient selection is mandatory.

Numerous operative procedures have been recommended for flexible flatfoot; the three most common are fusion of the navicular and the first and second cuneiform joints devised by Hoke, opening wedge osteotomy of the calcaneus described by Dillwyn-Evans, and medial sliding calcaneal osteotomy. The Hoke procedure corrects the talonavicular sag, but long-term follow-up reports indicate a high incidence of unsatisfactory results because of loss of motion in the midfoot. Opening wedge osteotomy of the calcaneus corrects the pronation and abduction of the forefoot but may not correct the secondary heel valgus. The medial sliding calcaneal osteotomy appears to correct heel valgus, maintain subtalar motion, and more adequately correct forefoot abduction and pronation (Fig. 6-3).

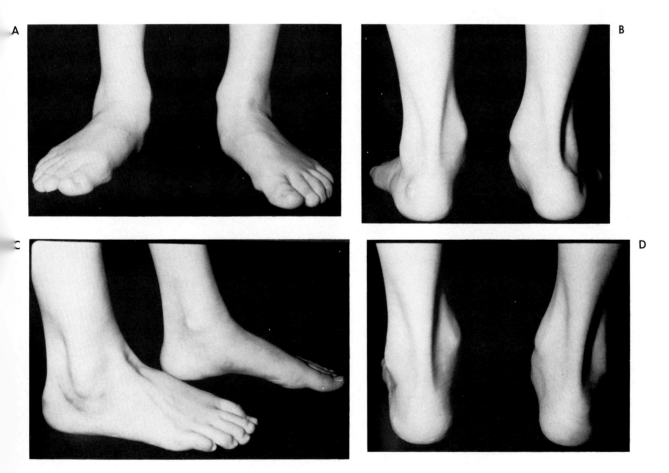

Fig. 6-3 Painful flexible flatfoot in 11-year-old boy. **A,** Frontal view. **B,** Posterior view. Note callus along medial arch and lateral aspect of calcaneus. **C** and **D,** After medial sliding calcaneal osteotomy. Note normal contour of medial arch and correction of excessive heel valgus on posterior view. (Courtesy Paul P Griffin, M.D.)

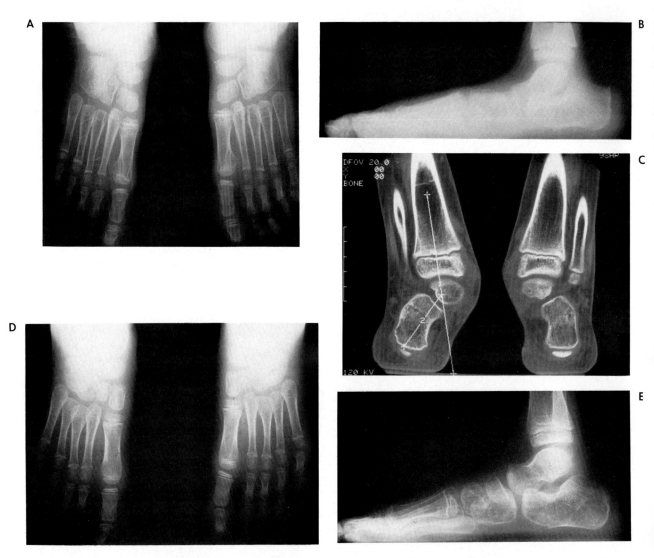

Fig. 6-4 Calcaneal osteotomy in flexible flatfoot. **A,** Standing anteroposterior view. Note increased talocalcaneal angle and forefoot abduction. **B,** Standing lateral view. Note increased talo–first metatarsal angle and talonavicular "sag." **C,** CT scan; by scale, 15 mm of displacement is needed for correction. **D** and **E,** After calcaneal osteotomy; note correction of talocalcaneal and talo–first metatarsal angles.

▶ *Technique.* Preoperative standing roentgenograms may be used for measurement of the talocalcaneal angle on anteroposterior and lateral views and the talo–first metatarsal angle on the lateral view. As an alternative, a CT scan in the frontal plane showing the long axis of the tibia, talus, and calcaneus can be used to determine the distance the calcaneus must be displaced medially to correct excessive valgus and to place the calcaneus in a neutral to slight valgus position in relation to the tibia (Fig. 6-4).

With the patient supine on the operating table and the tourniquet inflated, make an incision beginning near the lateral Achilles tuberosity and extending distally parallel and plantar to the sural nerve. Split the soft tissue directly down to the lateral wall of the calcaneus. Reflect the peroneal tendons and sural nerve superiorly. Insert a Kirschner wire on the lateral surface of the calcaneus, parallel to the plantar surface of the foot. Use image intensification or lateral roentgenograms to determine the exact level of the osteotomy. Begin the osteotomy just behind the posterior subtalar joint, and direct it plantarward towards the origin of the plantar aponeurosis. Place a retractor

anterior to the insertion of the tendo Achilles in the calcaneus and another beneath the calcaneus to protect the plantar fascia and short flexor musculature origin. A power saw can be used initially, but make the most medial cut with an osteotome. Since the medial extent of the osteotomy is not performed under direct vision, be careful not to penetrate the periosteum. After the osteotomy is completed, shift the loose proximal fragment medially to correct the lateral displacement of the calcaneus (Fig. 6-5). Insert a threaded Kirschner wire obliquely through the proximal fragment and across the distal fragment, but do not enter the subtalar joint. Because of the medial displacement of the calcaneus, closure of the surgical wound may cause some tension at the suture line. To prevent wound healing problems, use interrupted sutures. Insert a suction drain, and apply a short-leg cast.

▶ *Postoperative management.* If a Kirschner wire is used for internal fixation, the child is allowed to walk without bearing weight for 6 weeks, then the cast and wire are removed and a new short-leg walking cast is applied to be worn another 4 weeks.

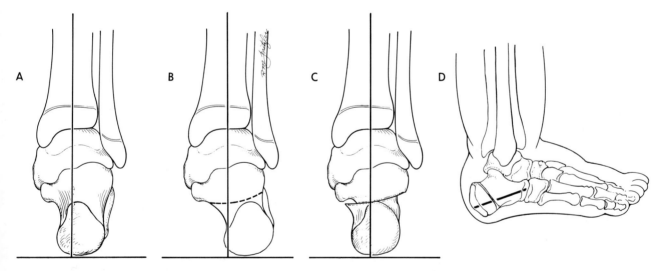

Fig. 6-5 Medial sliding calcaneal osteotomy. **A,** Normal foot. **B,** Crescenteric osteotomy for flexible flatfoot. **C,** Medial displacement after osteotomy. **D,** Fixation with axial Kirschner wire.

SKEWFOOT

Skewfoot consists of metatarsus adductus and excessive heel valgus with the tarsal navicular subluxated on the lateral aspect of the talar head. Skewfoot may be part of the spectrum of metatarsus adductus, but the excessive heel valgus is in contrast to simple metatarsus adductus. Skewfoot is not often detected in the newborn because accurate assessment of excessive heel valgus is difficult both clinically and roentgenographically.

Clinical Findings

The most common parental complaints are difficulty fitting the child's shoes and the child's intoed gait. Clinical examination usually reveals excessive heel valgus and forefoot adduction that is flexible to the midline but not beyond.

Roentgenographic Findings

If clinical examination suggests skewfoot, standing anteroposterior and lateral roentgenograms should be obtained in children old enough to cooperate. In children younger than 3 years the navicular may not be present to allow evaluation of lateral subluxation on the talar head. Metatarsus adductus of the forefoot is evident, with the first metatarsal appearing subluxated laterally to the long axis of the talus in the absence of an ossified navicular. The anteroposterior talocalcaneal angle is usually greater than 40 degrees, indicating excessive valgus of the hindfoot (Fig. 6-6).

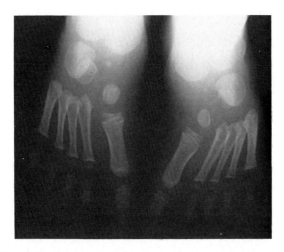

Fig. 6-6   Skewfoot deformity in 4-year-old boy: metatarsus adductus, lateral subluxation of forefoot, hindfoot valgus.

Orthopaedic Treatment

True skewfoot deformity is difficult to treat nonoperatively. Initial treatment is serial manipulation and casting for correction of the forefoot adduction, but special care must be taken to avoid placing the hindfoot in a more valgus position. Serial manipulation and casting for the metatarsus adductus of skewfoot in the child younger than walking age may require 3 to 6 months.

The goal of treatment of skewfoot deformity is a painless, plantigrade foot that can tolerate normal footwear. If this cannot be obtained in the older child with conservative methods, surgery is indicated. Most authors recommend that surgery be delayed until the child is older than 5 years, to determine the pattern of growth and development of the foot. The parents should be informed that a normal foot cannot be obtained by any procedure, but that shoe wear may be improved and pain relieved by surgical treatment.

The deformities that must be surgically corrected are (1) severe forefoot adduction, (2) short medial cuneiform, (3) lateral subluxation of the navicular on the talar head, and (4) excessive valgus of the hindfoot with lateral displacement of the calcaneus.

Occasionally a surgical option in the young child with a more flexible forefoot and hindfoot is tarsometatarsal capsulotomies, combined with medial capsulotomy of the talonavicular, naviculocuneiform, and cuneiform–first metatarsal joints to correct the forefoot adduction and the lateral displacement of the navicular on the head of the talus. This may be performed through dorsal and medial incisions. If necessary the Achilles, posterior tibialis, anterior tibialis, and flexor digitorum communis tendons may be lengthened as well.

More frequently, however, surgical correction is required for the deformity in a child older than 5 years with fixed hindfoot valgus and a forefoot that is no longer flexible. The treatment of choice for these children is metatarsal osteotomies to correct the forefoot (p. 77), combined with medial sliding calcaneal osteotomy to correct the hindfoot valgus (pp. 361 and 693). Even with these procedures, the navicular and midfoot generally remain subluxated on the head of the talus.

For the adolescent with fixed deformity of the forefoot and hindfoot, triple arthrodesis is recommended, combined with metatarsal osteotomies of the forefoot if necessary.

TORSIONAL PROBLEMS

Intoeing and outtoeing are common problems in growing children, primarily because of the many variations in gait among children, the concern of the parents, and the confusing information from various sources. Both the physician and the parents need to understand the location of the problem, its severity compared to other children, its natural history if untreated, and the treatment options available.

Intoeing

Femoral version refers to the normal angle between the femoral neck and the condyles of the distal femur. Tibial version is the angle between the axis of the knee and the transmalleolar axis of the normal tibia, which is rotated laterally. Abnormal amounts of rotation in the hip are referred to as excessive femoral anteversion or retroversion. In the tibia, abnormal rotation is most frequently medial or internal tibial torsion and rarely lateral or external tibial torsion. Frequently, deformities exist at the level of the hip and knee and may be associated with metatarsus adductus.

Studies of normal growth and development have shown that femoral anteversion gradually decreases from the range of 40 to 60 degrees in a newborn to approximately 15 degrees at skeletal maturity. Lateral tibial rotation increases from an average of ±5 degrees at birth to 15 degrees at skeletal maturity.

Many torsional problems in children are caused by the position of the fetus during limb development. Frequently the problem is not recognized until the child begins standing and attempting to walk, when parental concern or pressure from family or friends may initiate orthopaedic consultation.

Clinical Findings

The clinical history should include the age at which the child began walking, to rule out any neuromuscular disease, and any history of torsional problems in immediate relatives, especially if the parents have been given incorrect information regarding the long-term natural history and treatment of the problem. Any misconceptions held by the parents should be discussed before physical examination of the child.

Staheli described a detailed rotational profile that should be obtained as part of the screening examination of every child with potential torsional problems (Fig. 6-7). This profile includes four values: (1) the foot progression angle, (2) medial and lateral rotation of the hips, (3) the thigh-foot angle as a measurement of tibial torsion, and (4) the examination of the foot to detect any potential metatarsus adductus or

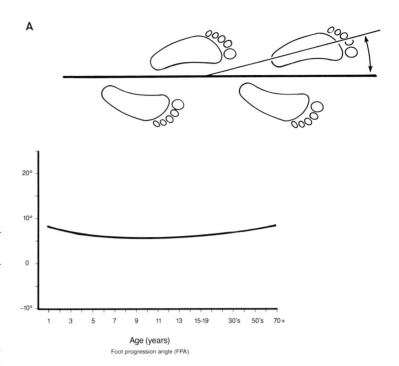

A

Foot progression angle (FPA).

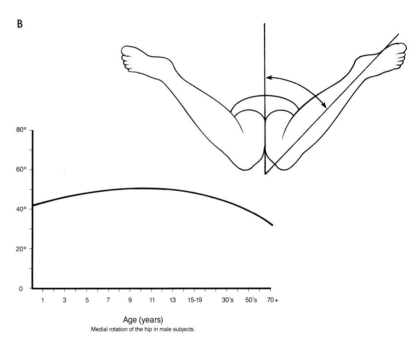

B

Medial rotation of the hip in male subjects.

Fig. 6-7 Rotational profile of Staheli. **A,** Foot progression angle (FPA). **B,** Medial rotation (MR) of hip in males. *Continued.*

C

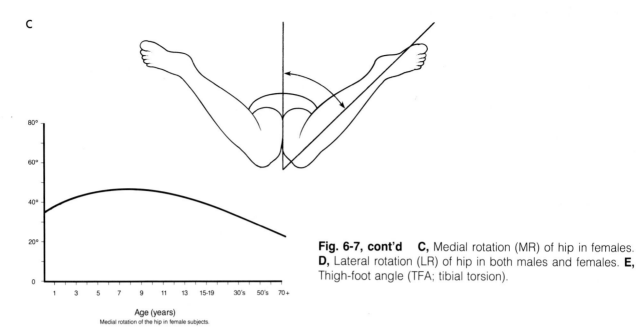

Age (years)

Medial rotation of the hip in female subjects.

Fig. 6-7, cont'd   C, Medial rotation (MR) of hip in females. **D,** Lateral rotation (LR) of hip in both males and females. **E,** Thigh-foot angle (TFA; tibial torsion).

D

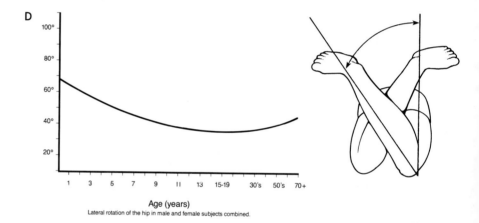

Age (years)

Lateral rotation of the hip in male and female subjects combined.

E

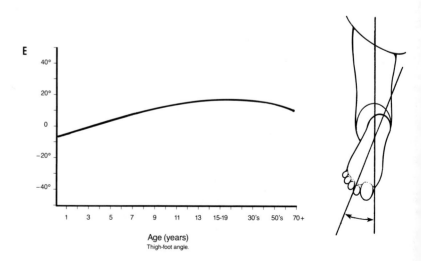

Age (years)

Thigh-foot angle.

skewfoot deformity. Staheli et al also outlined the normal rotational profile and degrees of deviation considered beyond the range of normal. From their studies, they concluded that the lack of impairment from most rotational problems and the apparent ineffectiveness of nonoperative treatment make observation the treatment of choice for most rotational problems in children. For the rare torsional problems that do not correct with growth and for children with severe cosmetic and functional problems, rotational osteotomy may be considered.

In a child younger than 4 years the examination frequently must be performed while the child sits in the parent's lap. For a cooperative child 4 years old and older the rotational profile is best obtained with the child in a prone position. Hip rotation is evaluated by flexing the child's knees to 90 degrees and al-

lowing gentle internal and external rotation of the hips to indicate internal and external rotation. Tibial torsion also may be evaluated with the child prone and the knees flexed to a right angle. The thigh-foot angle is estimated from an imaginary line along the posterior aspect of the thigh and the plantar aspect of the foot (Fig. 6-8). The transmalleolar axis may also be estimated by outlining the medial and lateral malleoli and evaluating this angle in comparison with the posterior aspect of the thigh longitudinally.

Examination of the foot frequently reveals metatarsus adductus and often flexible flatfoot. Metatarsus adductus can accentuate the intoeing when combined with excessive internal tibial torsion or femoral anteversion. Flexible flatfoot is frequently associated with external femoral torsion.

A

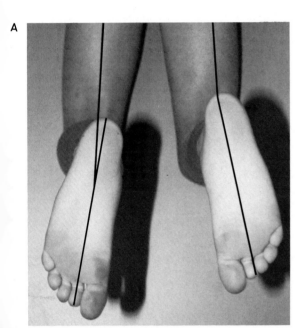

Fig. 6-8 Clinical measurement of tibial torsion. **A,** Thigh-foot angle (TFA). **B,** Transmalleolar axis. **C,** Normal increase in transmalleolar axis with age.

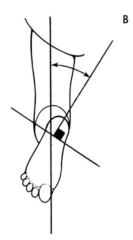

B

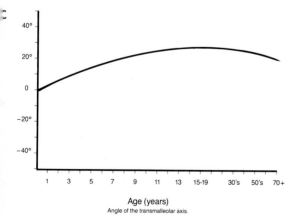

Age (years)

Angle of the transmalleolar axis.

Roentgenographic Findings

If examination of the foot reveals severe metatarsus adductus, roentgenograms may be obtained to detect any hip dysplasia, since these two conditions are frequently associated. If congenital hip dislocation or other anomalies are suggested by the physical examination, roentgenograms of the pelvis should be obtained. For the evaluation of older children with an uncorrected torsional deformity, CT scanning helps to assess the degree of femoral anteversion before considering corrective osteotomy (Fig. 6-9). CT scanning also may be used to assess tibial torsion, but the information obtained may be no more specific than that obtained by clinical examination.

Orthopaedic Treatment

The treatment of torsional problems in children can be difficult because of the necessity for proper identification of the level of deformity, the concerns of the family about future impairment, and the wide variety of treatment options available. No scientific studies have shown that any corrective devices, including corrective footwear, Denis Browne splints, or twister cable braces, are effective in correcting torsional problems in children.

The most commonly recommended approach is a detailed discussion of the natural history of the problem with the parents, an explanation of the available treatment options, and the suggestion that parents observe the child for spontaneous correction with growth. Parents also should be informed that there is a slight possibility that the deformity will not correct and that a very few adolescents require surgical correction if the deformity is not corrected with growth.

Intoeing caused by internal tibial torsion is most common in children between the ages of 12 and 36 months, and many parents request a Denis Browne splint. The effectiveness of night splinting is unproven scientifically, but many parents nonetheless opt to use the device. Intoeing in children older than 3 years generally is caused by femoral anteversion and usually is corrected by growth when the child is between the ages of 8 and 12 years old.

For adolescents with severe internal tibial torsion that has not corrected with growth and is causing cosmetic and functional problems, tibial osteotomy is occasionally indicated. The osteotomy can be performed either proximally or distally in these rare patients, but supramalleolar osteotomy is the treatment of choice in the young child, and proximal tibial osteotomy in the adolescent.

Just as infrequently, derotational osteotomy of the femur may be required in the child older than 8 years with severe cosmetic and functional deformity. Derotational osteotomy of the femur may be performed at any level. In the adolescent, the preferred site is the intertrochanteric-subtrochanteric region, with fixation by a plate–hip screw combination (Fig. 6-10). In the patient approaching skeletal maturity, closed femoral derotational osteotomy and intramedullary nail fixation may be performed.

A

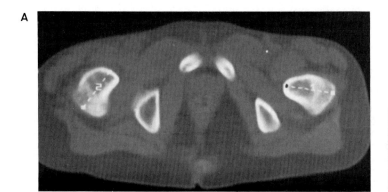

B

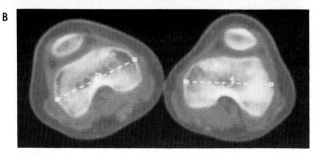

Fig. 6-9 CT scan to determine femoral anteversion of left hip. **A,** Plane of femoral necks. **B,** Femoral condyles.

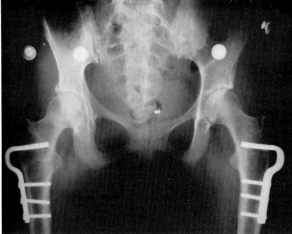

Fig. 6-10 Derotational osteotomy of proximal femur in 14-year-old girl for severe femoral anteversion.

Another less common torsional deformity is the windswept deformity, in which one extremity is in internal torsion and the other in external torsion. This is usually a combination of external femoral torsion in one extremity and femoral anteversion and internal tibial torsion in the contralateral limb. External femoral torsion also may be combined with pes planus. No treatment is indicated for either of these deformities because their natural history is to correct with growth.

GENU VARUM AND GENU VALGUM

Normal variations in the growth and development of children include genu varum and genu valgum. The orthopaedist frequently is consulted because of parental concern about the appearance of the child's bowlegs or knock-knees.

Clinical Findings

Clinical examination of children with genu varum or genu valgum should include a rotational profile to determine any rotational deformity that is commonly associated with angular deformity around the knee. It is important to distinguish physiologic genu varum and genu valgum from pathologic conditions that do not follow the natural history of physiologic bowlegs and knock-knees. Features for differential diagnosis are listed in the box at right.

From birth to approximately 18 months of age, many children have internal tibial torsion with physi-

---

DIFFERENTIAL DIAGNOSIS OF GENU VARUM AND GENU VALGUM

Genu Varum

1. Physiologic, uncorrected
2. Tibia vara (Blount's disease)
3. Rickets

Genu Valgum

1. Physiologic, uncorrected
2. Tibial metaphyseal fracture

Varus or Valgus

1. Trauma
    Malunion, physeal arrest
2. Metabolic
    Rickets
    Renal osteodystrophy
3. Miscellaneous
    Juvenile rheumatoid arthritis
    Osteogenesis imperfecta
    Infection

---

ologic bowlegs. Between the ages of 2 and 4 years, physiologic knock-knee becomes more prevalent. Between the ages of 3½ and 7 years, knock-knee improves rapidly and continues to improve slightly throughout the remainder of skeletal growth (Fig. 6-11).

A
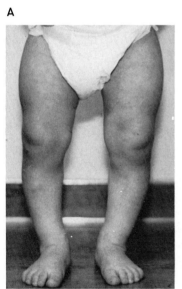

B
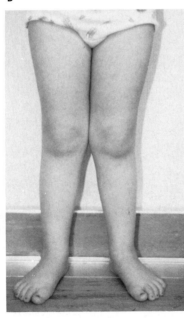

C
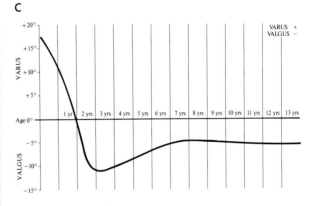

Fig. 6-11 Normal growth and development. **A,** Physiologic genu varum in 18-month-old boy. **B,** Physiologic genu valgum in 3-year-old girl. **C,** Spontaneous correction of femorotibial angle with growth. (From Salenius P and Vankka E: J Bone Joint Surg 57A:259, 1975.)

Roentgenographic Evaluation

If a pathologic cause of genu varum or genu valgum is suspected, roentgenograms should be obtained. In the child old enough to cooperate, a single standing anteroposterior roentgenogram of the pelvis and lower extremities allows measurement of the femoral-tibial and intermalleolar angles, which should also be determined clinically.

Orthopaedic Treatment

If no underlying pathologic process exists, true physiologic genu varum or genu valgum requires no treatment other than observation through several years of growth to make certain the alignment is correcting. Bracing does not appear to affect the natural history of physiologic genu varum or genu valgum and is not recommended. The most difficult problem is convincing the parents that observation is the best treatment for the child.

Although surgical correction frequently is required for pathologic conditions that cause genu varum and genu valgum, it rarely is required for physiologic genu varum and genu valgum. Surgical correction should be reserved for deformities beyond the range of normal by more than two standard deviations or those causing significant cosmetic and functional problems in adolescents. Prophylactic procedures occasionally may be indicated to prevent potential problems in adulthood.

Surgical correction of genu varum and genu valgum should produce extremities with physiologic angular measurements of the hip, knee, and ankle and a satisfactory overall alignment between the weight-bearing joints in both lower extremities. Specific procedures for correction of genu varum and genu valgum include osteotomy, hemiepiphysiodesis, and hemistapling. A standing anteroposterior roentgenogram showing the hip, knee, and ankle should be obtained before considering any surgical procedure.

Genu varum usually can be corrected by proximal tibial and fibular osteotomies and genu valgum by supracondylar femoral osteotomy. Occasionally, complex deformities require osteotomies of the distal femur and proximal tibia to achieve acceptable alignment of the hip, knee, and ankle. Although numerous osteotomy techniques are available, the most commonly performed is a closing wedge osteotomy with fixation by crossed Kirschner wires, avoiding the physes of the long bones (see p. 44). A long-leg cast is used for immobilization after osteotomy of the tibia and a hip-spica cast after supracondylar femoral osteotomy. Occasionally, external fixation of the osteotomies may be used in an older adolescent.

Hemiepiphysiodesis is an option for correction of severe genu varum or genu valgum in the older adolescent with remaining growth. Bowen, Leahey, Zhang, and MacEwen developed a useful variation of the Green-Anderson chart and described techniques for hemiepiphysiodesis around the distal femur and proximal tibia for correction of severe genu varum and genu valgum. The clinical deformity should correlate with the roentgenographic measurements. The width of the bone at the involved tibial or femoral physis is measured. The patient's skeletal age is determined from roentgenograms and the use of the *Greulich-Pyle Atlas,* and the growth percentile is determined from height charts.

The timing for hemiepiphysiodesis can be determined by using the chart shown in Fig. 6-12 as follows:

1. Choose the appropriate graph quadrant to represent the patient's sex and the area (distal femoral or proximal tibial) that is to undergo hemiepiphysiodesis.
2. Using the central portion of the chart, locate the physeal distance and find the angular deformity of the limb on the corresponding vertical line. Note that the degree values are marked just above the horizontal lines that represent them.

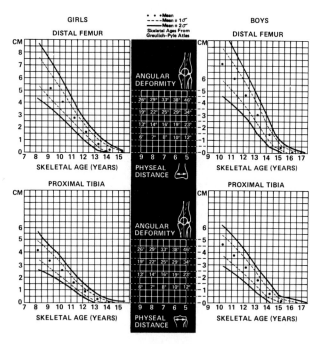

Fig. 6-12 Chart of Bowen, Leahey, Zhang, and MacEwen for calculation of angular deformity (genu varum or valgum) versus remaining growth (see text). (From Bowen JR et al: Clin Orthop 198:184, 1985.)

3. Draw a horizontal line from the point identifying physeal distance and angular deformity to the patient's percentile on the appropriate Green-Anderson quadrant.

4. Drop a vertical line from this point and read off the appropriate skeletal age at which the hemiepiphysiodesis should be performed.

As an example, a female with a 16-degree genu valgum deformity and a 7-cm tibial-physeal length who is in the 50th percentile for height should have a medial tibial physeal arrest at a skeletal age of 11 years.

Potential complications of this technique include overcorrection if hemiepiphysiodesis is performed too early or undercorrection if performed too late (Fig. 6-13).

▶ *Technique of hemiepiphysiodesis to correct angular deformity (Bowen, Leahey, Zhang, and MacEwen).* With the patient under general anesthesia, apply and inflate a tourniquet and prepare and drape the lower extremity. With the aid of image intensification, identify the most peripheral area of the physis. Make a 2-cm incision laterally or medially as indicated, and open the periosteum in a cruciate fashion. Using a square-box (White) osteotome or a 1-cm wide osteotome, remove a block of bone 0.5 cm deep from the center of the physis, taking care not to cut too deeply. Curet the periphery of the physis anteriorly and posteriorly to the bone block but no more than 0.5 cm deep. Reverse the bone block as in the Phemister technique, and insert it into the defect. If epiphysiodesis of the lateral part of the tibial physis is performed, epiphysiodesis of the proximal fibular physis should also be undertaken. Close the wound in layers and apply a knee immobilizer.

▶ *Postoperative management.* Ambulation with crutches is encouraged immediately after surgery, and range-of-motion exercises of the knee are begun within a few days. The knee immobilizer is discontinued at 4 weeks, and weight-bearing roentgenograms of the leg are obtained. After 3 to 6 months, partial physeal closure should be apparent. If complete correction of the deformity occurs while the remainder of the physis is open, complete epiphysiodesis of the remaining physis is indicated to prevent overcorrection.

• • •

Finally, hemistapling of the distal femur, proximal tibia, or both is indicated for correction of severe genu varum or genu valgum if the amount of remaining growth cannot be calculated. Potential problems with hemistapling are a second operation to remove the staples and overcorrection even after removal of the staples when the deformity is corrected.

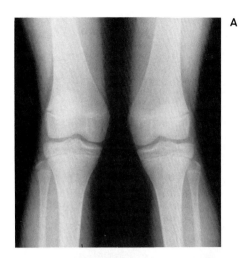

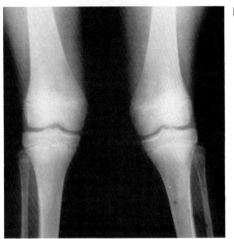

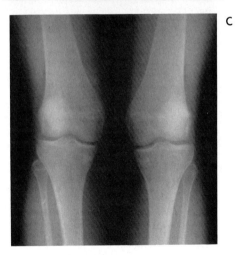

Fig. 6-13 Uncorrected physiologic genu valgum in 12-year-old girl. **A,** Preoperative roentgenogram. **B,** View 6 weeks after medial tibial hemiepiphysiodesis. **C,** Correction at age 15 years.

REFERENCES

Armstrong G: Evans elongation of lateral column of the foot for valgus deformity, J Bone Joint Surg 57A:530, 1975.

Barry RJ and Scranton PE Jr: Flat feet in children, Clin Orthop 181:68, 1983.

Bleck EE: The shoeing of children: sham or science? Dev Med Child Neurol 13:188, 1971.

Bleck EE: Developmental orthopaedics. III. Toddlers, Dev Med Child Neurol 24:533, 1982.

Bleck EE and Berzins UJ: Conservative management of pes valgus with plantar flexed talus, flexible, Clin Orthop 122:85, 1977.

Bordelon RL: Correction of hypermobile flat foot in children by molded insert, Foot Ankle 1:143, 1980.

Bordelon RL: Hypermobile flatfoot in children: comprehension, evaluation, and treatment, Clin Orthop 181:7, 1983.

Bowen JR et al: Partial epiphysiodesis at the knee to correct angular deformity, Clin Orthop 198:184, 1985.

Coleman SS: Complex foot deformity in children, Philadelphia, 1983, Lea & Febiger.

Cowell HR et al: Children's foot problems and corrections, Contemp Orthop 2:526, 1980.

Cowell HR: Flexible flatfoot, J Bone Joint Surg 71A:799, 1989 [editorial].

Evans D: Calcaneo-valgus deformity, J Bone Joint Surg 57B:270, 1975.

Fabry G, McEwen GD, and Shands AR Jr: Torsion of the femur: a follow-up study in normal and abnormal conditions, J Bone Joint Surg 55A:1726, 1973.

Gould N et al: Development of the child's arch, Foot Ankle 9:241, 1989.

Greulich WW and Pyle SL: Radiographic atlas of skeletal development of the hand and wrist, ed 2, Stanford, Calif, 1959, Stanford University Press.

Hoke M: An operation for correction of extremely relaxed flatfeet, J Bone Joint Surg 13:773, 1931.

Hubbard DD and Staheli LT: The direct radiographic measurement of femoral torsion using axial tomography: technic and comparison with an indirect radiographic method, Clin Orthop 86:16, 1972.

Hubbard DD et al: Medial femoral torsion and osteoarthritis, J Pediatr Orthop 8:540, 1988.

Knittel G and Staheli LT: The effectiveness of shoe modifications for intoeing, Orthop Clin North Am 7:1019, 1976.

Magilligan DJ: Calculation of the angle of anteversion by means of horizontal lateral roentgenography, J Bone Joint Surg 38A:1231, 1956.

Meehan PL: Other conditions of the foot. In Morrissy RT, editor: Lovell and Winter's pediatric orthopaedics, ed 3, Philadelphia, 1990, JB Lippincott Co.

Mereday C, Dolan CM, and Lusskin R: Evaluation of the University of California Biomechanics Laboratory: shoe insert in "flexible" pes planus, Clin Orthop 82:45, 1972.

Murphy SB et al: Femoral anteversion, J Bone Joint Surg 69A:1169, 1987.

Penneau K, Lutter L, and Winter R: Pes planus: radiographic changes with foot orthoses and shoes, Foot Ankle 2:299, 1982.

Pistevos G and Duckworth T: The correction of genu valgum by epiphyseal stapling, J Bone Joint Surg 59B:72, 1977.

Robertson WW Jr: Distal tibial deformity in bowlegs, J Pediatr Orthop 7:324, 1987.

Rydholm U et al: Stapling of the knee in juvenile chronic arthritis, J Pediatr Orthop 7:63, 1987.

Salenius P and Vankka E: The development of the tibiofemoral angle in children, J Bone Joint Surg 57A:259, 1975.

Scranton PE et al: Management of hypermobile flatfoot in the child, Contemp Orthop 2:645, 1981.

Staheli LT: Philosophy of care, Pediatr Clin North Am 33:1269, 1986.

Staheli LT: The lower limb. In Morrissy RT, editor: Lovell and Winter's pediatric orthopaedics, ed 3, Philadelphia, 1990, JB Lippincott Co.

Staheli, LT, Chew DE, and Corbett M: The longitudinal arch, J Bone Joint Surg 69A:426, 1987.

Staheli LT, Clawson DK, and Hubbard DD: Medial femoral torsion: experience with operative treatment, Clin Orthop 146:222, 1980.

Staheli LT and Engel GM: Tibial torsion: a method of assessment and a survey of normal children, Clin Orthop 86:183, 1972.

Staheli LT, Lippert F, and Denotter P: Femoral anteversion and physical performance in adolescent and adult life, Clin Orthop 129:213, 1977.

Staheli LT et al: Lower-extremity rotational problems in children: normal values to guide management, J Bone Joint Surg 67A:39, 1985.

Vanderwilde R et al: Measurements on radiographs of the foot in normal infants and children, J Bone Joint Surg 70A:407, 1988.

Wenger DR and Leach J: Foot deformities in infants and children, Pediatr Clin North Am 33:1411, 1986.

Wenger DR et al: Corrective shoes and inserts as treatment for flexible flatfoot in infants and children, J Bone Joint Surg 71A:800, 1989.

Wickstrom J and Williams RA: Shoe corrections and orthopaedic foot supports, Clin Orthop 70:30, 1970.

Winquist RA: Closed intramedullary osteotomies of the femur, Clin Orthop 212:155, 1986.

Zuege RC, Kempken TG, and Blount WP: Epiphyseal stapling for angular deformity at the knee, J Bone Joint Surg 61A:320, 1979.

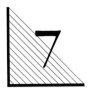

7 Metabolic and Endocrine Disorders

JAMES H. BEATY

Metabolic and endocrine abnormalities affect the osseous and cartilaginous growth of the immature skeleton and often interfere with the function of the musculoskeletal system. Because of the wide variety of causes and manifestations of metabolic bone diseases, endocrine disorders, and genetic dysplasias, there is no detailed classification of these disorders. This chapter includes only specific metabolic and endocrine disorders that occasionally require surgical intervention by the orthopaedic surgeon.

RICKETS AND OSTEOMALACIA

Rickets is a metabolic disorder of bone in which a relative decrease in calcium, phosphorus, or both is severe enough to interfere with the normal physeal growth and mineralization of the skeleton in the immature child. Osteomalacia is the adult form of this disorder and, although growth is not a factor as in the child, the overall effect on bone is identical.

Rickets and osteomalacia are manifested in the following five primary forms:

1. Vitamin D–resistant rickets
2. Vitamin D–deficient rickets
3. Renal osteodystrophy
4. Gastrointestinal disorders
5. Miscellaneous
   Seizure medication
   Fibrous dysplasia
   Neoplasm

Although vitamin D–resistant rickets has long been the most common form, an increasing number of children have rickets from gastrointestinal disorders, seizure medication, or renal osteodystrophy.

The development of vitamin D–deficient or vitamin D–resistant rickets is a complex process, but essentially the mechanism involves a decreased intake of vitamin D or a decrease in synthesis of 1,25-dihydroxy vitamin D, which causes a reduction in the absorption of calcium from the gastointestinal tract. This process leads to hypocalcemia, subsequent secondary hyperparathyroidism, and reduced tubular reabsorption of phosphate, which lowers the serum phosphate. The decreased concentrations of calcium and phosphorus and the secondary hyperparathyroidism cause the clinical and roentgenographic picture of rickets and osteomalacia. Serum and urine laboratory findings vary, depending on the cause of the rickets (Table 7-1). These findings allow differentiation among the various types of rickets, which is essential for determining the prognosis of the disorder, appropriate medical therapy, and occasionally surgical treatment.

Table 7-1 Laboratory values in rickets

Type of rickets	Serum						Urine		Miscellaneous
	Ca^{++}	P	Alk Phos	PTH	25(OH) Vit D	1,25(OH)$_2$ Vit D	% TRP	Ca^{++}	
Vitamin D–Resistant Rickets									
I. Phosphate diabetes	→	↓↓		→	→	→	↓↓	→	
II. ↓ 1,25 (OH)$_2$ vitamin D production	↓	↓	↑	↑	→	↓↓	↓	↓	
III. End organ intensitivity	↓	↓	↑	↑	↑ or →	↑ or →	↓	↓	
IV. Renal tubular acidosis	↓	↓	↑	↑	↑ or →	↑ or →	↓	↑	Na ↓, K ↓, Cl ↑; acidosis alkaline urine
Vitamin D–Deficient Rickets	↓ or →	↓	↑	↑	↓	↓	↑	↓	
Dietary Phosphate Deficiency	→	↓	↑	→	→	→	→	→	
Renal Osteodystrophy	↓	↑	↑	↑↑	↓↓	↓↓	?	↓↓	BUN ↑
Gastrointestinal Rickets	↓	↓	↑	↑	↓	↓ or →	↓	↓	↓ Absorption from gastrointestinal tract

Clinical Findings

In very young children with florid rickets the clinical signs are characteristic and severe. Prominence of the frontal bones with frontal bossing and delayed dentition are common. The costal cartilages of the chest are typically enlarged (rachitic "rosary"), occasionally with pectus carinatum. A long, smooth, dorsal kyphosis is the characteristic spinal deformity. Weakness of the abdominal musculature may cause the rachitic "pot belly."

More often, however, children have the more subtle findings of vitamin D–resistant rickets rather than those of the severe florid disease. Common signs are short stature with slight thickening of the joints, shortening of the long bones, and possibly bowing in the lower and upper extremities. Evaluation of bowed legs may give the first indication of the diagnosis.

Histologic Findings

The most significant feature in the histologic appearance of trabecular bone in rickets is unmineralized bone (osteoid seam) surrounding a mineralized segment of bone. Although this may occur in hyperparathyroidism and fibrous dysplasia, wide osteoid seams are typical of rickets and osteomalacia.

The most striking feature in the immature skeleton is mechanical alteration of the physis. The resting and proliferative zones are normal in appearance, but the zone of maturation is grossly distorted. The normal pattern of columnation is lost, and both the width and height of this zone are enlarged.

Roentgenographic Findings

The typical appearance of the physes, especially in the lower extremity and occasionally in the wrist and elbow, is pathognomonic for rickets. The physeal height is increased, and the physis and metaphysis are cupped or flared, particularly in the knee, ankle, and wrist. The normally dense zone of provisional calcification is either absent or subtle (Fig. 7-1).

Other roentgenographic features in children with rickets include the presence of Looser's lines, also known as Milkman's pseudofractures. These are not true fractures but represent localized collections of osteoid with mechanical weakening of the bone. Looser's lines have been reported in 20% of patients with all types of rickets, but are most commonly seen in vitamin D–resistant rickets and renal osteodystrophy.

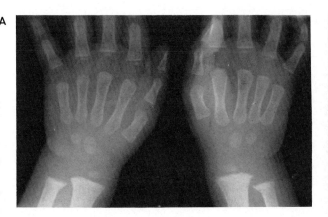 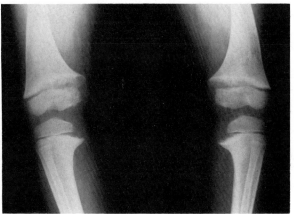

Fig. 7-1 Vitamin D–resistant rickets. **A,** Note widened metaphyseal flare of distal ulnar physes. **B,** Genu varum with widening of physes and metaphyseal flaring of femur and tibia.

Orthopaedic Treatment

The orthopaedic surgeon may be the first physician to diagnose the rickets. If appropriate, diagnostic consultation may be obtained with a pediatric endocrinologist or pediatric nephrologist. Medical treatment includes the use of vitamin D, 1,25-dihydroxy vitamin D, calcium, neutral phosphate solutions, and other treatment regimens designed to correct the metabolic disorder and assist more normal growth of the immature skeleton.

Even after medical treatment is well established, these children occasionally have angular deformities that are best treated surgically, especially in the lower extremities. Genu varum is the most common angular deformity requiring surgical correction, followed by varus deformity of the ankle. Rarely, severe coxa vara or genu valgum requires surgical correction in older adolescents.

The indications for osteotomy around the knee, ankle, and hip are similar to those for osteotomy of an angular deformity in other disorders. For severe genu varum, proximal tibial and fibular osteotomies are recommended. Occasionally, severe varus deformity of the ankle requires supramalleolar osteotomy, and rarely severe coxa vara requires subtrochanteric osteotomy (Fig. 7-2). The alignment of the entire extremity should be reviewed carefully before surgery to assess the effect of the osteotomy on the remaining joints. In addition, most authors recommend discontinuing medical treatment 2 to 4 weeks before surgery to prevent immobilization hypercalcemia during postoperative cast wear.

Because of the tendency of angular deformities to recur with growth, even after osteotomy, some authors recommend postponing surgery until near the end of skeletal growth. Continued medical management is imperative after osteotomy in young children, and yearly orthopaedic follow-up is necessary to evaluate the growth and development of the corrected extremity.

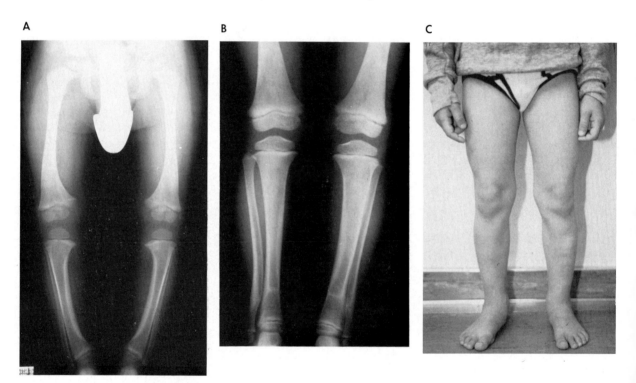

Fig. 7-2 Vitamin D–resistant rickets. **A,** Varus deformity of knee and ankle at age 4 years. **B,** After proximal and distal tibial osteotomies. **C,** Clinical appearance at age 6 years.

RENAL OSTEODYSTROPHY

Because of an imbalance in calcium and phosphorus homeostasis, children and young adults with chronic renal failure have significant skeletal abnormalities in addition to chronic medical illness. Dialysis systems and renal transplantation have increased the lifespan of children with chronic renal disease, and many of these patients require orthopaedic treatment well into young adulthood.

Although the pathophysiology of renal osteodystrophy is complex, the ultimate result is a combination of four pathophysiologic syndromes: (1) rickets and osteomalacia, (2) secondary hyperparathyroidism (osteitis fibrosa), (3) osteosclerosis, and (4) ectopic calcification and ossification.

Clinical Findings

The child with renal osteodystrophy is generally short, with delayed developmental milestones and skeletal age. The appearance of secondary centers of ossification and signs of sexual maturation are delayed also. Fractures occur quite frequently with minor trauma and can cause severe impairment. The increased incidence of slipped capital femoral epiphysis in children with renal osteodystrophy is attributed to the secondary hyperparathyroidism, with subsequent resorption of bone at the metaphyseal-physeal junction, in combination with the chronic nature of this disorder.

Roentgenographic Findings

Angular deformities in patients with renal osteodystrophy, particularly in the lower extremities, may be indistinguishable from those in patients with rickets. There may also be resorption of the ulna, resorption of the distal aspect of the distal phalanges in the hand, and subperiosteal resorption of the medial aspect of the proximal tibia. In young adults with chronic renal osteodystrophy, brown tumors may cause pathologic fractures in the pelvis and long bones.

Orthopaedic Treatment

Treatment of renal osteodystrophy generally is medical, with chronic renal problems controlled by dialysis or renal transplantation and appropriate serum and urine levels of calcium and phosphate maintained by medication. Occasionally parathyroidectomy is required for control of the secondary hyperparathyroidism.

Surgical treatment in patients with renal osteodystrophy occasionally is required for slipped capital femoral epiphysis, severe genu varum or genu valgum, or pathologic fracture of the femur or tibia (Fig. 7-3). Slipped capital femoral epiphysis should be treated as in other children; pinning in situ is appropriate in most cases. Tibial or femoral osteotomy may be indicated for severe angular deformities around the knee, and pathologic fractures through brown tumors may require excision, bone grafting, and internal fixation in the young adult patient.

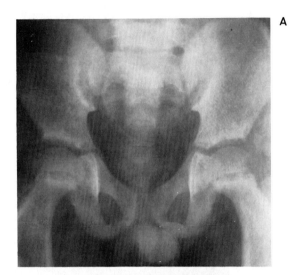

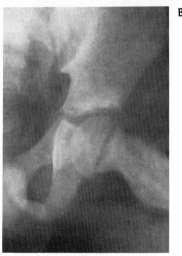

Fig. 7-3 Renal osteodystrophy. Bilateral slipped capital femoral epiphysis. **A,** Anteroposterior view shows widening of physes and diffuse osteopenia. **B,** Grade I slipped capital femoral epiphysis of left hip.

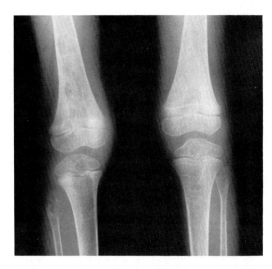

Fig. 7-4 Hypophosphatasia. Nine-year-old girl with generalized osteopenia, notching of margins of physes, and delayed ossification of fibular epiphyses.

HYPOPHOSPHATASIA

Hypophosphatasia is a metabolic disorder of bone characterized by a decrease in serum and leukocyte alkaline phosphatase and, in children with clinical disease, the presence of large concentrations of phosphoethanolamine in the urine. It is transmitted as an autosomal recessive disorder. There are some clinical and roentgenographic similarities between hypophosphatasia and rickets, but distinct differences exist in pathophysiology.

Clinical Findings

Hypophosphatasia is generally identified in infancy, with the florid syndrome causing growth retardation, failure to thrive, and multiple systemic problems. The mortality rate for the infantile form of hypophosphatasia is quite high, ranging from 50% to 70%. If these children survive, they usually have severe skeletal deformity and physical impairment.

Children or young adults with milder forms of hypophosphatasia are short and have varying degrees of orthopaedic problems. Common orthopaedic manifestations include enlargement near the joints of the lower extremity, angular deformity of the knee, prominent costochondral junctions, and kyphosis.

Roentgenographic Findings

Generalized osteopenia of the skeleton, most severe in the skull and metaphyseal regions of long bones, is characteristic of hypophosphatasia (Fig. 7-4). The physes may be cup shaped or wedge shaped, mainly at the center, with irregular notching at the margins. The epiphyses may be delayed in appearance but ultimately are normal in outline.

Orthopaedic Treatment

Pathologic fractures, particularly in the lower extremities, are frequent in children or young adults with hypophosphatasia. These fractures heal very slowly, and multiple pathologic fractures may present difficulties similar to those encountered in osteogenesis imperfecta. Intramedullary fixation and bone grafting are recommended for nonunion of pathologic fractures in young adults. In younger children with multiple pathologic fractures, treatment with either expanding Bailey nails or overlapping Rush rods, similar to the treatment of osteogenesis imperfecta, is recommended.

Fig. 7-5 Hypothyroidism. Slipped capital femoral epiphysis of right hip in 10-year-old girl.

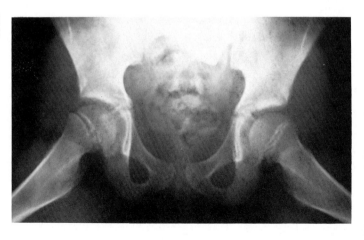

HYPOTHYROIDISM

The deficiency of thyroid hormone in children causes varying symptoms depending on the age of the child. In the newborn, it causes cretinism and delayed development. Neurologic development also is delayed, but if hypothyroidism is recognized and treatment is instituted, long-term damage to the central nervous system may be prevented. In adolescents and young adults, the symptoms and signs of hypothyroidism resemble those in adults. The diagnosis is made by measurement of the levels of thyroid hormone and thyroid-stimulating hormone.

Roentgenographic Findings

Bone age in children with hypothyroidism is generally delayed much more severely than in other endocrine disorders that affect maturation. The appearance of secondary ossification centers is delayed in all the epiphyses. In congenital hypothyroidism, roentgenograms of the knee show delay in ossification of the distal femoral epiphysis, which is normally present at birth.

There is a risk of slipped capital femoral epiphysis before diagnosis and during medical treatment. Some authors recommend endocrinologic evaluation of children under the skeletal age of 10 who have slipped capital femoral epiphyses (Fig. 7-5). If slipped capital femoral epiphysis does occur with hypothyroidism, it should be treated as in other children, generally with in situ pinning.

OSTEOGENESIS IMPERFECTA

Osteogenesis imperfecta is a syndrome in which an inherited disorder of connective tissue is associated with several metabolic abnormalities. Proposed classifications have differentiated between osteogenesis imperfecta congenita and osteogenesis imperfecta tarda based on the time of occurrence of the initial fracture. Sillence proposed a classification based on the pattern of inheritance and clinical features of each syndrome (Table 7-2).

Clinical Findings

Clinical features of osteogenesis imperfecta are variable and depend on the specific type. In general there is fragility of long bones, short stature, defective formation of the teeth, middle ear deafness, ligamentous laxity, and blue sclerae. Differential diagnoses include rickets, battered child syndrome, and juvenile osteoporosis.

Roentgenographic Findings

The long bones are diffusely osteopenic with thin cortices and an attenuated trabecular pattern. Angular deformity is common, particularly in the lower extremity, and fractures are frequent. Fractures can occur at any age from birth to late adolescence. Although the healing process is undisturbed, the often-abundant callus is quite plastic and easily deformed by subsequent weight bearing and minor trauma. In patients with severe osteogenesis imperfecta the metaphyses may appear cystic at birth, but this is seen more often during early childhood.

Table 7-2   Osteogenesis imperfecta

Type	Genetics	Clinical features
I	Autosomal dominant	Bone fragility, blue sclerae, onset of fractures after birth (most preschool age); type A, without dentinogenesis imperfecta; type B, with dentinogenesis imperfecta
II	Autosomal recessive	Lethal in perinatal period, dark blue sclerae, concertina femurs, beaded ribs
III	Autosomal recessive	Fractures at birth, progressive deformity, normal sclerae and healing
IV	Autosomal dominant	Bone fragility, normal sclerae, normal hearing; type A, without dentinogenesis imperfecta; type B, with dentinogenesis imperfecta

From Sillence D: Clin Orthop 159:11, 1981.

Orthopaedic Treatment

Currently no effective medical management exists for osteogenesis imperfecta.

The goal of orthopaedic treatment is to treat acute fractures and to provide long-term rehabilitation in an attempt to maintain ambulation through skeletal growth and development. When ambulatory status has been maintained and psychologic trauma minimized, these children have been shown to adapt as well as adults to their impairment and to be productive both socially and professionally.

Surgical intervention is recommended for several specific problems. Severe scoliosis occasionally develops in children with osteogenesis imperfecta. These curves tend to progress rapidly, and bracing is usually ineffective. Surgical fusion with internal fixation can be difficult because of the poor quality of bone, but newer methods of instrumentation have improved results of surgical fusion in patients with osteogenesis imperfecta. Surgery is recommended for progressive curves approaching 30 to 40 degrees in the skeletally immature child.

In children with severe angular deformity of the femur, tibia, or both, elective osteotomy with intramedullary internal fixation may be performed. Even though initial fractures may be treated by closed means, two or three fractures of the femur, tibia, or both are indications for implantation of an intramedullary device. Current internal fixation devices include the Bailey-Dubow telescoping intramedullary rod, overlapping Rush rods, or a single Rush rod in the very small child (Fig. 7-6). Numerous complica-

tions have been reported with the use of all of these devices. Single or overlapping Rush rods are generally preferred in very young children and the Bailey-Dubow rods in juveniles. In the young adult near skeletal maturity, an interlocking nail similar to that used for fractures in the femur or tibia may be considered.

▶ *Technique (Bailey-Dubow telescoping rod).* For the femur, place the patient in a 45-degree lateral decubitus position to allow access to the buttock and knee. After sterile preparation and draping, expose the angular deformities of the femur through one long lateral incision or through multiple small incisions. Expose the knee joint through a medial parapatellar incision; if necessary for adequate exposure of the intercondylar notch, dislocate the patella laterally.

For the tibia, use the same medial approach at the knee joint. Next, at the level of the ankle joint, make a transverse incision extending from the midline anteriorly to the posterior aspect of the medial malleolus. Transect the deep deltoid to allow exposure and insertion of a rod into the center of the distal tibial epiphysis.

After osteotomies have been performed in the metaphyses of the involved bone, perform multiple osteotomies so that the segments can be aligned when the rod is inserted (Fig. 7-7). When collapsed the rod should reach from the proximal to the distal end of the entire bone less 2 cm to allow a margin for error and for impaction of the shaft segments after surgery. Fit the tubular sleeve with the special detachable drill point, and drill through the medullary

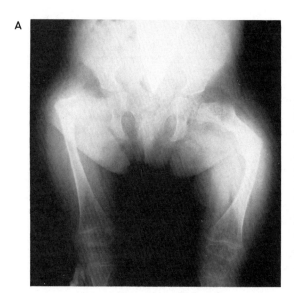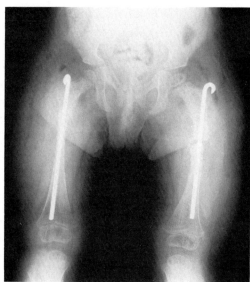

Fig. 7-6 Osteogenesis imperfecta. **A,** Severe malunion of bilateral femoral fractures in 18-month-old girl. **B,** View after osteotomy and Rush rod insertion.

canal of one metaphysis, through the bony epiphysis, and into the knee or ankle joint; repeat this at the opposite end of the bone. After drilling the medullary canal of all fragments with the same drill point attached to the tubular sleeve, replace the drill point with the T-shaped flange that screws on the end of the tubular sleeve. At the other end of the bone, insert the obturator rod through the articular cartilage and into the canal in the metaphysis. Thread the fragments of the shaft on the sleeve portion of the rod, and then place the other metaphysis in position with the obturator inside the tubular sleeve. Countersink the T-shaped end of the obturator through the articular cartilage and into the bony portion of the epiphysis. Then impact the sleeve end of the rod into the joint cartilage at the opposite end of the bone. Confirm alignment with roentgenograms and close the periosteum around the fragments. Close the incision sites and apply a hip-spica cast or long-leg cast, depending on the site of the osteotomies.

Technical points to assist in the use of Bailey-Dubow nails include the following.

For the femur:

1. Insert the sleeve proximally through the base of the neck of the femur or the top of the greater trochanter.
2. "Crimp" the attached T-piece at the proximal end of the sleeve to prevent loosening.
3. Insert the obturator in the central portion of the intercondylar notch.
4. Use the longest rod of the largest possible diameter for maximal overlap of the obturator and sheath.

For the tibia:

1. Insert the sleeve proximally and near the posterior aspect of the anterior tibial spine.
2. Insert the obturator distally in the central portion of the distal tibial epiphysis.

For both the femur and the tibia:

1. Countersink the T-ends of both the obturator and sleeve into the cartilage of the epiphysis or base of the femoral neck.
2. Carefully check the rotation of limbs before application of the cast to prevent rotational malunion.

▲ *Postoperative management.* After femoral osteotomy, a spica cast is worn for 8 to 12 weeks or until all osteotomies heal. After tibial osteotomy, a long-leg cast is worn for 8 to 12 weeks or until all osteotomies heal (Fig. 7-8). Polypropylene splints may be used after cast removal during the 12- to 24-month rehabilitation process. Patients should be evaluated at least once a year, and the rods should be revised if necessitated by growth or fracture.

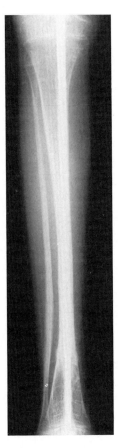

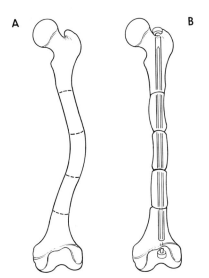

Fig. 7-7 Use of Bailey-Dubow rod in femur for osteogenesis imperfecta. **A,** Multiple osteotomies. **B,** Realignment and insertion of rod.

Fig. 7-8 Insertion of Bailey-Dubow rod after multiple fractures in tibia of 7-year-old boy with osteogenesis imperfecta.

OSTEOPETROSIS

Osteopetrosis is a rare disorder of the immature skeleton in which the failure of osteoclastic and chondroclastic resorption causes density of the skeletal bones (Fig. 7-9). Pathologic fractures and narrowing of the marrow space and foraminal openings in the skull by unresorbed masses of dense bone are the prominent clinical signs of this disorder.

Clinical Findings

Two clinical forms have been described. The milder form (osteopetrosis tarda) is transmitted as an autosomal dominant disorder, and the more severe form (osteopetrosis congenita) is transmitted as an autosomal recessive trait. The severe form is apparent in early infancy and causes faulty development of the medullary canals. Survival beyond age 20 years is unlikely. Patients with the autosomal dominant, more benign form of osteopetrosis generally have a normal life span with minimal skeletal involvement. Mild anemia may occur.

Histologically, osteopetrotic bone has thickened trabeculae and hypercellular cortices with a paucity of osteoblasts and virtually a complete absence of osteoclasts.

Orthopaedic Treatment

The autosomal recessive form of osteopetrosis in children has been successfully treated by allogenic bone transplantation or marrow transplantation from a human lymphocyte antigen (HLA)–mismatched donor after preoperative marrow ablation and total body irradiation.

Osseous involvement is asymmetric in the older adolescent or young adult with osteopetrosis. Occasionally, fractures recur in a particular area of the skeleton. Despite the thickness of the sclerotic bone, fractures occur more frequently in patients with osteopetrosis than in unaffected persons. Fractures generally heal with nonoperative management, but occasionally nonunion of the femur or tibia requires surgical intervention.

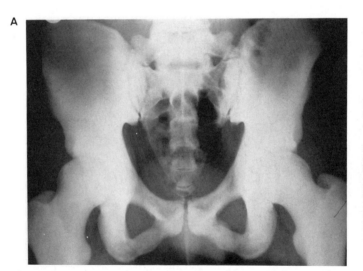
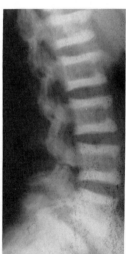

Fig. 7-9 Osteopetrosis. **A,** Obliteration of marrow space and dense bone on anteroposterior pelvic roentgenogram of 17-year-old boy. **B,** "Rugger jersey" spine, bone-within-bone appearance of lateral lumbar spine.

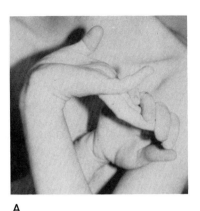

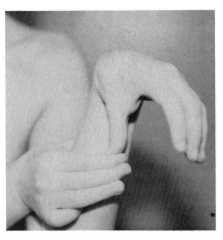

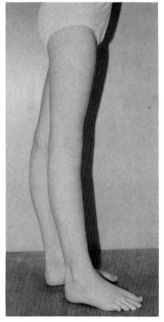

Fig. 7-10 Ehlers-Danlos syndrome, clinical features in 8-year-old girl. **A,** Wrist hyperextension. **B,** Placement of thumb on forearm with hyperflexion. **C,** Genu recurvatum. (From Beaty JH and Sloan M: J Pediatr Orthop 9:331, 1989.)

EHLERS-DANLOS SYNDROME

Ehlers-Danlos syndrome is a group of disorders characterized by hyperextensibility of the skin, hypermobility of the joints, susceptibility to bruising, and calcification of the soft tissues. Ehlers-Danlos syndrome has been classified into eight separate types based on the pattern of genetic transmission and the clinical features. Type VI is the classic type, characterized by a biochemical dysfunction in which levels of lysine hydroxylase are decreased and by a deficiency of hydroxylysine in collagen.

Clinical Findings

Most children and young adults with Ehlers-Danlos syndrome have variable signs and symptoms of the disorder. The skin may be mildly or severely hyperextensible. Joint hypermobility can include hyperextension of the knee and elbow, hyperdorsiflexion of the wrist, and the ability to place the thumb on the forearm during flexion of the wrist (Fig. 7-10).

Orthopaedic Treatment

Treatment should be directed toward the specific joint disorders. Recurrent dislocation of joints, most commonly the patella, the shoulder, and infrequently the hip and elbow, have been reported. Because of the underlying laxity of the skin and soft tissues, surgical treatment of these problems can be difficult. When surgery is considered, any underlying bone dysplasia should be evaluated carefully and included in the surgical correction if appropriate (Fig. 7-11).

Patients with Ehlers-Danlos syndrome may have occult bleeding disorders, and preoperative hematologic consultation is generally appropriate. Wound management should be meticulous after surgery, with hemostasis following the release of tourniquets and detailed skin closure. Skin sutures are left in place for a longer period of time than usual.

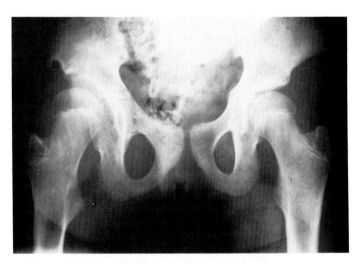

Fig. 7-11 Ehlers-Danlos syndrome after Pemberton osteotomy and anterior capsulorrhaphy for recurrent anterolateral dislocation of right hip. (From Beaty JH and Sloan M: J Pediatr Orthop 9:331,1989.)

MARFAN SYNDROME

Marfan syndrome is a genetic disorder with an associated connective tissue disorder and a variety of clinical manifestations. Marfan syndrome is transmitted as an autosomal dominant disorder.

Clinical Findings

Clinical features involve the skeletal, ocular, and cardiovascular systems. Arachnodactyly, dolichostenomelia, and scoliosis are skeletal manifestations (Fig. 7-12). Findings in the cardiovascular system may include aortic dilatation, aneurysms, or mitral valve prolapse. Pathologic conditions of the eye include myopia and superior displacement of the lens, unlike the ocular complications in homocystinuria, where inferior displacement of the lens occurs.

No clinical laboratory tests are available to establish the diagnosis of Marfan syndrome. Diagnosis generally is made on the basis of clinical and roentgenographic features.

Roentgenographic Findings

Although many roentgenographic findings in Marfan syndrome are specific for the disorder, there is considerable overlap between these findings and the variety seen in the normal population. Arachnodactyly can be determined on roentgenograms by the long, slender phalanges, metatarsals, and metacarpals

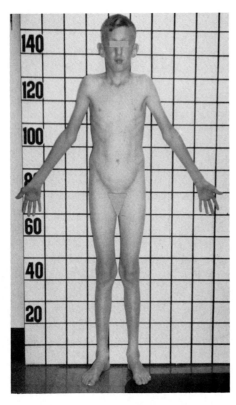

Fig. 7-12 Marfan syndrome. Note arachnodactyly and dolichostenomelia in 10-year-old boy.

and the increased ratio of length to width of the second to fifth metacarpals. Scoliosis is quite common and is similar to idiopathic scoliosis, but in some patients the vertebral height is markedly increased.

Orthopaedic Treatment

Before any surgical procedure in children or young adults with Marfan syndrome, consultations with a cardiologist and ophthalmologist are recommended. Scoliosis is the most common orthopaedic problem requiring treatment. In general, it should be treated similarly to idiopathic scoliosis, with the usual guidelines for bracing and surgical treatment. Occasionally, adolescents with Marfan syndrome have a painful flexible flatfoot that requires surgical correction for functional symptoms or difficulty with fitting shoes.

HOMOCYSTINURIA

Homocystinuria is a disorder of enzyme dysfunction with defects that lead to the accumulation of homocysteine and homocystine in the blood and homocysteine in the urine. The clinical and roentgenographic manifestations are similar to those of Marfan syndrome, and differentiation is mandatory for appropriate treatment. An ophthalmologic consultation is recommended because of potential dislocation of the lens.

Clinical Findings

Children with homocystinuria are tall, with long limbs, and may show arachnodactyly and scoliosis as do patients with Marfan syndrome. Dislocation of the lens is common, but unlike that in Marfan syndrome, the displacement is inferior. Severe osteoporosis is a common feature of type I homocystinuria but is not seen in Marfan syndrome. Type I homocystinuria also is associated with an abnormality in clotting, which can lead to venous and arterial thromboembolic incidents. The biochemical defect in type I homocystinuria is a deficiency of cystathionine synthetase. Screening for homocysteine in the urine differentiates between type I homocystinuria and Marfan syndrome.

Orthopaedic Treatment

Scoliosis is treated similarly to idiopathic scoliosis, with appropriate guidelines for bracing and surgery. Medical treatment of homocystinuria depends on the specific type. In type I, recommended treatment is methionine restriction and pyridoxine supplementation. In types II and III, restriction of methionine is not recommended. Vitamin B_{12} is used in the management of type II homocystinuria and folic acid for type III.

REFERENCES

Rickets and osteomalacia

Blockley NJ, Murphy AV, and Mocan H: Management of rachitic deformities in children with chronic renal failure, J Bone Joint Surg 68B:791, 1986.

Bosley AR, Verrier-Jones ER, and Campbell MJ: Aetiological factors in rickets of prematurity, Arch Dis Child 55:683, 1980.

Brighton CT: Longitudinal bone growth: the growth plate and its dysfunctions. In The American Academy of Orthopaedic Surgeons: Instructional Course Lectures, Vol 36, St. Louis, 1987, The CV Mosby Co.

Callenbach JC et al: Etiologic factors in rickets of very low-birth-weight infants; J Pediatr 98:800, 1981.

Chesney RW, Hamstra AJ, and DeLuca HF: Rickets of prematurity: supranormal levels of serum 1,25-dihydroxyvitamin D, Am J Dis Child 135:34, 1981.

Eke FU, Winterborn MH, and Robertson PW: Detection of early renal osteodystrophy, Child Nephrol Urol 9:33, 1988-89.

Fraser DR and Salter RB: The diagnosis and management of the various types of rickets, Pediatr Clin North Am 26:417, 1958.

Gefter WB et al: Rickets presenting as multiple fractures in premature infants on hyperalimentation, Radiology 142:371, 1982.

Greene WB and Kahler SG: Hypophosphatemic rickets: still misdiagnosed and inadequately treated, South Med J 78:1/79, 1985.

Loeffler RD and Sherman RC: The effect of treatment on growth and deformity in hypophosphatemic vitamin D–resistant rickets, Clin Orthop 162:4, 1982.

Mankin HJ: Review article: rickets, osteomalacia, and renal osteodystrophy, J Bone Joint Surg 56A:164, 1974.

Mankin HJ: Rickets, osteomalacia, and renal osteodystrophy: an update, Orthop Clin North Am 21:81, 1990.

Marie PJ et al: Histological osteomalacia due to dietary calcium deficiency in children, N Engl J Med 307:584, 1982.

Mason RS et al: Vitamin D metabolism in hypophosphatemic rickets, Am J Dis Child 136:909, 1982.

Norman ME: Vitamin D in bone disease, Pediatr Clin North Am 29:947, 1982.

Perry W and Stamp TC: Hereditary hypophosphatemic rickets with autosomal recessive inheritance and severe osteosclerosis: a report of two cases, J Bone Joint Surg 60B:430, 1978.

Rosier RN: Orthopaedic basic science: update, Orthopedics 10:1793, 1987.

Sheridan RM, Chiroff RT, and Friedman EM: Operative and nonoperative treatment of rachitic lower extremity deformities: a long-term study with 46-year average follow-up, Clin Orthop 116:66, 1976.

Timperlake RW et al: Effects of anticonvulsant drug therapy on bone mineral density in a pediatric population, J Pediatr Orthop 8:467, 1988.

Tsuru N, Chan JC, and Chinchilli VM: Renal hypophosphatemic rickets: growth and mineral metabolism after treatment with calcitriol (1,25-dihydroxy vitamin D_3) and phosphate supplementation, Am J Dis Child 141:108, 1987.

Zaleske DJ, Dopplet SH, and Mankin HJ: Metabolic and endocrine abnormalities of the immature skeleton. In Morrissy RT (editor): Lovell and Winter's pediatric orthopaedics, ed 3, Philadelphia, 1990, JB Lippincott Co.

Renal osteodystrophy

Blockley NJ, Murphy AV, and Mocan H: Management of rachitic deformities in children with chronic renal failure, J Bone Joint Surg 68B:791, 1986.

Chan JC: Vitamin D disorders in children with chronic renal failure, Va Med 109:255, 1982.

Chan JC and Hsu AC: Vitamin D and renal diseases, Adv Pediatr 27:117, 1980.

Chesney RW et al: Renal osteodystrophy in children: the role of vitamin D, phosphorus and parathyroid hormone, Am J Kidney Dis 7:275, 1986.

Donckerewolcke RA: Diagnosis and treatment of renal tubular disorders in children, Pediatr Clin North Am 29:895, 1982.

Hely D et al: Osteonecrosis of the femoral head and condyle in the post-transplantation courses of children and adolescents, Int J Pediatr Nephrol 3:297, 1982.

Hodson EM et al: Growth retardation and renal osteodystrophy in children with chronic renal failure, J Pediatr 103:735, 1983.

Hsu AC et al: Renal osteodystrophy in children with chronic renal failure: an unexpectedly common and incapacitating complication, Pediatrics 70:742, 1982.

Kricun ME and Resnick D: Patellofemoral abnormalities in renal osteodystrophy, Radiology 143:667, 1982.

Kricun ME and Resnick D: Elbow abnormalities in renal osteodystrophy, AJR 140:577, 1983.

Mankin HJ: Rickets, osteomalacia, and renal osteodystrophy. Part I. J Bone Joint Surg 56A: 101, 1974.

Mankin HJ: Rickets, osteomalacia and renal osteodystrophy. Part II. J Bone Joint Surg 56A:352, 1974.

Mehls O et al: Slipped epiphyses in renal osteodystrophy, Arch Dis Child 50:545, 1975.

Sundaram M et al: Terminal phalangeal tufts: earliest site of renal osteodystrophy findings in hemodialysis patients, AJR 133:25, 1979.

Sundaram M et al: Erosive azotemic osteodystrophy, AJR 136:363, 1981.

Watson AR et al: Renal osteodystrophy in children on CAPD: a prospective trial of 1-alpha-hydroxycholecalciferol therapy, Child Nephrol Urol 9:220, 1988-89.

Wolfson BJ and Capitanio MA: The wide spectrum of renal osteodystrophy in children, CRC Crit Rev Diagn Imaging 27:297, 1987.

Hypophosphatasia

Anderton JM: Orthopaedic problems in adult hypophosphatasia: a report of two cases, J Bone Joint Surg 61B:82, 1979.

Coe JD, Murphy WA, and Whyte MP: Management of femoral fractures and pseudofractures in adult hypophosphatasia, J Bone Joint Surg 68A:392, 1986.

Hypothyroidism

Aronson R et al: Growth in children with congenital hypothyroidism detected by neonatal screening, J Pediatr 116:33, 1990.

Birrell J, Frost GJ, and Parkin JM: The development of children with congenital hypothyroidism, Dev Med Child Neurol 25:512, 1983.

Crawford AH, MacEwen GD, and Fonte D: Slipped capital femoral epiphysis co-existent with hypothyroidism, Clin Orthop 122:135, 1977.

Hulse JA: Outcome of congenital hypothyroidism. Arch Dis Child 59:23, 1984.

Illig R et al: Sixty children with congenital hypothyroidism detected by neonatal thyroid: mental development at 1, 4 and 7 years: a longitudinal study, Acta Endocrinol [Suppl] 279:346, 1986.

LaFranchi S: Diagnosis and treatment of hypothyroidism in children, Compr Ther 13:20, 1987.

Lobovits A: Early recognition of congenital hypothyroidism, J Pediatr 103:662, 1990.

Lyon IC: Screening of congenital hypothyroidism: a three year experience, NZ Med J 97:175, 1984.

Rivkees S, Bode HH, and Crawford JD: Long-term growth in juvenile acquired hypothyroidism: the failure to achieve normal adult stature, N Engl J Med 318:599, 1988.

Zubrow AB, Lane JW, and Parks JS: Slipped capital femoral epiphysis occurring during treatment for hypothyroidism, J Bone Joint Surg 60A:256, 1978.

Osteogenesis imperfecta

Albright JA: Management overview of osteogenesis imperfecta, Clin Orthop 159:80, 1981.

Andersen PE Jr and Hauge M: Congenital generalized bone dysplasias: a clinical, radiological, and epidemiological survey, J Med Genet 26:37, 1989.

Bailey RW: Further clinical experience with the extensile nail, Clin Orthop 159:171, 1981.

Bailey RW and Dubow HI: Experimental and clinical studies of longitudinal bone growth utilizing a new method of internal fixation crossing the epiphyseal plate, J Bone Joint Surg 47A:1669, 1965.

Bailey RW and Dubow HI: Evolution of the concept of an extensible nail accommodating to normal longitudinal bone growth: clinical considerations and implications, Clin Orthop 159:157, 1981.

Benson DR and Newman DC: The spine and surgical treatment in osteogenesis imperfecta, Clin Orthop 159:147, 1981.

Bleck EE: Nonoperative treatment of osteogenesis imperfecta: orthotic and mobility management, Clin Orthop 159:111, 1981.

Bullough PG, Davidson DD, and Lorenzo JC: The morbid anatomy of the skeleton in osteogenesis imperfecta, Clin Orthop 159:42, 1981.

Burke TE, Crerand SJ, and Dowling F: Hypertrophic callus formation leading to high-output cardiac failure in a patient with osteogenesis imperfecta, J Pediatr Orthop 8:605, 1988.

DalMonte, A et al: Osteogenesis imperfecta: results obtained with the Sofield method of surgical treatment, Ital J Orthop Traumatol 8:43, 1982.

Finidori G: Treatment of osteogenesis imperfecta in children, Ann NY Acad Sci 543:167, 1988.

Gamble JG et al: Non-union of fractures in children who have osteogenesis imperfecta, J Bone Joint Surg 70A:439, 1988.

Gitelis S, Whiffen J, and DeWald RL: The treatment of severe scoliosis in osteogenesis imperfecta: case report, Clin Orthop 175:56, 1983.

Goldman AB et al: "Popcorn" calcifications: a prognostic sign in osteogenesis imperfecta, Radiology 136:351, 1980.

Habekost HJ and Zichner L: Experiences with the operative therapy of osteogenesis imperfecta, Z Orthop 120:673, 1982.

Herring JA: Indications, patient selection, and evaluation in pediatric orthopedics. In Luque ER (editor): Segmental spinal instrumentation, Thorofare NJ, 1984, Slack, Inc.

Huaux JP and Lokietek W: Is APD a promising drug in the treatment of severe osteogenesis imperfecta? J Pediatr Orthop 8:71, 1988.

King JD and Bobechko WP: Osteogenesis imperfecta: an orthopaedic description and surgical review, J Bone Joint Surg 53B:72, 1971.

Letts M, Monson R, and Weber K: The prevention of recurrent fractures of the lower extremity in severe osteogenesis imperfecta using vacuum pants: a preliminary report in four patients, J Pediatr Orthop 8:454, 1988.

McCall RE and Bax JA: Hyperplastic callus formation in osteogenesis imperfecta following intramedullary rodding, J Pediatr Orthop 4:361, 1984.

Middleton RW and Frost RB: Percutaneous intramedullary rod interchange in osteogenesis imperfecta, J Bone Joint Surg 69B:429, 1987.

Middleton RW: Closed intramedullary rodding for osteogenesis imperfecta, J Bone Joint Surg 66B:652, 1984.

Millar EA: Observation on the surgical management of osteogenesis imperfecta, Clin Orthop 159:154, 1981.

Morefield WG and Miller GR: Aftermath of osteogenesis imperfecta: a disease in adulthood, J Bone Joint Surg 62A:113, 1980.

Morel G and Houghton GR: Pneumatic trouser splints in the treatment of severe osteogenesis imperfecta, Acta Orthop Scand 53:547, 1982.

Niemann KM: Surgical treatment of the tibia in osteogenesis imperfecta, Clin Orthop 159:134, 1981.

Paterson CR, McAllion S, and Miller R: Osteogenesis imperfecta with dominant inheritance and normal sclera, J Bone Joint Surg 65B:35, 1983.

Pozo JL, Crockard HA, and Ransford AO: Basilar impression in osteogenesis imperfecta, J Bone Joint Surg 66B:233, 1984.

Rodriguez RP and Bailey RW: Internal fixation of the femur in patients with osteogenesis imperfecta, Clin Orthop 159:126, 1981.

Root L: Upper limb surgery in osteogenesis imperfecta, Clin Orthop 159:141, 1981.

Rush A and Burke SW: Hangman's fracture in a patient with osteogenesis imperfecta, J Bone Joint Surg 66A:778, 1984.

Shapiro F: Consequences of an osteogenesis imperfecta diagnosis for survival and ambulation, J Pediatr Orthop 5:456, 1985.

Sillence DO: Osteogenesis imperfecta: an expanding panorama of variance, Clin Orthop 159:11, 1981.

Sillence DO, Senn A, and Danks DM: Genetic heterogeneity in osteogenesis imperfecta, J Med Genet 16:101, 1979.

Stockley I, Bell MJ, and Sharrard WJ: The role of expanding intramedullary rods in osteogenesis imperfecta, J Bone Joint Surg 71B:422, 1989.

Tiley F and Albright JA: Osteogenesis imperfecta: treatment by multiple osteotomy and intramedullary rod insertion, J Bone Joint Surg 55A:701, 1973.

Williams PF: Fragmentation and rodding in osteogenesis imperfecta, J Bone Joint Surg 47B:23, 1965.

Wynne-Davies R and Gormley J: Clinical and genetic patterns in osteogenesis imperfecta, Clin Orthop 159:26, 1981.

Yong-Hing K and MacEwen GD: Scoliosis associated with osteogenesis imperfecta, J Bone Joint Surg 64B:36, 1982.

Ziv I, Rang M, and Hoffman HJ: Paraplegia in osteogenesis imperfecta: a case report, J Bone Joint Surg 65B:184, 1983.

Osteopetrosis

Aarskog D, Aksnes L, and Markestad R: Effect of parathyroid hormone on vitamin D metabolism in osteopetrosis, Pediatrics 68:109, 1981.

Andersen PE Jr and Hauge M: Congenital generalised bone dysplasias: a clinical, radiological, and epidemiological survey, J Med Genet 26:37, 1989.

Cameron HU and Dewar FP: Degenerative osteoarthritis associated with osteopetrosis, Clin Orthop 127:148, 1977.

Fischer A and Griscelli C: Allogeneic bone marrow graft in children, Arch Fr Pediatr 43:666, 1986.

Greene WB and Torre BA: Case report: femoral neck fracture in a child with autosomal dominant osteopetrosis, J Pediatr Orthop 5:483, 1985.

Hasenhuttl K: Osteopetrosis: review of the literature on comparative studies on a case with a 24-year follow-up, J Bone Joint Surg 44A:359, 1962.

Horton WA, Schimke RN, and Iyama T: Osteopetrosis: further heterogeneity, J Pediatr 97:580, 1980.

Kadota RP and Smithson WA: Bone marrow transplantation for diseases of childhood, Mayo Clin Proc 59:171, 1984.

Kaibara, N et al: Intermediate form of osteopetrosis with recessive inheritance, Skeletal Radiol 9:47, 1982.

Kaplan FS et al: Successful treatment of infantile malignant osteopetrosis by bone-marrow transplantation, J Bone Joint Surg 70A:617, 1988.

Marks SC Jr: Osteopetrosis: multiple pathways for the inception of osteoclast function, Appl Pathol 5:172, 1987.

Milgram JW and Jasty M: Osteopetrosis: a morphological study of twenty-one cases, J Bone Joint Surg 64A:912, 1982.

Milhaud G et al: Osteopetro-rickets: a new congenital bone disorder, Metab Bone Dis Relat Res 3:91, 1981.

Morrow G III et al: Calcium mobilization in osteopetrosis, Am J Dis Child 114:161, 1967.

Oliveria G et al: Osteopetrosis and rickets: an intriguing association, Am J Dis Child 140:377, 1986.

Seifert MF: The biology of macrophages in osteopetrosis: structure and function, Clin Orthop 182:270, 1984.

Shapiro F et al: Human osteopetrosis: a histological, ultrastructural, and biochemical study, J Bone Joint Surg 62A:382, 1980.

Sieff CA et al: Allogenic bone-marrow transplantation in infantile malignant osteopetrosis, Lancet 1:437, 1983.

Teitelbaum, SL et al: Malignant osteopetrosis: a disease of abnormal osteoclast proliferation, Metab Bone Dis Relat Res 3:99, 1981.

Zintl F et al: Status of allogeneic bone marrow transplantation in childhood in the GDR, Folia Haematol 116:389, 1989.

Ehlers-Danlos syndrome

Beaty JH and Sloan M: Recurrent voluntary anterior dislocation of the hip: case report and review of the literature, J Pediatr Orthop 9:331, 1989.

Beighton P and Horan F: Orthopedic aspects of the Ehlers-Danlos syndrome, J Bone Joint Surg 51B:444, 1969.

Hernandez A et al: Third case of a distinct variant of the Ehlers-Danlos syndrome, Clin Genet 20:222, 1981.

Igarashi M et al: Clinical features and an ultrastructural study of Ehlers-Danlos syndrome Type II, J Dermatol 9:309, 1982.

Matton MT et al: Unusual familial manifestation of Ehlers-Danlos syndrome, Prog Clin Biol Res 104:243, 1982.

Welbury RR: Ehlers-Danlos syndrome: historical review, report of two cases in one family and treatment needs, ASDC J Dent Child 56:220, 1989.

Wesley JR, Mahour H, and Wooley MM: Multiple surgical problems in two patients with Ehlers-Danlos syndrome, Surgery 87:319, 1980.

Marfan syndrome

Amis J and Herring JA: Iatrogenic kyphosis: a complication of Harrington instrumentation in Marfan's syndrome: a case report, J Bone Joint Surg 66:460, 1984.

Birch JG and Herring JA: Spinal deformity in Marfan syndrome, J Pediatr Orthop 7:546, 1987.

Boucek RJ et al: The Marfan syndrome: a deficiency in chemically stable collagen cross-links, N Engl J Med 305:988, 1981.

Brenton DP et al: Homocystinuria and Marfan's syndrome, J Bone Joint Surg 54B:277, 1972.

Chemke J et al: Homozygosity for autosomal dominant Marfan syndrome, J Med Genet 21:173, 1984.

Ellis DG: Chest wall deformities in children, Pediatr Ann 18:161, 1989.

Pennes DR, Braunstein EM, and Shirazi KK: Carpal ligamentous laxity with bilateral perilunate dislocation in Marfan syndrome, Skeletal Radiol 13:62, 1985.

Pyertiz RE and McKusick VA: The Marfan syndrome: diagnosis and management, N Engl J Med 300:772, 1979.

Robins PR, Moe JH, and Winter RB: Scoliosis in Marfan's syndrome: its characteristics and results of treatment in thirty-five patients, J Bone Joint Surg 57A:358, 1975.

Savini R, Cervellati S, and Beroaldo E: Spinal deformities in Marfan's syndrome, Ital J Orthop Traumatol 6:19, 1980.

Scherer LR et al: Surgical management of children and young adults with Marfan syndrome and pectus excavatum, J Pediatr Surg 23:1169, 1988.

Waters P et al: Scoliosis in children with pectus excavatum and pectus carinatum, J Pediatr Orthop 9:551, 1989.

Wenger DR et al: Protrusio acetabuli in Marfan's syndrome, Clin Orthop 147:134, 1980.

Winter RB: Severe spondylolisthesis in Marfan's syndrome: report of two cases, J Pediatr Orthop 2:51, 1982.

Homocystinuria

Bartholomew DW et al: Therapeutic approaches to cobalamin-C methylmalonic acidemia and homocystinuria, J Pediatr 112:32, 1988.

Brenton DP: Skeletal abnormalities in homocystinuria, Postgrad Med J 53:488, 1977.

Golden GS: Stroke syndromes in childhood, Neurol Clin 3:59, 1985.

Kurczynski TW et al: Maternal homocystinuria: studies of an untreated mother and fetus, Arch Dis Child 55:721, 1980.

MacCarthy JMT and Carey MC: Bone changes in homocystinuria, Clin Radiol 19:128, 1968.

Sepe SJ et al: Genetic services in the United States, JAMA 248:1733, 1982.

8 Hematologic Diseases

ALVIN H. CRAWFORD
F. STIG JACOBSEN

The primary treatment of diseases related to the hemopoietic system is medical, but as the longevity of these patients increases, the orthopaedic surgeon will become more involved in treating the musculoskeletal manifestations of these diseases.

LEUKEMIA

Leukemia is a neoplastic disorder of blood cells that mainly affects the leukocytes. It is the most common form of childhood cancer, accounting for one third of the 7000 childhood cancers per year in the United States. The peak incidence of leukemia is in children 3 to 4 years of age, with a poorer prognosis for those younger than 2 years or older than 10 years of age. Of those children with leukemia 70% have acute lymphocytic leukemia (ALL); the remainder have a form of leukemia that is nonlymphogenic in origin and occasionally is connected with conditions of chromosomal fragility as in Fanconi's anemia.

The symptoms of leukemia usually are nonspecific, and two thirds of patients have symptoms for less than 6 weeks before the diagnosis is made, by which time the disease usually is disseminated. The first clinical signs may be lethargy, bleeding, fever, or an infection from which the child does not completely recover. Joint pain is the initial symptom of ALL in about 10% of children. Pain usually occurs asymmetrically in the hips and knees and may mimic juvenile rheumatoid arthritis, rheumatic fever, or other arthropathies. Bone pain probably is caused by proliferation of the hemopoietic tissue within the medullary canal, but it may occur without apparent roentgenographic changes. Low back pain may be caused by osteoporosis and collapse of some of the vertebral bodies.

HEMATOLOGIC DISEASES

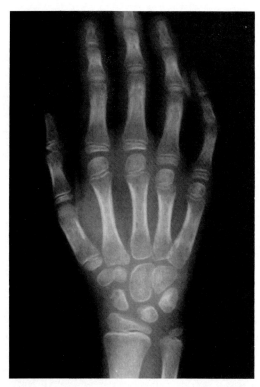

Fig. 8-1 Destruction of carpal bones and moth-eaten appearance of metacarpals in 6-year-old child with acute leukemia.

Roentgenographic changes appear initially in approximately 50% of all patients with ALL and in a higher percentage of children younger than 1 year of age. Changes are almost completely absent in patients older than 10 years of age. Roentgenographic changes in leukemia are osteoporosis, metaphyseal lucency, periosteal reaction, osteosclerosis, and osteolytic lesions. Most authors report that the presence of bone lesions in children with leukemia does not influence the prognosis, although Rajantie et al and Hughes and Kay reported a slightly better prognosis in patients with bone lesions. Roentgenographic changes usually do not persist in children who achieve remission and generally do not reappear at the time of relapse of the disease. Osteopenia (Fig. 8-1) is the most common roentgenographic finding, occurring in up to 25% of all patients. It may be caused by altered metabolism, direct marrow proliferation of leukemic infiltrates, inactivity, or possibly steroid treatment. Osteopenia is seen most often in the spine. Metaphyseal lucency (leukemic lines) (Fig. 8-2) is usually the first skeletal roentgenographic change and occurs in metaphyses of rapid growth, usually around the knee. Dense bands of calcification are present in the epiphysis and on the metaphyseal side,

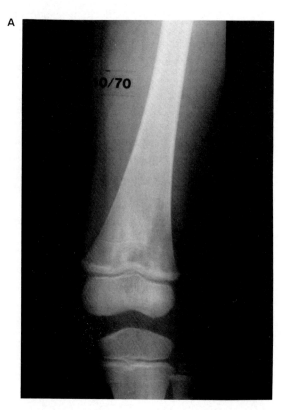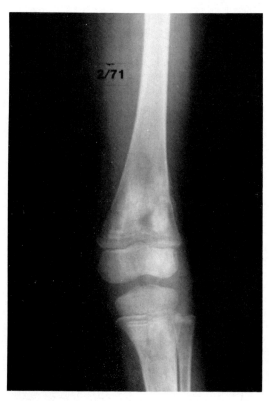

Fig. 8-2 Roentgenographic changes in 4-year-old child with acute lymphocytic leukemia. **A,** Note dense metaphyseal band with adjacent lucency in distal femoral physis, diffuse osteoporosis, and Harris growth arrest lines. **B,** Several months later. Note typical changes of acute leukemia with osteolytic and osteoblastic lesions, periosteal elevation, and diffuse osteoporosis.

a very clear lucent line. This is believed to represent a slow endochondral bone formation rather than leukemic infiltrations. This banding is a nonspecific sign that also appears in malnutrition, juvenile rheumatoid arthritis, and septicemia. Banding usually disappears as the disease is affected by treatment, but horizontal lines still may be present in the metaphysis, representing periods of slowed and accelerated growth during the process of the disease. These are similar to Harris growth arrest lines and give the bone a "zebra" appearance. Osteolytic areas (Fig. 8-3, *A*) may be focal or diffuse and usually represent aggressive, local tumor growth. Focal osteolysis gives the bone a "moth-eaten" appearance and usually is noted in the long bones or the pelvis. These areas of focal osteolysis persist even after remission of the disease (Fig. 8-3, *B*). Osteosclerosis is the least frequent roentgenographic finding, reported in approximately 10% of Silverman's patients. This may represent a concentration of tumor cells or bone changes after osteonecrosis. Periosteal elevation is not uncommon in the long bones of the lower extremity (Fig. 8-3, *C*) and is caused by tumor cells erupting through the periosteum, lifting it and initiating reactive bone formation.

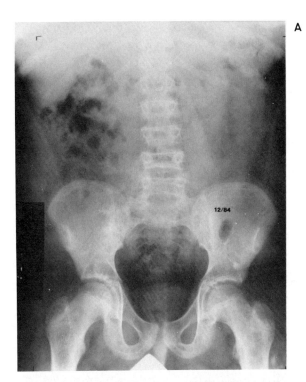

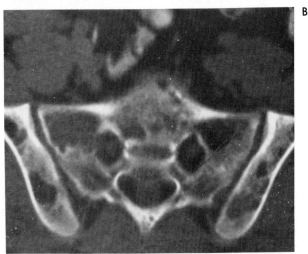

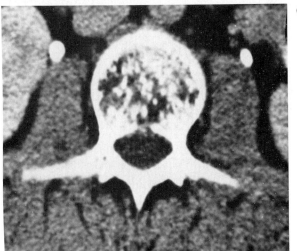

Fig. 8-3   Roentgenographic findings in 15-year-old boy treated 4 years previously for acute lymphocytic leukemia. **A,** Note pronounced osteoporosis in the vertebral bodies, with flattening of the vertebral body of L4, with lytic and sclerotic lesions scattered throughout the pelvis. **B,** CT scan shows large lytic lesions in the sacrum and ilium, illustrating the healing process. Disease is still in remission. **C,** CT scan of lumbar vertebral body reveals osteoporosis with rough trabeculae, which is similar to that in hemangioma.

Most patients with ALL have anemia, thrombocytopenia, and an elevated erthrocyte sedimentation rate. Approximately half have leukocyte counts of less than 3000/mm³. A low leukocyte count is the single most important factor for a favorable prognosis according to Miller and Ettinger. The diagnosis is confirmed by bone marrow aspiration. Skeletal survey and chest roentgenograms are necessary, and spinal tap may be required to determine central nervous system involvement. Technetium bone scanning does not correlate with painful areas or with the prognosis. Caudle et al reported negative findings in bone scans of patients with ALL, which they attributed to intramedullary packing of malignant cells or bone necrosis. When a "cold" bone scan is obtained, septic infarct of bone must be ruled out. A lytic lesion or periosteal elevation in the long bones may be seen on roentgenogram and must be differentiated from Ewing sarcoma, eosinophilic granuloma, infection, or metastasis from a neuroblastoma.

The treatment of ALL is medical. Survival rates in patients with ALL have greatly increased since better classification systems and treatment modalities have become available. Steroid-induced osteonecrosis is a frequent complication of treatment (Fig. 8-4). Prednisone, vincristine, and other chemotherapeutic agents are the treatment of choice. Vincristine, however, is neurotoxic and may cause peripheral nerve paralysis, most often of the peroneal nerve, which results in an equinovarus foot deformity. Most nerve

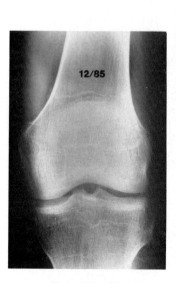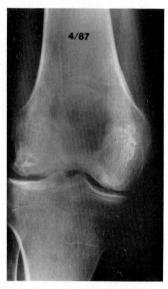

Fig. 8-4 Roentgenographic findings in 20-year-old man who had had acute lymphoblastic leukemia at the age of 14 years and who was originally treated with steroids and large doses of chemotherapy. Increasing knee pain developed and roentgenograms 14 months later revealed the development of osteonecrosis of the femoral condyles.

paralysis resolves spontaneously, but appropriate physical therapy and splinting are important to avoid a fixed deformity. Tendo achilles lengthening (p. 663) may be required for long-standing equinus deformity, and surgical treatment occasionally may be necessary for osteomyelitis or fractures in patients with ALL. Osteomyelitis may occur early or late in the course of the disease and can be difficult to detect in immunosuppressed children. Technetium and gallium scans are sometimes helpful in evaluating the area for aspiration. Gallium scan is especially helpful to evaluate soft tissue infection. Fractures are common in patients with ALL. Rogalsky et al reported that 12% of their patients had pathologic fractures, most commonly compression fractures of the spine; an additional 15% had fractures through apparently normal bone. All fractures healed uneventfully with conventional treatment.

SICKLE CELL DISEASE

Hereditary hematologic disorders are characterized by the presence of the abnormal hemoglobin S. The terms *sickle cell trait, sickle cell anemia,* and *sickle cell disease* have been used interchangeably, which has led to confusion. Sickle cell trait refers to the heterozygous genetic state for hemoglobin S in which both normal hemoglobin A and hemoglobin S are present. It is an essentially benign, asymptomatic, genetic characteristic. Sickle cell anemia refers to the homozygous state of hemoglobin S and is a chronic hemolytic anemia (sickle cell–hemoglobin S disease). Sickle cell disease refers to doubly heterozygous genetic conditions in which a variant gene for hemoglobin S is present along with another variant gene for either the production or structure of hemoglobin. Included in this group are sickle cell–hemoglobin C disease, sickle cell β-thalassemia disease, and sickle cell–hemoglobin D disease. Sickle cell disease states are chronic hemolytic anemias that may or may not be as severe clinically as sickle cell anemia.

The hemoglobin S gene is a mutant allele of hemoglobin A, which is found predominantly in the black race, although it may be found in other races, especially those of Mediterranean descent. Its incidence in nonblack persons in this country is approximately 0.80%. In Central Africa the sickle cell trait appears in approximately 20% of the population and sickle cell anemia in approximately 1% to 2%. The incidence of sickle cell disease and its variants is approximately 7.7% in the black population of the United States. Sickle cell anemia is one of the more common chronic illnesses of black children, occurring in approximately 1 in 500.

The basic changes in the skeletal system associated with sickle cell disease are thrombosis, marrow hyperplasia involving the long and short tubular bones and the axial skeleton, a tendency for spontaneous fracture, disturbance of bone growth, and osteomyelitis. The thrombosis is believed to be caused by the sickling phenomenon, chronic stasis, and infarction. The marrow hyperplasia is a response to the chronic hemolysis of red cells. Replacement of cancellous trabeculae by red marrow causes the widespread osteoporosis, accounting for the tendency to spontaneous fracture. Retardation of height and weight is not completely understood. The unique characteristics of osteomyelitis in sickle cell disease are discussed in a later section.

Roentgenographic changes are most apparent in the skull, vertebrae, and long bones. Common roentgenographic findings in the skull are a granular appearance of the bony texture, thickening of the calvarium, and widening of the diploic space. One third to one half of patients with sickle cell disease have roentgenographic changes in the skull, most often in the parietal and frontal regions. Vertebral changes are common; Caroll and Evans found changes in the trabecular pattern of the vertebral bodies in 70% of their 39 patients. The deformity in the vertebral column is diagnostic of sickle cell disease in that the center of the end plate is compressed ("step-deformity") whereas the periphery retains its normal flat contour, in contrast to the uniformly compressed appearance in such disorders as osteoporosis or multiple myeloma (Fig. 8-5). Vertebral changes usually occur when the child is older than 10 years of age. Changes in the long bones reflect the same pathologic processes active in the skull and vertebrae. Thinning of the cortex and widening of the medullary cavity may result from severe chronic local ischemia. Periosteal elevation occurs near the time of crisis and residual ossification after a crisis. Signs of marrow hyperplasia and thrombosis may be present, but those caused by infarction are more common: dense amorphous chalky zones and sclerosis. The combination of processes occasionally creates a "bone-within-a-bone" appearance (Fig. 8-6).

In mature patients, infarction is more common in long bones and occurs in 20% to 60% of patients with the hemoglobin C variant. The roentgenographic appearance varies with the size and location of the lesions and the frequency with which they occur. The vascular engorgement that results from this sickling and circulatory stagnation causes a rise in intramedullary pressure, resulting in the pain that commonly accompanies a crisis. Roentgenographic signs usually are not evident until 2 to 3 weeks after the onset of symptoms.

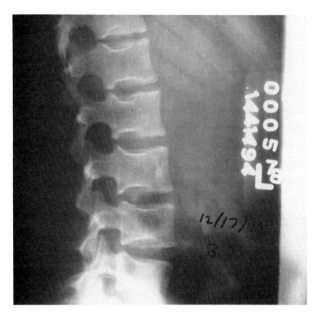

Fig. 8-5 Trabecular coarsening of vertebrae in sickle cell disease.

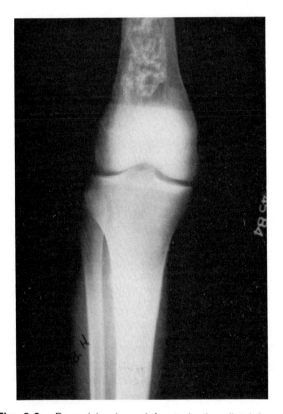

Fig. 8-6 Bone islands or infarcts in the distal femur and proximal tibia are located in the central portion of the medullary canal and do not affect the growth or articular regions. (Reprinted with permission from Crawford AH: Pediatric orthopaedic surgery, ed 2, Burbank, Calif, 1988, Science Image Communications.)

Avascular Necrosis

Bone infarction in older children and adults causes ischemia that tends to involve the epiphyses of the long bones. The femoral and humeral heads are the most common sites of involvement, which may range from homogenous increase in density to bizarre destruction and collapse. Sebes and Kraus reported that 28% of their 281 patients with sickle cell disease had avascular necrosis of the femoral head. The degree of anemia did not correlate with symptoms. Joint problems usually begin as synovitis, periostitis, or possibly a "bone crisis." Ultrasound examination will show evidence of joint effusion during the crisis. There is generally progressive destruction of the bony epiphysis with elevation of the periosteum of the metaphysis. The metaphysis survives the periostitis, but the effect on the bony epiphysis is more permanent, with occasional complete destruction (Fig. 8-7).

The most common pathologic change in the hip is avascular necrosis, which may result in severe arthritic changes and, rarely, osteochondritis dissecans and coxa vara. Spontaneous fractures also are rare. Avascular necrosis has been reported in patients with sickle cell thalassemia and hereditary persistence of fetal hemoglobin, but it is probably more common in those with hemoglobin C disease; it is rare in patients with hemoglobin S disease, possibly because of their shortened life expectancy. The lesions in sickle cell disease differ from those in Legg-Calvé-Perthes disease in that sickle cell arthropathy more commonly occurs late, just before physeal closure, and usually involves only a portion of the epiphyseal nucleus. Differentiation between Legg-Calvé-Perthes disease and hemoglobinopathic avascular necrosis is made on the basis of age, race, sex, and areas of involvement. Legg-Calvé-Perthes disease occurs in younger

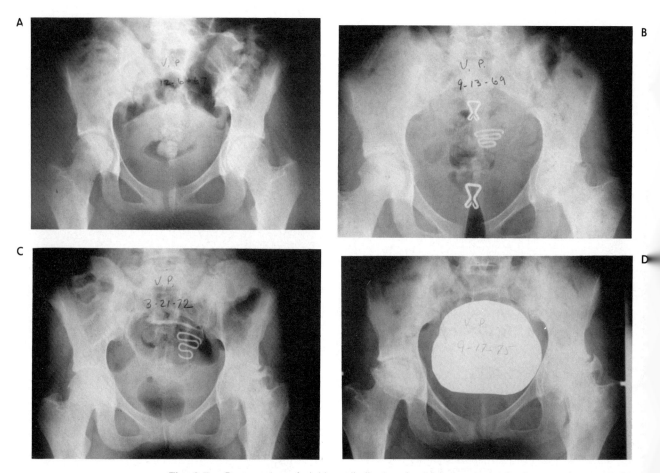

Fig. 8-7   Progression of sickle cell disease in adolescent who had avascular necrosis and progressive joint destruction of both hips during an 8-year period. **A,** At age 16, anteroposterior views of the pelvis with no evidence of disease. **B,** At age 19, evidence of early degenerative changes in the left hip and increased density in the femoral head on the right side. **C,** At age 22, severe destruction of the left hip with only increased density in the right hip. **D,** At age 25, severe destructive changes in the left hip and early destructive changes in the femoral head on the right side, as well as the acetabulum.

children, approximately 3 to 10 years of age, whereas hemoglobinopathic avascular necrosis occurs in children 10 years of age or older. Legg-Calvé-Perthes disease is ten times more common in white children than in black children and five times more common in boys; avascular necrosis from hemoglobinopathies has an equal sex distribution. Legg-Calvé-Perthes disease may involve the metaphysis, whereas involvement of the metaphysis almost never occurs in sickle cell disease.

Chung and Ralston categorized patients with sickle cell osteochondrosis into three groups according to roentgenographic and clinical criteria: group I, roentgenographic changes of total head infarction with involvement of the capital epiphysis similar to that in Legg-Calvé-Perthes disease; group II, localized involvement and infarction and the appearance of osteochondrosis or osteochondritis dissecans; and group III, hip deformities representing the late changes of femoral head infarction in older patients. This classification is somewhat oversimplified because characteristics of all three stages may exist simultaneously.

Although some authorities recommend total joint arthroplasty at a young age in these persons because of their decreased life expectancy, this course requires serious consideration. Infection, pulmonary problems, and sickle cell crises are potential complications of any surgical procedure in patients with sickle cell disease. Most can be prevented by presurgical transfusions to correct anemia, as well as by adequate hydration and the avoidance of hypoxia and acidosis during anesthesia.

Sickle Cell Dactylitis (Hand-Foot Syndrome)

Often the earliest manifestation of sickle cell disease in infancy is a painful, soft tissue swelling of the dorsum of the foot or hand, or both. This hand-foot syndrome, or sickle cell dactylitis, usually occurs during the first 2 years of life but may be seen in children up to 6 years of age. The clinical picture of hand-foot syndrome is that of a tourniquet placed around the proximal arm or leg to cause distal edema. Pseudoparalysis with pain usually is present, and the child is reluctant to use the extremity. Findings on initial roentgenograms are normal except for soft tissue swelling, but at about 10 to 14 days there usually is periosteal elevation or the appearance of subperiosteal new bone and lytic lesions around the diaphyseal cortex, which may be indistinguishable from osteomyelitis (Fig. 8-8). The tubular bones often acquire a rectangular appearance because of subperiosteal bone formation in the diaphysis. Bony resolution usually follows and is complete at 4 to 8 weeks. Hand-foot syndrome should be suspected in any child with a hemoglobin abnormality who has painful, symmetric hand and foot swelling. The condition is self-limiting and may be treated expectantly once osteomyelitis and bone crisis are ruled out.

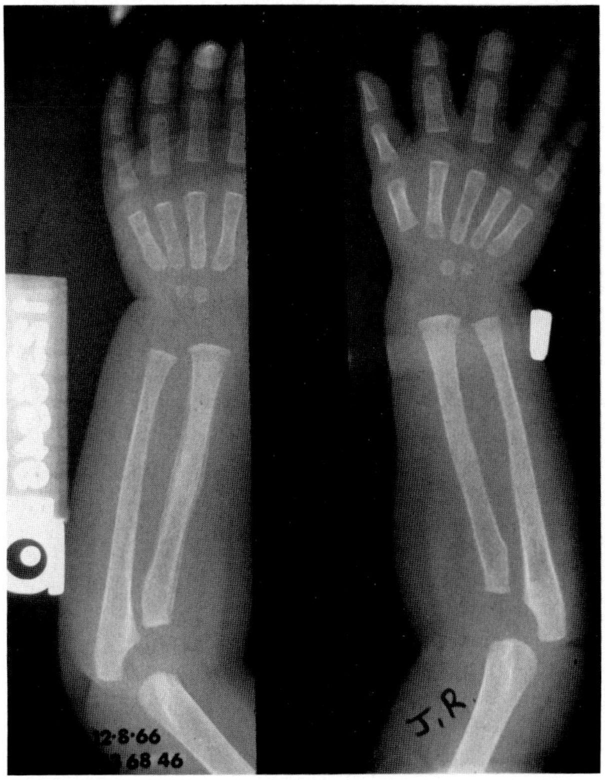

Fig. 8-8 Comparison views of the forearm in a patient with hand-foot syndrome demonstrate elevation of the periosteum along the midshaft of the radius of the left forearm.

Osteomyelitis

Osteomyelitis is a well-recognized complication of the sickle cell hemoglobinopathies, but it is difficult to distinguish clinically from a bone crisis. Both may involve multiple diaphyses of the long bones, and boys appear to be more susceptible to both. Both conditions cause fever and excruciating pain in a long bone, and both demonstrate positive findings on bone scans and elevated erythrocyte sedimentation rates. Differentiation is made by blood culture and/or bone aspiration. Patients with sickle cell disease are susceptible to the common infectious agents such as *Staphylococcus aureus, Haemophilus influenzae,* and *Escherichia coli* and are uniquely vulnerable to bone infection from the *Salmonella* group (Fig. 8-9).

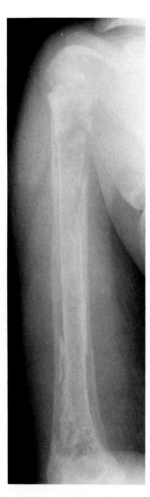

Fig. 8-9 *Salmonella* osteomyelitis of the entire humerus, with involucrum formation, in 14-year-old girl with sickle cell disease.

The roentgenographic findings of osteomyelitis in sickle cell hemoglobinopathies vary and often are indistinguishable from changes caused by infarcts and thrombosis: patchy radiolucency, subperiosteal new bone formation, and sclerosis. Engh et al described longitudinal intracortical fissuring of the diaphysis, with overabundant involucrum formation of multiple and often symmetric sites, as characteristic of osteomyelitis in sickle cell disease, especially when associated with persistent spiking of fever and leukocytosis.

Regardless of the causative organism, osteomyelitis produces changes that are nonspecific, and therapy often is instituted before bacteriologic confirmation, a policy much debated in the literature. Engh et al devised three treatment protocols for their patients with sickle cell disease in whom osteomyelitis or bone crisis was suspected:

1. Patients with low-grade fever and minimal bone tenderness believed to have a painful marrow crisis. For these patients, blood and stool cultures were obtained and antibiotics were given only if the cultures were positive.
2. Patients with symptoms similar to the first but with mild toxicity. These children were hospitalized, appropriate specimens for culture were obtained, and ampicillin therapy was initiated. Further treatment was modified by culture and sensitivity results.
3. Patients with obvious acute infection. For these patients, intravenous chloramphenicol therapy was begun before the results of culture and sensitivity were known.

Although the surgical management of these patients is controversial, the optimal treatment of any infection is open drainage (with decompression if necessary) and institution of antibiotic therapy on the basis of appropriate culture and sensitivity results. Multiple periosteal and marrow aspirations by large bore needles rather than by open drainage may be used for the initial bacteriologic diagnosis, but chronic infection with sequestrum formation requires an open procedure. After open drainage and removal of the sequestrum, immediate wound closure with closed suction perfusion irrigation rather than open drainage is recommended. The most common complication of open drainage in sickle cell patients is secondary contamination of the bone with *S. aureus.*

The use of tourniquets in patients with sickle cell disease has been questioned, but it has not been shown to increase the complication rate.

HEMOPHILIA

Hemophilia is a bleeding disorder caused by factor deficiencies in the clotting mechanism. In classic hemophilia or hemophilia A there is a deficiency of factor VIII; in hemophilia B, or Christmas disease, there is a deficiency of factor IX. The conditions are clinically indistinguishable and can be separated only by factor activity assay. The clinical severity of hemophilia varies considerably. The disease of patients with more than 30% factor VIII or IX levels may remain undiagnosed because excessive bleeding occurs only after major trauma or surgery. If all severities are included, hemophilia occurs in 1 in 10,000 of a known population. Hemophilia A accounts for 80% of hemophiliac disorders. Hemophilia has been shown to be inherited by a sex-linked recessive pattern. The gene is linked to the X chromosome and affects males almost exclusively. Members of the same family with hemophilia usually have similar severity of manifestations. Spontaneous mutations account for approximately 20% of cases.

The clinical manifestations of the hemophiliac disorders is abnormal bleeding. The severity of the bleeding correlates with the amount of factor deficiency. Patients with less than 1% of normal factor levels have severe hemophilia manifested by spontaneous joint and soft tissue bleeding. Patients with moderate hemophilia usually have factor levels between 1% and 5%, and pronounced bleeding follows minor trauma. Patients with factor levels over 30% usually lead normal lives but may experience excessive bleeding after surgery or major trauma.

The severe form of hemophilia may be obvious at birth because neither factor VIII nor factor IX can cross the placenta. Infants with the disease may have large cephalic hematomas, especially after difficult deliveries. If the mother is a known carrier, delivery by cesarean section should be strongly considered. Bleeding also may be seen from the umbilical cord or during circumcision. Bleeding episodes in the first year of life are rare until the patient becomes a toddler and begins to fall and bump into objects. Bleeding episodes then increase and probably correlate with the child's activity level. Because of more aggressive treatment, bleeding episodes generally decrease with age. With proper factor replacement therapy, the life expectancy of patients with hemophilia can approach normal.

Hemophilia can be diagnosed prenatally. If a pregnant woman is a known carrier and ultrasound or amniocentesis determines that the baby is a boy, a blood sample can be obtained from the fetus; however, this is not a risk-free procedure. If hemophilia is suspected, a blood sample should be obtained

from the umbilical cord just after delivery. In the older child recurrent bleeding episodes after falls, intramuscular bleeding after immunizations, gastrointestinal bleeding after aspirin ingestion, nose bleeds, tongue bleeds, or any abnormal soft tissue or joint bleeding should initiate complete hematologic evaluation. Basic hematologic screening should include evaluation of platelet levels, bleeding time, prothrombin time, and partial prothrombin time. Platelet levels are normal in the patient with hemophilia, but several cases of thrombocytopenia have been described in patients who are seropositive for HIV. Platelet function is abnormal in von Willebrand disease (factor X deficiency). The prothrombin time is sensitive to deficiencies of prothrombin, to factors V, VII, and X, and to fibrinogen, whereas the activated partial thromboplastin time screens all coagulation factors except factors VII and XIII. Prothrombin time and activated partial prothrombin time may differentiate between defects of the intrinsic and extrinsic pathways of coagulation, but both these screening tests allow only a preliminary diagnosis; factor levels must be established by specific assay techniques.

Detection of hemophilia carriers is important for genetic counseling, and hemophilia A usually can be recognized in 90% of carriers by determining the ratio between two of the factor VIII components. Carriers of hemophilia B are more difficult to detect because of the heterogeneity of factor IX.

Nonsurgical Treatment

A coordinated, multidisciplinary approach is necessary to obtain optimal benefits of treatment. The cornerstone of treatment is replacement therapy to supply a sufficient level of factor VIII or IX in the blood to allow hemostasis. Since the 1970s an intensive home care program has been established and the National Hemophiliac Foundation has produced a home treatment training module. This program involves earlier treatment, better prophylaxis, and less permanent joint disease. It also fosters independence in the patient and results in improved school attendance and performance and better psychosocial development. The patient and the family must be thoroughly taught to judge a bleeding situation and must be carefully educated about the treatment. Patients are encouraged to keep log sheets recording the frequency and dosage of treatment.

Concentrated preparations of factor VIII (cryoprecipitates) are prepared from fresh plasma, usually at the local blood banks from single units of donor plasma, or are commercially manufactured from a large pool of plasma from multiple donors. There is some risk of contracting both hepatitis and acquired immunodeficiency syndrome (AIDS), especially from commercial preparations.

Factor replacement therapy usually is necessary only when acute bleeding occurs. Generally for joint bleeding or major soft tissue bleeding, factor levels from 25% to 50% should be maintained for 5 to 10 days (25 units/kg). For surgery, bony procedures require 50 units/kg to maintain factors levels of 75% to 100% for the first 5 days, 50% to 75% for the second 5 days, and 25% to 50% for an additional 5 days. For soft tissue procedures each of these periods can usually be shortened by 2 days. During postoperative physical therapy, factor levels between 15% and 25% should be maintained. Kisker and Burke reported that steroids may decrease the amount of factor replacement needed and may decrease synovitis. They recommend a short course of treatment (1 week) with 1 to 2 mg/kg daily. In patients with hemophilia A in whom inhibitors against factor VIII develop (approximately 15% of patients) treatment consists of prothrombin complex concentrate (PCC) or activated prothrombin complex concentrate. Patients with hemophilia B are treated with factor IX from fresh frozen plasma or prothrombin complex concentrate. PCC entails a higher risk for thromboembolic complications, which seems to diminish with the addition of heparin. Production of factor VIII from cloned DNA is now undergoing clinical trials.

Hemophilia-related AIDS in the United States was first reported in 1981. In 1984 AIDS was found to be caused by the lymphadenopathy-associated virus (LAV)/human T-cell leukemia/lymphoma virus (HTLV) III, and antibodies against this virus have been found in most patients who receive clotting factor concentrations since the appearance of the disease. In 1984 Melbye et al reported the presence of AIDS antibodies in 17% of all patients with hemophilia from Scotland treated with locally produced factor concentrates and 57% of Danish patients with hemophilia treated with plasma products from the United States. In the United States, estimates of the number of patients with hemophilia who have antibodies against AIDS range from 30% to 90%. From 1981 to 1987, AIDS was diagnosed in approximately 400 patients with hemophilia, that is, about 1% of all patients with AIDS. Seropositivity has been found in 10% of the sexual partners of patients with hemophilia and AIDS. The infection probably is transmitted through commercially manufactured factor VIII, for which components are gathered from a large pool of donors. Since 1985 these products have been donor screened and heat treated, which should decrease the chances for infection.

All patients with severe hemophilia have some disuse muscle atrophy, and a continuing program of muscle strengthening exercise is mandatory. Isometric exercises, especially of the quadriceps muscles, are extremely helpful and may prevent atrophy of this muscle group, thus lessening the chance of knee injury. Isometric exercises usually are combined with some recreational therapy. Chambers found that swimming and gymnastics, after adequate warm-up, produce the fewest injuries. Greene and Wilson found decreased strength in the hamstrings, and they developed a home program without any special equipment for isokinetic strengthening of the knee.

Surgical Treatment
General Principles

Orthopaedic procedures in patients with hemophilia may be performed to decrease bleeding, such as synovectomy and removal of pseudotumors, or to improve function, such as total joint replacement, osteotomy, and arthrodesis. Surgery in patients with hemophilia is best done in institutions with a knowledgeable, multidisciplinary team that includes orthopaedists, hematologists, physical therapists, and social workers, as well as a reliable coagulation laboratory available at all times. As many procedures as possible should be performed at one time. Contraindications to surgery include inhibitors in the blood or acute hepatitis. Elective surgical procedures should be carefully considered in patients with hemophilia B because of the risk of thromboembolic complications with repeated doses of PCC.

Before surgery a hematologist should perform an evaluation of the patient, consisting especially of tests for the presence of inhibitors, liver function tests, HIV test, and blood type screening. A test dose of factor VIII is recommended 1 day before surgery to determine the half-life of the infused factor; this is a more sensitive method to detect low level in vivo inhibitors. If the patient's blood type is A, B, or AB, and long-term replacement therapy is planned, blood type–specific concentrates should be used to prevent hemolysis. Clotting factor should be given one-half hour before surgery with a bolus of 50 units/kg, and replacement treatment should continue every 12 hours to maintain the factor levels outlined in the preceding section.

During surgery a tourniquet should be used, and bleeding vessels should be cauterized or ligated. Before completion of the procedure, the tourniquet should be released and all bleeding vessels ligated. Meticulous closure with tight suture should be performed, and suction drains are recommended.

After surgery, pain medication should be administered intramuscularly or, preferably, orally. Analgesics that contain aspirin, antihistamines, or other medications known to inhibit platelet aggregation should not be used. Instead, proproxyphene (Darvon) or acetaminophen (Tylenol) is recommended. Factor replacement should be given at the time of removal of the drains and skin sutures. Postoperative complications include thromboembolic episodes and disseminated intravascular coagulation, which usually are caused by PCC treatment. Especially suspectible to thromboembolic complications are patients who are immobilized postoperatively or those with liver disease. Excessive bleeding after surgery may be caused by low factor levels, inhibitors, or other coagulopathy. Hemolytic anemia may occur in patients with A, B, or AB blood types because commercial factor concentrates use a high percentage of type O blood, resulting in significant titers of A and B isoagglutinins. This usually is evident 5 to 7 days after surgery and requires treatment with washed group O red cells or steroids until replacement therapy is discontinued.

Hepatitis always has been a risk for patients with hemophilia who frequently are exposed to blood products. Only about 80% of donors with hepatitis B antigen are detected with radioimmune assay, and patients with hemophilia who receive commercial factor concentrate have a high incidence of hepatitis. All patients with hemophilia scheduled for surgery should be screened for the presence of Australian antigen and, if present, special care must be taken in the operating room. Similarly, every precaution should be taken by the operating room personnel to avoid AIDS contamination from the patient.

Specific Procedures

Synovectomy. Synovectomy is the most common surgical procedure performed in patients with hemophilia. The rationale for removal of the synovium is both mechanical and biochemical. Mechanically, if a large amount of the boggy, proliferative synovium is removed, the joint is less vulnerable to bleeding from minor trauma. Biochemically, hemophiliac synovial tissue was shown by Storti et al to be highly fibrinolytic and by Arnold and Hilgartner to contain proteolytic enzymes destructive to cartilage. In 1969 Storti et al first reported the effectiveness of synovectomy in 16 patients, none of whom had recurrent bleeding 1 to 2 years after surgery. Since that time others have reported mostly favorable results with synovectomy. Dyszy-Laube et al, Post et al, and Canale et al, among others, reported decreased episodes of bleeding after synovectomy in patients with hemophilia, although the process of joint destruction did not seem to be altered. Postoperative complications, including hematoma, hemolytic anemia, and intraarticular adhesions, have been reported by several authors, as has

loss of joint motion after synovectomy. The effectiveness of the continuous passive motion machine for maintaining or improving joint motion after surgery has not been firmly established, although Greene and Canale et al reported improved motion in their patients who used the machine.

Indications for synovectomy are recurrent bleeding in a joint for more than 6 months and persistent synovial hypertrophy. Synovectomy is most beneficial for patients with Arnold and Hilgartner roentgenographic stage I involvement (p. 405). Patients with more advanced disease already have significant joint destruction that cannot be reversed by synovectomy (Fig. 8-10).

Synovectomy usually is performed surgically, although medical synovectomy by means of osmic acid or radioactive gold has been described. Gamba et al found chemical synovectomy less effective than surgical synovectomy. Osmic acid also may have a toxic effect on the articular surface, and radioactive gold may spread the isotope through the treated joint. Sledge et al reported the use of dysprosium-165-ferric hydroxide macroaggregates for synvectomy in patients with rheumatoid arthritis, but this technique has not been reported in patients with hemophilia.

Synovectomy of the knee

The knee is a frequent site of bleeding, which may result in significant disability if allowed to continue. Synovectomy of the knee is effective in preventing or reducing recurrent bleeding and in relieving pain, but significant decreases in motion after synovectomy have been reported in recent series. Although early synovectomy is recommended, before irreversible joint destruction occurs, the child should be old enough to cooperate in postoperative rehabilitation.

TECHNIQUE. Apply and inflate the tourniquet. Make a parapatellar incision, and then incise the capsule from the superior proximal portion of the incision to the meniscus. Inspect the joint. Protect the meniscus, and further expose the distal portion of the joint. Continue further dissection proximal and distal, dislocating and everting the patella. In a systematic fashion, excise as much synovium as possible from each of the four quadrants (superomedial, inferomedial, superolateral, and inferolateral). Remove all synovium from the lateral gutter and then the medial joint space, including over and around the medial meniscus and collateral ligaments. Then remove the synovium from the intercondylar notch, the anterior cruciate ligament, and the lateral joint space. Do not excise the meniscus or anterior cruciate ligament. Remove any pannus formation on the articular surfaces of the femoral condyles and patella and any loose pieces of cartilage. Release the tourniquet, and obtain

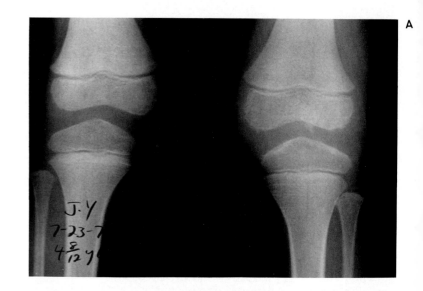

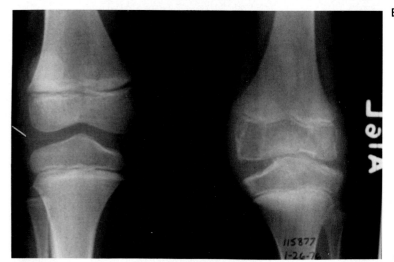

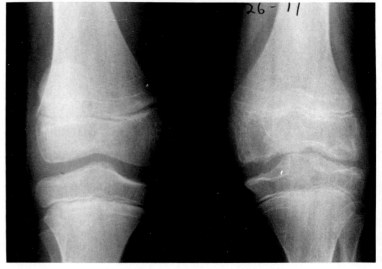

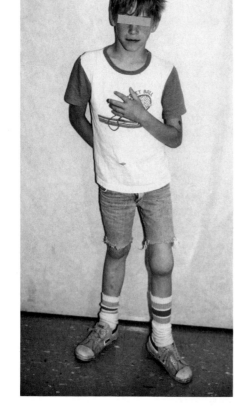

Fig. 8-10 Progressive destructive changes in knee of child with hemophilia. **A,** Significant soft tissue swelling of left knee at 4 years of age. **B,** Progressive destruction of left knee joint 3 years later. **C,** Widening of intercondylar notch of distal femur, as well as destructive lesions of articular surface of both femur and tibia. **D,** Clinical photograph shows significant chronic effusion and flexion contracture of the left knee.

meticulous hemostasis with ligation or electrocautery, which may require more time than the synovectomy itself. Allow 5 minutes of compression packing of the incision, and then secure hemostasis in each of the four quadrants; the superolateral quadrant and the lateral gutter are the most tedious and time-consuming. Close the capsule and soft tissues tightly in layers to obliterate any dead space, and insert a closed suction drain. If the medial capsule is redundant after synovectomy, oversew the capsule medially to prevent dislocation of the patella. Apply a bulky compressive dressing with the knee in as much extension as possible.

Montane et al apply a powdered gelfoam mixed with thrombin to all denuded areas before the tourniquet is released and then compress the joint for 5 minutes. The wound is then inspected, the bleeding vessels are cauterized, and the joint is irrigated to remove the gelfoam.

POSTOPERATIVE MANAGEMENT. The knee is immobilized for 24 hours, and then motion is begun with the aid of a physical therapist, supplemented by the continuous motion machine. Drains are removed 48 hours after surgery with adequate factor replacement. Full weight bearing is not allowed for 4 weeks. Factor levels are maintained as outlined on p. 396. If adhesions develop and motion is significantly decreased, the joint may be manipulated closed or open 3 weeks after synovectomy, but the possibility of iatrogenic fracture of the osteoporotic bone or fracture through the physis in the patient with hemophilia should be considered (Fig. 8-11).

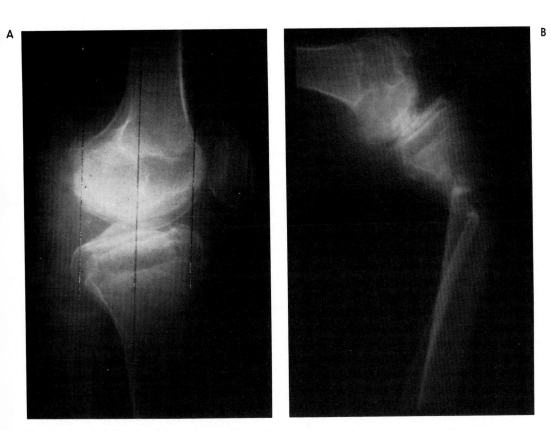

Fig. 8-11 **A,** Stiff knee joint in hemophilic patient 4 weeks after synovectomy. **B,** Fracture of proximal tibia produced by attempted closed manipulation.

Synovectomy of the elbow

In general, synovectomy of the elbow yields more consistently good results than does synovectomy of the knee. Kay et al reported a lower complication rate, a shorter hospital stay, and less loss of motion after elbow synovectomy than after knee synovectomy. In 23 elbow synovectomies in young patients with hemophilia LeBalc'h et al found increased motion and no roentgenographic evidence of deterioration in most patients and recurrent episodes of bleeding in only four patients.

TECHNIQUE. Apply and inflate the tourniquet. Make a lateral incision between the anconeus muscle and the extensor carpi radialis brevis. Develop the cleavage between the capsule and synovium, and remove as much synovium as possible. Do not remove the radial head unless it is destroyed and the patient is skeletally mature; it never should be removed in a skeletally immature patient. Perform any necessary cartilage debridement and lysis of adhesions. Apply gelfoam embedded in thrombin to all rough surfaces, compress the joint, and release the tourniquet. After 5 minutes of compression, obtain meticulous hemostasis with ligation or electrocautery and irrigate the joint to remove the gelfoam. Place a suction drain in the wound, close the capsule and skin, and apply a large compression dressing with a plaster splint holding the elbow in 90 degrees of flexion and neutral pronation and supination.

POSTOPERATIVE MANAGEMENT. The drains are removed 2 to 3 days after surgery with adequate factor replacement, and gentle range of motion exercises are begun 3 to 5 days after surgery. A commercial passive motion splint (Dynasplint) also may be used to decrease elbow flexion contracture.

Arthroscopic synovectomy

In recent years, arthroscopic synovectomy has become an attractive alternative to an open procedure. Arthroscopic synovectomy has several advantages: (1) a more complete synovectomy can be performed, which should reduce the chance of recurrent bleeding; (2) it is less traumatic to soft tissues, which should ensure an easier postoperative rehabilitation; and (3) a better range of motion may be obtained after surgery, especially if a constant passive motion machine is used. Several recent reports, including those by Wiedel, Limbird and Dennis, and Klein et al, have indicated good results and few complications with arthroscopic synovectomy. Disadvantages to arthroscopic synovectomy include longer operative time, the possibility of incomplete synovectomy, and the lack of hemostasis.

TECHNIQUE (ARTHROSCOPIC SYNOVECTOMY OF THE KNEE). Apply and inflate the tourniquet. Perform the synovectomy through the anteromedial and anterolateral portals (p. 818), placing the inflow supralaterally. First inspect the joint in the routine manner. This may be difficult because of the synovial hypertrophy, and complete inspection of the menisci, ligaments, and articular cartilage may be possible only after synovectomy. Remove the synovium with a high-speed synovial shaver beginning at the suprapatellar pouch, going from the medial gutter to the anterior portion of the knee. Change portals with the arthroscope and the shaver, and remove the synovium from the lateral side of the knee. Change portals with the scope and the shaver as many times as is necessary to remove as much synovium as possible. Perform partial meniscectomy, chondroplasty, and lysis of adhesions if necessary. Insert a suction drain, close the skin incisions, and apply a large bulky dressing with slight compression (Fig. 8-12, *A* to *E*).

POSTOPERATIVE MANAGEMENT. The drain is removed 48 hours after surgery. Straight leg-raising exercises are begun immediately. Limbird and Dennis and others recommend using the continuous passive motion machine in the recovery room with a range of flexion from 10 to 60 degrees; this is increased daily until a range from 0 to 100 degrees of flexion is obtained. Active range of motion exercises are begun 6 to 8 days after surgery. Adequate factor replacement therapy should be instituted for each stage of the surgery and rehabilitation (p. 396).

Osteotomy. Osteotomy may be necessary to correct joint deformities if more conservative measures have failed. Knee flexion contracture is common in patients with hemophilia and may become severe enough to interfere with ambulation. If conservative treatment with physical therapy, traction, and Quengel or drop-out casting (p. 407) has failed, supracondylar femoral extension osteotomy may be indicated. Arnold and Hilgartner recommend extension osteotomy for resistant knee contractures of more than 25 degrees if knee range of motion is 80 degrees or more. The anterior closing wedge osteotomy is performed in the supracondylar area proximal to the distal femoral physis and is held with crossed pins, staples, or an external fixator. If the physis is closed, angled plate fixation may be used. If the contracture is severe, a two-stage procedure may be required: posterior capsulotomy and hamstring lengthening followed by traction and then extension osteotomy. If extension osteotomy is performed for severe contracture without prior stretching of the soft tissues, the femur must be shortened significantly to avoid neurovascular compromise.

Varus or valgus deformity of the tibia may occur in young adults with unicompartmental hemophiliac arthropathy, but this is rare. In patients with closed

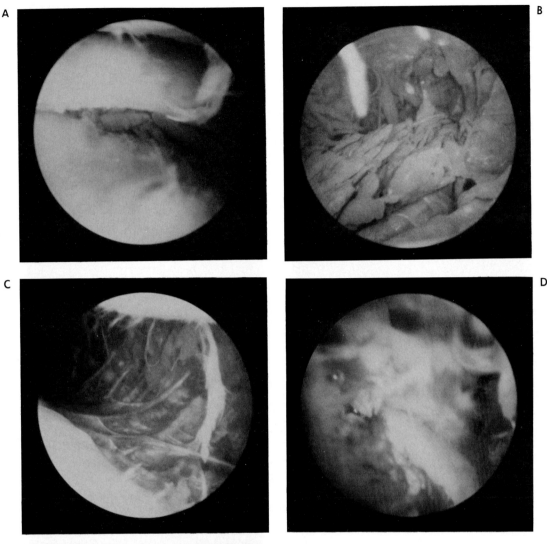

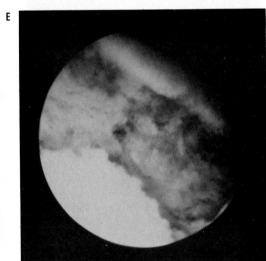

Fig. 8-12 Arthroscopic views of knee in patient with hemophilia. **A,** Pigmented hypertrophied synovium extruding from beneath posterior aspect of lateral meniscus. Articular cartilage shows moderate surface degenerative changes. **B,** Suprapatellar pouch of knee demonstrating hemophilic synovium with marked villonodular hypertrophy and hemosiderin pigmentation. **C,** Lateral recess of knee showing mild to moderate synovial hypertrophy with extensive hemosiderin pigmentation. Articular cartilage shows mild fibrillation. **D,** Extensive synovial hypertrophy and invasion of articular cartilage surface. **E,** After synovectomy and debridement a large erosion of the articular surface becomes visible. (**B** to **E,** Courtesy Jerome Wiedel, MD, Denver.)

physes, a high tibial osteotomy (p. 44) may correct the deformity. Smith et al (1981) reported good results in six knees treated with osteotomy for painful varus deformity. Their patients ranged in age from 19 to 32 years, and all had stage IV or V arthropathy. After osteotomy, all maintained their preoperative range of motion, and all had a dramatic decrease in bleeding episodes.

Joint replacement. Total joint replacement may be beneficial for adolescents or young adults with hemophilia who have incapacitating pain and severe joint destruction. The knee is the most commonly replaced joint, with hip and elbow replacement performed less frequently. Preoperative evaluation should determine that pain is caused by degenerative changes in the joint and not by recurrent bleeding. If replacement therapy (2 to 3 times a week), physical therapy, and a short course of steroid therapy are not effective, pain probably is caused by joint deterioration. Contraindications for joint replacement include an ankylosed joint, recent sepsis, narcotic dependency, and a high level of inhibitors in the blood. Appropriate factor levels should be obtained and maintained preoperatively and postoperatively (p. 396). Techniques for joint replacement in patients with hemophilia are essentially the same as for other joint disorders but should be combined with synovectomy to decrease postoperative bleeding. All general surgi-

cal principles applicable to patients with hemophilia should be followed.

Most authors report good results in pain relief and improvement of joint motion after total knee replacement, but complications are more frequent in patients with hemophilia than in those with osteoarthritis or rheumatoid arthritis. Wilson et al, Goldberg et al, Lachiewicz et al, Small et al, and McCollough et al reported complications of postoperative bleeding, peroneal and posterior tibial nerve palsies, superficial skin necrosis, subcutaneous hematoma, hemolytic anemia, and deep infection after total knee replacement in hemophiliac patients. Hip arthroplasty is performed much less frequently than knee arthroplasty and there are few reports in the literature; however, Wilson et al, Hoskinson and Duthie, and Hilgartner (1979) all report satisfactory results. Interposition arthroplasty of the elbow with the use of silicone was reported by Smith et al to be successful in six patients.

Arthrodesis. Arthrodesis may be required as a salvage procedure in the skeletally mature patient after failed total joint replacement, or it may be used as the primary procedure for a severely deteriorated ankle joint because joint replacement in this area has not been particularly successful. Houghton and Dickson reported 16 arthrodeses in patients with hemophilia; they used screws for fixation and discouraged pin fixation or Charnley compression arthrodesis because of the possibility of bleeding from the fixation pin. Patel et al, however, reported use of the Charnley compression apparatus for knee arthrodesis without complications, and Wilson et al used external pin fixation with good results.

Specific Problems

Soft tissue bleeding. Soft tissue bleeding may begin spontaneously or after trauma and usually is less painful than joint bleeding. Muscle bleeding most often occurs in the iliac muscle, the anterior thigh, the calf, the forearm, or the shoulder. The bleeding is usually visible, and the extremity is swollen and tender with some limitation of range of motion in the adjacent joints.

Iliopsoas bleeding

Bleeding in the iliopsoas muscle is common. Swelling usually is less pronounced than in other extremities, although occasionally a painful swelling can be felt in the iliac fossa or under the inguinal ligament. The extremity is held in flexion, and external rotation and forced extension cause pain, unlike joint bleeding. Femoral nerve palsy often is associated with iliopsoas bleeding, most commonly in patients between the ages of 15 and 20 years. Goodfellow et

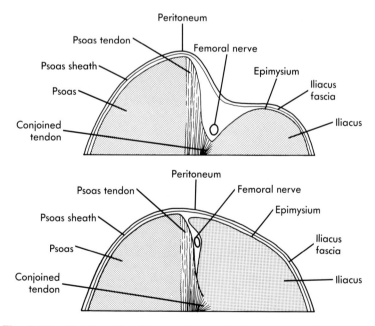

Fig. 8-13 Relationship of femoral nerve to iliopsoas tendon under normal circumstances *(top)* and after hemorrhage into iliac muscle *(bottom)*. (From Wells J and Templeton J: Clin Orthop 124:158, 1977.)

al, Nobel et al, and Wells and Templeton described the anatomic basis for femoral nerve entrapment in hematoma of the iliac muscle. Both the iliac and psoas muscles are covered separately with heavy muscle sheaths, with the femoral nerve lying in the gutter between the two muscles (Fig. 8-13). Increased pressure, such as bleeding, in the psoas muscle usually does not increase the pressure on the femoral nerve because this muscle is easily distensible in its upper part, but increased pressure in the iliac muscle creates a tense swelling that may compress the femoral nerve against the psoas tendon. The lateral cutaneous nerve and the genitofemoral nerve lie outside the fascia and are not compressed. Femoral nerve palsy can be difficult to diagnose, especially if the patient has contractures of the knee joint, but the usual symptoms are paralysis of the quadriceps mechanism and decreased sensation over the anterior and medial parts of the thigh and the medial side of the leg distally to the medial malleolus. The patellar tendon reflex is absent. The diagnosis can be made by a thorough physical examination and plain roentgenograms, which show a blurred psoas shadow. CT scanning and ultrasound are valuable to evaluate the size and subsequent resorption of the hematoma (Figs. 8-14 and 8-15).

Hematoma in the iliopsoas muscle is treated with analgesics and bed rest, followed by physical therapy to decrease hip flexion contracture. Gentle skin traction may be used for persistent hip flexion contracture. Any femoral nerve compromise usually resolves as the hematoma recedes, but this may be a lengthy process and bracing of the knee occasionally is required to maintain stability. Active assisted exercises for the quadriceps are instituted as early as possible.

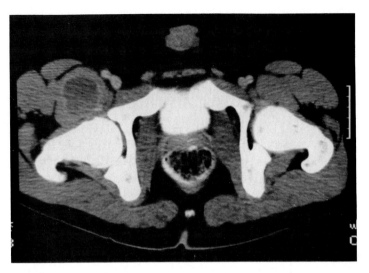

Fig. 8-14 Iliac hematoma in patient with hemophilia. Note hematoma in front of hip joint on left side.

Fig. 8-15 **A,** Ultrasound view of iliac hematoma, which is well defined in front of hip joint (lower portion of figure). **B,** Size of hematoma can be followed by ultrasound, and decrease in size can be appreciated.

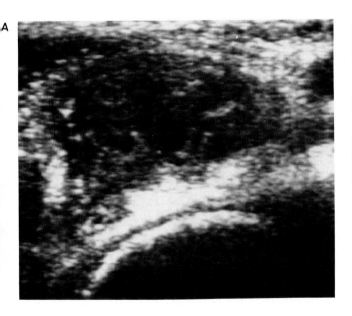

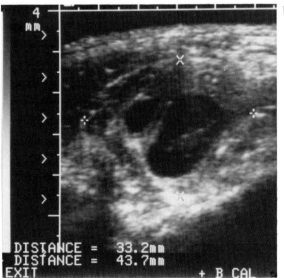

Gastrocsoleus bleeding

Hematoma in the gastrocsoleus muscle complex is a common cause of equinus deformity. A compartment syndrome may develop, especially in the anterior and deep posterior tibial compartments, and peroneal or tibial nerve involvement should be carefully evaluated.

In the acute stage bleeding in the calf area is treated with appropriate factor replacement therapy and a posterior splint with the ankle in maximum dorsiflexion. Range of motion exercises for the ankle are begun when soreness subsides. Equinus deformity may be treated with serial casting as recommended by Greene and Wilson.

Forearm bleeding

Bleeding in the volar aspect of the forearm results in a firm, tender mass palpable in the forearm with flexion of the wrists and fingers. Because of the limited capacity of the anterior forearm compartment, bleeding easily can give rise to a Volkmann's contracture and nerve compression should be carefully evaluated. The medial and ulnar nerves are the most frequently involved. Although nerve compression in the extremities usually is caused by direct pressure from a hematoma, it also may be caused by compression from joint bleeding, such as on the ulnar nerve from elbow bleeding. Rarely does bleeding in the neural sheath cause nerve compression. In a large series of 234 patients with hemophilia, Ehrmann et al found a 10.8% incidence of peripheral nerve compression; approximately one third of the involved nerves were femoral nerves. The prognosis is favorable with prompt treatment.

With any forearm hematoma, the possibility of a compartment syndrome must be considered. If compartment syndrome is suspected, intracompartmental pressures should be measured (after adequate factor replacement therapy) and, if indicated, fasciotomy should be performed. Mintzer et al reported that when fasciotomy was performed in less than 24 hours from onset of symptoms, recovery was complete, but when surgery was delayed, significant residual disability resulted. In the patient with hemophilia, however, fasciotomy is not a minor procedure because of the possibility of secondary bleeding and infection; adequate factor levels also must be maintained for later secondary closure or skin grafting. If there is only mild bleeding without signs of increased compartmental pressures, the treatment is factor replacement therapy, compression dressing, and immobilization, followed by physical therapy and possibly splinting.

Hemophiliac pseudotumors

A cyst may develop in an extremity when bleeding forms a pseudocapsule. The cyst may be subperiosteal or intraosseous, as well as in the soft tissues, and may compress adjacent structures. Subperiosteal or intraosseous cysts may erode into the bone, creating a so-called pseudotumor whose roentgenographic appearance may resemble a malignant tumor with areas of bone destruction and new bone formation and calcification or ossification of the surrounding tissue. Gilbert described two forms of pseudotumors; one affects the ilium and the femur and usually is seen in adults, and the other involves the more distal bones, is usually seen in children, and tends to indicate a better prognosis. With early, aggressive treatment of hemophilia the incidence of pseudotumors has decreased in recent years.

Pseudotumors in the distal extremities should be followed closely, both clinically and roentgenographically. If recurrent bleeding in the cyst is suspected, factor replacement therapy should be instituted and the limb should be immobilized until repeated evaluation confirms resolution of the cyst. Aspiration of the cyst should not be performed because of the possibility of fistula development followed by infection as described by Ahlberg. Pseudocysts in the pelvis and femur also should be observed closely for progression, spontaneous fracture, or impingement on vital structures, any of which may indicate the need for resection and bone grafting. If infection is present, amputation should be considered. Several authors have reported promising results with irradiation of pseudocysts, but the efficacy of this treatment modality has not been established.

Joint bleeding. Joint bleeding is most common in the knee, elbow, and ankle joints. Bleeding in the shoulder and hip joints is rare because these joints are protected in their muscular envelopes and have fewer synovial recesses. Joint bleeding rarely occurs in the first few years of life, but it is frequent when the child is older than 5 years of age, and most patients with severe hemophilia past their fifth year have obvious roentgenographic changes. The number and severity of bleeding episodes in a joint seem to correlate with the amount of joint destruction.

The mechanism by which joint bleeding causes joint destruction is not fully understood, but hemosiderin from the erythrocytes is known to have a toxic effect on cells, and the leukocyte fraction of autologous blood has been shown to provoke a severe inflammatory response in the synovium similar to rheumatoid arthritis. Bleeding usually starts in the synovium, triggering proliferation of the synovial cells and increased vascularity. Hemosiderin is deposited in the lining cells and subsynovial tissue, and a mild inflammatory response occurs (Fig. 8-16). If bleeding does not recur, the synovium returns to normal within 10 to 14 days. Repeated hemorrhages, however, produce changes that are irreversible. In the synovium, hemosiderin causes hypertrophy of the lining cells, which form two or three cell layers, and results in the characteristic villi and the deep chocolate-brown color of the synovium. In the deeper layers inflammatory infiltrates around the hemosiderin deposits, along with the hypervascularity, further increase the chance for recurrent bleeding. As the disease process continues, more and more fibrous tissue invades the synovium and replaces the lining cells, leading to pannus formation on the articular cartilage. Changes in synovial fluid composition deplete the articular cartilage nourishment, and proteolytic enzyme activity also may degrade the cartilage. As the quality of the articular cartilage diminishes, clefts form and further decrease the strength. Subchondral cysts frequently further weaken the articular cartilage and make it more susceptible to trauma. The articular cartilage becomes progressively thinner until it is destroyed, exposing the sclerotic and eburnated bone. The loss of articular surface and increasing fibrosynovium cause joint contractures that progress to typical hemophilic arthropathy (Figs. 8-17 and 8-18).

Roentgenographic changes in the joints correspond to the amount of joint deterioration. Loss of cartilage and narrowing of the joint space are the most important factors that affect range of motion. Arnold and Hilgartner divided the roentgenographic changes into the following five stages:

Stage I—only soft tissue swelling without other roentgenographic changes

Stage II—osteoporosis and overgrowth of the epiphysis (The overgrowth is believed to be caused by hypervascularity in the adjacent joint and usually is manifested as an increase in the size of the patella and medial femoral condyle in the knee or of the radius in the elbow. Overgrowth on one side of the joint can cause angular deformities.)

Stage III—subchondral cysts with typical widening and deepening of the intercondylar notch in the knee joint

Stage IV—cartilage destruction with joint space narrowing

Stage V—loss of joint space with fibrous joint contractures and complete disorganization of the joint

Pettersson et al developed a classification system in which each roentgenographic factor is assigned a numerical value and the values are totaled for each joint. This system may allow better correlation between clinical and roentgenographic evaluations.

The primary goals of treatment of hemarthrosis are arrest of the hemorrhage in the joint and restoration of function. Several treatment protocols have been developed, including those by Greene and Wilson, Arnold and Hilgartner, and Niemann. Their recommendations may be summarized as follows. Mild to moderate bleeding can be treated by the patient at home with replacement treatment to achieve between 25% and 50% normal factor levels for 48 hours. Mild analgesics are used for pain. For joint

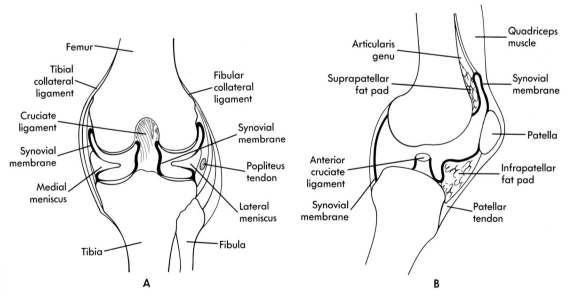

Fig. 8-16 **A,** Location of synovium *(heavy line)* in knee joint in anteroposterior projection. **B,** Lateral projection. (From Wilde AH: Orthop Clin North Am 2:191, 1971.)

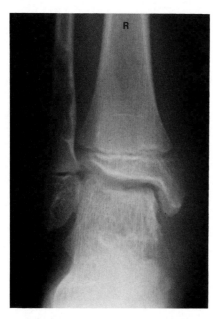

Fig. 8-17 Stage IV ankle arthropathy as result of hemophilia. Ankle joint has congruent incongruency. Scalloping defect can be seen in diaphyseal area of fibula as in pseudotumor.

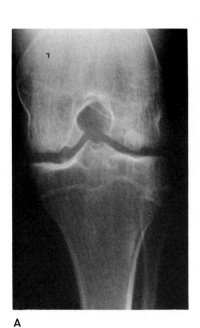
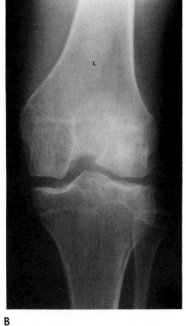

A   B

Fig. 8-18 Knee of adolescent patient with hemophilia. **A,** Subchondral erosions and flattening of both condyles and erosion in intercondylar notch. **B,** Complete flattening on the medial side of joint. Congruent incongruency is caused by long-standing disease.

bleeding that involves weight-bearing joints, the patient is encouraged to use crutches until pain subsides and 90 degrees of knee motion and full ankle dorsiflexion have been achieved. For major joint bleeding, replacement treatment is given for 48 hours and may be repeated at 48 and 96 hours. A compression dressing with plaster splint or a short period of casting (24 to 48 hours) also is recommended. Aspiration of the joint is done only for a very tense, acutely painful joint after replacement treatment has begun, but it always should be considered in the hip to avoid avascular necrosis or subluxation caused by increased pressure in the joint.

Once bleeding has occurred in a joint, the increased vascularity of the synovium makes it highly susceptible to repeated bleeding. Repeated bleeding 1 to 2 days after the primary episode is common and should be observed carefully. With repeated episodes of bleeding permanent changes in the joint result in subacute hemarthropathy characterized by a thickened synovium, a moderate decrease in range of motion, and muscle atrophy. Greene and Wilson defined subacute hemarthropathy as three bleeding episodes in the same joint within 6 weeks or persistent hypertrophy of the synovium 6 weeks after the previous episode. If there is no articular cartilage narrowing, the patient is treated with factor replacement and 3 weeks of cast immobilization. After cast removal, factor replacement is given three times a week for 3 weeks and then twice a week for an additional 3 weeks. A vigorous muscle strengthening program is begun. If episodes of bleeding or synovitis persist after cast removal, non–weight bearing is begun and prophylactic factor replacement is given to minimize the risk of recurrent bleeding. Prednisone is also given for 1 week. The joint is protected in a knee-ankle-foot orthosis, and strengthening exercises of appropriate muscle groups are continued. If hemarthrosis or synovitis persists after 4 to 6 months, synovectomy is considered.

Joint contractures. If joint destruction continues, the ultimate outcome is painful deformity. Treatment at this stage consists of continuing physical therapy, protective splinting to avoid further injury of the involved joint, and mild analgesics for pain. Upper extremity joint contractures are common in chronic hemarthropathy but usually cause little disability and rarely require treatment. Hip joint contractures usually are caused by iliopsoas bleeding and only rarely by hemarthropathy. Equinus deformity of the ankle may be caused by bleeding in the gastrocsoleus muscle complex. Initial treatment should include ice applications and range of motion exercises. Tendo achilles lengthening is indicated for persistent deformity or, if surgery is contraindicated, special shoes with built-up heel supports can be used. Knee flexion contractures are the most common contractures and usually are combined with external rotation of the tibia. Aggressive treatment is necessary to prevent compromise of ambulation. Physical therapy, protective splinting, and possibly short periods of steroid treatment to decrease synovitis may be used. The tibia is often posteriorly subluxed on the femur, and cast wedging may increase the subluxation.

Several conservative methods have been developed for treating knee flexion contractures in patients with hemophilia; regardless of the method chosen, factor replacement therapy should be instituted during any orthopaedic treatment.

The Quengel cast (Fig. 8-19) was originally described by Jordan and later modified by McDaniel. It has been used for severe knee flexion contractures up to 60 degrees. A below-the-knee cast is applied with a cast cuff around the thigh and a Quengel hinge incorporated in the cast. Thick padding is applied under the cast over bony pressure points. A ring nut on the hinge is turned one to four times a day to gradually extend the knee, usually to 20 to 30 degrees of flexion. Corrective cast wedging can then be applied, followed by a knee brace with a polycentric joint. Greene and Wilson reported good results with this technique except in patients with diminished articular cartilage.

The use of a drop-out cast (Fig. 8-20) also has been reported to be effective in treating knee contractures in patients with hemophilia. The cast is applied with the knee flexed and then is cut out dorsally to allow active extension but no further flexion. When sufficient extension has been gained, a new drop-out cast is applied to allow maximum extension of the knee.

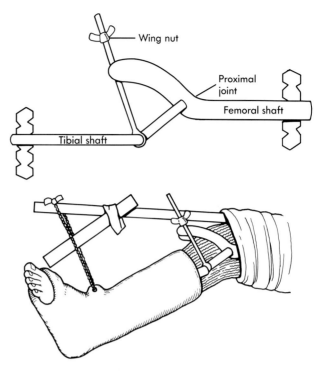

Fig. 8-19 Nonsurgical management of hemophilic arthropathy and muscle hemorrhage with Quengel antisubluxation hinge and cast. (Redrawn from Greene WB and Wilson FC: Instructional Course Lectures, vol 32, St Louis, 1983, The CV Mosby Co.)

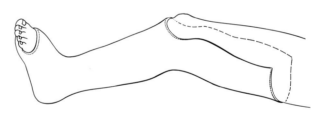

Fig. 8-20 Drop-out cast prevents flexion but allows extension.

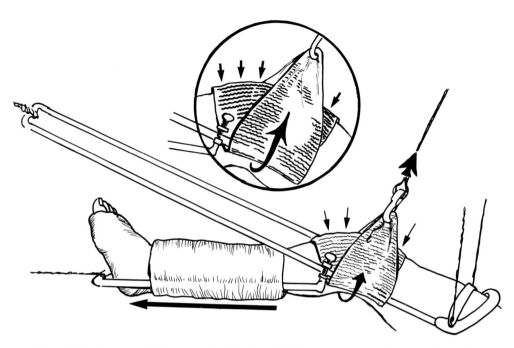

Fig. 8-21   Reversed dynamic sling for knee flexion contracture. (Redrawn from Stein H and Dickson RA: J Bone Joint Surg 57A:282, 1975.)

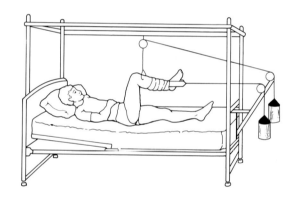

Fig. 8-22   90/90–degree traction for a knee contracture with subluxation. (Redrawn from Bianco AJ Jr and Peterson HA: Orthop Clin North Am 2:745, 1971.)

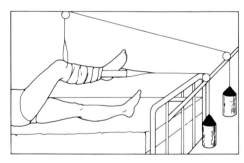

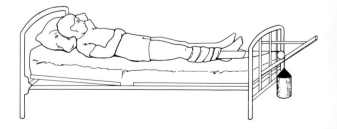

Stein and Dickson recommend traction with a half ring and Thomas splints with a Pearson knee attachment (Fig. 8-21). Leaving the distal part of the thigh free, a well-padded canvas sling is applied at the supracondylar level, threaded underneath the middle part of the splint on either side, and then connected to traction through a pulley. Longitudinal traction of 2 to 3 kilos is applied. Stein and Dickson reported better and more rapid response with this method than with cast wedging.

Nelson et al have recently described the use of a flowtron garment air-bag with intermittent compression for knee flexion contractures. Their early results are encouraging.

Bianco and Peterson use a 90/90–degree traction (Fig. 8-22) for knee flexion contractures in patients with juvenile rheumatoid arthritis, and this can be applied to some patients with hemophilia. Under adequate factor control, a skeletal pin is inserted in the proximal tibia, carefully avoiding the tibial tubercle. Traction is begun at 90 degrees of hip flexion and 90 degrees of knee flexion and, as the tibia is brought anteriorly and the subluxation reduced, the hip and knee gradually are extended until the contracture is corrected. During traction treatment the hips and knees are exercised daily to preserve the existing range of motion.

Septic arthritis. Septic arthritis is rare in patients with hemophilia, possibly because of the increased blood flow in the joint from chronic inflammation. Differentiation of septic arthritis from acute bleeding in the joint is difficult, but septic arthritis should be suspected if the patient has fever or does not respond to factor replacement therapy. Several treatment protocols have been proposed, including open irrigation followed by suction catheter irrigation, aspiration and body casting, and daily joint aspirations with appropriate antibiotics. Aggressive treatment is indicated in involved hip, knee, and ankle joints and should include open drainage followed by cast immobilization.

Fractures. Osteoporosis, limited joint motion, and muscle atrophy all predispose the patient with hemophilia to fractures. Pathologic fractures may be caused by hemophiliac pseudotumors or bone cysts. Patients with severe hemophilia may sustain fractures with only minimal trauma. Factor replacement therapy should be begun immediately to diminish the fracture hematoma. The rate of fracture healing in patients with hemophilia generally is agreed to be the same as in patients without the disease. Although most authors recommend nonoperative fracture treatment, using well-padded splints or bivalved casts until swelling subsides, Feil et al recommend internal fixation to prevent displacement with recurrent bleeding and pseudotumors. If adequate factor levels can be obtained, the indications for internal fixation of fractures in the patient with hemophilia are the same as in other patients. The use of traction has been discouraged because of the risk of hemorrhage at the pin sites, but Ahlberg and Nilsson, Patel et al, and Handelsman report good results with traction after adequate replacement therapy. Patients with in vivo inhibitors should be treated without surgery. Avascular necrosis is not infrequently seen, especially in the hip joint, where it is thought to be due to bleeding around the epiphyseal vessels.

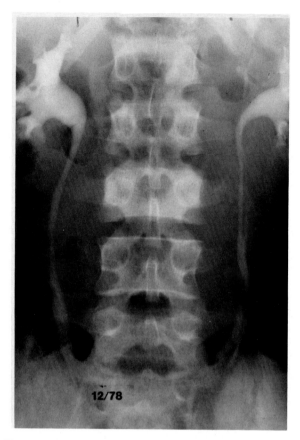

Fig. 8-23 The typical ivory vertebra of Hodgkin's disease is seen in L3, which is much denser than the adjacent vertebrae. These changes will disappear with successful treatment.

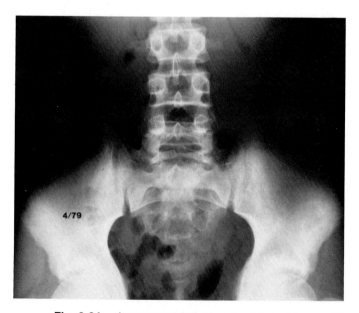

Fig. 8-24 Anteroposterior view of pelvis in 14-year-old patient shortly after Hodgkin's disease was diagnosed by biopsy of lesion on left side of pelvis. Biopsy is important to determine the stage of the disease.

LYMPHOMA

Lymphoma is divided into Hodgkin's lymphoma and non-Hodgkin's lymphoma, each with different manifestations, treatment, and prognosis. Hodgkin's lymphoma rarely is seen in children younger than 5 years of age, and its peak incidence occurs at approximately 20 years of age. Chan et al reported Hodgkin's lymphoma as an isolated primary bone tumor in four adolescents. The predominant clinical finding is enlargement of the lymph glands; other symptoms may include weight loss, fever, and sweating. Bone involvement in Hodgkin's lymphoma occurs in approximately 15% of adults and even fewer children. The spine and pelvis are most frequently involved with both lytic and blastic lesions and possibly periosteal elevation. Infiltration of a vertebra may cause a characteristic "ivory vertebra" appearance (Fig. 8-23), which usually disappears after successful treatment. Non-Hodgkin's lymphoma is more common in younger children, and approximately 20% of patients have bone involvement with features and distribution similar to those in Hodgkin's lymphoma. Neurologic manifestations are seen in both forms and are caused by extradural compression by direct bone involvement, lymph gland compression, or interference with the vascular supply to the spinal cord. The diagnosis is established by blood analysis and biopsy of the involved glands or bony lesions (Fig. 8-24).

Appropriate tumor staging should be done in every patient before treatment. The standard treatment of lymphoma is a combination of chemotherapy and irradiation, but increasing numbers of reports in the literature document sequelae after medical treatment. Avascular necrosis of the femoral or humeral head was reported by Prosnitz et al in 10% of patients with long-term survival periods. Radiation sarcoma of bone after treatment of Hodgkin's disease is rare but can occur.

GAUCHER DISEASE

Gaucher disease is a congenital metabolic disease in which a deficiency of β-glucosidase results in an accumulation of glucocerebroside in the reticuloendothelial system. This complex lipid is stored in the Gaucher cell, which is about 40 to 80 μ in diameter with a small, eccentrically placed nucleus and a wrinkled-appearing cytoplasm that contains lipid. The proliferation and expansion of the Gaucher cells cause enlargement of the spleen, liver, lymph nodes, and bone marrow.

The disorder has been classified into three types. Type I is the most common form with deposits in the spleen, liver, and bone marrow, without involvement of the central nervous system. Type II is an infantile or acute form, which is very rare and usually occurs at birth with hepatosplenomegaly, pulmonary problems, and severe involvement of the central nervous system; these patients usually die within the first 2 months of life. Type III is a poorly defined, subacute form manifesting in early adulthood; the central nervous system is involved, usually with seizures, ataxia, or mental deterioration. The disease is believed to be an autosomal recessive disorder. Types II and III are independent of race, whereas type I is about 10 times more frequent in Ashkenazi Jews than in the general population.

Skeletal changes in Gaucher disease are caused by deposits of the Gaucher cells in the bone marrow. Approximately 75% of patients with the disease have skeletal changes, but only half of these patients have musculoskeletal symptoms. Patients with advanced organ involvement have the most disabling bone disease. The femora, vertebrae, and humeri are most often involved, but lesions may occur in the ribs, pelvis, and other bones of the extremities. The metaphyses usually are involved, but the epiphyses usually are spared. Recent magnetic resonance imaging (MRI) studies by Rosenthal et al showed that the spine is always more involved and the proximal parts of the extremities are much more involved than the distal parts. Amstutz considers the femur to be the "skeletal barometer" of the disease.

The bony changes in Gaucher disease are osteoporosis with medullary expansion, fusiform widening of the bones, and cortical thinning (Fig. 8-25). Modeling processes are decreased, possibly because of osteoclastic depression that causes the characteristic Erlenmeyer flask deformity in the distal femur. The bone marrow displays cystic spaces mixed with sclerotic areas, and the periosteum may show an almost onion-skin elevation. Infarction of the bone and marrow with secondary repair are common. Avascular necrosis of the femoral head is typical; Amstutz reported avascular necrosis in 75% of his patients. It most often is bilateral and usually involves the whole femoral head; recurrent bone infarctions are common. Avascular necrosis also may involve the humeral head. Pathologic fractures are frequent in children with this disease and may be caused by osteoporosis, cortical thinning, or softening of the bone after the repair phase of avascular necrosis. These fractures occur most often in the femoral neck or distal femur.

Symptoms usually are present in early childhood but occasionally may not appear until adulthood. Clinical signs include patchy pigmentation of the skin, deposits in the sclerae (pingueculae), and varying degrees of hepatosplenomegaly, anemia, and bleeding tendencies. Bone pain is common in patients with Gaucher disease and usually is described as a dull ache involving the femur or proximal tibia. This pain may be caused by small bone infarcts. A more alarming syndrome is the "bone crisis" or pseudoosteomyelitis caused by sudden infarct of a larger bone segment. This syndrome is difficult to distinguish from osteomyelitis because it so closely mimics the symptoms of a bone infection: fever, tachycardia, pain, redness, swelling, elevated erythrocyte sedimentation rate, and mild leukocytosis. In the series of Bell et al of 49 patients with Gaucher disease, 5 of 11 patients hospitalized for bone pain had hematogenous osteomyelitis. Deep wound infections developed in six patients after elective orthopaedic sur-

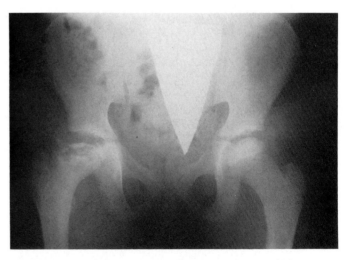

Fig. 8-25 Gaucher disease. Bilateral necrosis of hip; early changes in left hip, late changes in right hip.

gery. Several other reports in the literature describe the high incidence of infection after aspiration or surgical drainage for possible osteomyelitis.

Decreased amounts of glucocerebroside in the amnionic fluid can establish the diagnosis in utero as early as the seventeenth week of gestation. Postpartum bone marrow aspiration that shows Gaucher cells confirms the diagnosis. Laboratory analysis shows anemia, leukopenia, and thrombocytopenia caused partly by hypersplenism or, in later stages, bone marrow insufficiency. The nontartrate inhibitant acid phosphatase activity in the blood is increased. Measurement of glucocerebroside activity in the leukocytes gives an approximate index of the severity of the disease.

Roentgenographic signs of the disease are present in approximately 75% of patients with Gaucher disease. Rosenthal et al reported that MRI scanning revealed skeletal abnormalities in all of their patients. They found MRI useful for evaluating the extent of the lesions and for determining the presence of avascular necrosis. Technetium scanning may show increased or decreased activity, depending on the stage of the osteonecrosis.

Nonsurgical Treatment

Bone pain usually can be treated with analgesics, bed rest, and immobilization. Treatment of the patient with systemic and local manifestations is more difficult; the differentiation between bone infarct and osteomyelitis must be made first. Several authors, including Noyes and Smith and Stowens et al, have emphasized that surgery in these patients is particularly risky with high incidences of infection and bleeding. The diagnosis, then, must be established as early as possible by noninvasive methods. Blood cultures are useful if results are positive, but only 50% of blood cultures are positive for Gaucher disease in patients with osteomyelitis. Decreased uptake on technetium bone scanning indicates a bone crisis rather than osteomyelitis. CT scanning may show soft tissue changes, and MRI is helpful to determine the extent of the lesion. If blood cultures are negative and bone and CT scanning are inconclusive, needle biopsy should be done under strict aseptic conditions. Administration of systemic antibiotics should be delayed until a bacteriologic diagnosis has been established. If infection is diagnosed, a longer period of antibiotic treatment than normal should be anticipated because the infection usually is in avascular bone and is difficult to control. Several authors have reported patients whose infection necessitated amputation.

Avascular necrosis of the femoral head usually is bilateral and can be treated like Legg-Calvé-Perthes disease. A Scottish Rite brace is recommended to contain the femoral head in the acetabulum during ambulation, and night traction is recommended for joint stiffness. The healing process in avascular necrosis usually is longer than in Legg-Calvé-Perthes disease, probably because of the repeated and more severe infarctions. Core decompression or vascular grafting is not indicated because of the high risk of infection.

Fractures in patients with Gaucher disease occur most often in the base of the femoral neck or the distal femur, followed by the proximal tibia and the spine. Callus formation is extremely slow, and prolonged immobilization is necessary. Amstutz and Katz et al reported that union of femoral neck fractures requires from 1 to 2 years with conservative treatment and that all fractures heal in some degree of varus angulation. Distal femoral fractures can be treated with a non–weight-bearing cast brace. Spine fractures usually are treated with bed rest and bracing.

Surgical Treatment

In any operative procedure on a child with Gaucher disease complications can compromise a good technical result. Careful preoperative planning is mandatory. Because the patients often have anemia and thrombocytopenia with abnormal liver function, platelet counts and bleeding and coagulation times always should be evaluated before surgery, and fresh frozen plasma and platelets should be available during surgery. Prophylactic antibiotics should be given, and any procedure should be done under strictly aseptic conditions to diminish the risk of infection.

Needle biopsy for suspected osteomyelitis has a lower risk of causing infection than does open biopsy. Image intensification is helpful for needle biopsy of the sacroiliac joint or spine. Internal fixation of femoral neck fracture in a patient with Gaucher disease has been reported only once in the literature. Avascular necrosis of the femoral head developed as it did in many patients treated conservatively, but the fracture healed without varus deformity. Fixation of all displaced fractures of the femoral neck is recommended, with the pins crossing the physis if necessary to prevent varus deformity and lengthy immobilization. Non–weight bearing is continued until solid callus is visible. Increasing kyphosis may necessitate spinal fusion. Hip replacement may be performed in the adult with Gaucher disease, but the risk of intraoperative bleeding and later loosening of the femoral component is increased. Lachiewicz et al reported hip replacement in a child with Gaucher disease in whom loosening of the femoral component occurred 3 years after surgery.

NIEMANN-PICK DISEASE

Niemann-Pick disease is a rare metabolic disorder in which a lack of the lysosomal enzyme, sphingomyelinase, results in an accumulation of phosolipid in the reticuloendothelial system. As in Gaucher disease the spleen, liver, and bone marrow are primarily involved. There is no sex predilection, and the disease is believed to be an autosomal recessive disorder with predominance among Ashkenazic Jews.

Several subgroups of Niemann-Pick disease have been identified. Subgroup A is the most frequent and manifests in the first months of life with hepatosplenomegaly, slow physical development, mental retardation, and possibly icterus. In Videbaek's study of 72 children with subgroup A Niemann-Pick disease, half of the children died before 9 months of age and only 5% survived longer than 18 months. In subgroup B there is hepatosplenomegaly but no neurologic involvement. Patients with this form of the disease usually live into adulthood, although with significant skeletal changes. Subgroups C and D represent more juvenile forms of the disease.

Roentgenographic skeletal changes rarely are described, probably because they have little time to develop because most of these children die at a very early age. In the more prolonged form of Niemann-Pick disease, roentgenographic changes occur in approximately half of the patients. These changes are caused by the accumulation of lipid-loaded histiocytes in the bone marrow. The femur and humerus show the same expansion as in Gaucher disease, with a lack of the modeling process resulting in the deformities of Erlenmeyer flask. Most patients also have osteoporosis and coxa valga. Kyphosis may result from the osteoporosis, and widening of the metacarpal bones has been reported in approximately one half of patients with subgroup B disease. Avascular necrosis and fractures do not routinely occur in Niemann-Pick disease.

All patients with Niemann-Pick disease have a slight degree of anemia, thrombocytopenia, and possibly leukopenia. Microscopic examination of bone marrow shows the foam histiocytes that contain sphingomyelin, and examination by phase microscopy distinguishes Niemann-Pick disease from Gaucher disease. Deficiency of sphingomyelinase in the peripheral blood or leukocytes or in cultured fibroblasts further identifies the disease, allowing prenatal diagnosis by amniocentesis.

Successful bone marrow transplantation has been reported in mice with Niemann-Pick disease, but no specific treatment in humans has been established. No surgical treatment of the musculoskeletal system is indicated.

MASSIVE OSTEOLYSIS OF BONE

Osteolysis, also known as disappearing bone disease, massive osteolysis, primary idiopathic osteolysis, hemangiomatosis, Gorham disease, or phantom bone disease, is an extremely rare condition manifested by spontaneous and massive osteolysis in apparently normal bone. It usually is unicentric and associated with hemangiomatosis. Another form is idiopathic multicentric osteolysis, also known as acroosteolysis or carpal-tarsal osteolysis, which involves primarily the bones of the wrist and ankle. No metabolic or endocrine abnormality has been associated with osteolysis; however, carpal-tarsal osteolysis frequently is hereditary.

Osteolysis is not clearly defined, and no classification system has been developed, although Tyler and Rosenbaum limit Gorham disease to a unicentric osteolysis that usually develops around the shoulder or pelvic girdle. Carpal-tarsal osteolysis can be divided into two forms: hereditary, either dominant or recessive, and nonhereditary, associated with severe nephropathy, with no genetic trend, that leads to early death.

Gorham unicentric osteolysis is most common in adolescents and young adults and affects both sexes. Involved bones usually are the upper portion of the humerus, scapula, clavicle, ribs, upper portion of the femur with adjacent acetabulum, and more rarely the spine. Patients usually have pain that increases if the osteolytic bone fractures. Increasing bone resorption leads either to bizarre abnormal motion or to severe joint contractures. Spontaneous arrest of the disease after several years is usual, but there is no evidence of reossification after resorption has ceased. During the active disease process, invasion of adjacent soft tissues may occur; more rarely, there is involvement of the lungs and mediastinum, and if they become involved, the prognosis is poor. Death can be caused by pulmonary complications from rib cage collapse or by paraplegia from spine collapse.

Symptoms of carpal-tarsal osteolysis usually appear in children between the ages of 2 and 7 years. Many patients appear to have Marfan syndrome, and the symptoms usually begin with swollen, deformed, and painful wrist or ankle joints. As the disease progresses, osteolysis occurs in the phalanges, radius, and ulna and also may involve the elbow joint, causing bizarre joint destruction. In some patients the disease stops in adolescence but then reappears at a later age. In the nonhereditary form, nephropathy usually leads to proteinuria, causing early death from renal failure and malignant hypertension.

The earliest roentgenographic change usually is a lucent area close to the cortex. The osteolysis progresses without regard for joints or physes and can affect bones on either side of the joint. In the later stages of the disease the cortex is only a thin shell and the diaphysis may have a tapered appearance. Muscle weakness and atrophy often are present. The histologic appearance of Gorham disease is proliferation of thin-walled capillaries within the disappearing bones. The anastomosing network of vascular channels usually is filled with red blood cell elements. Bone trabeculae are present early but later are replaced by vascular fibrous tissue, a process usually attributed to lymphangioma or hemangioma. Osteoclasts rarely are seen on histologic examination, but studies have confirmed that mononuclear perivascular cells in contact with bone take part in the resorption. No bone restoration or rebuilding is evident either histologically or roentgenographically.

The diagnosis is based on a combination of clinical, roentgenographic, and histopathologic findings. Many diseases are similar in appearance and must be systematically ruled out. Results of blood tests usually are normal, and only occasionally is the alkaline phosphatase level slightly elevated. Results of bone scan usually are normal or show only slightly increased uptake because there is no significant osteoblastic activity. Biopsy of the involved area generally is necessary to confirm the diagnosis. The usual precautions for tumor biopsy must be observed, and the biopsy site must be protected because of the possibility of pathologic fracture after biopsy.

There is no specific treatment for this disease. Steroids, chemotherapy, and calcitonin all have been tried with limited success. Radiation therapy has seemed to benefit some patients, but it is difficult to determine if improvement is the result of treatment or the spontaneous remission of the disease. Radiation therapy has been reported to induce osteogenesis in the involved bone, which usually does not occur spontaneously. Treatment should first be directed at symptoms and should include bed rest, traction if necessary, gentle physical therapy, and possibly orthoses to prevent contractures and provide stability. Local resection and bone grafting have been tried, but the bone graft usually is invaded and resorbed in a manner similar to that which occurs in the primary bone. Butler et al reported successful strut grafting after the destructive process has ceased. Removal of the diseased bone and replacement with a metallic prosthesis have been reported by Aston and by Poirier to give good results in adult patients. Amputation should be considered if well-defined involvement causes severe disability.

FANCONI ANEMIA

In 1927, Fanconi of Italy described three brothers with multiple congenital anomalies who, between the ages of 5 and 7 years, developed increasing brownish pigmentation and hypoplastic anemia combined with pancytopenia. (Fanconi anemia should not be confused with Fanconi syndrome, which is a renal tubular insufficiency.) The hematologic features are the result of bone marrow hypoplasia with subsequent reduction of all cellular elements in the bone marrow and increasing infiltration of fat into the bone marrow. Fanconi anemia is a rare disease, and only about 600 cases have been described in the literature. It is believed to be an autosomal recessive disorder with a low degree of penetrance and occurs twice as often in boys as in girls.

The underlying defect in Fanconi anemia is unknown, but patients with this disorder have cells that are hypersensitive to agents that damage DNA. The number of chromosomes is normal, but the chromosomes are much more fragile and have a higher breakage rate than normal when exposed to DNA-damaging agents. This fragility is the key to diagnosis of the disease and can be determined prenatally because amniotic fluid cells have the same chromosomal abnormality.

The hematologic disorders of Fanconi anemia usually are not present before the child is 6 to 8 years of age, and the onset in boys slightly precedes that in girls. Patients usually are of short stature and low birth weight, and an olive-brown melanin skin pigmentation subsequently develops, especially concentrated around the trunk and skin folds in the axilla and groin. Other frequent findings are mental retardation, hypogonadism, and deafness. About 40% of patients have skeletal abnormalities. The upper extremities are much more involved than the lower extremities. The thumb and adjacent carpal bones may be aplastic or hypoplastic, and a supernumerary thumb sometimes is present. The radius may be hypoplastic or absent (radial clubhand). When there is complete radial aplasia, the corresponding thumb is usually absent also (Fig. 8-26). Atrophy of the thenar muscles, radial head dislocation, or radioulnar synostosis occasionally may occur. Much less frequent roentgenographic features are Klippel-Feil syndrome, Sprengel deformity, congenitally dislocated hips, clubfoot, toe abnormalities, osteoporosis, and delayed bone age. Approximately one third of these patients have renal abnormalities such as an absent or horseshoe-shaped kidney. The hematologic disorder becomes evident when the child is approximately 7 years of age, with the occurrence of anemia and fatigue, shortness of breath, and because of thrombocytopenia, an increased bleeding tendency, with easy bruising, epistaxis, and possibly gastrointestinal bleeding. There is a higher than normal incidence of leukemia and malignant tumors among patients with Fanconi's anemia, but most patients die either of hemorrhage or of infection.

Laboratory evaluation with peripheral blood values identifies thrombocytopenia and leukopenia, followed later by anemia. The bone marrow is hypoplastic with an increased amount of fat. Patients with characteristic malformations or involved siblings can be diagnosed in the preanemic state by chromosomal studies. Fanconi's anemia recently has been redefined to include patients with the characteristic chromosomal response to clastogenic stress who may or may not have a normal physical examination or evidence of hematologic disease.

In the past the only treatment for Fanconi anemia with bone marrow failure was blood transfusion, and the majority of patients died within a few years. Androgens combined with corticosteroids have been found to be of benefit, and recently bone marrow transplantation has been moderately successful. Associated congenital dislocation of the hip can be treated in the routine manner with flexion-abduction bracing. Nonsurgical treatment should be the first choice for radial clubhand in patients with Fanconi anemia. If surgery is necessary, it should be done early and before pancytopenia manifests itself, usually when the child is 6 to 8 years of age. Careful presurgical evaluation of the hematologic studies is vital. (The technique for surgical treatment of radial clubhand is described on p. 267.)

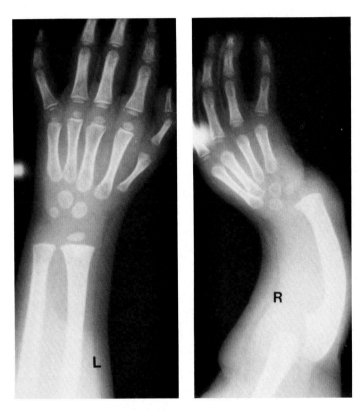

Fig. 8-26   Right and left forearm and wrist of a patient with Fanconi anemia. *Right,* Patient has complete aplasia of the radius together with the first ray. *Left,* Normal radius but deficient first ray. These differences are typical of Fanconi anemia.

THROMBOCYTOPENIA–ABSENT RADIUS SYNDROME

Thrombocytopenia–absent radius syndrome (TAR) is a rare disorder that consists of thrombocytopenia and absent radii, but all five fingers are present. It is an autosomal recessive disease consistent with a predominant defect in the amebakaryocytic (white cell) precursors. Thrombocytopenia develops in most patients with TAR within the first few weeks of life, with hemorrhagic manifestations such as petechiae and melena or intracranial bleeding. About 30% of patients die within the first year of life as a result of massive gastrointestinal or central nervous system hemorrhage. In the surviving patients there is a spontaneous increase in platelets and a decreased chance of bleeding after the child is 1 year of age. Although all phalanges are present, because of deficient extensor tendons the thumb is acutely flexed and clasped, and partial syndactyly may be present in the fingers. Several recent reports describe extensive involvement of the lower extremity in these patients, such as pronounced angular or torsional deformities of the tibia. Platelet counts usually are below 50,000 in patients with symptoms of TAR. Anemia may occur as a result of bleeding. Diagnosis is possible in utero with ultrasound.

Platelet transfusions during acute bleeding episodes usually are necessary only within the first year of life. Treatment of the radial clubhand should begin early with very careful stretching exercises and splinting. If stretching causes bleeding, it should be postponed until the thrombocytes are elevated and bleeding tendencies are lessened. Surgical correction of radial clubhand, when the thrombocytes have returned to normal, results in a good prognosis. Knee problems are especially critical when the patient begins to walk. Varus deformity usually is combined with internal tibial torsion, and bracing should be instituted. MRI may be helpful to evaluate the ligaments and menisci, which may be hypoplastic or absent. Fourteen of 19 patients in the series of Shoenecker et al required proximal tibial osteotomy and soft tissue release to realign the lower extremity. Recurrence of the deformity is frequent and, although there seems to be no correlation with the timing or location of the osteotomy, there usually is minimal progression of the deformity after skeletal maturity.

REFERENCES

Leukemia

Appell RG et al: Absence of prognostic significance of skeletal involvement in acute lymphocytic leukemia and non-Hodgkin lymphoma in children, Pediatr Radiol 15:245, 1985.

Aur RJA, Wesbrook HW, and Riggs W: Childhood acute lymphocytic leukemia, Am J Dis Child 124:653, 1972.

Baehner RL and Miller DR: Hematologic malignancies: leukemia and lymphoma. In Blood diseases of infancy and childhood, St Louis, 1984, The CV Mosby Co.

Behrman RE and Vaughan VC: Neoplasms and neoplasm-like lesions. In Nelson Textbook of Pediatrics, Philadelphia, 1983, WB Saunders Co.

Blatt J, Martini SL, and Penchansky L: Characteristics of acute lymphoblastic leukemia in children with osteopenia and vertebral compression fractures, J Pediatr 105:280, 1984.

Bos GD et al: Childhood leukemia presenting as a diaphyseal radiolucency, Clin Orthop 135:66, 1978.

Caudle RJ et al: Childhood acute lymphoblastic leukemia presenting as "cold" lesions on bone scan: a report of two cases, J Pediatr Orthop 7:93, 1987.

Clausen N et al: Skeletal scintigraphy and radiography at onset of acute lymphocytic leukemia in children, Med Pediatr Oncol 11:291, 1983.

Epstein BS: Vertebral changes in childhood leukemia, Radiology 68:65, 1957.

Hughes RG and Kay HEM: Major bone lesions in acute lymphoblastic leukaemia, Med Pediatr Oncol 10:67, 1982.

Miller JH and Ettinger LJ: Gallium citrate Ga 67 scintigraphic detection of chronic osteomyelitis in children with leukemia, Am J Dis Child 140:230, 1986.

Newman AJ and Melhorn DK: Vertebral compression in childhood leukemia, Am J Dis Child 125:863, 1973.

Nixon GW and Gwinn JL: The roentgen manifestations of leukemia in infancy, Radiology 107:603, 1973.

Pear BL: Skeletal manifestations of the lymphomas and leukemias, Semin Roentgenol 9:229, 1974.

Rajantie J et al: Prognostic significance of primary bone changes in children with acute lymphoblastic leukemia, Pediatr Radiol 15:242, 1985.

Rogalsky RJ, Black GB, and Reed MH: Orthopaedic manifestations of leukemia in children, J Bone Joint Surg 68A:494, 1986.

Rokicka-Milewska R, et al: Children cured of acute lymphoid leukemia, Am J Pediatr Hematol Oncol 8:208, 1986.

Rosenfield NS and McIntosh S: Prospective analysis of bone changes in treated childhood leukemia, Radiology 123:413, 1977.

Ryan JR and Emami A: Vincristine neurotoxicity with residual equinocavus deformity in children with acute leukemia, Cancer 51:423, 1983.

Samuda GM, Cheng MY, and Yeung CY: Back pain and vertebral compression: an uncommon presentation of childhood acute lymphoblastic leukemia, J Pediatr Orthop 7:175, 1987.

Saulsbury FT and Sabio H: Acute leukemia presenting as arthritis in children, Clin Pediatr 24:625, 1985.

Silverman FN: The skeletal lesions in leukemia, Am J Roentgenol 59:819, 1948.

Simmons CR, Harle TS, and Singleton EB: The osseous manifestations of leukemia in children, Radiol Clin North Am 6:115, 1968.

Van Slyck EJ: The bony changes in malignant hematologic disease, Orthop Clin North Am 3:733, 1972.

Sickle cell disease

Burko H, Watson J, and Robinson M: Unusual bone changes in sickle cell disease in childhood, Radiology 80:957, 1963.

Caroll DS and Evans JW: Roentgenographic findings in sickle cell anemia, Radiology 53:834, 1949.

Catterall A: The natural history of Perthes disease, J Bone Joint Surg 533:37, 1971.

Chung SMK and Ralston EL: Necrosis of the femoral head associated with sickle cell anemia and its genetic variants. A review of the literature and study of 13 cases. J Bone Joint Surg 51A:33, 1969.

Cockshott WP: Some radiological aspects of the S-hemoglobinapthies as seen in Ibadan. In Jonxis JHP, editor: Abnormal hemoglobins in Africa, Philadelphia, 1965, FA Davis Co.

Conn HO: Sickle cell trait and splenic infarction associated with high altitude flying, N Engl J Med 251:417, 1954.

Diggs LW: Bone and joint lesions in sickle cell disease, Clin Orthop 52:119, 1967.

Dresbach R: Elliptical human red corpuscles, Science 19:469, 1904.

Engh CA et al: Osteomyelitis in the patient with sickle cell disease, J Bone Joint Surg 53A:1, 1971.

Golding JSR: The bone changes in sickle cell anemia, Ann R Coll Surg Engl 19:296, 1956.

Golding JSR, MacIver JE, and Went LN: The bone changes in sickle cell anemia and its genetic variants, J Bone Joint Surg 41B:711, 1959.

Gunderson C, D'Ambrosia RD, and Shoji H: Total hip replacement in patients with sickle cell disease, J Bone Joint Surg 59A:760, 1977.

Hahn EV and Gillespie EB: Sickle cell anemia: report of a case greatly improved by splenectomy. Experimental study of sickle cell formation. Arch Intern Med 39:233, 1927.

Herrick JB: Peculiar elongated and sickle shaped red blood corpuscles in a case of severe anemia, Arch Intern Med 6:517, 1910.

Ingram VM: A special chemical difference between globins of normal human and sickle cell anemia hemoglobin, Nature 178:792, 1956.

Middlemiss JH and Raper AB: Skeletal changes in the hemoglobinopathies, J Bone Joint Surg 48B:693, 1966.

Murphy JR: Sickle cell hemoglobin (Hb A5) in black football players, JAMA 225:981, 1973.

Nachmie BA and Dorfman HD: Ischemic necrosis of bone in sickle cell trait, Mt Sinai J Med 41:527, 1974.

Nelson WE, editor: Textbook of pediatrics, ed 13, Philadelphia, 1987, WB Saunders Co.

Pauling L, et al: Sickle cell anemia: a molecular disease, Science 110:543, 1949.

Reynolds J: A reevaluation of the "fish vertebrae" found in sickle cell hemoglobinopathy, Am J Roentgenol 97:693, 1966.

Robbins JB and Pearson HA: Normal response of sickle cell anemia patients to immunization with salmonella vaccine, J Pediatr 66:877, 1965.

Scott RB: Health care priority in sickle cell anemia, JAMA 214:731, 1962.

Sebes JI and Kraus AP: Avascular necrosis of the hip in the sickle cell hemoglobinopathies, J Can Assoc Radiol 34:136, 1983.

Shahidi NT and Diamond LK: Skull changes in infants with chronic iron deficiency anemia, N Engl J Med 262:137, 1960.

Sherman M: Pathogenesis of disintegration of the hip in sickle cell anemia, South Med J 52:632, 1959.

Stein RE and Urbaniak J: Use of the tourniquet during surgery in patients with sickle cell hemoglobinopathies, Clin Orthop 151:231, 1980.

Whitten CF: Growth status of children with sickle cell anemia, Am J Dis Child 102:101, 1961.

Hemophilia

Abildgaard CF, Penner JA, and Watson-Williams EJ: Anti-inhibitor coagulant complex (Autoplex) for treatment of factor VIII inhibitors in hemophilia, Blood 56:978, 1980.

Ahlberg A and Nilsson IM: Fractures in haemophiliacs with special reference to complications and treatment, Acta Chir Scand 133:293, 1967.

Ahlberg A and Pettersson H: Synoviorthesis with radioactive gold in hemophiliacs, Acta Orthop Scand 50:513, 1979.

Ahlberg AKM: On the natural history of hemophilic pseudotumor, J Bone Joint Surg 57A:1133, 1975.

Arnold WD and Hilgartner MW: Hemophilic arthropathy, J Bone Joint Surg 59A:287, 1977.

Aronstam A, Rainsford SG, and Painter MJ: Patterns of bleeding in adolescents with severe haemophilia A, Br Med J 1:469, 1979.

Aronstam A et al: The identification of high-risk elbow hemorrhages in adolescents with severe hemophilia A, J Pediatr 98:776, 1981.

Aronstam A et al: The clinical features of early bleeding into the muscles of the lower limb in severe haemophiliacs, J Bone Joint Surg 65B:19, 1983.

Bianco AJ Jr and Peterson HA: Juvenile rheumatoid arthritis, Orthop Clin North Am 2:745, 1971.

Boardman KP and English P: Fractures and dislocations in hemophilia, Clin Orthop 148:221, 1980.

Boldero JC and Kemp HS: The early bone and joint changes in haemophilia and similar blood dyscrasias, Br J Radiol 39:172, 1966.

Brighton CT, Bigley EC, and Smolenski BI: Iron induced arthritis in immature rabbits, Arthritis Rheum 13:849, 1970.

Brower TD and Wilde AH: Femoral neuropathy in hemophilia, J Bone Joint Surg 48A:487, 1966.

Brumfield RH and Resnick CT: Synovectomy of the elbow in rheumatoid arthritis, J Bone Joint Surg 67A:16, 1985.

Bryan RS and Peterson LFA: Synovectomy of the knee, Orthop Clin North Am 2:705, 1971.

Bussi L et al: Results of synovectomy of the knee in haemophilia, Haematologica 59:81, 1974.

Caffey J and Schlesinger ER: Certain effects of hemophilia on the growing skeleton, J Pediatr 16:549, 1940.

Canale ST, Dugdale M, and Howard BC: Synovectomy of the knee in young patients with hemophilia, South Med J 81:1480, 1988.

Casscells CD: Commentary: the argument for early arthroscopic synovectomy in patients with severe hemophilia, Arthroscopy 3:78, 1987.

Chambers RB: Orthopaedic injuries in athletes, Am J Sports Med 7:195, 1979.

Chen YF: Bilateral hemophilic pseudotumors of the calcaneus and cuboid treated by irradiation, J Bone Joint Surg 47A:517, 1965.

Clark MW: Knee synovectomy in hemophilia, Orthopedics 1:285, 1978.

Cohen S and Jones R: An evaluation of the efficacy of arthroscopic synovectomy of the knee in rheumatoid arthritis: 12-24 month results, J Rheumatol 14:452, 1987.

Colombo M et al: Transmission of non-A, non-B hepatitis by heat-treated factor VIII concentrate, Lancet 2(1):1, 1985.

Coventry MB et al: Survival of patient with hemophilia and fracture of femur, J Bone Joint Surg 41A:1392, 1959.

Davis KC et al: Acquired immunodeficiency syndrome in a patient with hemophilia, Ann Intern Med 3:284, 1983.

DePalma AF and Cotler J: Hemophilic arthropathy, Clin Orthop 8:163, 1956.

DeValderrama, JAF and Matthews JM: The haemophilic pseudotumor or haemophilic subperiosteal haematoma, J Bone Joint Surg 47B:256, 1965.

Dyszy-Laube B et al: Synovectomy in the treatment of hemophilic arthropathy, J Pediatr Surg 9:123, 1974.

Eagleton MC et al: Relationship of clinical and immunological abnormalities in haemophilia A to F VIII therapy and HIV exposure: a longitudinal study, Eur J Haematol 40:35, 1988.

Ehrmann L et al: Peripheral nerve lesions in haemophilia, J Neurol 225:175, 1981.

Eichenblat M, Hass A, and Kessler I: Synovectomy of the elbow in rheumatoid arthritis, J Bone Joint Surg 64A:1074, 1982.

Evatt BL et al: Coincidental appearance of LAV/HTLV-III antibodies in hemophiliacs and the onset of the AIDS epidemic, N Engl J Med 312:8, 1985.

Ewald B, Myers M, and Crooks J: Synovectomy in hemophilia—a preliminary report, J Bone Joint Surg 57A:139, 1975.

Eyster ME et al: Development and early natural history of HTLV-III antibodies in persons with hemophilia, JAMA 253:15, 1985.

Feil E, Bentley G, and Rizza CR: Fracture management in patients with haemophilia, J Bone Joint Surg 56B:643, 1974.

Floman Y and Niska M: Dislocation of the hip joint complicating repeated hemarthrosis in hemophilia, J Pediatr Orthop 3:99, 1983.

Gamba G, Grignani G, and Ascari E: Synoviorthesis versus synovectomy in the treatment of recurrent haemophilic haemarthrosis: long-term evaluation, Thromb Haemost 45:127, 1981.

Ghormley RK and Clegg RS: Bone and joint changes in hemophilia, J Bone Joint Surg 30A:589, 1948.

Gilbert MS: Characterizing the hemophilic pseudotumor, Ann NY Acad Sci 240:313, 1975.

Goldberg VM et al: Total knee arthroplasty in classic hemophilia, J Bone Joint Surg 63A:695, 1981.

Goldsmith JC et al: High prevalence and high titers of LAV/HTLV-III antibodies in healthy hemophiliacs in the midwestern United States, Am J Med 81:579, 1986.

Goodfellow J, Fearn CB, and Matthews JM: Iliacus haematoma, J Bone Joint Surg 49B:748, 1967.

Greene WB: Use of continuous passive slow motion in the postoperative rehabilitation of difficult pediatric knee and elbow problems, J Pediatr Orthop 3:419, 1983.

Greene WB et al: Treatment of hypertrophic synovitis and recurrent hemarthrosis in children with severe hemophilia, Dev Med Child Neurol 25:112, 1983.

Greene WB and Wilson FC: Nonoperative management of hemophilic arthropathy and muscle hemorrhage, Instr Course Lect 32:223, 1983.

Handelsman JE: The knee joint in hemophilia, Orthop Clin North Am 10:139, 1979.

Harrison JF: Haemophilic pseudotumor after fractured femur, Br Med J 1:544, 1964.

Hasiba U et al: Liver dysfunction in Pennsylvania's multitransfused hemophiliacs, Dig Dis Sci 25:776, 1980.

Heim M et al: Haemophiliac hands—a three year follow-up study, Hand 14:333, 1982.

Heim M et al: Iliopsoas hematoma—its detection and treatment with special reference to hemophilia, Arch Orthop Trauma Surg 99:195, 1982.

Highgenboten CL: Arthroscopic synovectomy, Orthop Clin North Am 13:399, 1982.

Hilgartner MW: Home care for hemophilia: current state of the art, Scand J Hematol 30:58, 1977.

Hilgartner MW: Managing the child with hemophilia, Pediatr Ann 8:68, 1979.

Hilgartner MW and Arnold WD: Hemophilic pseudotumor treated with replacement therapy and radiation, J Bone Joint Surg 57A:1145, 1975.

Hoaglund FT: Experimental hemarthrosis, J Bone Joint Surg 49A:285, 1967.

Hofmann A, Wyatt R, and Bybee B: Septic arthritis of the knee in a 12-year-old hemophiliac, J Pediatr Orthop 4:498, 1984.

Hofmann P, Menge M, and Brackmann HH: Reconstructive surgery in the lower limb in hemophiliacs, Isr J Med Sci 13:988, 1977.

Hoskinson J and Duthie RB: Management of musculoskeletal problems in the hemophilias, Orthop Clin North Am 9:455, 1978.

Houghton GR: Septic arthritis of the hip in a hemophiliac, Clin Orthop 129:223, 1977.

Houghton GR and Dickson RA: Lower limb arthrodesis in haemophilia, J Bone Joint Surg 60B:387, 1978.

Houghton GR and Duthie RB: Orthopedic problems in hemophilia, Clin Orthop 138:197, 1979.

Hutcheson J: Peripelvic new bone formation in hemophilia, Radiology 109:529, 1973.

Hutchinson RJ, Penner JA, and Hensinger RN: Anti-inhibitor coagulant complex (Autoplex) in hemophilia inhibitor patients undergoing synovectomy, Pediatrics 71:631, 1983.

Ikkala E et al: Changes in the life expectancy of patients with severe hemophilia A in Finland in 1930-79, Br J Haematol 52:7, 1982.

Ingram GIC, Mathews JA, and Bennett AE: A controlled trial of joint aspiration in acute haemophilic haemarthrosis, Br J Haematol 23:649, 1972.

Jackson RW: Current concepts review: arthroscopic surgery, J Bone Joint Surg 65A:416, 1983.

Jackson S: Femoral neuropathy secondary to heparin-induced intrapelvic hematoma, Orthopedics 10:1049, 1987.

Johnson RP and Babbitt DP: Five stages of joint disintegration compared with range of motion in hemophilia, Clin Orthop 201:36, 1985.

Jordan HH: Orthopedic appliances, ed 2, Springfield, Ill, 1963, Charles C Thomas, Publisher.

Karthaus RP and Novakova IRO: Total knee replacement in haemophiliac arthropathy, J Bone Joint Surg 70B:382, 1988.

Kasper CK: Postoperative thromboses in hemophilia B, N Engl J Med 289:160, 1973.

Kay L et al: The role of synovectomy in the management of recurrent haemarthroses in haemophilia, Br J Haematol 49:53, 1981.

Kelly PJ, Martin WJ, and Coventry MB: Bacterial (suppurative) arthritis in the adult, J Bone Joint Surg 52A:1595, 1970.

Kemp HS and Matthews JM: The management of fractures in haemophilia and Christmas disease, J Bone Joint Surg 50B:351, 1968.

Key JA: Hemophilic arthritis, Ann Surg 95:198, 1932.

Kisker CT and Burke C: Double blind studies on the use of steroids in the treatment of acute hemarthrosis in patients with hemophilia, N Engl J Med 282:639, 1970.

Klein KS et al: Long term follow-up of arthroscopic synovectomy for chronic hemophilic synovitis, Arthroscopy 3:231, 1987.

Krill CE and Mauer AM: Pseudotumor of calcaneus in Christmas disease, J Pediatr 77:848, 1970.

Kurczynski EM and Penner JA: Activated prothrombin concentrate for patients with factor VIII inhibitors, N Engl J Med 291:164, 1974.

Lachiewicz PF et al: Total knee arthroplasty in hemophilia, J Bone Joint Surg 67A:1361, 1985.

Lancourt JE, Gilbert MS, and Posner MA: Management of bleeding and associated complications of hemophilia in the hand and forearm, J Bone Joint Surg 59A:451, 1977.

Large DF, Ludlam CA, and MacNicol MF: Common peroneal nerve entrapment in a hemophiliac, Clin Orthop 181:165, 1983.

Lazarovits P and Griem ML: Radiotherapy of hemophilia pseudotumors, Radiology 91:1026, 1968.

LeBalc'h T et al: Synovectomy of the elbow in young hemophilic patients, J Bone Joint Surg 69A:264, 1987.

Leipnitz G et al: AIDS-related thrombocytopenia, Vox Sang 56:57, 1989.

Levy JA, Mitra G, and Mozen MM: Recovery and inactivation of infectious retroviruses from factor VIII concentrates, Lancet 2:722, 1984.

Lewis JH, Cottington, GM, and Brower TD: The use of plasma fraction I to maintain hemostasis following amputation for hemorrhagic cyst of the thigh in a severe hemophiliac, J Bone Joint Surg 47A:333, 1965.

Limbird TJ and Dennis SC: Synovectomy and continuous passive motion (CPM) in hemophiliac patients, Arthroscopy 3:74, 1987.

Lofthouse RN: Bone changes in haemophilia, J Bone Joint Surg 39B:794, 1957.

Lusher JM et al: Autoplex versus Proplex: a controlled, double-blind study of effectiveness in acute hemarthrosis in hemophiliacs with inhibitors to factor VIII, Blood 62:1135, 1983.

Madigan RR, Hanna WT, and Wallace SL: Acute compartment syndrome in hemophilia, J Bone Joint Surg 63A:1327, 1981.

Marder VJ and Shulman NR: Major surgery in classic hemophilia using fraction I, Am J Med 41:56, 1966.

Matsen FA III, Winquist RA, and Krugmire RB: Diagnosis and management of compartmental syndromes, J Bone Joint Surg 62A:286, 1980.

McCollough NC III: Orthotic management. In Lovell WW and Winter RB, editors: Pediatric orthopedics, ed 2, Philadelphia, 1986, JB Lippincott Co.

McCollough NC III et al: Synovectomy or total replacement of the knee in hemophilia, J Bone Joint Surg 61A:69, 1979.

McDaniel WJ: A modified subluxation hinge for use in hemophilic knee flexion contractures, Clin Orthop 103:50, 1974.

McMillan CW et al: The management of musculoskeletal problems in hemophilia, Instr Course Lect 32:210, 1983.

McMillan CW et al: Continuous intravenous infusion of factor VIII in classic haemophilia, Br J Haematol 18:659, 1970.

Melbye M et al: HTLV-III seropositivity in European haemophiliacs exposed to factor VIII concentrate imported from the USA, Lancet 2:1444, 1984.

Miller EH, Flessa HC, and Glueck HI: The management of deep soft tissue bleeding and hemarthrosis in hemophilia, Clin Orthop 82:92, 1972.

Mintzer DM, Cotler JM, and Shapiro SS: Compartment syndromes in hemophilia, Contemp Orthop 9:77, 1984.

Moneim MS and Gribble TJ: Carpal tunnel syndrome in hemophilia, J Hand Surg 9:580, 1984.

Montane I, McCollough NC III, and Lian ECY: Synovectomy of the knee for hemophilic arthropathy, J Bone Joint Surg 68A:210, 1986.

Mubarak SJ et al: Acute compartment syndromes: diagnosis and treatment with the aid of the Wick catheter, J Bone Joint Surg 60A:1091, 1978.

Nathan DG and Oski FA: Hematology in infancy and childhood, Philadelphia, 1987, WB Saunders Co.

Nelson IW, Atkins RM, and Allen AL: The management of knee flexion contractures in haemophilia: brief report, J Bone Joint Surg 71B:327, 1989.

Nelson MG and Mitchell ES: Pseudotumour of bone in haemophilia, Acta Haemat 28:137, 1962.

Nicol RO and Menelaus MB: Synovectomy of the knee in hemophilia, J Pediatr Orthop 6:330, 1986.

Niemann, KMW: Surgical correction of flexion deformities in hemophilia, Am Surg 37:685, 1971.

Niemann, KMW: Management of lower extremity contractures resulting from hemophilia, South Med J 67:437, 1974.

Nobel W, Marks SC, and Kubik S: The anatomical basis for femoral nerve palsy following iliacus hematoma, J Neurosurg 52:533, 1980.

Oleske J et al: Immune deficiency syndrome in children, JAMA 249:2345, 1983.

Parsons JR, Zingler BM, and McKeon JJ: Mechanical and histological studies of acute joint hemorrhage, Orthopedics 10:1019, 1987.

Patel MR, Pearlman HS, and Lavine LS: Arthrodesis in hemophilia, Clin Orthop 86:168, 1972.

Paton RW and Evans DIK: Silent avascular necrosis of the femoral head in haemophilia, J Bone Joint Surg 70B:737, 1988.

Pettersson H, Ahlberg A, and Nilsson IM: A radiologic classification of hemophilic arthropathy, Clin Orthop 149:153, 1980.

Pietrogrande V, Dioguardi N, and Mannucci PM: Short-term evaluation of synovectomy in haemophilia, Br Med J 2:378, 1972.

Post M and Telfer M: Surgery in hemophilic patients, J Bone Joint Surg 57A:1136, 1975.

Post M, Watts G, and Telfer M: Synovectomy in hemophilic arthropathy, Clin Orthop 202:139, 1986.

Ragni MV et al: Acquired immunodeficiency–like syndrome in two haemophiliacs, Lancet 1:213, 1983.

Richardson ML et al: Skeletal changes in neuromuscular disorders mimicking juvenile rheumatoid arthritis and hemophilia, Am J Roentgenol 143:893, 1984.

Rosenthal RL, Graham JJ, and Selirio E: Excision of pseudotumor with repair by bone graft of pathological fracture of femur in hemophilia, J Bone Joint Surg 55A:827, 1973.

Rosner SM and Rabinder SB: Infectious arthritis in a hemophiliac, J Rheumatol 8:519, 1981.

Roy S: Ultrastructure of articular cartilage in experimental hemarthrosis, Arch Pathol 86:69, 1968.

Roy S and Ghadially FN: Ultrasound of synovial membrane in human hemarthrosis, J Bone Surg 49A:1636, 1967.

Shapiro SS: Antibodies to blood coagulation factors, Clin Haematol 8:207, 1979.

Sheppeard H, Aldin A, and Ward DJ: Osmic acid versus yttrium-90 in rheumatoid synovitis of the knee, Scand J Rheumatol 10:234, 1981.

Shibata T, Shiraoka K, and Takubo N: Comparison between arthroscopic and open synovectomy for the knee in rheumatoid arthritis, Arch Orthop Trauma Surg 105:257, 1986.

Silverstein A: Neuropathy in hemophilia, JAMA 190:162, 1964.

Sjamsoedin, LJM et al: The effect of activated prothrombin-complex concentrate (FEIBA) on joint and muscle bleeding in patients with hemophilia A and antibodies to factor VII, N Engl J Med 305:717, 1981.

Sledge CB et al: Synovectomy of the rheumatoid knee using intra-articular injection of dysprosium-165-ferric hydroxide macroaggregates, J Bone Joint Surg 69A:970, 1987.

Small, M et al: Total knee arthroplasty in haemophilic arthritis, J Bone Joint Surg 65B:163, 1983.

Smith MA, Savidge GF, and Fountain EJ: Interposition arthroplasty in the management of advanced haemophilic arthropathy of the elbow, J Bone Joint Surg 65B:436, 1983.

Smith MA, Urquhart DR, and Savidge GF: The surgical management of varus deformity in haemophilic arthropathy of the knee, J Bone Joint Surg 63B:261, 1981.

Sneppen O, Beck H, and Holsteen V: Synovectomy as a prophylactic measure in recurrent haemophilic haemarthrosis, Acta Paediatr Scand 67:491, 1978.

Soeur R: The synovial membrane of the knee in pathological conditions, J Bone Joint Surg 31A:317, 1949.

Soreff J: Joint debridement in the treatment of advanced hemophilic knee arthropathy, Clin Orthop 191:179, 1984.

Soreff J and Blomback M: Arthropathy in children with severe hemophilia A, Acta Paediatr Scand 69:667, 1980.

Speer DP: Early pathogenesis of hemophilic arthropathy, Clin Orthop 185:250, 1984.

Steel WM, Duthie RB, and O'Connor BT: Haemophilic cysts, J Bone Joint Surg 51B:614, 1969.

Stehr-Green JK et al: Hemophilia-associated AIDS in the United States, 1981 to September 1987, Am J Public Health 78:4, 1988.

Stein H and Dickson RA: Reversed dynamic slings for knee-flexion contractures in the hemophiliac, J Bone Joint Surg 57A:282, 1975.

Stein H and Duthie RB: The pathogenesis of chronic haemophilic arthropathy, J Bone Joint Surg 63B:601, 1981.

Steven MM et al: Radio-isotopic joint scans in haemophilic arthritis, Br J Rheumatol 24:263, 1985.

Storti E and Ascari E: Surgical and chemical synovectomy, Ann NY Acad Sci 240:316, 1975.

Storti E et al: Synovectomy, a new approach to haemophilic arthropathy, Acta Haematol (Basel) 41:193, 1969.

Sullivan JL et al: Hemophiliac immunodeficiency: influence of exposure to factor VIII concentrate, LAV/HTLV-III, and herpesvirus, J Pediatr 108:504, 1986.

Sundaram M et al: Case report 13, Skeletal Radiol 6:54, 1981.

Swanton MC: Hemophilic arthropathy in dogs, Lab Invest 8:1269, 1959.

Tabor DC and Votaw ML: Fatal myocardial hemorrhagic infarction in hemophilia A after factor IX and Autoplex therapy, Blood 62:278, 1983.

Thomas HB: Some orthopaedic findings in ninety-four cases of hemophilia, J Bone Joint Surg 18:140, 1936.

Update: Acquired immunodeficiency syndrome (AIDS) in persons with hemophilia, MMWR 33:42, 1984.

VanCreveld S et al: Degenerations of joints in haemophiliacs under treatment by modern methods, J Bone Joint Surg 63B:296, 1971.

Vas W et al: Myositis ossificans in hemophilia, Skeletal Radiol 7:27, 1981.

Wells J and Templeton J: Femoral neuropathy associated with anticoagulant therapy, Clin Orthop 124:155, 1977.

Wiedel JD: Arthroscopic synovectomy for chronic hemophilic synovitis of the knee, Arthroscopy 1:205, 1985.

Wilkins RM and Wiedel JD: Septic arthritis of the knee in a hemophilic J Bone Joint Surg 65A:267, 1983.

Wilson FC, Mahew DE, and McMillan CW: Surgical management of musculoskeletal problems in hemophilia. Instructional course lecture XXXII, St Louis, 1983, The CV Mosby Co.

Wolf CR and Mankin HJ: The effect of experimental hemarthrosis on articular cartilage of rabbit knee joints, J Bone Joint Surg 47A:1203, 1965.

Wood K, Omer A, and Shaw MT: Haemophilic arthropathy, Br J Radiol 42:498, 1969.

Wood WI et al: Expression of active human factor VIII from recombinant DNA clones, Nature 312:330, 1984.

Lymphoma

Appell RG, Oppermann HC, and Brandeis WE: Skeletal lesions in Hodgkin's disease, Pediatr Radiol 11:61, 1981.

Beachley MC, Lau BP, and King ER: Bone involvement in Hodgkin's disease, Am J Roentgenol 114:559, 1972.

Braunstein EM: Hodgkin disease of bone: radiographic correlation with the histological classification, Radiology 137:643, 1980.

Chan KW et al: Hodgkin's disease in adolescents presenting as a primary bone lesion, Am J Pediatr Hematol Oncol 4:11, 1982.

Engel IA et al: Osteonecrosis in patients with malignant lymphoma: a review of twenty-five cases, Cancer 48:1245, 1981.

Hancock BW, Huck P, and Ross B: Avascular necrosis of the femoral head in patients receiving intermittent cytotoxic and corticosteroid therapy for Hodgkin's disease, Postgrad Med J 54:545, 1978.

Hertz M, Solomon A, and Aghai E: Ivory vertebra in Hodgkin's disease, JAMA 238:2402, 1977.

Hope-Stone HF: The diagnosis of osteonecrosis in Hodgkin's disease—active disease or infarction? Br J Radiol 52:580, 1979.

Hustu HO and Pinkel D: Lymphosarcoma, Hodgkin's disease and leukemia in bone, Clin Orthop 52:83, 1967.

Ihde DC and DeVita VT: Osteonecrosis of the femoral head in patients with lymphoma treated with intermittent combination chemotherapy (including corticosteroids), Cancer 36:1585, 1975.

Kay CJ, Rosenberg MA, and Burd R: Hypertrophic osteoarthropathy and childhood Hodgkin's disease, Radiology 112:177, 1974.

Lecanet D et al: Les localisations osseuses de la maladie de Hodgkin, Ann Radiol (Paris) 14:845, 1971.

Mould JJ and Adam NM: The problem of avascular necrosis of bone in patients treated for Hodgkin's disease, Clin Radiol 34:231, 1983.

Mullins GM and Lenhard RE: Digital clubbing in Hodgkin's disease, Johns Hopkins Med J 128:153, 1971.

Newcomer LN et al: Bone involvement in Hodgkin's disease, Cancer 49:338, 1982.

Niebrugge D et al: Osteogenic sarcoma following Hodgkin's disease, Cancer 48:416, 1981.

Prosnitz LR et al: Avascular necrosis of bone in Hodgkin's disease patients treated with combined modality therapy, Cancer 47:2793, 1981.

Smith J et al: Hodgkin's disease complicated by radiation sarcoma in bone, Br J Radiol 53:314, 1980.

Sweet DL, Roth DG, and Desser RK: Avascular necrosis of the femoral head with combination therapy, Ann Intern Med 85:67, 1976.

Timothy AR et al: Osteonecrosis in Hodgkin's disease, Br J Radiol 51:328, 1978.

Gaucher disease

Amstutz HC: The hip in Gaucher's disease, Clin Orthop 90:83, 1973.

Bell RS, Mankin HJ, and Doppelt SH: Osteomyelitis in Gaucher disease, J Bone Joint Surg 68A:1380, 1986.

Cheng TH and Holman BL: Radionuclide assessment of Gaucher's disease, J Nucl Med 19:1333, 1978.

Davies FWT: Gaucher's disease in bone, J Bone Joint Surg 34B:454, 1952.

DeNardo GL and Volpe JA: Detection of bone lesions with the strontium-85 scintiscan, J Nucl Med 7:291, 1966.

Gelfand G and Bienenstock H: Hemorrhagic bursitis and bone crises in chronic adult Gaucher's disease: a case report, Arthritis Rheum 25:1369, 1982.

Goldblatt J, Sacks S, and Beighton P: The orthopedic aspects of Gaucher disease, Clin Orthop 137:208, 1979.

Greenfield GB: Miscellaneous diseases related to the hematologic system, Semin Roentgenol 4:241, 1974.

Holder LE and O'Mara RE: Bone/joint IV: osteomyelitis, J Nucl Med 6:977, 1986.

Katz JF: Recurrent avascular necrosis of the proximal femoral epiphysis in the same hip in Gaucher's disease, J Bone Joint Surg 49:514, 1967.

Katz K et al: Fractures in children who have Gaucher disease, J Bone Joint Surg 69A:1361, 1987.

Lachiewicz PF: Gaucher's disease, Orthop Clin North Am 15:765, 1984.

Lachiewicz PF, Lane JM, and Wilson, PD: Total hip replacement in Gaucher's disease, J Bone Joint Surg 63:602, 1981.

Lau MM et al: Hip arthroplasties in Gaucher's disease, J Bone Joint Surg 63:591, 1981.

Marks C, Ram MD, and Zaas R: Surgical considerations in Gaucher's disease, Surg Gyncol Obstet 132:609, 1971.

Matsubara T et al: Histologic and histochemical investigation of Gaucher cells, Clin Orthop 166:244, 1982.

Merkel KD et al: Comparison of indium-labeled–leukocyte imaging with sequential technetium-gallium scanning in the diagnosis of low-grade musculoskeletal sepsis, J Bone Joint Surg 67A:465, 1985.

Miller JH, Ortega JA, and Heisel MA: Juvenile Gaucher disease simulating osteomyelitis, Am J Roentgenol 137:880, 1981.

Nishimura RN and Barranger JA: Neurologic complications of Gaucher's disease, type 3, Arch Neurol 37:92, 1980.

Noyes FR and Smith WS: Bone crises and chronic osteomyelitis in Gaucher's disease, Clin Orthop 79:132, 1971.

Rose JS et al: Accelerated skeletal deterioration after splenectomy in Gaucher type I disease, Am J Roentgenol 139:1202, 1982.

Rosenthal DI et al: Evaluation of Gaucher disease using magnetic resonance imaging, J Bone Joint Surg 68A:802, 1986.

Ruff ME, Weis LD, and Kean JR: Acute thoracic kyphosis in Gaucher's disease, Spine 9:835, 1984.

Schein AJ and Arkin AM: The classic: hip-joint involvement in Gaucher's disease, Clin Orthop 90:4, 1973.

Schneider EL et al: Infantile (type II) Gaucher's disease: in utero diagnosis and fetal pathology, Pediatrics 81:1134, 1972.

Schubiner H, Letourneau M, and Murray DL: Pyogenic osteomyelitis versus pseudo-osteomyelitis in Gaucher's disease, Clin Pediatr 20:667, 1981.

Silverstein MN and Kelly PJ: Osteoarticular manifestations of Gaucher's disease, Am J Med Sci 253:569, 1967.

Stowens DW et al: Skeletal complications of Gaucher disease, Medicine 64:310, 1985.

Niemann-Pick disease

Basson MG and French JH: Recent advances in the cerebromacular degenerations, J Natl Med Assoc 63:412, 1971.

Beaudet AL: Lysosomal storage diseases. In Petersdorf RG, editor: Harrison's principles of internal medicine, ed 10, New York, 1983, McGraw-Hill

Bondy PK and Rosenberg LE: The sphingolipidoses. In Metabolic control and disease, ed 8, Philadelphia, 1980, WB Saunders Co.

Crocker AC and Farber S: Niemann-Pick disease: a review of eighteen patients, Medicine 37:1, 1958.

Gilbert EF et al: Niemann-Pick disease type C, Eur J Pediatr 136:263, 1981.

Kampine JP, Brady RO, and Kanfer JN: Diagnosis of Gaucher's disease and Niemann-Pick disease with small samples of venous blood, Science 155:86, 1967.

Lachman R et al: Radiological findings in Niemann-Pick disease, Radiology 108:659, 1973.

Sakiyama T et al: Bone marrow transplantation for Niemann-Pick mice, J Inherited Metab Dis 6:129, 1983.

Sakiyama T et al: Bone marrow transplantation in Niemann-Pick mice, J Inherited Metab Dis 9:305, 1986.

Wenger DA, Barth G, and Githens JH: Nine cases of sphingomyelin lipidosis, a new variant in Spanish-American children, Am J Dis Child 131:955, 1977.

Wenger DA, Kudoh T, Sattler M: Niemann-Pick disease type B: prenatal diagnosis and enzymatic and chemical studies on fetal brain and liver, Am J Hum Genet 33:337, 1981.

Videbaek A: Niemann-Pick's disease: acute and chronic type? Acta Paediatr Scand 37:95, 1949.

Osteolysis

Aston JN: A case of "massive osteolysis" of the femur, J Bone Joint Surg 40:514, 1958.

Beals RK and Bird CB: Carpal and tarsal osteolysis, J Bone Joint Surg 57A:681, 1975.

Butler RW, McCance RA, and Barrett AM: Unexplained destruction of the shaft of the femur in a child, J Bone Joint Surg 40:487, 1958.

Edwards WH, Thompson RC, and Varsa EW: Lymphangiomatosis and massive osteolysis of the cervical spine, Clin Orthop 177:222, 1983.

Fornasier VL: Haemangiomatosis with massive osteolysis, J Bone Joint Surg 52B:444, 1970.

Gherlinzoni F and Rocco M: Progressive teleangiomatous osteolysis, Ital J Orthop Traumatol 9:515, 1983.

Gorham LW and Stout AP: Massive osteolysis (acute spontaneous absorption of bone, phantom bone, disappearing bone), J Bone Joint Surg 37:985, 1955.

Gorham LW et al: Disappearing bones: a rare form of massive osteolysis, Am J Med 17:674, 1954.

Gutierrez RM and Spjut HJ: Skeletal angiomatosis, Clin Orthop 85:82, 1972.

Halliday DR et al: Massive osteolysis and angiomatosis, Radiology 82:637, 1964.

Hardegger F, Simpson LA, and Segmueller G: The syndrome of idiopathic osteolysis, J Bone Joint Surg 67B:89, 1985.

Hejgaard N and Olsen PR: Massive Gorham osteolysis of the right hemipelvis complicated by chylothorax: report of a case in a 9-year-old boy successfully treated by pleurodesis, J Pediatr Orthop 7:96, 1987.

Heyden G, Kindblom LG, and Nielsen JM: Disappearing bone disease, J Bone Joint Surg 59A:57, 1977.

Johnson PM and McClure JG: Observations on massive osteolysis, Radiology 17:28, 1958.

Jones GB, Midgley RL, and Smith GS: Massive osteolysis—disappearing bones, J Bone Joint Surg 40:494, 1958.

Joseph J and Bartal E: Disappearing bone disease: a case report and review of the literature, J Pediatr Orthop 7:584, 1987.

Koblenzer PJ and Bukowski MJ: Angiomatosis (hamartomatous hemolymphangiomatosis), Pediatrics 65:28:65, 1961.

Kohler E et al: Hereditary osteolysis, Radiology 108:99, 1973.

Lagier R and Rutishauser E: Osteoarticular changes in a case of essential osteolysis, J Bone Joint Surg 47B:339, 1965.

Milner SM and Baker SL: Disappearing bones, J Bone Joint Surg 40:502, 1958.

Poirier H: Massive osteolysis of the humerus treated by resection and prosthetic replacement, J Bone Joint Surg 50:158, 1968.

Sacristan HD et al: Massive osteolysis of the scapula and ribs, J Bone Joint Surg 59:405, 1977.

Thompson JS and Schurman DJ: Massive osteolysis, Clin Orthop 103:206, 1974.

Tookman AG, Paice EW, and White AG: Idiopathic multicentric osteolysis with acro-osteolysis, J Bone Joint Surg 67B:86, 1985.

Torg JS and Steel HH: Sequential roentgenographic changes occurring in massive osteolysis, J Bone Joint Surg 51:1649, 1969.

Tyler T and Rosenbaum HD: Idiopathic multicentric osteolysis, Am J Radiol 126:23, 1976.

Fanconi anemia

Altay C, Sevgi Y, and Pirnar T: Fanconi's anemia in offspring of patients with congenital radial and carpal hypoplasia, N Engl J Med 293:155, 1975.

Auerbach AD, Sagi M, and Adler B: Fanconi anemia: prenatal diagnosis in 30 fetuses at risk, Pediatrics 76:794, 1985.

Deeg HJ et al: Fanconi's anemia treated by allogeneic marrow transplantation, Blood 61:954, 1983.

Erslev AJ: Hematology ed 2, New York, 1977, McGraw-Hill Book Co.

Gellis SS and Feingold M: Special feature: picture of the month, Am J Dis Child 113, 1967.

Glanz A and Fraser FC: Spectrum of anomalies in Fanconi anaemia, J Med Genet 19:412, 1982.

Gluckman E et al: Bone marrow transplantation in Fanconi anaemia, Br J Haematol 45:557, 1980.

Goldberg M: The dysmorphic child, New York, 1987, Raven Press.

Juhl JH, Wesenberg RL, and Gwinn JL: Roentgenographic findings in Fanconi's anemia, Radiology 89:646, 1967.

McDonald R and Goldschmidt B: Pancytopenia with genital defects (Fanconi's anaemia), Arch Dis Child 35:367, 1960.

Minagi H and Steinbach HL: Roentgen appearance of anomalies associated with hypoplastic anemias of childhood: Fanconi's anemia and congenital hypoplastic anemia (erythrogenesis imperfecta), Am J Radiol 97:100, 1966.

Nathan DG and Oski FA: Hematology of infancy and childhood, Philadelphia, 1987, WB Saunders Co.

Perkins J, Timson J, and Emery AE: Clinical and chromosome studies in Fanconi's aplastic anaemia, J Med Genet 6:28, 1969.

Riley E, Caldwell R, and Swift M: Comparison of clinical features in Fanconi anemia probands and their subsequently diagnosed siblings, Am J Hum Genet 31:82A, 1979.

Silver HK, Blair WC, and Kempe CH: Fanconi syndrome, Am J Dis Child 83:14, 1952.

Varela MA and Sternberg WH: Preanaemic state in Fanconi's anaemia, Lancet 2:566, 1967.

Wood VE and Adams B: Personal communication, 1988.

Thrombocytopenia–absent radius syndrome

Adeyokunnu AA: Radial aplasia and amegakaryocytic thrombocytopenia (TAR syndrome) among Nigerian children, Am J Dis Child 138:346, 1984.

Dell PC and Sheppard J: Thrombocytopenia, absent radii, Clin Orthop 162:129, 1982.

Fayen WT and Harris JW: Thrombocytopenia with absent radii (TAR syndrome), Am J Med Sci 280:95, 1980.

Goldberg M: The dysmorphic child, New York, 1987, Raven Press.

Luthy DA et al: Prenatal ultrasound diagnosis of thrombocytopenia with absent radii, Am J Obstet Gynecol 141:350, 1981.

Nathan DG and Oski FA: Hematology of infancy and childhood, Philadelphia, 1987, WB Saunders Co.

Ray R et al: Brief clinical report: lower limb anomalies in the thrombocytopenia absent–radius (TAR) syndrome, Am J Med Genet 7:523, 1980.

Schoenecker PL et al: Dysplasia of the knee associated with the syndrome of thrombocytopenia and absent radius, J Bone Joint Surg 66A:421, 1984.

Shaw S and Oliver RAM: Congenital hypoplastic thrombocytopenia with skeletal deformities of siblings, Blood 14:374, 1958.

Tolo VT: Congenital absence of the menisci and cruciate ligaments of the knee, J Bone Joint Surg 63A:1022, 1981.

9 Cervical Spine Anomalies

WILLIAM C. WARNER, JR.

ANOMALIES OF ODONTOID

Although congenital anomalies of the odontoid are rare, they can cause significant atlantoaxial instability. These anomalies usually are detected as incidental findings following trauma or when symptoms occur spontaneously. The atlantotoaxial instability may cause a compressive myelopathy, vertebral artery compression, or both.

Congenital anomalies of the odontoid can be divided into three groups: aplasia, hypoplasia, and os odontoideum. Aplasia or agenesis is complete absence of the odontoid. Hypoplasia is partial development of the odontoid, and the bone may vary from a small peglike projection to almost normal size. In os odontoideum, the odontoid is an oval or round ossicle with a smooth, sclerotic border. It is separated from the axis by a wide transverse gap, leaving the apical segment without support (Fig. 9-1). The ossicle can be of variable size and usually is located in the position of the normal odontoid (orthotopic), although occasionally it appears near the basal occiput in the area of the foramen magnum (dystopic). Because this lesion is frequently asymptomatic and remains undiscovered until brought to the physician's attention by trauma or the onset of symptoms, the exact incidence of os odontoideum is not known, but it is probably more common than appreciated. Odontoid anomalies have been reported to be more common in patients with Down syndrome, Klippel-Feil syndrome, Morquio syndrome, and spondyloepiphyseal dysplasia.

Knowledge of the embryology and vasculature of the odontoid is essential to understanding the etiologic theories of congenital anomalies of the odontoid. The odontoid is derived from mesenchyme of the first cervical vertebra. During development it becomes separated from the atlas and fuses with the axis. A vestigial disc space between C1 and C2 forms a synchondrosis within the body of the axis. The apex or tip of the odontoid is derived from the most caudal occipital sclerotome or proatlas. This separate ossification center, called ossiculum terminale, appears at age 3 years and fuses by age 12 years. Anomalies of this terminal portion are rarely of clinical significance.

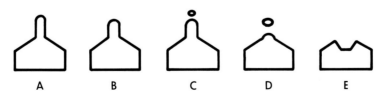

Fig. 9-1 Types of odontoid anomalies. **A,** Normal odontoid. **B,** Hypoplastic odontoid. **C,** Ossiculum terminale. **D,** Os odontoideum. **E,** Aplasia of odontoid. (Redrawn from Hensinger RN and Fielding JW. In Morrissy RT, editor: Lovell and Winter's pediatric orthopaedics, ed 3, Philadelphia, 1990, JB Lippincott Co.)

The arterial blood supply to the odontoid is derived from the vertebral and carotid arteries (Fig. 9-2). The vertebral artery gives off an anterior ascending artery and a posterior ascending artery that begin at the level of C3 and ascend anterior and posterior to the odontoid, meeting superiorly to form an apical arcade. The most rostral portion of the extracranial internal carotid artery gives off "cleft perforators," which supply the superior portion of the odontoid. This peculiar arrangement of blood supply is necessary because of the embryologic development and anatomic function of the odontoid. The synchondrosis prevents direct vascularization of the odontoid from C2, and vascularization from the blood supply of C1 cannot occur because of the synovial joint cavity surrounding the odontoid.

Both congenital and acquired causes for odontoid anomalies have been suggested. The congenital causes include failure of fusion of the apex or ossiculum terminale and failure of fusion of the odontoid to the axis, neither of which explains all the findings in os odontoideum. The ossiculum terminale is usually too small to influence stability significantly, and the theory of failure of fusion of the odontoid to the axis does not explain the fact that the space between the ossicle and the axis is at the level of the articulating facets of C2 rather than below the level of the articulating facets where the synchondrosis occurs during development. Os odontoideum can be acquired after infection, trauma, or avascular necrosis. Fielding suggests that an unrecognized fracture at the base of the odontoid is the most common cause. A distraction force by the alar ligament pulls the tip of the fractured odontoid away from its base to produce a nonunion. Tredwell and O'Brien documented 13 patients with acquired os odontoideum resulting from avascular necrosis after halo-pelvic traction.

The presentation of os odontoideum is variable. Signs and symptoms can range from minor to frank compressive myelopathy or vertebral artery compression. Presenting symptoms may be neck pain, torticollis, or headache caused by local irritation of the atlantoaxial joint. Neurologic symptoms vary from transient episodes of paresis following trauma to complete myelopathy caused by cord compression. Symptoms may consist of weakness and loss of balance with upper motor neuron signs, although upper motor neuron signs may be completely absent. Proprioceptive and sphincter disturbances are common findings. Vertebral artery compression causes cervical and brainstem ischemia resulting in seizures, syncope, vertigo, and visual disturbances. Lack of cranial nerve involvement helps differentiate os odontoideum from other occipitovertebral anomalies, since the spinal cord impingement occurs below the foramen magnum.

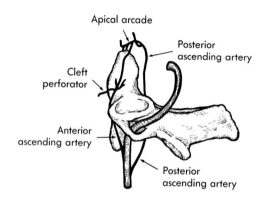

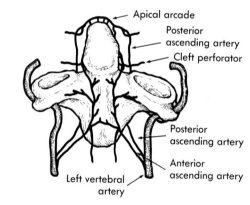

Fig. 9-2 Blood supply to odontoid: posterior and anterior ascending arteries and apical arcade. (Redrawn from Schiff DC and Parke WW: J Bone Joint Surg 55A:1450, 1973.)

Roentgenographic Findings

Odontoid anomalies can be diagnosed on a routine cervical spine roentgenographic series that includes an open-mouth odontoid view. Anteroposterior and lateral tomograms may be helpful in making the initial diagnosis of os odontoideum, and lateral flexion and extension roentgenograms and tomograms can detect any instability. Odontoid aplasia appears as a slight depression between the superior articulating facets on the open-mouth odontoid view. Odontoid hypoplasia is seen as a short bony remnant. With os odontoideum there is a space between the body of the axis and a bony ossicle. The free ossicle of os odontoideum is usually half the size of a normal odontoid and is oval or round with smooth, sclerotic borders. The space differs from that of an acute fracture, in which the space is thin and irregular instead of wide and smooth. This space should not be confused with the neurocentral synchondrosis in children younger than 5 years. The amount of instability can be documented by lateral flexion and extension plain films or tomograms that allow measurement of the amount of anterior and posterior displacement of the atlas on the axis. In children, motion between the odontoid and the body of the axis must be demonstrated before instability with os odontoideum can be diagnosed, since the ossicle is fixed to the anterior arch of C1 and moves with it during flexion and extension. Measurement of the relation of C1 to the free ossicle is of little value, since this moves as one unit. A more significant measurement is made by projecting a line superiorly from the body of the axis to a line projected inferiorly from the posterior border of the anterior arch of the atlas. Measurements of this angle greater than 3 mm in adults and 4 to 5 mm in children indicate significant instability. The space available for the spinal cord is also a very helpful measurement. This is determined by measuring the distance from the posterior aspect of the odontoid or axis to the nearest posterior structure. Fielding reported that the majority of symptomatic patients in his study had an average of 1 cm of movement. Cineradiography also may be helpful in determining motion around the C1-C2 articulation.

The prognosis of os odontoideum depends on the clinical presentation. The prognosis is good if only mechanical symptoms (torticollis or neck pain) or transient neurologic symptoms exist. It is poor if there is a slow progression of neurologic deficits.

Treatment

The primary concern in congenital anomalies of the odontoid is that an already abnormal atlantoaxial joint may subluxate or dislocate and cause permanent neurologic damage or even death with minor trauma. Patients with local symptoms usually recover with conservative treatment such as cervical traction, plaster immobilization, or a cervical orthosis. The indications for surgical stabilization are (1) neurologic involvement (even if this is transient), (2) instability greater than 5 mm anteriorly or posteriorly, (3) progressive instability, and (4) persistent neck complaints associated with atlantoaxial instability and not relieved by conservative treatment.

Prophylactic surgical stabilization of asymptomatic patients with instability less than 5 mm is controversial. Because restriction of a child's activities may be difficult if not impossible, the safety of stability without restriction of activity must be weighed against the possible complications of surgery. The decision concerning prophylactic fusion must be made after discussion with the patient and family concerning potential risks of both surgical and nonsurgical treatment.

In patients with neurologic deficits, skull traction should be used for 1 to 2 weeks before surgery to achieve reduction, allow recovery of neurologic function, and decrease spinal cord irritation. Achieving and maintaining reduction is probably the most important aspect in the treatment of this anomaly. If prophylactic fusion is performed and no reduction is needed, skull traction is applied at the time of surgery.

Before C1-C2 fusion the integrity of the posterior arch of C1 must be documented. Incomplete development of the posterior ring of C1 is uncommon (3 cases in 1000) but is reported to occur with increased frequency in patients with os odontoideum.

Atlantoaxial Fusion

There are many variations of two basic techniques of atlantoaxial fusion. The Gallie and Brooks techniques have been the most frequently used for posterior atlantoaxial fusion. The Gallie technique has the advantage of using only one wire passed beneath the lamina of C1, but tightening the wire can cause the unstable C1 vertebra to displace posteriorly and fuse in a dislocated position (Fig. 9-3). The Brooks technique has the disadvantage of requiring sublaminar wires at C1 and C2 but gives greater resistance to rotational movement, lateral bending, and extension. The size of the wire used varies from 22- to 18-gauge, depending on the age of the patient and the size of the spinal canal. In children younger than 6 years of age, wire fixation should not be used; instead the graft is placed along the decorticated fusion site and a halo or Minerva cast is used for postoperative immobilization.

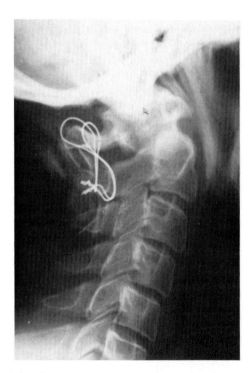

Fig. 9-3   Posterior translation of atlas after C1-C2 posterior Gallie-type fusion.

▲ *Technique (Gallie).* Carefully intubate the patient in the supine position while the patient is on a stretcher. Place the patient on the operating table in a prone position with the head supported by traction, maintaining the head-thorax relationship at all times during turning. Make a lateral cervical spine roentgenogram to ensure proper alignment before surgery.

Prepare and drape the skin in a sterile fashion, and inject a solution of epinephrine (1:500,000) intradermally to aid hemostasis. Make a midline incision from the lower occiput to the level of the lower end of the fusion, extending it deeply within the relatively avascular midline structures, the intermuscular septum or ligamentum nuchae. Take care not to expose any more than the area to be fused to decrease the chance of spontaneous extension of the fusion. By subperiosteal dissection, expose the posterior arch of the atlas and the lamina of C2. Remove the muscular and ligamentous attachments from C2 with a curet, taking care to dissect laterally along the atlas to prevent injury to the vertebral arteries and vertebral venous plexus that lie on the superior aspect of the ring of C1, less than 2 cm lateral to the midline. Expose the upper surface of C1 no farther laterally than 1.5 cm from the midline in adults and 1 cm in children. Decortication of C1 and C2 generally is not necessary. From below, pass a wire loop of appropriate size upward under the arch of the atlas either directly or with the aid of a merseline suture. The merseline suture can be passed with an aneurysm needle. Pass the free ends of the wire through the loop, grasping the arch of C1 in the loop.

Take a corticocancellous graft from the iliac crest and place it against the lamina of C2 and the arch of C1 beneath the wire. Then pass one end of the wire through the spinous process of C2, and twist the wire on itself to secure the graft in place. Irrigate the wound and close it in layers with suction drainage tubes.

Fielding has described several modifications of the Gallie fusion, as shown in Fig. 9-4.

▲ *Postoperative management.* Skeletal traction may be maintained immediately after surgery until lack of significant swelling is ensured. The patient is then immobilized in a Minerva jacket, halo vest, or a cervicothoracic orthosis. Immobilization usually is continued for 12 weeks.

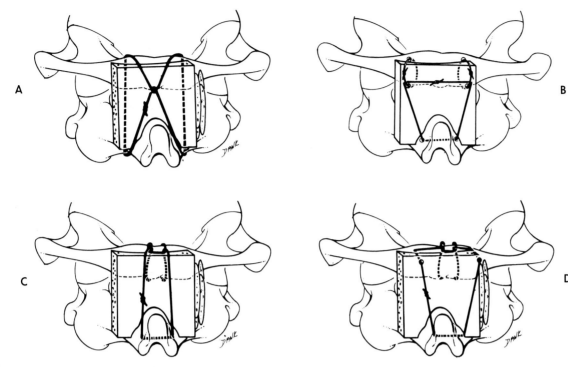

Fig. 9-4   Fielding's modifications of using wire to hold graft in place. **A,** Wire passes under lamina of atlas and axis and is tied over graft. **B,** Wire passes through holes drilled in lamina of atlas and through spine of axis; holes are drilled through graft. **C,** Wire passes under lamina of atlas and through spine of axis and is tied over graft. This method is most frequently used. **D,** Wire passes under lamina of atlas and through spine of axis; holes are drilled through graft. (From Fielding JW, Hawkins RJ, and Ratzan SA: J Bone Joint Surg 58-A:400, 1976.)

▶ *Technique (Brooks-Jenkins).* Intubate and turn the patient onto the operating table as for the Gallie technique. Prepare and drape the operative site as described. Expose C1 and C2 through a midline incision. Using an aneurysm needle, pass a merseline suture from cephalad to caudal on each side of the midline under the arch of the atlas and then beneath the lamina of C2 (Fig. 9-5, *A*). These serve as guides to introduce two doubled 20-gauge wires. The size of the wire used varies depending on the size and age of the patient. Obtain two full-thickness bone grafts approximately 1.25 by 3.5 cm from the iliac crest, and bevel them so that the apex of the graft fits in the interval between the arch of the atlas and the lamina of the axis (Fig. 9-5, *B*). Fashion notches in the upper and lower cortical surfaces to hold the circumferential wires and prevent them from slipping. Tighten the doubled wires over the graft and twist them on each side (Fig. 9-5, *C* and *D*). Irrigate and close the wound in layers over suction drains.

Postoperative management is the same as described for the Gallie technique.

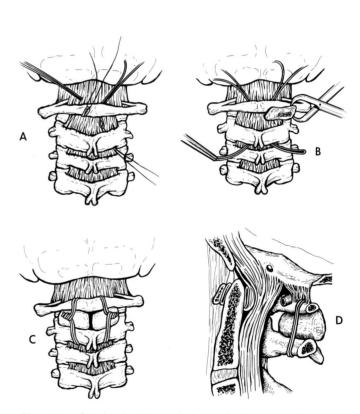

Fig. 9-5   Brooks-Jenkins technique of atlantoaxial fusion. **A,** Insertion of wires under atlas and axis. **B,** Wire in place with graft being inserted. **C** and **D,** Bone grafts secured by wires (anteroposterior and lateral views). (Redrawn from Brooks AL and Jenkins EB: J Bone Joint Surg 60A:279, 1978.)

Occipitocervical Fusion

When other bony anomalies occur at the occipitocervical junction, such as absence of posterior arch of C1, the fusion may extend up to the occiput. The following technique for occipitocervical fusion includes features of techniques described by Cone and Turner, Rogers, and Willard and Nicholson.

▶ *Technique.* Approach the base of the occiput and the spinous processes of the upper cervical vertebrae through a longitudinal midline incision, extending it deeply within the relatively avascular intermuscular septum. Expose the entire field subperiosteally. Dissect the posterior occiput laterally to the level of the external occipital protuberance. Make two burr holes in the posterior occiput about 7 mm from the foramen magnum and 10 mm lateral to the midline (Fig. 9-6). Separate the dura from the inner table of the skull by blunt dissection with a right-angled dissector. Pass short lengths of wire through the holes in the occiput and through the foramen magnum. Next pass wires beneath the posterior arch of C1 on either side if the arch is intact. Drill holes in the outer table of the spinous processes of C2 and C3, completing them with a towel clip or Lewin clamp, and pass short lengths of wire through the holes.

Obtain a corticocancellous graft from the iliac crest and make holes at appropriate intervals to accept the ends of the wires. Pass the wires through the holes in the graft and lay the graft against the occiput and the lamina of C2 and C3. Tighten the wires to hold the graft firmly in place (Fig. 9-6, *inset*). Lay thin strips of cancellous bone around the cortical grafts to aid in fusion. Inspect the graft and wires to ensure that they do not impinge on the dura or vertebral arteries. Irrigate and close the wound in layers over suction drains.

Robinson and Southwick pass individual wires beneath the lamina of C2 and C3 instead of through the spinous processes.

▶ *Postoperative management.* Some form of external support is recommended. This may vary from a Minerva jacket or halo vest to a cervicothoracic brace, depending on the degree of preoperative instability and the stability of fixation.

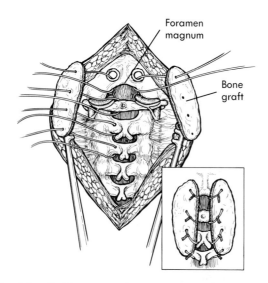

Fig. 9-6   Robinson and Southwick method of occipitocervical fusion. (Redrawn from Robinson RA and Southwick WO. The American Academy of Orthopaedic Surgeons: Instructional course lectures, vol 17, St Louis, 1960, The CV Mosby Co.)

• • •

Wertheim and Bohlman described a technique of occipitocervical fusion similar to that described by Grantham et al in which wires are passed through the outer table of the skull at the occipital protuberance instead of through both the inner and outer tables of the skull near the foramen magnum. Superior to the foramen magnum the occipital bone is very thin, but at the external occipital protuberance it is thick and allows passage of wires without passing through both tables. The transverse and superior sagittal sinuses are cephalad to the protuberance and thus are out of danger.

▲ *Technique (Wertheim and Bohlman).* Stability of the spine is obtained preoperatively with cranial skeletal traction with the patient on a turning frame or cerebellar head rest. Place the patient prone and obtain a lateral roentgenogram to document proper alignment. Prepare the skin and inject the subcutaneous tissue with a solution of epinephrine (1:500,000). Make a midline incision extending from the external occipital protuberance to the spine of the third cervical vertebra. Sharply dissect the paraspinous muscles subperiosteally with a scalpel and a periosteal elevator to expose the occiput and cervical laminae, taking special care to stay in the midline to avoid the para-

median venous plexus. At a point 2 cm above the rim of the foramen magnum, use a high-speed diamond burr to create a trough on either side of the protuberance, making a ridge in the center (Fig. 9-7, *A*). With a towel clip, make a hole in this ridge through only the outer table of bone. Loop a 20-gauge wire through the hole and around the ridge, and then loop another 20-gauge wire around the arch of the atlas. Pass a third wire through a drill hole in the base of the spinous process of the axis and around this structure, giving three separate wires to secure the bone grafts on each side of the spine (Fig. 9-7, *B*).

Expose the posterior iliac crest and obtain a thick, slightly curved graft of corticocancellous bone of premeasured length and width. Divide this horizontally into two pieces, and place three drill holes in each graft (Fig. 9-7, *C*). Decorticate the occiput and anchor the grafts in place with the wires on both sides of the spine (Fig. 9-7, *D*). Pack additional cancellous bone around and between the two grafts. Close the wound in layers over suction drains.

▲ *Postoperative management.* Either a rigid cervical orthosis or a halo cast is worn for 6 to 16 weeks, followed by a soft collar that is worn for an additional 6 weeks.

• • •

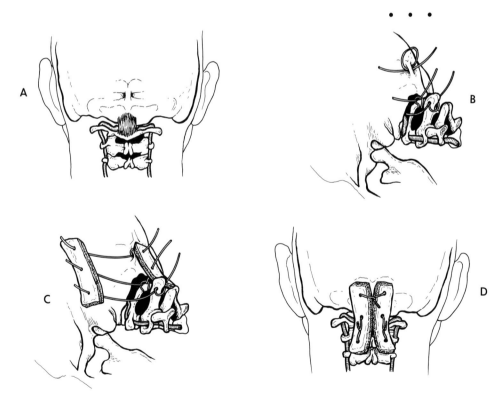

Fig. 9-7 Wertheim and Bohlman method of occipitocervical fusion. **A,** Burr is used to create ridge in external occipital protuberance, then hole is made in ridge. **B,** Wires passed through outer table of occiput, under arch of atlas, and through spinous process of axis. **C,** Grafts placed on wires. **D,** Wires tightened to secure grafts in place. (Redrawn from Wertheim SB and Bohlman HH: J Bone Joint Surg 69A:833, 1987.)

Koop, Winter, and Lonstein described a technique of occipitocervical arthrodesis without internal fixation for use in children. The spine is decorticated and autogenous corticocancellous iliac bone is placed over the area to be fused. In children with vertebral arch defects, an occipital periosteal flap is reflected over the bone defect to provide an osteogenic tissue layer for the bone grafts. A halo cast is used for postoperative stability.

▲ *Technique (Koop et al).* After the administration of endotracheal anesthesia, apply a halo with the child supine. Turn the child prone and secure the head with the neck in slight extension by securing the halo to a traction frame. Make a midline incision. In patients with intact posterior elements, expose the vertebrae by sharp dissection. Decorticate the exposed vertebral elements and lay strips of autogenous cancellous iliac bone over the decorticated bone. Take care to expose just the vertebrae to be included in the fusion. In patients with defects in the posterior elements, take care not to expose the dura if possible. At the level of the occiput, dissect the nuchal tissue from the periosteum and retract it laterally (Fig. 9-8, *A*). Then elevate the occipital periosteum in a triangular-based flap attached near the margin of the foramen magnum. Reflect this flap caudally to cover the defects in the posterior vertebral elements, and suture it in place (Fig. 9-8, *B*). Decorticate the occiput and the remaining exposed vertebral elements with an air drill (Fig. 9-8, *C*). Lay strips of autogenous cancellous bone in place over the entire area (Fig. 9-8, *D*). Close the wound in layers over a suction drain. Turn the child supine and apply a halo cast.

▲ *Postoperative management.* The halo cast is worn until union is roentgenographically evident, usually about 5 months. When union is documented by lateral flexion and extension roentgenograms, the halo cast is removed and a soft collar is worn for 1 month.

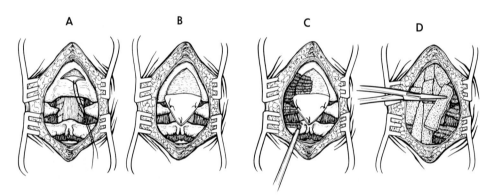

Fig. 9-8 Koop, Winter, and Lonstein method of occipitocervical fusion used when posterior arch of C1 is absent. **A,** Exposure of occiput, atlas, and axis. **B,** Reflection of periosteal flap to cover defect in atlas. **C,** Decortication of exposed vertebral elements. **D,** Placement of autogenous cancellous iliac bone grafts. (Redrawn from Koop SE, Winter RB, and Lonstein JE: J Bone Joint Surg 66A:403, 1984.)

Anterior Cervical Approaches

C1-C2 subluxation or dislocation sometimes cannot be reduced with traction. If the patient has no neurologic deficits, a simple in situ posterior fusion can be performed with little increase in risk. Posterior decompression by laminectomy has been associated with increased morbidity and mortality. Posterior decompression increases C1-C2 instability unless accompanied by fusion from the occiput to C2 or C3. If reduction of the C1-C2 dislocation is necessary, or if posterior stabilization cannot be performed because of the clinical situation, an anterior approach should be considered. A lateral retropharyngeal or a transoral approach can be used. The retropharyngeal approach usually is preferred because of the high incidence of wound complications and infection associated with the transoral approach.

Transoral approach

L *Technique (Fang).* Parenteral prophylactic antibiotics are given based upon preoperative nasopharyngeal cultures. Endotracheal intubation is achieved using a noncollapsible tube and cuff. If extensive dissection is anticipated, then a tracheostomy should be performed.

Place the patient in the Trendelenburg position, and insert a mouth gag to provide retraction. Identify the vertebral bodies by palpation. The ring of the first vertebra has a midline anterior tubercle, and the disc between the second and third vertebrae is prominent, providing another localizing landmark. Make a longitudinal incision in the midline of the posterior pharynx (Fig. 9-9, *A*). The soft palate can be divided in the midline, making postretraction paresis less likely, or it can be folded back on itself. Continue the midline dissection down to bone, and reflect the tissue laterally to the outer margin of the lateral masses of the axis (Fig. 9-9, *B*). Beyond these margins are the vertebral arteries, and care should be taken not to harm them. The soft tissue flap can be retracted using long stay sutures. After the procedure is complete, irrigate and close the wound loosely with interrupted absorbable sutures. Continue antibiotics for at least 3 days after surgery.

Fang and Ong achieved fusion by placing rectangular grafts into similarly shaped graft beds extending from the lateral mass of the atlas to the lateral mass and body of the axis. If only an anterior decompression is performed, it should be followed by a posterior fusion.

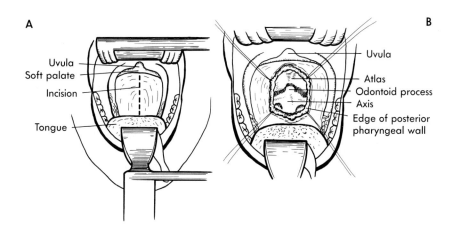

Fig. 9-9 Transoral approach to upper cervical spine for exposure of anterior aspect of atlas and axis (see text). (Redrawn from Fang HSY and Ong GB: J Bone Joint Surg 44A:1588, 1962.)

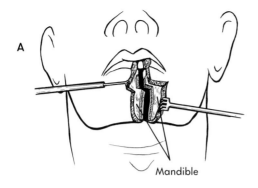

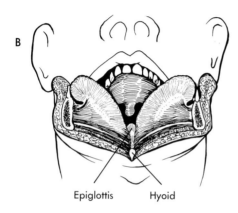

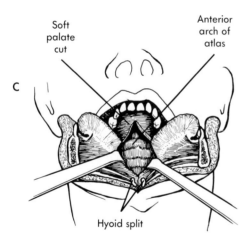

Fig. 9-10   Mandible and tongue-splitting transoral approach (see text). (Redrawn from Sherk HH and Pratt L. In Cervical Spine Research Society: The cervical spine, Philadelphia, 1983, JB Lippincott Co.)

Transoral, mandible and tongue-splitting approach

Hall, Denis, and Murray described a mandible and tongue-splitting, transoral approach to the cervical spine that gives more extensive exposure of the upper cervical spine than the approach of Fang and Ong.

▶ *Technique (Hall, Denis, and Murray).* Apply a halo cast preoperatively and perform tracheostomy through the fourth tracheal ring. Then with the patient under general anesthesia, prepare the operative field with betadine solution and drape it to exclude the halo cast and tracheostomy tube. Make an incision from the anterior gum margin through both surfaces of the lower lip and down over the middle of the mandible to the hyoid cartilage (Fig. 9-10, *A*). Divide the tongue in the midline with an electrocautery. Place traction sutures to allow better exposure of the midline raphe. Remove the lower incisor and make a step cut with an oscillating saw in the mandible. Split the tongue longitudinally to the epiglottis through its central raphe (Fig. 9-10, *B*). Fold the uvula on itself and suture it to the roof of the soft palate; retract the mandible and tongue down on each side to improve exposure. Open the mucosa over the posterior wall of the oral pharynx to expose the anterior cervical spine from the first cervical vertebra to the upper portion of the fifth cervical vertebra (Fig. 9-10, *C*). Divide the anterior longitudinal ligament in the midline and reflect it laterally to allow enough exposure for removal of the anterior portion of the cervical spine and placement of bone grafts for fusion. Fix the posterior pharyngeal flap with 3.0 chromic suture. Thread a suction drain through the nose and insert it deep into the pharyngeal flap. Repair the tongue with 2.0 and 3.0 chromic sutures and fix the mandible with wires inserted through drill holes on each side of the osteotomy. Close the infralingual mucosa with 3.0 chromic sutures, and then close the subcutaneous tissue and skin. Preoperative and postoperative antibiotics are recommended.

▶ *Postoperative management.* The halo cast is worn until fusion is evident on roentgenograms. Then the halo cast is removed and a soft collar is worn for 1 month.

Lateral retropharyngeal approach

The lateral retropharyngeal approach described by Whitesides and Kelly is an extension of the classic approach of Henry to the vertebral artery. In this approach the sternocleidomastoid muscle is everted and retracted posteriorly. The remainder of the dissection follows a plane posterior to the carotid sheath.

▶ *Technique (Whitesides and Kelly).* Make a longitudinal incision along the anterior margin of the sternocleidomastoid muscle. At the superior end of the muscle, carry the incision posteriorly across the base of the temporal bone. Divide the muscle at its mastoid origin. Partially divide the splenius capitis muscle at its insertion in the same area. At the superior pole of the incision is the external jugular vein, which crosses the anterior margin of the sternocleidomastoid; ligate and divide this vein. Branches of the auricular nerve may also be encountered and may require division. Evert the sternocleidomastoid muscle and identify the spinal accessory nerve as it approaches and passes into the muscle. Divide and ligate the vascular structures that accompany the nerve. Develop the approach posterior to the carotid sheath and anterior to the sternocleidomastoid muscle (Fig. 9-11, *A*). The transverse processes of all of the exposed cervical vertebrae are palpable in this interval. Using sharp and blunt dissection, develop the plane between the alar and prevertebral fascia along the anterior aspect of the transverse processes of the vertebral bodies. The dissection plane is anterior to the longus colli and capitis muscles, as well as the overlying sympathetic trunk and superior cervical ganglion. (An alternative approach is to elevate the longus colli and capitis muscles from their bony insertion on the transverse processes and retract the muscles anteriorly, but this approach can disrupt the sympathetic rami communications and cause Horner syndrome.) When the vertebral level is identified, make a longitudinal incision to bone through the anterior longitudinal ligament. Dissect the ligament and soft tissues subperiosteally to expose the vertebral bodies. For fusion, place corticocancellous strips in a longitudinal trough made in the vertebral bodies. Irrigate and close the wound in layers over a suction drain in the retropharyngeal space.

▶ *Postoperative management.* Because of the potential for postoperative edema and airway obstruction, the patient should be monitored closely. Traction may be required for 1 to 2 days after surgery. When the traction is removed, the patient is immobilized in a cervicothoracic brace or halo vest.

• • •

De Andrade and Macnab described an approach to the upper cervical spine that is an extension of the approach described by Robinson and Southwick and Bailey and Badgley. This approach is anterior to the sternocleidomastoid muscle (Fig. 9-11, *B*), but the dissection is anterior to the carotid sheath rather than posterior. This approach carries an increased risk of injury to the superior laryngeal nerve.

McAfee et al used a superior extension of the anterior approach of Robinson and Smith to the cervical spine. This approach provides exposure from the atlas to the body of the third cervical vertebra without the need for posterior dissection of the carotid sheath or entrance into the oral cavity and gives adequate exposure for insertion of iliac or fibular strut grafts.

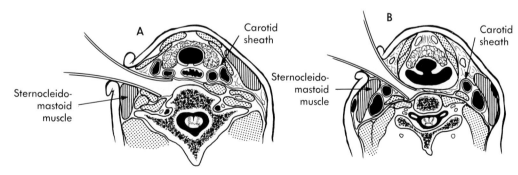

Fig. 9-11 Anterior approach to cervical spine. **A,** Whitesides and Kelly approach anterior to sternocleidomastoid muscle and posterior to carotid sheath. **B,** Approach anterior to sternocleidomastoid muscle and anteromedial to carotid sheath. (Redrawn from Whitesides TE Jr and Kelly RP: South Med J 59:879, 1966.)

▶ *Technique (McAfee et al).* Place the patient on an operative-wedge turning frame in the supine position and perform neurologic examination. Monitor the spinal cord during the operation using cortically recorded somatosensory evoked potentials. Apply Gardner-Wells tongs with 4.5 kg of traction, if not already in place. Carefully extend the neck with the patient awake. Mark the maximum point of safe extension and do not exceed this at any time during the operative procedure.

Perform fiberoptic nasotracheal intubation with the patient under local anesthesia. When the airway has been secured, place the patient under general anesthesia. Keep the mouth free of all tubes to prevent any depression of the mandible inferiorly that may compromise the operative exposure.

Make a modified transverse submandibular incision (the incision can be made on the right or left side depending on the surgeon's preference) (Fig. 9-12, *A*). As long as the dissection does not extend caudal to the fifth cervical vertebra, this exposure is sufficiently superior to the right recurrent laryngeal nerve to prevent damage to this structure. Carry the incision through the platysma muscle, and mobilize the skin and superficial fascia in the subplatysmal plane of the superficial fascia.

Locate the marginal mandibular branch of the facial nerve with the aid of a nerve stimulator and by ligating and dissecting the retromandibular veins superiorly. Branches of the mandibular nerves usually cross the retromandibular vein superficially and superiorly. By ligating this vein as it joins the internal jugular veins and by keeping the dissection deep and inferior to the vein as the exposure is extended superiorly, the superficial branches of the facial nerve are protected.

Free the anterior border of the sternocleidomastoid muscle by longitudinally transecting the superficial layer of deep cervical fascia. Locate the carotid sheath by palpation. Resect the submandibular salivary gland, and suture its duct to prevent a salivary fistula. Identify the posterior belly of the digastric muscle and the stylohyoid muscle. Divide and tag the digastric tendon for later repair. Division of the digastric and stylohyoid muscles allows mobilization of the hyoid bone and the hyopharynx medially (Fig. 9-12, *B*). Free the hypoglossal nerve from the base of the skull to the anterior border of the hypoglossal muscle, and retract it superiorly throughout the remainder of the procedure (Fig. 9-12, *C*).

Continue the dissection between the carotid sheath laterally and the larynx and pharynx anteromedially. Beginning inferiorly and progressing superiorly, the following arteries and veins may need to be ligated for exposure: the superior thyroid artery and vein, the lingual artery and vein, and the facial artery and vein. Free the superior laryngeal nerve from its origin near the nodose ganglion to its entrance into the larynx.

Transect the alar and prevertebral fascia longitudinally to expose the longus colli muscles (Fig. 9-12, *D*). Ensure orientation to the midline by noting the attachment of the right and left longus colli muscles as they converge toward the anterior tubercle of the atlas. Then detach the longus colli muscles from the anterior surface of the atlas and axis. Divide the anterior longitudinal ligament, and expose the anterior surface of the atlas and axis. Take care not to carry the dissection too far laterally and damage the vertebral artery.

McAfee shapes a fibular or bicortical iliac strut graft into the shape of a clothespin. The anterior body of C2 and the disc of C2 and C3 can be removed. Place the two prongs of the clothespin superiorly to straddle the anterior arch of the atlas. Tamp the inferior edge of the graft into the superior aspect of the body of C3, which is undercut to receive the graft. If the anterior aspect of the atlas must be removed, the superior aspect of the graft can be secured to the clivus.

Begin closure by approximation of the digastric tendon. Place suction drains in the retropharyngeal space and the subcutaneous space. Then suture the platysma and skin in the standard fashion. If the spine has been made unstable by the anterior decompression, perform a posterior cervical or occipitocervical fusion. If the hypopharynx has been inadvertently entered, have the anesthesiologist insert a nasogastric tube intraoperatively. Close the hole in two layers with absorbable sutures.

▶ *Postoperative management.* Parenteral antibiotics effective against anaerobic organisms should be added to the routine postoperative prophylactic antibiotics. The nasogastric tube is left in place for 7 to 10 days. Skull traction is maintained with the head elevated 30 degrees to reduce hypopharyngeal edema. Nasal intubation is maintained for 48 hours. If extubation is not possible in 48 to 72 hours, then a tracheostomy can be performed. Two or 4 days after surgery the Gardner-Wells tongs are removed and a halo vest is applied and is worn for about 3 months. When the halo vest is removed, a cervical collar is worn for an additional month.

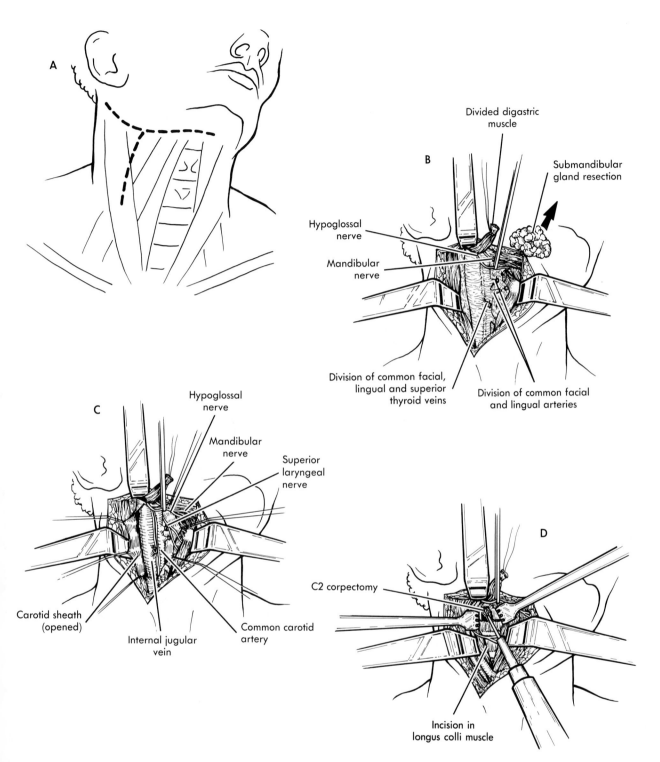

Fig. 9-12 Anterior retropharyngeal approach to upper cervical spine described by McAfee et al. **A,** Submandibular incision. Lower limb of incision is used only if midcervical vertebrae must be exposed. **B,** Submandibular gland is resected and digastric tendon is divided. Superior thyroid artery and vein also are divided. **C,** Hypoglossal nerve and superior laryngeal nerve are mobilized. Contents of carotid sheath are mobilized laterally, and hypopharynx is mobilized medially. **D,** Longus colli muscle is dissected laterally to expose anterior aspect of atlas and axis. (Redrawn from McAfee PC et al: J Bone Joint Surg 69A:1371, 1987.)

BASILAR IMPRESSION

Basilar impression (basilar invagination) is a rare deformity in which the tip of the odontoid is more cephalad than normal. The odontoid may protrude into the foramen magnum and encroach upon the brainstem, causing neurologic symptoms because of the limited space available for the brainstem and spinal cord. Neurologic damage can be caused by direct pressure from the odontoid or from other constricting structures around the foramen magnum, circulatory compromise of the vertebral arteries, or impairment of cerebrospinal fluid flow. It is important that the orthopaedist be familiar with basilar impression and its presentation because this spinal deformity is often unrecognized or misdiagnosed as a posterior fossa tumor, bulbar palsy of polio, syringomyelia, amyotrophic lateral sclerosis, spinal cord tumor, or multiple sclerosis.

Basilar impression may be either primary (congenital) or secondary (acquired). Primary basilar impression is a congenital structural abnormality of the craniocervical junction that is often associated with other vertebral defects (atlantooccipital fusion, Klippel-Feil syndrome, odontoid anomalies, hypoplasia of the atlas, and bifid posterior arch of the atlas). Secondary basilar impression is an acquired deformity of the skull resulting from systemic disease that causes softening of the osseous structures at the base of the skull, such as Paget disease, osteomalacia, rickets, osteogenesis imperfecta, rheumatoid arthritis, neurofibromatosis, and ankylosing spondylitis. Basilar impression also is frequently associated with Arnold-Chiari malformation, syringomyelia, atlantooccipital fusion, and abnormalities of the odontoid; these associated conditions may cause the predominant symptoms.

Basilar impression causes neurologic symptoms because of crowding of the neural structures as they pass through the foramen magnum. Clinical presentation is varied, and patients with severe basilar impression may be totally asymptomatic. Symptoms usually appear during the second and third decades of life, probably because of increased ligamentous laxity and instability with age and decreased tolerance to compression of the spinal cord and vertebral arteries.

Most patients with basilar impression have a short neck, asymmetry of the face or skull, and torticollis, but these findings are not specific for basilar impression and can be seen in patients with other congenital vertebral anomalies. Headache in the distribution of the greater occipital nerve is a frequent complaint. DeBarros et al divided the signs and symptoms into two categories: those caused by pure basilar impression and those caused by the Arnold-Chiari malformation. They found that symptoms caused by pure basilar impression were primarily motor and sensory disturbances, such as weakness and paresthesia in the limbs, whereas patients with Arnold-Chiari malformation had symptoms of cerebellar and vestibular disturbances, such as ataxia, dizziness, and nystagmus. Involvement of the lower cranial nerves also occurs in basilar impression. The trigeminal, vagus, glossopharyngeal, and hypoglossal nerves may be compressed as they emerge from the medulla oblongata. DeBarros et al also noted sexual disturbances, such as impotence and reduction in libido, in 27% of their patients.

Compression of the vertebral arteries as they pass through the foramen magnum is another source of symptoms. Bernini et al found a significantly higher incidence of vertebral artery anomalies in patients with basilar impression and atlantooccipital fusion. Symptoms caused by vertebral artery insufficiency, such as dizziness, seizures, mental deterioration, and syncope, can occur singly or in combination with other symptoms of basilar impression. Children with occipitocervical anomalies may be more susceptible to vertebral artery injury and brainstem ischemia; if skull traction is applied, it may further compromise the abnormal vertebral vessels.

Roentgenographic Findings

Numerous measurements have been suggested for diagnosing basilar impression, reflecting the difficulty of evaluating this area of the spine roentgenographically, and several methods of evaluation (plain roentgenograms, tomography, computed tomography [CT] scan, and magnetic resonance imaging [MRI]) may be needed to confirm the diagnosis. The most commonly used measurements are the lines of Chamberlain, McGregor, McRae, and Fischgold and Metzger. The Chamberlain, McGregor, and McRae lines are made on a lateral roentgenograms of the skull; the Fischgold and Metzger line are made on an anteroposterior view.

Chamberlain's line (Fig. 9-13) is drawn from the posterior edge of the hard palate to the posterior border of the foramen magnum. Symptomatic basilar impression may occur when the odontoid tip extends above this line. There are two disadvantages to Chamberlain's line: the posterior tip of the foramen magnum is difficult to define on the standard lateral view, and the posterior tip of the foramen magnum is often invaginated. McGregor modified Chamberlain's line by drawing a line from the upper surface of the posterior edge of the hard palate to the most caudal point of the occipital curve, which is much easier to identify on a standard lateral roentgenogram. The position of the tip of the odontoid is measured in relation to McGregor's line, and a distance of 4.5 mm above this line is considered the upper limit of normal. McRae's line determines the anteroposterior dimension of the foramen magnum and is formed by drawing a line from the anterior tip of the foramen magnum to the posterior tip. McRae observed that if the tip of the odontoid is below this line, the patient usually is asymptomatic.

The lateral lines of McGregor and Chamberlain have been criticized because the anterior reference point (the hard palate) is not part of the skull, and measurements can be distorted by an abnormal facial configuration or a high-arched palate. To prevent these problems, Fischgold and Metzger described a more accurate method of assessing basilar impression that uses an anteroposterior tomogram (Fig. 9-14). This assessment is based on a line drawn between the two digastric grooves (the junction of the medial aspect of the mastoid process at the base of the skull). Normally the digastric line passes above the odontoid tip (10.7 mm) and the atlantooccipital joint (11.6 mm).

McGregor's line is used as a routine screening test because the landmarks for this line can be defined easily on a standard lateral roentgenogram. If more information is needed, the Fischgold and Metzger digastric line is used to confirm the diagnosis of basilar impression, and McRae's line is helpful in assessing its clinical significance. McAfee recommends CT scanning and MRI for evaluation of spinal cord compression of the upper cervical spine. He states that these are complementary studies, the CT scan providing better osseous detail and the MRI providing superior soft tissue resolution. A "functional" MRI obtained with the cervical spine in flexion and then extension shows the dynamics of spinal cord compression caused by vertebral instability or anomaly.

Treatment

Conservative treatment of symptomatic patients with a collar or cervical orthosis has not been successful. Many patients with basilar impression have no neurologic symptoms, and some have minimal symptoms with no sign of progressive neurologic damage. These patients should be observed and examined periodically; surgery is indicated only if the clinical picture becomes worse. The indications for surgery are based on the clinical symptomatology and not on the degree of basilar impression. DeBarros et al found that once a patient becomes symptomatic, progression of the disease is likely.

If symptoms are caused by anterior impingement from the odontoid, stabilization in extension by an occipital C1-C2 fusion is indicated. If the odontoid cannot be reduced, an anterior excision of the odontoid can be performed after posterior stabilization. Posterior impingement requires suboccipital craniectomy and laminectomy of C1 and possibly C2 to decompress the brainstem and spinal cord. The dura should be opened during this procedure so as not to overlook a tight posterior dural band that may be causing the symptoms instead of the bony abnormalities. Posterior fusion is recommended in addition to decompression if stability is in question.

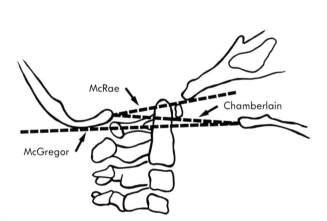

Fig. 9-13 Base of skull and upper cervical spine showing location of McRae's, McGregor's, and Chamberlain's lines. (Redrawn from Hensinger RN: Section 23, Cervical spine: pediatric. In American Academy of Orthopaedic Surgeons: Orthopaedic knowledge update I. Home study syllabus, Chicago, 1984, The Academy.)

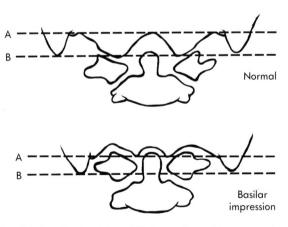

Fig. 9-14 Fischgold and Metzger lines. Line was originally drawn from lower pole of mastoid process (B), but because of variability in size of mastoid processes, they recommend line between digastric grooves (A). (Redrawn from Fielding JW, Hensinger R, and Hawkins RJ: The cervical spine. In Lovell WW and Winter RB, editors: Pediatric orthopaedics, ed 1, Philadelphia, 1978, JB Lippincott.)

ATLANTOOCCIPITAL FUSION

Atlantooccipital fusion (occipitalization) is a partial or complete congenital fusion between the atlas and the base of the occiput ranging from a complete bony fusion to a bony bridge or even a fibrous band uniting one small area of the atlas and occiput. This condition can lead to chronic atlantoaxial instability and can produce a wide range of symptoms because of spinal cord impingement and vascular compromise of the vertebral arteries. The incidence of atlantooccipital fusion has been reported to be 1.4 to 2.5/1000 children, affecting males and females equally. Symptoms usually appear in the third and fourth decades of life. Atlantooccipital fusion frequently is associated with congenital fusion between C2 and C3 (reportedly in as many as 70% of patients). Approximately half of patients with atlantooccipital fusion develop atlantoaxial instability. Kyphosis and scoliosis also are frequently associated with this deformity. Other associated congenital anomalies, such as anomalies of the jaw, incomplete cleft of the nasal cartilage, cleft palate, external ear deformities, cervical ribs, and urinary tract anomalies, occur in 20% of patients with atlantooccipital fusion.

Patients with atlantooccipital fusion commonly have a low hairline, torticollis, a short neck, and restricted neck movement. Spillane et al found that none of their patients with atlantooccipital fusion had a normal-appearing neck. Many patients complain of a dull, aching pain in the posterior occiput and the neck, with episodic neck stiffness, but symptoms vary depending on the area of spinal cord impingement. If the impingement is anterior, pyramidal tract signs and symptoms predominate; if the impingement is posterior, posterior column signs and symptoms predominate.

McRae and Barnum believe that the shape and the position of the odontoid are the keys to neurologic symptoms. When the odontoid lies above the foramen magnum, a relative or actual basilar impression is present. If the odontoid lies below the foramen magnum, the patient is usually asymptomatic. McRae found that in this condition the odontoid was excessively long and angulated posteriorly, thus decreasing the anteroposterior diameter of the spinal canal. Autopsy findings showed that the brainstem was indented by the abnormal odontoid. Anterior spinal cord compression with pyramidal tract irritation causes muscle weakness and wasting, ataxia, spasticity, pathologic reflexes (Babinski and Hoffman), and hyperreflexia. Posterior compression causes loss of deep pain, light touch, proprioception, and vibratory sensation. Nystagmus is a common finding. Cranial nerve involvement can cause diplopia, dysphagia, and auditory disturbances. Disturbances of the vertebral artery result in syncope, seizures, vertigo, and an unsteady gait.

Neurologic symptoms generally begin in the third and fourth decades of life, possibly because the older patient's spinal cord and vertebral arteries become less resistant to compression. Symptoms may be initiated by trauma or infection in the pharynx or nasopharynx.

Roentgenographic Findings

Because this anomaly ranges from complete incorporation of the atlas into the occiput to a small fibrous band connecting part of the atlas to the axis, routine roentgenograms usually are difficult to interpret, and tomograms may be needed to demonstrate the occipitocervical fusion. Most commonly the anterior arch of the atlas is assimilated into the occiput and displaced posteriorly relative to the occiput. About half of patients have a relative basilar impression caused by loss of height of the atlas. Posterior fusion is usually a small bony fringe or a fibrous band that frequently is not evident on roentgenogram. This fringe is directed downward and into the spinal canal and may cause neurologic symptoms. Flexion and extension lateral cervical spine views should be part of the initial evaluation because of the frequency of atlantoaxial instability. McRae and Barnum measured the distance from the posterior aspect of the odontoid to the posterior arch of the atlas or the posterior lip of the foramen magnum, whichever was closer. When the distance was 19 mm or less, a neurologic deficit usually was present. This measurement should be made on a flexion view because maximum narrowing of the canal usually occurs in flexion. Myelography helps detect areas of encroachment on the spinal cord or medulla and is especially useful when a constricting fibrous band occurs posteriorly. MRI also can be used to detect fibrous bands or areas of encroachment.

Treatment

Patients who have minor symptoms or become symptomatic following minor trauma or infection can be treated nonoperatively with immobilization in plaster, traction, or cervical orthosis. When neurologic symptoms occur, cervical spine fusion or decompression is indicated. Anterior symptoms usually are caused by a hypermobile odontoid; preliminary reduction of the odontoid with traction, followed by fusion from the occiput to C2, relieves the symptoms. If the odontoid is irreducible, then the appropriateness of either in situ fusion without reduction or fusion with excision of the odontoid, with its associated risks and complications, must be determined. Posterior signs and symptoms are usually caused by bony compression or compression from a dural band. When this is documented by MRI or myelogram, suboccipital craniectomy, excision of the posterior arch of the atlas, and removal of the dural band are indicated. Results from surgery have been variable.

KLIPPEL-FEIL SYNDROME

Klippel-Feil syndrome is a congenital fusion of the cervical vertebrae and can involve two segments, a congenital block vertebra, or the entire cervical spine. Congenital cervical fusion is a result of failure of normal segmentation of the cervical somites during the third to eighth week of life. The skeletal system may not be the only system affected during this time, and cardiorespiratory, genitourinary, and auditory systems frequently are involved. In most patients, the exact cause is not known. Gunderson et al showed that in a few patients this is an inherited condition, and recently maternal alcoholism has been suggested as a causative factor.

Occipitalization of the atlas, hemivertebrae, and basilar impression occur frequently in patients with Klippel-Feil syndrome, but their isolated occurrence is not considered part of this syndrome. The classic features of Klippel-Feil syndrome are a short neck, low posterior hairline, and limited range of neck motion. Patients may consult an orthopaedist because of neurologic problems, signs of instability of the cervical spine, or cosmetic reasons; however, neurologic problems and cervical instability are rare. Because many patients are asymptomatic, the actual incidence of this condition is not known, but estimates in the literature range from 1 in 42,400 births to 3 in 700. Males and females are equally affected.

Feil classified the syndrome in three types: type I, block fusion of all cervical and upper thoracic vertebrae; type II, fusion of one or two pairs of cervical vertebrae; and type III, cervical fusion in combination with lower thoracic or lumbar fusion. Minimally involved patients with Klippel-Feil syndrome lead a normal, active life with no significant restrictions or symptoms. More severely involved patients have a good prognosis if genitourinary, cardiopulmonary, and auditory problems are treated early.

Neurologic symptoms usually appear between the second and third decades of life and are caused by occipitocervical anomalies, instability, or degenerative joint and disc disease. Instability and degenerative joint disease are frequent when two fused areas are separated by a single open interspace. Patients with multiple short areas of fusion (three or more vertebrae) separated by more than one open interspace do not develop instability or degenerative joint

disease as frequently, possibly because of a more equal distribution of stress in the cervical spine. Fielding and Hensinger identified three patterns of cervical spine fusion with a potentially poor prognosis because of late instability or degenerative joint disease. Pattern 1 is fusion of C1 and C2 with occipitalization of the atlas. This pattern concentrates the motion of flexion and extension at the atlantoaxial joint; the odontoid becomes hypermobile and may dislocate posteriorly, narrowing the spinal canal and causing neurologic compromise. Pattern 2 is a long fusion with an abnormal occipitocervical junction, concentrating the forces of flexion, extension, and rotation through an abnormal odontoid or poorly developed C1 ring; with time, this abnormal articulation becomes unstable. This pattern should be differentiated from a long fusion with a normal C1-C2 articulation and occipitocervical junction. Patients with pattern 2 fusions are not at high risk for instability and neurologic problems and have a normal life expectancy. Pattern 3 is a single open interspace between two fused segments with cervical spine motion concentrated at the single open interspace, which becomes hypermobile and causes instability and degenerative joint disease. On lateral roentgenogram the cervical spine with this pattern appears to hinge at an open segment.

Associated Conditions

A variety of congenital problems have been associated with congenital fusion of the cervical vertebrae, most commonly scoliosis, renal abnormalities, Sprengel deformity, deafness, synkinesis, and congenital heart defects.

Scoliosis

The most frequent orthopaedic anomaly is scoliosis. Hensinger found that 60% of patients with Klippel-Feil syndrome had scoliosis (curves greater than 15 degrees), kyphosis, or both. Most of these patients require treatment and should be followed closely until growth is complete. If deformity is recognized early, bracing may be effective; if bracing fails, spinal stabilization is indicated. Two types of scoliosis have been identified. The first is congenital scoliosis caused by vertebral anomalies. The second occurs in a normal-appearing spine below an area of congenital scoliosis or cervical fusion; this type of curve tends to be progressive. Roentgenograms of the entire spine should be obtained, since a progressive curve may not be appreciated until significant deformity has occurred if attention is focused just on the congenital scoliosis or cervical fusion.

Renal Anomalies

About one third of patients with Klippel-Feil syndrome have urogenital anomalies. Because the cervical vertebrae and genitourinary tract differentiate at the same time and location in the embryo, fetal maldevelopment between the fourth and eighth weeks of development may produce both genitourinary anomalies and Klippel-Feil syndrome. These renal anomalies are usually asymptomatic, and children with Klippel-Feil syndrome should be evaluated with an ultrasound or intravenous pyelogram since the renal problems can be life-threatening. The most common renal anomaly is unilateral absence of the kidney. Other anomalies include absence of the hemitrigone, absence of both kidneys, absence of the ureter, ectopic kidney, horseshoe kidney, and hydronephrosis from ureteral pelvic obstruction.

Cardiovascular Anomalies

The reported incidence of cardiovascular anomalies in children with Klippel-Feil syndrome ranges from 4.2% to 14%. Ventricular septal defects, either alone or in combination, are the most frequent anomaly. Patients may have significant dyspnea and cyanosis. Other reported cardiovascular anomalies include mitral valve insufficiency, coarctation of the aorta, right-sided aorta, patent ductus arteriosus, pulmonic stenosis, dextrocardia, atrial septal defect, aplasia of the pericardium, patent foramen ovale, single atrium, single ventricle, and bicuspid pulmonic valve.

Deafness

Approximately 30% of children with Klippel-Feil syndrome have some degree of hearing loss. Several reports document conduction defects with ankylosis of the ossicles, foot plate fixation, or absence of the external auditory canal. Other reports suggest a sensorineural defect. There is no common anatomic lesion, and the hearing loss may be conductive, sensorineural, or mixed. All patients with Klippel-Feil syndrome should have audiometric testing. Early detection of hearing defects in the young child may improve speech and language development by permitting early initiation of speech and language training.

Synkinesis

Synkinesis (mirror movements) are involuntary paired movements of the hands and occasionally arms. One hand is unable to move without a similar reciprocal motion of the opposite hand. Synkinesis can be observed in normal children younger than 5 years and is present in 20% of patients with Klippel-Feil syndrome. Synkinesis may be so severe as to restrict bimanual activities. The mirror movements become less obvious with increasing age and usually are not clinically obvious after the second decade of life.

In autopsy studies, Gunderson et al observed that there was incomplete decussation of the pyramidal tract in the upper cervical spinal cord, suggesting that an alternate extrapyramidal path is required to control motion in the upper extremity. Using electromyography Baird et al showed that clinically normal patients with Klippel-Feil syndrome had electrically detectable paired motion in the opposite extremity. These patients may be more clumsy in two-handed activities and can benefit from occupational therapy to improve bimanual dexterity.

Respiratory Anomalies

Pulmonary complications involving failure of lobe formation, ectopic lungs, or restrictive lung disease resulting from a shortened trunk, scoliosis, rib fusion, and deformed costovertebral joints have been reported.

Sprengel Deformity

Sprengel deformity occurs in about 20% of patients with Klippel-Feil syndrome and can be unilateral or bilateral. Descent of the scapula coincides with the period of development of Klippel-Feil anomalies, and maldevelopment during this time (third to eighth week) may cause both anomalies. Sprengel deformity increases the unsightly appearance of an already short neck and may affect the range of shoulder motion.

Clinical Findings

The classic clinical presentation of Klippel-Feil syndrome is the triad of a low posterior hairline, a short neck, and limited neck motion (Fig. 9-15). This triad indicates almost complete cervical involvement and may be clinically evident at birth; however, fewer than half of patients with Klippel-Feil syndrome have all parts of the triad. Many patients with Klippel-Feil syndrome have a normal appearance, and the syndrome is diagnosed through incidental roentgenograms. Shortening of the neck and a low posterior hairline are not constant findings and may be overlooked; webbing of the neck (pterygium colli) is seen in severe involvement. The most constant clinical finding is limitation of neck motion. Rotation and lateral bending are affected more than flexion and extension. If fewer than three vertebrae are fused, or if the lower cervical vertebrae are fused, motion is only slightly limited. Hensinger reported that some of his patients had almost full flexion and extension through only one open interspace.

Symptoms usually are not caused by the fused cervical vertebrae but by open segments adjacent to areas of synostosis that become hypermobile in response to increased stress placed on the area. Symptoms can be caused by mechanical or neurologic problems. Mechanical problems are caused by stretching of the capsular and ligamentous structures near the hypermobile segment, resulting in early degenerative arthritis with pain localized to the neck. Neurologic problems result from direct irritation of or impingement on a nerve root or from compression of the spinal cord. Involvement of the nerve root alone causes radicular symptoms; spinal cord compression may cause spasticity, hyperreflexia, muscle weakness, and even complete paralysis.

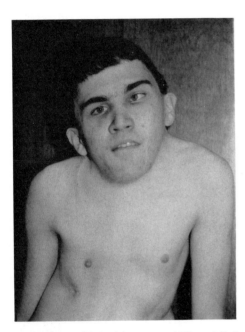 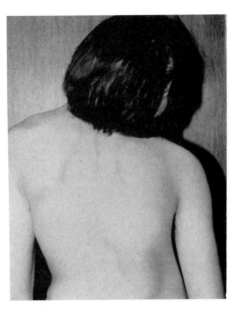

Fig. 9-15   Clinical features of Klippel-Feil syndrome in adolescent.

Roentgenographic Findings

Routine roentgenograms, tomography, cineradiography, CT scanning, and MRI may be useful in evaluation of Klippel-Feil syndrome. Adequate roentgenograms may be difficult to obtain in severely involved children, but initial examination should include anteroposterior, odontoid, and lateral flexion and extension views of the cervical spine. Lateral flexion-extension views are the most important to identify atlantoaxial instability or instability near an open segment between two congenitally fused areas (Fig. 9-16). If routine lateral roentgenograms are difficult to interpret, lateral flexion-extension tomograms should be obtained. Except for narrowing by degenerative osteophytes, the diameter of the spinal canal is normal. If there is enlargement of the spinal canal on roentgenograms, syringomyelia, hydromyelia, or Arnold-Chiari malformation should be suspected. In young patients with Klippel-Feil syndrome, serial lateral flexion-extension views should be obtained to evaluate instability at the atlantoaxial joint or at an open interspace between fused areas. Development of congenital or idiopathic scoliosis should be documented by roentgenographic examination of the entire spine. Cineradiography also is helpful in determining the amount of vertebral instability. Besides vertebral fusion, flattening and widening of involved vertebral bodies and absent disc spaces are common findings. In young children the spine may appear normal because of the lack of ossification. The posterior elements are usually the first to ossify and fuse, which aids in early diagnosis of Klippel-Feil syndrome. CT scanning is helpful for diagnosis of nerve root and spinal cord impingement by osteophyte formation. To evaluate instability and the risk of neurologic compromise, Bohlman uses a functional MRI in which images are obtained with the patient's neck flexed and extended to give much better soft tissue definition than plain roentgenograms.

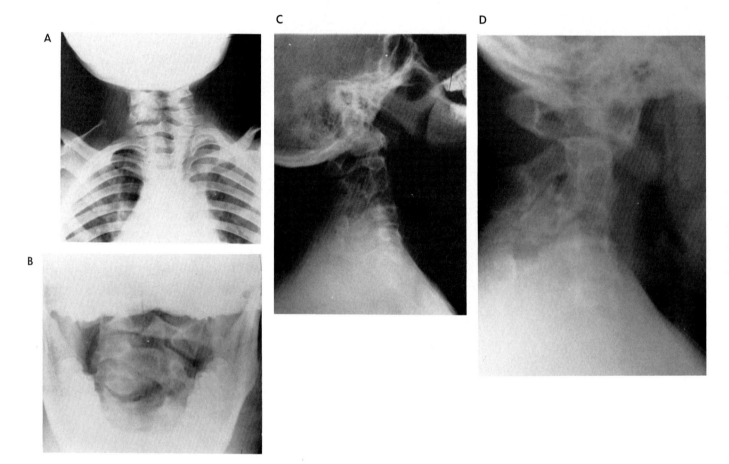

Fig. 9-16 Roentgenographic features of Klippel-Feil syndrome in adolescent. **A,** Posteroanterior view shows congenital anomalies of cervical spine and Sprengel deformity. **B,** Open-mouth odontoid view shows bony anomalies of cervical spine. **C,** Extension view shows odontoid in normal position. **D,** Flexion view shows increased atlanto-dens interval.

Treatment

Mechanical symptoms caused by degenerative joint disease usually respond to traction, a cervical collar, and analgesics. Neurologic symptoms should be carefully evaluated to locate the exact pathologic condition; surgical stabilization with or without decompression may be required. Prophylactic fusion of a hypermobile segment is controversial. The risk of neurologic compromise must be weighed against the further reduction in neck motion, and this decision must be made for each patient individually. Cosmetic improvement after surgery has been limited, but surgical correction of Sprengel deformity can significantly improve appearance, and occasionally soft tissue procedures such as Z-plasty and muscle resection improve cosmesis. Bonola described a method of rib resection to obtain an apparent increase in neck length and motion, but this is an extensive procedure with significant risk. The partial thoracoplasty is performed as a two-stage procedure: removal of the upper four ribs on one side and, after the patient has recovered from the first surgery, removal of the upper four ribs on the other side.

Posterior Fusion of C3-C7

▶ *Technique* (Fig. 9-17). Administer general anesthesia with the patient in a supine position. Turn the patient prone on the operating table, taking care to maintain traction and proper alignment of the head and neck. The head may be positioned in a head rest or maintained in skeletal traction. Obtain roentgenograms to confirm adequate alignment of the vertebrae and to localize the vertebrae to be exposed. There is a high incidence of extension of the fusion mass when extra vertebrae or spinous processes are exposed in the cervical spine. Make a midline incision over the chosen spinous processes, and expose the spinous process and lamina subperiosteally to the facet joints. If the spinous process is large enough, make a hole in the base of the spinous process with a towel clip or Lewin clamp. Pass 18-gauge wire through this hole, loop it over the spinous process, and pass it through the hole again. Make a similar hole in the base of the spinous process of the inferior vertebra to be fused. Pass the wire through this hole, loop it under the inferior aspect of the spinous process, and then pass it back through the same hole. Tighten the wire together and place corticocancellous bone grafts along the exposed lamina and spinous processes. Close the wound in layers. If the spinous process is too small to pass wires, then an in situ fusion can be performed and external immobilization used.

▶ *Postoperative management.* The patient should wear a rigid cervical orthosis until a solid fusion is documented radiographically.

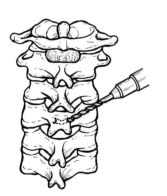
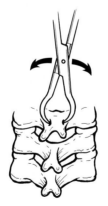
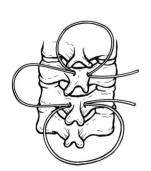
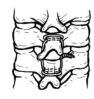
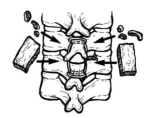

Fig. 9-17 Modified Rogers wiring of cervical spine (see text). (Redrawn from Murphy MJ and Southwick WO. In Cervical Spine Research Society: The cervical spine, Philadelphia, 1983, JB Lippincott Co.)

Rib Resection

▶ *Technique (Bonola).* Bonola performed his partial thoracoplasty with the use of local anesthesia, but general anesthesia can be used. Through a right paravertebral incision midway between the spinous processes and the medial margin of the scapula, divide the trapezius and rhomboid muscles to expose the posterior aspect of the first four ribs (Fig. 9-18, *A*). Cut these ribs with a rib cutter a few centimeters from the costovertebral joint. Continue dissection anteriorly along the ribs, dividing and removing the ribs as far anteriorly as dissection allows (Fig. 9-18, *B*). Close the wound in layers.

▶ *Postoperative management.* A cervical collar is fitted to help mold the resected area. The second stage of the procedure is performed on the opposite side after the patient has recovered from the initial surgery.

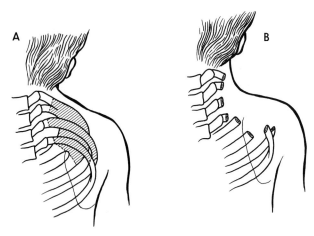

Fig. 9-18 Bonola partial thoracoplasty for treatment of short neck in Klippel-Feil syndrome (see text). (Redrawn from Bonola A: J Bone Joint Surg 38B:440, 1956.)

ATLANTOAXIAL ROTATORY SUBLUXATION

Atlantoaxial rotatory subluxation is a common cause of childhood torticollis, but the subluxation and torticollis usually are temporary. Rarely do they persist and become what is best described as atlantoaxial rotatory fixation. Atlantoaxial rotatory subluxation occurs when normal motion between the atlas and axis becomes limited or fixed and can occur spontaneously, be associated with minor trauma, or follow an upper respiratory tract infection. The cause of this subluxation is not completely understood. Watson-Jones suggested that hyperemic decalcification of the arch of the atlas causes attachments of the transverse ligaments to be inadequate, thus allowing rotatory subluxation. Coutts believes that synovial fringes become inflamed and act as an obstruction to reduction of subluxation. Firrani-Gallotta and Luzzatti believe that subluxation is caused by disruption of one or both of the alar ligaments with an intact transverse ligament. Kawabe et al recently reported a meniscus-like synovial fold in the C1-C2 facet joints that caused subluxation. They believe anatomic differences in the dens facet angle in children and adults account for this condition's appearance primarily in children. Most authors now agree that the subluxation is related to increased laxity of the alar and transverse ligaments and capsular structures caused by inflammation or trauma.

Fielding classified atlantoaxial rotatory subluxation into four types (Fig. 9-19): type I, simple rotatory displacement without anterior shift of C1; type II, rotatory displacement with an anterior shift of C1 on C2 of 5 mm or less; type III, rotatory displacement with an anterior shift of C1 on C2 greater than 5 mm; and type IV, rotatory displacement with a posterior shift. Type I displacement is the most common and occurs primarily in children. Type II is less common but has a greater potential for neurologic damage. Types III and IV are rare but have a high potential for neurologic damage.

Atlantoaxial rotatory subluxation usually occurs in children after an upper respiratory tract infection or minor or major trauma. The head is tilted to one side and rotated to the opposite side with the neck slightly flexed (the "cock robin" position). The sternocleidomastoid muscle on the long side is often in spasm in an attempt to correct this deformity. When the subluxation is acute, attempts to move the head cause pain. Patients are able to increase the deformity but cannot correct the deformity past the midline. With time, muscle spasms subside and the torticollis becomes less painful, but the deformity persists. A careful neurologic examination should determine any neurologic compression or vertebral artery compromise.

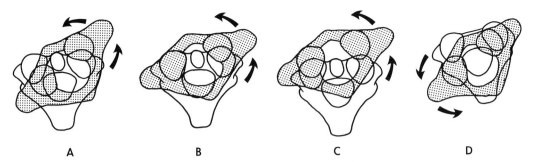

Fig. 9-19 Fielding and Hawkins classification of rotary displacement. **A,** Type I, simple rotary displacement without anterior shift; odontoid acts as pivot. **B,** Type II, rotary displacement with anterior displacement of 3 to 5 mm; lateral articular process acts as pivot. **C,** Type III, rotary displacement with anterior displacement of more than 5 mm. **D,** Type IV, rotary displacement with posterior displacement. (Redrawn from Fielding JW and Hawkins RJ Jr: J Bone Joint Surg 59A:37, 1977.)

Roentgenographic Findings

Adequate roentgenograms of the cervical spine may be difficult to obtain in children with torticollis. Initial examination should include anteroposterior and odontoid views of the cervical spine. On the open-mouth odontoid view the lateral mass that is rotated forward appears wider and closer to the midline, and the opposite lateral mass appears narrower and farther away from the midline (Fig. 9-20). One of the facet joints of the atlas and axis may be obscured by apparent overlapping. On the lateral view the anteriorly rotated lateral mass appears wedge-shaped in front of the odontoid. The posterior arch of the atlas may appear to be assimilated into the occiput because of the head tilt. Lateral flexion and extension views should be obtained to document any atlantoaxial instability. If the atlantoaxial articulation cannot be seen on routine roentgenograms, tomograms should be obtained. Cineradiography confirms the diagnosis by demonstrating the movement of atlas and axis as a single unit but is difficult to perform during the acute stage because movement of the neck is painful. Some recent reports advocate the use of dynamic CT scans in which the head is rotated as far to the left and right as possible during scanning to confirm the loss of normal rotation at the atlantoaxial joint.

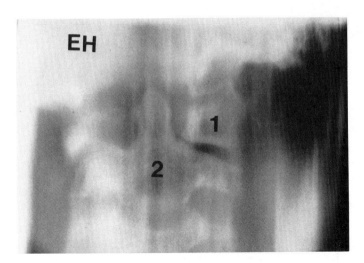

Fig. 9-20 Atlantoaxial rotatory subluxation. Note lateral masses.

Treatment

Phillips and Hensinger base their treatment plan on the duration of the subluxation. If rotatory subluxation has existed less than 1 week, immobilization in a soft collar, analgesics, and bed rest for 1 week are recommended. If reduction does not occur spontaneously, hospitalization and traction are indicated. When rotatory subluxation is present for more than 1 week but less than 1 month, hospitalization and cervical traction are indicated. Head halter traction generally is used, but when torticollis persists longer than 1 month, skeletal traction may be required. Traction is maintained until the deformity corrects, and then a cervical collar is worn for 4 to 6 weeks. Nonoperative treatment should be used only if no significant anterior displacement or instability is seen on roentgenographic evaluation.

Fielding listed as indications for operative treatment (1) neurologic involvement, (2) anterior displacement, (3) failure to achieve and maintain correction if the deformity exists for longer than 3 months, and (4) recurrence of the deformity following an adequate trial of conservative management consisting of at least 6 weeks of immobilization. When operative treatment is indicated, a C1-C2 posterior fusion is performed (Fig. 9-21). Fielding and Hawkins recommend preoperative traction for 2 to 3 weeks to correct the deformity as much as possible. Fusion is performed with the head in a neutral position. Fielding and Hawkins recommend 6 weeks of traction after surgery to maintain correction while the fusion becomes solid. This can also be accomplished with a halo cast or vest. Immobilization is continued until there is roentgenographic evidence of fusion.

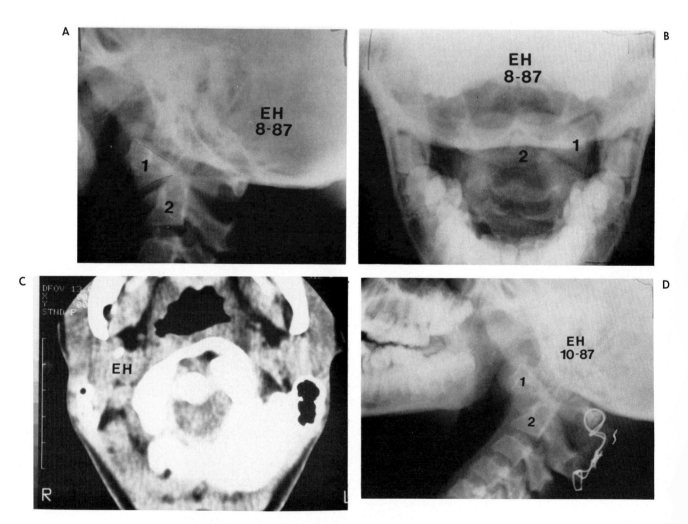

Fig. 9-21 Atlantoaxial rotatory fixation. **A,** Lateral roentgenogram shows wedge-shaped mass anterior to odontoid. **B,** Open-mouth odontoid view. **C,** CT scan. **D,** After C1-C2 in situ fusion.

REFERENCES

Surgical approaches

Bailey RW and Badgley CE: Stabilization of the cervical spine by anterior fusion, J Bone Joint Surg 42A:565, 1960.

Bonney G and Williams JPR: Trans-oral approach to the upper cervical spine: a report of 16 cases, J Bone Joint Surg 67B:691, 1985.

Brooks AL and Jenkins EB: Atlanto-axial arthrodesis by the wedge compression method, J Bone Joint Surg 60A:279, 1978.

Callahan RA et al: Cervical facet fusion for control of instability following laminectomy, J Bone Joint Surg 59A:991, 1977.

Cone W and Turner WG: The treatment of fracture-dislocation of the cervical vertebrae by skeletal traction and fusion, J Bone Joint Surg 19:584, 1937.

deAndrade JR and Macnab I: Anterior occipito-cervical fusion using an extra-pharyngeal exposure, J Bone Joint Surg 51A:1621, 1969.

Griswold DM et al: Atlanto-axial fusion for instability, J Bone Joint Surg 60A:285, 1978.

Hall JE, Denis F, and Murray J: Exposure of the upper cervical spine for spinal decompression by a mandible and tongue-splitting approach: case report, J Bone Joint Surg 59A:121, 1977.

Mayfield FH: Cervical spondylosis: a comparison of the anterior and posterior approaches, Clin Neurosurg 13:181, 1966.

Robinson RA: Fusions of the cervical spine, J Bone Joint Surg 41A:6, 1959.

Robinson RA and Smith GW: Anterolateral cervical disc removal and interbody fusion for cervical disc syndrome, Bull Johns Hopkins Hosp 96:223, 1955 [abstract].

Robinson RA and Southwick WO: Indications and technics for early stabilization of the neck in some fracture dislocations of the cervical spine, South Med J 53:565, 1960.

Rogers WA: Treatment of fracture-dislocation of the cervical spine, J Bone Joint Surg 24:245, 1942.

Rogers WA: Fractures and dislocations of the cervical spine: an end result study, J Bone Joint Surg 39A:341, 1957.

Southwick WO and Robinson RA: Surgical approaches to the vertebral bodies in the cervical and lumbar regions, J Bone Joint Surg 39A:631, 1957.

Southwick WO and Robinson RA: Recent advances in surgery of the cervical spine, Surg Clin North Am 41:1661, 1961.

White AA et al: Biomechanical analysis of clinical stability in the cervical spine, Clin Orthop 109:85, 1975.

Whitesides TE Jr and Kelly RP: Lateral approach to the upper cervical spine for anterior fusion, South Med J 59:879, 1966.

Willard D and Nicholson JT: Dislocation of the first cervical vertebra, Ann Surg 113:464, 1941.

Anomalies of the odontoid

Ahlback S and Collert S: Destruction of the odontoid process due to atlanto-axial pyogenic spondylitis, Acta Radiol [Diagn] 10:394, 1970.

Bailey DK: The normal cervical spine in infants and children, Radiology 59:712, 1952.

Bassett FH III and Goldner JL: Aplasia of the odontoid process, J Bone Joint Surg 50A:833, 1968 (abstract).

Blaw ME and Langer LO: Spinal cord compression in Morquio-Brailsford's disease, J Pediatr 74:593, 1969.

Brooks AL and Jenkins EB: Atlanto-axial arthrodesis by the wedge compression method, J Bone Joint Surg 60A:279, 1978.

Burke SW et al: Chronic atlanto-axial instability in Down syndrome, J Bone Joint Surg 67A:1356, 1985.

Callahan RA, Lockwood R, and Green B: Modified Brooks fusion for an os odontoideum associated with an incomplete posterior arch of the atlas: case report, Spine 8:107, 1983.

Davidson RG: Atlantoaxial instability in individuals with Down's syndrome: a fresh look at the evidence, Pediatrics 81:857, 1988.

Dawson EG and Smith L: Atlanto-axial subluxation in children due to vertebral anomalies, J Bone Joint Surg 61A:582, 1979.

Dyck P: Os odontoideum in children: neurological manifestations and surgical management, Neurosurgery 2:93, 1978.

Evarts CM and Lonsdale D: Ossiculum terminale: an anomaly of the odontoid process: report of a case of atlanto-axial dislocation with cord compression, Clev Clin Q 37:73, 1970.

Fang HSY and Ong GB: Direct anterior approach to the upper cervical spine, J Bone Joint Surg 44A:1588, 1962.

Fielding JW: Disappearance of the central portion of the odontoid process, J Bone Joint Surg 47A:1228, 1965.

Fielding JW: The cervical spine in the child, Curr Pract Orthop Surg 5:31, 1973.

Fielding JW and Griffin PO: Os odontoideum: an acquired lesion, J Bone Joint Surg 56A:187, 1974.

Fielding JW, Hawkins RJ, and Ratzan S: Fusion for atlantoaxial instability, J Bone Joint Surg 58A:400, 1976.

Fielding JW, Hensinger RN, and Hawkins RJ: Os odontoideum, J Bone Joint Surg 62A:376, 1980.

Ford FR: Syncope, vertigo and disturbances of vision resulting from intermittent obstruction of the vertebral arteries due to defect in the odontoid process and excessive mobility of the second cervical vertebra, Bull Johns Hopkins Hosp 91:168, 1952.

Freiberger RH, Wilson PD Jr, and Nicholas JA: Acquired absence of the odontoid process: a case report, J Bone Joint Surg 47A:1231, 1965.

French HG et al: Upper cervical ossicles in Down syndrome, J Pediatr Orthop 7:69, 1987.

Gamble JG and Rinsky LA: Combined occipitoatlantoaxial hypermobility with anterior and posterior arch defects of the atlas in Pierre-Robin syndrome, J Pediatr Orthop 5:475, 1985.

Garber JN: Abnormalities of the atlas and axis vertebrae: congenital and traumatic, J Bone Joint Surg 47A:1782, 1964.

Giannestras NJ et al: Congenital absence of the odontoid process: a case report, J Bone Joint Surg 46A:839, 1964.

Granger DK and Rechtine GR: Os odontoideum: a review, Orthop Rev 16:909, 1987.

Grantham SA et al: Occipitocervical arthrodesis: indications, technic, and results, Clin Orthop 65:118, 1969.

Hawkins RJ, Fielding FW, and Thompson WJ: Os odontoideum: congenital or acquired, J Bone Joint Surg 58A:413, 1976.

Hensinger RN: Osseous anomalies of the craniovertebral junction, Spine 11:323, 1986.

Koop SE, Winter RB, and Lonstein JE: The surgical treatment of instability of the upper part of the cervical spine in children and adolescents, J Bone Joint Surg 66A:403, 1984.

McAfee PC et al: The anterior retropharyngeal approach to the upper part of the cervical spine, J Bone Joint Surg 69A:1371, 1987.

Nicholson JS and Sherk HH: Anomalies of the occipitocervical articulation, J Bone Joint Surg 50A:295, 1968.

Pueschel SM and Scola FH: Atlantoaxial instability in individuals with Down's syndrome: epidemiologic, radiographic, and clinical studies, Pediatrics 80:555, 1987.

Robinson RA and Southwick WO: Surgical approaches to the cervical spine. In The American Academy of Orthopaedic Surgeons: Instructional course lectures, vol 17, St Louis, 1960, The CV Mosby Co.

Sherk HH and Pratt L: Transoral approaches. In Cervical Spine Research Society: The cervical spine, Philadelphia, 1983, JB Lippincott Co.

Swischuk LE, Hayden CK, and Sarwar M: The posteriorly tilted dens: a normal variation mimicking a fractured dens, Pediatr Radiol 8:27, 1979.

Tredwell SJ and O'Brien JP: Avascular necrosis of the proximal end of the dens: a complication of halo-pelvic distraction, J Bone Joint Surg 57A:332, 1975.

VanGilder JC and Menezes AH: Craniovertebral abnormalities and their treatment. In Schmidek HH, Sweet WH, editors: Operative neurosurgical techniques, ed 2, New York, 1988, Grune & Stratton.

Wertheim SB and Bohlman HH: Occipitocervical fusion: indications, technique, and long-term results in thirteen patients, J Bone Joint Surg 69A:833, 1987.

Whitesides TE Jr and Kelly RP: Lateral approach to the upper cervical spine for anterior fusion, South Med J 59:879, 1966.

Basilar impression

Adam AM: Skull radiograph measurements of normals and patients with basilar impression: use of Landzert's angle, Surg Radiol Anat 9:225, 1987.

Bernini F et al: Angiographic study on the vertebral artery in cases of deformities of the occipitocervical joint, AJR 107:526, 1969.

Bull J, Nixon WLB, and Pratt RTC: The radiological criteria and familial occurrence of primary basilar impression, Brain 78:229, 1955.

Chakrabarti AK et al: Osteomalacia, myopathy and basilar impression, J Neurol Sci 23:227, 1974.

Chamberlain WE: Basilar impression (platybasia): a bizzare developmental anomaly of the occipital bone and upper cervical spine with striking and misleading neurologic manifestations, Yale J Biol Med 11:487, 1939.

DeBarros MC et al: Basilar impression and Arnold-Chiari malformation: a study of 66 cases, J Neurol Neurosurg Psychiatry 31:596, 1968.

DeBarros MC et al: Disturbances of sexual potency in patients with basilar impression and Arnold-Chiari malformation, J Neurol Neurosurg Psychiatry 38:598, 1975.

DirHeimeri Y and Babin E: Basilar impression and hereditary fragility of the bones, Neuroradiology 3:41, 1971.

Dolan KD: Cervico-vasilar relationships, Radiol Clin North Am 15:155, 1977.

Epstein BS and Epstein JA: The association of cerebellar tonsillar herniation with basilar impression incident to Paget's disease, Am J Roentgenol 107:535, 1969.

Fielding JW, Hensinger R, and Hawkins RJ: The cervical spine. In Lovell WW and Winter RB: Pediatric orthopaedics, ed 2, Philadelphia, 1986, JB Lippincott Co.

Fischgold H and Metzger J: Etude radiotomographique de l'impression basilaire, Rev Rhum Mal Osteoartic 19:261, 1952.

Hensinger RN: Osseous anomalies of the craniovertebral junction, Spine 11:323, 1986.

Hensinger RN, Lang JR, and MacEwen GD: The Klippel-Feil syndrome: a constellation of related anomalies, J Bone Joint Surg 56A:1246, 1974.

Hensinger RN and MacEwen GD: Congenital anomalies of the spine. In Rothman RH and Simeone FA, editors: The spine, ed 2, Philadelphia, 1982, WB Saunders Co.

Hinck VC, Hopkins CE, and Savara BS: Diagnostic criteria of basilar impression, Radiology 76:572, 1961.

Kulkarni MV et al: Magnetic resonance imaging in the diagnosis of the cranio-cervical manifestations of the mucopolysaccharidoses, MRI 5:317, 1987.

Lee CK and Weiss AB: Isolated congenital cervical block vertebrae below the axis with neurological symptoms, Spine 6:118, 1981.

McAfee PC et al: Comparison of nuclear magnetic resonance imaging and computed tomography in the diagnosis of upper cervical spinal cord compression, Spine 11:295, 1986.

McGregor M: The significance of certain measurements of the skull in the diagnosis of basilar impression, Br J Radiol 21:171, 1948.

Raynor RB: Congenital malformations of the base of the skull. In Cervical Spine Research Society: The cervical spine, Philadelphia, 1983, JB Lippincott Co.

Teodori JB and Painter MJ: Basilar impression in children, Pediatrics 74:1097, 1984.

Atlantooccipital fusion

Bharucha EP and Dastur HM: Craniovertebral anomalies (a report of 40 cases), Brain 87:469, 1964.

Hensinger RN: Atlantooccipital fusion. In Cervical Spine Research Society: The cervical spine, Philadelphia, 1983, JB Lippincott Co.

McRae DL: Bony abnormalities in the region of the foramen magnum: correlation of the anatomic and neurologic findings, Acta Radiol 40:335, 1953.

McRae DL: The significance of abnormalities of the cervical spine, Am J Roentgenol 84:3, 1960.

McRae DL and Barnum AS: Occipitalization of the atlas, Am J Roentgenol 70:23, 1953.

Nicholson JT and Sherk HH: Anomalies of the occipito-cervical articulation, J Bone Joint Surg 50A:295, 1968.

Spillane JD, Pallis C, and Jones AM: Developmental abnormalities in the region of the foramen magnum, Brain 80:11, 1957.

Watson AG and Mayhew IG: Familial congenital occipitoatlantoaxial malformation (OAAM) in the Arabian horse, Spine 11:334, 1986.

Klippel-Feil syndrome

Avery LW and Rentfro CC: The Klippel-Feil syndrome: a pathologic report, Arch Neurol Psych 36:1068, 1936.

Baga N, Chusid EL, and Miller A: Pulmonary disability in the Klippel-Feil syndrome, Clin Orthop 67:105, 1969.

Baird PA, Robinson CG, Buckler WSJ: Klippel-Feil syndrome, Am J Dis Child 113:546, 1967.

Bonola A: Surgical treatment of the Klippel-Feil syndrome, J Bone Joint Surg 38B:440, 1956.

Cattell HS and Filtzer DL: Pseudosubluxation and other normal variations in the cervical spine in children, J Bone Joint Surg 47A:1295, 1965.

Drvaric DM et al: Congenital scoliosis and urinary tract abnormalities: are intravenous pyelograms necessary? J Pediatr Orthop 7:441, 1987.

Dubousset J: Torticollis in children caused by congenital anomalies of the atlas, J Bone Joint Surg 68A:178, 1986.

Feil A: L'absence et la dimunution des vertebres cervicales (etude clinique et pathogenique): le syndrome de reduction numerique cervicale, Theses de Paris, 1919.

Fielding JW, Hensinger RN, and Hawkins RJ: The cervical spine. In Lovell WW and Winter RB, editors: Pediatric orthopaedics, ed 2, Philadelphia, 1986, JB Lippincott Co.

Gheehr RB, Rothman SLG, and Kier EL: The role of computed tomography in the evaluation of upper cervical spine pathology, Comput Tomogr 2:79, 1978.

Gunderson CH and Soltaire GB: Mirror movements in patients with the Klippel-Feil syndrome: neuropathic observations, Arch Neurol 18:675, 1968.

Gunderson CH et al: Klippel-Feil syndrome: genetic and clinical reevaluation of cervical fusion, Medicine 46:491, 1967.

Hensinger RN: Congenital anomalies of the atlantoaxial joint. In Cervical Spine Research Society: The cervical spine, Philadelphia, 1983, JB Lippincott Co.

Hensinger RN: Congenital anomalies of the odontoid. In Cervical Spine Research Society: The cervical spine, Philadelphia, 1983, JB Lippincott Co.

Hensinger RN, Fielding JW, and Hawkins RJ: Congenital anomalies of the odontoid process, Orthop Clin North Am 9:901, 1978.

Hensinger RN, Lang JR, and MacEwen EG: Klippel-Feil syndrome: a constellation of associated anomalies, J Bone Joint Surg 56A:1246, 1974.

Klippel M and Feil A: Un cas d'absence des vertebres cervicales avec cage thoracique remontant jusqu'a la base du crane, Nouv Icon Salpetriere 25:223, 1912.

Kulkarni MV et al: Magnetic resonance imaging in the diagnosis of the cranio-cervical manifestations of the mucopolysaccharidoses, MRI 5:317, 1987.

Lee CK and Weiss AB: Isolated congenital cervical block vertebrae below the axis with neurological symptoms, Spine 6:118, 1981.

MacEwen GD, Winter RB, and Hardy JH: Evaluation of kidney anomalies in congenital scoliosis, J Bone Joint Surg 54A:1451, 1972.

Michie I and Clark M: Neurological syndromes associated with cervical and craniocervical anomalies, Arch Neurol 18:241, 1968.

Moore WB, Matthews TJ, and Rabinowitz R: Genitourinary anomalies associated with Klippel-Feil syndrome, J Bone Joint Surg 57A:335, 1975.

Nagashima C: Atlanto-axial dislocation due to agenesis of the os odontioideum or odontoid, J Neurosurg 33:270, 1970.

Pizzutillo PD: Klippel-Feil syndrome. In Cervical Spine Research Society: The cervical spine, Philadelphia, 1983, JB Lippincott Co.

Pizzutillo PD, Woods MW, and Nicholson L: Risk factors in the Klippel-Feil syndrome, Orthop Trans 11:473, 1987 Co.

Raynor RB: Congenital malformations of the base of the skull. In Cervical Spine Research Society: The cervical spine, Philadelphia, 1983, JB Lippincott Co.

Roach JW et al: Atlanto-axial instability and spinal cord compression in children: diagnosis by computerized tomography, J Bone Joint Surg 66A:708, 1984.

Sherk HH and Dawoud S: Congenital os odontoideum with Klippel-Feil syndrome and fatal atlanto-axial instability: report of a case, Spine 6:42, 1981.

Sherk HH, Shut L, and Chung S: Iniencephalic deformity of the cervical spine with Klippel-Feil anomalies and congenital elevation of the scapula: report of three cases, J Bone Joint Surg 56A:1254, 1974.

Shoul MI and Ritvo M: Clinical and roentgenological manifestations of the Klippel-Feil syndrome (congenital fusion of the cervical vertebrae, brevicollis): report of eight additional cases and review of the literature, Am J Roentgenol 68:369, 1952.

Southwell RB et al: Klippel-Feil syndrome with cervical cord compression resulting from cervical subluxation in association with an omovertebral bone Spine 5:480, 1980.

Spierings ELH and Braakman R: The management of os odontoideum: analysis of 37 cases, J Bone Joint Surg 64B:422, 1982.

Tori JA and Dickson JH: Association of congenital anomalies of the spine and kidneys, Clin Orthop 148:259, 1980.

Tredwell SJ et al: Cervical spine anomalies in fetal alcohol syndrome, Spine 7:331, 1982.

Whittle IR and Besser M: Congenital neural abnormalities presenting with mirror movements in a patient with Klippel-Feil syndrome: case report, J Neurosurg 59:891, 1983.

Yousefzadeh DK, El-Khoury GY, and Smith WL: Normal sagittal diameter and variation in the pediatric cervical spine, Pediatr Radiol 144:319, 1982.

Atlantoaxial rotatory subluxation

Coutts MB: Atlanto-epiphyseal subluxations, Arch Surg 29:297, 1934.

Fielding JW: The cervical spine in the child, Curr Pract Orthop Surg 5:31, 1973.

Fielding JW and Hawkins RJ: Atlanto-axial rotatory fixation (fixed rotatory subluxation of the atlanto-axial joint); J Bone Joint Surg 59A:37, 1977.

Fielding JW, Hawkins RJ, and Ratzan S: Fusion for atlantoaxial instability, J Bone Joint Surg 58A:400, 1976.

Firrani-Gallotta G and Luzzatti G: Sublussazione laterale e sublussazione rotatorie dell'atlante, Arch Orthop Trauma Surg 70:467, 1957.

Georgopoulos G, Pizzutillo PD, and Lee MS: Occipito-atlantal instability in children: a report of five cases and review of the literature, J Bone Joint Surg 69A:429, 1987.

Hensinger RN, DeVito PD, and Ragsdale CG: Changes in the cervical spine in juvenile rheumatoid arthritis, J Bone Joint Surg 68A:189, 1986.

Hohl M and Baker HR: The atlantoaxial joint: roentgenographic and anatomical study of the normal and abnormal motion, J Bone Joint Surg 46A:1739, 1964.

Kawabe N, Hirotani H, and Tanaka O: Pathomechanism of atlanto-axial rotatory fixation in children, J Pediatr Orthop 9:569, 1989.

Phillips WA and Hensinger RN: The management of rotatory atlantoaxial subluxation in children, J Bone Joint Surg 71A:664, 1989.

Watson-Jones R: Spontaneous hyperaemic dislocation of the atlas, Proc R Soc Med 25:586, 1931.

10 The Pediatric Spine

Barney L. Freeman III

This chapter discusses deformities and diseases that involve mainly the thoracic and lumbar spine regions. The deformities and diseases are for the most part organized according to the outline prepared by the Terminology Committee of the Scoliosis Research Society. The various surgical and casting techniques are discussed in association with the condition for which they generally are performed.

Scoliosis

Scoliosis is a lateral curvature of the spine. Structural curves are those in which lateral bending of the spine is asymmetric or the involved vertebrae are fixed in a rotated position, or both. The patient either is unable to correct the curve or is unable to maintain correction. Lateral bending is asymmetric when the long, gentle curve formed by the entire spine on bending to either side is asymmetric in some way, either in the areas that bend or in the degree of bending. Nonstructural curves, in contrast, are those in which intrinsic changes in the spine or its supporting structures are absent. In these curves lateral bending is symmetric and the involved vertebrae are not fixed in a rotated position. Generally, a nonstructural curve requires no treatment; if any is required, treatment is directed toward the cause, which is not located in the spine itself. This chapter discusses structural problems involving the spine.

INFANTILE IDIOPATHIC SCOLIOSIS

Infantile idiopathic scoliosis is a structural, lateral curvature of the spine with its onset occurring in patients before 3 years of age. James is credited with the use of the term *infantile idiopathic scoliosis.* He noted that these curves occurred before 3 years of age and were more frequent in boys than in girls and that the curves were primarily thoracic and convex to the left.

Wynne-Davies noted plagiocephaly in 97 children in whom curves developed in the first 6 months of life; the flat side of the head was on the convex side of the curve. She also found the occurrence of mental retardation in 13% and inguinal hernias in 7.4% of boys with progressive scoliosis and congenital dislocation of the hip in 3.5% and congenital heart disease in 2.5% of all patients. This led her to believe that the etiologic factors of infantile idiopathic scoliosis are likely to be multiple, with a genetic tendency that is either "triggered" or prevented by external factors.

There are two types of infantile idiopathic scoliosis: progressive, which usually increases rapidly, and resolving (or structural resolving), which resolves spontaneously within a few years with or without treatment. The resolving type occurs in 70% to 90% of patients with infantile idiopathic scoliosis. Unfortunately, when a curve is mild, no absolute criteria are available for differentiating the two types. According to James, when compensatory or secondary curves develop or when the curve measures more than 37 degrees by the Cobb method when first seen, the scoliosis is probably progressive. Conversely, if the curve measures only 10 to 15 degrees when first seen, it probably is resolving scoliosis. Mehta developed a method for differentiating resolving from progressive curves in infantile idiopathic scoliosis. Her method is based on the development of the rib-vertebral angle (RVA). The RVA is measured by drawing one line perpendicular to the apical vertebral end plate and another from the midneck to the midhead of the corresponding rib. The angle formed by the intersection of these lines is the RVA (Fig. 10-1). The RVA difference (RVAD) is the difference between the values of the RVAs on the concave and the convex sides of the curve. Mehta found the RVAD was consis-

tently greater in progressive curves. Any curve with an initial RVAD of 20 degrees or more is considered progressive until proved otherwise. Thus whether or not a given curve is progressive can be determined by observing it for only a few months.

Treatment

Treatment of infantile scoliosis is determined by the type of curve. Resolving curves (with an RVAD of less than 20 degrees) and flexible curves (with an RVAD of less than 20 degrees) require observation only, with examination and roentgenograms every 4 to 6 months until the curve resolves.

If the RVAD is greater than 20 degrees and the curve is not flexible on clinical examination, it is considered progressive until proved otherwise. Frequently, an efficient orthotist can make a satisfactory Milwaukee brace for a child younger than 3 years of age. If the Milwaukee brace is fitted satisfactorily, progression of many infantile curves can be prevented and significant improvement often can be obtained during the early period of skeletal growth. If the curve is severe or increases despite the use of a Milwaukee brace, a relatively short fusion, including only the structural or primary curve, probably is the best treatment. The spine still must be controlled by a Milwaukee brace until growth is complete. Moe et al described the use of a subcutaneous Harrington rod without fusion followed by a full-time external orthosis in certain flexible curves in growing children. With the use of the "shortening formula" (0.07 times the number of segments fused times the number of years of growth), the average shortening in their patients would have been 4.5 cm had fusion been performed. The authors noted an average length gain in the instrumented area of 3.8 cm for nine patients who ultimately underwent fusion. Complications, most frequently hook dislocation and rod breakage, occurred in 50% of patients.

Subcutaneous Harrington Instrumentation

◣ *Technique (Moe et al).* Place the patient prone on the operating table or frame; prepare and drape the back in the routine sterile fashion. Take care to select the neutral vertebrae at both ends of the curve, and make two small incisions over the lamina after infiltration of 1:500,000 epinephrine. Make a single, long, straight incision into the subcutaneous tissue to facilitate placement of the rod. With roentgenographic guidance, carry the dissection down to the lamina and spinous process of the vertebra on the concave side of the curve. Strip the periosteum from the concave lamina out to the facet joint at each of the two sites selected for hook insertion. Strip the ligamentum flavum from the underside of the lamina se-

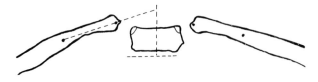

Fig. 10-1 Construction of rib-vertebral angle (RVA). (From Mehta MH: J Bone Joint Surg 54B:232[2], 1972.)

lected to receive the appropriate hook at each end. In small children a special pediatric hook is used; otherwise, the No. 1254 hook, which is not sharp, is preferred. Then place a subcutaneous rod of the estimated length with one nut attached to each end for future lengthening deep in the subcutaneous tissues, superficial to the erector muscles of the spine. Before insertion, bend the rod to fit the natural contours of thoracic kyphosis and lumbar lordosis. After the subcutaneous rod is placed through the hole in each hook, tighten the nuts over the ends of both hooks, applying distraction. Destroy the threads adjacent to the nuts to prevent the nuts from spinning down, causing loss of correction. For very soft bones or deficient laminae, add bone chips at the decorticated hook sites to allow solid bone block formation and to prevent disruption of the laminae. A "wake-up" test or spinal cord monitoring is used.

▶ *Postoperative management.* The patient is placed in a previously prescribed and manufactured Milwaukee brace for full-time external support. Ambulation is begun within 48 hours, and the patient usually is discharged on the following day.

Anteroposterior and lateral roentgenograms are obtained 4 to 6 months after insertion of the subcutaneous rod. If the curve has outgrown the rod with a loss of correction of 10 degrees or more, the rod is lengthened. When the Moe modified subcutaneous rod is used, a short incision is made at one or both ends, and after thorough cleaning of the surface of the rod, lengthening is performed by further tightening the nuts. The threads immediately behind the nut are destroyed to avoid nut slippage and loss of correction. Roentgenograms are again obtained 4 to 6 months after rod lengthening. If maximum lengthening of the initial rod has been reached, it is removed, leaving the hooks intact. A new, longer rod is inserted through the same subcutaneous channel into both hooks and is tightened. The threads adjacent to the nuts are destroyed to prevent slippage and loss of correction. Subsequently, rods are lengthened or replaced as required while the Milwaukee brace is adjusted according to growth. The brace is worn full-time until spinal fusion with Harrington rod instrumentation is performed.

JUVENILE IDIOPATHIC SCOLIOSIS

Juvenile idiopathic scoliosis appears between the ages of 4 and 10 years and affects approximately 15% of all patients with idiopathic scoliosis. Multiple curve patterns can occur, but the convexity of the thoracic curve is usually to the right.

The treatment of juvenile idiopathic scoliosis follows guidelines similar to those for adolescent idiopathic scoliosis. For curves of less than 20 degrees, observation is indicated, with examination and standing posteroanterior roentgenograms every 4 to 6 months. The success of nonoperative treatment is variable. In the series of Figueiredo and James, 44% of patients were successfully managed conservatively; 56% required spinal fusion. In Tolo's series, 27% of patients required surgical fusion for progressive curves. Tolo and Gillespie found that it was not possible to predict which curves would increase from the curve pattern, the degree of curvature, or the patient's age at the time of diagnosis. Although they found the initial RVAD measurement of only limited value, serial measurements were useful to evaluate brace treatment. From their experience they formulated the following guidelines. If the RVAD does not go below more than 10 degrees during brace wear, progression can be expected. If the RVAD values decline as treatment continues, a part-time Milwaukee brace wear should be adequate. Those curves with RVAD values near or below 0 at the time of diagnosis generally require only a relatively short period of full-time brace wear before part-time brace wear is begun. Tolo and Gillespie recommend that, unless the curve is quite advanced when the juvenile patient is first seen, evidence of progression be obtained before a Milwaukee brace is applied because some curves, even in the range of 20 to 30 degrees, did not progress over a period of several months.

If orthotic treatment does not halt curve progression, surgical stabilization is indicated. If the curve progresses beyond 60 degrees despite orthotic treatment, fusion of the major curve should be performed. A solid fusion usually prevents curve progression, although protection of the immature fusion mass by a brace may be necessary to prevent deformation with growth. The area of the fusion is selected as described for adolescent idiopathic scoliosis, and a Moe fusion with Harrington distraction instrumentation usually is performed (p. 478).

ADOLESCENT IDIOPATHIC SCOLIOSIS
Incidence and Natural History

A knowledge of the natural history and incidence of idiopathic scoliosis is essential to determine if and when treatment is necessary. Three important questions need to be answered:

1. What is the incidence of idiopathic scoliosis in the general population?
2. What is the likelihood of curve progression necessitating treatment in the adolescent with scoliosis?
3. What problems may occur in adult life if scoliosis is left untreated and the curve progresses?

Kane summarized the prevalence of larger curves in the normal population: on the average the incidence of curves greater than 20 degrees is 5:1000 adults; curves greater than 30 degrees, 2:1000; and curves greater than 40 degrees, 1:1000. The importance of these findings is that small degrees of scoliosis are very common, but most curves do not require treatment. In younger patients with small curves, the incidence is almost equal in boys and girls. Beyond 10 or 11 years of age, however, 80% of patients with significant curves (greater than 20 degrees) are girls.

Once scoliosis is discovered in the adolescent, the curve must be evaluated for the probability of progression. Prognostic factors have been summarized by Rogala et al and by Bunnell. Spontaneous improvement occurs in 3% of adolescents with idiopathic scoliosis, the majority of whom have curves of less than 11 degrees. Treatment in the form of bracing or surgery is required in 2.75:1000 students screened. Progression is far more likely in girls than in boys. In Bunnell's series of 123 patients with curves averaging 33 degrees, the risk of progression greater than 5 degrees is 77% for patients with thoracic curves, 67% for those with thoracolumbar curves, 30% for those with lumbar curves, and 66% for those with double curves. The larger the curve when first seen, the more likely is progression. The most significant prognosticators of curve progression are those related to the patient's growth potential: the age at onset, the occurrence of menarche in girls, and skeletal age as determined by the Risser sign. Curves diagnosed in patients younger than 10 years of age have an 88% risk of progression, whereas those diagnosed in patients older than 15 years of age have a 29% risk. Of curves diagnosed in patients before the onset of menses, 53% progress 10 degrees or more, whereas only 11% of those diagnosed after menarche progress 10 degrees or more. A patient with a Risser sign of 0 at the time of diagnosis has a 68% risk of curve progression of 10 degrees or more. This risk is decreased to 18% for those with a Risser sign of 3 or 4.

The effect of progressive curves on adults with untreated scoliosis has been studied by several investigators, including Ponseti and Friedman, Nilsonne and Lundgren, Nachemson, Ascani et al, and Weinstein and Ponseti. These studies indicate that larger curves, particularly those between 50 and 80 degrees, can be expected to progress in adult life. Back pain is common in adults with untreated idiopathic scoliosis, but whether it is disabling is arguable. Recently, however, there has been an increase in the number of adults with untreated idiopathic scoliosis who complain of increasingly disabling back symptoms, especially those with thoracolumbar and lumbar curves. Smaller curves, particularly those less than 30 to 40 degrees, usually can be expected to have a benign natural history.

Patient Evaluation

The original evaluation of the patient should include a thorough history, complete physical and neurologic examinations, and roentgenograms of the spine. After the general physical examination the spine should be examined carefully, and the characteristics of the deformity should be recorded. The height of the patient while standing and while sitting should be measured and recorded; these measurements are compared with later ones to determine changes in the patient's total height and whether any change is due principally to growth of the lower extremities or to an increase or a decrease in the height of the trunk. A thorough neurologic examination should be performed to determine if an intraspinal neoplasm or a neurologic disorder is the cause of scoliosis.

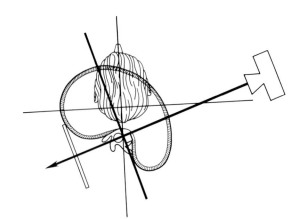

Fig. 10-2 Diagramatic representation of Stagnara derotation view. (From Bradford DS et al: Moe's textbook of scoliosis and other spinal deformities, ed 2, Philadelphia, 1987, WB Saunders Co.)

Radiographic Evaluation

Posteroanterior and lateral roentgenograms of the spine, including the iliac crest distally and most of the cervical spine proximally, should be made with the patient standing. Faster roentgenographic film and rare earth screens reduce the patient's exposure to radiation, and breast irradiation is reduced by obtaining the roentgenogram from a posteroanterior direction. Right and left bending films as described by Schmidt can be made, but as a rule they are obtained

only when evaluation for surgery is appropriate. A spot lateral roentgenogram of the lumbosacral joint should be made to screen for spondylolisthesis. An anteroposterior roentgenogram of the hand and wrist should be made to determine skeletal age, which is considered in addition to other signs of maturation, including ossification of the vertebral ring apophyses, iliac apophyses excursion, and physical signs of maturity such as breast development and pubic hair appearance.

In larger curves the posteroanterior roentgenogram does not show the true magnitude of the deformity because of severe spinal rotation. Stagnara described a roentgenographic technique to eliminate this rotational component of the curve. In this technique an oblique roentgenogram is made with the cassette parallel to the medial aspect of the rotational rib prominence and the roentgen beam positioned at right angles to the cassette (Fig. 10-2). This view gives a much more accurate measurement of the curve's size and better assesses vertebral anatomy (Fig. 10-3).

Measurement of Curves

The Cobb method of measurement recommended by the Terminology Committee of the Scoliosis Research Society (Fig. 10-4) consists of three steps: (1) locating the superior end vertebra, (2) locating the inferior end vertebra, and (3) drawing intersecting perpendicular lines from the superior surface of the superior end vertebra and from the inferior surface of the inferior end vertebra. The angle of deviation of these perpendiculars from a straight line is the angle

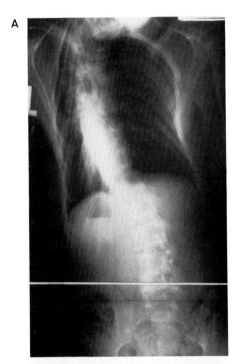

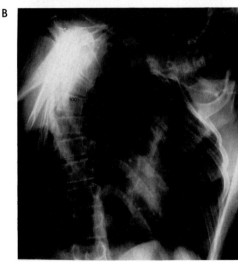

Fig. 10-3   **A,** Standard posteroanterior view of spine in severe thoracic scoliosis. **B,** Derotated view of spine better shows anatomy of vertebral bodies and curve.

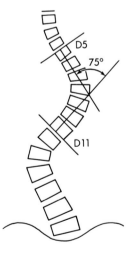

Fig. 10-4   Diagram of Cobb method. (Redrawn from Cobb JR. In The American Academy of Orthopaedic Surgeons: Instructional course lectures, vol 5, Ann Arbor, Mich, 1948, JW Edwards Co.)

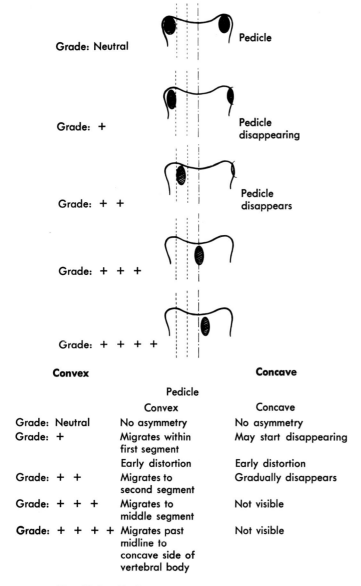

	Pedicle	
Convex		**Concave**
Grade: Neutral	No asymmetry	No asymmetry
Grade: +	Migrates within first segment	May start disappearing
	Early distortion	Early distortion
Grade: + +	Migrates to second segment	Gradually disappears
Grade: + + +	Migrates to middle segment	Not visible
Grade: + + + +	Migrates past midline to concave side of vertebral body	Not visible

Fig. 10-5 Pedicle method of determining vertebral rotation. Vertebral body is divided into 6 segments and grades from 0 to 4+ are assigned, depending on location of pedicle within segments. Because pedicle on concave side disappears early in rotation, pedicle on convex side, easily visible through wide range of rotation, is used as standard. (From Nash CL Jr and Moe JH: J Bone Joint Surg 51A:223, 1969.)

of the curve. The end vertebra of the curve is the one that tilts the most into the concavity of the curve being measured. Generally, as one moves away from the apex of the curve, the next intervertebral space below the inferior end vertebra or above the superior end vertebra is wider on the concave side of the curve. Within the curve the intervertebral spaces usually are wider on the convex side and narrower on the concave side. When significantly wedged, the vertebrae themselves, rather than the intervertebral disk spaces, may be wider on the convex side of the curve and narrower on the concave side.

Vertebral Rotation

The position of the pedicles on the initial postero-anterior roentgenogram indicates the degree of vertebral rotation, which Nash and Moe divided into five grades (Fig. 10-5). If the pedicles are equidistant from the sides of the vertebral bodies, there is no vertebral rotation (0 rotation). The grades then are increased up to grade IV rotation, which indicates that the pedicle is past the center of the vertebral body.

Curve Patterns

Idiopathic scoliosis curves were found by Ponseti and Friedman to form five main patterns that behaved differently (Fig. 10-6). A sixth curve pattern was described by Moe.

Single major lumbar curve. Ponseti and Friedman found 23.6% of patients had this curve pattern, usually involving five vertebrae, T11 to L3, with the apex at L1 or L2 (Fig. 10-7). The average increase in this curve (after skeletal maturity) was 9 degrees; curves greater than 31 degrees increased an average of 18 degrees, but curves of less than 31 degrees did not increase. Cosmetically, these curves can cause a marked distortion of the waistline.

Single major thoracolumbar curve. This curve pattern was seen in 16% of patients. Six to eight vertebrae usually were included, extending from T6 or T7 to L1 or L2 with the apex at T11 or T12 (Fig. 10-8). This pattern frequently is associated with decompensation of the spine from the midline and often produces a severe cosmetic deformity.

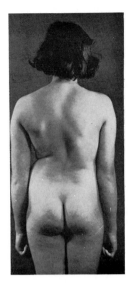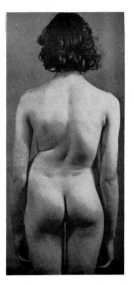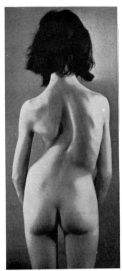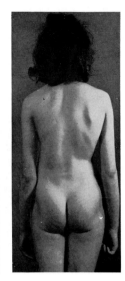

Fig. 10-6 Scoliosis deformity varies with pattern of curve. In each patient shown, angle of primary curve or curves is 70 degrees, but pattern of curve is different. *Left to right:* Lumbar, thoracolumbar, thoracic, and combined thoracic and lumbar curves. (From James JIP: J Bone Joint Surg 36B:36, 1954.)

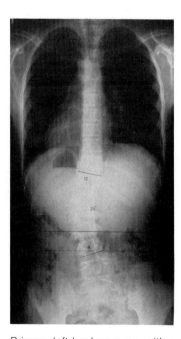

Fig. 10-7 Primary left lumbar curve with apex at L2.

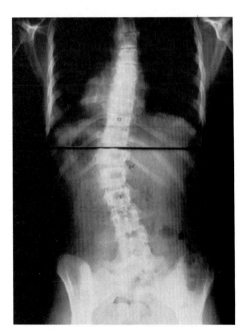

Fig. 10-8 Single major thoracolumbar curve with apex at T12.

Combined thoracic and lumbar curves (double major curves). This curve pattern was found in 37% of patients. The thoracic curve usually was to the right and included five or six vertebrae from T5 or T6 to T10 or T11 with the apex at T7 or T8. The lumbar curve usually was to the left and included five or six vertebrae from T10 to T11 to L3 or L4 with the apex at L1 or L2. Because the curves were of nearly the same degree and rigidity (Fig. 10-9), the trunk usually was balanced and the deformity was not as cosmetically apparent as other curve patterns.

Single major thoracic curve. This curve pattern occurred in 22% of patients. Six vertebrae from T5 or T6 to T11 or T12 usually were included with the apex at T8 or T9 (Fig. 10-10). Because of the thoracic loca-

tion of this curve, rotation of the involved vertebrae usually was marked. The curve produced prominence of the ribs on the convex side, depression of the ribs on the concave side, and elevation of one shoulder, resulting in an unsightly deformity (Fig. 10-5). Twenty years later Collis and Ponseti found that those single major thoracic curves that measured between 60 and 80 degrees increased an average of 28 degrees after skeletal maturity. Backache was less common in patients with this curve pattern than in the group as a whole, but they had the most severe cardiopulmonary symptoms. The severity of the cardiopulmonary symptoms and the decrease in the vital capacity correlated with the severity of the curves, especially in curves of greater than 80 degrees.

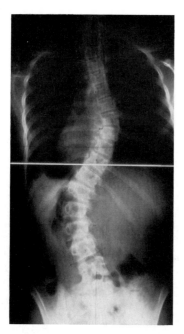

Fig. 10-9 Combined thoracic and lumbar curves with thoracic curve convex to right and lumbar curve convex to left.

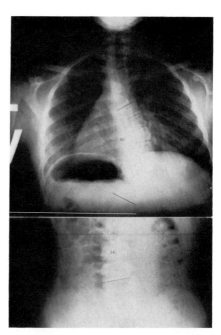

Fig. 10-10 Right major thoracic curve with apex at T9.

Single major high thoracic curve. There were only five patients with this curve pattern in the series of Ponseti and Friedman. Although none of these curves ever became large, the deformity was unsightly because of the elevated shoulder and deformed thorax. The apex of the curve was usually at T3 with the curve extending from C7 or T1 to T4 or T5.

Double major thoracic curve. This pattern was described by Moe and consists of a short upper thoracic curve, often extending from T1 to T5 or T6 with considerable rotation of the vertebrae and other structural changes in combination with a lower thoracic curve extending from T6 to T12 or L1. The upper curve usually is to the left, and the lower usually is to the right (Fig. 10-11, *A*). Deformity in patients with this curve pattern usually is not as severe as in those with a single thoracic curve, but because of asymmetry of the neckline produced by the upper curve, this pattern is more deforming than combined thoracic and lumbar curves. In this curve pattern the highly structural upper curve may be overlooked if the roentgenograms, especially the bending films, do not include the lower part of the cervical spine. If only the lower thoracic curve is corrected by fusion and Harrington instrumentation, the upper curve may not be flexible enough to allow for erect posture. Consequently, both curves should be corrected and fused (Fig. 10-11, *B*).

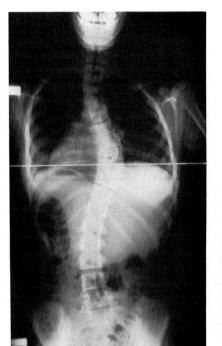
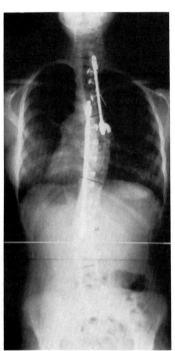

Fig. 10-11   A, Double major thoracic curve with high thoracic curve convex to left and lower thoracic curve convex to right. **B,** Postoperative roentgenogram after instrumentation for both thoracic structural curves.

Nonsurgical Management

Nonsurgical treatment of adolescent idiopathic scoliosis may include observation, or orthoses.

Observation

Although some degree of scoliosis is frequent in the general population, few individuals have curves that require treatment. Unfortunately, however, there is no reliable method for accurately predicting at an initial evaluation which curves will progress; thus observation is the primary treatment of all curves. At present a roentgenogram of the spine is the only definitive documentation of curve size and curve progression. Attempts have been made to monitor external contours with measurement of the rib hump, measurement of the trunk rotation angle with a "scoliometer," and use of contour devices such as a moiré topography. These methods may be useful in certain small curves and for low-risk patients, but periodic evaluation of the spine with roentgenograms still is necessary.

In general, young patients with mild curves can be examined every 6 to 12 months. Adolescents with larger degrees of curvature should be examined every 3 to 4 months. Each physician has his or her own protocol for observation, but these are the generally accepted guidelines. If the patient has not reached skeletal maturity and has a curve of less than 20 degrees, follow-up roentgenograms are made every 6 months. Skeletally mature patients with curves of less than 20 degrees generally do not require further evaluation. A curve of greater than 20 degrees in a patient who has not reached skeletal maturity demands more frequent examination, usually every 3 to 4 months, with a standing posteroanterior roentgenogram. If progression of the curve is beyond 25 degrees, orthotic treatment is considered. For curves of 30 to 40 degrees in a skeletally immature patient, orthotic treatment is recommended at the initial evaluation. Curves of 30 to 40 degrees in skeletally mature patients generally do not require treatment, but in view of recent studies indicating the potential for progression in adult life, these patients should be followed with standing posteroanterior roentgenograms for 2 to 3 years after skeletal maturity.

Orthotic Treatment

The use of orthoses for the nonsurgical treatment of idiopathic adolescent scoliosis by Blount et al, Moe, and others has been effective in skeletally immature patients. As described by Edmonson and Morris, an efficient Milwaukee brace, conscientiously worn, halts the progress of most mild or moderate curves. When the orthosis is worn until skeletal maturity, an average decrease of 6 degrees (or about 20%) can be obtained. Observation of an increasing curve until skeletal maturity or until the curve becomes severe enough to justify fusion is rarely, if ever, appropriate.

For the orthosis to be effective, forces must be ap-

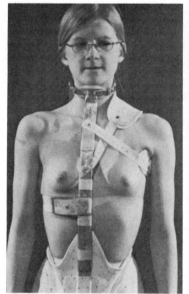 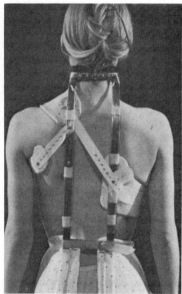

Fig. 10-12 Milwaukee brace for patient with double thoracic curve pattern. (From Winter RB and Moe JH: Clin Orthop 102:84, 1974.)

plied indirectly to the spinal deformity. These forces are applied to the thoracic spine using the ribs as levers. In the lumbar spine, the orthosis decreases lordosis and derotates the lumbar curve. There are two basic types of orthoses: cervical-thoracic-lumbar-sacral orthosis (CTLSO) and thoracic-lumbar-sacral orthosis (TLSO). An example of the CTLSO is the Milwaukee brace as introduced by Blount and Schmidt (Fig. 10-12). The TLSO is an underarm orthosis such as the Boston or Miami brace (Fig. 10-13). Curves with the apex below T8 usually can be managed with the TLSO. If the apex is higher than T8, a CTLSO is generally recommended.

Orthotic treatment of adolescent idiopathic scoliosis is indicated for a mild and flexible curve in a growing child, a curve of 25 degrees or more with documented progression, or a curve between 30 and 40 degrees at initial evaluation. Most reports indicate that orthotic treatment is not successful in curves greater than 60 degrees. In addition to the actual curve measurements, other factors such as thoracic hypokyphosis, osteopenia, obesity, skin disorders, curve flexibility, emotional stability, and family cooperation must be considered before deciding on orthotic treatment, especially in curves between 40 and 60 degrees.

Scoliosis associated with certain conditions such as neurofibromatosis, congenital kyphosis, and a unilateral unsegmented bar should not be treated with an orthosis, and, there is no indication for orthotic treatment of adolescent idiopathic scoliosis in skeletally mature patients.

Once the appropriate orthosis has been fitted, it is checked by the physician and roentgenograms are made with the orthosis in place. At 3- to 4-month intervals, standing posteroanterior roentgenograms of the spine are made without the brace, and the brace is checked. Additional roentgenograms with the patient in the brace are obtained only if modifications of the brace are needed. Weaning from the orthosis is begun when there is objective evidence of skeletal maturity. The weaning schedule is individualized for each patient, but generally the time out of the brace is increased by 4-hour increments at each visit. Nighttime-only brace wear usually is continued for an additional year.

The orthosis primarily is used as a holding device. Most curves show some initial improvement and then lose some correction during the weaning process but ultimately stabilize at about the original degree of curvature. If, in spite of an adequate orthosis and complete compliance, the curve continues to progress beyond 40 degrees, surgery is recommended.

Surface electrical stimulation recently has been proposed as a possible replacement for orthotic treatment of idiopathic scoliosis; however, on the basis of results of several reports, the Milwaukee brace and the Boston-type underarm brace are more reliable and predictable.

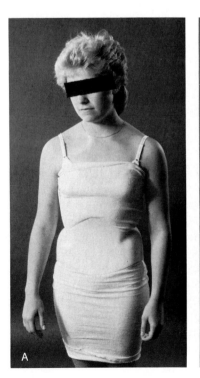 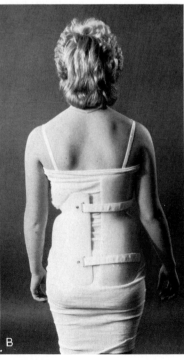

Fig. 10-13 **A** and **B,** TLSO for left lumbar scoliosis. (From Bradford DS et al: Moe's textbook of scoliosis and other spinal deformities, ed 2, Philadelphia, 1987, WB Saunders Co.)

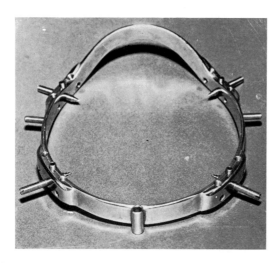

Fig. 10-14 Halo (anterior view) for stabilizing head and neck. (From Perry J and Nickel VL: J Bone Joint Surg 41A:37, 1959.)

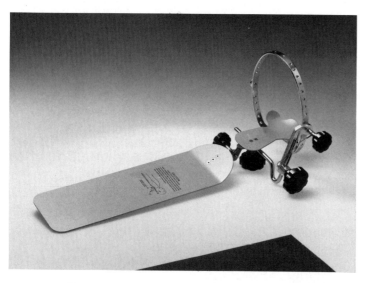

Fig. 10-15 Halo ring positioning fixture. (Courtesy Durr-Fillauer.)

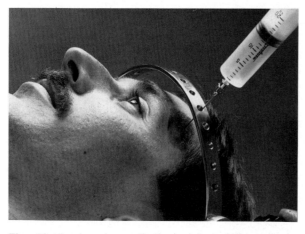

Fig. 10-16 Local anesthetic is injected through selected screw hole. (Courtesy Durr-Fillauer.)

Surgical Techniques
Distraction Techniques

Halo. In 1959 Perry and Nickel introduced the halo (Fig. 10-14), a device that provides stable fixation and comfort for the patient. The halo is useful for selected patients in whom preoperative traction is needed. With the improved spinal instrumentation and spinal cord monitoring, the need for supplemental traction correction of severe stiff curves and for monitoring spinal and pulmonary function of an unanesthetized patient is greatly diminished, but the halo device still is useful in certain situations: (1) in the preoperative evaluation of flexible paralytic curves in patients with severe pulmonary insufficiency (if preoperative traction improves the patient's pulmonary function, then surgery may be indicated), (2) as a halo cast or vest for added external immobilization in cervical and upper thoracic deformities in which surgery does not offer sufficient inherent stability to maintain correction for stabilization of the spine until the fusion consolidates, and (3) in cervical spine fractures.

▶ *Technique.* General anesthesia may be necessary in young children, but local anesthesia routinely is used in most older patients. The halo should be used very carefully in children younger than 4 years because of the possibility of poor cranial bone stock. Six standard sizes of halos are available and should accommodate the cranial circumferences of most patients. Determine the appropriate size before application and sterilize the halo and pins. Place the patient supine with the head supported by an assistant or a narrow metal extension that is cupped to cradle the head (Fig. 10-15). Shave the immediate areas of pin insertion and prepare the skin with antiseptic solution. Infiltrate the skin and the periosteum in the selected areas of pin insertion with a local anesthetic (Fig. 10-16). Support the halo around the patient's head with the application device or an assistant's help. The halo must be held below the area of greatest diameter of the skull, just above the eyebrows and about 1 cm above the tips of the ears.

After anesthetizing the skin and periosteum, choose the anterior pin sites, usually the most medial halo channels. Some surgeons prefer to keep the pin insertions within the hairline, but this requires a more posterior location in the temporalis muscle where the bone is also thinner. Posteriorly, the central channels are usually the best site for the pins. Introduce the pins and tighten two diagonally opposed pins simultaneously. Continue this until all four pins just engage the skin and bone. It is important that, as the pins are being tightened, the patient keep his eyes closed to ensure that the skin on the forehead is not anchored in such a way as to prevent the eyelids from closing after application of the halo (Fig. 10-17). Continue tightening diagonally opposite pins with a torque screwdriver to about 4 lb-in for children (Fig. 10-18). Some authors recently have reported superior results with tightening of the screws to 7 to 8 lb-ft in adults, but the screws should not be tightened that much in children. Alternate the tightening of diagonal pins to prevent an asymmetric halo. Finally secure the pins to the halo with appropriate lock nuts or set screws.

▶ *Postoperative management.* The pins are cleansed daily at the skin interface with hydrogen peroxide, or a small amount of povidone-iodine (Betadine) ointment can be applied and the pins simply inspected daily. The pins are not tightened daily. The pins rarely enter the skull more than 2 mm but rather act as a wedge, forcing the halo from the skull. The indications for changing the pins are excessive drainage, inflammation, or a clicking sensation; otherwise they should remain undisturbed.

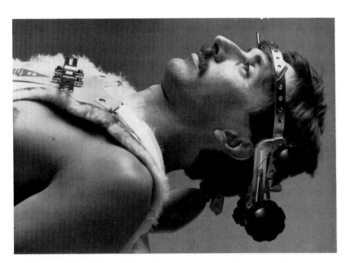

Fig. 10-17 Halo position is checked and patient's eyes are closed before final tightening of halo pins. (Courtesy Durr-Fillauer.)

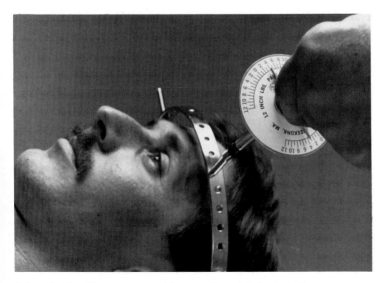

Fig. 10-18 Torque screwdriver applies 4 lb-in to halo pin. (Courtesy Durr-Fillauer.)

Halo vest. Semirigid plastic vests with shoulder straps and metal attachments for a skull halo are available commercially. They are fitted by measurements and are usually lined with a synthetic sheepskin (Fig. 10-19). The immobilization these devices provide is not as secure as a halo cast that includes the pelvis. In certain patients, the halo vest may control bending and rotational stresses on the spine but is only as secure as the patient permits because all straps and adjustments are accessible and can be loosened by the patient. If secure immobilization is needed, and especially if it is necessary to counteract compressive forces of gravity, a halo cast, well molded to the iliac crest, is necessary.

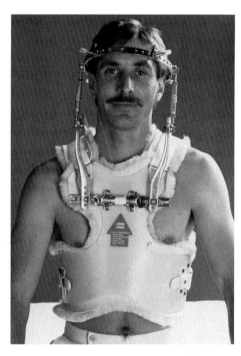

Fig. 10-19 Anterior view of halo vest. (Courtesy Durr-Fillauer.)

Halo cast

▲ *Technique.* The halo is applied as previously described. Place the patient supine on the Risser table, attach the halo to the table, and apply traction. With the patient resting on a canvas strap tied to the rectangular plaster frame, stretch a stockinette over the patient from the head to the knees. Place felt padding over the shoulders and around the iliac crest. Pass muslin straps around the waist over the stockinette but just beneath the felt. Position the straps above the iliac crest and tie them on the opposite side at the level of the greater trochanter. Next, attach the straps to the end of the frame and, using the windlass, apply longitudinal traction. These straps lie between the felt and the stockinette, allowing their removal when the patient is removed from the table. With the cross bar at the level of the axilla, apply extra strong, resin-reinforced plaster, which provides better long-term durability and also requires fewer layers of plaster. Apply the plaster over the shoulders but do not encompass the neck. Mold the plaster snugly and carefully around the iliac crest, the anterosuperior iliac spines, the sacrum, and the symphysis pubis. After the cast has hardened, trim it to relieve any areas of excess pressure. Trim the pelvic section above the pubis and laterally over the thighs to just below the anterosuperior iliac spine to allow 100 degrees of hip flexion. Trim the posterior aspect much like a Milwaukee brace to relieve pressure over the sacral prominence, while still allowing purchase over the pelvis posteriorly. Generally, the most posterior extent of the cast over the buttocks is level with the greater trochanter. Cut a window over the abdomen so that the upper portion of the abdomen and lower costal margin are free. Contour the halo shoulder supports with bending irons to fit the shoulder straps and attach them with plaster. Apply the connecting rods to the shoulder straps into the halo itself (Fig. 10-20). By loosening these adjustments, very fine movements can be performed to control the position of the head and neck. It may be necessary to readjust the position of the halo once the patient is ambulatory in the cast.

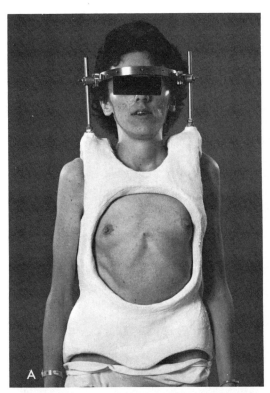

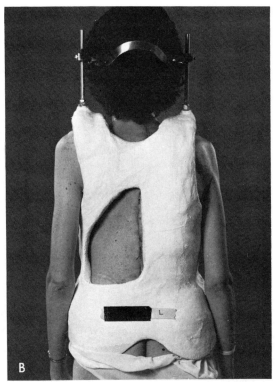

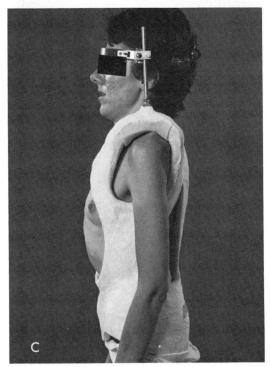

Fig. 10-20   A to **C,** Anterior, posterior, and lateral views of halo cast. (From Bradford DS et al: Moe's textbook of scoliosis and other spinal deformities, ed 2, Philadelphia, 1987, WB Saunders Co.)

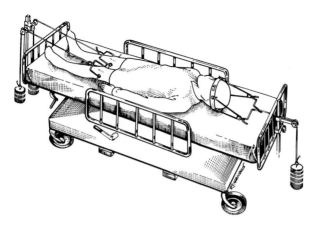

Fig. 10-21   Halo-femoral traction for severe scoliosis curvatures.

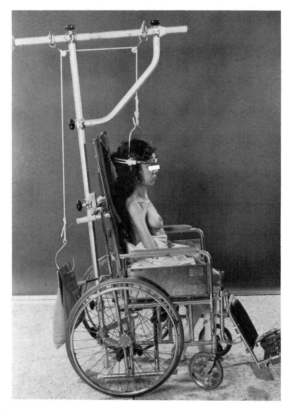

Fig. 10-22   Halo wheelchair as advocated by Stagnara. (From Bradford DS et al: Moe's textbook of scoliosis and other spinal deformities, ed 2, Philadelphia, 1987, WB Saunders Co.)

Halo femoral distraction. Halo femoral traction, which exerts strong distraction forces on the spine, is used much less frequently since the development of superior spinal instrumentation and spinal cord monitoring. Cummine et al described its use in a two-stage corrective procedure for failed scoliosis fusion. They used halo femoral distraction after the initial stage of surgery, which consisted of multiple osteotomies through the posterior fusion mass or resection of the pseudarthrosis. The technique, however, must be carefully monitored. Twice-daily neurologic examinations are mandatory and should include evaluation of the function of the cranial nerves, as well as evaluation of the neurologic status of the lower extremities.

▲ *Technique.* The halo is applied as previously described. Prepare and drape both knees in a sterile field. Introduce a large, smooth Steinmann pin through a stab wound into each distal femoral diaphyseal area, well above the epiphysis. Begin traction with about 6 kg or a 3-kg weight on each leg. Gradually and equally add weights up to a total of 12 kg on each leg (Fig. 10-21). The use of traction for more than 10 days has not been shown to improve angular correction. For pelvic obliquity, most of the lower extremity weight can be applied on the high side limb.

Rather than confine the patient to bed, a halo wheelchair as designed by Stagnara can be used during the day (Fig. 10-22).

Halo pelvic distraction. DeWald and Ray first reported the pelvic halo in 1970; it was designed for patients with severe pulmonary restriction, pressure sores from a cast, soft tissue contractures, or inability to control pelvic tilt and rotation. The complications of this procedure include skin intolerance with pin tract infections, bowel perforation, nerve palsy and paraplegia, hip subluxation, and degenerative cervical arthritis. Furthermore, the areas for obtaining bone grafts are poorly accessible. For these reasons, as well as improvements in segmental spinal instrumentation and other internal spinal fixation devices, the halo pelvic distraction only rarely is used now. The technique is presented here for completeness.

▲ *Technique (O'Brien et al).* With the patient under general anesthesia, insert the pelvic pin at a point on the iliac crest anteriorly opposite the rough gluteal tubercle so that it emerges posteriorly just medial to the posterior superior iliac spines (Fig. 10-23, *A* and *B*). This placement of pins is very important to prevent pin tract infections. Use the drilling jig to ensure the proper path of penetration, and introduce the self-tapping pelvic pin with a carpenter's brace.

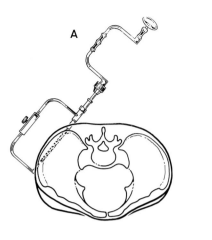
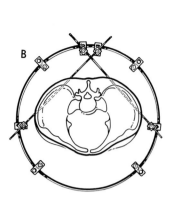
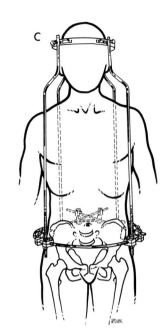

Fig. 10-23 Halo-pelvic distraction device. **A** and **B,** Pelvic pin insertion. **C,** Extension bars fitted between cranial and pelvic halos.

▶ *Postoperative management.* Postoperatively, the patient should have no more than minor discomfort from either the skull halo or the pelvic halo. Continuing severe pain indicates that something is wrong, especially with regard to the pelvic halo.

After several days, extension bars are fitted between the cranial and pelvic halos with the patient awake (Fig. 10-23, *C*). O'Brien et al used large spring balances with an upward distracting force of 20 to 30 pounds (9 to 13.5 kg). The protruding pins in the pelvic region are covered with dry dressing; if drainage begins, appropriate antibiotics are given. Distraction is increased at the rate of 2 or 3 mm/day. If neck pain develops, the distraction is discontinued for several days. A daily neurologic examination and careful clinical examination of those nerves most prone to injury are performed each day. This evaluation includes not only the lower extremities but the upper extremities and cranial nerves as well.

Spinal Fusion
General Principles

Although nonsurgical treatment is the most frequently used treatment for idiopathic scoliosis, it is important to recognize the necessity for surgical intervention. The indications for surgery are not always definite, but the primary ones are (1) an increasing curve in a growing child, (2) a severe deformity with asymmetry of the trunk in an adolescent, regardless of whether growth of the spine has ceased, and (3)

pain that cannot be controlled by conservative measures in older patients.

The success of any surgical procedure for scoliosis depends on the achievement of a solid spinal arthrodesis and stability of the spine. Recently there has been a wave of enthusiasm for new and perhaps better methods of instrumentation, some of which necessitate modifications of the basic fusion technique. Although preliminary reports are encouraging, the long-term goal of spinal surgery should not be overlooked: a solid spinal arthrodesis.

An essential part of successful spinal fusion and instrumentation is patient orientation. Harrington noted that successful surgery includes (1) spending time with the patient to gain his or her confidence and allay hidden fears, (2) showing the patient examples of the expected results and providing the names of other patients with whom to confer, and (3) explaining the use of instrumentation and its limitations as well as its benefits.

The first aim in the treatment of scoliosis by spinal fusion is restoration of the symmetry of the trunk by centering the first thoracic vertebra above the sacrum while keeping the pelvis and shoulders level. The second and equally important aim is to straighten the structural curves, primarily in the thoracic area, enough to halt the deterioration of pulmonary function and to minimize the unsightly deformity of the thorax.

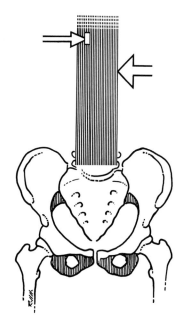

Fig. 10-24 Stable zone for inferior vertebra as described by Harrington.

Preoperative preparation. Preoperative evaluation of the spinal levels to be fused by careful roentgenographic study is essential. A thorough physical examination and any necessary preoperative tests should be completed before surgery. In addition to the standard preoperative tests, other studies such as pulmonary function tests, bleeding studies, myelograms, computed tomography (CT) scans, and magnetic resonance imaging (MRI) may be needed before complicated procedures. For patients who qualify, the use of autologous blood is recommended as a safe and effective way of decreasing or eliminating the need for bank blood with all its potential problems. This technique requires the patient to give staged donations of autologous blood for several weeks before surgery. In most spine surgery, spinal cord monitoring is recommended. The occipital electrodes are applied preoperatively and a baseline reading is obtained, then the spinal cord monitoring is done continuously during surgery (see p. 508).

A   B   C

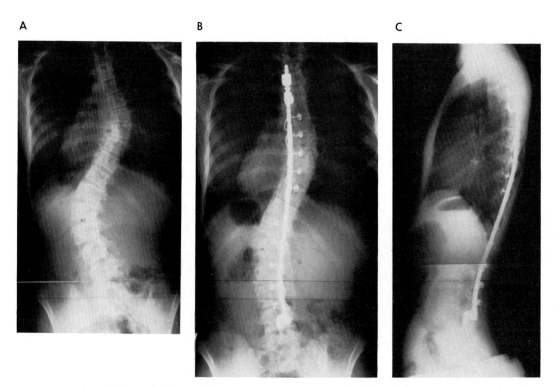

Fig. 10-25 **A,** Posteroanterior view of King type I curve in idiopathic scoliosis. **B,** Postoperative posteroanterior view showing both curves instrumented and fused. **C,** Postoperative lateral view. Note contoured Harrington distraction rods used to maintain lumbar lordosis.

Selection of fusion levels

Fusion levels are selected by identifying the major curve or curves, the neutrally rotated end vertebrae for each major curve, and the relationship of the curves to a vertically drawn midsacral line.

The major curve or curves are identified by determining curve flexibility on side-bending roentgenograms. The stiffer curves, and therefore the more structural curves, are the major curves. Two curves with nearly identical flexibility imply a double major curve pattern. The rotation of the individual vertebra is determined by the relationship of the pedicle and the vertebral body margins on the posteroanterior roentgenogram, as described by Nash and Moe (see Fig. 10-5). As a general rule, fusion should extend from one end vertebra to the other. Harrington suggested that the fusion extend from one vertebra above the curve to two vertebrae below in primary thoracic and primary thoracolumbar curves. He also suggested that if the centroid of function of the lower hook does not fall within the stable zone, the instrumentation must be supplemented (Fig. 10-24) by overlapping distraction rods or by using a "dollar sign" rod application for both curves.

King et al reviewed their experience in the surgical treatment of idiopathic thoracic scoliosis or combined thoracic and lumbar scoliosis with Harrington distraction rods and formulated guidelines for determining the necessity for instrumentation of the lower curve. They divided the combined curve patterns into five types. Type I is an S-shaped curve in which both the thoracic and lumbar curves cross the midline. The lumbar curve is larger than the thoracic curve on the standing roentgenogram, and the thoracic curve

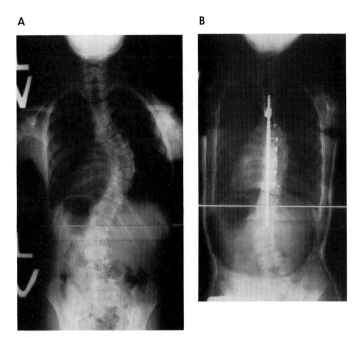

Fig. 10-26   A, Posteroanterior view of King type II curve. **B,** Postoperative posteroanterior view of instrumentation of thoracic curve only, with lower hook in stable vertebra.

is more flexible than the lumbar curve on side bending (Fig. 10-25). Type II curves are S-shaped curves in which the thoracic and lumbar curves both cross the midline, but the thoracic curve is greater than the lumbar curve, and the lumbar curve is more flexible on the bending films (Fig. 10-26). The type III curve is a thoracic curve in which the compensatory lumbar curve does not cross the midline (Fig. 10-27). Type IV

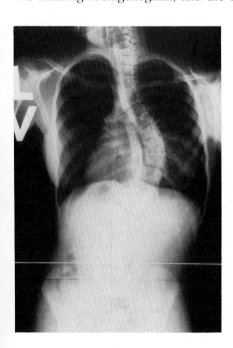
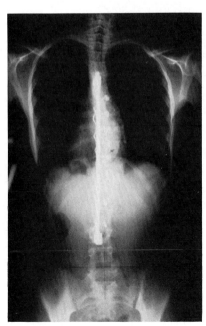

Fig. 10-27   A, Preoperative posteroanterior view of King type III thoracic curve. **B,** Postoperative posteroanterior view. Note inferior hook in L3, which was bisected by center sacral line in preoperative roentgenogram.

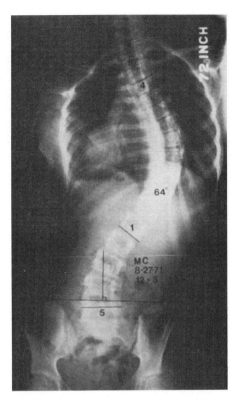

Fig. 10-28   King type IV curve. (From King HA et al: J Bone Joint Surg 65A:1306, 1983.)

A

B

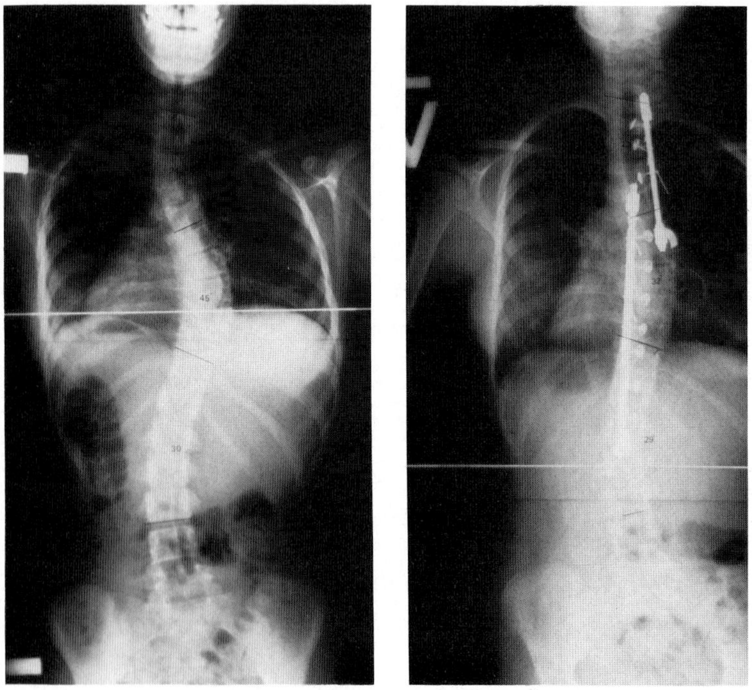

Fig. 10-29   **A,** Posteroanterior view of King type V double thoracic curve. **B,** Postoperative view of instrumentation of both thoracic curves.

is a long thoracic curve in which L5 is centered over the sacrum, but L4 tilts into the long thoracic curve (Fig. 10-28). Type V is a double thoracic curve with T1 tilted into the convexity of the upper curve, which is structural on side bending (Fig. 10-29).

In type I curves it is necessary to fuse both the thoracic and the lumbar curves (Fig. 10-25, *B* and *C*); there is no indication to fuse below L4. In type II curves a selective thoracic fusion can be performed (Fig. 10-26, *B*), but the stable vertebra must be selected for the lower hook. The stable vertebra is that vertebra that is bisected or most closely bisected by a single line drawn through the center of the sacrum perpendicular to the iliac crest (Fig. 10-30). If the neutral vertebra is not the stable vertebra, fusion must be to the stable vertebra. In types III and IV curves the fusion should include the thoracic curve with the lower level of the fusion at the first vertebra that is most closely bisected by the center sacral line (Fig. 10-27, *B*). Type IV curves are longer than type III curves, and the fusion usually must be carried farther into the lumbar spine. In type V curves both thoracic curves should be fused; failure to treat the upper thoracic curve can lead to a disfigured shoulder line and loss of balance. The lower level of this fusion should include the vertebra that is most closely bisected by the center sacral line (Fig. 10-31). In single major thoracolumbar and lumbar curves, fusion above and below the end vertebrae is best. It usually is necessary to extend the fusion to L4, but there is no indication for continuing fusion to the sacrum in an adolescent with this curve pattern.

Positioning of the patient

Because spinal surgery requires extensive dissection, which may result in severe blood loss, a large-bore intravenous line, as well as an arterial line, is necessary. Relton and Hall first emphasized the role of intraabdominal pressure on blood loss, and they designed a frame to eliminate some of this intraabdominal pressure and consequently reduce blood loss (Fig. 10-32, *A*). The patient is positioned on the Relton-Hall frame with the arms carefully supported and the elbows padded. The shoulders should not be abducted more than 90 degrees to avoid pressure or stretch on the brachial plexus. The upper pads of the frame rest on the chest and not in the axilla, again to relieve pressure on any nerves from the brachial plexus (Fig. 10-32, *B*). When the patient is positioned on the frame with the hips flexed, the lumbar lordosis is partially eliminated. If the fusion is to be extended into the lower lumbar spine, then the knees and thighs should be elevated so that the patient lies with the hip joints extended to maintain the lumbar lordosis.

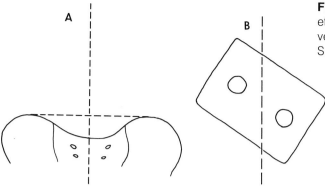

Fig. 10-30 **A,** Center sacral line as described by King et al. **B,** Vertebra most closely bisected by line is stable vertebra. (Redrawn from King HA et al: J Bone Joint Surg 65A:1303, 1983.)

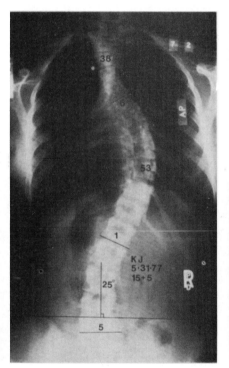 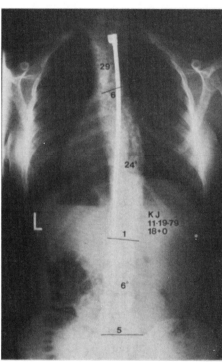

Fig. 10-31 **A,** Preoperative postero-anterior view of King type V curve. **B,** Postoperative view of instrumentation of upper thoracic curve with dollar-sign rod. (From King HA et al: J Bone Joint Surg 65A:1306, 1983.)

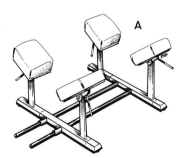 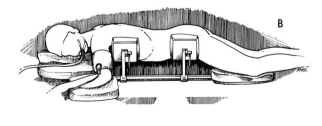

Fig. 10-32 **A,** Relton-Hall frame for reduction of intraabdominal pressure. **B,** Positioning of patient on Relton-Hall frame with hips in extension to maintain lumbar lordosis.

Preparation and draping

First scrub the patient's back with a surgical soap solution for 5 to 10 minutes, then prepare it with antiseptic solution, such as a diluted iodine solution followed by alcohol. Drape the area of the operation using a plastic sterile drape.

Surgical exposure. The skin incision is best made in a straight line from one to two vertebrae above the proposed fusion area to one vertebra below it. A straight scar improves the postoperative appearance of the back (Fig. 10-33, *A*). Make the initial incision through the dermal layer only, and infiltrate the intradermal and subcutaneous area with an epinephrine solution (1:500,000). Deepen the incision to the level of the spinous processes. Use self-retaining Weitlaner retractors to retract the skin margins. Control bleeding with electrocautery. Identify the interspinous ligament between the spinous processes (Fig. 10-33, *B*). This often is seen as a "white line." As the incision is deepened, keep the Weitlaner retractors tight to aid exposure and minimize bleeding. Now incise the cartilaginous cap overlying the spinous process as close to the midline as possible. This midline may vary because of rotation of the spinous processes in many spinal deformities. Using a Cobb elevator, expose the spinous processes subperiostally after the cartilaginous caps are moved to either side. After several of the spinous processes have been exposed, the Weit-

laner retractors can be moved to a deeper level and tension maintained for retraction and hemostasis. After exposure of all the spinous processes, obtain a localizing roentgenogram. While the roentgenogram is being developed, reopen the wound and continue subperiosteal exposure of the entire area to be fused, with the retractors tight at all times (Fig. 10-33, *C*). It is generally easier to dissect distally to proximally because of the oblique attachments of the short rotator muscles and ligaments of the spine. Extend the subperiosteal dissection first to the facet joints on one side and then the other side.

Continue lateral dissection to the ends of the transverse processes on both sides to allow exposure and coagulation of a branch of the segmental vessel just lateral to each facet joint (Fig. 10-34). Place the self-retaining retractors deeper to hold the entire incision open. Sponges soaked in the 1:500,000 epinephrine solution help maintain hemostasis. Now use a curet and a small pituitary rongeur to completely clean the interspinous ligament and the lateral facets of all ligament attachments and capsule in the lumbar area. Using a Cobb curet and working from the midline and proceeding laterally (Fig. 10-35) make it less likely that the curet will slip and penetrate the spinal canal. The entire spine now has been exposed from one transverse process to the other with all soft tissue removed and is ready for instrumentation or decortication.

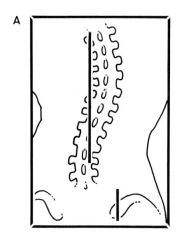
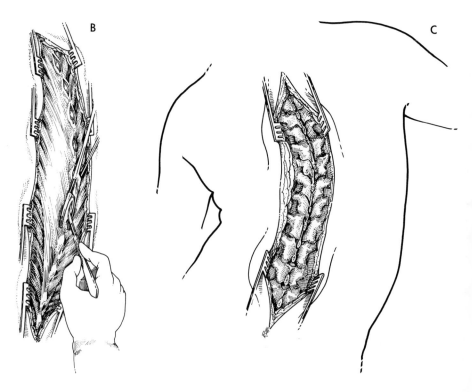

Fig. 10-33 **A,** Skin incisions for posterior fusion and autogenous bone graft. **B,** Incisions over spinous processes and interspinous ligaments. **C,** Weitlaner retractors used to maintain tension and exposure of spine during dissection.

Bone grafting. Before decortication is performed, a bone graft is taken from the outer table of the ilium. Although some studies indicate that the use of bone bank allograft results in acceptable fusion rates, a large amount of autogenous bone graft should be used whenever possible. If the autogenous bone graft is deficient or cannot be used for other reasons, then the graft is supplemented with allograft, preferably from a bone bank femoral head.

Make an incision over the iliac crest (Fig. 10-33, *A*); if the original incision was made far enough distally into the lumbar spine, the iliac crest can be exposed through the same incision. Infiltrate the intradermal and subcutaneous area with 1:500,000 epinephrine solution. Expose the cartilaginous apophysis overlying the posterior iliac crest, and split this cartilaginous cap through its midline. Using a Cobb elevator, expose the ilium subperiosteally. The superior gluteal artery emerges from the area of the sciatic notch (Fig. 10-36, *A*) and should be carefully avoided during this bone grafting procedure. At this point the posterior crest of the ilium can be exposed on the inner side. Using a large gouge, obtain two or three strips of bicortical graft, which may be placed anterior to the transverse processes in the lumbar spine if desired. Otherwise, take cortical and cancellous strips of bone from the outer table of the ilium (Fig. 10-36, *B*). Place these bone grafts in a kidney basin, and cover them with a sponge soaked in saline or blood. Control bleeding from the iliac crest with bone wax. Approximate the cartilaginous cap of the posterior crest of the ilium with an absorbable suture. Leave a suction drain in place at this bone graft site, and connect it to a separate reservoir so that postoperative bleeding in both the bone graft and spinal fusion sites can be monitored. Use the bone grafts as quickly as possible after obtaining them.

▲ *Postoperative management.* There are many different types of postoperative casts, as well as postoperative immobilization regimens, after surgical fusion for scoliosis. The stability of the fixation, the type of curve, and the surgeon's preference determine the type of immobilization used. Polypropylene body jackets may be successfully used in adults and older children, but in younger children cast immobilization is more secure because they will remove any type of brace that can be removed. For most patients a simple underarm cast provides sufficient immobilization.

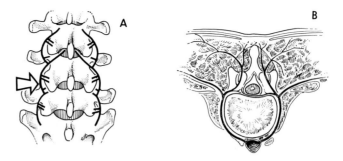

Fig. 10-34 **A,** Posterior view of segmental vessels just lateral to each facet joint. **B,** Axial view of arteries supplying posterior spinal muscles. (**A** redrawn from MacNab I and Dall D: J Bone Joint Surg 53[13]: 628, 1971; **B** redrawn from Wagoner G: J Bone Joint Surg 19:469, 1937.)

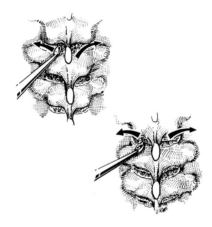

Fig. 10-35 Cobb curets used to clean the facets of ligament attachments.

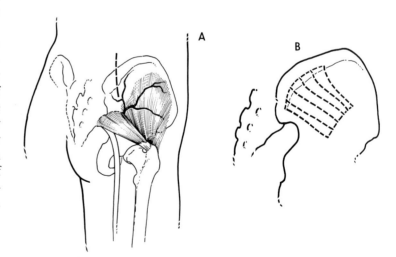

Fig. 10-36 **A,** Superior gluteal artery as it emerges from area of sciatic notch. **B,** Cortical and cancellous strips removed from outer table of ilium for autogenous bone graft.

Underarm cast

With improvements in internal fixation, it usually is not necessary to apply a full Risser-Cotrel cast, which incorporates the neck. More frequently, an underarm cast is used for any necessary external immobilization (Fig. 10-37).

▲ *Technique.* Place the patient on the Risser table, and apply a stockinette so that it extends from over the head to the knees. Position the removable cross-bar at the level of the upper portion of the shoulders. Use felt to pad the canvas strap on which the patient is resting. Pass muslin straps around the waist over the stockinette, and tie them at the level of the greater trochanter on the opposite side. Then pass these muslin straps through the windlass at the end of the table, and apply a slight amount of traction. Now apply felt over the iliac crest, and carefully hold it in place with adhesive tape. Use extra-strong, resin-reinforced plaster. Extend the cast to the sternum anteriorly and the upper portion of the back posteriorly. Mold the cast well around the pelvis and iliac crest. As the cast dries, trim it at the level of the pubic symphysis anteriorly, extending proximally to about the level of the anterosuperior iliac spine to allow 100 degrees of hip flexion. Posteriorly, trim low over the buttocks, generally the distalmost level being at the level of the greater trochanters, and then trim proximally to relieve pressure over the sacral promi-

nence. Remove an abdominal window to free the upper portion of the abdomen, the lower costal margin, and the xiphoid process.

Risser "localizer cast"

With improved techniques of internal fixation of the spine, the Risser localizer cast is rarely necessary; however, it can be useful in patients in whom fusion must extend into the upper thoracic and lower cervical spine and in whom internal fixation is not possible, making the rigid immobilization of the halo cast necessary.

▲ *Technique (Risser).* Place the patient supine on the Risser table (Fig. 10-38) and resting on the canvas strap. Place a stockinette from the head to the knees. Then apply the cast in stages. Apply a plaster girdle over felt padding and the previously applied stockinette. Mold this plaster snugly and carefully about the iliac crest, the anterosuperior iliac spines, the sacrum, and the symphysis pubis. After this section has hardened, apply traction with a head halter and a pelvic belt attached over the plaster girdle. Adjust the traction with the windlass at both ends of the table. Begin with a well-molded neck and shoulder part that includes the chin and occiput, and finish incorporating the entire trunk with plaster applied snugly over the felt to maintain the corrected position. Place the localizer plate over the ribs on the convex side of the

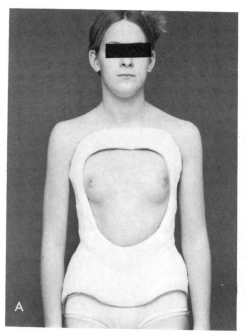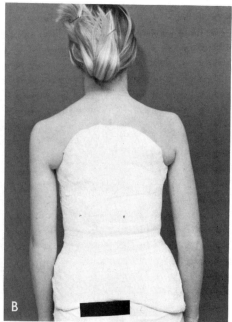

Fig. 10-37 **A** and **B,** Underarm cast for postoperative immobilization in idiopathic scoliosis. (From Bradford DS et al: Moe's textbook of scoliosis and other spinal deformities, ed 2, Philadelphia, 1987, WB Saunders Co.)

chest, pressing in an anterolateral direction. After the cast has hardened, trim it to relieve any excess pressure at the side of the localizer or on the point of the chin. At the bottom, trim the cast to the groin, leaving it relatively low over the buttocks. Then cut a window over the abdomen, so that the upper portion of the abdomen, the lower costal margin, and the xiphoid process are free.

Modified Cotrel cast

Moe uses the Risser table or the Risser attachments for the Bell table to apply a cast patterned after those used by Cotrel in France. The cast is applied in one piece, with the use of two fabric slings looped around the waist, superior to the iliac crest, and crossed anterior and posterior so that as distal traction is applied to the slings and thus to the pelvis, the waistline is molded well proximal to the iliac crest. A disposable halter is used for head traction. The fabric slings are placed between the two layers of stockinette so that they will not adhere to the plaster and can be removed after the cast is applied. Cotrel applied the cast over the two layers of stockinette only. Moe usually applies, in addition, thin felt padding around the neck, shoulder, and pelvis. When the cast is used to correct curves before surgery, Moe recommends that a heavy layer of felt or other padding be applied to the entire anterior aspect of the pelvic and shoulder girdles so that minimal pressure is placed on localized areas of the skin during the several hours the patient is prone on the operating table.

◣ *Technique (Moe).* Place the patient supine on a Risser or Bell table. Apply the two layers of stockinette, the fabric slings for pelvic traction, the halter for head traction, and any padding desired. Then apply strong pelvic and head traction, and rapidly apply a cast similar to the Risser localizer cast. Next place a canvas strap 15 to 10 cm wide transversely across the table beneath the patient's back at the level of the axillae; attach it to the table frame on the side of the body opposite the rib prominence. Apply it smoothly around the thorax over the rib prominence, and turn it 90 degrees to rise vertically to the overhead winch of the Bell table or to the overhead attachment of the Risser table. Just before the plaster dries, tighten the straps securely against the outside of the cast for corrective molding. After the cast is dried, remove the halter and the pelvic traction straps and trim the cast as desired over the abdomen and chest; window it posteriorly if it is to be left in place during surgery.

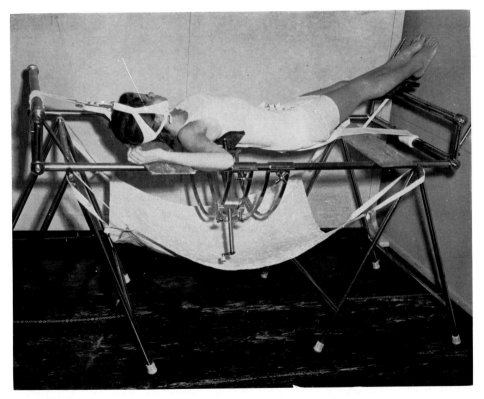

Fig. 10-38   Application of Risser localizer cast (see text). (From Risser JC. In The American Academy of Orthopaedic Surgeons: Instructional course lectures, vol 10, Ann Arbor, Mich, 1953, JW Edwards Co.)

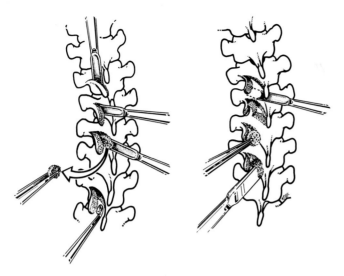

Fig. 10-39 Moe technique of thoracic facet fusion (From Bradford DS et al: Moe's textbook of scoliosis and other spinal deformities, ed 2, Philadelphia, 1987, WB Saunders Co.)

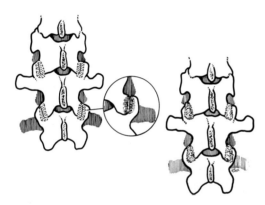

Fig. 10-40 Moe technique for lumbar facet fusion.

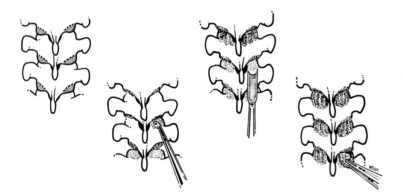

Fig. 10-41 Hall technique of facet fusion. (Redrawn in part from Bradford DS et al: Moe's textbook of scoliosis and other spinal deformities, ed 2, Philadelphia, 1987, WB Saunders Co.)

Posterior Fusion

Techniques. The long-term success of any surgical procedure for scoliosis depends on a solid arthrodesis. The classic Hibbs technique is essentially an extraarticular fusion and generally has been replaced by a modification of the intraarticular fusion described by Moe and the meticulous dissection around the transverse processes recommended by Goldstein. Improvements in surgical techniques over the past 20 years have increased the fusion rate and decreased the infection rate to 1% or less and the pseudarthrosis rate to 2% or less. The higher fusion rate probably has resulted from more complete facet joint excision, replacement with autogenous iliac bone graft, thorough decortication of the entire laminal area, and inclusion of the transverse processes in the fusion mass.

▶ ***Technique (Moe).*** Expose the spine to the tips of the transverse processes as previously described (p. 472). Begin a cut over the cephalad lateral articular process at the base of the lamina, and carry it along the transverse process almost to its tip. Bend this fragment laterally to lie between the transverse processes, leaving it hinged if possible. Thoroughly remove the cartilage from the superior articular process. Now make another cut in the area of the superior articular facet with the Cobb gouge, beginning medially and working laterally to produce another hinged fragment. Place cancellous bone graft in the defect created (Fig. 10-39). In the lumbar spine the facet joints are oriented in a more sagittal direction, and a facet fusion is best accomplished by removing the adjoining joint surfaces with a small osteotome or a needle-nose rongeur. This creates a defect, which is packed with cancellous bone (Fig. 10-40).

As the next step, carry out decortication with Cobb gouges over the entire exposed spine. Again, it is best to use the gouge from the midline, progressing laterally so that if the gouge slips, it is moving away from the spinal canal. Then add cancellous bone graft. Concentrate the bone graft on the thoracolumbar and lumbar areas inasmuch as these are the areas with the highest incidence of pseudarthrosis. Also, concentrate the bone graft on the concave side of the curve because the bone will be subjected to compressive forces on this side of the curve as opposed to tension forces on the convex side.

Close the deep tissues with a running absorbable suture. Place a suction drain in the subcutaneous tissue, and keep its reservoir separate from the reservoir for the bone graft to allow monitoring of bleeding from the individual sites. If the patient has little subcutaneous tissue, the suction drain can be left in the deep layer. Approximate the subcutaneous tissues with 2-0 absorbable sutures, and approximate skin edges with either skin staples or a running subcuticular 3-0 absorbable stitch. Apply a bulky dressing.

▲ *Technique (Hall).* Hall described another technique of facet joint fusion. In the first step, cut the inferior facet sharply with a gouge. Remove this bone fragment, exposing the superior facet cartilage. Remove this cartilage with a sharp curet. Create a trough by removing the outer cortex of this superior facet, and add cancellous bone graft (Fig. 10-41). Proceed with decortication and wound closure as described in the Moe technique.

▲ *Postoperative management.* The patient is transferred to the bed from the operating table. Intravenous fluids are continued until the patient is able to tolerate oral intake and no longer requires any intravenous medication. Prophylactic preoperative, intraoperative, and postoperative intravenous antibiotics are given. Most patients have a Foley catheter inserted at the time of surgery; this is removed about 48 to 72 hours after surgery. Other postoperative treatment, such as casting, bracing, or ambulation, depends on the type of internal fixation, if any, used with the individual procedure.

Spinal instrumentation. There are numerous techniques of instrumentation of the scoliotic spine, but the goal of treatment of each is to achieve a balanced, stable spine with as little residual deformity as is safely possible. Instrumentation serves as both a correction device and an internal fixation device. The fusion mass in a well-corrected spine is subjected to much lower bending moments and tensile forces than is the fusion mass in an uncorrected spine (Fig. 10-42). Many authors have noted a higher incidence of pseudarthrosis in spinal arthrodesis without instrumentation. In a long-term study, however, Moskowitz et al found that patients with a solid spine fusion rarely had progression of their scoliosis and that they had no more low back pain than persons of their same age without scoliosis. The purpose of instrumentation therefore is to lower the incidence of pseudarthrosis and improve the amount of correction obtained at surgery.

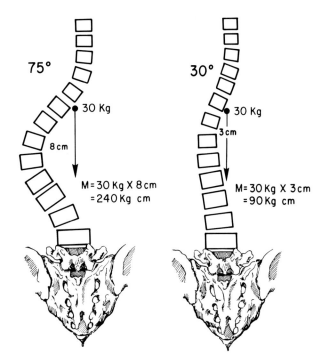

Fig. 10-42 Comparative bending forces exerted at apexes of 75-degree curve and 30-degree curve. (From Dunn HK. In The American Academy of Orthopaedic Surgeons: Instructional course lectures, vol 32, St Louis, 1983, The CV Mosby Co.)

Harrington instrumentation and variations of his original technique have proved successful in the treatment of most patients with adolescent idiopathic scoliosis, but recently several authors have reported problems with instrumentation of thoracolumbar and lumbar idiopathic scoliosis curves. They have found that distraction of the lumbar spine may reduce the normal lumbar lordosis and that extension of the fusion distally decreases the number of open segments between the end of the fusion mass and the pelvis. To combat these problems, anterior fusion with Zielke or Dwyer instrumentation has been recommended to limit the distal extent of the fusion and save one or two vertebral levels as well as to maintain normal lumbar lordosis. With the Harrington instrumentation it is important that the lower hook not be placed distal to L4. Because lumbar lordosis must be contoured into the rod, Moe square-ended rods should be used. In addition, a compression system used in the lumbar spine to provide segmental fixation helps to maintain lumbar lordosis, or the spinous processes of the lower two vertebrae can be wired together as described by Lagrone (Fig. 10-43).

A 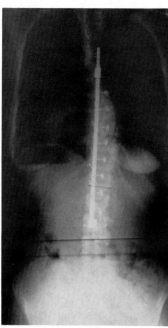 **B**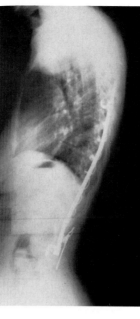

Fig. 10-43 **A,** Postoperative posteroanterior view of instrumentation and fusion into lumbar spine for idiopathic scoliosis. **B,** Lateral view of contoured Moe rod with wiring of spinous processes of lower two vertebrae to maintain lumbar lordosis.

Harrington instrumentation

In 1962 Harrington introduced an instrumentation system for spinal deformities. The Harrington distraction rod is a stainless steel rod that is connected to the posterior elements of the spine; distraction is adjusted by the ratchet principle (Fig. 10-44). The distraction rod is available in lengths of 0.5-inch increments. Some rods have eleven ratchets and some six; each requires a different distractor as well as a different length rod. A variety of hooks are available for securing the ratchet end of the rod to the spine (Fig. 10-45) and for use at the collared end of the rod (Fig. 10-46); the ratchet hooks and collar hooks are not interchangeable. Several basic instruments are needed to insert the distraction rod (Fig. 10-47).

Moe modified Harrington rods by squaring the collar end and using corresponding square hooks (Fig. 10-48). These are used when contouring of the rods is necessary to maintain lumbar lordosis or thoracic kyphosis. Without the squared ends the rod would rotate, causing the contouring to end up in a different plane from that intended. The instrumentation was designed to apply forces of distraction and compres-

Table 10-1 Expectation of representative strengths of fixation

	Thoracic vertebrae	Lumbar vertebrae
Facet and lamina	70 kgf	140 kgf
Base of transverse process	35 kgf	7 kgf
Tip of transverse process	7 kgf	
Base of spinous process	15 kgf	

From Dunn, HK. In The American Academy of Orthopaedic Surgeons: Instructional course lectures, vol 32, St Louis, 1983, The CV Mosby Co.
kgf, Kilogram-force.

sion over several segments of the spine in the area of the posterior elements and thus hold the correction until fusion occurs and the spine is stable. Although the major force is provided by the distraction system, the compression system is integral to the effectiveness of the total system. The principal limiting factor on the amount of force that can be placed on the spine is the strength of the bone into which the instruments are inserted. Dunn developed a table of the relative strengths of fixation in longitudinally applied forces through the midthoracic and lumbar vertebrae (Table 10-1). It should be emphasized that these forces are for longitudinally applied forces and not posteriorly directed forces. No more than half the force estimated to cause failure of the weakest link of the system should be applied. Thus, from 80 to 100 lb (36.3 to 45.4 kg) is the safe range of force applied to a distraction hook; force on the compression hook rarely is more than 25 lb (11.3 kg). The majority of hook failures consist of the hook's cutting out posteriorly when the lamina fails. The strength of the bone in the thoracic lamina and facet area to these posteriorly directed forces is considerably less than resistance to longitudinally directed forces.

Seating of a hook requires utmost care to prevent instrument failure, particularly lateral rotation. Rotation may be prevented in three ways: (1) seating the distraction hook in the pedicle at the described angle, (2) using a No. 1262 hook, the keel of which will prevent rotation and lateral slipping, or using a bifid hook to encircle a pedicle on either side, or (3) introducing the whole shoe of a No. 1253 hook into the spinal canal; the lower hook always is placed in the spinal canal.

Fig. 10-44 Harrington distraction rod. (Courtesy Zimmer.)

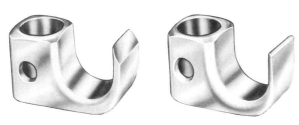

Fig. 10-45 Examples of ratchet end hooks used with Harrington distraction rod. (Courtesy Zimmer.)

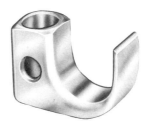

Fig. 10-46 Examples of collar-end hooks used with Harrington distraction rod. (Courtesy Zimmer.)

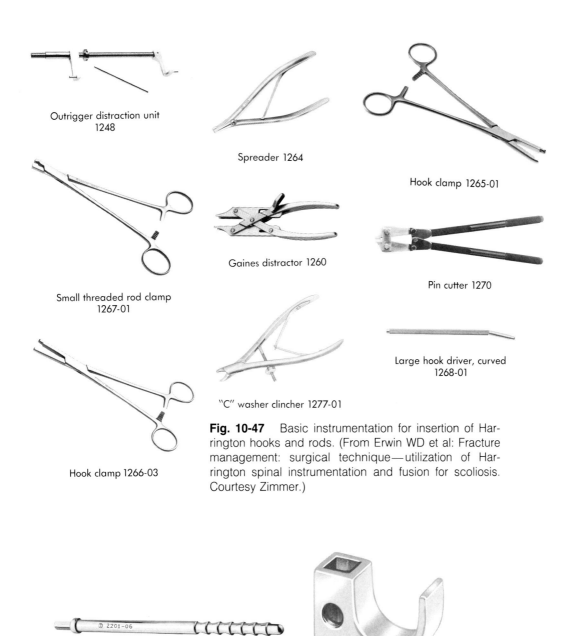

Outrigger distraction unit
1248

Spreader 1264

Hook clamp 1265-01

Small threaded rod clamp
1267-01

Gaines distractor 1260

Pin cutter 1270

"C" washer clincher 1277-01

Large hook driver, curved
1268-01

Hook clamp 1266-03

Fig. 10-47 Basic instrumentation for insertion of Harrington hooks and rods. (From Erwin WD et al: Fracture management: surgical technique—utilization of Harrington spinal instrumentation and fusion for scoliosis. Courtesy Zimmer.)

2201-06

Fig. 10-48 Moe square-ended rod with corresponding square-ended collar hook. (Courtesy Zimmer.)

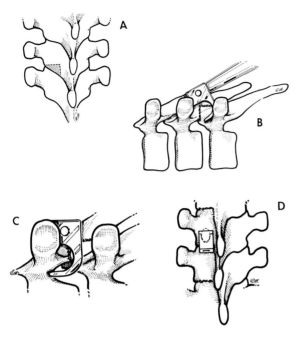

Fig. 10-49 **A** to **D,** Insertion of superior hook for Harrington distraction rod.

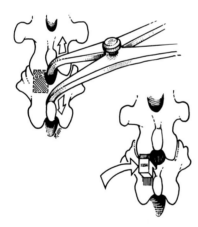

Fig. 10-50 Insertion of inferior distraction hook for Harrington distraction instrumentation.(Redrawn from Bradford DS et al: Moe's textbook of scoliosis and other spinal deformities, ed 2, Philadelphia, 1987, WB Saunders Co.)

▶*Technique.* After the initial exposure (p. 472), prepare the site for the upper hook by removing a small piece of the inferior facet (Fig. 10-49, *A*). This allows the hook to be securely seated into the stronger portion of the facet and into the pedicle or around the pedicle. Using the hook inserter, insert a sharp-edged, plain, large Harrington hook (No. 1251) without excessive force, making sure that the blade of the hook actually goes between the two joint surfaces and not within the medulla of the lamina of the vertebra above. When the location for the hook has been established, withdraw this hook and insert a large, dull-flanged hook (No. 1262) in its place. The vertical flange is designed to prevent the blade in the hook from slipping laterally out of the joint or the unlikely possibility of its slipping medially toward the spinal canal. The proper seating angle for this hook is shown in Fig. 10-49, *B* and *C*. Alternatively, a bifid hook can be used, incorporating the pedicle to prevent lateral displacement (Fig. 10-49, *D*). Once the hook is fully seated, check its stability by forcing it superiorly to ensure that an adequate distraction force can be applied.

The inferiormost distraction hook usually is placed in a lumbar vertebra, although it may be placed under the lamina of T12 when the posterior elements of this vertebra are similar to those of a lumbar vertebra. Do not place the hook through the lamina of a higher thoracic vertebra. Remove the ligamentum flavum from the superior portion of the lamina of the lumbar vertebra to undergo instrumentation. A lamina spreader or an Enge retractor used to spread the spinous processes makes this portion of the procedure a little easier (Fig. 10-50). Once the ligamentum flavum has been removed, remove portions of the lateral part of the lamina with a Kerrison rongeur to allow insertion of a dull hook (No. 1254 or No. 1279-001 if there is room enough in the patient's canal to accommodate this). If the compression system is to be used, insert it at this time (this technique is described in the next section).

Now use the Harrington outrigger to allow decortication while the spine is in the corrected position (Fig. 10-51), or insert the distraction rod on the concave side of the curve and perform decortication around the distraction rod. Performing the decortication with the distraction rod in place does not prevent an adequate intraarticular fusion, and the surgeon avoids having to carry out the distraction in the face of active bleeding from decortication. Select a distraction rod of suitable length, and insert its notched end through the superior hook while holding the hook in place with a hook holder. Then while the superior hook and hook holder are held by an assistant, grasp the inferior hook with a hook holder and feed the inferior end of the rod into the eye of that hook. If Moe square-ended rods and squared hooks are used and the rod is contoured to allow lumbar lordosis, this can be difficult. The rod-holding device and a pushing device (Fig. 10-52) facilitate this portion of the procedure. Next fit the spreader between the superior hook and the notch of the rod just inferior to it. By repeated speading of the instrument, force the superior hook up the notched part of the rod (Fig. 10-53, *A*). When the six ratchet rods are used, a Gaines distractor must be used (Fig. 10-53, *B*). Make every effort to keep the superior hook as close to the ratchet transition region of the solid rod as possible. This hook placement results in a much longer service life for the rod and much less fatigue for the system. As the distance between the hooks at each end of the rod is increased with each successive click of the instrument, distraction is applied. Proceed carefully with the distraction while observing the stability of both hooks. As the distraction becomes more difficult and the instruments tighten, any evidence of fracture or tearing of the posterior elements indicates that the distraction should be stopped and that the correction obtained at that point should be accepted. At the completion of the distraction, apply a C-washer distal to the upper hook to prevent loss of distraction. The correction obtainable varies considerably, depending on the age and maturity of the patient and the hardness of the bone. When the bone is mature, the distraction usually can be continued until the rod begins to bow. It always must be remembered that considerably more force can be exerted with the Harrington distractor than can be tolerated by any of the posterior elements.

After insertion of the distraction rod, complete the decortication and intraarticular fusion as described on p. 476 and close the wound as described on p. 477.

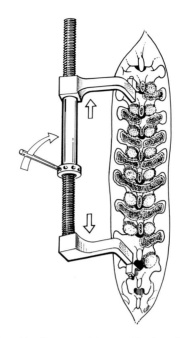

Fig. 10-51   Harrington outrigger allowing decortication of spine in corrected position.

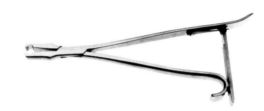

Fig. 10-52   Rod clamp used to hold and manipulate distraction rods. (Courtesy Zimmer.)

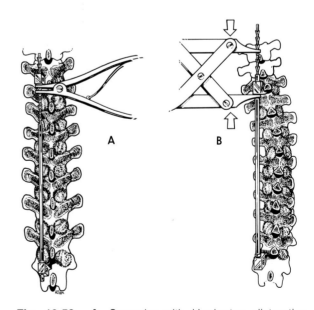

Fig. 10-53   **A,** Spreader with Harrington distraction rod. **B,** Gaines distractor with six-ratchet Harrington distraction rods.

Harrington distraction instrumentation to the sacrum

Distraction implants to the sacrum should be avoided if at all possible. Distraction in this area produces a loss of lumbar lordosis, sacral malrotation, a high likelihood of pseudarthrosis, implant failure, and hook dislodgment. In idiopathic scoliosis, fusions distal to L4 rarely are needed. Fusion to the sacrum generally is used for neuromuscular scoliosis. If instrumentation to the sacrum is required, the upper hook site is prepared as previously described and the ala of the sacrum is exposed. Square-ended Harrington rods and a square-ended sacral alar hook are used. The alar hook is placed around the ala of the sacrum, and the appropriate length square-ended rod is inserted. Appropriate contouring of the lumbar lordosis must be performed during instrumentation to the sacrum. Then fusion is carried out (see p. 476).

Harrington compression instrumentation

Harrington considers the compression rod assembly an integral part of his system although other surgeons have used the Harrington distraction rod with external immobilization or segmental fixation such as interspinous or sublaminar wires. The compression rod applies a significant corrective force for any kyphotic deformity and should be used whenever there is a significant kyphotic component. Compression is useful in the correction of Scheuermann's disease and helps maintain lumbar lordosis if the fusion extends lower into the spine. The insertion of the compression assembly is somewhat complex and also decreases the amount of bone available for decortication and subsequent fusion. The basic equipment consists of two threaded rods, the larger of which is ³⁄₁₆ inch in diameter (4.8 mm) and requires a No. 1256 hook. The smaller threaded compression rod is ⅛ inch in diameter (3.2 mm) and requires a No. 1259 compression hook. The smaller threaded rod is used most often because it is easier to insert and more easily adapts to the shape of the spine.

▶ *Technique.* Prepare the compression rod with three hooks facing distally and three proximally (Fig. 10-54, *A*). Cut the costotransverse ligaments around the transverse processes, using the sharp No. 1259 hook introduced beneath the transverse process with the hook holder (Fig. 10-54, *B*). The No. 1251 sharp distraction hook also may be used; it is a larger distraction hook with a sharp end that will provide a larger area for subsequent insertion of the No. 1259 hooks. Direct these hooks caudad on all vertebrae above the apex of the curve and cephalad on all vertebrae below the apex of the curve. Caudal to T11 the transverse processes generally are inadequate, so place the hooks under the lamina (Fig. 10-54, *C*). Grasp the compression assembly with hook holders, and beginning cranially, place all the hooks beneath the trans-

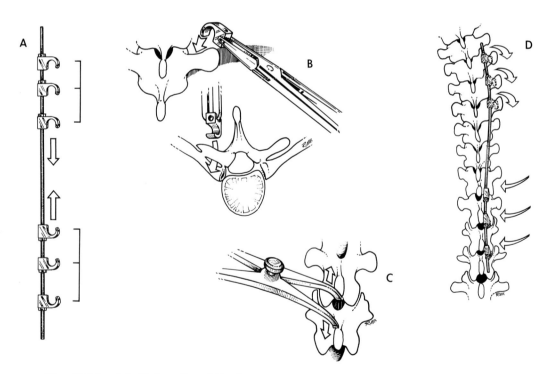

Fig. 10-54   **A** to **D,** Insertion of Harrington compression rod on convex side of thoracic spine for idiopathic scoliosis (see text). (Redrawn from Bradford DS et al: Moe's textbook of scoliosis and other spinal deformities, ed 2, Philadelphia, 1987, WB Saunders Co.)

verse processes. Place the caudal hooks beneath the transverse processes or lamina, as indicated (Fig. 10-54, *D*). Tighten the system by using the spreader between a rod holder and hook holder (Fig. 10-55). Use a wrench to tighten the nuts. This device produces a lordosis, and tightening should cease when this begins to occur. If the compression assembly is used in conjunction with the distraction rod for scoliosis, the compression assembly usually is tightened before the distraction is applied.

Now pack the wound open with sponges, and obtain a bone graft from the posterior iliac crest as described on p. 473. After the bone graft is obtained, perform a Moe intraarticular decortication (p. 476) combined with meticulous decortication of the lamina and transverse processes. Then pack the bone graft in the area of the fusion, and close the wound as previously described.

Harrington distraction system plus compression system with transverse loading device

The transverse loading device connects between the Harrington distraction rod and the Harrington compression system (Fig. 10-56). The basic principle of this device is reduction of the distance from the apex of the curve to the midline to produce a more stable spine and provide additional support on the convex side of the curve at the apex through the linkage to the compression rod. In large curves longitudinally applied distraction force is biomechanically effective, but in smaller curves it becomes much less effective and transverse loading becomes more effective. Dunn has shown that in a 90-degree scoliotic curve about 70% of the distraction force is acting to correct the curve. In a 45-degree curve only 35% of the force is corrective. In the smaller curve, however, transversely applied force acts almost exclusively for correction. The transverse traction device has been used successfully for many years, but it should be pointed out that the Harrington system was not originally designed for use with this type of load, and hook cut-out can occur in the use of these transverse loads. Armstrong and Connock used a modified Harrington distraction system in their transverse traction device.

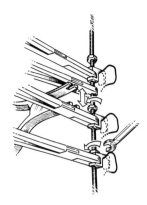

Fig. 10-55 Distractor and rod clamps for applying compression to Harrington compression system. (Redrawn from Bradford DS et al: Moe's textbook of scoliosis and other spinal deformities, ed 2, Philadelphia, 1987, WB Saunders Co.)

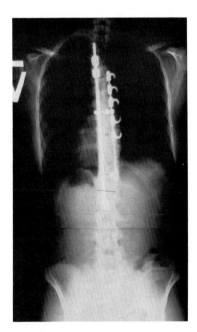

Fig. 10-56 Transverse loading device connecting Harrington distraction and compression rods.

Segmental spinal instrumentation

Segmental spinal instrumentation simply denotes a technique that allows fixation of the instrumentation to vertebral components at multiple levels. Technically, this includes the Harrington compression system, the Harrington rods augmented with sublaminar or interspinous wiring, and anterior techniques such as the Dwyer or Zielke instrumentation. Recently, however, the term *segmental spinal instrumentation* has come to imply the use of sublaminar wires on each side of the spinous process with a long L-shaped rod, a technique introduced by Eduardo Luque of Mexico City in 1973. The rods can be contoured, and the spine is corrected as the wires are tightened. Internal fixation is more rigid than that obtained with the Harrington distraction instrumentation. This technique has been developed and standardized in the United States by Allen and associates. Many spine surgeons believe that the fixation provided by this system is secure enough so that external immobilization is not needed postoperatively, but there have been some reports to the contrary, and external immobilization often is used with the Luque rods.

Neurologic complications, apparently from passage or manipulation of the wire in the spinal canal, have been reported frequently enough so that use of the procedure only for neuromuscular scoliosis seems prudent, especially in patients in whom external immobilization must be limited or eliminated entirely. Some centers do use the procedure in neurologically normal patients, but this should be performed only by spine surgeons experienced with this technique and in medical centers where spinal cord monitoring can be carried out.

The basic instrumentation for the system consists of ³⁄₁₆-inch (4.8 mm) diameter rods of stainless steel or a nickel-chrome (MP-35-N) alloy; ¼-inch (6.3 mm) diameter rods are also available. Wires are available in diameters of 16 and 18 gauge. If the alloy rods are used, compatible alloy wires should be used with them.

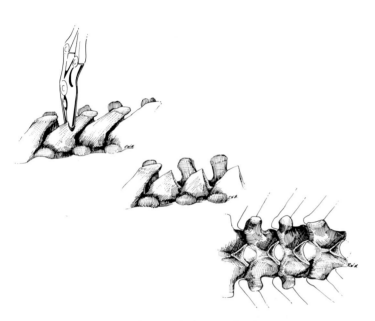

Fig. 10-57   Removal of caudally slanting spinous processes to expose ligamentum flavum. (From Segmental spinal fixation and correction using Richards' L-rod instrumentation, Memphis, Richards Mfg Co.)

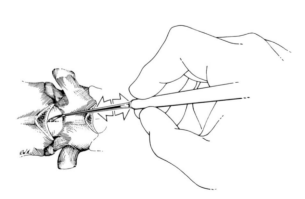

Fig. 10-58   Penfield No. 4 dissector for freeing deep surfaces of ligamentum flavum. (From Segmental spinal fixation and correction using Richards' L-rod instrumentation, Memphis, Richards Mfg Co.)

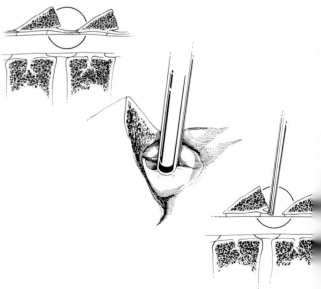

Fig. 10-59   Kerrison punch for removing remainder of ligamentum flavum. (From Segmental spinal fixation and correction using Richards' L-rod instrumentation, Memphis, Richards Mfg Co.)

▶ *Technique.* Expose the spine in the routine manner as described on p. 472, and excise the ligamentum flavum. Using a needle-nose rongeur, gradually thin the ligamentum flavum until the midline cleavage plane is visible. In the thoracic spine the spinous processes slant distally, and the spinous processes must be removed before the ligamentum flavum can be adequately seen (Fig. 10-57). Once the midline cleavage plane is visible, carefully sweep a Penfield No. 4 dissector across the deep surface of the ligamentum flavum on the right and left sides (Fig. 10-58). Use a Kerrison punch to remove the remainder of the ligamentum flavum (Fig. 10-59). Take care during this step to avoid damaging the dura or the epidural vessels. Shape 16- or 18-gauge wire as shown in Fig. 10-60. The major diameter of the bend should be slightly larger than the lamina. Several studies have shown that the depth of penetration of the wire as it is passed around the lamina can be significant. Although the cerebral spinal fluid that bathes the spinal cord probably cushions it from the trauma of the passage of these wires, this portion of the surgical procedure is the most critical and dangerous as far as causing a neurologic injury. It is important that both surgeon and assistant be completely prepared for each step before passage of the wire and that they are careful about sudden movements and inadvertent touching or hitting of the wires that have already been passed. Gently place the tip of the wire into the neural canal at the inferior edge of the lamina in the midline. Hold the long end of the doubled wire in one hand, and advance the tip with the other. Rest the hand advancing the tip firmly on the patient's back. Lift the tails of the wire slightly, pulling them to

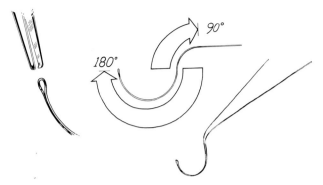

Fig. 10-60   Shape of double wire before it passes under lamina. (From Segmental spinal fixation and correction using Richards' L-rod instrumentation, Memphis, Richards Mfg Co.)

keep the wires snugly against the undersurface of the lamina, and roll the tip so that it emerges on the upper end of the lamina (Fig. 10-61). As the tip of the wire emerges, grab it with a needle holder or wire holder that will not spring off the loop. An alternative is a Kocher clamp with the tooth placed into the loop of the wire. Take the clamp from the assistant, and pull the wire with the clamp until it is positioned beneath the lamina with half its length protruding above and half below the lamina. As the clamp is pulled, gently feed from the long end of the wire. At this point cut the tip off the wire and place one length of the wire on the right side and the other on the left side of the lamina. An alternative is to leave double wires on one side and pass another wire to have double wires on both sides. Crimp each wire

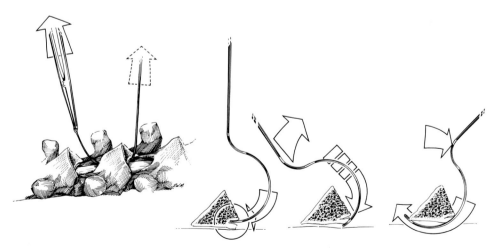

Fig. 10-61   Passage of segmental wire beneath lamina. (From Segmental spinal fixation and correction using Richards' L-rod instrumentation, Memphis, Richards Mfg Co.)

onto the surface of the lamina to prevent any from being pushed accidently into the neural canal (Fig. 10-62). As more wires are passed, it becomes easy to accidently hit other wires; be very careful not to do this even though the wires are crimped over the lamina. Crimp the superior wire toward the midline and the inferior wire laterally. Use double wires at the cephalad and caudal lamina of the segment undergoing instrumentation. Two rods are implanted for most scoliosis corrections, with the first rod applied either to the convex or to the concave side of the curve. Lumbar scoliosis generally is more easily corrected by the concave rod technique.

► *Technique (convex rod).* The convex rod technique is most useful in the correction of thoracic curves. Fasten the initial rod to the upper region of the scoliotic curve, with the short limb placed transversely across the lamina of the second vertebra above the curve. Tighten the second and third wires on the convex side, then tighten wires sequentially from proximal to distal as the rod is levered toward the spine (Fig. 10-63). After about half the convex wires have been tightened, apply the concave rod. Place the L portion of this rod distal to the lamina that is to undergo instrumentation through a hole cut in the spinous process to accommodate the rod. Place the L portion underneath the convex rod distally. Then tie this rod down over the distal lamina, working distally

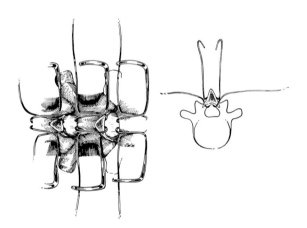

Fig. 10-62 Following division of wire, wire is crimped on laminar surface of each side of spinous process. (From Segmental spinal fixation and correction using Richards' L-rod instrumentation, Memphis, Richards Mfg Co.)

to proximally. Tighten the wires sequentially. At the proximal end the long end of the concave rod (Fig. 10-63) should lie over the short L leg of the convex rod. Cut the ends of the wire, and bend them toward the midline.

► *Technique (concave).* The concave technique is preferable for lumbar scoliosis, with the appropriate amount of lordosis or kyphosis bent into the rods with the rod bender. Place the initial rod with its short limb passing transversely across the lamina of the lowermost vertebra to undergo instrumentation. Pass it through a hole at the base of the spinous process, and tighten the inferior double-end wire on the concave side to supply firm fixation at the distal level. Now tighten the wires to the lamina above the vertebra of the curve. Loosely attach the convex rod proximally after the short end is placed loosely under the long limb of the concave rod. Once the concave rod is completely tightened, it is quite difficult to pass this short limb under the long limb of the concave rod. Reduce the spine to the rod, using either manual correction or a wire tightener. An assistant can apply appropriate manual correction by pressure on the trunk as wires are tightened beneath the apex of the curvature (Fig. 10-64). Securely fasten the convex rod, tightening wires from cephalad to caudad. Once in position, both rods usually can be brought into firm contact with the lamina by squeezing them together with a rod approximator. As the rods are approximated, the concave wires will loosen and must be tightened again. Trim the wires to about 0.5 inch in length, and bend them toward the midline.

► *Technique (fusion).* By virtue of the internal fixation device itself, there is very little exposed bone for decortication and facet excision. A large volume of bone graft is necessary, and cancellous bone is harvested from the posterior iliac crest. If the procedure is performed for neuromuscular scoliosis, bone bank bone also may be needed. Place the graft lateral to the rods on both sides of the spine and out to the tips of the transverse processes.

PELVIC FIXATION. Because the Luque-rod system is used primarily for neuromuscular conditions, most of which involve curves that include the sacrum, pelvic fixation is an important part of this system. Fixation can be obtained by passing the short arm of the rod through the posterior iliac spine. Allen and Ferguson, however, described a technique known as the Galveston technique, which obtains better fixation to the pelvis.

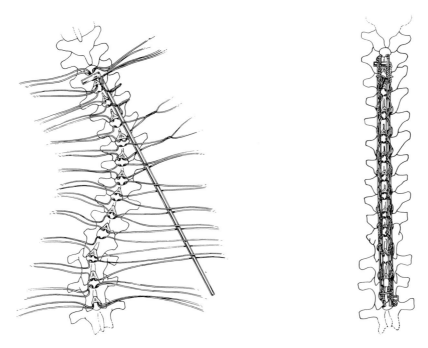

Fig. 10-63 Convex rod technique for correction of thoracic scoliosis. (From Segmental spinal fixation and correction using Richards' L-rod instrumentation, Memphis, Richards Mfg Co.)

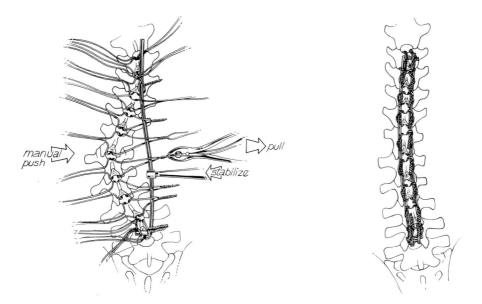

Fig. 10-64 Concave rod technique for correction of lumbar scoliosis. (From Segmental spinal fixation and correction using Richards' L-rod instrumentation, Memphis, Richards Mfg Co.)

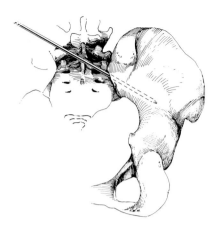

Fig. 10-65 Insertion of guide pin just posterior to sacroiliac joint at level of posterior iliac spine. (From Segmental spinal fixation and correction using Richards' L-rod instrumentation, Memphis, Richards Mfg Co.)

▶ *Technique (Allen and Ferguson).* Expose both iliac crests to the sciatic notches. Drill a guide pin, the same diameter as the rod to be used, along the transverse bar of the ilium, with the entrance site just posterior to the sacroiliac joint at the level of the posterosuperior iliac spine. Drill this pin into a depth of approximately 6 to 9 cm (Fig. 10-65). Contour the rod in three different planes. Using two sleeve benders, make the first bend at a 90-degree angle, leaving the short-arm approximately 12 cm in length. Make a second bend about 2 cm lateral to the first bend, using a pelvic rod-bending clamp and a sleeve bender in combination; this angle generally is between 50 and 75 degrees but basically is contoured to fit the angle of the ilium to the patient's midsagittal plane. Using a French rod bender, bend the lordosis into the long limb of the rod. As this lordosis is applied to the rod, the short limb of the rod approximates angle of the pin in its caudal tilt (Fig. 10-66). Remove the pelvic pin, and drive the iliac portion of the rod into the prepared hole (Fig. 10-67). Tighten the sublaminar wires, and perform fusion as described previously.

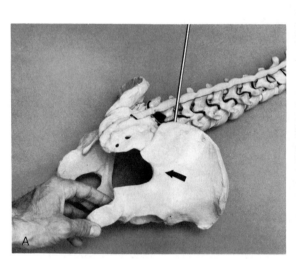
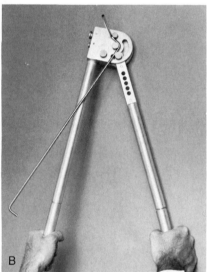

Fig. 10-66 **A** to **E,** Contouring of L-rod to maintain lumbar lordosis. (From Bradford DS et al: Moe's textbook of scoliosis and other spinal deformities, ed 2, Philadelphia, 1987, WB Saunders Co.)

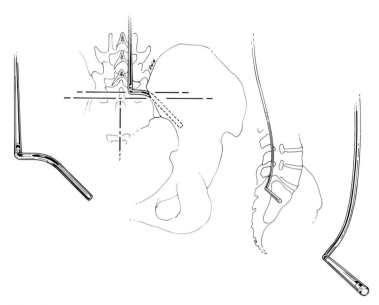

Fig. 10-67 Insertion of L-rod into previously prepared hole in ilium. (From Segmental spinal fixation and correction using Richards' L-rod instrumentation, Memphis, Richards Mfg Co.)

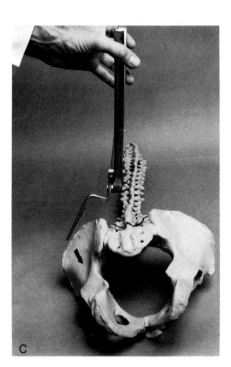

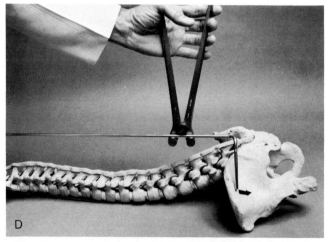

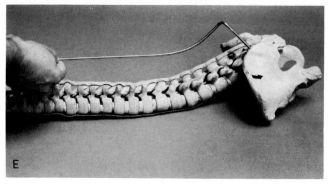

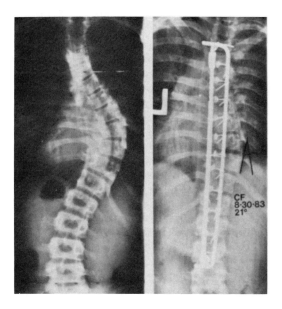

Fig. 10-68 Preoperative and postoperative roentgenograms of patient who underwent interspinous segmental spinal instrumentation. (From Guadagni J et al: J Pediatr Orthop 4:405, 1984.)

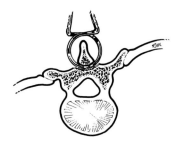

Fig. 10-69 Lewen clamp to make hole in base of spinous process for Drummond wires.

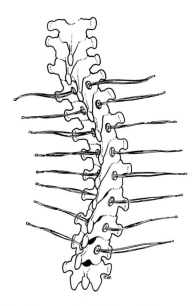

Fig. 10-70 Placement of buttons of Drummond wires.

Harrington rod instrumentation with Drummond interspinous segmental wiring

Drummond developed an interspinous segmental wiring technique that provides the stability afforded by segmental spinal instrumentation without the risk of passing sublaminar wires. The technique uses a paired, button-wire implant that is anchored to the base of the spinous processes (Fig. 10-68). Drummond's laboratory tests have shown that the base of the spinous process provides a good purchase site for fixation. The spinal buttons consist of 16- or 18-gauge stainless steel wire welded at the free ends to form a bead for easy passage and to prevent penetration of surgical gloves. The button attached to the wire is 0.6 mm thick and 8 mm in diameter.

▶ *Technique (Drummond).* Select the levels for fusion as for Harrington distraction instrumentation. After the spine has been exposed, insert the upper hook as previously described. Drummond recommends the use of a bifid hook to grasp the pedicle (see Fig. 10-49, *D*). Using an awl or a Lewen clamp, create a hole at the base of the spinous processes (Fig. 10-69). Pass two wires in opposite directions through the hole in the spinous process. Then pass the wires through the hole in the opposite button, and pull the buttons snugly to the base of the spinous processes (Fig. 10-70). Tamp the buttons into position with a mallet and a tamp. Insert only one button wire from the concave to the convex side at the uppermost and lowermost

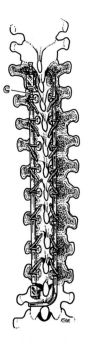

Fig. 10-71 Completed interspinous segmental spinal instrumentation.

segments. Using a square-ended Harrington rod carefully contoured to preserve physiologic kyphosis and lordosis, pass the rod through the open loops of wire implants on the concave side of the curve. Insert the rod in the upper and lower hooks in a routine manner. Accomplish initial correction by distraction. Contour a ³⁄₁₆-inch L-rod to preserve physiologic kyphosis and lordosis, and make right angle bends at the upper and lower ends of the rod. Pass the upper limb of the rod under the ratchet system of the distraction rod to prevent rotation of this rod. At this point, decortication of the convex side can be performed; only the posterior elements lateral to the button should be decorticated. Pass the contoured L-rod through the open wire loops of the implants on the convex side of the curve while an assistant presses the rod against the spine. To obtain correction, tighten each loop with a wire tightener. Tighten the apical wire first and then each proximal and distal level alternatively. The Harrington distraction rod then can be distracted further if possible. Place a C-clamp just below the upper hook to prevent loss of distraction. Tighten the wires on the Harrington rod but not so tightly as to rotate the hooks on the distraction rod (Fig. 10-71). Now obtain a bone graft from the iliac crest, complete the decortication, and insert the graft. Ambulation is allowed on the third or fourth day after surgery without any external immobilization.

Harrington distraction rods with Drummond wires alone

Contoured, square-ended Harrington distraction rods also can be used in combination with Drummond wires without the addition of the L-rod on the convex side of the curve. This obtains excellent segmental fixation and offers the advantages of a facet fusion, more complete decortication, and a larger area for bone graft incorporation. This technique does not, however, offer sufficient fixation to allow ambulation without external support, and a cast or brace should be used postoperatively.

▶ *Technique.* Expose the spine in the routine manner, and pass Drummond wires from the convex to the concave side of the curve with the button on the convex side and the wire on the concave side (Fig. 10-72). Place the Harrington distraction rod through the concave wires and apply distraction. Tighten the concave wires with a wire tightener. Apply a C-clamp just below the upper hook. Decorticate the spine (emphasizing a facet fusion), the lamina, and transverse processes lateral to the buttons (Fig. 10-73). If the patient has a significant rib hump, osteotomy of the transverse processes on the convex side can be performed.

▶ *Postoperative management.* A Risser cast is applied about 1 week after surgery (Fig. 10-74). The Risser cast is worn for about 4 months if the fusion is strictly in the thoracic area. If the fusion extends significantly down into the lumbar spine, the cast is maintained for 6 months.

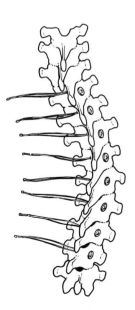

Fig. 10-72 Drummond wires passed from convex to concave side of curve.

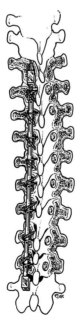

Fig. 10-73 Decortication along lamina and transverse processes lateral to buttons allows more complete decortication on convex side.

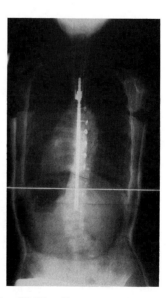

Fig. 10-74 Posteroanterior roentgenogram of patient in underarm cast after instrumentation with Harrington distraction rod and Drummond segmental wires.

Fig. 10-75 Cotrel-Dubousset rod with diamond-shaped irregularities allows strong fixation of vertebral hooks or screws at any level, with any degree of rotation, and in distraction and compression. Rod can be bent its entire length. (From Cotrel Y, Dubousset J, and Guillaumat M: Clin Orthop 227:10, 1988.)

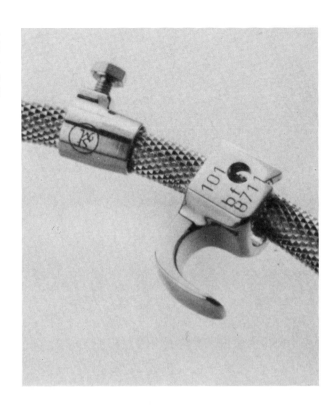

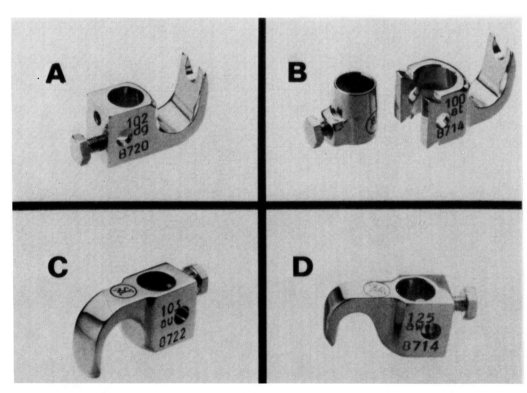

Fig. 10-76   Hooks used in Cotrel-Dubousset instrumentation. **A,** Pedicular hook with closed body. **B,** Pedicular hook with opened body and cylindroconic ring. **C,** Lumbar laminar hook with closed body. **D,** Thoracic laminar hook with closed body. (From Cotrel Y, Dubousset J, and Guillaumat M: Clin Orthop 227:10, 1988.)

Cotrel-Dubousset instrumentation

The concept of segmental instrumentation with the use of hooks was introduced by Cotrel and Dubousset in 1981. This method has achieved rapid, widespread use because of several advantages. (1) The system has the ability to distract and compress between segments with multiple hooks, whereas the Harrington distraction system distracts only on the end hooks. (2) Three-dimensional correction is possible because of the more lateral placement of the pedicle hooks together with prebending of the Cotrel-Dubousset concave rod. (3) Shufflebarger and Dubousset have shown a more normal sagittal contour of the spine after Cotrel-Dubousset instrumentation. (4) Because of the stability provided by multiple segmental fixation sites, no postoperative brace or cast is required. There are, however, several disadvantages of the system. (1) The surgical technique is much more difficult and time-consuming than the Harrington distraction system. (2) Much more experience is necessary to apply this system because of the multiple options of hook placement. (3) Because of the longer time between decortication and closure, blood loss is increased. (4) The system implants are significantly more expensive than the Harrington systems. (5) Although still quite low the neurologic complication rate is higher than with the Harrington system alone. As for any new procedure, further experience and longer follow-up are needed before the definite role of this system can be determined. The early results are encouraging although Hall et al noted some design problems with the present system.

The Cotrel-Dubousset rods are solid 7-mm rods with a knurled, diamond-point surface that allows rigid hook fixation at any location along the rod (Fig. 10-75). There are three basic hook types: pedicle, lumbar laminar, and thoracic laminar. Each is available in either an "open" or "closed" style (Fig. 10-76). A transverse loader rod, ⅛-inch in diameter, serves to interlock the two rods (Fig. 10-77). The rod is held into the open hooks by a hook blocker. Set screws prevent the rod from rotating once the position has been set.

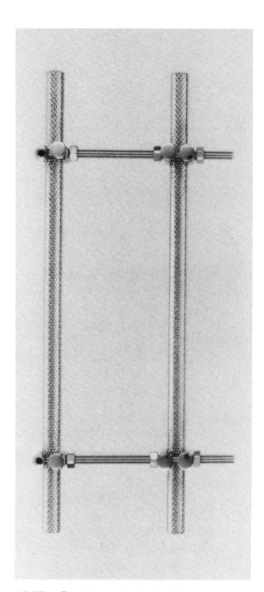

Fig. 10-77 Double rods locked by two transverse loading rods, resulting in strong framelike setup. (From Cotrel Y, Dubousset J, and Guillaumat M: Clin Orthop 227:10, 1988.)

HOOK SITE SELECTION. The end vertebrae to be included in the fusion are determined in a manner similar to the Harrington system, although some recent reports indicate that this is not always true for the inferior hook, and many instances of decompensation of the spine with selective fusion of the thoracic curve in King type II curves have been reported. The lowermost vertebra to undergo instrumentation usually is the neutral vertebra. Care must be taken to be certain that the lower hooks are within the stable zone of Harrington. The lateral film should also show that the inferior hook is well into the lordotic segment of the spine, and the superior hook should not stop at the apex of the kyphotic segment. Preoperative standing and bending films are necessary to determine the apical vertebra and the intermediate vertebrae levels. The apical vertebra is the vertebral body with the most rotation on the plain standing film. The intermediate vertebrae are selected on the bending films and generally are one to two vertebral bodies on either side of the apical vertebra and show the least mobility on side bending (Fig. 10-78). Planned hook placement should be marked on the preoperative films (Table 10-2). Distraction is achieved on the concave side of the curve with a closed pedicle hook on the proximalmost vertebra and a closed laminar hook, either thoracic or lumbar, in the distalmost vertebra. An open pedicle hook is placed in the uppermost intermediate vertebra and an open thoracic laminar in the lowermost rigid vertebra on the concave side. On the convexity a closed laminar hook is used in the transverse process of the uppermost vertebra and a closed pedicle hook in the

facet joint. An open pedicle hook is placed into the facet joint of the apical vertebra on the convex side. At the distal end of the convexity a closed laminar hook is placed if the hook is in the lumbar spine, or a closed pedicle hook is used if the distal vertebra is in the thoracic spine (Fig. 10-79).

▶ *Technique.* After the patient is anesthetized and placed on the operating table in the prone position, head halter and leg traction may be used if desired. Expose the spine through a posterior approach as described on p. 472. Prepare the hook sites, and insert the hooks according to preoperative planning. Insert the concave hooks first. Prepare the pedicle hook sites with an osteotome and a pedicle seeker. Once the hooks are in place, contour the concave rod using a malleable rod as a template, which also determines the length of the concave rod. Contour the concave rod to conform to the scoliotic curve in the anteroposterior plane. At this point in the procedure, obtain an iliac crest bone graft. Carry out decortication on the concave side before placing the rod in position. Insert the concave rod, and push hook blockers into the open pedicle and laminar hooks on the concave side of the intermediate vertebra. Distract these hooks, and hold them in position by temporarily tightening the C-rings but not tightening the set screws of the bushings within the open hooks. If these set screws are tightened, rotation of the rod will not be possible. Accomplish this segmental distraction at the intermediate open hooks, using a spreader between appropriate open rings and locally applied rod grippers. If traction has been applied, release it at this time. Using rod holders, derotate the

Table 10-2 Hook placement in the Cotrel-Dubousset technique

Instrumented vertebra	Concave hook	Convex hook
Uppermost instrumented vertebra = proximal		Closed laminar (transverse process)
Neutral or end vertebra	Closed pedicular	Closed pedicular
Uppermost vertebra of most rigid curve	Open pedicular	
Apical vertebra		Open pedicular
Lowermost vertebra of most rigid curve	Open thoracic laminar	
Lowermost instrumented vertebra = distal neutral or end vertebra	Closed laminar facing caudally	Closed laminar facing cranially

From Farcy J, Weidenbaum M, and Roye DP Jr: Surg Rounds for Orthopaedics 5:11, 1987.

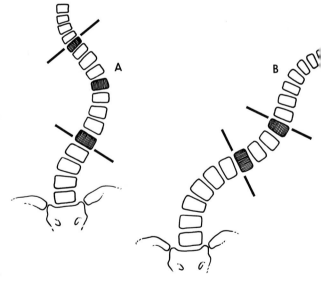

Fig. 10-78 **A,** Anteroposterior diagrams of uppermost and lowermost instrumented vertebrae. **B,** Upper and lower rigid vertebral bodies are shown on bending films.

spine approximately 90 degrees, correcting scoliosis and producing a physiologic kyphosis (Fig. 10-80). During this procedure the length of the spine is increased slightly, and the intermediate hooks are slightly loosened; seat them more snugly with an open hook pusher. Examine the upper and lower hooks to be certain they are seated snugly, and tighten the set screws to prevent the rod from derotating. Remove the two C-rings from the intermediate hook sites. Apply the convex hooks as determined on preoperative films. Using the malleable template, contour and insert a convex rod. Load the convex rod with a single hook blocker, oriented to fit the open pedicular hook on the convex side. Insert the proximal end of the convex rod into the two proximal end hooks, which are held together with hook holders. Place the rod into the open pedicular hook. Insert the distal end of the rod into the closed hook using the rod driver. Gently move the rod distally with the rod gripper or apply compression, causing distal migration of the rod through the distal hook. Squeeze the upper hooks together with a hook compressor to create a pediculotransverse claw-type fixation. Tighten the hexagonal screws of these hooks. Then apply compression between the proximal hooks and the intermediate open hook. During this procedure the distal hook must be held in place with a hook holder to prevent dislodgment of the hook while rod migration occurs as a result of the compression. Then apply the gripper distally, and with a hook compres-

sor compress the distal hook and provide segmental compression between the apical vertebra and the lowermost instrumented vertebra. Tighten the set screw.

The final step is application of the device for transverse traction (DTT), which converts the system into a more rigid, four-sided frame. Place the DTT as far proximal and distal as possible. Tighten the hexagonal set screws. Perform a Stagnara wake-up test (p. 508). After the wake-up test is performed, overtighten the set screws until they shear off, locking the system into place and preventing loss of fixation. Perform further decortication, and apply copious autogenous bone graft. Close the wound over drains in a routine manner.

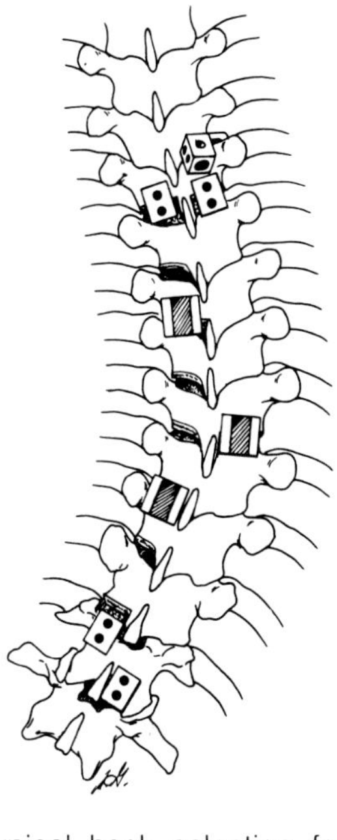

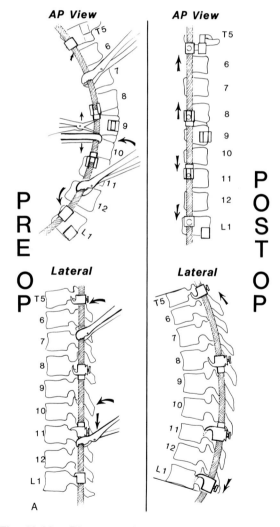

Fig. 10-80 Diagrammatic representation of rotation of Cotrel-Dubousset rods in anteroposterior plane to correct anteroposterior deformity and restore normal kyphosis in sagittal plane. (From Bradford DS et al: Moe's textbook of scoliosis and other spinal deformities, ed 2, Philadelphia, 1987, WB Saunders Co.)

Fig. 10-79 Typical hook selection for right thoracic curve, T4 to T12. (From Denis F: Orthop Clin North Am 19:291, 1988.)

▲ *Postoperative management.* The patient is log-rolled in bed for 2 to 3 days, and mobilization and ambulation are begun when the drains are removed. No postoperative immobilization is needed. Most patients are dismissed from the hospital on the sixth or seventh day after surgery. The patient's activities gradually are increased, but full release to normal activities is not allowed for one year while the bone graft matures (Fig. 10-81).

This technique applies only to thoracic curve patterns. Double-curve patterns, with either thoracic and lumbar curves, are more complex and require more hooks at more fixation sites. The technique is complex and places considerable demands on the surgeon. Because extensive decortication is performed before the fixation is inserted, blood loss can be excessive. Clinical training, especially with hands-on experience, should be obtained before this procedure is attempted. Its ultimate success, of course, depends on a solid bony fusion. Whether this system will ultimately prove to be superior to the Harrington system still is open to question.

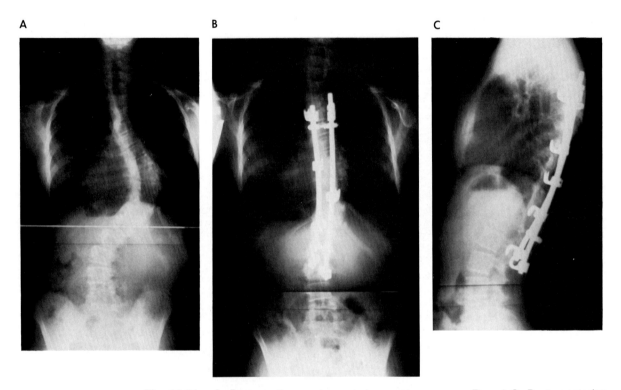

A   B   C

Fig. 10-81　**A,** Preoperative posteroanterior roentgenogram. **B** and **C,** Posteroanterior and lateral roentgenograms after Cotrel-Dubousset instrumentation.

Anterior Fusion

With the posterior approach for correction of spinal deformities well established, more attention in recent years has been placed on the anterior approach to the spinal column. Advances in anesthesia and intensive care have made it possible to perform anterior spinal surgery with acceptable safety. The anterior approach to spinal surgery seldom was used until the 1950s. Leaders in the anterior approach to the cervical and lumbar areas include Cloward, Southwick and Robinson, Bailey and Badgley, Harmon, and Wiltberger. Although Nachlas and Borden, Smith, von Lackum, and Wylie were among the first to report their experiences with the transthoracic approach to the thoracic spine, its major proponents were Hodgson et al of Hong Kong. The development of the Dwyer and Zielke anterior instrumentation has greatly enhanced the treatment of various deformities of the thoracic and lumbar spine.

Although the majority of spine deformities can be approached posteriorly, many are better approached anteriorly. Hall's indications for an anterior approach to the spine are outlined in the box. Correction of spinal deformities by the anterior approach has several risks, including excessive angulation or compression of the spinal cord by too rapid correction of the deformity, intolerable distraction of the cord with an opening wedge procedure, and interference of the circulation of the spinal cord because of ligation of the segmental vessels and perhaps the artery of Adamkiewicz. The anterior approach to the spine should be limited to those conditions in which it is absolutely indicated.

When the anterior approach to the spine is used, the aid of a thoracic or general surgeon can be enlisted during both the intraoperative exposure and the postoperative management. The orthopaedic surgeon, however, must be aware of the basic anatomy and approaches and should guide the thoracic surgeon in the exposure needed for the spinal procedure.

INDICATIONS FOR ANTERIOR APPROACH

I. Absolute
  A. Scoliosis with deficient posterior spinal elements
    1. Congenital—myelomeningocele
    2. Acquired—after extensive laminectomy
  B. Severe rigid congenital scoliosis
    1. Unilateral unsegmented bar
    2. Hemivertebrae
  C. Severe kyphosis
    1. Congenital
       Anterior hemi- or microvertebrae
       Anterior unsegmented bar
    2. Acquired
       Posttraumatic
       Inflammatory (tuberculosis)
       Postirradiation
  D. Hyperlordosis
     After lumboperitoneal shunts with tethered spinal cord
II. Relative
  A. Cervical spondylosis
  B. Some paralytic curves with lordosis (cerebral palsy)
  C. Thoracolumbar scoliosis
  D. Spondylolisthesis (without neurologic deficit)
  E. Thoracic idiopathic scoliosis

From Hall JE: Orthop Clin North Am 3:81, 1972.

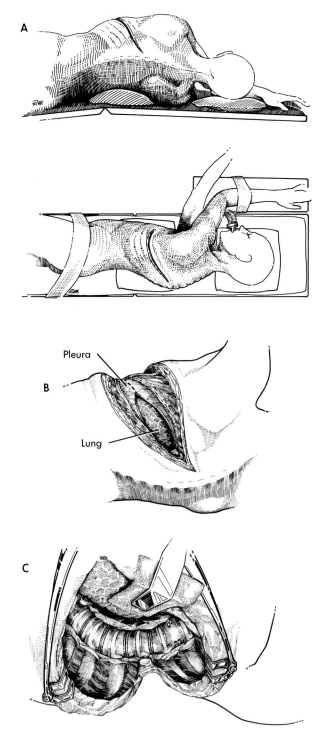

Fig. 10-82   A, Positioning of patient and incision for transthoracic approach. **B,** Rib removal and division of pleura, exposing lung. **C,** Exposure of spine and division of segmental vessels over one of the vertebral bodies.

Approaches
Transthoracic

The thoracic spine can be approached from either the right or the left side. The spine generally is approached from the convex side of the curvature, but in the absence of a significant scoliosis most surgeons prefer to enter the chest on the left side because the aorta tolerates handling better than the thin-walled vena cava.

The level of exposure is determined by the deformity to be corrected and should be two ribs above the vertebral level sought. For example, if T7 is to be exposed, the fifth rib on the left is removed. This is necessary because of the caudad inclination of the ribs. It is possible to go cephalad as high as the third rib by careful mobilization of the scapula upward and forward.

▶ *Technique.* Place the patient in a lateral decubitus position. Prepare and drape the skin in the routine sterile manner. Make an incision from the posterior angle of the rib to the tip of the costocartilage (Fig. 10-82, *A*). Expose the rib subperiostally, and detach it anteriorly from the costochondral junction and posteriorly as close to the costotransverse articulation as possible. Many thoracic surgeons prefer entry through an intercostal space, but rib resection affords a larger working aperture and the rib provides any necessary bone graft (Fig. 10-82, *B*). If possible use a retropleural approach. If this is not possible, incise the parietal pleura along the rib bed. Use rib spreaders to expose the chest cavity. Pack off the lung, and every 20 to 30 minutes aerate the lung to remove all cyanotic spots.

Using blunt and sharp dissection, mobilize the areolar tissue between the great vessels and the vertebral bodies. This serves as a protective layer in which to place retractors. Identify the segmental vessels as they adhere to the waist of each vertebra. Clamp and ligate each of these vessels, and section them near the midline (Fig. 10-82, *C*). Do not ligate them near the distribution point of Dommisse at the foramen. If they are ligated too far laterally, the collateral vessels from the foramen may be disrupted and the segmental feeder vessels to the spinal cord may be damaged. At this point the spine can be exposed either subperiosteally or extraperiosteally (depending on the procedure to be performed); the extraperiosteal exposure will minimize bleeding. If the procedure is simple disk excision, then extraperiosteal dissection is adequate. If the procedure is strut grafting, then the subperiosteal approach is preferable.

Thoracoabdominal

▶ *Technique.* Place the patient in the lateral decubitus position with the side to be entered elevated. Make a curvilinear incision along the tenth rib extending distally along the anterolateral abdominal wall just lateral to the rectus abdominis muscle (Fig. 10-83, *A*). Excise the tenth rib and identify the diaphragm as a separate structure; it tends to closely approximate the wall of the thoracic cage. The diaphragm can be removed in two ways. It can be removed from the chest cavity, and then retroperitoneal dissection is continued distally. Alternatively, the retroperitoneum can be entered below the diaphragm, and then the diaphragm can be divided. To remove the diaphragm from the chest cavity, enter the chest cavity transpleurally through the bed of the tenth rib. Then divide the diaphragm close to the chest wall, using electrocautery (Fig. 10-83, *B*). Leave a small tag of diaphragm for reattachment. Once the diaphragm has been reflected, expose the retroperitoneal space. Dissect the peritoneal cavity from underneath the internal oblique muscle in the abdominal musculature. Split the internal oblique and the transverse abdominal muscles in line with the skin incisions, and extend the exposure distally as far as necessary.

An alternative method of releasing the diaphragm is to divide it retroperitoneally. With the tenth rib removed, enter the abdominal cavity retroperitoneally. This is facilitated by dissection with the fingertips between the cut edges of the rib cartilage, peeling off the peritoneum from the underside of the diaphragm (Fig. 10-83, *C*). Because the transversalis fascia and the peritoneum do not diverge, dissect with caution and then identify the two cavities on either side of the diaphragm. Once both cavities have been identified, the diaphragm can be reflected from the origin on the lower ribs and the crus from the side of the spine.

Once the two cavities have been combined and the retroperitoneal space entered, identify the vertebral bodies and carefully dissect the psoas muscle laterally off the intervertebral disk spaces. Divide the prevertebral fascia in the direction of the spine. Identify the segmental arteries and veins over the waist of each vertebral body, and isolate and ligate them in the midline. Expose the bone either extraperiosteally or subperiosteally, as previously described (p. 498). The exposure from T10 to L2 or L3 with this approach is simple but as one proceeds more distally, the iliac vessels overlie the L4 and L5 vertebrae, and exposure in this area requires much more meticulous dissection and displacement of these vessels.

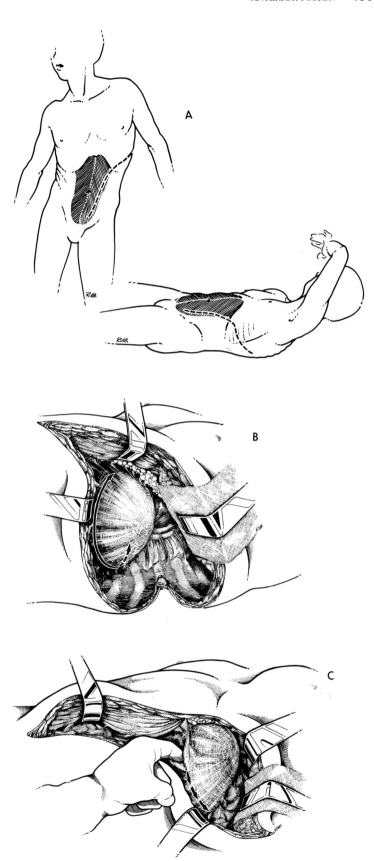

Fig. 10-83   A, Skin incision for thoracoabdominal approach to spine. **B,** Transthoracic detachment of diaphragm. **C,** Retroperitoneal detachment of diaphragm.

Lumbar extraperitoneal

▶ *Technique.* Place the patient in the right lateral decubitus position, and make the approach from the left. If scoliosis is present, make the approach from the convex side of the curve. Make a midflank incision from the midline anteriorly to the midline posteriorly (Fig. 10-84, *A*). Divide the abdominal oblique muscles in line with the incision (Fig. 10-84, *B* and *C*). As the dissection proceeds laterally, identify the latissimus dorsi muscle as it adds another layer: the transverse fascia and the peritoneum. The transverse fascia and the peritoneum diverge posteriorly as the transverse fascia lines the trunk wall; the peritoneum turns anteriorly to encase the viscera. Posterior dissection in this plane allows access to the spine without entering the abdominal cavity. Any inadvertent entry into the peritoneum should be repaired immediately because it may not be identifiable later. Reflect all the fat containing areolar tissue back to the transverse fascia and the lumbar fascia, reflecting the ureter along with the peritoneum (Fig. 10-84, *D*). Locate the major vessels in the midline, divide the lumbar fascia, and carefully retract the great vessels. Divide segmental arteries and veins as they cross the waist of the vertebra in the midline, and ligate them to control hemorrhage.

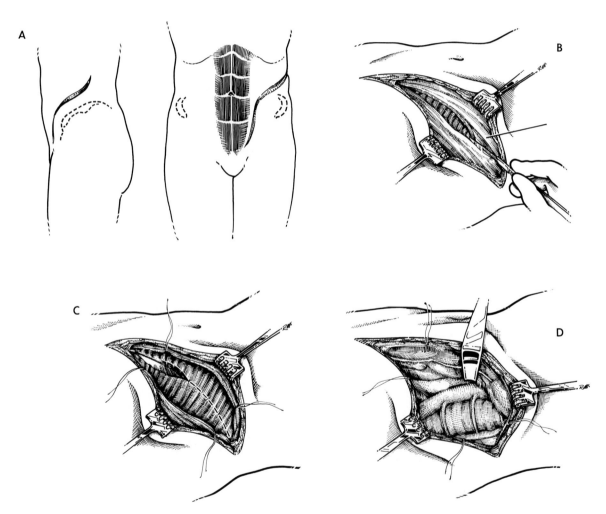

Fig. 10-84   A, Skin incision for extraperitoneal approach to lumbar and lumbosacral spine. **B,** Incision of fibers of external oblique muscle. **C,** Incision into fibers of internal oblique muscle. **D,** Exposure of spine before ligation of segmental vessels.

Transperitoneal

The anterior transperitoneal approach, as described by Freebody et al, is useful for surgical procedures in the L4 to S1 area. The major disadvantage of the transperitoneal approach at the lumbosacral level is that upward extension and exposure cannot be accomplished without generous mobilization of the vessels so that the surgeon can alternatively work above and below them. The second vascular obstacle is the middle sacral artery, which originates from the bifurcation and transverses distally over the midline of the spine; it can cause considerable hemorrhage if not identified. The patient should have presurgical bowel preparation and insertion of a Foley catheter.

▲ *Technique.* Make a midline or a Pfannenstiel's incision (Fig. 10-85, *A*). Divide the rectus muscle, enter the peritoneum, and pack the bowel out of the operative field. Identify the retroperitoneum and incise it along the midline. Identify the middle sacral artery along with its vein and ligate them (Fig. 10-85, *B*). Displace the presacral plexus bluntly to avoid damage to the nerve supply to the bowel, bladder, and genitalia.

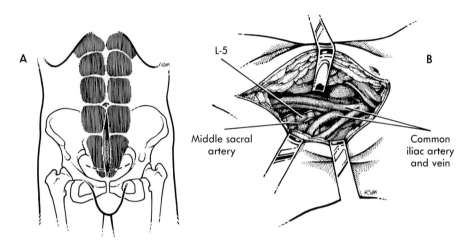

Fig. 10-85 **A,** Median longitudinal incision for transperitoneal approach to lumbar spine. **B,** Exposure of L5 vertebral body and middle sacral artery.

Techniques for anterior arthrodesis. Once the anterior portion of the spine has been exposed, various techniques may be used to perform an anterior arthrodesis with or without instrumentation. The disk may be removed and fusion obtained with an interbody technique, or an anterior strut-type fusion can be performed. The type of fusion, of course, depends on the condition for which the surgery is being performed.

Disk excision and interbody fusion

▲ *Technique.* Expose desired levels of the spine as previously described and identify the disks. The disks can be felt as soft, rounded, protuberant areas of the spine compared with the concave surface of the vertebral body. Divide the anulus sharply with a scalpel. Remove the anulus and the nucleus pulposus with rongeurs and curets. Once the disk excision has been completed, remove the cartilage end plates with an osteotome or a sharp periosteal elevator (Fig. 10-86, *A*). The posterior aspects of the cartilage end plates are more easily removed with angled curets. Control hemostasis with Gelfoam soaked in thrombin. Cut the rib removed for the thoracotomy into small pieces, and apply the bone graft into the disk space (Fig. 10-86, *B*). It usually is not necessary with this approach

to remove the posterior anulus of the disk; thus the chance of injury to the spinal cord is lessened. Place any remaining portions of the rib in a trough along the lateral aspect of the vertebral body. Suture the parietal pleura over the vertebral bodies, and close the wound in the routine manner.

Alternatively, cut a trough in the lateral aspect of the vertebral body, and place several complete rib-strut grafts in the trough to function as supporting bone (Fig. 10-86, *C*). Undercut the trough posteriorly back toward the subchondral bone to better lock the strut grafts in place. Iliac bone graft may be necessary to provide additional cancellous bone along the strut graft and in the disk spaces.

Strut graft

▲ *Technique.* If the patient has a severe angular kyphosis that is not correctable, strut grafts may be placed anterior to the vertebral bodies. If possible, the strut should extend from end vertebra to end vertebra of the kyphosis. The exposure must be subperi-

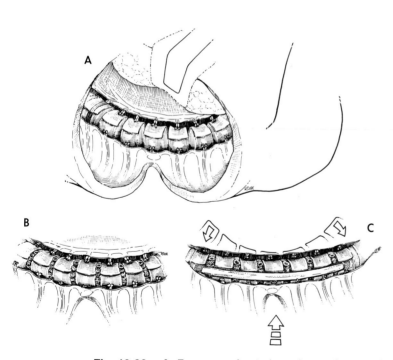

Fig. 10-86   A, Exposure of anterior spine and removal of disks and end plates before insertion of bone graft. **B,** Insertion of cancellous bone and rib struts in disk space anteriorly. **C,** Use of rib as strut graft within confines of vertebral body with cancellous bone graft in disk spaces. (Redrawn from Bradford DS et al: Moe's textbook of scoliosis and other spinal deformities, ed 2, Philadelphia, 1987, WB Saunders Co.)

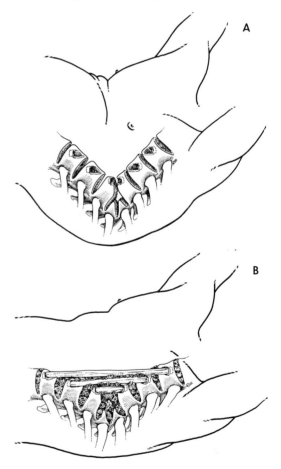

Fig. 10-87   A, Preparation of tunnels for strut grafts. **B,** Insertion of strut grafts into pre-prepared tunnels with cancellous bone graft in disk spaces. (Redrawn from Bradford DS et al: Moe's textbook of scoliosis and other spinal deformities, ed 2, Philadelphia, 1987, WB Saunders Co.)

osteal because the bone grafts are placed against the vertebral body rather than within the axis of the vertebral bodies. Fashion a tunnel proximally and distally (Fig. 10-87, *A*), and place the strut in position (Fig. 10-87, *B*). If there is a significant kyphosis that requires greater strength than is provided by a rib, a fibular graft may be used instead. Place pressure over the apex of the kyphos to obtain some correction, position the strut, and then release the pressure. Pack the space between the strut graft and the vertebral bodies with bone graft. Place Gelfoam over the lateral aspect of the graft at the completion of the procedure to prevent bone chips from dislodging into the thoracic or retroperitoneal space. Close the wound in the routine manner.

Anterior vascular rib bone grafting. Bradford noted a frequent fracture of strut grafts when the grafts were not in contact with the vertebral bodies and simply spanned an open area between vertebrae. It is known that a rib or fibular graft may take up to 2 years for replacement and that it is weakest approximately 6 months after surgery. To avoid graft fracture Bradford developed a technique of vascular pedicle bone graft for the treatment of kyphosis. He credits Rose et al with first describing the technique in 1975.

◣ *Technique (Bradford).* Plan the thoracotomy to remove enough rib to bridge the kyphosis. For a kyphosis with an apex from T2 to T5, remove a rib two to three segments below the apex of the kyphosis and rotate the distal rib segment to the superior vertebral body to be fused. If the kyphosis is at an apex of T6 or below, remove a rib two to three segments more proximal to the apex of the kyphosis and rotate the distal segment to the distal vertebral body to be fused. Make a skin incision as in the routine transthoracic exposure (see Fig. 10-80, *A*). Take care to identify the appropriate rib and avoid use of electrocautery over the rib periosteum. Perform the thoracotomy first without removing the rib by cutting through the intercostal musculature 0.5 to 1 cm above the rib. Divide the rib at the costochondral junction. Next divide the intercostal musculature inferiorly to the rib, distally to proximally, leaving a margin of intercostal muscle to avoid damage to the artery and vein complex (Fig. 10-88, *A*). Once the angle of the rib has been reached, place the chest retractors in the wound to allow better exposure of the thorax and better identification of the intercostal vasculature. Again, taking great care, proceed with the dissection proximally to the rib–transverse process junction and divide the rib. The rib now is mobilized with its intact intercostal musculature and artery and vein complex. Dissect and mobilize the vessels to the junction of the intervertebral foramen. Dissect 1 cm of rib subperiostally, proximally and distally, to allow bone-to-bone contact when the rib is locked into the

vertebral body. Identify the intervertebral body to be fused, taking care to prevent the rib graft from kinking the vessels. Make a hole with a curet into the anterior aspect of the vertebral body above and below to accept the end of the rib graft. Trim the rib so that the ends will match the length of the spine to be fused. Segmental vessels overlying the vertebrae need not be divided, and the intervetebral disks need not be excised if an in situ fusion is planned. If, on the other hand, mobilization of each intervertebral disk space to obtain some correction of the kyphosis is desired, ligate the segmental vessels and prepare the spine for an interbody fusion at each level as described on p. 502. It is important, however, not to violate or jeopardize the segmental vessels supplying the intercostal vessels of the rib that have been mobilized. Once the slots into the vertebral bodies have been cut out and the rib has been fashioned to a correct length, rotate the rib on its axis approximately 90 degrees and then wedge it into the vertebrae above and below (Fig. 10-88, *B*). Close the chest in a routine fashion over chest tubes.

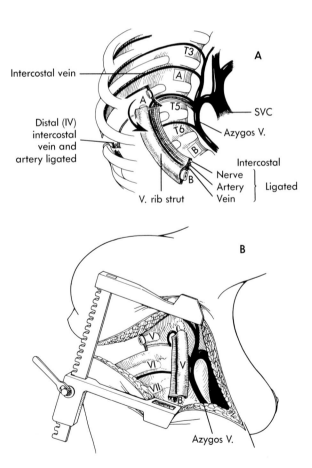

Fig. 10-88   Thoracotomy. **A,** Wide margin of intercostal muscle left attached to rib to ensure intact blood supply. **B,** Rib graft rotated 90 degrees on its axis and keyed into vertebral bodies over length of kyphosis to be fused. (Redrawn from Bradford DS: Spine 5:318, 1980.)

Anterior instrumentation
Dwyer instrumentation

In 1964, Dwyer, in cooperation with Newton and Sherwood, developed instrumentation for spinal correction and fixation through an anterior approach. Dwyer instrumentation uses large metal staples of several sizes that are attached to each vertebral body with a large screw. The screws have a large head with a hole for passage of a cable that is tightened at each level and then fixed by crimping the screw heads. By placing the staples more anteriorly, lordosis can be corrected. By placing the staples and screws in the same location in each vertebral body, regardless of the position of the body, rotation also can be corrected as the curve straightens. Dwyer instrumentation is contraindicated in kyphosis.

There are several advantages of Dwyer instrumentation and fusion: (1) disk removal results in marked mobilization with increased correction and sound fixation of the curve obtained at every level; (2) excellent correction of lordosis is obtained; and (3) correction of rotation, as well as curvature, is possible. The Dwyer procedure has the following disadvantages: (1) the procedure is time-consuming; (2) because instrumentation of the sacrum is difficult, correction of the pelvic obliquity is difficult; (3) instrumentation above the T6 level is difficult; (4) the internal fixation strength of the Dwyer system is extremely poor because the strength of fixation directly depends on the strength of the bone-screw interface; (5) the flexible, braided, titanium cable can resist forces only in tension. Flexion, extension, lateral bending toward the cable, and rotation are resisted only by the impacted vertebral end plates; and (6) the Dwyer system tends to pull the spine into kyphosis and therefore is contraindicated in a preexisting kyphotic condition.

Complications of the Dwyer procedure include those common to any major anterior surgical exposure of the spine: pneumothorax, hemothorax, aspiration pneumonia, and paralytic ileus. In addition, there is the possibility of mechanical damage to the spinal cord by a screw or vascular damage to the cord from extensive exposure with division of multiple segmental arteries. In addition, cable breakage and loss of fixation at one level are common, and even with an intact apparatus, solid interbody fusion does not always occur. With the Dwyer procedure alone for rigid paralytic curves, the group at Rancho Los Amigos Hospital noted a pseudarthrosis rate of more than 50% and consequently recommend that the anterior Dwyer fusion be supplemented by a posterior fusion.

Indications for a Dwyer procedure are (1) lumbar curves in patients with deficient posterior elements such as in myelomeningocele, (2) thoracolumbar curves with extreme lordosis, and (3) rigid thoracolumbar paralytic curves for which a combined anteroposterior fusion in two stages is required. Hall reported excellent results with the Dwyer procedure for thoracolumbar curves in patients with idiopathic scoliosis. An absolute contraindication to the Dwyer procedure is kyphosis in the area to be treated. The Dwyer procedure also is not recommended for children younger than 10 years because of the small size of the vertebral bodies.

∟ *Technique.* Position the patient in the lateral decubitus position with the convex aspect of the curve uppermost. Approach the spine anteriorly as previously described. Excise the disks as described in the interbody fusion technique (Fig. 10-89, *A*).

Instrumentation proceeds from above downward on the convex side of the curve. Incise the anulus of the intact disk of the uppermost body to allow the flange of the staple to grip just over the end plate. During placement of the screws, check and recheck the direction to avoid penetration of the posterior cortex into the spinal canal. The ideally placed screw runs horizontally across the body, just engaging the opposite cortex and lying safely in front of the neural foramen. Measure the width of the vertebral body, select a staple of the same width, and place it into the staple holder. Place the staple holder along the convex aspect of the vertebra, and using a mallet place the staple around the vertebral body (Fig. 10-89, *B*). When the staple holder is removed, a hole is left in the vertebral body made by the spike of the staple holder. Measure the width of the vertebral body, and insert an appropriate Dwyer screw through this staple and into the vertebral body, trying to engage the opposite cortex but avoiding the neural canal (Fig. 10-89, *C*). After the first two staples and screws have been placed, insert rib chips into the disk space. Introduce the cable through the two screws and apply a tensioner. Obtain correction by pressure with the screwdriver on the convex side. Use the tensioner to take up the slack in the cable (Fig. 10-89, *D*). If the tensioner is used for correction, the screws can pull out. When correction is obtained, crimp the screw head onto the cable (Fig. 10-89, *E*). Perform the same procedure on adjacent disk spaces. Apply a collar over the cable before cutting the cable. Crimp this collar on the cable below the final screw (Fig. 10-89, *F*). At the conclusion of the procedure cover the cables and screws if possible by suturing over the pleura or the psoas muscle in the thoracic or lumbar area, respectively.

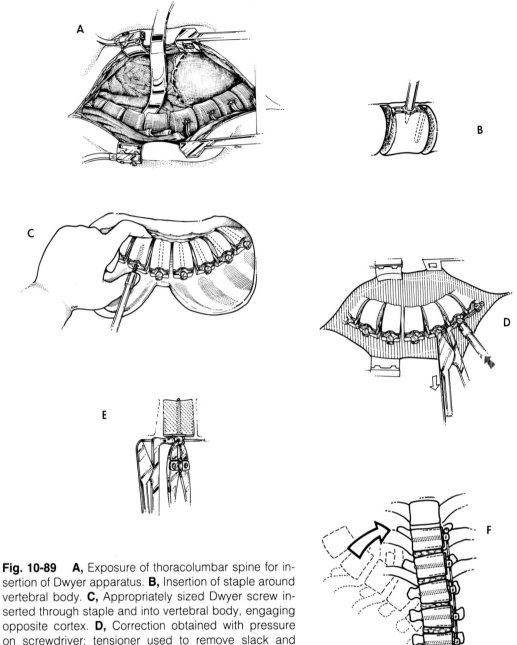

Fig. 10-89 **A,** Exposure of thoracolumbar spine for insertion of Dwyer apparatus. **B,** Insertion of staple around vertebral body. **C,** Appropriately sized Dwyer screw inserted through staple and into vertebral body, engaging opposite cortex. **D,** Correction obtained with pressure on screwdriver; tensioner used to remove slack and tighten cable between vertebral screws. **E,** Crimper used to fix shortened cable in screw head. **F,** Diagramatic representation of correction obtained at each instrumented level with Dwyer instrumentation.

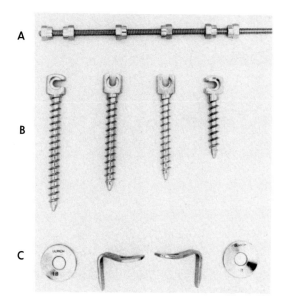

Fig. 10-90 **A,** Compression rod fitted with Ventral Derotation Spondylodesis hexnuts. **B,** Screws; insertion slit for rod points upward or laterally; shorter screws have deeper thread. **C,** Sharp-bladed angle plates and washers. (From Bradford DS and Hensinger RM: The pediatric spine, New York, 1985, Thieme Inc.)

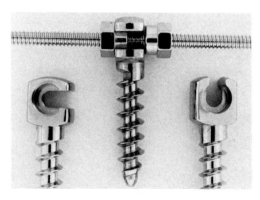

Fig. 10-91 Detail of screw head; cylindrical process of left nut is inserted to corresponding part of screw head to prevent displacement. (From Bradford DS and Hensinger RM: The pediatric spine, New York, 1985, Thieme Inc.)

Zielke instrumentation

In 1975 Zielke modified the Dwyer system and called it the *Ventral Derotation Spondylodesis (VDS) System*. This system is different from the Dwyer system in that the implants are made of stainless steel instead of titanium. The screw heads are slotted instead of cannulated and the slots have either a top opening or a side opening (Fig. 10-90). The screws are implanted into the vertebral bodies through convex circular washers or angled plates. Instead of cable, a 3.2-mm diameter solid flexible rod is used. Collared hexnuts are used to lock the rod in the screw heads and provide compression and fixation (Fig. 10-91). The solid rod allows the anterior instrumentation to be used in kyphotic areas of the spine and is reported to be superior in its ability to derotate the spine. Experienced spine surgeons in some medical centers have been successful with this type of anterior instrumentation, primarily for curves in patients with deficient posterior elements such as in myelomeningocele or in selected idiopathic lumbar curves.

▶ *Technique.* The appropriate levels for instrumentation are identified preoperatively. As a general rule, all vertebral bodies adjacent to intervertebral disk spaces that are wedged open into the convexity of the curve should undergo instrumentation.

Remove the disks as described in the interbody fusion technique. The opposite outer fibers of the anulus on the concave side may be left intact to act as a hinge and prevent overcorrection. Measure the transverse diameter of the vertebral body with a caliper, and use an awl to make a hole in the side of the vertebral body at its midlateral portion. Insert the appropriate size Zielke screw with an attached double-bladed staple across the midportion of the end vertebral body. Except for the end vertebra, all other screws are inserted with washers (Fig. 10-92, *A*). Use the index finger of the opposite hand to tell when the screw has engaged the opposite cortex. As the spine undergoes instrumentation at each more distal level, place the screw sites more posteriorly in the vertebral body. This lessens the tendency for postoperative kyphosis and helps with derotation of the spine.

Also direct the screws in a slightly more posterior than anterior direction across the midportion of the vertebral body to enhance the derotation effect. The most proximal and distal screws should be inserted approximately 1 cm more anteriorly than the apical screws. This will form a C-shaped curve when viewed laterally. As the spine is derotated, the rod will assume a straight position, which facilitates derotation.

Insert a flexible, stainless steel, threaded rod of appropriate length into the screw heads. The most distal and proximal screws should be side opening, and the middle screws should be top opening (Fig. 10-92, *B*). The most proximal and distal screws should have double nuts, one facing the other, but the intervening screws need only have one locking nut facing the apex of the deformity. After the rod is in place, apply the derotator, using a handle for additional leverage. Derotate the spine toward a more normal anatomic position (Fig. 10-92, *C*), producing a lordosis. At this stage cut the rib into 1 to 2 cm pieces, and wedge these anteriorly between each vertebral body at the anteriormost lip. This also helps prevent instrumentation kyphosis and facilitates the production of lumbar lordosis. Roughen the vertebral end plates, and pack the remaining portion of rib bone, cut into very small pieces, loosely, into the intervertebral disk space. With the spine held in the derotated position, sequentially tighten the locking nuts, approximating the vertebral bodies and correcting the curve. The weakest link of this chain is similar to that of the Dwyer procedure: the interspace of the most cephalad level undergoing instrumentation. To prevent screw pullout Zielke advocates additional instrumentation of one vertebra above and a block fusion across the disk space without disk excision.

Crimp the threads of the compression rod to prevent the locked nuts from unwinding. Approximate the soft tissues over the instrumentation, and be certain that the great vessels are not lying over the implant, which might cause vessel rupture. Close the wound in the routine manner.

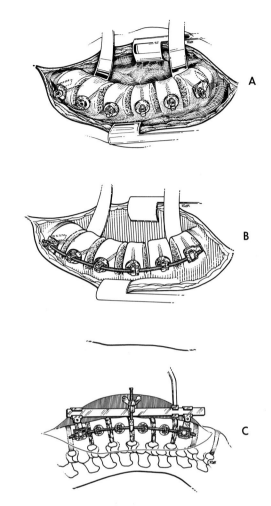

Fig. 10-92 **A,** Zielke screw and washers inserted through appropriate vertebral bodies. **B,** Threaded rod applied through screw heads; notice C-shaped curve of rod. **C,** Spine derotated and lordosis applied.

Complications of Scoliosis Surgery

The surgical treatment of scoliosis is formidable, and significant complications are possible. Complications may occur at any stage of treatment, from the application of a corrective cast until convalescence after surgery is complete.

Complications in the Cast

In the cast, pressure sores may develop over any improperly padded bony prominence. Any complaint of localized pain under the cast should be investigated immediately, and usually a part of the cast should be removed and repadded or the entire cast should be removed and reapplied. Meticulous technique in applying casts will minimize or eliminate pressure sores.

Compression of the duodenum in its third portion by the superior mesenteric artery was described by von Rokitansky more than 100 years ago. This condition may appear in two forms—acute and chronic (designated Wilkie's syndrome)—and has been observed in various pathologic states. The cast syndrome described by Dorph in 1950 is the acute form of this syndrome, which consists of vascular compression of the duodenum, leading to acute duodenal obstruction and gastric dilatation. Pernicious and often projectile vomiting ensues, and a potentially dangerous situation exists. A high index of suspicion must be maintained when vomiting, abdominal distention, and mild pain occur. Because this is a partial obstruction, flatus will continue to be passed and symptoms may be intermittent. The diagnosis is based on the roentgenographic finding of a dilated duodenum. Contrast studies show a linear obstruction at the level where the superior mesenteric vessels cross the duodenum. A lateral decubitus examination of the abdomen with the patient's right side up reveals a dilated duodenal loop and a long air-fluid level. When combined with the appropriate history and physical findings, this is virtually a pathognomonic sign. Treatment consists of prompt removal of the cast and early nasogastric suction. Other measures include position changes, particularly to a prone position, restriction to a liquid diet, and ambulation if possible. General surgical consultation should be sought early because patients who face prolonged immobilization may require surgical correction of the obstruction.

Evarts et al reported 30 cases of vascular compression of the duodenum, properly termed *superior mesenteric artery syndrome*. Eighteen occurred with surgical correction of scoliosis; 12 occurred with only the application of body casts. The authors emphasize that correction of the curvature increases the angle of the superior mesenteric artery with the aorta and results in compression of the duodenum and symptoms of partial intestinal obstruction.

Intraoperative Complications

Some complications were included in the discussion of surgical techniques, but neurologic sequelae remain the most feared and unpredictable. Neurologic injury may occur from direct injury to the cord or nerves or from excessive traction during correction. Reporting its use in 124 patients Vauzelle et al described a method of anesthesia to sufficiently disassociate pain from consciousness while permitting spontaneous motion on command after instrumentation. By observing motion of the patient's hands and feet, the surgeon can determine the neurologic function distal to the spinal surgery. If motor power does not clearly appear in the lower extremities but does so in the hands, instrumentation is immediately removed and the request repeated. The success of this technique depends on careful and controlled anesthesia. Engler et al pointed out real hazards in arousing a prone, intubated patient from anesthesia: (1) raising the head may cause accidental extubation, which could be disastrous, and reintubation is difficult with the patient prone; (2) a sudden, deep inhalation during awakening could lead to air embolism through aspiration of air into the open vessels of the wound; and (3) a violent movement could dislodge the spinal instrumentation or intravenous tubing or could result in laminar fractures. As Brown and Nash also pointed out, this test documents only that spinal cord function has not suffered a major compromise at the time the test is performed. Because the time at which the test is performed during the surgical procedure is quite critical, multiple wake-up tests have been advocated to increase safety.

Electrical monitoring of spinal cord function is based on the principle that stimulation of a peripheral nerve produces an evoked response or electrical potential that sophisticated electronic equipment can detect proximally in the spinal cord itself or from the cerebral cortex. The spinal-evoked potentials from the cord and cortical-evoked potentials from the brain frequently are referred to as *somatosensory evoked potentials*. It generally is accepted that these potentials and their transmissions effectively reflect function of the dorsal columns only. The degree to which they reflect anterior cord function is not yet well established.

Interpretation of recordings obviously is critical and requires both skill and experience. When competently performed, spinal cord monitoring, by demonstrating changes in evoked potentials, may provide some measure of early warning of spinal cord pathology and add one more safety factor to those already available for spinal surgery. Spinal cord monitoring can indicate that spinal cord function is impaired but, even in expert hands, does not relay with certainty this information before irreversible spinal cord damage occurs, and, regardless of monitoring findings, movement by the patient on command is the ultimate test of neurologic function and obviously must be basic to clinical decision making when monitoring findings are uncertain or confusing.

Complications Immediately After Surgery

Ileus is a common complication after spinal fusion for scoliosis. Withholding oral feedings until the bowel sounds return, usually in 36 to 72 hours after surgery, is recommended. Until then, intravenous fluids must be administered.

Atelectasis is a common cause of fever after surgery. Frequent turning of the patient and deep breathing and coughing usually control or prevent serious atelectasis. Inhalation therapy with intermittent positive pressure breathing may be beneficial in cooperative patients, but inflation of the stomach during this type of breathing must be avoided. Incentive spirometry is now commonly used instead.

A deep wound infection after scoliosis fusion is a major complication but rarely is disastrous. The tissues in the area of fusion are vascular in the posterior elements of the spine, and the autogenous cancellous bone grafts seem to be extremely resistant to most infections. The extensive dissection, the lengthy time required for the operation, the use of metallic implants, and the closure of the wound over freely bleeding bone are all factors common to most surgery for scoliosis and theoretically make infection more likely. Infection rates also are high in patients with myelodysplasia or urinary tract infections. Among the general factors important in preventing infection in the operating room are careful control of the circulating air and of the circulating personnel, frequent evaluation of the equipment used for sterilizing instruments and linen, and proper surgical technique. The skin must be carefully prepared both on the ward and in the operating room. The drapes must be carefully applied, and the wound must be carefully closed to avoid leaving dead spaces, especially in the subcutaneous tissues. Suction drainage and careful closure of the subcutaneous tissues and the skin help prevent subcutaneous hematomas or seromas. Certainly, hematomas are always present around the fusion mass, and a large hematoma is usually present between the skin and the deep fascia overlying the spinal muscles. Suction drainage with one tube in the fusion area should be left in place for 48 hours.

Moe et al reported two types of wound infections after surgery. The first is quite obvious in that a high fever develops, usually within 2 to 5 days after surgery, and the wound almost always appears infected. In the second type the temperature is elevated only slightly or moderately, and the wound appears relatively normal. Diagnosis of this latter type of wound sepsis may be difficult. Patients often have a postoperative temperature elevation of up to 102° F, which should decline gradually during the first 4 postoperative days. Any spike of temperature above 102° F should raise strong suspicion of a deep wound infection, especially if a steady improvement in the patient's general condition is not seen. The appearance of the wound usually is deceiving, with no significant swelling, erythema, or tenderness. Moe et al recommend prompt aspiration of the wound in several sites. Cultures should be submitted, but results should not be awaited, and reoperation should be planned immediately.

The treatment of such an established infection requires an antibiotic for penicillin-resistant *Staphylococcus aureus* inasmuch as it is the most common offending organism. With additional blood transfusions available and the patient under general anesthesia, all infected necrotic tissue is removed by careful debridement. The bone grafts and instrumentation are left in place, and the wound is closed over two plastic ingress-egress tubes. Antibiotic wound irrigation is carried out for about 5 days and is discontinued when the patient is afebrile and laboratory evidence of infection is decreasing. Intravenous antibiotics are administered for approximately 10 days, with oral administration continuing for a minimum of 6 weeks. Most fusion masses become solid even after an infection, but occasionally a draining sinus persists until the instruments are removed. After removal of the instruments the wound should be closed and irrigated.

Another treatment for deep wound infections after spinal instrumentation is the time-honored technique of opening the wound widely and allowing it to close secondarily. This may be satisfactory, but morbidity is much greater than with debridement and irrigation and the cosmetic result is less desirable. Regardless of the treatment used, Moe et al emphasize that procrastination must be avoided; exploring a suspicious but clean wound is better than procrastinating in the exploration of an infected wound.

Late Complications

The most common late complications are pseudarthrosis and recurrence of the deformity. A pseudarthrosis represents a failure of the operation to accomplish its purpose. Recurrence of the deformity usually is caused by one or more pseudarthroses, but it can be caused by bending of the fusion mass, traumatic fracture of the fusion mass, or the addition to the curve of one or more adjacent vertebrae superior or inferior to the fusion so that the curve is lengthened. The frequency of the last three causes can be decreased by good judgment in evaluating the maturity of the fusion mass and by correctly locating the fusion area at the time of surgery and including in the fusion all vertebrae that are rotated in the same direction as the vertebrae in the curve. An additional safeguard against the addition of more vertebrae to the curve is to include in the fusion one unrotated vertebra at each end of the curve.

Improvements in the treatment of scoliosis have produced a steady decrease in the rate of pseudarthrosis. The protection of the fusion mass after surgery, the development of both corrective and fixation devices, and the development of better surgical technique, including meticulous removal of the soft tissues, intraarticular fusion of the lateral articulations, and the addition of much autogenous cancellous bone to the fusion mass, have all been helpful. The intelligent use of instrumentation for internal fixation probably has been one of the most important factors in preventing pseudarthroses.

A spinal fusion for scoliosis usually is considered successful if the correction obtained is not lost. A loss of correction then is the only indication for repair of a suspected pseudarthrosis. Late breakage of internal fixation devices usually is presumptive evidence that the fusion is not solid. If there is no significant loss of correction, however, this is not a definite indication for reoperation. Pain or other symptoms caused by pseudarthrosis in the absence of demonstrable loss of correction are extremely rare. In years past, scoliosis fusions were explored routinely in several centers during the first 6 months after surgery. Although an extremely high incidence of defects in the fusion mass was reported, exploration is indicated only if correction is being lost. Pseudarthrosis frequently can be demonstrated on anteroposterior and right and left oblique roentgenograms, but if the correction is being maintained, then the fusion mass is functioning successfully and a diagnosis of pseudarthrosis is of no practical significance.

Several techniques are helpful in confirming pseudarthrosis. Routine posteroanterior and especially oblique roentgenograms of the involved fusion area may show the pseudarthrosis; if not, tomograms or CT scans may be necessary. Bone scans also are helpful in indicating areas of increased uptake that may indicate a pseudarthrosis. Many times, however, the pseudarthrosis cannot be confirmed, even with the most sophisticated roentgenographic evaluation, and can be detected only by surgical exploration.

The roentgenographic finding of a wedged or "open" interspace, an unfused lateral articulation, or a defect in the fusion mass is helpful in locating a pseudarthrosis. At exploration the cortex usually is smooth and firm over the mature and intact areas of the fusion mass and the soft tissues strip away easily. Conversely, at a pseudarthrosis, the soft tissues usually are adherent and continuous into the defect; however, a narrow pseudarthrosis may be extremely difficult to locate, especially if motion in it is only slight. In this instance, decortication of the fusion mass in suspicious areas is indicated, and a search always should be made for several pseudarthroses. When one or more have been identified, they are cleared of fibrous tissue and the curves again are corrected by instrumentation. When the loss of correction has been significant, osteotomy of one or more intact areas of the fusion mass sometimes is justified to obtain additional correction. When most or all the correction has been lost and the spine is explored late, a solid fusion mass often is found, and several osteotomies may be indicated to permit correction of the curve. These osteotomies and any pseudarthroses are treated as ordinary joints to be fused, and their edges are freshened and decorticated. If the fusion mass is thick and of good quality, it may be decorticated throughout to obtain additional bone for grafting. If necessary, fresh autogenous iliac bone is added. Halo-femoral traction may be used to regain correction after multiple osteotomies, but instrumentation can be used if spinal cord function is monitored. The same criteria are used in judging the maturity of the fusion mass after repair of a pseudarthrosis as after the original fusion. After the repair, however, the period of immobilization usually is shorter than after a primary correction and fusion. This is especially true when the pseudarthrosis is discovered and repaired during convalescence before the fusion mass is completely matured. According to most reports, pseudarthroses are most common at the thoracolumbar junction, in the lumbar area, and at the extreme ends of the fusion mass. Cobb pointed out that the success of any fusion depends on good surgical technique, the use of a large mass of good bone in the fusion area, sufficient immobilization for a time long enough to permit the fusion mass to mature, and a good bone metabolism. A heavier fusion mass than usual generally is necessary to maintain correction when the deformity has been severe, especially in patients with neurofibromatosis, or when the deformity includes a kyphosis.

NEUROMUSCULAR SCOLIOSIS

Neuromuscular scoliosis may be caused by an array of underlying disorders, and patients have varying sensory abnormalities, asymmetric or symmetric paralysis, and progressive or nonprogressive disease. Common to all, however, is a paralytic state that results in limb and spinal deformities. The Scoliosis Research Society classifies neuromuscular spinal deformity as neuropathic or myopathic (see box).

O'Brien and Yau, James, and others have emphasized the differences between paralytic and idiopathic scoliosis. The paralytic curves are longer and usually develop at a younger age than the idiopathic type. Small curves may progress beyond skeletal maturity and throughout life. Pelvic obliquity often exists, and muscle imbalance affects the curve. Hip joint contractures and other lower extremity asymmetry can affect the lumbar spine. A larger percentage of these curves are progressive.

Management

Many neuromuscular spinal deformities ultimately require surgical intervention. The basic treatment modalities, however, are similar to those for idiopathic scoliosis: observation, orthotic treatment, and surgery.

Observation

Not all neuromuscular spinal deformities require immediate bracing or surgery. Small curves less than 20 to 25 degrees may be followed carefully for progression before treatment is instituted. Similarly, large curves in very retarded patients in whom the curve is not causing any functional disability or hindering nursing care in any manner can be observed. If curve progression is noted, or if the functional abilities of the child are compromised, treatment is begun.

Orthotic Treatment

Bunch stated that the indication for the use of a Milwaukee brace as a passive device in neuromuscular scoliosis is a paralytic, flexible curve in a child in whom fusion is not yet desirable. The child may need several brace changes as trunk height increases with growth. Bunch described the contraindications to brace treatment as obesity or inability of the parents to manage the brace. In 1980 Nash presented an excellent review of the current concept of scoliosis bracing in which he recommended that mild to moderate neuromuscular scoliosis be managed with a total contact thoracolumbosacral orthosis, frequently with a removable front half. Patients with severe neuromuscular scoliosis may do best in a chair-insert seating-type of orthosis, frequently with anterior

---

CLASSIFICATION OF NEUROMUSCULAR SPINAL DEFORMITY

A. Neuropathic
1. Upper motor neuron
    a. Cerebral palsy
    b. Spinocerebellar degeneration
        i. Friedreich's ataxia
        ii. Charcot-Marie-Tooth
        iii. Roussy-Levy
    c. Syringomyelia
    d. Spinal cord tumor
    e. Spinal cord trauma
2. Lower motor neuron
    a. Poliomyelitis
    b. Other viral myelitides
    c. Traumatic
    d. Spinal muscle atrophy
        i. Werdnig-Hoffmann
        ii. Kugelberg-Welander
    e. Dysautonomia (Riley-Day syndrome)
B. Myopathic
1. Arthrogryposis
2. Muscular dystrophy
    a. Duchenne
    b. Limb-girdle
    c. Facioscapulohumeral
3. Fiber-type disproportion
4. Congenital hypotonia
5. Myotonia dystrophica

---

shells added. All agree that the orthosis functions as a purely passive body container. As Brown et al. indicated, the bracing provides the flaccid patient with trunk support, allowing the use of the upper extremities for purposeful activities. The orthosis also may delay progression of the spinal deformity. A custom-molded, total contact thoracolumbosacral orthosis may be used for children whose trunk contour will not accommodate the more standard braces or for older children who have poor voluntary trunk muscle control. Those patients who have more voluntary control can be treated in a Boston brace or a more conventional type of orthosis. Patients with severe involvement and no head control frequently require custom-fabricated seating devices combined with orthoses or head control devices.

Orthotic treatment of these children requires a major commitment on the part of the physician, the orthotist, and the patient's family. The brace must be very carefully fitted and frequently checked. If any pressure sores develop, they must be treated immediately and the brace modified accordingly.

Surgical Treatment

In paralytic scoliosis the aim of surgery is not only correction of the curves and prevention of their recurrence but also secure stabilization of the weakened trunk and a balanced spine in both the frontal and sagittal planes over a level pelvis. Consequently, the indications for fusion and the determination of the fusion area are different from those in idiopathic scoliosis. To stabilize the trunk effectively in a patient with paralytic scoliosis or with an unstable spine, a much longer fusion is necessary than usually is indicated for idiopathic scoliosis. Although in idiopathic scoliosis only the primary curve need be fused, in paralytic scoliosis the area that includes the primary and secondary curves often must be fused. This area generally extends from a horizontal vertebra in the upper portion of the spine to a horizontal vertebra or the pelvis in the lower portion of the spine.

The patient with paralysis presents additional problems such as (1) significant pulmonary deficits caused by intercostal paralysis, (2) more osteoporotic bone and the possibility of failure of instrumentation, (3) atrophied pelvis with insufficient bone for grafting, (4) an increased blood loss in a patient with an initially smaller blood volume, (5) prolonged postoperative immobilization, (6) more postoperative pulmonary complications, and (7) immobilization pressure sores, especially in those with altered skin sensation. In view of these potential problems, preoperative evaluation should be extensive, with consultation of any appropriate subspecialty physicians. Careful evaluation of the pulmonary function is critical. Nickel et al reported that patients with vital capacities of less than 30% of predicted normal require respiratory support postoperatively, and those with a similar decrease of vital capacity and without a voluntary cough reflex require a tracheostomy. Bradford prefers to use an endotracheal tube postoperatively for respiratory assistance as long as necessary. A combination of these techniques can be formulated on the basis of close consultation with a pulmonary specialist before the patient's surgery.

The anesthesiologist should be aware of the problems that can occur intraoperatively. The patient usually requires an arterial line, a Foley catheter to monitor urine output, a rectal probe, and on occasion a central venous line. Excessive blood loss can be expected, and the use of warming blankets, cell savers, and hypotensive anesthesia should be considered. Because chronic anemia and poor nutrition are common in patients with neuromuscular scoliosis, most are not candidates for preoperative autodonation of blood. Because of the long fusion required and the insufficient iliac bone available, most will require augmentation of the fusion by bone bank allograft.

Because of the extremely complicated nature of this surgery and the possibility of significant complications, a thorough discussion with the patient's family is necessary. The surgical procedure, with its indications, risks, benefits, and alternative therapies, should be discussed and documented before surgery.

Bonnett et al, reporting the Rancho Los Amigos experience with paralytic scoliosis in 351 patients, provided the following indications for surgery: (1) a collapsing and unstable paralytic deformity, (2) progressive increase in the scoliosis, (3) decreasing cardiorespiratory function, (4) decreased independence necessitating the use of hands for more stable sitting, and (5) back pain or loss of sitting balance coincident with increasing pelvic obliquity.

As experience has increased and technologic advances have appeared, the results of surgery have improved, primarily because of improved skeletal fixation. The Dwyer anterior operation (p. 504) has proved excellent for improving the percentage of correction but inadequate in that the fusion mass is too short. The Harrington posterior distraction rod allows greater correction above and below the apex of the curve. The combined anterior and posterior approaches therefore permit improved correction and have decreased the pseudarthrosis rate. Recently the use of posterior segmental instrumentation (p. 484), with extension to the pelvis as performed by Allen and Ferguson, has become the most widely used method of posterior stabilization for neuromuscular deformity.

The potential for complications is great. Death can result from anesthesia problems or more frequently from postoperative pulmonary deterioration. Other major complications include paralysis, pulmonary complications, infection, and pseudarthrosis with failure of instrumentation.

Cerebral Palsy

Scoliosis in patients with cerebral palsy frequently is progressive and is best managed by early recognition and control of the curve before the deformity becomes severe. Unfortunately, however, scoliosis often is overlooked in these patients and many do not seek orthopaedic treatment until a severe and progressive spinal deformity has developed. Unlike idiopathic scoliosis, scoliosis caused by cerebral palsy often is painful. Bonnett et al found that a majority of their cerebral palsy patients with scoliosis complained of back pain. If the scoliosis is left untreated, the patient may suffer loss of function in addition to pain. If the patient is ambulatory, the trunk may become so distorted that standing erect becomes impossible. Sitting may become more difficult, with increasing pelvic obliquity, and if supplemental support by the hands is needed to sit, the patient will lose the ability to perform activities that require use of the upper extremity. With a severe lumbar deformity, pelvic obliquity may predispose to dislocation of the hip.

The incidence of spinal deformities in cerebral palsy varies, depending on the degree of neuromuscular involvement. Bleck found the incidence of scoliosis to be less than 10% in ambulatory patients with spastic hemiplegia. Madigan and Wallace found an incidence of almost 70% in a population of persons with spastic quadriplegia who required total care. Most studies have shown an incidence greater than in the normal population, with the highest incidence in nonambulatory patients.

The goals of scoliosis treatment in patients with cerebral palsy have been divided into seven areas by Bonnett et al: (1) improvement in assisted sitting to make positioning and transfer easier for nursing attendants and family, (2) relief of pain in the hips and back, (3) increased independence because of decreased need for assistance, both for the positioning required to relieve pain and to prevent pressure areas and for feeding, (4) improvement in upper extremity function and table-top activities by eliminating the need to use the upper extremities for trunk support, (5) reduction of the equipment needed, making possible the use of other equipment, (6) placement of the patient in a different facility, one in which less care is provided, and (7) improved eating ability made possible by a change in position. Each patient must be evaluated individually to determine the potential for these rehabilitation goals.

Observation

If the curve is small, careful observation is indicated. If the curve progresses or is greater than 30 degrees in a growing child who is an independent ambulator or sitter, treatment should be instituted. If the child is skeletally mature, bracing is not likely to be effective and surgery is indicated if the curve is 50 to 60 degrees or greater. If neurologic involvement is extreme and the patient is severely mentally retarded and if the curve is not causing any significant change in functional status, observation is appropriate.

Orthotic Treatment

Bunnell and MacEwen reported the use of a removable plastic jacket in 48 patients with cerebral palsy. In 35 the curvature was held within 5 degrees of the initial measurement. Most authors believe that if the curve is progressive, the orthotic device may be helpful as a temporizing device but will not offer permanent control of the curve. The brace is helpful in the ambulatory child and in the patient capable of independent or assisted seating. Often the orthosis provides enough trunk support to free the upper extremities for functional use. If the curve progresses in spite of the orthosis, surgery is indicated.

Surgical Treatment

The surgical treatment of scoliosis in cerebral palsy is extremely complex. It is difficult to decide not only which type of surgery is needed but also whether any surgical procedure is warranted. Before the introduction of newer techniques and instrumentation, the surgical treatment of these patients was prone to failure, but the ability to treat these individuals has greatly improved.

The indications for surgical stabilization depend on the degree of mental involvement and the functional state of the individual with cerebral palsy. Allen and Ferguson state that all patients who have functional abilities that would likely be lost were the scoliosis left untreated are surgical candidates and that it is acceptable to permit the deformity to run its natural course in functionless persons. Determining what functional abilities would be helped by surgery is not always easy. Certainly in ambulatory children and in those of near normal intelligence surgical indications are similar to those for idiopathic scoliosis. In children with more severe involvement the indications are more conservative. If the curve affects the child's sitting ability, for instance, surgery is indicated to stabilize the spine.

When surgery is indicated, the type of surgery and instrumentation must be determined. MacEwen found a pseudarthrosis rate of 20% in patients with posterior spine fusion and Harrington instrumenta-

tion. Bonnett et al concluded that only the combined anterior and posterior procedure gave adequate correction and a low incidence of pseudarthrosis. This also was the recommendation of Moe et al.

Lonstein and Akbarnia classified cerebral palsy curves into two groups (Fig. 10-93). Group I curves, double curves with both a thoracic and a lumbar component, occurred in 40% of their patients. These curves, which are similar to curves of idiopathic scoliosis, occurred more commonly in patients with only mental retardation who were ambulatory and lived at home. Group II curves were present in 58% of patients; these are more severe lumbar or thoracolumbar curves that extend into the sacrum with marked pelvic obliquity. Patients with these curves usually were nonambulatory with spastic quadriplegia, generally were not cared for at home, and were more likely to have classic cerebral palsy rather than mental retardation alone.

According to Lonstein and Akbarnia, group I patients usually require only a posterior fusion, with fusion to the sacrum rarely needed. They suggested that the combined anterior and posterior approach to group I curves is needed only when where is a significant lumbar component, in which case an anterior release and fusion, together with posterior instrumentation, add correction and reduce the rate of pseudarthrosis. They stressed that anterior instrumentation is used in these curves only when there is

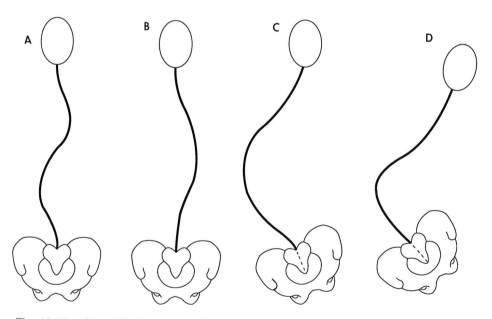

Fig. 10-93 **A** and **B,** Group I double curves with thoracic and lumbar component and little pelvic obliquity. **C** and **D,** Group II large lumbar or thoracolumbar curves with marked pelvic obliquity. (Redrawn from Lonstein JE and Akbarnia BA: J Bone Joint Surg 65A:43, 1983.)

no danger of overcorrecting the lumbar curve, with a resultant loss of balance and decompensation.

Group II patients usually require a long fusion to the sacrum because the sacrum is part of the curve and pelvic obliquity is present. Lonstein and Akbarnia found that the combined approach gave better correction of the scoliosis, slightly greater correction of the pelvic obliquity, and a lower rate of pseudarthrosis. Studies by Gersoff and Renshaw and by Allen and Ferguson have shown superior results and fixation with Luque-rod segmental instrumentation. They reported 33 and 10 cases, respectively, and found no pseudarthrosis. This technique improves fixation and is the instrumentation of choice for patients with cerebral palsy (Fig. 10-94).

Lonstein and Renshaw presented a management protocol for group II curves in which they recommended traction roentgenograms made with the patient on the Risser-Cotrel frame, and with the use of a head halter, pelvic straps, and a lateral convex Cotrel strap. If a level pelvis and balanced spine can be obtained, a one-stage posterior approach is indicated. If, however, the traction roentgenogram shows residual pelvic obliquity or if the torso is not balanced over the pelvis, a two-stage approach is best. In general the larger the lumbar curve, the more severe the pelvic obliquity, and the more rigid the curve, the more likely a two-stage procedure will be needed. With improved posterior instrumentation, anterior instru-mentation usually is not needed; however, it may be useful in patients with severe spasticity or athetosis in whom the additional internal fixation is helpful.

Gersoff and Renshaw found several technical points to be important: (1) 0.25-inch Luque rods are used if the patient is large enough (usually a weight of more than 80 pounds) to accept them; (2) whenever possible, two doubled 16-gauge wires are passed under each lamina; (3) facet joints are excised before the wire is passed; (4) the spinous processes are morcelized and the transverse processes are decorticated; and (5) bone-bank bone also is necessary. Allen and Ferguson reported equally good results, although in fewer patients, without decortication and facet excision. Their technique emphasizes removal of soft tissue from the posterior elements and the addition of a large volume of bone graft. They believe the $\frac{3}{16}$-inch rod is strong enough if it is made of MP-35-N alloy rather than stainless steel and if the curve is flexible. The 0.25-inch rod is used only in patients with athetosis, large body mass, seizure disorders, or unusual activity demands and in those patients whose condition cannot be corrected to a compensated position even after anterior release. The 0.25-inch rods are much stiffer and bulkier, and they make less bone surface available for fusion.

If the two-stage approach is used, the anterior disk excision and fusion proceed as described on p. 502. The Luque-rod technique is described on p. 484, and

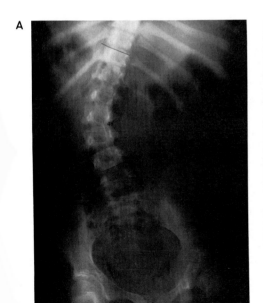
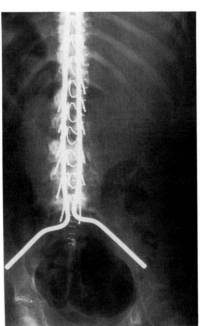

Fig. 10-94   A, Group II 49-degree thoracolumbar curve in child with cerebral palsy.
B, After Luque instrumentation with fixation to pelvis (Galveston technique).

fusion to the sacrum, which usually is necessary, is by the Galveston technique of pelvic fixation as described on p. 488.

Most authors have found that traction does not aid in the treatment of these curves either preoperatively or between the anterior and posterior procedures. Lonstein and Akbarnia still occasionally use halofemoral traction for selected, uncooperative patients to help control the patient or to facilitate nursing care, but not for curve correction. Postoperative immobilization after the spinal fusion depends on the activity level of the child and the security of the internal fixation. If the child can tolerate external support without any detrimental effect on function, it is used on all patients, no matter how secure the internal fixation, usually for 9 to 12 months or until the fusion is solid. If, however, the external support would significantly hinder the patient's functional ability and the internal fixation is secure, no support is used.

Complications of Surgery

With improved techniques of instrumentation and preoperative and postoperative management, the complication rate is decreasing although it is still significant in these patients. Lonstein and Akbarnia reported an 81% complication rate. Their complication rate has improved with greater experience and improved instrumentation, but a much higher complication rate should be expected with this type of scoliosis surgery than that for idiopathic curves. Some complications such as pressure sores have been eliminated with improved posterior instrumentation. In their study Gersoff and Renshaw found an incidence of infection of 15%, which was comparable to the average of 19% for other studies. The patients in whom a deep infection developed were treated by removal of all sutures down to the instrumentation and graft, irrigation and debridement, administration of systemic antibiotics, packing of the wound, and frequent changes of dressing until granulation tissue covered the instrumentation and the graft. Delayed primary closure then was accomplished. All infections cleared in this manner without removal of the instrumentation. The incidence of pseudarthrosis has been reported to be as high as 52%. Recent studies indicate that this has been significantly decreased with the Luque-rod segmental instrumentation, but longer follow-up is needed before this is proved. Pulmonary complications often develop in these patients because they cannot cooperate in performing deep breathing and coughing exercises. Appropriate prophylactic pulmonary measures are therefore needed. It should be noted that all three patients in Lonstein and Akbarnia's series who died after surgery succumbed to bronchial pneumonia 5 to 9 months after

surgery. If the upper limit of the fusion is not carefully selected, kyphosis cephalad to the upper limit of the fusion can occur. Other possible complications are those inherent in any spinal operation, such as urinary infection, ileus, and blood loss.

Although the complications can be significant in the management of these cases, the functional improvement or prevention of deterioration of function is well worth the effort and the risks of surgery. Complications should be expected and planned for; prompt treatment will lessen their severity. Avoidance of surgery for scoliosis in these patients who already have serious problems in walking and in trunk stability and function is unreasonable.

Friedreich's Ataxia

Friedreich's ataxia is a recessively inherited condition characterized by spinocerebellar degeneration. The clinical onset takes place in persons between the ages of 6 and 20 years. Affected children frequently are wheelchair bound in the first and second decades of life and have a cardiomyopathy that often leads to death in the third or fourth decade of life. There have been few reports in the literature concerning the incidence of spinal deformity in these patients. The largest reported series to date is that of Labelle et al who followed up 56 patients with typical Friedreich's ataxia in accordance with the criteria of Geoffrey et al. They found the prevalence of scoliosis in Friedreich's ataxia to be 100%. The most common pattern of scoliosis was a double structural thoracic and lumbar curve (57%) whereas the typical neuromuscular thoracolumbar curve with pelvic obliquity was found in only 14%. Similar findings were reported by Cady and Bobechko in 38 patients. Because no significant correlation could be established between the overall muscle weakness and curve progression, as would be expected in a neuromuscular scoliosis, they postulated that the pathogenesis of scoliosis in Friedreich's ataxia may be a disturbance of equilibrium and postural reflexes rather than muscle weakness. Labelle et al also found that not all curves in Friedreich's ataxia were progressive and the onset of the disease at an early age and the presence of a scoliosis before puberty were major factors in progression; they concluded that scoliosis appearing in the late teens or early twenties is less likely to be progressive.

Most authors have found bracing for progressive curvatures in Friedreich's ataxia to be a failure. Labelle et al recommended that curves of less than 40 degrees be observed; curves of more than 60 degrees be treated surgically, and curves of between 40 and 60 degrees be observed or treated surgically, depending on the age of the patient at onset of the disease and such characteristics of the scoliosis as the patient's age when it is recognized and evidence of the progression of the curve (Fig. 10-95).

Before any consideration of surgery for these patients, a cardiologic evaluation is recommended. Patients with Friedreich's ataxia frequently are unable to walk with a postoperative cast or brace. Preoperative traction and prolonged bed rest during the postoperative period must be kept to a minimum; otherwise a rapid increase in weakness can occur. For this reason the ideal instrumentation for these patients is segmental spinal instrumentation by the Luque technique, with early ambulation postoperatively without external support (see p. 484).

Charcot-Marie-Tooth Disease

Classic Charcot-Marie-Tooth disease is a demyelinating neuropathy. The condition is dominantly inherited, with considerable variation in severity (see p. 724). Hensinger and MacEwen studied 69 patients with Charcot-Marie-Tooth disease of whom seven (10%) had kyphoscoliosis. Two patients had mild degrees of curvature and did not require treatment, two were successfully treated with the Milwaukee brace, and three underwent posterior spine stabilization and fusion. Daher et al, in a study of 12 patients with Charcot-Marie-Tooth disease and scoliosis, also found that nonoperative treatment with the brace was well tolerated without any special problems. Both these reports emphasize that Charcot-Marie-Tooth disease and spinal deformity may be managed with the same techniques used for idiopathic scoliosis, including bracing and surgery.

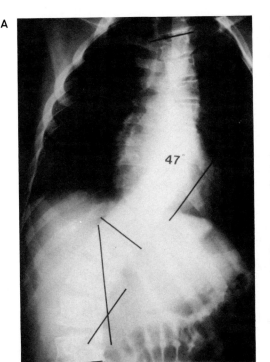 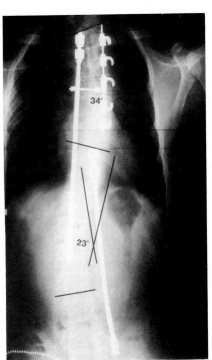

Fig. 10-95   A, Patient with Friedreich's ataxia and progressive scoliosis. **B,** After posterior instrumentation and fusion.

Syringomyelia

Syringomeylia is a tubular cavity that contains fluid within the spinal cord. Scoliosis may be the first manifestation of a syringomyelia. Huebert and MacKinnon reported scoliosis in 63% of 43 children with syringomyelia. Scoliosis was found in 82% of children whose symptoms had been noted before the age of 16 years. Certain physical findings may indicate the possibility of a syringomyelia, including neurologic deficits with the scoliosis, as noted by Nordwall and Wikkelso, and a left thoracic curvature. If the diagnosis of syringomyelia is suspected, magnetic resonance imaging (MRI) should be performed.

The association of a syringomyelia with the scoliosis may have a significant influence on treatment. Huebert and MacKinnon reported one patient in whom a spinal fusion after laminectomy was fatal when a large cyst in the cord ruptured. The other patient in whom they performed surgery with Harrington rods without laminectomy was stable and without complaints 3 years after surgery. Nordwall and Wikkelso noted delayed onset of paraplegia in a patient with syringomyelia who was treated with Harrington rod instrumentation. Obviously, the rate of progression of the neurologic deficit and the prognosis of the curve should be considered before any extensive operations are considered for patients with this disease. Bradford advocates initial treatment of this condition with drainage of the cyst followed by observation to determine the subsequent curve status. If curvature progresses, surgical stabilization and

fusion should be carried out. He believes that sublaminar wiring poses additional risks to the dilated spinal cord and favors the use of Harrington instrumentation alone, with intraoperative spinal cord monitoring and the wake-up test.

Spinal Cord Injury

Several series in the literature have demonstrated a significant incidence of spine deformity after spinal cord injuries in children. Kilfoyle et al found that spinal curvature and pelvic obliquity developed in 97 in 104 children with spinal trauma. Lancourt et al reported that scoliotic curves of more than 20 degrees developed in 31 of 50 patients and, more significantly, that scoliosis developed in all patients who were younger than 10 years of age at the time of injury. In a study of 40 children with spinal cord injury, Mayfield et al found that paralytic spinal deformity developed in all 25 patients who were injured before the adolescent growth spurt (Fig. 10-96). In 96% of these patients it was progressive. In the preadolescent period scoliosis was the most common deformity and kyphosis was second. In contrast, the postadolescent patients rarely had a paralytic spinal deformity and their spine deformities were those associated with instability of the fracture itself.

Increasing curvature with pelvic obliquity in the child with spinal cord injury can lead to loss of sitting balance that requires the use of the upper extremities for trunk support rather than for functional tasks (Fig. 10-97). Pressure sores may arise on the downside of the ischium, and hip subluxation can occur on the

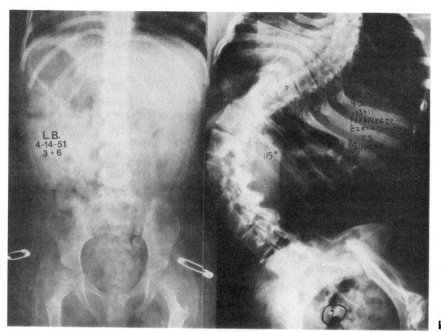

Fig. 10-96   A, Spine of paraplegic infant with T5 lesion. **B,** Development of significant scoliosis at age 14. (From Mayfield JK et al: J Bone Joint Surg 63A:1401, 1981.)

A

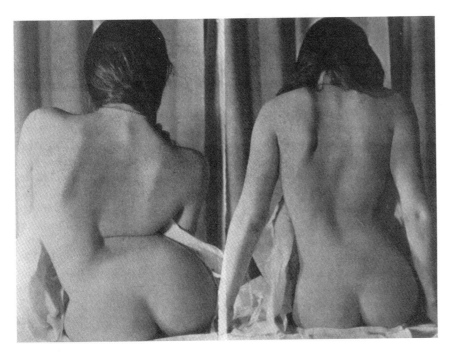

Fig. 10-97 Impairment of sitting balance by pelvic obliquity. (From Mayfield JK et al: J Bone Joint Surg 63A:1401, 1981.)

high side of the pelvic obliquity. The physician should therefore be constantly vigilant for any sign of development of a paralytic spine deformity.

Orthotic Treatment

Although Lancourt et al state that it does not appear possible to alter the natural progression of scoliosis with devices such as braces or corsets, other authors such as Mayfield et al, Bonnett, and Lonstein and Renshaw indicate that orthotic treatment does have a place in the management of scoliosis in the preadolescent patient with spinal cord injury. They believe that, although orthotic treatment is difficult, it can be effective in delaying progression of the curvature and allowing for further spinal growth before fusion is necessary. Orthotic treatment requires close cooperation among the physician, the family, and the patient. A custom-fitted, well-padded, plastic total-contact bivalved body jacket (TLSO) generally is used (Fig. 10-98). Close attention must be paid for any evidence of pressure changes on the skin. The brace may be removed at night and used only during sitting.

Surgical Treatment

Most preadolescent children with spinal cord injury ultimately require surgical stabilization of their scoliosis. In the series of Mayfield et al 68% of the patients ultimately required stabilization and fusion. If the curve progresses in spite of orthotic treatment,

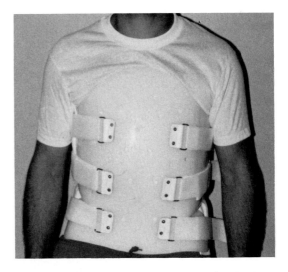

Fig. 10-98 Bivalved thoracolumbosacral orthosis used for external support in children with paralytic deformity of spine. (From Mayfield JK et al: J Bone Joint Surg 63A:1401, 1981.)

surgical intervention is indicated. Children with curves greater than 60 degrees should be considered for immediate surgery. Curves treated with an orthosis are considered for surgery if the curve progresses beyond 40 degrees, and curves between 40 and 60 degrees are considered individually. If the scoliosis or the kyphosis is large when the physician first sees the patient, surgery should be strongly considered at that time.

Poliomyelitis

With the advent of the Salk and Sabin vaccines, poliomyelitis in children is rare in the United States. Consequently, most recent experience in treating postpolio spinal deformities is with adult patients. The basic principles of treatment, however, are no different from those for spinal deformities as a result of neuromuscular disease. Bonnett et al outlined the indications for correction and posterior spine fusion in patients with polio: (1) collapsing spinal deformity because of marked paralysis, (2) progressive spinal deformity that does not respond to nonoperative treatment, (3) reduction of cardiorespiratory function associated with progressive restrictive lung disease, (4) decreasing independence in functional activities because of spinal instability, which necessitates use of the upper extremities for trunk support rather than for table-top activities, and (5) back pain and loss of sitting balance associated with pelvic obliquity, which frequently causes ischial pain and pressure necrosis on the downside of the gluteal region. It appears that these indications are still valid. As in any other neuromuscular curve the length of fusion will be much greater in a patient with poliomyelitis than in one with idiopathic scoliosis. Segmental instrumentation is recommended. In the evaluation of the distal extent of the fusion in a patient with poliomyelitis it must be determined whether the pelvic obliquity is due to the spinal curvature itself or to other factors such as iliotibial band contractures.

Infantile Spinal Muscle Atrophy

Infantile spinal muscle atrophy (Werdnig-Hoffmann disease) is an autosomal recessive condition in which atrophy of the anterior horn cells occurs throughout the spinal cord. Because of the clinical variations in the condition, it has been subdivided into groups I, II, and III, depending on the extent of involvement and the time within the first 2 years of life when the diagnosis becomes apparent. Group I patients are diagnosed within the first 2 months of life, remain severely hypotonic, and often die within the first year or two of life. Group II patients are diagnosed between the ages of 2 and 12 months, and group III patients are diagnosed between the ages of 1 and 2 years. As noted by Schwentker and Gibson and by Evans et al, scoliosis develops in virtually all patients with this condition. The onset usually occurs in childhood and the majority of the curves are progressive. The scoliosis often is the most severe problem in patients who survive childhood.

Orthotic Treatment

Schwentker and Gibson and Riddick et al believe that bracing can slow the progression of curvature and also allow sitting for longer periods of time. When the scoliosis in a skeletally immature patient reaches 20 degrees in the sitting position, orthotic treatment should be considered, usually a total-contact bivalved body jacket (TLSO), used only during sitting to minimize the rate of progression of the curve and to provide an extremely weak child with a stable sitting support. When the curve approaches 40 to 50 degrees, surgical intervention is recommended.

Surgical Treatment

Surgical treatment is posterior spinal fusion with posterior instrumentation and adequate bone grafting. Because fusion to the sacrum is needed for many of these patients, Luque-rod fixation with sublaminar wires and fixation to the pelvis by the Galveston technique (p. 488) provides optimal internal fixation. Augmentation of the fusion with bone-bank allograft bone usually is necessary. If the vertebrae are extremely osteoporotic, external support, such as a bivalved body jacket, may be used. If the curve has progressed to greater than 100 degrees and the patient has a severe fixed lumbar curve with pelvic obliquity, it may be necessary to combine an anterior fusion with the posterior instrumentation. As indicated by Shapiro and Bresnan, the anterior fusion adds considerably to the risks of the procedure. The anterior approach almost invariably involves "taking down" the diaphragm, which is the main respiratory muscle in these patients.

Complications in this group of patients are frequent and should be expected. Pulmonary complications are the most common, and postoperative management requires respiratory support for longer than normal. The patient should be mobilized as rapidly as possible. As indicated by Kepes et al, the patient with spinal muscle atrophy may be particularly sensitive to medications that depress the respiratory center, and the use of these drugs in the postoperative period should be minimal. As indicated by Lonstein and Renshaw, if the pulmonary involvement is such that the forced vital capacity is less than 20% of that predicted, the patient is at great risk for postoperative death. A vigorous preoperative and postoperative physical therapy program is mandatory. Bradford discourages the routine use of traction in these patients and encourages early mobilization.

Kugelberg-Welander Disease

Kugelberg-Welander disease is an atrophy of anterior horn cells similar to Werdnig-Hoffmann disease, but it becomes apparent in an older age-group (2 to 17 years). These patients are able to walk for several years, which complicates the management of the scoliosis deformity. Many of these patients assume a hyperlordic posture when walking to maintain balance, and orthotic management in the face of this spinal lordosis is quite difficult. If the lumbar spine is braced in flexion, as is common in most scoliotic conditions, the patient will fall forward and lose balance when walking. Because bracing generally is not tolerated, the spine must be assessed frequently. When the curve has progressed to approximately 50 degrees, surgery should be considered. The patient and family should be warned of the possibility of some loss of function because of the decrease in spinal flexibility. The curve, however, should not be allowed to progress to a more rigid and severe curve, which is more difficult to treat.

Familial Dysautonomia

Familial dysautonomia (Riley-Day syndrome) was first described in 1949 by Riley and Day. It is an autosomal recessive disorder found mostly in Jewish children of Eastern European extraction. The disease is caused by a reduction in the number of neurons in the posterior root ganglion, in the sympathetic ganglion, and in the lateral columns of the spinal cord. Most patients die in childhood or early adolescence, most often because of pulmonary disease. Yoslow et al found scoliosis in 39 of 65 patients and indicated that it is the major orthopaedic problem in patients with this disease. Although the scoliosis may be a significant progressive problem in these patients, Yoslow et al. warn that the features of the syndrome, such as the vasomotor and thermal instability, can give rise to troublesome and sometimes fatal operative or postoperative complications. These patients also may have dysphagia, which frequently leads to aspiration pneumonia. The use of a Milwaukee brace is complicated by the tendency for pressure ulcers to develop. When these potential complications are combined with the fact that most patients die before the age of 20 years with pulmonary complications, the advisability of treating the scoliosis must be carefully weighed. Hensinger and MacEwen reported the long-term result after spine fusion in one patient with this form of progressive neurologic disease. Eight years after spine fusion her trunk stability and alignment were improved, as was her ability to walk. Multiple problems, however, were encountered, including difficulty with heat exchange and pressure sores. Because the patient was unable to tolerate a cast, it was removed and she was nursed in recumbency on a turning frame for 6 months. Bradford has performed few spine fusions in these patients and emphasizes that the risks and complications are high and should be well appreciated before any surgical correction is undertaken.

Arthrogryposis Multiplex Congenita

Arthrogryposis multiplex congenita is a syndrome of persistent joint contractures that are present at birth. The etiology of the disorder is uncertain. Herron et al found a 20% incidence of scoliosis in patients with arthrogryposis multiplex congenita. They also found that most of these curves are progressive and become rigid and fixed at an early age. The scoliosis usually is detected at birth or within the first few years of life. If after that time no scoliosis occurs, the deformity does not develop. Most series have indicated that brace treatment is rarely successful and should be used only in patients with flexible curves. The onset of pelvic obliquity is a serious problem. If treatment of the pelvic obliquity by release of contractures in the hip area does not halt progression of the curve, spinal fusion to the sacrum is necessary. Similarly, as indicated by Daher et al, the onset of thoracic lordosis requires prompt treatment. Because of the severity and rigidity of the curves, postoperative complications are frequent. The connective tissue is tough, and the bones are osteoporotic. Daher et al reported the average blood loss to be 2000 ml. Herron et al obtained a maximum correction of only 25%. Herron et al and Daher et al reported the use of Harrington instrumentation and posterior fusion alone, but segmental fixation with Luque instrumentation may have significant advantages for these patients, with its improved fixation and improved instrumentation to the pelvis; however, there have been no reports of Luque instrumentation in this condition.

Duchenne Muscular Dystrophy

Scoliosis develops in a significant number of patients with Duchenne muscular dystrophy (Fig. 10-99). According to Bunch, spinal deformity seldom occurs in ambulatory patients with muscular dystrophy but rather develops after the patient becomes confined to a wheelchair. Robin and Brief reported spinal deformity in 24 of 27 patients with muscular dystrophy. The curves were predominantly long thoracolumbar curves with pelvic obliquity, the collapse of which were caused by absence of muscles and not by asymmetric muscle activity or contracture. The curves increased with advancing age to a severe deformity. Wilkins and Gibson identified five major types of curvature in Duchenne muscular dystrophy and reported that patients with extended spines had little scoliotic deformity, which they attributed to the maintainance of the facet joints in a locked position.

Orthotic Treatment

Orthotic treatment of scoliosis in patients with muscular dystrophy has been attempted, but with little success. Renshaw found that 77% of patients continued to show curve progression in spite of orthotic treatment. Although the average progression was 15 degrees per year in the orthosis-treated group versus 31 degrees per year in patients not treated with orthoses, the important fact is that the curve still progressed.

In patients with Duchenne muscular dystrophy, pulmonary function deteriorates approximately 4%

A   B   C

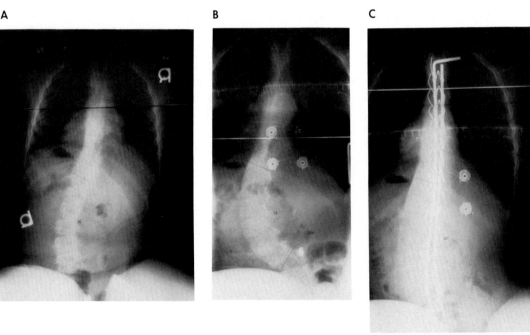

Fig. 10-99   **A** to **C,** Progressive scoliosis (from 35 to 79 degrees) in patient with muscular dystrophy. Luque instrumentation and fusion corrected curve to 45 degrees.

per year after 12 years of age, and if orthotic treatment is continued until pulmonary function deteriorates significantly, surgical stabilization may become impossible. The slowly increasing scoliosis also decreases pulmonary function. The importance of pulmonary function was emphasized by Sakai et al, who recommended prophylactic tracheostomy for patients with vital capacities less than 40% of predicted normal or with a poor functional cough. If vital capacity is decreased below 25% of predicted normal, they believe surgery is contraindicated. Lonstein and Renshaw emphasize that orthotic treatment of scoliosis in Duchenne muscular dystrophy must not delay surgery until the patient is at greater operative and postoperative risk.

Surgical Treatment

Lonstein and Renshaw's indications for spinal fusion in patients with muscular dystrophy are curves greater than 30 degrees, a forced vital capacity greater than 30% of normal, and a prognosis of at least 2 years of life remaining. The patient should have a functional cough, little or no cardiomyopathy, and should have stopped ambulating independently because a long spinal fusion in an independent ambulator with severe neuromuscular disease often removes the compensatory balance mechanisms necessary for walking. In fact, however, the majority of patients with scoliosis in Duchenne muscular dystrophy already have stopped walking and therefore this latter factor frequently is of little concern.

Luque-rod instrumentation with sublaminar wires (p. 484) is the ideal instrumentation for these patients. If there is no fixed pelvic obliquity, the fusion and instrumentation can be stopped at the level of L5. If a significant fixed pelvic obliquity is present, then fusion to the pelvis with Galveston-type pelvic fixation (p. 488) is indicated (Fig. 10-100). The fusion must extend into the high upper thoracic spine at T2 or T3. The sagittal contours of the patient's spine, especially the lumbar lordosis, should be maintained for good sitting balance. As in any other neuromuscu-

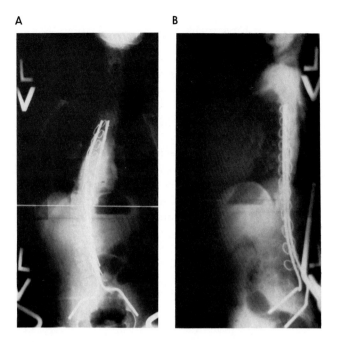

Fig. 10-100   A and **B,** Patient with muscular dystrophy after Luque segmental instrumentation and Galveston-type fixation to pelvis.

lar condition, adequate preoperative consultations and tests should be obtained. Large amounts of blood loss should be expected, and bone-bank allograft is needed because massive amounts of bone graft will be necessary. Adequate postoperative pulmonary care is essential. As a result of pulmonary compromise these patients are unable to tolerate any postoperative external immobilization, and rapid postoperative mobilization is important.

Lonstein and Renshaw summarized the benefits of spinal fusion in patients with Duchenne muscular dystrophy: (1) preservation of sitting balance, (2) avoidance of back pain, (3) improvement of spinal decompensation, (4) freeing the arms of the necessity of trunk support, (5) improvement of body image, and (6) possibly slowing of the deterioration of pulmonary function.

Variants of Muscular Dystrophy Other Than Duchenne

Spinal curvature in association with non-Duchenne muscular dystrophy is uncommon. The occurrence of scoliosis depends on the specific type of dystrophic disease, and its progress is related to the severity of the primary disease. Siegel found that childhood dystrophia myotonica is not associated with spinal curvature. The onset of limb girdle dystrophy usually occurs in middle or late adolescence, and weakness often is symmetric and progression slow. Patients usually are ambulatory into the second or third decade and seldom show scoliosis severe enough to warrant treatment. Facioscapulohumeral dystrophy is more rapidly progressive when the onset occurs in childhood. Frequently it is also asymmetric in distribution, and structural scoliosis can occur and interfere with balance and walking. These patients fortunately are amenable to more traditional forms of treatment because of the slow progression of their disease and relative maintenance of their strength. The use of an orthosis in the juvenile years can control the curve until the pubertal growth spurt. Thoracic lordosis, however, tends to develop, and the Milwaukee brace is contraindicated in its presence.

Congenital myopathies only recently have become distinguishable, primarily on the basis of enzyme histochemistry and electron microscopic studies of involved muscles. Various types have been described: central core disease, nemaline myopathy, myotubular myopathy, congenital fiber-type disproportion, and mitochondrial myopathy. The main orthopaedic problems in patients with these diseases are related to congenital dislocation of the hip, coxa valga, and hip subluxation that develops with time, as described by Ramsey and Hensinger.

Daher et al, in a review of 11 patients with spinal deformities caused by muscular dystrophy other than Duchenne muscular dystrophy, found that patients with these conditions generally had slowly evolving curves and that the use of an orthosis in the juvenile years controlled the curve until the pubertal growth spurt. Surgical treatment consisting of posterior instrumentation and fusion was successful in stabilizing the deformities (Fig. 10-101). Thoracic lordosis was frequent in these patients, requiring careful observation and management.

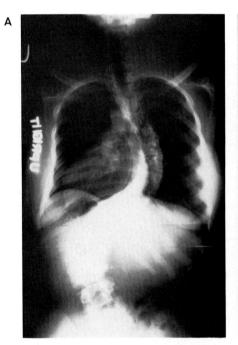 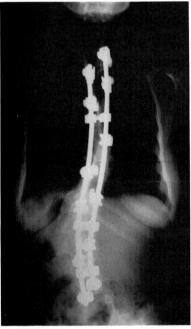

Fig. 10-101 **A,** Scoliosis in adolescent with congenital myopathy. **B,** After posterior spinal fusion with Cotrel-Dubousset instrumentation.

CONGENITAL SCOLIOSIS

Congenital scoliosis is a lateral curvature of the spine caused by the presence of vertebral anomalies that result in an imbalance in the longitudinal growth of the spine. These anomalies develop during the first 6 weeks of intrauterine life when the anatomic pattern of the spine is formed in mesenchyme. Some type of anomaly must be visible on the roentgenograms of the spine before a diagnosis of congenital scoliosis can be made. A congenital scoliosis often is rigid, and correction can be difficult. It is therefore important to detect these curves early and to institute appropriate treatment while the curve is small rather than to attempt the dangerous salvage-type procedures that are necessary when the deformity is severe.

Classification

The classification proposed by MacEwen et al and later modified by Winter et al is the one most uniformly accepted. This classification divides the malformations into three basic types:
A. Failure of formation (Fig. 10-102)
   1. Partial failure of formation (wedge vertebra)
   2. Complete failure of formation (hemivertebra)
B. Failure of segmentation (Fig. 10-103)
   1. Unilateral failure of segmentation (unilateral unsegmented bar)
   2. Bilateral failure of segmentation (block vertebra)
C. Miscellaneous

The congenital curvature also should be classified according to the area of spine involved because this is indicative of prognosis of the specific deformity. The generally accepted areas to distinguish are those involving the cervicothoracic spine, thoracic spine, thoracolumbar spine, and lumbosacral spine.

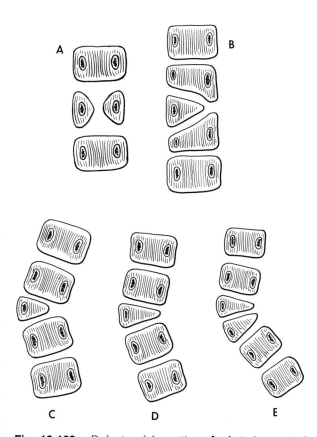

Fig. 10-102 Defects of formation. **A,** Anterior central defect. **B,** Incarcerated hemivertebra. **C,** Free hemivertebra. **D,** Wedge vertebra. **E,** Multiple hemivertebrae. (Redrawn from Bradford DS and Hensinger RM: The pediatric spine, New York, 1985, Thieme Inc.)

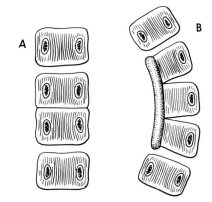

Fig. 10-103 **A,** Block vertebra. **B,** Unilateral unsegmented bar. (Redrawn from Bradford DS and Hensinger RM: The pediatric spine, New York, 1985, Thieme Inc.)

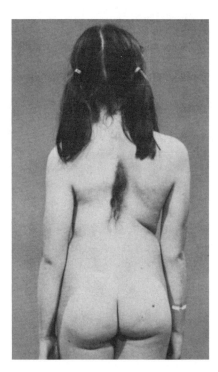

Fig. 10-104   Hair patch associated with diastematomyelia and congenital scoliosis. (From Winter RB et al: J Bone Joint Surg 56A:27, 1974.)

Patient Evaluation

In addition to routine spinal evaluation, there are some specific physical findings to be sought in congenital scoliosis. The skin of the back should be carefully examined for such signs as hair patches, lipomata, dimples, and scars (Fig. 10-104). The presence of any of these deformities may indicate an underlying anomalous vertebra. The neurologic evaluation also should be very thorough. Evidence of neurologic involvement such as clubfoot, calf atrophy, absent reflexes, and atrophy of one lower extremity compared with the other should be noted carefully. There is a high incidence of other anomalies in children with congenital scoliosis. MacEwen et al emphasized the importance of a complete evaluation of the genitourinary system: 18% of their patients had coexisting urologic anomalies, including 2.5% who had obstructive disease that could be life threatening. The incidence of congenital heart disease is reported to be 7% and diastematomyelia (Fig. 10-105) occurs in approximately 5% of patients.

A high-quality series of routine roentgenograms is essential to evaluate the deformity. The type of congenital curve should be classified as to a failure of segmentation or a failure of formation, and the roentgenograms should be examined carefully for any evidence of widening of the pedicles or midline bony defects that may indicate an underlying cord anomaly. Careful measurements with the use of the Cobb system should be made of all the congenital curves, including the compensatory or secondary ones in the seemingly normal parts of the spine. Measurements should include each end of the anomalous area, as well as each end of the entire curve generally considered in treatment, that is, from the vertebra maximally tilted at each end. Measuring the anomalous area separately is a more accurate way to determine if growth is asymmetric or if the curve is increasing because the vertebrae are being added to the curve. Tomograms sometimes are helpful to further delineate the type of congenital curve that can be difficult to determine on plain films. Myelography must be used if there is a suspicion of a diastematomyelia or if any neurologic abnormality exists in the lower extremities (Fig. 10-106). Gillespie et al emphasized the high risk of congenital intraspinal anomalies with congenital scoliosis and the lack of cutaneous manifestations in a significant number of patients. If correction of the curve is anticipated, either by bracing or surgery, then a myelogram is indicated. CT or MRI may be helpful to delineate any anomalies. An intravenous pyelogram certainly should be considered in view of the high incidence of associated genitourinary abnormalities.

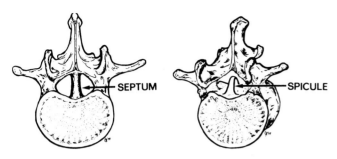

Fig. 10-105 Diastematomyelia spicule invaginates dura and divides spinal cord, either partially or completely. (From Hood RW et al: J Bone Joint Surg 62A:520, 1980.)

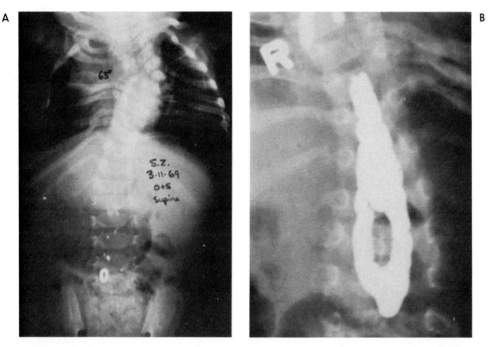

Fig. 10-106 **A,** Widening of spinal canal from T12 to L5. **B,** Myelogram shows classic midline defect at L2 of diastematomyelia. (From Winter RB et al: J Bone Joint Surg 56A:27, 1974.)

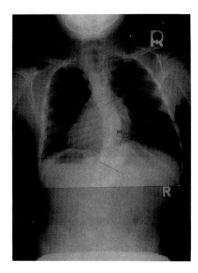

Fig. 10-107 Left-sided, unsegmented bar with resulting 50-degree congenital scoliosis.

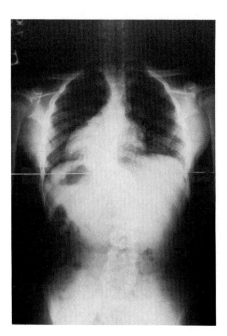 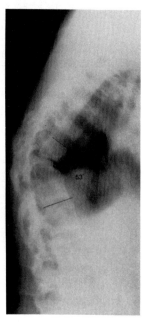

Fig. 10-108 Congenital kyphoscoliosis caused by hemivertebra.

Natural History

There have been several excellent studies on the natural history of congenital scoliosis. The most recent study by McMaster and Ohtsuka followed up 216 untreated patients for 5 years. The early study by Kuhns and Hormell found only 15% of congenital curves to be progressive, but later studies emphasize the significant potential for progression of these congenital curves if left untreated. Several characteristics of the natural history of this condition are agreed on by all authors. The type of anomaly that causes the most severe scoliosis in any region of the spine is a unilateral unsegmented bar with a contralateral hemivertebra at the same level. This is followed in severity by scoliosis caused by a unilateral unsegmented bar (Fig. 10-107). The least severe scoliosis is caused by a block vertebra. Congenital scoliosis that appears in the thoracic and thoracolumbar regions of the spine carries a worse prognosis than do lumbar and cervicothoracic curves. The rate of deterioration is not constant, but if the curve is present before the patient is 10 years of age, it usually increases, especially during the adolescent growth spurt. The mean rate of deterioration, however, in patients who are younger than 10 years of age is about 5 degrees per year.

The deformity produced by failure of formation is much more difficult to predict than that caused by failure of segmentation. A hemivertebra produces scoliosis by acting as an enlarging wedge on the affected side of the spine, whereas in patients with a unilateral unsegmented bar, there is retarded growth on the affected side. The growth imbalance in patients with hemivertebrae is never as severe as in those with a unilateral unsegmented bar. Winter reported that a hemivertebra can exist tucked into the spine between adjacent normal vertebrae and not cause a corresponding malformation. He called this an *incarcerated hemivertebra*. If, however, the hemivertebra is separated from either of the adjacent vertebra by a disk, it is a segmented hemivertebra, which infers two functioning growth plates on either side of the hemivertebra that in all likelihood will cause a slowly progressive curve (Fig. 10-108).

The natural history of congenital scoliosis caused by mixed anomalies is virtually impossible to predict, and treatment must be based on continued follow-up evaluations.

Orthotic Treatment

The Milwaukee brace, which provides the most effective nonsurgical treatment available, is used primarily for the more flexible secondary curve below the congenital one. If the brace maintains the curve in an acceptable position, it can be continued; however, if the curve begins to deteriorate despite faithful brace wearing, fusion is indicated. Winter et al in 1976 found that the best results with Milwaukee brace treatment were in mixed anomalies with a progressive secondary curve. No attempt should be made to brace a scoliosis that is completely rigid or any curve that exceeds 50 degrees. If nonsurgical treatment is elected, careful measurement and comparison of spine roentgenograms at 6-month intervals must be made. Because of the slow progression of curves (approximately 5 degrees a year), it is important to compare current roentgenograms with all previous films to detect curve progression.

Surgical Treatment

Because 75% of congenital scoliosis curves are progressive, surgery remains the fundamental treatment. Fusion for congenital scoliosis may be performed in the very young child to eliminate growth on the convex side of the curve and prevent its progression. A Milwaukee brace is not used routinely after fusion in a young patient, but the brace may be required to control the secondary curves until growth is complete. Without bracing, the secondary curves in the previously normal area of the spine may become structural and more than double the angle of the congenital curve. There are several surgical approaches to congenital curves, and the selection depends on the type of curve, its location, and its severity.

Fusion in Situ

Fusion in situ is appropriate for minor curves detected early and for stiff, rigid curves in which progression is inevitable, such as a unilateral unsegmented bar. Fusion is performed through a posterior exposure. If enough autogenous bone is unavailable because of the child's young age, bone-bank bone is used. The top and bottom of the fused area can be marked with a wire suture or metal clip for postoperative observation. Postoperative immobilization is obtained in a Risser cast, and the patient remains ambulatory. Winter et al found that posterior spine fusion without instrumentation gave predictably good results in patients with congenital scoliosis. Although

they found some improvement in curve measurements, they emphasized that the main goal of this procedure is stabilization of the curve and prevention of progression. Of 163 patients having posterior fusion without rods, paralysis or infection did not develop in any. Bending of the fusion mass was the most common reason for loss of correction and occurred in 14% of patients. Winter et al attributed this bending to a growth discrepancy between the convex and concave sides of the curve. Bending of a solidly united mass fusion did not occur after cessation of growth.

Posterior Fusion and Cast Correction

Posterior fusion and cast correction are useful in curves flexible enough to allow cast correction but in which instrumentation is impractical or dangerous. The posterior fusion (p. 476) always should encompass one vertebra above and below the measured curve, and all vertebra should be rotated in the same direction as those in the apex of the curve. Maximum cast correction is obtained with longitudinal traction and localizer force, with the patient on the Risser table. In the past the patient was kept in bed for 6 months, but now most children are encouraged to begin ambulation 1 or 2 days after surgery. Cast immobilization for 9 to 10 months usually is required.

Halo-Femoral Traction and Fusion

Halo-femoral traction and fusion are rarely used in congenital curves and are reserved for more rigid curves (90 degrees or greater) for which cast correction is inadequate and in which a greater degree of correction is desired. As a general rule the amount of traction weight used should not exceed 50% of the patient's total body weight. Weights are added gradually each day, with careful monitoring of the neurologic status; an inability to void is the first sign of neurologic dysfunction of the cord. Cranial and peripheral nerve function should be evaluated. Any sudden pain, numbness, or weakness mandates removal of all weights, which are reapplied gradually after symptoms have disappeared. Usually a period up to 3 weeks is necessary to gain maximum correction with the slow addition of weights. A posterior fusion (p. 476) without instrumentation is performed with the patient in traction with the weight reduced by 50%. The weights gradually are brought back up to the preoperative level between 24 and 72 hours after surgery, and a halo cast is applied.

Harrington Instrumentation and Fusion

Complications of Harrington instrumentation and fusion in congenital scoliosis are far more frequent and serious than in idiopathic scoliosis. Spinal cord monitoring is highly desirable in these patients and, if unavailable, a wake-up test is mandatory. Even if spinal cord monitoring is used, the wake-up test also should be done. Letts and Hollenberg reported that congenital scoliosis is the most common condition in which paraplegia occurs after Harrington instrumentation. Winter found that the Harrington rods gave slightly better correction than fusion alone but were directly related to the only two cases of paralysis in his series. Infection developed in four of his patients, all of whom had Harrington instrumentation. Therefore the selection of patients in whom to use Harrington instrumentation for congenital scoliosis must be made very carefully. Before instrumentation a metrizamide myelography must be performed to rule out a tethered cord. Larger curves in older children are more appropriate for instrumentation because it is more difficult to obtain and maintain correction of these curves with a plaster cast alone. Instrumentation may be used mainly as a stabilizing strut, with reliance on halo-femoral traction or casting for correction of the curve.

Combined Anterior and Posterior Convex Fusion

In 1981 Winter reported 10 patients with progressive congenital scoliosis treated by convex anterior and posterior epiphysiodesis and arthrodesis. His criteria for effective correction with this procedure are (1) epiphysiodesis of the entire curve, not merely the apical segments, (2) both anterior and posterior fusions, (3) arthrodesis of the involved segment, which accompanies the epiphysiodesis, (4) rigid immobilization of the spine until the arthrodesis is solid, and (5) performance of the procedure at an early age. He reported excellent early results but stated that several more years of follow-up are necessary before definitive conclusions can be reached.

▶ *Technique (Winter).* Position the patient on the concave side in the straight lateral position, and prepare and drape the back and side together in the same field. Make two incisions, a midline posterior and a second one along the rib to be removed (the rib leading to the upper end of the curve).

Expose the vertebrae anteriorly by a transpleural, retropleural, or retroperitoneal approach, depending on the area involved. Identify the proper levels by a roentgenogram obtained in the operating room. Ligate segmental vessels. Remove the lateral half of the disk along with the lateral half of the growth plate and the bony end plate. Insert an autogenous bone graft (usually the rib), and close the wound. Posteriorly, expose only the convexity of the curve. Excise the facet joints, decorticate the lamina and transverse process, and insert an autogenous graft.

A corrective cast is applied while the child is still under anesthesia to avoid a second anesthetization for cast application. Casting is continued for 6 months, followed by a brace for 6 more months.

Wedge Resection (Hemivertebra Excision)

Wedge resection usually is reserved for patients with pelvic obliquity uncorrectable by other means (Fig. 10-109) or with a fixed lateral translation of the thorax that cannot be corrected by other means. The safest level at which to perform such excision is at the L3, L4, or lumbosacral level, below the level of the conus medullaris. Wedge resection in the T4 to T9 area should not be performed because this area of the spinal canal is the narrowest and has the least blood supply. Hemivertebra excision is best performed as a two-stage procedure, as described by Leatherman and Dickson, in which the vertebral body is removed by an anterior exposure initially. Two weeks later a posterior approach and excision of the remainder of the hemivertebra are carried out. The defect then can be closed with a Harrington compression rod. This procedure always must be accompanied by a fusion of the appropriate length. Postoperative care consists of cast immobilization in the supine position for 6 months, followed by an ambulatory cast for another 4 months or until fusion is completely solid.

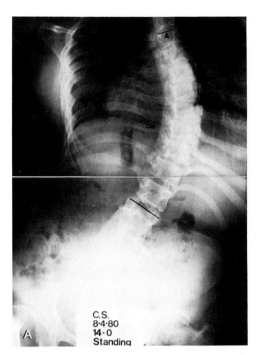

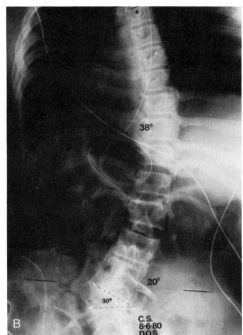

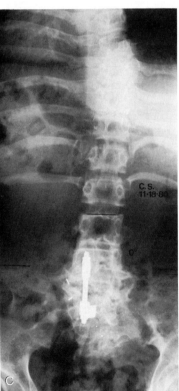

Fig. 10-109 **A,** Thoracolumbar scoliosis secondary to hemivertebra at L5. **B,** Anterior wedge of bone removed through left retroperitoneal exposure. **C,** Posterior Harrington compression rod closing wedge on convex side. (From Bradford DS et al: Moe's textbook of scoliosis and other spinal deformities, ed 2, Philadelphia, 1987, WB Saunders Co.)

Kyphosis

SCHEUERMANN'S DISEASE

In 1920 Scheuermann described a fixed kyphosis and vertebral wedging in adolescents. In 1964 Sorenson suggested that the diagnosis be made if three central vertebrae are wedged 5 degrees or more. This disorder is relatively common, with an incidence of 0.4% to 8.3% of the adolescent population.

Etiology

The true cause of Scheuermann's disease remains a puzzle. Scheuermann proposed that the kyphosis was the result of avascular necrosis of the ring apophysis of the vertebral body. The entity would therefore be classified with the other osteochondroses. Bick and Copel demonstrated that the ring apophysis actually lies outside of the true cartilaginous growth plate and therefore contributes nothing to the longitudinal growth of the body; thus a disturbance in the ring apophysis should not affect the growth potential of the vertebra and lead to vertebral wedging. In 1930 Schmorl suggested that the vertebral wedging was due to herniation of disk material into the vertebral body. These herniations now are known as *Schmorl's nodes*. As the disk material is extruded into the bony spongiosum, the height of the intervertebral disk is diminished, which causes increased pressure anteriorly and disturbances of enchondral growth of the vertebral body and subsequent wedging. Schmorl's nodes, however, are relatively common and frequently occur in patients with no evidence of Scheuermann's disease. Ferguson implicated the persistence of anterior vascular grooves in the vertebral bodies of preadolescents and adolescents. He believes that these vascular defects create a point of structural weakness in the vertebral body, which leads to wedging and kyphosis.

Present investigation into etiologic factors is centered on endocrine abnormalities, hereditary characteristics, malnutrition, osteoporosis, and mechanical factors. Bradford and Moe investigated the gross and histologic changes in two patients with Scheuermann's kyphosis and found that the anterior longitudinal ligament was thickened and created a bowstring across the apex of the kyphosis. Disk material had been pushed out anteriorly under this ligament, the bodies had become severely compressed, and the disk space was narrowed. Histologic and electron microscopic examination showed normal bone, cartilage, and disk. The ring apophysis showed no definite avascular necrosis. Protrusion of disk material into the bony spongiosa of the vertebral body was noted. The authors postulated that patients with Scheuer-

mann's kyphosis may have a mild form of juvenile osteoporosis. Because Scheuermann's kyphosis is seen in a high percentage of patients with Turner's syndrome or cystic fibrosis and these conditions are associated with osteoporosis, it is conceivable that an episode of juvenile osteopenia may be the preliminary event in this disorder. Lopez et al. correlated densitometric evidence of decreased bone with the presence of Scheuermann's disease. In spite of multiple attempts to definitely determine the cause of this condition, it still is unknown.

Patient Evaluation

Most patients seek evaluation of Scheuermann's disease because of deformity, but many are totally unaware of their deformity and are encouraged to come in for evaluation by family or friends. Pain is present in 20% to 60% of patients. Hensinger et al and Sorenson noted a higher incidence of pain in patients with thoracolumbar kyphosis than in those with thoracic kyphosis. This pain is localized over the kyphosis and is nonradiating.

Physical examination shows an increased kyphosis, with angulation in the area of the kyphosis and an increased compensatory lordosis below. In the thoracic spine the kyphosis is sharply angular. This kyphosis is quite apparent and does not correct with the prone extension test (Fig. 10-110, *A* to *C*). Kyphosis in the thoracolumbar and lumbar areas is not as easily visible. The lumbar lordosis below the kyphosis usually is flexible and corrects with forward bending. Tight hamstring and pectoral muscles are commonly seen in this disorder. On forward bending a minimal structural scoliosis can be seen in as many as 30% of these patients. The neurologic examination usually is normal except in the rare patient with secondary cord compression.

Roentgenographic Findings

Roentgenographic evaluation includes a 2-m standing lateral film taken with the patient's arms horizontal to determine the presence of vertebral wedging, Schmorl's nodes, and irregular end plates. The angle of kyphosis is measured by marking the end vertebrae, which are maximally tilted into the concavity of the curve. This angle is measured just as in scoliosis. Vertebral wedging is measured from angles created by lines parallel to the end plates. A standing 2-m posteroanterior roentgenogram also is made to rule out an associated scoliosis, which is present in 30% of these patients. On posteroanterior view the pedicles should be evaluated carefully for any evidence of increased interpedicular distance, such as would be seen in a patient with spinal epidural cysts that can

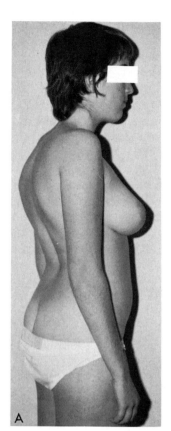

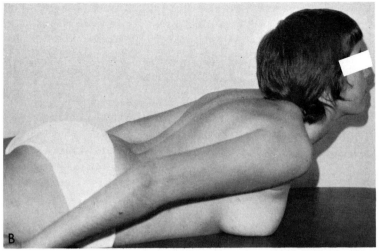

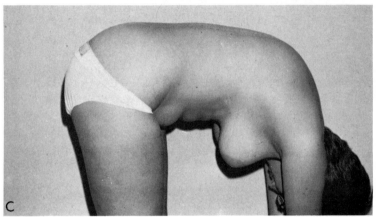

Fig. 10-110   A, Increased thoracic kyphosis. **B,** Thoracic kyphosis does not fully correct on thoracic extension, indicating structural kyphosis. **C,** On forward bend test, angular kyphosis is evident in thoracic spine; lumbar lordosis corrects on forward bending. (From Bradford DS et al: Moe's textbook of scoliosis and other spinal deformities, ed 2, Philadelphia, 1987, WB Saunders Co.)

cause a deformity much like that in Scheuermann's disease.

Mobility of the spine is evaluated by a supine hyperextension lateral roentgenogram, for which a plastic wedge is placed at the apex of the curvature. Skeletal age is determined from a bone age roentgenogram, and this is combined with the status of the iliac crest apophyses and the vertebral ring apophyses to determine skeletal maturity. Bradford found that the best roentgenographic criteria for the diagnosis of Scheuermann's disease are (1) irregular vertebral end plates, (2) apparent narrowing of the vertebral disk space, (3) one or more vertebrae wedged 5 or more degrees, and (4) an increase in the normal thoracic kyphosis above 45 degrees (Fig. 10-111).

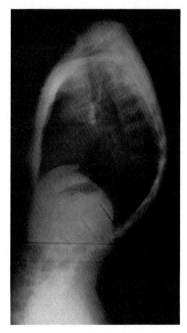

Fig. 10-111   Kyphosis of 81 degrees in patient with Scheuermann's disease.

Differential Diagnosis

The most common entity that must be differentiated from Scheuermann's disease is postural round-back deformity. This deformity characteristically produces a slight increase in the thoracic kyphosis, which seems to be quite mobile clinically and is easily correctable on the prone extension test. Roentgenograms show normal vertebral body contours without vertebral wedging. This kyphosis is more gradual than the angular kyphosis commonly seen in Scheuermann's disease. The presence of a normal roentgenogram, however, may not rule out the presence of Scheuermann's disease because roentgenographic changes may not be apparent until the child is 10 to 12 years of age.

If pain is a presenting symptom, infectious spondylitis must be considered. This usually can be excluded, however, by clinical and laboratory studies and tomograms or bone scans of the spine. Occasionally traumatic injuries can present problems in the differential diagnosis, but usually the wedging caused by a compression fracture involves only a single vertebra rather than the three or more found in true Scheuermann's kyphosis. Osteochondrodystrophies, such as Morquio's and Hurler's syndromes, as well as tumors and congenital deformities, especially congenital kyphosis, also must be considered. If the patient is a young man, ankylosing spondylitis must be ruled out, and this may require a human leukocyte antigen (HLA) B27 blood test.

Management

The treatment of Scheuermann's disease is somewhat controversial, probably because of the lack of a clear, concise, long-term study of the natural history of untreated Scheuermann's disease. Sorenson indicated that thoracic Scheuermann's disease has a favorable prognosis, but Bradford reported many adults with disabling thoracic pain caused by Scheuermann's disease. Bradford also reported that neurologic complications, although rare, may occur in Scheuermann's disease. Cord compression may develop as a result of the angle of deformity alone or in association with a herniated thoracic intervertebral disk at the apex of the curvature.

The potential for pain in adult life may be a controversial indication for treatment, but cosmesis also should be considered. Although curves of 40 degrees are difficult to detect clinically, a 70-degree deformity with resultant cervical and lumbar hyperlordosis can be deforming. Treatment of Scheuermann's disease in a growing child is a worthwhile procedure, certainly to improve cosmesis and also perhaps to lessen the chance of pain from this deformity.

Orthotic Treatment

Treatment in the past often consisted of serial casting, but in 1965 Moe reported that the Milwaukee brace was of greater benefit. Bradford et al later studied 194 patients with kyphosis and vertebral body wedging and 29 patients with kyphosis without wedging deformities. They found that with kyphosis greater than 35 degrees and at least one vertebra wedged more than 5 degrees, correction was obtained within 6 to 12 months. The curve correction improved 40% overall, the wedging improved 41%, and the lordosis 36%. If the kyphosis exceeded 75 degrees and the wedging of the vertebral bodies was greater than 10 degrees, and if the patient was near or past skeletal maturity, the results were much poorer. Sach et al reported that in patients followed up for 5 or more years, improvement was maintained in more than 60%.

For a supple kyphosis without wedging exercises and observation are recommended. These patients may well have a postural kyphosis, and bracing is not routinely recommended for postural problems. If the kyphosis angle increases or if wedging of the vertebral bodies appears, then a Milwaukee brace is indicated. Patients with vertebral body wedging when first examined should be braced immediately. Surgery rarely is necessary and is reserved for a severe deformity after completion of growth, for severe pain in the kyphotic area unresponsive to long-term rehabilitative efforts, and for those patients with neurologic signs or symptoms.

Surgical Treatment

In 1965 Moe presented his early experience with posterior fusion alone for the management of kyphosis. Bradford et al reported posterior Harrington compression instrumentation and fusion in 22 patients with Scheuermann's kyphosis. Loss of correction occurred in 16 of these patients and was caused by the presence of severe initial deformity, inadequate length of the fusion, severe wedging of the vertebral bodies, and probably a contracted anterior longitudinal ligament. They noted the difficulty of obtaining a solid posterior arthrodesis over a kyphosis because the fusion mass posteriorly is placed under tension rather than compression. Kostuik and Lorenz in 1983 also noted a high percentage of pseudarthroses from posterior arthrodesis alone.

In a later report Bradford et al reported 24 patients with an average age of 21 years who underwent combined anterior and posterior fusion for Scheuermann's disease. Their indications for combined anterior and posterior fusion include a kyphosis of more than 70 degrees in a patient who is skeletally mature and who has pain that cannot be controlled by conservative means. They also consider as good surgical candidates patients who are physiologically immature but in whom the kyphosis has not been controlled by a brace, as well as patients with early spastic paraparesis caused by the kyphosis. This recommendation does not include patients with neurologic changes caused by a sharply angular kyphotic component or a localized anterior cord compression. They did not find preoperative traction beneficial and do not recommend it in this later report. Bradford et al, as well as Taylor et al, reported loss of correction when the posterior fusion and instrumentation were not extended to the lowermost and uppermost vertebrae of the kyphosis. The end vertebra should be the last vertebra from the apex that is tilted maximally into the concavity of the curve; at least one vertebra above

and one vertebra below should be added to the fusion. Anteriorly the fusion should include the most rigid apical segment of the curve as identified by comparison of the standing lateral roentgenogram with a supine hyperextension roentgenogram. This usually involves six or seven apical vertebrae that can be conveniently exposed through a single thoracotomy incision with the removal of a single rib. Using a combined anterior and posterior approach, Bradford et al were able to obtain more than 50% correction (Fig. 10-112). Sturm et al reported good results with posterior fusion using large threaded compression rods rather than small ones. Coscia et al found long-term problems such as junctional kyphosis with Luque rods and segmental wires even when combined with anterior fusion, and they do not believe this type of instrumentation should be used.

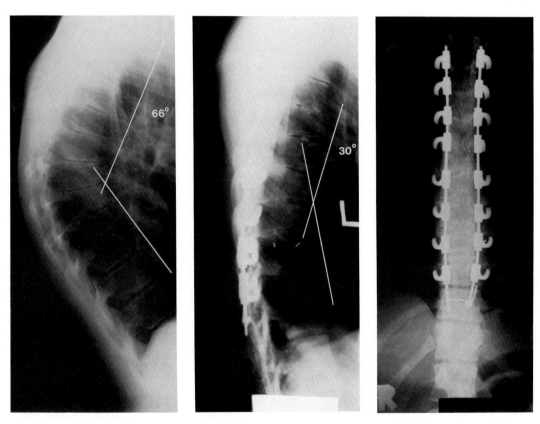

Fig. 10-112   Before and after combined anterior diskectomy and posterior compression instrumentation for Scheuermann's disease in 24-year-old woman. (From Bradford DS et al: J Bone Joint Surg 57A:439, 1975.)

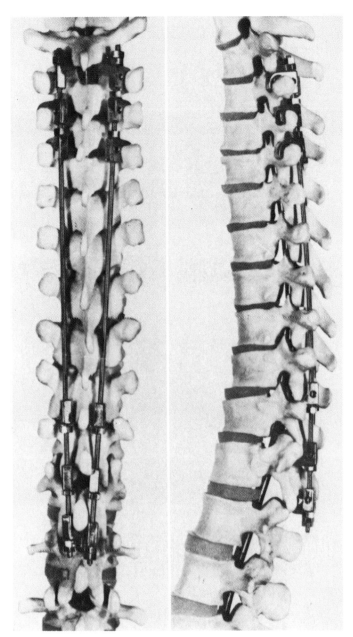

Fig. 10-113 Second stage of operative treatment of severe kyphosis: posterior instrumentation and fusion. (From Bradford DS et al: J Bone Joint Surg 57A:439, 1975.)

▲ *Technique (posterior fusion).* Place the patient prone on the Hall frame. Prepare and drape the skin in a routine sterile manner. Make a midline incision over the area to be fused, and expose the spine subperiostally as previously described (p. 472). Use two Harrington compression rods posteriorly. Prepare the hook sites for the No. 1259 hooks in the routine manner (p. 482). Extend the upper hook as high as T2 or T3. Place the compression hooks distal to the apex of the kyphosis beneath the lamina. The more levels to undergo instrumentation above and below the kyphosis the more stable the system will be. Use autogenous cancellous bone graft to supplement the fusion.

▲ *Postoperative management.* External immobilization with an underarm Risser cast or a molded plastic jacket is used for 9 to 12 months or until the fusion is solid.

▲ *Technique (anterior and posterior fusion).* Through an anterior approach, excise the entire disk and cartilaginous end plate, leaving only the posterior portion of the anulus and the posterior longitudinal ligament. Do not remove the bony end plate. Loosen or mobilize each joint, using a Blount or lamina spreader, and then pack each joint temporarily, preferably with Gelfoam or Surgicel to minimize blood loss. When all the desired joints have been cleared, remove the packing as each joint is grafted with short transverse segments of rib or other bone. Autogenous iliac bone or preferably bone strips from the exposed vertebral bodies may be added if the single rib is not sufficient. This approach and fusion is described in more detail on p. 502. About 2 weeks later perform the posterior fusion, placing the top no. 1259 hooks as high as T2 or T3 and engaging the transverse processes, with the lower three hooks engaging the caudal aspect of the appropriate laminae (Fig. 10-113). Use autogenous cancellous bone to supplement the fusion. This procedure is described in greater detail on p. 482.

▲ *Postoperative management.* External immobilization by an underarm Risser cast or a molded plastic jacket is used for 9 to 12 months or until the fusion is solid.

CONGENITAL KYPHOSIS

Kyphosis of the spine caused by congenital vertebral anomalies is uncommon, but significant deformities and disabilities can result. In a classic article Winter et al reported 130 patients with congenital kyphosis and classified congenital kyphosis into three types. In type I there is congenital failure of vertebral body formation. In type II there is a failure of vertebral body segmentation. Type III represents a combination of both these conditions (Fig. 10-114). This classification is extremely important in predicting the natural history of these congenital kyphotic deformities.

Type I deformities (defects of formation) are more common than type II deformities and generally are in the thoracic or thoracolumbar area. The deformities caused by this type of kyphosis are more severe and progress more rapidly. Winter et al emphasized that paraplegia was seen in only those patients with type I deformity (defects of formation). Left untreated, the kyphosis will progress relentlessly, averaging 7 degrees per year. The progression reaches a maximum during the adolescent growth spurt. Type II deformities (failure of segmentation) are less common. In a follow-up article in 1980, Mayfield et al reported the natural history and treatment of kyphosis caused by defects of anterior segmentation. They found that this deformity progresses with vertebral growth at an average rate of 5 degrees per year. The deformity is most frequent in the thoracic spine, followed by the thoracolumbar spine. The kyphosis is a symmetric, midline, mesenchymal defect, and, unlike the asymmetric defects, it is not commonly associated with other congenital anomalies. The deformity is not as severe as type I deformity. Paraplegia was not observed in their patients with type II kyphosis. Low back pain and cosmetic deformities were, however, significant problems to these patients. The authors believed the pain was related to the compensatory lumbar hyperlordosis below the defect. Thus this deformity, although less progressive than type I deformity and unassociated with paraplegia, has significant deleterious effects on the patient, and early treatment is warranted in this condition as well as in type I deformity.

Surgical Treatment

As shown by Winter et al, treatment of either type of congenital kyphosis with an orthosis is ineffective; the natural history is not affected by any means other than surgery. The surgical procedure depends on the type of deformity, the severity of the deformity, the age of the patient, and the presence or absence of neurologic symptoms.

Mayfield et al outlined a treatment plan for congenital kyphosis caused by defects of anterior segmentation (type II). In younger children with a progressive deformity, a posterior fusion extending from one vertebral segment above to one below the measured curve can be expected to halt progression of this kyphosis. In the adolescent age-group, mild deformities (to a maximum of 50 degrees) can be stabilized by posterior fusion (p. 482) combined with a Harrington compression system. If the instrumentation is not possible because of the patient's size, rigid immobilization in a cast for at least 1 year is recommended. In the adolescent in whom compression instrumentation can be used, immobilization in a plaster cast for

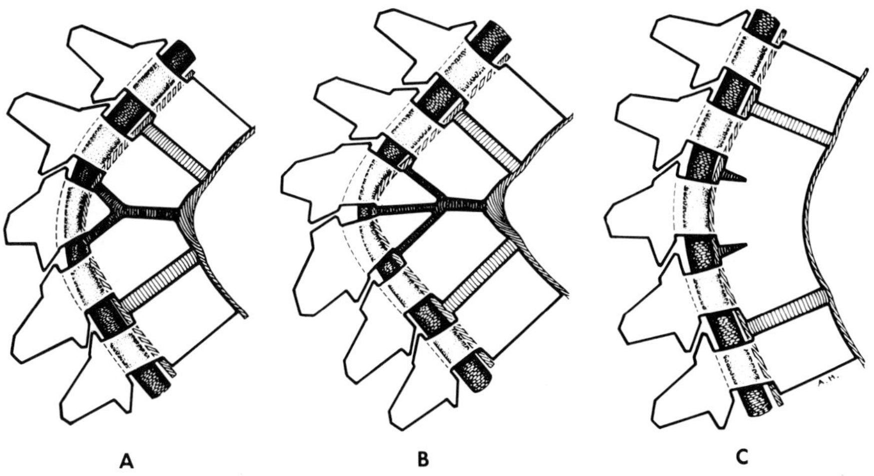

Fig. 10-114 Classification of congenital kyphosis. **A** and **B,** Type I. **C,** Type II. (Type III not shown.) (From Winter RB et al: J Bone Joint Surg 55A:223, 1973.)

6 to 9 months is recommended. Patients with severe, unacceptable kyphotic deformities require a combined anterior and posterior approach, including osteotomies of all levels of the anterior bar and anterior and posterior arthrodesis. The anterior osteotomies and interbody fusions extend the length of the kyphotic curve. In a second stage a posterior fusion is performed, combined with Harrington compression instrumentation. The posterior fusion should extend one to two levels beyond the ends of the kyphotic curve. For patients with a severe deformity, halo traction can be used for correction between the stages. It should be emphasized, however, that halo-femoral traction can be used only in type II kyphosis; in type I deformities it has an unacceptably high incidence of neurologic complications.

The treatment of type I deformities is somewhat different. Because they are more severe and can lead to paraplegia, prompt treatment is extremely important. Ideally, if the patient is seen early (between the ages of 1 and 3 years), a Moe-type posterior fusion is performed with no instrumentation (p. 476). In these young children it frequently is necessary to use allograft bone-bank bone. Postoperative casting or bracing is continued for 12 months with changes as necessitated by growth. Winter has noticed some actual decrease in the angle of kyphosis after successful posterior fusion in these patients and believes therefore that anterior fusion should not be performed in this age-group.

For children older than 5 years with type I deformities, posterior fusion alone can be successful if the kyphosis is not greater than 50 degrees. If posterior fusion is performed, dual Harrington compression rods usually are used (p. 482). For those patients with type I deformities and kyphosis greater than 50 degrees, a combined anterior and posterior arthrodesis is necessary. Halo-femoral or halo-pelvic traction should not be used because it is associated with a very high incidence of paraplegia.

Anterior osteotomy

▶ *Technique (Winter et al).* Expose the spine through an anterior approach appropriate for the vertebral level sought. Ligate the segmental vessels, and expose the spine by subperiosteal stripping (Fig. 10-115, *A*). Divide the thickened anterior longitudinal ligament at one or more levels. It is important that circumferential exposure all the way to the opposite foramen is performed before beginning the osteotomy. Divide the bony bar using a sharp osteotome or high-speed drill, starting the division anteriorly and working posteriorly until the remaining disk material is entered. Once the remaining disk material is seen, use a laminar spreader and excise the disk material back to the level of the posterior longitudinal ligament (Fig. 10-115, *B*). If the bony bar is complete, the osteotomy must be completed all the way through the posterior cortex. Take great care in the area of the posterior longitudinal ligament because the ligament may be absent. Once the osteotomy and decompression are complete, insert strut grafts, slotting them into bodies above and below the area of the kyphos. Hollow out the cancellous bone of each body with a curet. Using rib, fibula, or iliac crest grafts of sufficient length, insert the upper end into the slot first. As manual pressure is applied posteriorly against the kyphos, use an impactor to tap the lower end of the graft in place. Place additional grafts in the disk space defects, and close the pleura over them if possible.

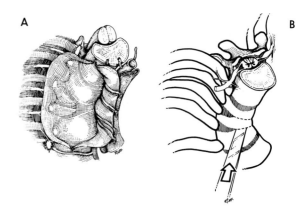

Fig. 10-115 A, Anterolateral exposure of spine in preparation for anterior osteotomy. **B,** Completion of osteotomy with osteotome. (Redrawn from Bradford DS et al: Moe's textbook of scoliosis and other spinal deformities, ed 2, Philadelphia, 1987, WB Saunders Co.)

Lonstein et al reviewed 42 patients with kyphosis and neurologic deficits and found that, except for a few flexible (and noncongenital) kyphoses, anterior decompression and fusion followed by a staged posterior fusion gave the best results. They indicated that patients with paraparesis or paraplegia should have hyperextension roentgenograms to differentiate a flexible from a rigid kyphosis. If the kyphosis is flexible, the patient may be placed in halo-femoral traction, with careful neurologic monitoring. It should be noted, however, that in the series of Lonstein et al most patients in this category had neurofibromatosis and not a type I congenital kyphosis. If the kyphosis is rigid, as is usually the case in type I kyphosis, the best approach is an anterior spinal cord decompression and fusion followed by a posterior fusion.

Anterior cord decompression and fusion

▲ *Technique (Winter and Lonstein).* Expose the spine through an anterior approach appropriate for the vertebral level sought. Identify the apical vertebra and the site of compression, and completely remove the intervertebral disk on each side of the vertebral body or bodies. Remove the vertebral body laterally at the apex of the kyphosis, using curets, rongeurs, or high-speed drills. Remove the cancellous bone back to the posterior cortex of the vertebral body from pedicle to pedicle, removing a wedge-shaped area of bone (Fig. 10-116, *A*). Beginning on the side far away from the apex, remove the posterior cortical shell, using angled curets. In this manner the bone farthest away is removed first, preventing the spinal cord from falling into the defect and blocking vision on the far side (Fig. 10-116, *B*). Then remove the closest bony shell, working toward the apex. Control epidural bleeding with thrombin-soaked Gelfoam. Once the cord is decompressed, perform an anterior strut graft fusion (Fig. 10-116, *C*). Close and drain the incision in the routine manner.

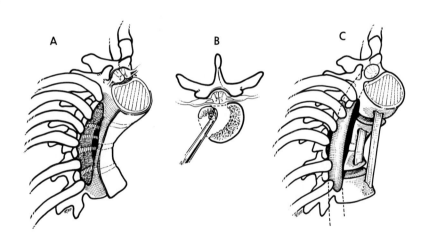

Fig. 10-116   **A,** Anterolateral exposure of spine and partial removal of apex of kyphosis. **B,** Posterior cortex is removed, allowing decompression of spinal cord. **C,** Cord is decompressed and strut grafts are in place. (Redrawn from Bradford DS et al: Moe's textbook of scoliosis and other spinal deformities, ed 2, Philadelphia, 1987, WB Saunders Co.)

At a second stage a posterior fusion with or without instrumentation is performed. As in any patient with a congenital spine deformity, if any surgical intervention is considered, a myelogram is necessary to rule out conditions such as tethered cord and diastematomyelia. In congenital kyphosis with neurologic change it also is helpful to definitely localize the area of cord compression (Fig. 10-117).

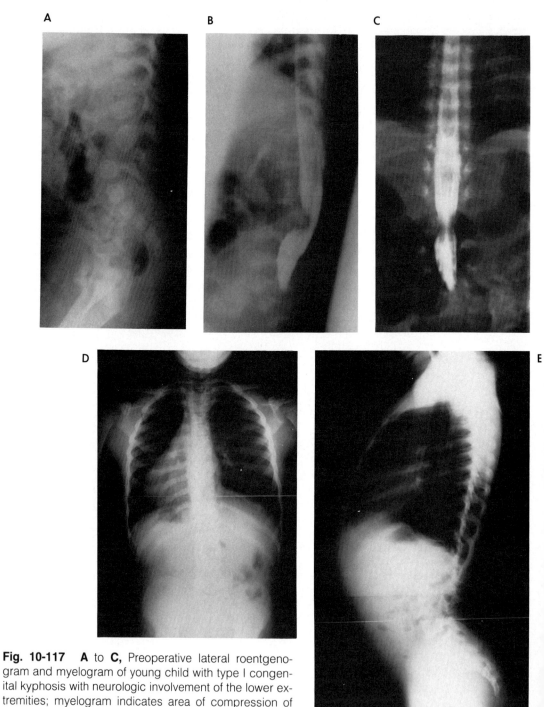

Fig. 10-117 **A** to **C,** Preoperative lateral roentgenogram and myelogram of young child with type I congenital kyphosis with neurologic involvement of the lower extremities; myelogram indicates area of compression of cauda equina. **D** and **E,** Solid anterior fusion 8 years after excision of hemivertebra and anterior strut grafting.

SPONDYLOLISTHESIS

Herbiniaux, a Belgian obstetrician, generally is credited with the first description of spondylolisthesis. The term *spondylolisthesis* was used by Kilian in 1854 and is derived from the Greek *spondylos,* meaning vertebra, and *olisthesis,* meaning to slip or slide down a slippery path. Spondylolisthesis generally is defined as anterior or posterior slipping or displacement of one vertebra on another.

Classification

The most generally accepted classification is that developed by Wiltse et al (Fig. 10-118):

Type I, dysplastic. Congenital abnormalities of the upper sacrum or arch of L5 permit slipping of L5 on S1; there is no pars interarticularis defect in this type.

Type II, isthmic. There is a lesion in the pars interarticularis that allows the forward slipping of L5 on S1; three types of this spondylolisthesis are recognized.

   A. Lytic—a stress fracture of the pars interarticularis

   B. An elongated but intact pars interarticularis

   C. An acute fracture of the pars interarticularis

Type III, degenerative. This lesion results from intersegmental instability of a long duration with subsequent remodeling of the articular processes at the level of involvement.

Type IV, traumatic. This type results from fractures in areas of the bony hook other than in the pars interarticularis.

Type V, pathologic. This type results from generalized or localized bone disease such as osteogenesis imperfecta.

The types most commonly seen in children are the isthmic and dysplastic types.

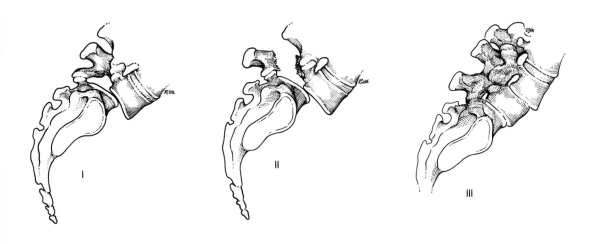

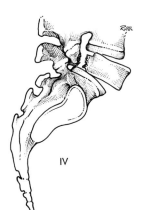

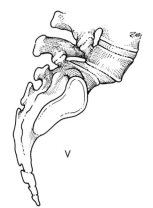

Fig. 10-118 Five types of spondylolisthesis: type I, dysplastic; type II, isthmic; type III, degenerative; type IV, traumatic; type V, pathologic. (Redrawn from Hensinger RN: Spondylolysis and spondylolisthesis in children. In the American Academy of Orthopaedic Surgeons: Instructional course lectures, vol 32, St Louis, 1983, The CV Mosby Co.)

Anatomy and Biomechanics

Isthmic spondylolisthesis is characterized by bilateral defects in the pars interarticularis of a vertebra and the resultant anterior displacement of the body of this vertebra and the rest of the spine on the vertebra below. This type of spondylolisthesis most frequently occurs at the level of the L5 vertebra, which is displaced anteriorly on the sacrum. Normally, the inferior articular facets of L5 prevent the body of this vertebra from being displaced anteriorly on the sacrum. In isthmic spondylolisthesis the bilateral defects in the pars interarticularis make the neural arch a loose fragment, cause a loss in osseus continuity between the inferior articular facets and the body of the L5 vertebra, and allow the body of the vertebra gradually to become displaced anteriorly.

The defect in the pars interarticularis may be either unilateral or bilateral. When it is bilateral, the L5 vertebra may become displaced anteriorly; when it is unilateral, it is displaced little if any. As Scaglietti et al indicated, spondylolisthesis basically is a kyphosis. The anterior slipping of the L5 vertebra is followed by contracture of the hamstrings, which tends to rotate the pelvis and bring the sacrum to a more vertical plane. The kyphosis thus formed at the lumbosacral junction is responsible for the stretching of the distal end of the dural sac and kinking of the L5 and S1 nerve roots (Fig. 10-119).

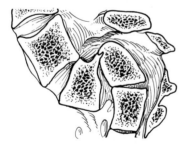

Fig. 10-119   Illustration of spondylolisthesis by Neugebauer. (From Leslie IJ and Dickson RH: J Bone Joint Surg: 63B:266, 1981.)

Etiology and Natural History

The incidence of spondylolisthesis in the general population is approximately 5% and is about equal in women and men. Spondylolisthesis seems to result from a stress fracture that occurs in children with a genetic predisposition for the defect. The defect has not been noted to be present at birth. The most common age of onset is between 5 and 7 years. It is not seen in chronic invalids and is more common in certain types of athletes. All these factors indicate that the condition is acquired rather than congenital, although there is a definite variation among races that indicates a genetic predisposition. As many as 50% of Eskimos are reported to have spondylolisthesis, whereas Rowe and Roche found an incidence of only 2.8% in black children. Increased slipping of spondylolisthesis usually occurs between the ages of 9 and 15 years and seldom after the age of 20 years.

Risk Factors

Hensinger described several risk factors for the progression of spondylolisthesis during adolescence and divided these into clinical factors and roentgenographic factors.

Clinical progression of spondylolisthesis occurs primarily in the growth years (9 to 15 years of age). Girls seem to be at greater risk of further slipping and more severe grades of spondylolisthesis. Children who have had an episode of back pain because of spondylolisthesis of any grade have a higher incidence of recurrent episodes.

Children with dysplastic (type I) spondylolisthesis more frequently show progressive slip on roentgenographic examination, and they have more persistent symptoms than those with type II. Children with a dome-shaped, vertical sacrum and a trapezoid-shaped L5 vertebral body have a greater propensity for further slip. Those who have a buttress because of degenerative changes on the anterior lip of the sacrum are less likely to have further displacement. Children with 50% or greater spondylolisthesis (types III and IV) are at high risk of further deformity. Sagittal rotation of L5 on the sacrum is an accurate indication of the potential risk for further progression. Finally, if flexion-extension views demonstrate instability or excessive motion, further displacement is more likely. Hensinger also noted that if the dysplastic spondylolisthesis does not fracture, there is a greater likelihood of neurologic compression.

Clinical Findings

The most common symptom of spondylolistheses is pain that varies from mild to severe, and most patients are first seen during adolescence when the pain becomes worse. In most patients with mild spondylolisthesis, the predominant complaint is backache, with only occasional leg pain. The pain is mechanical in nature; it worsens with high activity levels or competitive sports and decreases with activity restriction and rest. The back pain probably results from instability of the affected segment, and the leg pain usually is related to the L5 nerve root. In children with more severe slips the pain is more severe and radiates into the posterior aspect of both thighs. Frequently the parents report an abnormal gait pattern and posture in the child.

The physical findings vary with the severity of the symptoms. With significant symptoms there is a palpable step-off at the lumbosacral junction, motion of the lumbar spine is restricted, and there is significant hamstring tightness on straight leg raising. As the vertebral body displaces anteriorly, the patient assumes a lordotic posture above the level to compensate for this displacement. The sacrum will become more vertical, and the buttocks will appear "heart shaped" because of the sacral prominence (Fig. 10-120). With more severe slips the trunk becomes shortened and can lead to complete absence of the waistline. These children walk with a peculiar spastic gait described as a "pelvic waddle" by Newman because of the hamstring tightness and the lumbosacral kyphosis. Various neurologic deficits may exist.

Scoliosis is a relatively common finding in younger patients with spondylolisthesis. Fortunately most of these curves are not structural; they occur as C-shaped curves that extend to the spondylistic area. These nonstructural curves tend to resolve after treatment of the spondylolisthesis. Severe curves, however, may become structural and treatment more complicated.

A
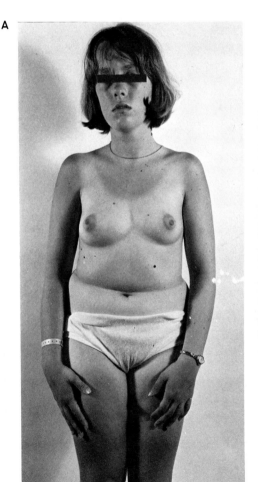

B
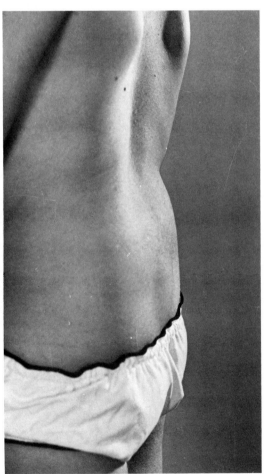

Fig. 10-120 Typical posture **(A)** and back contours **(B)** in adolescent with type III or IV spondylolisthesis. (From Hensinger RN. In The American Academy of Orthopaedic Surgeons: Instructional course lectures, vol 32, St Louis, 1983, The CV Mosby Co.)

Fig. 10-121 Percentage of slipping calculated by measuring distance from line parallel to posterior portion of first sacral vertebral body to line parallel to posterior portion of body of L5; anteroposterior dimension of L5 inferiorly is used to calculate percentage of slipping. (From Boxall D et al: J Bone Joint Surg 61A:479, 1979.)

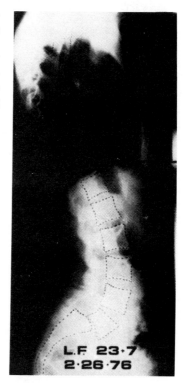 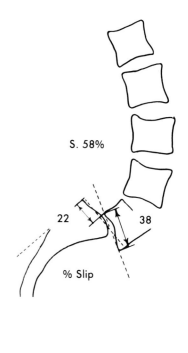

Fig. 10-122 Angle of slipping, formed by intersection of line drawn parallel to inferior aspect of L5 body and line drawn perpendicular to posterior aspect of body of S1. (From Boxall D et al: J Bone Joint Surg 61A:479, 1979.)

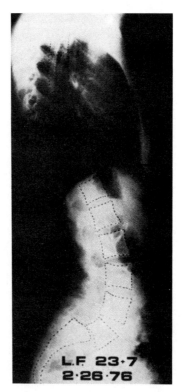 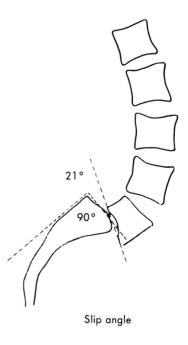

Roentgenographic Findings

The key to diagnosis of spondylolisthesis lies in routine roentgenograms. The initial evaluation should include anteroposterior, lateral, and oblique views. If spondylolisthesis is present, a routine lateral view will show the defect. In spondylolysis without slippage, the pars interarticularis defect is best seen on the oblique view. The lateral view should be taken with the patient standing because Lowe has shown a 26% increased slip on standing films compared with recumbent films.

The two most helpful roentgenographic measurements are the percentage of slip and the slip angle. The percentage of slip is calculated by measuring the ratio between the anteroposterior diameter of the top of the first sacral vertebra and the distance the L5 vertebra has slipped anteriorly (Fig. 10-121). Meyerding classified spondylolisthesis into grades I, II, III, and IV, depending on the severity of this displacement of the L5 vertebra on the sacrum below. Grade I displacement is 25% or less, grade II between 25% and 50%, grade III between 50% and 75%, and grade IV greater than 75%.

According to Boxall et al, the angular relationships are the best predictors of instability or progression of the deformity. These relationships are expressed as the slip angle. This angle is calculated by drawing a line parallel to the inferior aspect of the L5 vertebra and a line drawn perpendicular to the posterior aspect of the body of the S1 vertebra (Fig. 10-122). These roentgenograms, as for the percentage of slip, should be made in the standing position. Boxall et al found an associated incidence between a higher slip angle and progression of the deformity.

Nonsurgical Treatment

Surgery is not always necessary in spondylolisthesis. Often restriction of the patient's activities, spinal and abdominal muscular rehabilitation, and other conservative measures, including the intermittent use of a rigid back brace, are sufficient. If symptoms improve, progressive increases in activity are permitted. If the patient has simply a spondylolysis or a very small degree of spondylolisthesis and remains symptom free routine restriction of activities is not necessary. For the symptom-free patient with a slip of greater than 25% but less than 50%, the avoidance of contact sports is recommended.

Surgical Treatment

In children with persistent symptoms in spite of adequate conservative treatment, no matter what the degree of slip, surgical treatment is indicated. If the child has a significant slip of 50% or greater with symptoms, surgical treatment also is indicated. More controversial is the treatment of symptom-free children with slips greater than 50%. Harris and Weinstein reported 12 patients with greater than 50% slips followed for as long as 25 years. They concluded that although many of these patients function well, those with a spinal fusion seemed to do better. Most authors agree that slips greater than 50%, even if asymptomatic, are best treated surgically.

For patients with slipping of less than 50% whose symptoms remain in spite of conservative treatment, fusion between L5 and the sacrum usually is sufficient. Laminectomy, as described by Gill, as an isolated technique in a growing child is contraindicated because further slipping will occur in many. Wiltse believes that extremely tight hamstrings, decreased Achilles reflexes, and even a footdrop can improve after a solid arthrodesis. When neurologic deficits are present, a posterior decompression may be considered in rare instances with the fusion, but the most important part of this combined procedure is the fusion itself.

▲ *Technique (Watkins).* Make two longitudinal skin incisions along the lateral borders of the paraspinal muscles, curving medially at the distal end across the posterior crest of the ilium (Fig. 10-123, *A*). Divide the lumbothoracic fascia, and establish the plane of cleavage between the border of the paraspinal muscles and the fascia overlying the transverse abdominal muscle. The tips of the transverse processes now can be palpated in the depths of the wound (Fig. 10-123, *B*). Release the iliac attachments of the muscles with an osteotome, taking a thin layer of the ilium. Continue the exposure of the posterior crest of the ilium by subperiosteal dissection, and remove the crest almost flush with the sacroiliac joint, taking enough bone to provide one or two grafts. Removal of the iliac crest increases exposure of the spine. Retract the sacrospinalis muscle toward the midline, and denude the transverse processes of their dorsal muscle and ligamentous attachments; expose the articular facets

by excising the joint capsule. Remove the cartilage from the facets with an osteotome, and level the area to allow the graft to fit snugly against the facets, the pars interarticularis, and the base of the transverse process at each level. Comminute the facets with a small gouge or osteotome, and turn bone chips up and down from the facet area, the upper sacral area, and the transverse processes. Now split the resected iliac crest longitudinally into two grafts. Shape one to fit into the prepared bed, and impact it firmly in place with its cut surface against the spine (Fig. 10-123, *C*). Preserve the remaining graft for use on the opposite side, with or without additional bone from the opposite iliac crest. Now pack additional ribbons and chips of cancellous bone from the ilium about the graft. Allow the paraspinal muscles to fall into position over the fusion area, and close the wound over drains.

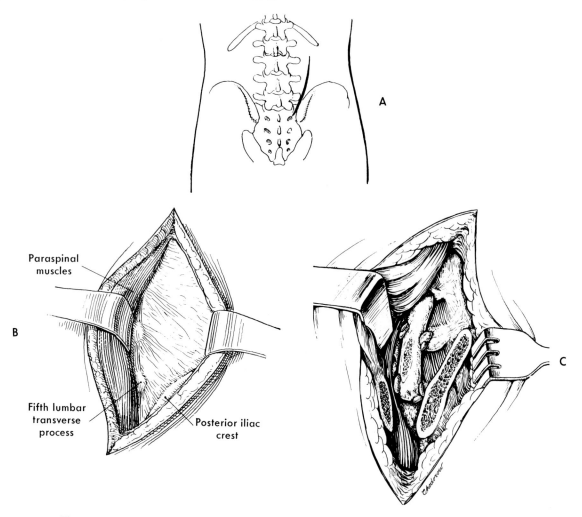

Fig. 10-123 Watkins posterolateral fusion. **A,** Incision. **B,** Lumbothoracic fascia has been incised, paraspinal muscles have been retracted medially, and tips of transverse processes are now palpable. **C,** Split iliac crest and smaller grafts have been placed against spine. (**A** and **B** from Watkins MB: J Bone Joint Surg 35A:1014, 1953; **C** from Watkins MB: Clin Orthop 35:80, 1964.)

▶ *Technique (Wiltse)*. Place the patient prone on the Hall frame. Make curved incisions through the skin and subcutaneous tissue, about three fingerbreadths lateral to the midline and just medial to the postero-superior iliac spine (Fig. 10-124, *A*); curve both incisions slightly inward at their caudal ends. Alternatively, one midline incision can be made and the skin retracted to either side to allow the fascial incisions. Make similar incisions in the fascia at about the same distance lateral to the spinous processes, also curving these fascial incisions toward the midline on their distal ends. This transverse portion of the fascial incision allows adequate retraction. Use the index finger to dissect through the sacrospinalis muscle mass down to the sacrum and forward on the back of the sacrum to the articular processes of L5 and S1, as well as to the space between the transverse process of L5 and the ala of the sacrum. If the spondylolisthesis is greater than 50%, it may be necessary also to expose the L4, L5 facet and the transverse process and the lamina of the L4 vertebral body. Two long Gelpi retractors are good instruments for retracting the muscle (Fig. 10-124, *B*). Expose the lamina of the vertebra to be fused to the bases of the spinous processes. Denude the lumbar transverse processes of soft tissue all the way to their tips (Fig. 10-124, *C*). If dissection is not carried anterior to the transverse processes, the spinal nerve roots will not be injured. Only the lateral surface of the superior articular process of the topmost vertebra to be included should be denuded to avoid damage to the facet joint above the level of the fusion. Within the fusion area, denude of soft tissue the lateral surface of the superior articular process, the lamina as far medially as the base of the spinous processes, and the pars interarticularis. Do not expose the spinous processes to preserve their ligamentous attachments and blood supply. Carefully expose the intervertebral joints within the fusion area, and remove the articular cartilage in the posterior two thirds of each joint.

Prepare the graft bed as for a classic Hibbs fusion. Turn an anteriorly based flap of bone from the top of the ala of the sacrum forward and cephalad to form a bridge to the transverse process of L4 or L5. Obtain iliac grafts from one or both sides of the pelvis through the ipsilateral skin incision. Ordinarily, one iliac crest will supply enough graft. Take the bone graft from the outer part of the ilium, leaving the inner cortex intact. Tamp cancellous bone between the denuded articular processes, and tamp strips of iliac cancellous and cortical bone into place over the area to be fused (Fig. 10-124, *D*). Close the deep fascia with an absorbable stitch, and close wound over drains.

▶ *Postoperative management.* The postoperative treatment for spondylolisthesis after a bilateral lateral fusion is varied, based on the preference of the individual surgeon. In most patients with grade I, II, or III slips, an underarm Risser cast is used. For those patients with more severe slips, such as grade IV or for those with a significantly high slip angle that is considered unstable, an underarm cast is used, with extension down the thigh on one side to better immobilize the lumbosacral joint. This pantaloon-type cast is worn for 3 months, followed by another 3 months in an underarm Risser cast. After 6 months in a cast the patient then wears a lumbosacral corset for another 6 months. At the end of 12 months all immobilization is discontinued.

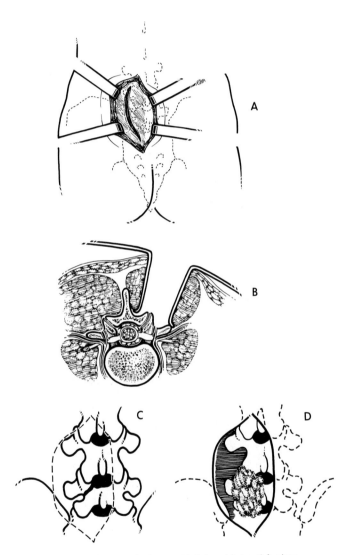

Fig. 10-124 Wiltse technique of bilateral lateral fusion. **A,** Skin incision and fascial incision. **B,** Axial view of paraspinal sacrospinalis splitting approach to lumbar spine. **C,** Lateral portion of lamina of L4, L5, and ala of sacrum exposed. **D,** Bone graft applied in lateral position after decortication of lamina and transverse processes. (Redrawn from Wiltse LL et al: J Bone Joint Surg 50A: 921, 1968.)

A
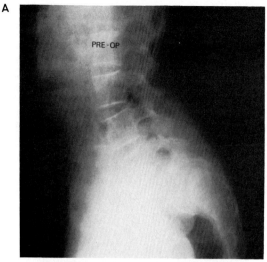

B
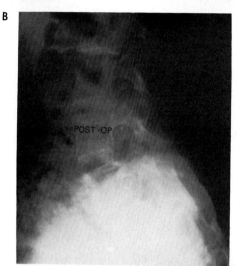

C
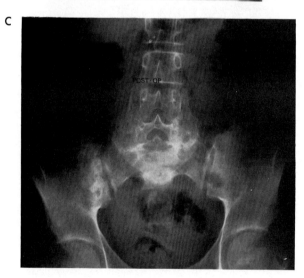

Severe Spondylolisthesis

Surgical treatment for slips greater than 50% is much more controversial. Most authors agree that slipping of this degree or greater should be fused, but there are many surgical options, including bilateral lateral fusion, anterior fusion and release with posterior fusion, posterior interbody fusion, cast reduction and fusion, and posterior surgical reduction and fusion.

Bradford noted that reduction of spondylolisthesis is difficult and that the indications and risks must be carefully weighed. His indications include (1) 50% slip or greater, (2) necessity for decompression, (3) satisfactory bone stock, (4) unacceptable sagittal alignment, and (5) adult patient. In most circumstances children and adolescents do not meet these indications for open reduction techniques (Fig. 10-125). Often the deformity is flexible enough that posterolateral fusion followed by cast correction is possible.

Although the cosmetic appeal of reduction of the spondylolisthesis is important, the complications and risks of this procedure compared with the more standard in situ bilateral lateral fusion should be considered. Johnson and Kerwin reported decreased pain, decreased hamstring tightness, improvement in straight leg raising, and no progression in 16 of 17 patients with greater than 50% slips treated with in situ fusion. Wiltse noted excellent results in 24 patients with bilateral lateral fusion and found no postoperative change in the average percentage of slip. Freeman and Donati found similar results in 12 patients who returned for follow-up examination and roentgenograms an average of 12 years after in situ

Fig. 10-125 A, Adolescent with grade IV isthmic spondylolisthesis. **B,** After bilateral lateral fusion. **C,** Solid fusion between L4 and sacrum. Patient was symptom free, with very acceptable clinical and cosmetic results.

fusion. No patient had a pseudarthrosis, seven had absolutely no pain, and five had occasional mild pain with strenuous activities. No patient complained of severe pain, and none believed that activities were significantly restricted. Six were unaware of any cosmetic deformity, four were aware of some deformity but were satisfied with their clinical appearance, and only two patients were dissatisfied with the appearance of their back. The only neurologic complications encountered in the series of Freeman and Donati were in the two patients in whom reduction was attempted with Harrington distraction instrumentation. Until posterior instrumentation techniques improve, bilateral lateral fusion in situ, even for severe degrees of slip, is a satisfactory and safe surgical procedure for the majority of patients with this deformity. With significant degrees of spondylolisthesis the fusion should extend from L4 to the sacrum by means of the posterolateral fusion technique as described by Wiltse (p. 547).

Scoliosis Associated with Spondylolisthesis

Scoliosis associated with spondylolisthesis may be either structural or functional. Functional scoliosis is caused by pain from the spondylolisthesis, and the curve disappears when the patient is supine. Treatment of the spondylolisthesis is sufficient for this type of curve. Structural idiopathic scoliosis associated with spondylolisthesis should be managed separately. For thoracolumbar or lumbar curves the lumbosacral joint should be fused in a corrected position at the time of scoliosis correction.

Kyphoscoliosis

MYELOMENINGOCELE

Treatment of patients with myelomeningocele spinal deformities is the most challenging in spine surgery. It requires a team effort with the cooperation of consultants in several subspecialties. These children probably are best treated at centers with experience in managing their complex problems.

The exact cause of myelomeningocele deformity has not been determined. The deformity develops early in embryonic life, on or before day 19 when the neural folds meet to form the neural tube. If the neural tube does not close, the adjacent mesodermal structures do not develop normally and the vertebral laminae fail to fuse posteriorly.

Incidence and Natural History

The natural history and incidence of spinal deformities associated with myelomeningocele have been studied extensively. Raycroft and Curtis reviewed 130 patients with myelomeningocele and distinguished two types of deformities: developmental (paralytic) and congenital (with congenitally malformed vertebrae). They also divided these deformities into scoliosis, lordosis, and kyphosis (Table 10-3). Congenital scoliosis consists of lateral structural disorganization of the vertebrae with asymmetric growth and includes all the congenital anomalies associated with congenital scoliosis: hemivertebrae, unilateral unsegmented bars, and various combinations of the two. In developmental scoliosis the spine is straight at birth and gradually develops a progressive curvature because of the neuromuscular problems. Raycroft and Curtis reported spinal deformity in 52% of the 103 patients without vertebral body abnormalities; 41 patients had scoliosis, 30 had lordosis, and 12 had kyphosis. Of the 27 patients with vertebral body abnormalities, 100% had a congenital spinal deformity.

Table 10-3 Spinal deformities in myelomeningocele

I. Scoliosis
A. Congenital
B. Developmental (paralytic)
C. Combination
II. Kyphosis
A. Congenital
B. Developmental (paralytic)
III. Lordosis
Usually found in combination with scoliosis or kyphosis

From Brown HP: Orthop Clin North Am 9:392, 1978.

Mackel and Lindseth reported a 66% incidence of spine deformity in 82 patients. Of those patients with a T12-level paralysis, 100% had deformity. In their study all curves were progressive.

Clinical Findings

Thorough patient evaluation is critical for determining appropriate management of the individual spinal deformity. The following areas are investigated: the presence of hydrocephalus, any surgical procedures for shunting, bowel and bladder function, the frequency of urinary tract infections, the use of an indwelling catheter or intermittent catheterization, current medications, the patient's mental status, method of ambulation, the level of the defect, and any noticable progression of the curve. All patients should be examined carefully for any evidence of pulmonary compromise, contractures in the lower extremities, and neurologic problems such as hydrocephalus. The spine is examined to determine the type and flexibility of the deformity, as well as any evidence of pressure sores or lack of sitting balance. Hydromyelia or other tethering lesions may be responsible for continued neurologic deterioration or progression of the scoliosis, or both.

Roentgenographic Findings

Plain roentgenographic views are extremely important. Films should be taken with the patient upright as well as supine. If the patient can ambulate, standing films should be made. If the patient is nonambulatory, sitting films should be made. The upright films allow better evaluation of the actual deformity of the spine when the patient is functioning, and the supine films show better detail of various associated spinal deformities. The flexibility of the curves can be determined with traction films.

Various specialized roentgenograms may be helpful. Myelography and MRI are extremely useful for evaluating such conditions as hydromyelia, tethered cord, diastematomyelia, and Arnold-Chiari malformation. Intravenous pyelography is needed at regular intervals according to the urologist's recommendation.

Scoliosis and Lordosis
Orthotic Treatment

Spinal fusion is not necessary for all scoliosis associated with myelomeningocele. One goal of nonsurgical treatment is to delay spinal fusion until adequate spinal growth has occurred. Bracing can delay the progression of developmental curves but will not affect congenital curves. The brace also may improve sitting balance and free the hands for other activities. Custom-fitted body jackets, usually bivalved, are used, which require very close and frequent observation by the parents. The skin must be examined frequently for pressure areas; any sign of pressure requires immediate brace adjustment. If the curve fails to respond to bracing, or if bracing becomes impossible because of pressure sores or noncompliance, surgery is indicated.

Surgical Treatment

Sriram et al reported 33 spinal fusions in patients with myelomeningocele, with 16 good results, 8 fair, and 9 poor. The surgical procedures varied considerably, but some observations could be made. Posterior spinal fusion is fraught with many difficulties, primarily because of densely scarred and adherent soft tissue. Spinal exposure often is lengthy and hemorrhagic. The deformity often is rigid, and proper correction is impossible. The quality of the bone often provides poor seating for the Harrington hooks, and the inadequacy of the posterior bone mass provides a poor bed for grafting. Osebold et al reported that in 40 patients with myelomeningocele and paralytic scoliosis, posterior spine fusion and Harrington instrumentation extending to the sacrum, combined with anterior fusion by means of either Dwyer or Zielke instrumentation, gave the best results. The combined fusion method reduced the incidence of pseudarthrosis to 23% compared with 46% when only posterior fusion and instrumentation were used. Prophylactic antibiotics were an important part of their regimen and reduced the infection rate to 8%. Posterior fusion or anterior fusion alone was inadequate even with instrumentation. Early mobilization was allowed, with the use of bivalved polypropylene body jackets.

A combined anterior and posterior fusion, if possible, is desirable. The lack of posterior bony elements makes the reliability of a posterior fusion uncertain even with the newer forms of segmental instrumentation. If the patient is large enough, an anterior fusion and instrumentation are performed with the Dwyer or Zielke apparatus, followed by a posterior fusion with segmental instrumentation posteriorly.

Preoperative evaluation is critical. Every report of surgery for this condition emphasizes the many problems and complications that make these deformities so difficult to treat. Thorough evaluations should be performed by the orthopaedist, the neurosurgeon, the urologist, the pediatrician, the plastic surgeon, and the anesthesiologist. Any neurosurgical problem, such as hydrocephalus and shunt function, should be corrected. Ideally the urine should be sterile, but if this is not possible, the infecting organism should be identified and the appropriate prophylactic antibiotics begun at the time of surgery. Prophylactic antibiotics are essential because the infection rate in these patients is quite high. Death has occurred from postoperative sepsis caused by a urinary tract infection. If inadequate skin coverage is present, the appropriate plastic surgery procedures should be performed either preoperatively or certainly at the time of scoliosis correction.

The area to be fused is determined from preoperative sitting, supine, and traction roentgenograms. Virtually all patients with myelomeningocele require fusion from the upper portion of the thoracic region to the sacrum; pelvic obliquity is not affected without fusion to the sacrum. Instrumentation of the lumbosacral area is the most difficult problem.

There are as many techniques of surgery for myelomeningocele as there are surgeons. There is no one best system for correcting these curves, and correction often requires a combination of techniques. Bone-bank bone usually is necessary because of the hypoplastic iliac crest. The technique described here is a representative technique that has been found useful in patients with this difficult problem. Because there are many different physical deformities and degrees of severity, the surgeon should be ready to modify any technique to accommodate the patient's deformity.

▶ *Technique.* Place the patient prone on the Hall frame. Prepare and drape the back in a sterile manner. Make a midline incision from the area of the superior vertebra to undergo instrumentation down to the sacrum (Fig. 10-126, *A*). In the area of the normal spine carry out subperiosteal dissection as previously described (p. 472). Avoid the midline area in the area of the sac as there are no useful bony elements for fusion in that area. Carry the dissection laterally over the convex and concave facet areas and down to the ala of the sacrum (Fig. 10-126, *B*). Now expose the area of normal spine to be fused and the bony elements of the abnormal sac area. Because the fusion will extend to the sacrum, contour a lumbar lordosis into the rod. To prevent rod rotation use square-ended Harrington rods and a square-ended hook. Apply a square-ended sacral alar hook over the ala on the concave side of the lumbar curve. Prepare the site for the upper Harrington distraction hook in a routine manner and insert the hook. Pass sublaminar wires beneath the lamina of the normal vertebra above the sac area. In the area of the defect attempt to achieve segmental fixation. Pass a wire around a pedicle and twist it on itself to secure fixation (Fig. 10-126, *C*). Pass wires on both the concave and the convex sides of the curve. Contour the square-ended Harrington distraction rod to maintain lumbar lordosis; insert this rod and perform distraction (Fig. 10-126, *D*). Secure the rod in place by tightening the segmental wires. On the convex side contour a Luque rod to fit the sagittal curves of the spine (Fig. 10-126,

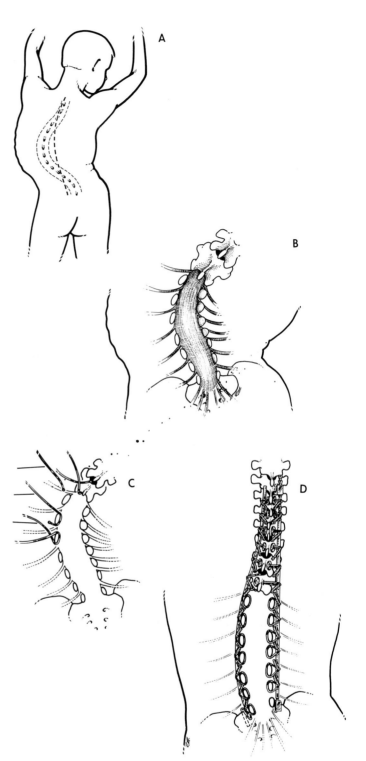

Fig. 10-126 Correction of scoliosis in myelomeningocele. **A,** Skin incision. **B,** Spinal exposure; dural sac is not dissected. **C,** Sublaminar wires placed in normal spine; in area of spina bifida, wires encircle pedicle for segmental fixation. **D,** Contoured Harrington distraction rod inserted on concave side of spine. Luque rod applied to convex side of curve and instrumented to sacrum with Dunn technique; segmental wires are tightened to provide more correction and stability.

D). Because of the frequently hypoplastic iliac crest in the patient with myelomeningocele, the Luque rods are fixed to the sacrum with the technique described by Dunn (Fig. 10-127). Prebend the Luque rod to curve over the sacral ala; pass it anterior to the sacrum and hold it in place with segmental wires. Decorticate any areas of exposed bone that can be decorticated without compromising the fixation device. Cut bone bank femoral heads into small pieces, and place these along the entire area of the spine, especially in the lateral gutters. The lateral bone graft is especially important in the lumbar spine because it is the only area for bony fusion (Fig. 10-128).

If the patient has lumbar lordosis with no evidence of kyphosis, and has bones large enough and strong enough to accept a Dwyer or Zielke apparatus, the posterior fusion should be performed in conjunction with an anterior fusion (Fig. 10-129). Anterior instrumentation should be performed to the sacrum, if possible, to allow a 360-degree fusion and a more stable spine. Frequently, however, anterior instrumentation to the sacrum is very difficult, especially in a severely lordotic portion of the curve; if instrumentation to this level cannot be achieved, it should be performed as far distally as possible. A bivalved, plastic body jacket is worn postoperatively for 12 months. It usually is unnecessary to immobilize the hips. The bivalved jacket allows frequent inspection of the skin, which is important because of the possibility of problems relating to insensitive skin.

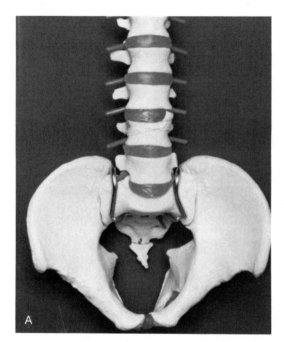
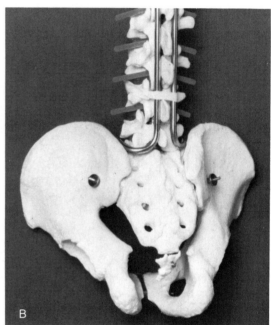

Fig. 10-127 A and **B,** Dunn technique for contouring Luque rod for alar purchase on sacrum. (From Bradford DS et al: Moe's textbook of scoliosis and other spinal deformities, ed 2, Philadelphia, 1987, WB Saunders Co.)

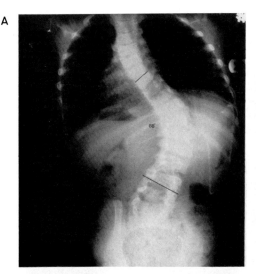

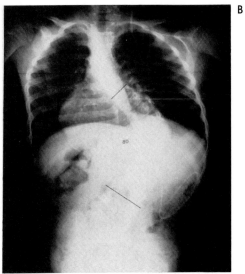

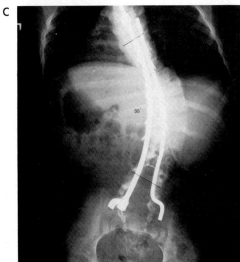

Fig. 10-128 **A** and **B,** Progression of paralytic scoliosis from 68 to 80 degrees in patient with myelomeningocele. **C,** Posterior instrumentation and fusion to sacrum using combined Harrington and Luque rod instrumentation with segmental wires.

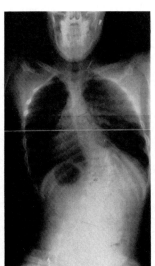

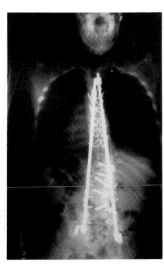

Fig. 10-129 **A,** Paralytic scoliosis in patient with myelomeningocele. **B,** After anterior Dwyer instrumentation and posterior instrumentation with dual Harrington distraction rods and segmental wires.

Kyphosis
Incidence and Natural History

Kyphosis in the patient with myelomeningocele can be either developmental or congenital. Developmental kyphosis is not present at birth and progresses slowly. It is a paralytic kyphosis that is aggravated by the lack of posterior stability. Congenital kyphosis, which is a much more difficult problem, usually measures 80 degrees or more at birth. The level of the lesion usually is T12, with total paraplegia. The kyphosis is rigid and progresses rapidly during infancy. Children with severe kyphosis are unable to wear braces and often have difficulty sitting in a wheelchair because their center of gravity is displaced forward. An ulceration may develop over the prominent kyphus and may make skin coverage quite difficult. Progression of the kyphosis may lead to respiratory difficulty because of incompetence of the inspiratory muscles, crowding of the abdominal contents, and upward pressure on the diaphragm. Increased flexion of the trunk can interfere with urinary drainage and also may cause problems if urinary diversion or ileostomy becomes necessary.

Hoppenfeld described the anatomy of this condition and noted that the pedicles are widely spread and the rudimentary laminae actually are everted. The anterior longitudinal ligament is short and thick. The paraspinal muscles are present but are displaced far anterolaterally (Fig. 10-130). All muscles therefore act anteriorly to the axis of rotation, which tends to worsen the kyphosis.

Surgical Treatment

The surgical correction of kyphosis is more demanding and difficult than that of the scoliotic deformity. Apical vertebral ostectomy, as proposed by Sharrard, facilitates closure of the skin in the neonate but provides only short-term improvement, and the kyphotic deformity invariably recurs. Lindseth and Selzer reported 23 children with myelomeningocele whose kyphosis was treated with vertebral excision. Their most consistent results were obtained with partial resection of the apical vertebra and the proximal lordotic curve, which was performed in 12 patients. If only the apical vertebra and the vertebrae on either side of the apex were excised, correction of the kyphotic prominence was lost. Their goals of kyphosis treatment were (1) to straighten and stabilize the spine to allow balance in sitting, (2) to decrease the prominence of the bone, and (3) to allow an increase in the height of the abdominal wall. The age of the patients at the time of surgery did not seem to influence the results, although the smaller degree of kyphosis at the time of surgery, the smaller the degree of kyphosis at follow-up and the better the overall correction. The youngest child in their series was 1 year and 11 months of age. They emphasized that the operation is a major undertaking and is technically difficult. A considerable loss of blood and frequent complications are to be expected.

▲ *Technique (Lindseth and Selzer).* Use a midline posterior incision (Fig. 10-131, *A*), which may be varied somewhat depending on local skin conditions. Ex-

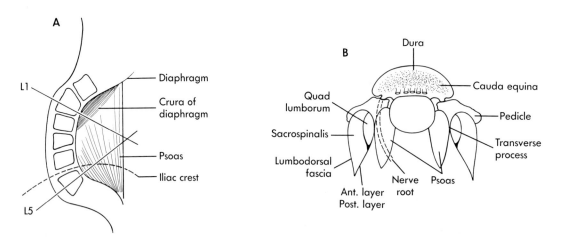

Fig. 10-130 **A,** Sagittal diagram showing deforming effect of psoas muscle on kyphosis. **B,** Transverse section of lumbar spine and attached muscles in region of kyphosis. Pedicles and laminae of vertebrae are splayed laterally; erector spinae muscles enclosed in thoracolumbar fascia lie lateral to vertebral bodies and act as flexors. (Redrawn from Sharrard WJW and Drennan JC: J Bone Joint Surg 54B:50, 1972.)

pose subperiosteally the more normal vertebra superiorly and the area of the abnormality, continuing the exposure past the lateral bony ridges.

At this point, remove the sac. Dissect inside the lamina until the foramina are exposed on each side of the spine. Exposed, divide, and coagulate the nerve, artery, and vein within each foramen, exposing the sac distally where it is scarred down and thin. At its distal level cross-clamp the sac with Kelly clamps and divide it between the clamps (Fig. 10-131, *B*). Close the scarred ends with a running stitch. Now dissect the sac proximally. As this proximal dissection is performed, large venous channels connecting the sac to the posterior vertebral body will be encountered; control the bleeding from the bone with bone wax and from the soft tissue with electrocautery. Dissect the sac up to the level of more normal-appearing dura (Fig. 10-131, *C*).

At this point the sac can be transected. If this is done, the dura should be closed with a purse-string suture. The cord itself should not be sutured shut but left open so that the spinal fluid can escape from the central canal of the cord to the arachnoid space. If the sac is not removed, it can be used at the completion of the procedure to further cover the area of the resected vertebra.

Once the sac has been reflected proximally, continue dissection around the vertebral bodies, exposing only the area to be removed. If the entire area of the spine is exposed subperiostally, there is the potential for avascular necrosis of these vertebral bodies. At this point remove the vertebrae between the apex of the lordosis and the apex of the kyphosis (Fig. 10-131, *D*). Generally the vertebra at the apex of the kyphosis is removed first by removing the intervertebral disk with a Cobb elevator and curets. Take care to leave the anterior longitudinal ligament intact to act as a stabilizing hinge. Once this one vertebra is removed, the spine can be preliminarily corrected as an indication as to how many more vertebrae should be removed (Fig. 10-131, *E*). Remove enough vertebrae to correct the kyphosis as much as possible but not so many that reapproximation is impossible. Morcellation of these vertebral bodies provides additional bone graft.

There have been many techniques described for fixation of the kyphotic deformity, but Luque rod instrumentation to the pelvis (Dunn technique) with segmental wires (Fig. 10-131, *F*) is recommended. Alternatively the right angle bend in the rod can be passed through the S1 foramen rather than around the ala of the sacrum. Move the distal segment to the proximal segment, and tighten the segmental wires. Apply additional allograft bone graft. Irrigate the wound and close it over suction drains. Antibiotics are given intravenously for several days before and after surgery.

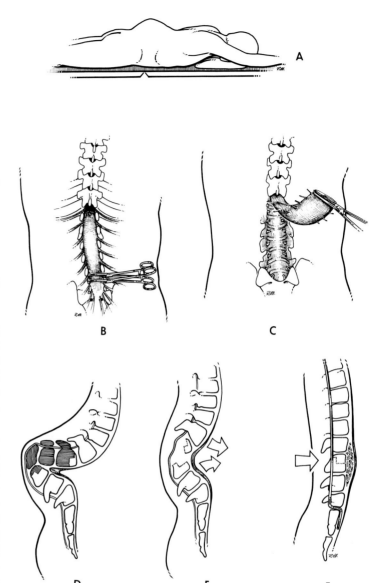

Fig. 10-131   Technique of vertebral excision (Lindseth and Selzer). **A,** Skin incision. **B,** Exposure of area of kyphosis and dural sac. **C,** Sac is divided distally and dissected proximally. **D,** Vertebrae between apex of lordosis and apex of kyphosis are removed. **E,** Kyphosis is reduced. **F,** Reduction is maintained with stable internal fixation (in this instance with Luque rods and segmental wires).

▶ *Postoperative management.* When the patient is stable after surgery, a plaster model is taken for a bivalved, plastic body jacket; it is not necessary to immobilize the hips. The patient is returned to the sitting position as soon as the jacket is available. Some patients, in whom bone is too osteoporotic and the stability of the internal fixation is in doubt, may be kept at bed rest for several months or allowed to sit only in an inclined chair. The fusion usually is solid in 6 to 9 months.

The postoperative care of these patient requires close observation by all subspecialty consultants involved. A high incidence of postoperative infections, urinary tract problems, skin problems, and pseudarthrosis can be expected. The improved function of these patients, however, and the prevention of progression of the curve make surgery worth the risks (Fig. 10-132).

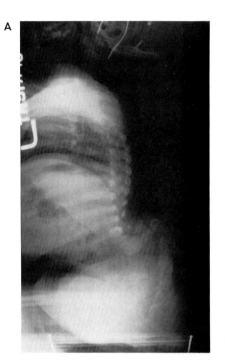
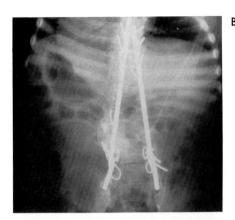
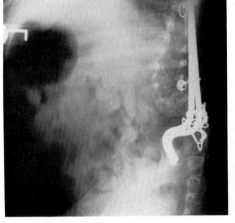

Fig. 10-132   A, Congenital kyphosis in child with myelomeningocele. **B** and **C,** After kyphectomy and instrumentation with Luque rods and segmental wires.

SACRAL AGENESIS

Sacral agenesis is a rare lesion. Since its description by Hohl in 1852, there have been only review articles and occasional case reports about the condition.

Etiology

The etiologic factors of sacral agenesis still are unknown. Renshaw postulated that the condition is teratogenically induced or is a spontaneous genetic mutation. To support his thesis he cites (1) the association of sacral agenesis with a high incidence of maternal diabetes mellitus, (2) the known association of insulin-dependent diabetes mellitus with the major histocompatibility system, (3) the recording of sacral agenesis as an inherited defect in at least four families, (4) the consistent relationships between neurologic findings and skeletal defects, and (5) certain recent developments in genetics and embryology. This genetic mutation then predisposes to or causes failure of embryonic induction of the caudal notochord sheath and ventral spinal cord. The dorsal ganglia and the dorsal (sensory) portion of the spinal cord continue to develop. The vertebrae and motor nerves are not subsequently induced, and the sacral agenesis results. Sensation remains intact because the dorsal ganglia and dorsal portion of the spinal cord have been derived from neural crest tissue. This disturbance in the normal sequence of development explains the observation that the lowest vertebral body with pedicles corresponds closely to the motor level, whereas the sensory level is distal to the motor level.

Classification

Renshaw studied 23 patients with sacral agenesis and proposed the following working classification:

Type I, Either total or partial unilateral sacral agenesis (Fig. 10-133, *A*)

Type II, Partial sacral agenesis with partial but bilaterally symmetric defects in the stable articulation between the ilia and a normal or hypoplastic S1 vertebra (Fig. 10-133, *B*)

Type III, Variable lumbar and total sacral agenesis with the ilia articulating with the sides of the lowest vertebra present (Fig. 10-133, *C*).

Type IV, Variable lumbar and total sacral agenesis with caudal end plate of the lowest vertebra resting above either fused ilia or an iliac amphiarthrosis (Fig. 10-133, *D*)

The type II defect is the most common and type I the least common. Types I and II defects usually have a stable vertebral-pelvic articulation, whereas types III and IV show instability and possibly a progressive kyphosis.

Text continued on p. 562.

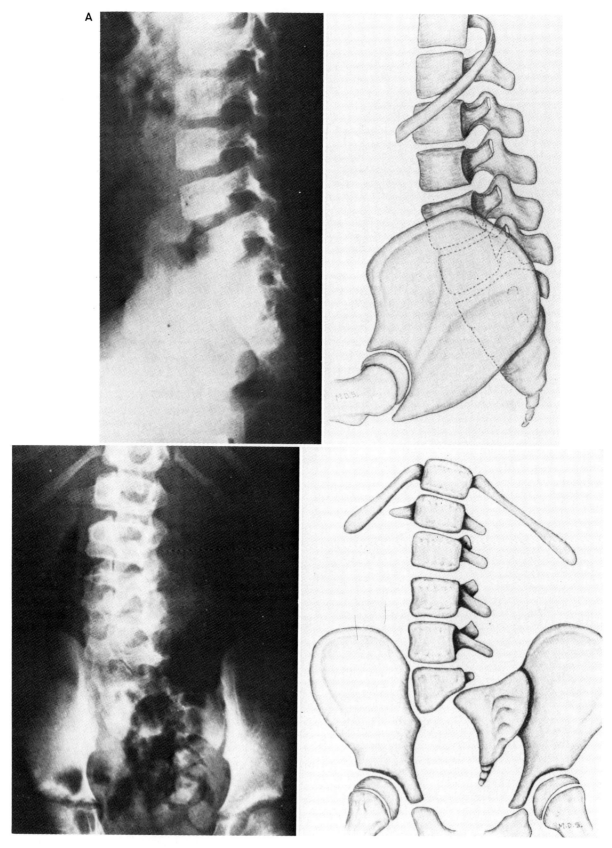

Fig. 10-133   Types of sacral agenesis (see text). **A,** Type I, total or partial unilateral sacral agenesis. (From Renshaw TS: J Bone Joint Surg: 60A:373, 1978.)

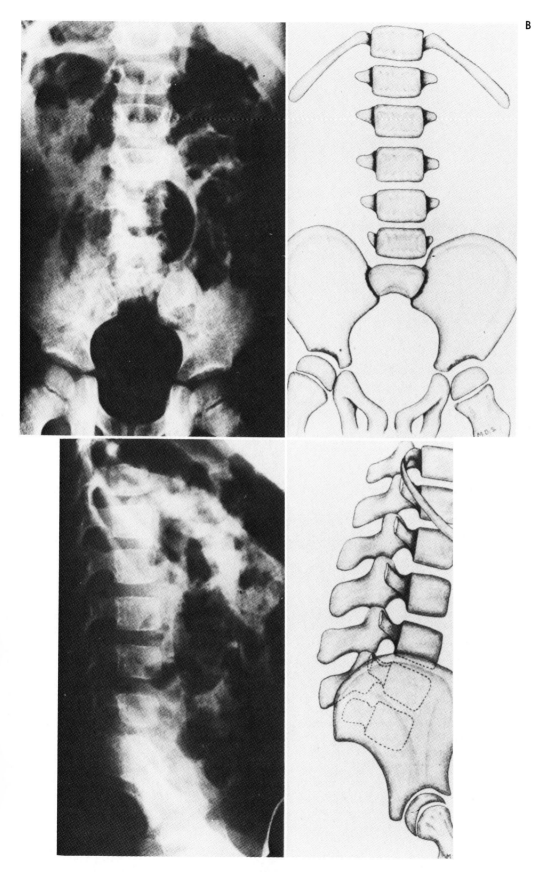

Fig. 10-133, cont'd   **B,** Type II, partial sacral agenesis with partial, bilateral symmetric defects in stable articulation between ilia and normal or hypoplastic S1 vertebra.

C

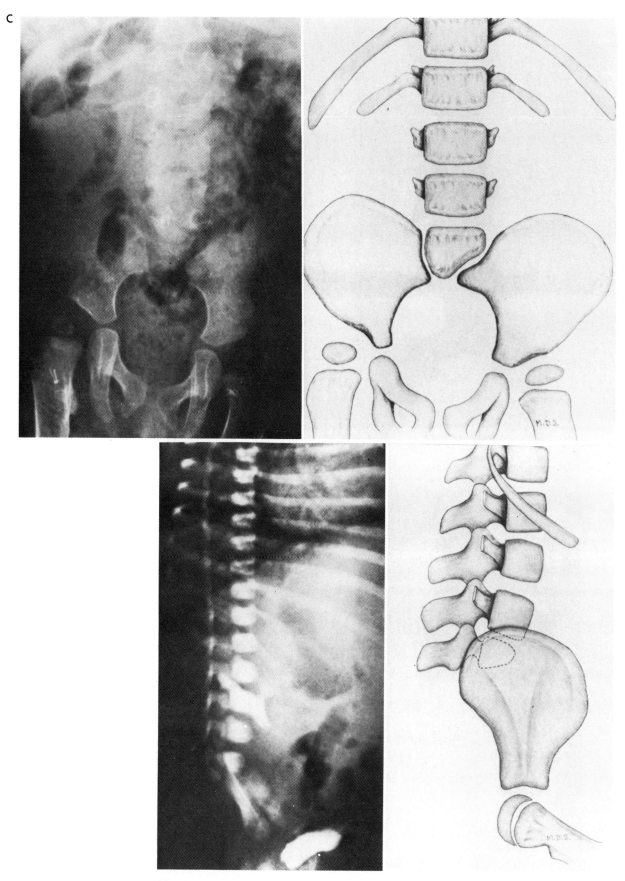

Fig. 10-133, cont'd   **C,** Type III, variable lumbar and total acral agenesis; ilia articulate with lowest vertebra.

D

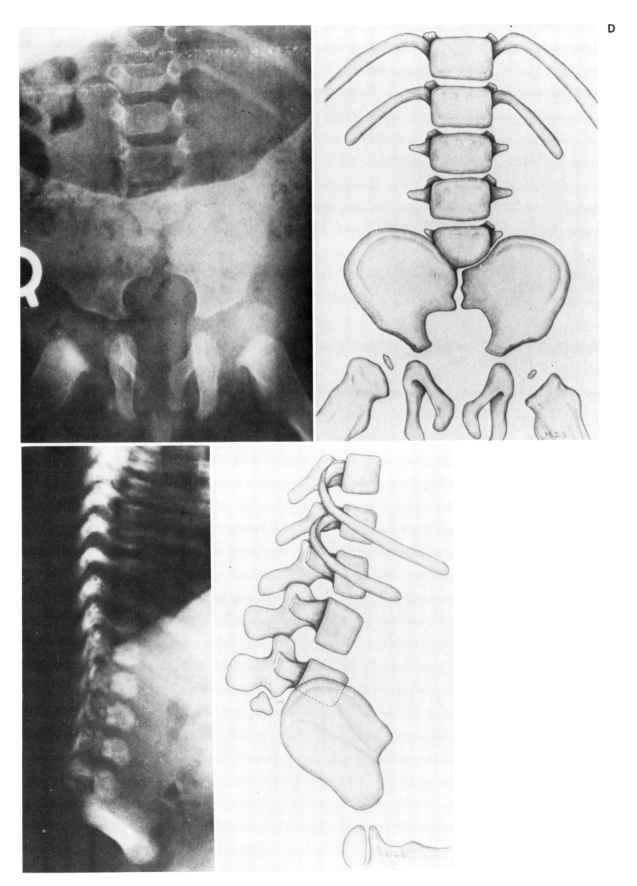

Fig. 10-133, cont'd   **D,** Type IV, variable lumbar and total sacral agenesis; caudal end plate of lowest vertebra rests above fused ilia or iliac amphiarthrosis.

Clinical Findings

The clinical appearance of a child with sacral agenesis ranges from one of severe deformities of the pelvis and lower extremities to no deformity or weakness whatsoever. Those with a partial sacral or coccygeal agenesis may be symptom free. Those with lumbar or complete sacral agenesis may be severely deformed with multiple musculoskeletal abnormalities, including foot deformities, knee-flexion contractures with popliteal webbing, hip-flexion contractures, dislocated hips, spinal-pelvic instability, and scoliosis. The posture of the lower extremities has been compared with a "sitting Buddha" (Fig. 10-134). Anomalies of the viscera, particularly in the genitourinary system and in the rectal area, often are seen as well. Inspection of the back reveals a bony prominence representing the last vertebral segment. There often is gross motion between this vertebral prominence and the pelvis. Flexion and extension may occur at the junction of the spine and the pelvis rather than at the hips.

Neurologic examination usually reveals that motor power is intact down to the level of the lowest vertebral body that has pedicles. Sensation, however, is present down to more caudal levels. Even patients with the most severe involvement may have sensation to the knees and spotty hypesthesia distally. Bladder and bowel control is often impaired, however.

Management

In an excellent article Phillips et al in 1982 reviewed the orthopaedic management of lumbosacral agenesis. They concluded that all patients with partial or complete absence of the sacrum only (type I and type II) have an excellent chance of becoming community ambulators. Management of more severe deformities (type III and type IV) is more controversial. On the basis of their experience Phillips et al recommend that management of lumbosacral agenesis in a child includes a careful assessment of the strength and sensation in the lower extremities in order to set appropriate goals for treatment, periodic examinations of the spine, and assessment of the function of the viscera, particularly the urinary tract. At least one intravenous pyelogram should be obtained in search of anatomic abnormalities.

Scoliosis is the most common spinal anomaly associated with sacral agenesis. There is no correlation between the type of defect and the likelihood of scoliosis. The scoliosis may be associated with congenital anomalies, such as hemivertebra, or with no obvious spinal abnormality above the level of the vertebral agenesis. Progressive scoliosis or kyphosis necessitates surgical stabilization as indicated for similar scoliosis without the presence of sacral agenesis.

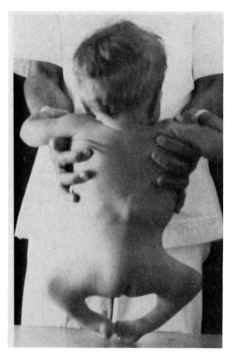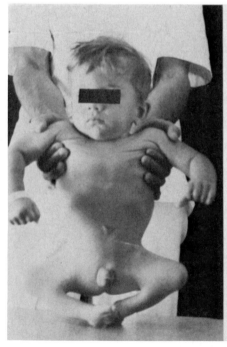

Fig. 10-134 Severe knee-flexion contractures with popliteal wedging and hip-flexion deformities or contractures as a result of lumbosacral agenesis at T12 level. (From Phillips WA et al: J Bone Joint Surg 64A:1282, 1982.)

The treatment of spinal-pelvic instability is more controversial. Excessive motion between the end of the spine and the pelvis makes stretching of hip-flexion contractures difficult. When the patient is sitting, the spine collapses toward the pelvis, increasing compression of the viscera by the poorly supported upper part of the body. Perry et al believe the key to rehabilitation of a patient with an unstable spinal-pelvic junction is establishment of a stable vertebral-pelvic complex about which lower extremity contractures can be stretched or surgically released. The stability also frees the upper extremities from the necessity of supporting an unstable collapsing back and protects the viscera from physiologically abnormal compression and angulation. Renshaw also believes that patients with type III or IV defects must be observed closely for signs of progressive kyphosis or instability. If progressive deformity is noted, he recommends lumbopelvic arthrodesis as early as is consistent with successful fusion. In his series, fusion was performed in patients 4 years of age or older. He noted that after fusion the patients were better sitters, had improved conditions at the ilial conduits and better respiratory reserve, and could use their orthoses or prostheses more efficiently. Phillips et al, however, found that spinal-pelvic instability was not a problem in 18 of the 20 surviving patients at long-term follow-up. Proper care of patients with sacral agenesis is best provided by a treatment team, including an orthopaedic surgeon, a urologist, a neurosurgeon, a pediatrician, a physical therapist, and an orthotist-prosthetist. Only with this team approach can appropriate, intelligent decisions be made about surgical treatment in these very complicated cases.

Unusual Causes of Scoliosis

NEUROFIBROMATOSIS

Frederick von Recklinghausen is given credit for establishing neurofibromatosis as a clinical entity. He recognized the neural element in the abnormal tissues, as well as the hereditary nature of the disease. The disease is inherited as an autosomal dominant trait with variable penetration and has a multiplicity of clinical manifestations as described by McCarroll.

Neurofibromatosis involves both ectodermal and mesenchymal tissues. These hamartomatous tissues may appear in any organ system of the body. The incidence of skeletal involvement ranges from 29% to 51%. The association of neurofibromatosis with scoliosis is well known. Chaglassian et al found a 26% incidence of scoliosis in 141 patients.

Natural History

Two basic types of scoliosis occur in association with neurofibromatosis: with or without dystrophic bony changes. Winter et al reviewed 102 patients with neurofibromatosis and spine deformity and found 80 to have curvatures associated with dystrophic changes in the vertebrae and ribs. They recognized the progressive tendency of the dystrophic curves compared with the nondystrophic curves. The nondystrophic curves behaved according to their causative factors (e.g., idiopathic, congenital, and Scheuermann's disease), and the neurofibromatosis did not appear to have any influence on the curve or its treatment. The natural history of dystrophic curves was much less benign. Winter et al emphasized that although a few patients reached adult life with minor curves and without disability, they were the exception. They believe that observation of progression of a spinal deformity in neurofibromatosis is unjustified. Winter et al also noted that spinal deformity caused paraplegia only in those patients with dystrophic kyphoscoliosis compared with those with dystrophic scoliosis alone and that laminectomy alone worsened spinal cord compression caused by kyphoscoliosis.

Clinical Findings

Crowe and Schull described the classic clinical criteria for the diagnosis of neurofibromatosis, two or more of which are necessary for diagnosis: (1) a minimum of six café au lait spots larger than 1.5 cm in diameter, (2) multiple subcutaneous neurofibromas, (3) elephantiasis neuromatosa, (4) positive results of a biopsy specimen, (5) a family history of the disease, and (6) specific osseous dystrophic manifestations of the disease.

Roentgenographic Findings

Roentgenographic findings were delineated by Hunt and Pugh and include (1) the classic, sharply angulated curve of five to eight vertebrae with an acute kyphosis in the same area (these vertebrae are typically dystrophic, whereas those in nonkyphotic curves are less so), (2) "penciling" of the ribs at the apical portion of the curve, (3) scalloped vertebrae, with invaginations on myelographic examination that are probably caused by meningoceles, (4) dystrophic vertebrae, which are less common in patients with more skin manifestations, (5) occasional idiopathic-type curve or congenital vertebral abnormalities, and (6) occasional enlarged intervertebral foramina (Fig. 10-135). The exact cause of these changes in the spine is still unknown. Severe kyphoscoliosis can occur, even without visible neurofibromatosis tissue in or around the spine.

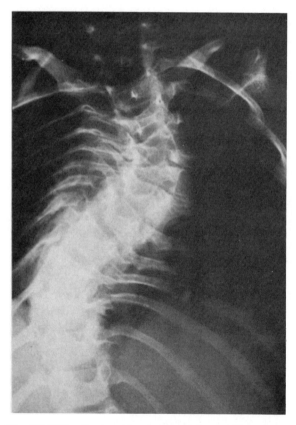

Fig. 10-135 Dystrophic changes of neurofibromatosis in scoliosis of thoracic spine: rib penciling, splindling of transverse processes, scalloping of vertebral bodies, foraminal enlargement, and paravertebral soft tissue tumor. (From Winter RB et al: J Bone Joint Surg 61A:677, 1979.)

Management

The treatment of the scoliosis necessitates differentiating the dystrophic from the nondystrophic curves. Nondystrophic curves can be treated according to the primary cause. Dystrophic curves generally require surgical treatment because of unrelenting progression.

Orthotic Treatment

Winter et al attempted brace treatment in 10 of 80 patients with dystrophic curves. The brace was worn for at least 12 months; the curves averaged 27 degrees of progression during brace treatment and none was improved. Eight of the 10 patients subsequently underwent fusion. They believe that brace treatment is not indicated for the typical dystrophic curve of neurofibromatosis.

Surgical Treatment

Appropriate surgical treatment is determined by the presence or absence of a kyphotic deformity in addition to the scoliosis.

Scoliosis. In patients without a significant kyphotic deformity, posterior fusion alone produces satisfactory results (Fig. 10-136). Unless contraindicated (e.g., young age, osteoporotic bone, or peculiar anatomic configurations), Harrington instrumentation provides greater correction and permits ambulation with a well-fitting Risser-Cotrel cast without significant loss of correction. In patients with scoliosis alone but with severe dystrophic changes Winter et al recommended reexploration and augmentation of the fusion mass 6 months after posterior fusion. Hsu et al, however, reported that all their patients with scoliosis alone had a good result with no loss of correction after Harrington instrumentation and fusion.

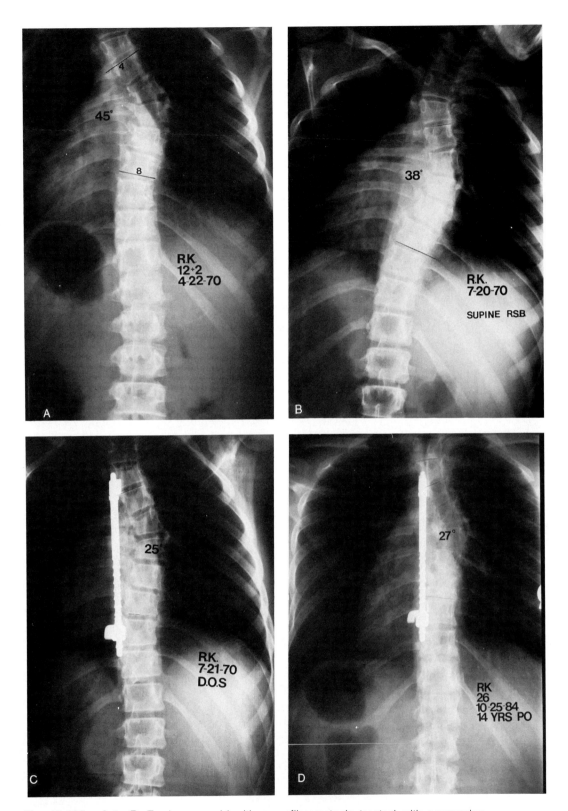

Fig. 10-136 **A** to **D,** Twelve-year-old with neurofibromatosis treated with aggressive surgical approach for management of dystrophic curve. (From Bradford DS et al: Moe's textbook of scoliosis and other spinal deformities, ed 2, Philadelphia, 1987, WB Saunders Co.)

Kyphoscoliosis. Winter et al and Hsu et al emphasize that dystrophic patients with an angular kyphosis respond very poorly to a posterior fusion alone and that good results were consistently obtained only in those patients who underwent combined anterior and posterior fusion. They also emphasized that not every patient had a solid fusion initially even with both anterior and posterior procedures (Fig. 10-137). Winter et al believe that the common reason for failure is too little bone and too limited a fusion area. They emphasize that the entire structural area of the deformity must be fused anteriorly, with complete disk excision and strong strut grafts, preferably from the fibula, as well as the rib and iliac bone, if needed. All anterior grafts must be in contact throughout with other grafts or with the spine. Hsu et al, however, note that an "adequate" anterior procedure can be difficult to achieve in severely angulated dystrophic curves. They emphasize the importance of early diagnosis and treatment by combined anterior and posterior fusion with internal fixation if possible.

Whether the anterior or posterior procedure is performed first depends on the flexibility of the spine as determined by preoperative bending, hyperextension, or traction roentgenograms. If the curve is rigid, the anterior procedure should be performed first to obtain optimal correction. If the kyphosis can be corrected by traction or extension, the posterior fusion is performed first with Harrington compression and bent distraction rods plus fusion with abundant autogenous bone graft. Two weeks later the anterior fusion is performed. Winter et al believe the anterior strut grafts are far less likely to be displaced if posterior instrumentation is already in place.

In severe deformities, halo-femoral traction or halo-wheelchair traction can be of great benefit. If the kyphosis is flexible, pulmonary compromise or spinal cord compression often can be lessened with traction. The technique of anterior strut grafting is described on p. 502, and the Harrington distraction and compression rod is described on pp. 478 to 482.

Postoperative management generally consists of a halo cast. After 6 to 9 months the halo cast may be removed, but external support should be continued until strong vertical trabecular patterns can be seen in the fusion mass, which may occur at any time from 9 to 24 months after surgery.

Kyphoscoliosis with spinal cord compression. In the series of Winter et al 16 patients had spinal cord or cauda equina compression; eight had cord compression as a result of spinal angulation, five had neural signs caused by tumor, and three had problems caused both by tumor and by angulation. They noted that scoliosis without kyphosis, no matter how severe, never resulted in cord compression; cord compression in a purely scoliotic spine was always due to an

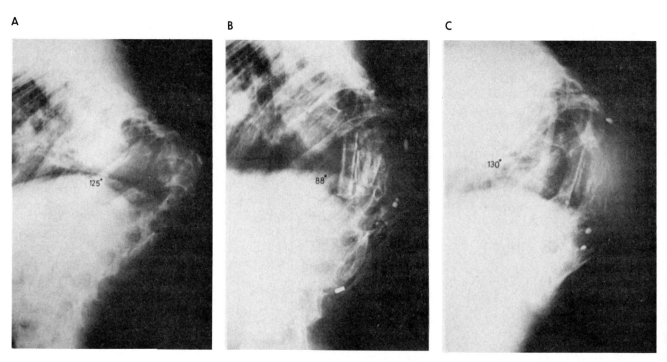

A   B   C

Fig. 10-137   A, Nineteen-year-old patient with kyphoscoliosis and neurofibromatosis. **B,** Correction to 88 degrees after fusion. **C,** Maturation of fusion but increase of kyphosis 7 years after surgery. (From Hsu LCS, Lee PC, and Leong JC: J Bone Joint Surg 66B:498, 1985.)

intraspinal tumor. All six of their patients who underwent laminectomy without spine fusion had unsatisfactory results. If the cord compression is from kyphoscoliotic deformity, laminectomy is absolutely contraindicated. Removal of the posterior elements adds a postlaminectomy kyphosis and also removes valuable bone surface for a posterior fusion. If the spinal cord compression is minor, preoperative curve correction with halo-femoral traction or cast application may improve the alignment of the spinal canal and eliminate compression. Anterior and posterior fusion then can be performed without the need for direct observation of the cord. If, however, the cord compression is significant and the patient exhibits a severe structural kyphoscoliosis, anterior cord decompression is required. The cord should be decompressed anteriorly through either a thoracotomy or a costotransversectomy approach; thoracotomy appears to provide better exposure of this area. Anterior fusion (p. 502) must be done with this decompression, and posterior fusion is performed as a second stage. If laminectomy is necessary for removal of a spinal cord tumor, fusion should be performed at the time of the decompression to prevent a rapidly increasing kyphotic deformity and neurologic injury.

Complications of Surgery

In addition to the complications inherent in any major spinal surgery, there are several complications relative to the neurofibromatosis. McCarroll pointed out that a plexiform venous anomaly may be encountered in the soft tissues surrounding the spine, which can impede the operative approach to the vertebral bodies and lead to excessive bleeding. The increased vascularity of the neurofibromatous tissue itself also may lead to increased blood loss. Hsu et al noted that a pheochromocytoma, a tumor arising from chromaffin cells, can be associated with neurofibromatosis.

The angular deformity of the neurofibromatosis itself can lead to significant mechanical problems with the anterior strut graft. The apical bodies may have subluxated into bayonet apposition or be so rotated that they no longer are in alignment with the rest of the spine. This malalignment does not allow the anterior strut grafts to be placed in the concavity of the kyphosis and makes them mechanically less effective in preventing its progression. Winter et al and Hsu et al emphasize the difficulty, as well as the necessity, of an adequate anterior fusion.

Many patients with neurofibromatosis and scoliosis also have cervical spine abnormalities (Fig. 10-138). Curtis et al reported deformities in the cervical spine to be the cause of cord compression in four of their eight patients who had paraplegia with neurofibromatosis. Yong-Hing et al found that 44% of their patients with scoliosis or kyphoscoliosis had associated cervical lesions, which they classified into two groups: abnormalities of bone structure and abnormalities of vertebral alignment. The highest incidence of cervical anomalies was in patients with short kyphotic curves or thoracic or lumbar curves that measured more than 65 degrees. This also is the group of patients more apt to require anesthesia, traction, and surgical stabilization of the spine. Yong-Hing et al therefore recommend routine roentgenography of the cervical spine in all patients with neurofibromatosis who are to have general anesthesia for any reason or traction for treatment of the scoliosis.

Winter et al reported postoperative paralysis in two patients as a result of contusion of the spinal cord by the periosteal elevator during exposure. Both these patients had unsuspected areas of laminae erosion because of dural ectasia. This, together with the high incidence of cervical spine abnormalities, has led Winter et al to suggest that patients with dystrophy should have a complete, high-volume myelogram series in the prone, lateral, and supine positions before treatment, either by surgery or traction.

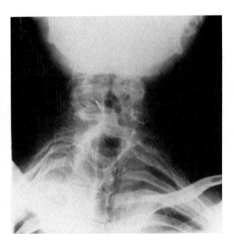 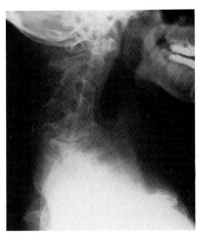

Fig. 10-138 A, Cervical spine of patient with neurofibromatosis. **B,** Cervical kyphosis and subluxation after anterior body excision and grafting.

B

MARFAN SYNDROME

Marfan syndrome is a hereditary disorder of connective tissue inherited as an autosomal dominant trait. Studies by Boucek et al have implicated a possible defect in collagen cross-links.

Diagnosis

Classic Marfan syndrome is characterized by arachnodactyly, ectopia lentis, and cardiovascular mitral value insufficiency. Because there is no specific chemical test to identify Marfan syndrome, the diagnosis can be made only clinically. According to McKusick a diagnosis cannot be made without the presence of ectopia lentis or a familial occurrence, or both, combined with other stigmata of Marfan syndrome. Other skeletal manifestations include dolichomorphism, dolichocephaly, pectus excavatum, pectus carinatum, high-arched palate, generalized ligamentous laxity, and various spinal deformities. Many patients exhibit fewer or questionable criteria for the diagnosis of Marfan syndrome and frequently are described as having "forme fruste" Marfan syndrome.

Scoliosis and kyphosis are frequent and potentially severe manifestations of Marfan syndrome. The incidence of scoliosis is reported to be between 40% and 60% in patients with true Marfan syndrome. Certainly, routine follow-up spinal examinations are indicated in all patients being treated for Marfan syndrome. The curve patterns of scoliosis in Marfan syndrome are similar to those in idiopathic scoliosis. Double major curves are more frequent. Scoliosis appears more frequently in the infantile and juvenile age-groups. Disabling back pain is more frequently a presenting complaint in patients with Marfan scoliosis than in patients with idiopathic scoliosis. Thoracic lordosis is common and may be associated with lumbar or thoracolumbar kyphosis. This sagittal plane configuration is extremely important in the consideration of appropriate surgical intervention.

Management
Observation

Because not all scoliosis in Marfan syndrome is progressive, observation every 3 to 4 months is indicated for the young patient with a small curve of less than 25 degrees. The family should be made aware, however, that many of these curves do become progressive.

Orthotic Treatment

The Milwaukee brace generally has been unsuccessful in the treatment of scoliosis associated with Marfan syndrome. Birch and Herring found brace treatment successful in only one of nine patients. Robins et al treated 14 patients with the Milwaukee brace and found three curves were improved and three did not increase. They concluded that the effectiveness of the Milwaukee brace for the treatment of Marfan scoliosis is limited. In spite of these relatively poor results, a trial of Milwaukee brace treatment still is indicated in patients in whom the scoliosis is less than 45 degrees, is flexible, and is not associated with thoracic lordosis or lumbar kyphosis. The brace is not indicated for rigid, large curves or curves associated with thoracic lordosis.

Surgical Treatment

Surgery is indicated for scoliosis greater than 40 to 45 degrees or a progressive curve that cannot be managed with a Milwaukee brace. Before surgical intervention is considered, a complete cardiovascular evaluation is mandatory. Any evidence of cardiovascular insufficiency must be completely evaluated and treated either medically or by cardiovascular surgery before surgical treatment of the scoliosis.

Robins et al concluded that correction and fusion of Marfan scoliosis can be accomplished with no more morbidity than in patients with idiopathic scoliosis and that solid fusion and maintenance of correction can be anticipated. Birch and Herring, however, note the high complication rate in these patients, reporting a 44% pseudarthrosis rate as well as postoperative loss of correction. They emphasize that these patients require a massive bone graft, secure segmental internal fixation, and careful postoperative observation for pseudarthrosis. They also emphasize the importance of a kyphotic deformity and recommend anterior fusion and posterior instrumentation when kyphosis is present.

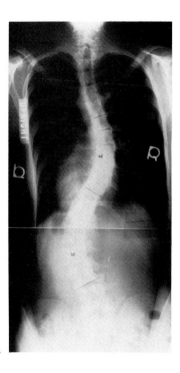
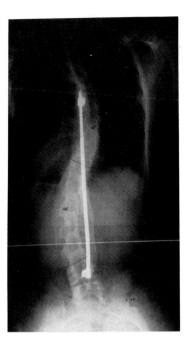

A

B

Fig. 10-139 **A,** Progressive scoliosis in patient with Marfan disease. **B,** Solid fusion and no progression of curve 5 years after Harrington rod instrumentation of both curves.

The treatment recommendations of Robins et al are used with the techniques appropriate for similar curve patterns in patients with adolescent idiopathic scoliosis (Fig. 10-139). Fusion to the sacrum generally is not needed. The patient is immobilized postoperatively in a snug-fitting Risser cast. If a thoracolumbar or lumbar kyphosis is present, bending films should be obtained. If the kyphotic deformity is flexible, then anterior surgery usually is not performed. If the kyphosis is rigid, then anterior release and fusion without instrumentation is indicated, followed by a second procedure for posterior instrumentation and fusion. If posterior fusion alone is performed, the upper or lower hook must not lie at the apex of the kyphosis; the entire area of the kyphosis must be included in the fusion (Fig. 10-140). For a significant thoracic lordosis, sublaminar wiring with the use of square-ended Moe-Harrington rods contoured into kyphosis or contoured Luque rods is the only effective procedure.

The life expectancy of patients with Marfan syndrome has been of some concern in consideration of treatment of the spinal deformities. Bowers found that most patients with Marfan syndrome live to be approximately 45 years of age. Considering the early onset of scoliosis in these patients and the severe deformity and pain that can occur, treatment is indicated. Unless there is a medical contraindication, surgical correction and stabilization are indicated for scoliosis in most patients with Marfan syndrome. Correction of the deformity in the sagittal plane, as well as the frontal plane, is essential in these patients.

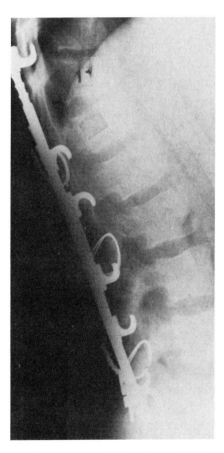

Fig. 10-140 Rod dislodgement and increased kyphosis in patient with Marfan syndrome after Harrington instrumentation. Fusion was not extended far enough proximally. (From Amis J and Herring JA: J Bone Joint Surg 66A:460, 1984.)

VERTEBRAL COLUMN TUMORS

Because their presentation can be variable, tumors of the vertebral column often present diagnostic problems. A team composed of a surgeon, diagnostic radiologist, pathologist, and often a medical oncologist and radiotherapist is necessary to treat the spectrum of tumors that involve the spine. This section discusses the most common primary tumors of the vertebral column in children.

Clinical Findings

A complete history is the first step in the evaluation of any patient with a tumor. The initial complaint of patients with a tumor involving the spine generally is pain. The exact type of pain or distribution of the pain varies with the anatomic location of the pathologic process. In general the pain caused by a neoplasm is not significantly relieved by rest and often is worse at night, interfering with sleep. Occasionally, constitutional symptoms such as anorexia, weight loss, or fever may be present. The age and sex of the patient may be important in the differential diagnosis. The physical examination should include a general evaluation in addition to careful examination of the spine. The tumor may produce local tenderness, muscle spasm, scoliosis, and limited spine motion. A careful neurologic examination is essential. Laboratory studies performed routinely should include a complete blood count level; urinalysis; sedimentation rate; serum calcium, phosporus, and alkaline phosphatase concentrations; and protein level. As the evaluation continues, further laboratory studies may be indicated.

Roentgenographic Findings

Roentgenograms of the spine should be made in at least two planes at 90-degree angles. Oblique views and tomograms often are helpful. A bone scan is of value in certain tumors of the spine, especially osteoid osteoma, which bone scan frequently will locate when the lesion is not visible on routine roentgenograms. CT has greatly enhanced assessment of the extent of the lesion and the presence of any spinal canal compromise. Arteriographic examination may be indicated to evaluate the extent of the tumor and localize major feeder vessels to the tumor; it has been reported to be helpful in embolization of the feeder vessels for vertebral tumors in selected cases. MRI has proved helpful in evaluating the extent of soft tissue involvement of the tumor.

Biopsy

Biopsy is the ultimate diagnostic technique for evaluating neoplasms and may be accomplished either by needle aspiration or by surgical sampling. The surgical sampling may be incisional (removal of a small portion of the tumor) or excisional (removal of the entire tumor).

Needle biopsy performed by experienced personnel using image intensification or CT to guide needle placement, and with a capable histologist and cytologist to interpret the material, can yield accurate diagnoses in two thirds of bone lesions and three fourths of soft tissue lesions. In many ways needle biopsy techniques are more demanding and possibly more hazardous than open procedures. Even if the technique is carried out satisfactorily, there is the possibility of tissue sampling error because of the small amount of tissue recovered. To a large extent the decision as to whether to obtain a needle biopsy of the lesion or to perform an open surgical biopsy depends on the experience and capabilities of the personnel available to the surgeon. Dunn recommends closed biopsy techniques for lesions in the lumbar spine and open biopsy techniques in the thoracic spine.

Valls et al described needle biopsy of dorsal and lumbar vertebrae, and if an experienced radiologist is not available, this may be appropriate, but needle biopsy probably is best used in the lumbar spine.

Needle biopsy of lumbar spine

▶ *Technique (Valls et al).* Administer general anesthesia, and intubate the patient. Identify the spinous process of the involved vertebra. Make a small incision 6.5 cm from the midline of this spinous process on the side most involved by the tumor in the vertebral body. Place the exploring needle (18-cm long, 1 mm in diameter, and containing a stylet) within the heavier and shorter aspiration needle that is marked to show the distance in centimeters from its point. Insert this combination of needles at an angle of 145 degrees from the horizontal and 6.5 cm from the midline, using the guide bar designed for this purpose (Fig. 10-141). If the angle is more than 145 degrees, the dura may be entered, and if less the vertebral body will not be encountered. Introduce the exploring needle to a depth of 6 or 7 cm so that its tip is at the level of the vertebral body. Check the position of the needle with anteroposterior and lateral roentgenograms, or use fluoroscopy with an image intensifier. Remove the stylet, and apply suction to ensure that the needle is not in a vessel or in the dural sac. When the needle is in the proper position, advance the large biopsy needle over the exploring needle until it touches the vertebra. Remove the ex-

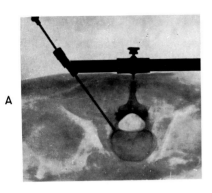
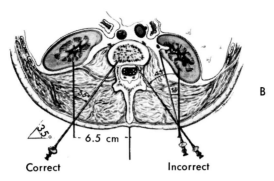

Fig. 10-141 Needle biopsy of T10 through T12 vertebrae and lumbar vertebrae. **A,** Correct angle for insertion of needle is determined by guide bar. **B,** Correct and incorrect angles of insertion of needle. (From Ottolenghi CE: J Bone Joint Surg 37A:443, 1955.)

ploring needle and guide bar. While maintaining a partial vacuum in the biopsy needle with a syringe, gradually advance it into the vertebral body, but no more than a total of 9 cm or the aorta may be punctured. If considerable resistance is encountered, move the tip of the needle slightly to find a softer area for aspiration.

Open biopsy of thoracic vertebra

▶ *Technique (Michele and Krueger).* Place the patient in the prone position. Make an incision over the side of the spinous process of the involved vertebra. Retract the muscles, and expose the transverse process. Perform an osteotomy at the base of the transverse process at its junction with the lamina (Fig. 10-142, *A*). By depressing or retracting the transverse process, expose the isthmus of the vertebra, revealing the cancellous nature of its bone structure. Roentgenographic verification of the level is very important. Insert a ³⁄₁₆-inch trephine with ¼-inch markings through the fenestra, and guide it downward with slight pressure so that a mere twisting action leads the trephine into the pedicle and finally into the body (Fig. 10-142, *B*). Remove the trephine repeatedly, and in each instance check that the contents consist of cancellous bone, which indicates that the trephine is within the medullary substance of the pedicle and thus has created a channel from the posterior elements directly into the vertebral body. Remove the pathologic tissue with a small blunt curet.

Alternatively, after the osteotomy of the base of the transverse process, expose the vertebral body by retracting the transverse process and depressing the adjacent rib to expose the junction of the pedicle and the body. Use the trephine to penetrate this junction at an angle of 45 degrees toward the midline, and remove the material with a curet (Fig. 10-142, *C*).

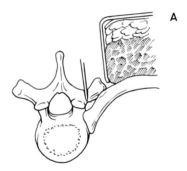
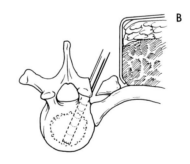
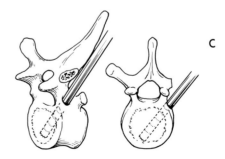

Fig. 10-142 **A,** Transverse osteotomy at base of thoracic transverse process. **B,** Trephine through fenestra of isthmus, into pedicle and body. **C,** Trephine inserted into body at junction of pedicle. (Redrawn from Michele AA and Krueger FJ: J Bone Joint Surg 31A:873, 1949.)

Benign Tumors of the Vertebral Column

The most common benign tumors of the vertebral column in children are osteoid osteoma, osteoblastoma, aneurysmal bone cyst, eosinophilic granuloma, and hemangioma.

Osteoid Osteoma

In 1935 Jaffee first described the tumor he called *osteoid osteoma.* Jackson et al, in a review of 860 osteoid osteomas collected from the English literature, found that 10% were located in the spine. Osteoid osteoma is a benign growth that consists of a discrete osteoid nidus and reactive sclerotic bone thickening around the nidus. No malignant change of these tumors ever has been documented. The lesion is seen more frequently in males than females. Spinal lesions occur predominantly in the posterior elements of the spine, especially the lamina and pedicles. Osteoid osteoma of the vertebral body has been reported but is quite rare. The lumbar spine is the most frequently involved area.

Typically, the patient with a spinal osteoid osteoma has pain that is worse at night and is relieved by aspirin. The pain increases with activity and often localizes to the site of the lesion. Radicular symptoms are especially common in lesions of the lumbar spine.

Physical examination reveals muscle spasm in the involved area of the spine. The patient's gait may be abnormal because of pain, and there may be moderate to severe localized tenderness over the tumor.

Osteoid osteoma is the most common cause of painful scoliosis in adolescents. Excellent studies by Marsh et al, Mehta, and Pettine and Klassen have shown a high incidence of scoliosis with involvement of the vertebral column. Classically, the scoliosis associated with osteoid osteoma is described as a C-shaped curve. Pettine, however, noted that only 23% of the scoliotic curves in his series had this classic curve pattern. The osteoid osteoma usually is located on the concave side of the curve and in the area of the apical vertebra.

When the osteoid osteoma is visible on plain roentgenograms, its appearance is diagnostic: a central radiolucency with surrounding sclerotic bony reaction (Fig. 10-143). Often, however, the lesion is not visible on plain films, especially in the spine, and a technetium bone scan should be considered in any adolescent with a painful scoliosis (Fig. 10-144). Negative results of a bone scan in a patient with osteoid osteoma of the spine have not been reported. CT also has been helpful in further delineating the lesion in preparation for surgery (Fig. 10-145).

A
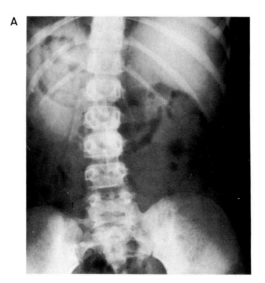
B
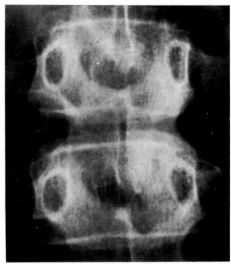

Fig. 10-143 Osteoid osteoma of lumbar vertebra in 9-year-old patient with back pain and mild scoliosis. **A,** Sclerotic lesion in pedicle of L3 on concave side of curve. **B,** Lesion more clearly seen in enlarged view of vertebra. Removal of lesion relieved pain, and scoliosis disappeared.

Mehta and Murray suggested that patients with spinal tumors and scoliosis reach a critical point after which the continuation of painful stimuli results in structural changes in the spine. Pettine and Klassen found that 15 months is the critical duration of symptoms if antalgic scoliosis is to undergo spontaneous correction after excision of the tumor. They noted improvement or complete correction of the scoliosis in 11 of 12 patients in whom the lesion was removed before 15 months of symptoms. In 10 of 11 patients with symptoms for more than 15 months, there was no improvement in the scoliosis after removal of the lesion.

Treatment of the osteoid osteoma is complete removal; recurrence is likely after incomplete removal. If pain and deformity persist after removal of the lesion, incomplete removal or perhaps a multifocal lesion should be suspected. Exact localization of the tumor is imperative; in the series of Pettine and Klassen, five patients had the initial surgical procedure on the wrong location. Rinsky and Israeli et al reported intraoperative localization of the lesion by skeletal scintigraphy.

Although excision of these lesions does not generally require a spinal fusion, if removal of significant portions of the facet joints and pedicles makes the spine unstable, spinal fusion may be performed at the time of tumor removal. Eleven of 31 patients in Pettine and Klassen's series required this concomitant fusion.

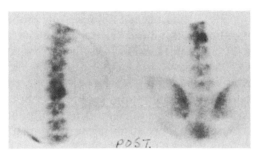

Fig. 10-144   Technetium bone scan of lumbar spine indicating increased activity on right side of L2 consistent with osteoid osteoma. (From Israeli A et al: Clin Orthop 175:194, 1983.)

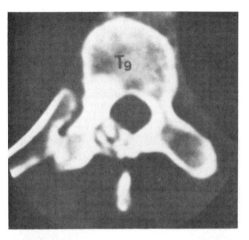

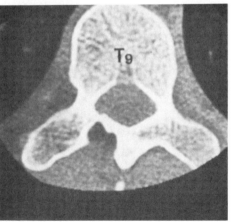

Fig. 10-145   CT scans used before and after surgery to localize tumor and avoid extensive skeletal resection. (From Pettine KA and Klassen RA: J Bone Joint Surg 68A:354, 1986.)

Osteoblastoma

Benign osteoblastoma is an uncommon primary bone tumor that accounts for fewer than 1% of all bone tumors. Of these reported tumors, however, 40% have been located in the spine, and more than half were associated with scoliosis. Marsh et al reported 197 cases of osteoblastomas, 41% of which were in the spine. More than half the patients whose tumor arose in the thoracolumbar spine or the ribs had an associated scoliosis.

As indicated by Akbarnia and Rooholamini, most of these patients have scoliosis and pain as presenting symptoms. The condition occurs more frequently in boys than in girls.

In contrast to osteoid osteoma, plain roentgenograms often are sufficient to confirm the diagnosis. Tomograms and bone scans, however, can be helpful (Fig. 10-146), and CT is useful for cross-sectional evaluation and localization of the tumor before surgical excision. The tumor generally is located at the apex of the curve on the concave side. Marsh et al indi-

cated that the tumor is more common in the laminae and the pedicles, and this was confirmed by Akbarnia and Rooholamini.

The treatment of this condition is complete surgical excision, although Marsh et al reported a high cure rate even if curettage was incomplete because of the location of the tumor. Recurrences after incomplete curettage, however, are not rare, and there have been several reports of apparent malignant change after incomplete curettage; therefore complete excision is advised whenever possible. Because of evidence of late sarcomatous changes after irradiation, irradiation of this lesion is not recommended.

If the diagnosis is made early and treatment undertaken, the scoliosis usually is reversible after excision. Akbarnia and Rooholamini found the scoliosis improved in three patients who had had symptoms for 9 months or less before surgery. The scoliosis did not improve in the two patients whose symptoms had been present for longer periods of time.

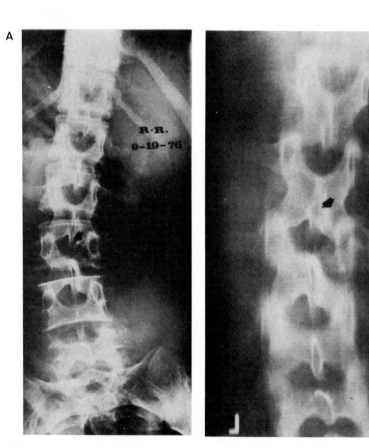

Fig. 10-146   **A,** Anteroposterior roentgenogram showing lumbar scoliosis. **B,** Tomogram defining osteoblastoma involving right transverse process, pedicle, and lamina of L3. (From Akbarnia BA and Rooholamini SA: J Bone Joint Surg 63A:1146, 1981.)

Aneurysmal Bone Cyst

Aneurysmal bone cyst probably is a nonneoplastic, vasocystic tumor originating on either a previously normal bone or a preexisting lesion. It is most common in children and young adults, and vertebral involvement is common. Its roentgenographic appearance usually is characteristic, consisting of an expansile lesion confined by a thin rim of reactive bone. The lesion can be found either in the vertebral body or in the posterior elements of the spine (Fig. 10-147). Unlike other vertebral tumors, aneurysmal bone cyst may involve adjacent vertebrae.

Pain in the spine is the most common symptom, and radicular symptoms can be present if cord compression is occurring.

Treatment is surgical excision whenever possible. Reported recurrence after curettage is about 25%. Because of the dangers of postirradiation sarcoma, radiotherapy rarely is indicated. Dick et al described arterial embolization as an adjuvant therapy in the surgical treatment of certain primary bone tumors. Because the vascular nature of the aneurysmal bone cyst may lead to profuse hemorrhage with the primary surgical approach, this may be a useful adjunct. Dick et al emphasize that this treatment is in addition to surgical excision and that the embolization of vessels that supply important segments of the spinal cord and brain should not be performed. If a significant spinal deformity is present or if the lesion is extensive, a combined approach followed by internal fixation and spinal fusion may be necessary.

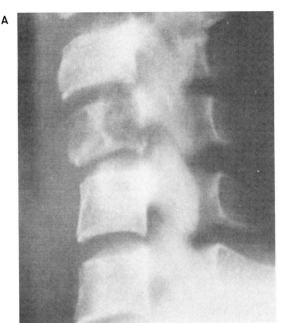 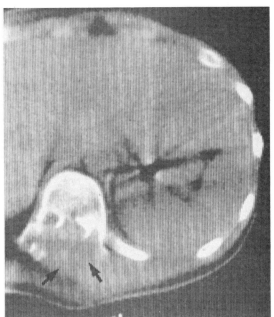

Fig. 10-147   A, Aneurysmal bone cyst arising in C4. **B,** Computed tomographic scan of aneurysmal bone cyst arising in posterior elements. (From Rothman RH and Simeone FA: The spine, ed 2, Philadelphia, 1982, WB Saunders Co.)

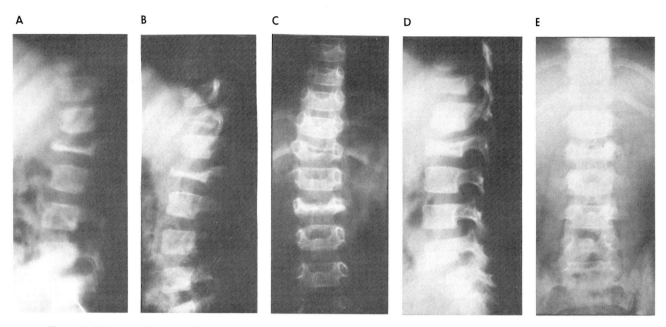

A, B, C, D, E

Fig. 10-148 **A,** Eosinophilic granuloma of spine in 3½-year-old patient. **B,** Sudden collapse of T12 3 weeks later, in addition to vertebra plana at L2. **C,** Collapse of T12 and L2. **D** and **E,** Considerable reconstitution of the vertebral height of T12 and L2 16 months later. (From Seimon LP: J Pediatr Orthop 1:371, 1981.)

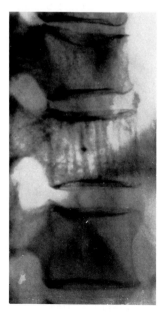

Fig. 10-149 Hemangioma of vertebral body.

Eosinophilic Granuloma

The term *eosinophilic granuloma* was introduced in 1940 by Lichtenstein and Jaffe. Eosinophilic granuloma in childhood usually is a solitary lesion. The cause of this lesion, which may not represent a true neoplasm, is unknown. Patients often have pain, and roentgenograms show collapse of a vertebra called *vertebra plana.* Considerable collapse of the vertebral body may occur without neurologic compromise, and significant reconstitution in height frequently follows treatment (Fig. 10-148). If the lesion does not have the characteristic roentgenographic appearance, then biopsy may be necessary. The treatment for vertebra plana generally focuses on amelioration of symptoms, and spontaneous healing of the lesion usually can be expected. In most cases of vertebra plana, chemotherapy, surgery, or radiation therapy is not needed.

Hemangioma

Hemangioma is the most common benign vascular tumor of bone. Most hemangiomas involve the vertebral bodies (Fig. 10-149) or skull, and involvement of other bones is rare. Vertebral involvement usually is an incidental finding and requires treatment only when neurologic function is compromised. Hemangioma has been reported in as many as 12% of spines studied by autopsy. The lesion usually produces a characteristic, vertical, striated appearance. If pain is the only symptom, low-dose radiation may be useful, but great caution is needed in recommending irradiation for lesions that most often are incidental findings. If neurologic dysfunction and anterior collapse occur, surgical excision of the lesion and anterior spinal fusion are recommended, perhaps with adjunctive embolization as described by Dick et al.

Primary Malignant Tumors of the Vertebral Column

Primary malignant tumors of the vertebral column are uncommon. In children the most common are Ewing's sarcoma and osteogenic sarcoma.

Ewing's Sarcoma

Ewing's sarcoma is a relatively rare, primary, malignant tumor of bone of uncertain histogenesis. The tumor occurs most frequently in males in the second decade of life. All bones, including the spine, may be affected. The tumor, however, much more commonly begins in the pelvis or long bone and then rapidly metastasizes to other skeletal sites, including the spine, especially the vertebral bodies and pedicles.

The currently recommended treatment for Ewing's sarcoma is radiotherapy and adjuvant chemotherapy. There is little role for surgery in the treatment of Ewing's sarcoma that involves the spine. Occasionally, surgery may be necessary to stabilize the spine in the presence of neural element compression and an unstable bony situation. If decompression of the neural elements becomes necessary, stabilization may be needed at the same time.

Osteogenic Sarcoma

Osteogenic sarcoma is the most common primary malignant bone tumor (excluding multiple myeloma), but fewer than 2% have their origin in the spine. It is a malignant tumor of bone in which tumor cells form neoplastic osteoid or bone, or both. Classic osteogenic sarcoma is most common in boys aged 10 to 15 years. This is a rapidly progressive malignancy, and multiple metastatic lesions to the vertebral column are more common than primary involvement.

At this time treatment for osteogenic sarcoma is controversial, although most authorities recommend surgery for local control. The controversy exists largely in the role of adjuvant chemotherapy for systemic control. The role of surgery for vertebral involvement is based on whether the spinal lesion is solitary, primary, or metastatic. When a cure is not possible, treatment usually consists of local radiation and systemic chemotherapy. If decompression of the spinal cord becomes necessary, or if structural integrity of the vertebral column is compromised, then stabilizing procedures usually are required.

POSTIRRADIATION SPINE DEFORMITY

Perthes in 1903 first demonstrated inhibition of osseous development by irradiation. Later studies by Hinkel, Barr et al, and Reidy et al indicated that the physis is particularly sensitive to radiation. It was found that a physis exposed to 600 rad or more shows some growth retardation, whereas complete inhibition of growth was produced by doses greater than 1200 rad. Bick and Copel reviewed histologic sections of fresh autopsy material of vertebral bodies taken from subjects varying in age from 14 weeks of fetal development to 23 years. They demonstrated that the longitudinal growth of a vertebral body takes place by means of true physeal cartilage, similar to the longitudinal growth of the metaphysis of long bones. In 1939 Engel implanted radium seeds unilaterally, adjacent to the vertebral bodies of goats, rabbits, and dogs, and produced experimentally a scoliosis with the concavity on the side of the implant. In 1948 Arkin and Simon expanded Engel's work and produced experimental scoliosis by means of asymmetric external radiation. They found that the bone wedging was not the result of pressure from contractural scarring on the concavity of the curve but was rather of unilateral suppression of the physis of the vertebra. In the same year Arkin et al reported the first known case of radiation-induced scoliosis in a human being. Since that time many other authors also have documented spinal deformity occurring after radiation therapy in children.

Incidence

Mayfield et al studied spinal deformity in children treated for neuroblastoma, and Riseborough et al studied spinal deformity in children treated for Wilms' tumor. Several principles can be summarized from these studies. There seems to be a direct relationship between the amount of irradiation and the severity of the spinal deformity. In general a dose of less than 2000 rad is not associated with a significant deformity, a dose between 2000 and 3000 rad is associated with a mild scoliosis, and a dose of more than 3000 is associated with a more significant scoliosis. Irradiation in younger children, especially those 2 years of age or younger, produces the most serious disturbance in vertebral growth. Radiation treatment in children older than 4 years of age less frequently is associated with spinal deformity. Asymmetric irradiation is associated with more frequent and also more severe deformities. In most patients the scoliosis remains slight until the adolescent growth spurt, at which time progression may occur. Scoliosis is the most frequent deformity, and the direction of the curve most commonly is concave toward the side of the irradiation. Kyphosis may occur in association with the scoliosis, or kyphosis alone may be present, most frequently at the thoracolumbar junction. The child who requires a laminectomy because of epidural spread of tumor is especially prone to development of moderate to severe spinal deformity. Similarly, those children whose disease causes paraplegia also are prone to rapid progression of the deformity. Any child undergoing radiation therapy to the spine should have orthopaedic consultation and regular follow-up until skeletal maturity.

Roentgenographic Findings

Neuhauser and associates described the roentgenographic changes in previously irradiated spines, and Riseborough et al divided the roentgenographic findings into four groups. The earliest noted changes were alterations in the vertebral bodies within the irradiated section of the spine, which are expressions of irradiation impairment of physeal endochondral growth at the vertebral end plates. The most obvious features of these lesions were growth arrest lines that subsequently led to the "bone-in-bone" picture (Fig. 10-150). This occurred in 28% of the patients in the study of Risenborough et al. End-plate irregularity with altered trabecular pattern and decreased vertebral body height were seen most frequently, being noted in 83% of patients. Contour abnormalities, causing anterior narrowing and beaking of the vertebral bodies much as one sees in Morquio's disease (Fig. 10-151), were present in 20% of patients. Asymmetric or symmetric failure of vertebral body development was apparent on the anteroposterior roentgenograms of all 81 patients studied. The second group of roentgenographic changes included alterations in spinal alignment. Scoliosis was present in 70% of patients and kyphosis in 25%. The third group of roentgenographic findings included skeletal alterations in bones other than the vertebral column, the most common of which were iliac-wing hypoplasia in 68% and osteochondromas in 6%. The fourth group consisted of patients with no evidence of deformity of the axial skeleton (27%).

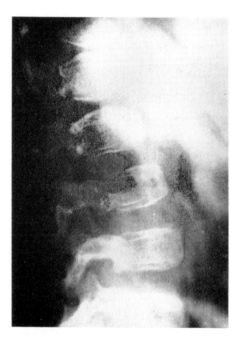

Fig. 10-150 "Bone-in-bone" appearance of irradiated spine, the equivalent of growth arrest line in long bone. (From Katzman H et al: J Bone Joint Surg 51A: 825, 1969.)

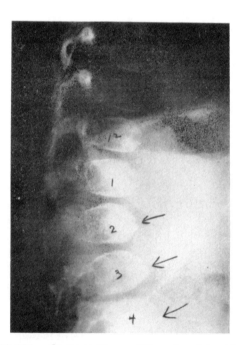

Fig. 10-151 Contour abnormalities of vertebral bodies after radiotherapy for Wilms' tumor in 8-month-old patient. (From Katzman H et al: J Bone Joint Surg 51A: 825, 1969.)

Management

Most studies indicate that the curves usually remain slight until the adolescent growth spurt when progression can be severe and rapid. Although there is no evidence that a Milwaukee brace will affect the progression of the curve, Ogilvie recommends its use when the curve reaches 20 degrees as measured by the Cobb method. He notes that the orthosis generally is not effective in reducing the curvature but may delay progression. A Milwaukee brace may be used in this situation unless there is extensive soft tissue scarring or contracture in the concavity of the curve that makes use of the brace impossible. Riseborough et al, however, found that all three of their patients treated with Milwaukee braces subsequently required surgical treatment. They believe the Milwaukee brace to be ineffective in the correction of postirradiation spinal deformity because of the severity of the changes in the architecture of the vertebrae and the excessive soft tissue scarring.

If curve progression continues, spinal instrumentation and fusion are indicated. Riseborough et al outlined the difficulties in obtaining adequate correction and fusion of these curves, which frequently are very rigid. Extensive soft tissue scarring may further complicate the surgery. Healing can be prolonged, and pseudarthrosis is a common problem, occurring in three of eight patients in the series of Riseborough et al, as is infection, which occurred in two of eight patients. Because all three pseudarthroses occurred in patients with kyphotic deformities in addition to scoliotic deformities, the authors recommend a two-stage procedure for patients with kyphoscoliosis. First, through an anterior approach, the soft tissues are excised and the intervertebral disks are removed and replaced with autogenous bone (p. 502). Then craniofemoral traction is used for 2 weeks to obtain correction (p. 466), after which a posterior fusion with Harrington rods and autogenous bone grafting is performed. Because of the kyphotic element of this deformity, the Harrington compression-distraction system (p. 482) may be effective. A Risser cast is worn for 6 months after surgery.

Posterior fusion with Harrington distraction instrumentation and autogenous bone graft may be adequate for a progressive scoliotic deformity without a significant kyphotic component. Ogilvie suggested exploration of the bone graft 6 months after surgery for repeated bone grafting of any developing pseudarthrosis. The choices of fusion limits and techniques for a purely scoliotic deformity are the same as for idiopathic scoliotic curves (p. 454).

OSTEOCHONDRODYSTROPHY
Diastrophic Dwarfism

Diastrophic dwarfism is inherited as an autosomal recessive disease. The dwarfing is severe, and the patients almost invariably have scoliosis. Bethem et al found the Milwaukee brace to be useful in treating scoliosis in these patients only when instituted while the curve is small. If the curve cannot be braced successfully, fusion is indicated and generally is successful in correcting the scoliosis. Cervical kyphosis occurs commonly, and although it usually resolves with age, it has the potential to cause to quadriplegia if untreated. These patients require roentgenographic evaluation of the cervical spine.

Spondyloepiphyseal Dysplasia

Orthopaedic aspects of spondyloepiphyseal dysplasia are discussed in Chapter 5. The spinal problems most commonly associated with this condition are scoliosis, kyphoscoliosis, and odontoid hypoplasia with atlantoaxial instability (Fig. 10-152). If the scoliosis and kyphoscoliosis are progressive, Milwaukee brace treatment sometimes is useful in delaying the fusion until the patient is older. Bethem et al found that the Milwaukee brace was more successful in managing the kyphotic deformity than the scoliotic deformity. In their patients the kyphosis decreased from an average 51 degrees to an average 25 degrees after 4 to 5 years of Milwaukee brace treatment; however, two of three patients with scoliosis eventually required fusion despite brace treatment. Progressive atlantoaxial instability should be treated by fusion.

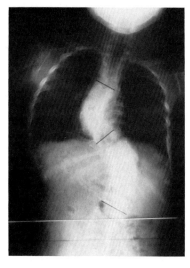

Fig. 10-152 Scoliosis in patient with spondyloepiphyseal dysplasia.

OSTEOGENESIS IMPERFECTA

The reported incidence of scoliosis in patients with osteogenesis imperfecta ranges from 40% to 90%. The natural history of scoliosis in osteogenesis imperfecta is one of continued progression. Benson et al found that the scoliosis present at a young age was almost always progressive. Moorefield and Miller reported that progression may continue into adulthood. King and Bobechko found severe and disabling spinal deformities in many adults with osteogenesis imperfecta. With improved methods of spinal instrumentation and fusion, early treatment of spinal curvature in these patients has become more feasible.

Treatment recommendations for scoliosis in patients with osteogenesis imperfecta have been based on several small series of patients. The largest series to date was reported by Yong-Hing and MacEwen: 121 patients treated by 51 different orthopaedic surgeons. They found that brace treatment was ineffective in stopping progression of scoliosis in patients with osteogenesis imperfecta even if the curves were small. They agree with Benson et al that the decision to fuse the spine should depend on the extent of the curvature and the presence of progression rather than on the age of the patient, and they recommend spinal fusion for curves greater than 50 degrees regardless of the age of the patient, provided there are no medical contraindications. Moderate or severe kyphosis should be treated by early spinal fusion. There was a high incidence of complications with spinal fusion and Harrington instrumentation in their group of patients, usually related to the size of the curves and especially to an associated kyphosis. In the absence of a pseudarthrosis or kyphosis, late bending of the fused spine did not occur.

Most authors agree that bracing does not control progressive scoliosis in these patients and that posterior spinal instrumentation and fusion are indicated. The autogenous bone graft may require supplemental bone-bank allograft. All the literature to date reports the use of Harrington instrumentation, but Bradford has performed segmental instrumentation with Luque rods and sublaminar wires (p. 484) in several patients with osteogenesis imperfecta. Although there are no reported series with this technique, because of the multiple purchase sites on the spine, the most appropriate procedure appears to be segmental instrumentation supplemented by an external orthosis or cast until fusion is solid. Osteogenesis imperfecta also is associated with spondylolisthesis as a result of elongation of the pedicle, which is treated as outlined on p. 541.

Unusual Causes of Kyphosis

POSTLAMINECTOMY SPINAL DEFORMITY
Incidence

Laminectomies most often are performed in children for the diagnosis and treatment of spinal cord tumors, although they also may be needed in other conditions such as neurofibromatosis and syringomyelia. Several authors, including Haft et al, Tachdjian and Matson, and Lonstein et al, have indicated a significant incidence of postlaminectomy spinal deformities in children. The incidence of deformity ranged from 33% in the series of Haft et al to 100% in the 32 patients studied by Lonstein et al.

Kyphosis is the most common deformity after multiple-level laminectomies. Yasuoka et al found that the incidence of spinal deformity after laminectomy was greater in children younger than 15 years of age. They also found, as did Fraser et al, that the higher the level of the laminectomy, the greater the likelihood of spinal deformity or instability. Yasuoka et al found that all cervical or cervicothoracic laminectomies were followed by deformity. Lonstein et al described two basic types of kyphosis: depending on the status of the facet joints posteriorly, the kyphosis can be sharp and angular or long and gradually rounding.

Scoliosis may also occur after laminectomy and generally is in the area of the laminectomy and associated with the kyphotic deformity. Scoliosis may occur at levels below the laminectomy, but this is caused by the paralysis that results from the cord tumor or its treatment rather than the laminectomy itself.

The causes of instability of the spine after multiple laminectomies include skeletal and ligamentous deficiencies, neuromuscular imbalance, progressive osseous deformity, and radiation therapy. Yasuoka et al noted increased wedging or excessive motion in children rather than subluxation as would occur in adults. They postulated that after laminectomy there is increased pressure on the cartilaginous end plates of vertebral bodies anteriorly, and with time there is decreased cartilage growth and wedging of the vertebrae (Fig. 10-153). Panjabi et al have shown that with loss of posterior stability caused by removal of the interspinous ligaments, spinous processes, and laminae

the normal flexion forces produce a kyphosis. Lonstein et al emphasized the importance of the facet joints posteriorly in these deformities. They showed that when the facet joint is completely removed at one level, gross instability results with maximal angulation at that level, causing a sharp, angular kyphus, enlargement of the intervertebral foramen, and opening of the disk space posteriorly. If this complete removal is on one side only, the angular kyphosis is accompanied by a sharp scoliosis with the apex at the same level. If all the facets are preserved, a gradual rounding kyphus results in the area of the laminectomy. Many authors, including Kilfoyle et al and Brown and Bonnett, have reported an extremely high incidence of spinal deformity in children younger than 10 years of age with complete paralysis. Brown and Bonnett found that a collapsing paralytic deformity develops in 100% of these patients. The child with an extensive laminectomy and paralysis as a result of the spinal cord tumor or the treatment is very likely to have an increasing spinal deformity. Radiation therapy, used to treat many spinal tumors, has been associated with injury to the vertebral physes and subsequent spine deformity (see p. 577). The cause of postlaminectomy spinal deformity is therefore multifactorial.

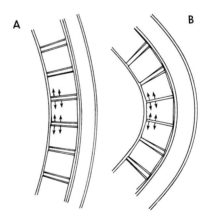

Fig. 10-153 Increased pressure on cartilaginous end plate of vertebra anteriorly after laminectomy **(A)** causes wedging of the vertebra **(B)**. (Redrawn from Yosuoka S et al: Neurosurgery 9:145, 1981.)

Management

When laminectomy is necessary, the facet joints should be preserved whenever possible. After surgery the child should be seen regularly by the orthopaedic surgeon. If a spinal deformity is detected, treatment is begun immediately with a Milwaukee brace. Lonstein et al found that results of nonsurgical treatment usually are temporary and provide lasting control in only a few patients.

If the deformity progresses in spite of brace treatment or if the child has a marked deformity, a spinal fusion should be performed. Of course, if the patient has a very limited life span because of a highly malignant tumor, there is no reason to subject this child to surgical procedures.

Most authors recommend combined anterior and posterior fusion for this condition, which is similar to spinal deformity in patients with myelomeningocele in that there is a very small amount of bone surface posteriorly after a wide laminectomy and many of these deformities have a kyphotic component. As shown by Bradford in Scheuermann's disease, an anterior spinal fusion can be more successful biomechanically than a posterior fusion because the area of the fusion mass is under compressive rather than distractive forces. Lonstein reviewed 45 patients and found a pseudarthrosis rate of 33% with posterior fusion alone, 22% with anterior fusion alone, and 9.5% with combined anterior and posterior fusion. At the first stage, an anterior fusion is performed by removing all of the disk space and taking special care to remove the entire disk back to the posterior longitudinal ligament to prevent growth in the posterior aspect of the vertebral end plate with increasing kyphotic deformity. The fusion also is reinforced with inlay strut grafts (p. 502). As a second stage 1 to 2 weeks later a posterior fusion is performed, and if possible, instrumentation is used. Often the extent of the deformity and the absence of the posterior elements make instrumentation impossible, and in these patients it may be necessary to use a halo cast after surgery (Fig. 10-154, A to C).

With improved treatment, including surgery, radiation therapy, and chemotherapy, more children with intraspinal tumors are surviving, and the orthopaedic surgeon must be aware of the likelihood that a progressive deformity of the spine will develop and require treatment. As stated by Lonstein et al, observation of a progressing deformity is not acceptable treatment.

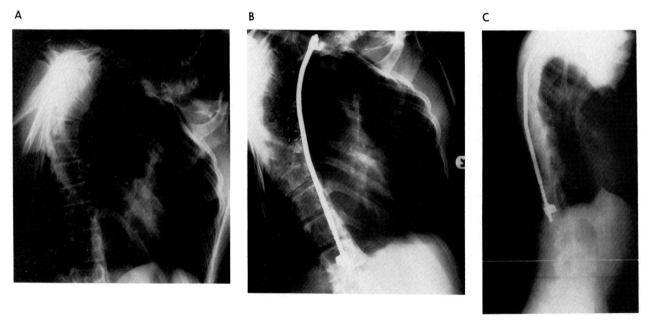

Fig. 10-154 **A,** Adolescent with progressive kyphoscoliosis after wide laminectomy for excision of arteriovenous malformation of spinal cord. **B,** After anterior disk excision and posterior distraction instrumentation. **C,** Harrington rod contoured because of kyphosis. Because internal fixation was not secure, halo cast was used for postoperative immobilization.

SKELETAL DYSPLASIAS
Achondroplasia

Achondroplasia is the most common of the bony dysplasias. The most frequent spinal deformity associated with this condition is thoracolumbar kyphosis that is present at birth. As muscle tone develops and walking begins, the kyphotic deformity usually resolves. Bailey found that approximately 30% of patients have a persistent kyphosis and that 36% of these curves become severe. This kyphosis is very poorly tolerated by the patient with achondroplasia because of the decreased size of the spinal canal related to a marked decrease in the interpedicular distance in the lower lumbar region and to shortened pedicles, which cause a reduction in the anteroposterior dimensions.

Hensinger and Bethem et al emphasized awareness of the possibility of persistent or progressive thoracolumbar kyphosis in these patients. Early bracing to prevent progression and correction of any associated hip-flexion contractures to prevent a hyperlordosis below the kyphosis are recommended. If the kyphosis is progressive in spite of brace treatment, surgical stabilization is indicated. A staged anterior and posterior fusion is recommended if the deformity is 60 degrees or greater. If the kyphosis is associated with paraparesis, anterior cord decompression followed by posterior spine fusion is indicated. Usually, however, during the childhood and adolescent years the patient with achondroplasia is free of any spine-related neurologic problems; it generally is the adult in whom symptoms of neurologic compression and spinal stenosis develop (Fig. 10-155). When posterior fusion is performed, instrumentation usually is impossible because of the extremely narrow spinal canal. Tolo reported good results with combined anterior and posterior fusions in these patients but also found a high incidence of neurologic injury when instrumentation was attempted.

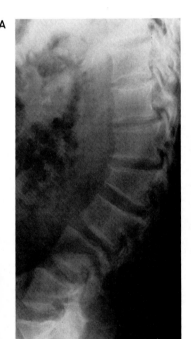 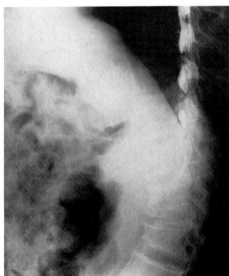

Fig. 10-155 **A,** Adult achondroplastic dwarf with persistent thoracolumbar kyphosis and increasing neurologic changes in lower extremities. **B,** Myelogram indicating total block at thoracolumbar junction.

Fig. 10-156   Kyphosis at thoracolumbar junction in patient with Hurler's syndrome.

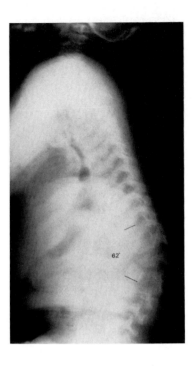

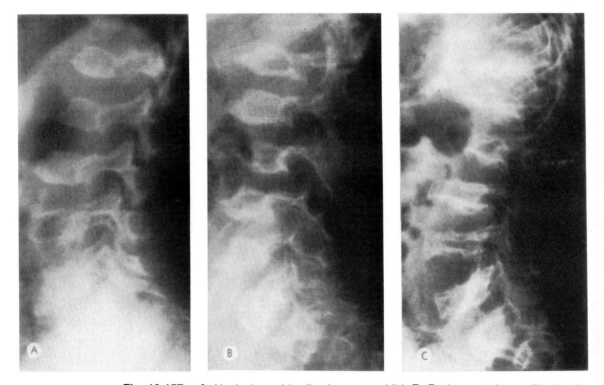

Fig. 10-157   **A,** Hook-shaped bodies in young child. **B,** Further anterior ossification in older child. **C,** Flattened, rectangular-shaped vertebral bodies in adult. (From Langer LO and Carey LS: Am J Roentgenol Rad Ther Nucl Med 97:1, 1966.)

Mucopolysaccharidoses

Of the many types of mucopolysaccharidoses, Morquio's, Hurler's, and Maroteaux-Lamy syndromes are the types most commonly associated with structural changes of the spine. Other orthopaedic problems associated with these diseases are discussed in Chapter 5. The deformity commonly seen in these conditions is a kyphosis, usually in the thoracolumbar junction (Fig. 10-156). The treatment of the condition depends on the degree of deformity, as well as the child's prognosis. Hurler's syndrome usually is rapidly progressive, and affected children usually die before 10 years of age.

Morquio's syndrome is the most common of the mucopolysaccharidoses (Fig. 10-157). Children with this condition may well live into adult life and have normal mentality. Many authors, including Blaw and Langer, Kopits, Langer, and Lipson, have emphasized the frequent occurrence of atlantoaxial instability in patients with Morquio's syndrome. This instability may result from either an anomalous development of the odontoid or laxity of the transverse atlantal ligament. Blaw stated that neurologic problems in the first two decades of life usually are related to odontoid abnormalities. In later life symptoms caused by kyphosis or gibbus tend to predominate. The treatment of atlantoaxial instability is discussed on p. 446. Blaw recommended that the developing gibbus during childhood be treated with an appropriate spinal orthosis to prevent late complications of neurologic deficit as a result of the gibbus deformity. Bethem et al used a Milwaukee brace with kyphosis pads in four patients younger than 10 years; three of the four were successfully maintained in the brace.

Infections of the Spine

Before the use of antibiotics, the mortality rate from infections of the spine and contiguous tissues was 40% to 70%. Advances in chemotherapy over the past 40 years have dramatically altered the natural history of these serious diseases. Today spinal infections are relatively rare, accounting for only 2% to 4% of all osteomyelitis, and the major problems are delay in diagnosis and a long recovery period.

The mechanism of infection of the vertebral bodies and the intervertebral disks in children still is debated. The intervertebral disk of the embryo and the young child receives its nutrition by blood vessels from the surfaces of adjacent vertebral bodies. Blood vessels pass through the hyaline cartilage of the disk proper to permit perfusion of nutrients to the disk cartilage. These vessels gradually disappear with maturation of the vertebral body and disk. Coventry et al demonstrated that the intervertebral disk has this blood supply until the individual is 30 years of age. Subsequent studies of Wiley and Trueta, Hassler, and most recently Crock and Yoshizawa confirmed the absence of a blood supply to the intervertebral disk in the adult but the presence of a good blood supply at the periphery of the disk and in all other areas of the spine. Infection may begin in the vertebral body at any age, with secondary disk involvement.

That most infective agents of the vertebral body are hematogenous has long been recognized, but the precise anatomic pathway to the vertebra is controversial. The drainage system of the pelvis through the venous plexus of Batson has been postulated to be the primary reason for the high percentage of lumbar vertebral infections caused by urinary tract infections. Wiley and Trueta have shown that the arterial route to bone is more easily accessible than the venous route. They noted that vertebral osteomyelitis begins in the metaphyseal area of the vertebra close to the anterior longitudinal ligament and spreads quickly across the periphery of the disk to involve the metaphysis of the adjacent vertebra above. They believe this distribution suggests an arterial spread through ascending and descending nutrient branches of the posterior spinal arteries.

Although the vertebral metaphysis is the primary focus for septic deposits, the intervertebral disk can be a separate site of infection as shown by Kemp et al and Menelaus. Stauffer emphasizes the importance of distinguishing vertebral osteomyelitis from true disk space infection. In the former the disk space is involved secondarily as a result of a hematogenous seeding in the subchondral bone of the vertebral body after a bacteremia. Disk space infection, on the other hand, most commonly occurs after surgical excision of the disk.

PYOGENIC OSTEOMYELITIS

As described by Wenger et al, diskitis, intervertebral disk space infection, and vertebral osteomyelitis form a spectrum of disorders with a probable common bacterial cause. Symptomatic narrowing of the disk space in a child with associated fever and an elevated sedimentation rate is a well-recognized syndrome that has been described as diskitis, spondyloarthritis, nonspecific spondylitis, disk space inflammation, intervertebral disk space infection, benign osteomyelitis of the spine, and pyogenic vertebral osteomyelitis. Most authors believe that the cause is a bacterial infection, although some have suggested that the process is more likely traumatic. The largest series of patients with this syndrome (45 children) was reported by Spiegel et al. Based on their biopsy results, as well as those in the literature, they believe that infection is the most likely etiologic factor. Wenger et al, reporting on 41 children with disk space infections, also believe that the condition is infectious in origin. Most positive culture reports have implicated *Staphylococcus aureus* as the causative organism.

Clinical Findings

The mean age of onset in the series of Spiegel et al was 6 years and 5 months and in that of Wenger et al, 7 years and 6 months. The duration of symptoms before hospitalization was approximately 4 weeks. Wenger et al noted three distinct groups, according to the presenting symptoms. In younger children, mean age 22 months, the presenting complaint frequently was difficulty in walking or standing. The child usually had a fever and general malaise, often associated with upper respiratory infections that preceded the rather sudden inability to stand or walk comfortably. On examination, the child cried when held in a standing position. A high index of suspicion is necessary in this group of patients because physical findings that concern the back frequently are not noted. The diagnosis often is delayed because the initial work-up is oriented toward the neurologic system. Once the diagnosis is confirmed, either by bone scan or roentgenograms showing disk space narrowing, examination reveals localized back tenderness, decreased spine motion, and hamstring tightness.

In children slightly older (mean age 7.8 years) abdominal pain was the main presenting symptom. The usual history was of a gradual onset of pain radiating from the subchondral region to either the umbilicus or symphysis pubis. Because of the abdominal symptoms, the orthopaedic surgeon frequently is not consulted until an extensive diagnostic work-up has been performed. Once the condition has been discovered, the local spine symptoms become apparent.

The third group of children had back pain or abnormal posture of the back, or both. Because the primary complaints were localized to the back, the physical findings in the back were noted much earlier, including localized tenderness, decreased motion of the spine, loss of lumbar lordosis, and hamstring tightness. In older children the symptoms were less marked, and often the localized tenderness and decreased motion of the spine were barely perceptible.

Laboratory Findings

The only laboratory finding with a positive result usually is an elevated sedimentation rate. Blood cultures may be helpful early in the disease.

Roentgenographic Findings

In the early stages of the disease the results of plain roentgenograms frequently are negative. Later in the course of the disease the disk infection produces narrowing of the disk space, which can be seen roentgenographically.

A technetium bone scan should be obtained if a disk space infection is suspected and results of initial radiographs are negative (Fig. 10-158). The scan is particularly useful in young children who are unable to localize their symptoms and show minimal or negative roentgenographic findings. It may allow an earlier diagnosis and thus a more prompt initiation of therapy. Marked uptake of isotope is visible in the region of involvement.

Management

The primary treatment of pyogenic vertebral osteomyelitis in children is rest, either with bed rest or rigid immobilization in a plaster jacket. Spiegel et al and Boston et al do not recommend antibiotics unless the patient does not respond to immobilization or has persistent pain and spasm and a high erythrocyte sedimentation rate in spite of treatment. Wenger et al, on the other hand, recommend intravenous administration of cephalothin once the diagnosis has been confirmed and blood cultures have been performed. The child is placed at bed rest, and the antibiotic is continued intravenously until the patient can walk and move about comfortably. Oral antibiotics then are used for an additional 3 weeks. Whether the spine is immobilized on discharge is determined by the severity of symptoms. Wenger et al do not recommend immobilization for the young child who has responded to antibiotics and who walks and moves the spine comfortably. A plaster jacket or back brace may be needed, however, in older children, who tend to have a more protracted course of symptoms. Most studies have shown at long-term follow-up that patients are symptom free, with minimal residual roentgenographic changes. Spontaneous fusion occurs in approximately 25% of patients. Only rarely does residual pain dictate spinal fusion. Disk space aspiration is not recommended unless the patient does not improve with standard clinical care or if tuberculosis is suspected.

Aggressive surgical treatment of pyogenic vertebral osteomyelitis in children is rarely, if ever, needed.

Infantile Pyogenic Osteomyelitis

Eismont et al described vertebral osteomyelitis in infants and emphasized that the symptoms are different from those of children with diskitis. Infants with vertebral osteomyelitis are systemically ill. There is almost complete dissolution of the involved vertebral bodies, with either normal or nearly normal adjacent vertebral end plates. The syndrome occurs in infants younger than 6 months, and recurrence of the infection is common; thus a 3-month course of antibiotics is recommended, with parenteral antibiotics given for the first 3 weeks. No neurologic deficit developed in any of the infants in the series of Eismont et al despite a severe degree of bone destruction. Years later the roentgenographic appearance of these children's spines may be identical to that of congenital scoliosis with either anterior failure of segmentation or posterior hemivertebrae. Treatment is the same as for congenital kyphosis, with early bracing and early fusion for progressive kyphosis. Eismont et al reviewed 61 patients with vertebral osteomyelitis; paralysis did not develop in any patient younger than 37 years of age. Therefore they believe that youth offers some protection against the development of a neural deficit.

A

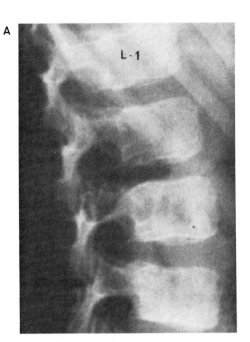

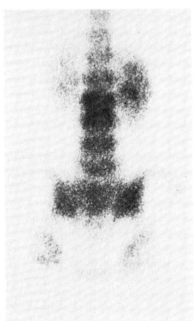

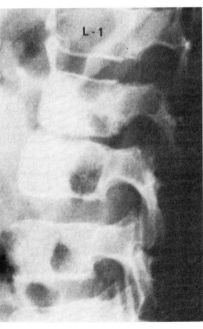

C

Fig. 10-158 **A,** Lateral roentgenogram of spine of 6-year-old girl with 2-week history of abdominal pain. **B,** Radioactive bone scan shows increased uptake in bodies of L2 and L3. **C,** Lateral roentgenogram 3 months later shows marked narrowing at level of disk space between L2 and L3. (From Wenger DR et al: J Bone Joint Surg 60A:100, 1978.)

TUBERCULOSIS

Tuberculosis of the spine is a granulomatous inflammation caused by *Mycobacterium tuberculosis*. It first was described by Sir Percivall Pott as a painful kyphotic deformity associated with paraplegia. It is a localized and destructive disease that usually is blood borne from a primary focus. In developed countries the disease is almost extinct, but in other parts of the world, especially Asia and Africa, it still is prevalent and most commonly affects children.

Pathogenesis

The infection usually begins in the cancellous bone of the vertebral body, eventually forming an abscess that spreads to involve two or more adjacent vertebrae by extension beneath the anterior longitudinal ligament or directly across the intervertebral disk (Fig. 10-159). The avascular vertebral bodies lose their mechanical stability and finally collapse, causing kyphosis.

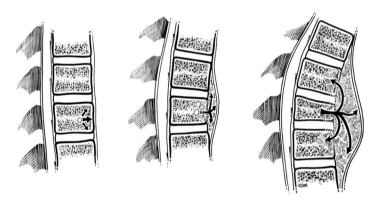

Fig. 10-159 Pathophysiology of vertebral body infection with *Mycobacterium tuberculosis* (see text).

Clinical Findings

The onset of symptoms usually is insidious. A history of a chronic illness with developing spinal symptoms, with or without neurologic involvement, is common, and afternoon or evening fever often is reported.

Physical examination reveals muscle spasm in the affected region of the spine and limited spinal motion. Spinal deformities, such as kyphosis, soft tissue masses, or draining sinuses, may be present. The neurologic examination is variable, depending on whether there is spinal cord involvement. Clonus is the most prominent early sign of developing Pott's paraplegia.

Roentgenographic Findings

The findings on the routine roentgenograms depend on the extent of involvement. A paravertebral abscess may be visible. Early in the disease the vertebral body exhibits loss of the bone trabecular pattern; later the intervertebral disk becomes narrowed and eventually totally obliterated. CT is valuable for detection of the extent of soft tissue spread.

Laboratory Findings

The diagnosis is confirmed by the growth of the causative organism in culture. Tuberculosis skin testing and sputum and gastric washings also are helpful. If a subcutaneous abscess is present, aspiration of the material is performed. Needle biopsy is dangerous in the thoracic spine because of the risk of hemorrhage, and open biopsy is preferable. If there is minimal bone involvement a costotransversectomy allows retrieval of material and drainage of the lesion. If there is extensive bone destruction, then anterolateral thoracotomy permits more adequate debridement and bone grafting.

Management

During the past few decades, treatment of tuberculosis of the spine has tended toward more radical surgery, although there have been many reports of successful treatment with drug therapy alone. After nearly 20 years of research following hundreds of patients, the Medical Research Council's Working Party on Tuberculosis of the Spine recommended surgical treatment whenever possible. The primary treatment of tuberculous spondylitis in children is medical. Only rarely is surgical debridement needed. The reader is referred to the work of Hodgson if surgery is deemed necessary.

REFERENCES

Infantile idiopathic scoliosis

Ceballos T et al: Prognosis in infantile idiopathic scoliosis, J Bone Joint Surg 62A:863, 1980.

Conner AN: Developmental anomalies and prognosis in infantile idiopathic scoliosis, J Bone Joint Surg 51B:711, 1969.

James JIP: Infantile idiopathic scoliosis, Clin Orthop 21:106, 1961.

James JIP: The management of infants with scoliosis, J Bone Joint Surg 57B:422, 1975.

James JIP, Lloyd-Roberts GC, and Pilcher, MF: Infantile structural scoliosis, J Bone Joint Surg 41B:719, 1959.

McMaster MJ and Macnicol MF: The management of progressive infantile idiopathic scoliosis, J Bone Joint Surg 61B:36, 1979.

Mehta MH: The rib-vertebra angle in the early diagnosis between resolving and progressive infantile scoliosis, J Bone Joint Surg 54B:230, 1972.

Moe JH et al: Harrington instrumentation without fusion plus external orthotic support for the treatment of difficult curvature problems in young children, Clin Orthop 185:35, 1984.

Morgan TH and Scott JC: Treatment of infantile idiopathic scoliosis, J Bone Joint Surg 38B:450, 1956.

Scott JC and Morgan TH: The natural history and prognosis of infantile idiopathic scoliosis, J Bone Joint Surg 37B:400, 1955.

Thompson SK and Bentley G: Prognosis in infantile idiopathic scoliosis, J Bone Joint Surg 62B:151, 1980.

Walker GF: An evaluation of an external splint for idiopathic structural scoliosis in infancy, J Bone Joint Surg 47B:524, 1965.

Wynne-Davies R: Infantile idiopathic scoliosis: causative factors, particularly in the first six months of life, J Bone Joint Surg 57B:138, 1975.

Juvenile idiopathic scoliosis

Figueiredo UM and James JIP: Juvenile idiopathic scoliosis, J Bone Joint Surg 63B:61, 1981.

Koop SE: Infantile and juvenile idiopathic scoliosis, Orthop Clin North Am 19:331, 1988.

Tolo VT and Gillespie R: The characteristics of juvenile idiopathic scoliosis and results of its treatment, J Bone Joint Surg 60B:181, 1978.

Incidence and natural history of adolescent idiopathic scoliosis

Ascani E et al: Natural history of untreated idiopathic scoliosis after skeletal maturity, Spine 11:784, 1986.

Brooks HL et al: Scoliosis: a perspective epidemiological study, J Bone Joint Surg 57A:968, 1975.

Bunnell WP: A study of the natural history of idiopathic scoliosis. Paper presented at the 19th Annual Meeting of the Scoliosis Research Society, Orlando, Fla, 1984.

Bunnell WP: The natural history of idiopathic scoliosis before skeletal maturity, Spine, 11:773, 1986.

Bunnell WP: The natural history of idiopathic scoliosis, Clin Orthop 229:20, 1988.

Bjure J and Nachemson A: Non-treated scoliosis, Clin Orthop 93:44, 1973.

Collis DK and Ponseti IV: Long-term follow-up of patients with idiopathic scoliosis not treated surgically, J Bone Joint Surg 51A:425, 1969.

Dickson RA: Scoliosis in the community, Br Med J 286:615, 1983.

Dickson RA et al: School screening for scoliosis: cohort study of clinical course, B Med J 281:265, 1980.

Kane WJ: Scoliosis prevalence: a call for statement of terms, Clin Orthop 126:43, 1977.

Kane WJ and Moe JH: A scoliosis-prevalence survey in Minnesota, Clin Orthop 69:216, 1970.

Lonstein JE: Screening for spinal deformities in Minnesota schools, Clin Orthop 126:33, 1977.

Lonstein JE: Natural history and school screening for scoliosis, Orthop Clin North Am 19:227, 1988.

Lonstein JE et al: Voluntary school screening for scoliosis in Minnesota, J Bone Joint Surg 64A:481, 1982.

Nachemson A: A long-term follow-up study of nontreated scoliosis, Acta Orthop Scand 39:466, 1968.

Nachemson A: A long-term follow-up study of nontreated scoliosis, J Bone Joint Surg 50A:203, 1969.

Nilsonne U and Lundgren KD: Long-term prognosis in idiopathic scoliosis, Acta Orthop Scand 39:456, 1968.

Picault C et al: Natural history of idiopathic scoliosis in girls and boys, Spine 11:777, 1986.

Renshaw TS: Screening school children for scoliosis, Clin Orthop 229:26, 1988.

Rogala EH, Drummond DS, and Gurr J: Scoliosis: incidence and natural history—a prospective epidemiological study, J Bone Joint Surg 60A:173, 1978.

Shands AR and Eisberg HB: The incidence of scoliosis in the state of Delaware: a study of 50,000 minifilms of the chest made during a survey for tuberculosis, J Bone Joint Surg 37A:1243, 1955.

Weinstein SL: Idiopathic scoliosis: natural history, Spine 11:780, 1986.

Weinstein SL and Ponseti IV: Curve progression in idiopathic scoliosis, J Bone Joint Surg 65A:447, 1983.

Weinstein SL, Zavala DC, and Ponseti IV: Idiopathic scoliosis: long-term follow-up and prognosis in untreated patients, J Bone Joint Surg 63A:702, 1981.

Willner S: Prospective prevalence study of scoliosis in southern Sweden, Acta Orthop Scand 53:233, 1982.

Patient evaluation in idiopathic scoliosis

Aaro S and Dahlborn M: Vertebral rotation: estimation of vertebral rotation and spinal and rib cage deformity in scoliosis by computerized tomography, Spine 6:460, 1981.

Binstadt DH, Lonstein JE, and Winter RB: Radiographic evaluation of the scoliotic patient, Minn Med 61:474, 1978.

Board R: Radiography of the scoliotic spine, Radiol Technol 38:219, 1967.

Bunnell WP: Vertebral rotation: a simple method of measurement in routine radiographs, Orthop Trans 9:114, 1985.

Cobb JR: Outline for the study of scoliosis in instructional course lectures. In The American Academy of Orthopaedic Surgeons: Instructional course lectures, vol 5, Ann Arbor, Mich, 1948, JW Edwards Co.

DeSmet A, Fritz SL, and Asher MA: A method for minimizing the radiation exposure from scoliosis radiographs, J Bone Joint Surg 63A:156, 1981.

DeSmet A et al: A clinical study of the differences between the scoliotic angles measured on the PA versus the AP radiographs, J Bone Joint Surg 64A:489, 1982.

Drummond D et al: Radiation hazards and scoliosis management, Spine 8:741, 1983.

Farren J: Routine radiographic assessment of the scoliotic spine, Radiography 47:92, 1981.

Ferguson AB: Roentgen interpretations and decisions in scoliosis. In The American Academy of Orthopaedic Surgeons: Instructional course lectures, vol 7, Ann Arbor, Mich, 1950, JW Edwards Co.

Gray JE, Hoffman AE, and Peterson HA: Reduction of radiation exposure during radiography for scoliosis, J Bone Joint Surg 65A:5, 1983.

Hopkins R, Grundy M, and Sherr-Mehl M: X-ray filters in scoliosis x-rays, Orthop Trans 8:148, 1984.

James JIP: Idiopathic scoliosis: the prognosis, diagnosis, and operative indication related to curve patterns and the age at onset, J Bone Joint Surg 36B:36, 1954.

Kleinman RE et al: A radiographic assessment of spinal flexibility in scoliosis, Clin Orthop 162:47, 1982.

Lonstein JE and Carlson JM: The prediction of curve progression in untreated idiopathic scoliosis during growth, J Bone Joint Surg 66A:1061, 1984.

Marshall WA and Tanner JM: Variations in pattern of pubertal changes in girls, Arch Dis Child 44:291, 1969.

Marshall WA and Tanner JM: Variation in pattern of pubertal changes in boys Arch Dis Child 45:13, 1970.

McAlister W and Shackelford G: Measurement of spinal curvatures, Radiol Clin North Am 13:113, 1975.

Mehta MH: Radiographic estimation of vertebral rotation in scoliosis, J Bone Joint Surg 55B:513, 1973.

Nash CL et al: Risk of exposure to x-rays in patients undergoing long term treatment for scoliosis, J Bone Joint Surg 61A:371, 1979.

Nash C and Moe J: A study of vertebral rotation, J Bone Joint Surg 51A:223, 1969.

Ponseti IV and Friedman B: Prognosis in idiopathic scoliosis, J Bone Joint Surg 32A:381, 1950.

Risser JC: Important practical facts in the treatment of scoliosis. In The American Academy of Orthopaedic Surgeons: Instructional course lectures, vol 5, Ann Arbor, Mich, 1948, JW Edwards Co.

Risser JC: The iliac apophysis: an invaluable sign in the management of scoliosis, Clin Orthop 11:111, 1958.

Risser JC and Ferguson AB: Scoliosis: its prognosis, J Bone Joint Surg 18:667, 1936.

Stagnara P: Examen du scoliotique. In Deviations laterales du rachis: scolioses, Encyclopedie mediocochirurgicale, vol 7, Paris, 1974, Appareil Locomoteur.

Nonsurgical management

Aaro S, Burstrom R, and Dahlborn M: The derotating affect of the Boston brace: a comparison between computer tomography and a conventional method, Spine 6:477, 1981.

Anderson S and Bradford DS: Low-profile halo, Clin Orthop 103:72, 1974.

Andriacchi TP et al: Milwaukee brace correction of idiopathic scoliosis: a biomechanical analysis and a retrospective study, J Bone Joint Surg 58A:806, 1976.

Apter A et al: The psychological sequelae of the Milwaukee brace in adolescent girls, Clin Orthop 131:156, 1978.

Axelgaard J and Brown JC: Lateral electrode surface stimulation for the treatment of progressive idiopathic scoliosis, Spine 8:242, 1983.

Bancel P et al: The Boston brace: results of a clinical and radiologic study of 401 patients, Orthop Trans 8:33, 1984.

Benson DR, Wolf AW, and Shoji, H: Can the Milwaukee patient participate in competitive athletics? Am J Sports Med 5:7, 1977.

Bjerkreim I, Carlsen B, and Korsell E: Preoperative Cotrel traction in idiopathic scoliosis, Acta Orthop Scand 53:901, 1982.

Blount WP, Schmidt AC, and Bidwell RG: Making the Milwaukee brace, J Bone Joint Surg 40A:526, 1958.

Blount WP et al: Milwaukee brace and the operative treatment of scoliosis, J Bone Joint Surg 40A:511, 1958.

Bradford DS, Tanguy A, and Vanselow J: Surface electrical stimulation in the treatment of idiopathic scoliosis: preliminary results in 30 patients, Spine 8:757, 1983.

Bunnell WP: Treatment of idiopathic scoliosis, Orthop Clin North Am 10:813, 1979.

Bunnell WP: Non-operative of spinal deformity: the case for observation. In The American Academy of Orthopaedic Surgeons: Instructional course lectures, vol 34, St Louis, 1985, The CV Mosby Co.

Carr WA et al: Treatment of idiopathic scoliosis in the Milwaukee brace, J Bone Joint Surg 62A:599, 1980.

Clark JA, Hsu LC, and Yau AC: Viscoelastic behavior of deformed spines under correction with halo-pelvic distraction, Clin Orthop 110:90, 1975.

Cochran T and Nachemson A: Long-term anatomic and functional changes in patients with adolescent idiopathic scoliosis treated with the Milwaukee brace, Spine 10:27, 1985.

Cummine JL et al: Reconstructive surgery in the adult for failed scoliosis fusion, J Bone Joint Surg 61A:1151, 1979.

DeWald RL, Mulcahy TM, and Schultz AB: Force measurement studies with the halo-hoop apparatus in scoliosis Orthop Rev 2:17, 1973.

DeWald RL and Ray RD: Skeletal traction for the treatment of severe scoliosis: the University of Illinois halo-hoop apparatus, J Bone Joint Surg 52A:233, 1970.

Dove J, Hsu LC, and Yau AC: The cervical spine after halo-pelvic traction: an analysis of the complications of 83 patients, J Bone Joint Surg 62B:158, 1980.

Edgar MA, Chapman RH, and Glasgow MM: Preoperative correction in adolescent idiopathic scoliosis, J Bone Joint Surg 64A:530, 1982.

Edmonson AS and Morris JT: Follow-up study of Milwaukee brace treatment in patients with idiopathic scoliosis, Clin Orthop 126:58, 1977.

Edmonson AS and Smith GR: Long-term follow-up study of Milwaukee brace treatment in patients with idiopathic scoliosis. Proceedings of the Scoliosis Research Society, Denver, Sept 22-29, 1982.

Fallstrom K, Cochran T, and Nachemson A: Long-term affects on personality development in patient with adolescent idiopathic scoliosis: influence of type of treatment, Spine 11:756, 1986.

Galante J et al: Forces acting in the Milwaukee brace on patients undergoing treatment for idiopathic scoliosis, J Bone Joint Surg 52A:498, 1970.

Hall JE et al: Boston brace system treatment of idiopathic scoliosis: follow-up in 400 patients finished treatment, Orthop Trans 8:148, 1983.

Hassan J and Bjerkreim I: Progression in idiopathic scoliosis after conservative treatment, Acta Orthop Scand 54:88, 1983.

Houtkin S and Levine DB: The halo yoke: a simplified device for attachment of the halo to a body cast, J Bone Joint Surg 54A:881, 1972.

Humbyrd DE et al: Brain abscess as a complication of halo traction, Spine 6:364, 1981.

Jonassen-Rajala E et al: Boston thoracic brace in the treatment of idiopathic scoliosis, Clin Orthop 183:37, 1984.

Kahanovitz N, Levine DB, and Lardone J: The part-time Milwaukee brace treatment of juvenile idiopathic scoliosis: long-term follow-up, Clin Orthop 167:145, 1982.

Kahanovitz N and Weiser S: LESS compliance in adolescent female scoliosis patients. Procedings of the Scoliosis Research Society, Coronado, Calif, 1985.

Kalamchi A et al: Halo-pelvic distraction apparatus: an analysis of 150 consecutive patients, J Bone Joint Surg 58A:1119, 1976.

Kazarian LE: Creep characteristics of the human spinal column, Orthop Clin North Am 6:3, 1975.

Kehl OK and Morrissy RT: Brace treatment in adolescent idiopathic scoliosis: an update on concepts and technique, Clin Orthop 229:34, 1988.

Keiser RP and Shufflebarger HL: The Milwaukee brace in idiopathic scoliosis: evaluation of 123 completed cases, Clin Orthop 118:19, 1976.

Kuhn RA and Garrett A: The halo in the management of cervical spine lesions, Orthop Rev 1:25, 1972.

Laurnen EL, Tupper JW, and Mullen MP: The Boston brace in thoracic scoliosis: a preliminary report, Spine 8:388, 1983.

Leider LL Jr, Moe JH, and Winter RB: Early ambulation after the surgical treatment of idiopathic scoliosis, J Bone Joint Surg 55A:1003, 1973.

Leslie IJ et al: A prospective study of deep vein thrombosis of the leg in children on halo-femoral traction, J Bone Joint Surg 63B:168, 1981.

Letts RM, Palakar G, and Bobechko WP: Preoperative skeletal traction in scoliosis, J Bone Joint Surg 57A:616, 1975.

Lindh M: The affect of sagittal curve changes on brace correction of idiopathic scoliosis, Spine 5:26, 1980.

Lonstein JE: Cast techniques. In Bradford DS et al, editors: Moe's textbook of scoliosis and other spinal deformities, Philadelphia, 1987, WB Sanders Co.

Lonstein JE and Winter RB: Adolescent idiopathic scoliosis: nonoperative treatment, Orthop Clin North Am 19:239, 1988.

McCollough NC et al: Miami TLSO in the management of scoliosis: preliminary results from 100 cases, J Pediatr Orthop 1:141, 1981.

Mellencamp DD, Bount WP, and Anderson AJ: Milwaukee brace treatment of idiopathic scoliosis: late results, Clin Orthop 126:47, 1977.

Miller JAA, Nachemson AL, and Schultz AB: Effectiveness of braces in mild idiopathic scoliosis, Spine 9:632, 1984.

Moe JH: Methods of correction and surgical techniques in scoliosis, Orthop Clin North Am 3:17, 1972.

Moe JH and Kettleson DN: Idiopathic scoliosis, J Bone Joint Surg 52A:1509, 1970.

Mulcahy T et al: A follow-up study of forces acting on the Milwaukee brace on patients undergoing treatment for idiopathic scoliosis, Clin Orthop 93:53, 1973.

Nachemson AL and Nordwall A: Effectiveness of preoperative Cotrel traction for idiopathic scoliosis, J Bone Joint Surg 59A:504, 1977.

Nachemson AL et al: Somatic, social and psychologic effects of treatment for idiopathic scoliosis, Orthop Trans 7:508, 1983.

Nash CL: Current concepts review: scoliosis bracing, J Bone Joint Surg 62A:848, 1980.

Nickel VL et al: The halo: a spinal skeletal traction fixation device, J Bone Joint Surg 50A:1400, 1968.

O'Brien JP: The halo-pelvic apparatus: a clinical, bio-engineering, and anatomical study, Acta Orthop Scand 163(suppl), 1975.

O'Brien JP, Yau AC, and Hodgson AR: Halo-pelvic traction: a technic for severe spinal deformities, Clin Orthop 93:179, 1973.

O'Brien JP et al: Halo-pelvic traction: a preliminary report on a method of external skeletal fixation for correcting deformities and maintaining fixation of the spine, J Bone Joint Surg 53B:217, 1971.

O'Donnell CS et al: Electrical stimulation in the treatment of idiopathic scoliosis, Clin Orthop 229:107, 1988.

Park J et al: A modified brace (prenyl) for scoliosis, Clin Orthop 126:67, 1977.

Perry J: The halo in spinal abnormalities: practical factors and avoidance of complications, Orthop Clin North Am 3:69, 1972.

Perry J and Nickel VL: Total cervical-spine fusion for neck paralysis, J Bone Joint Surg 41A:37, 1959.

Pieron AP and Welply WR: Halo traction, J Bone Joint Surg 52B:119, 1970.

Ransford AO and Manning CW: Complications of halo-pelvic distraction for scoliosis, J Bone Joint Surg 57A:131, 1975.

Renshaw TS: Orthotic treatment of idiopathic scoliosis and kyphosis. In The American Academy of Orthopaedic Surgeons: Instructional course lectures, vol 34, St Louis, 1985, The CV Mosby Co.

Risser JC: The application of body casts for the correction of scoliosis. In The American Academy of Orthopaedic Surgeons: Instructional course lectures, vol 12, Ann Arbor, Mich, 1955, JW Edwards Co.

Risser JC: Plaster body-jackets, Am J Orthop 3:19, 1961.

Risser JC et al: Three types of body casts. In The American Academy of Orthopaedic Surgeons: Instructional course lectures, vol 10, Ann Arbor, Mich, 1953, JW Edwards Co.

Rudicel S and Renshaw TS: The effect of the Milwaukee brace on spinal decompensation in idiopathic scoliosis, Spine 8:385, 1983.

Schmidt AC: Halo-tibial traction combined with Milwaukee brace, Clin Orthop 77:73, 1971.

Schultz A, Haderspeck K, and Takashima S: Correction of scoliosis by muscle stimulation: biomechanical analyses, Spine 6:468, 1981.

Swank SM, Winter RB, and Moe JH: Scoliosis and cor pulmonale, Spine 7:343, 1982.

Toledo LC, Toledo CH, and MacEwen GD: Halo traction with the circolectric bed in the treatment of severe spinal deformities: a preliminary report, J Pediatr Orthop 2:554, 1982.

Tredwell SJ and O'Brien JP: Avascular necrosis of the proximal end of the dens: a complication of halo-pelvic distraction, J Bone Joint Surg 57A:332, 1975.

Uden A and Willner S: The effect of lumbar flexion and Boston thoracic brace on the curves in idiopathic scoliosis, Spine 8:846, 1983.

Watts HG: Bracing spinal deformities, Orthop Clin North Am 10:769, 1979.

Watts HG, Hall JE, and Stanish W: The Boston brace system for the treatment of low thoracic and lumbar scoliosis by the use of a girdle without superstructure, Clin Orthop 126:87, 1977.

White AA and Panjabi MM: The clinical biomechanics of scoliosis, Clin Orthop 118:100, 1976.

Wickers F, Bunch W, and Barnett P: Psychological factors in failure to wear the Milwaukee brace for treatment of idiopathic scoliosis, Clin Orthop 126:62, 1977.

Wilkins C and MacEwen GD: Halo-traction affecting cranial nerves, J Bone Joint Surg 56A:1540, 1974.

Wilkins C and MacEwen GD: Cranial nerve injury from halo traction, Clin Orthop 126:106, 1977.

Willner S: Effect of the Boston thoracic brace on the frontal and sagittal curves of the spine, Acta Orthop Scand 55:457, 1984.

Winter RB and Carlson JM: Modern orthotics for spinal deformities, Clin Orthop 126:74, 1977.

Winter RB and Moe JH: Orthotics for spinal deformity, Clin Orthop 102:72, 1974.

Young R and Thomassen EH: Step-by-step procedure by applying halo ring, Orthop Rev 3:62, 1974.

Zwerling MT and Riggins RS: Use of the halo apparatus in acute injuries of the cervical spine, Surg Gynecol Obstet 138:189, 1974.

Surgical treatment of idiopathic scoliosis

Aaro S and Dahlborn M: The effect of Harrington instrumentation on the longitudinal axis rotation of the apical vertebra and on the spinal and rib-cage deformity and idiopathic scoliosis studied by computer tomography, Spine 7:456, 1982.

Aaro S and Ohlen G: The effect of Harrington instrumentation on the sagital configuration and mobility of the spine in scoliosis, Spine 8:570, 1983.

Akbarnia BA: Selection of methodology in surgical treatment of adolescent idiopathic scoliosis, Orthop Clin North Am 19:319, 1988.

Allen BL Jr: The place for segmental instrumentation in the treatment of spine deformity, Orthop Trans 6:21, 1982.

Allen BL Jr: Segmental spinal instrumentation. In The American Academy of Orthopaedic Surgeons: Instructional course lectures, vol 32, St Louis, 1983, The CV Mosby Co.

Allen BL Jr and Ferguson RL: The Galveston technique for L-rod instrumentation of the scoliotic spine, Spine 7:119, 1982.

Allen BL Jr and Ferguson RL: Neurologic injuries with the Galveston technique of L-rod instrumentation for scoliosis, Spine 11:14, 1986.

Allen BL Jr and Ferguson RL: A 1988 perspective on the Galveston technique of pelvic fixation, Orthop Clin North Am 19:409, 1988.

Allen BL Jr and Ferguson RL: The Galveston experience with L-rod instrumentation for adolescent idiopathic scoliosis, Clin Orthop 229:59, 1988.

Arkin AM: Correction of structural changes in scoliosis by corrective plaster jackets and prolonged recumbency, J Bone Joint Surg 46A:33, 1964.

Armstrong GWD and Connock SHG: A transverse loading system applied to a modified Harrington instrumentation, Clin Ortho 108:70, 1975.

Aurori BF et al: Pseudarthrosis after spinal fusion for scoliosis: a comparison of autogeneic and allogenic bone grafts, Clin Orthop 199:153, 1985.

Bailey TE and Mahoney OM: The use of banked autologous blood in patients undergoing surgery for spinal deformity, J Bone Joint Surg 69A:329, 1987.

Baily RW and Badgley CE: Stabilization of the cervical spine by anterior fusion, J Bone Joint Surg 42A:565, 1960.

Barnes J: Rib resection in infantile idiopathic scoliosis, J Bone Joint Surg 61B:31, 1979.

Ben-David B: Spinal cord monitoring, Orthop Clin North Am 19:427, 1988.

Bennett SH, Hoye RC, and Riggle GC: Intra-operative autotransfusion: preliminary report of a new blood suction device for anticoagulation of autologous blood, Am J Surg 123:257, 1972.

Bernard TN et al: Late complications due to wire breakage in segmental spinal instrumentation, J Bone Joint Surg 65A:1339, 1983.

Bieber E, Tolo V, and Uematsu S: Spinal cord monitoring during posterior spinal instrumentation and fusion, Clin Orthop 229:121, 1988.

Birch JG et al: Cotrell-Dubousset instrumentation in idiopathic scoliosis: a preliminary report, Clin Orthop 227:24, 1988.

Bradford DS: Anterior spinal surgery in the management of scoliosis: indications, techniques, results, Orthop Clin North Am 10:801, 1979.

Bradford DS: Anterior vascular pedicle bone grafting for the treatment of kyphosis, Spine 5:318, 1980.

Bradford DS: Techniques of surgery. In Bradford DS et al, editors: Moe's textbook of scoliosis and other spinal deformities, Philadelphia, 1987, WB Sanders Co.

Bradford DS et al: Techniques of anterior spine surgery for the management of kyphosis, Clin Orthop 128:129, 1977.

Bradford DS et al: Anterior strut grafting for the treatment of kyphosis, J Bone Joint Surg 64A:680, 1982.

Bradshaw K, Webb JK, and Faser AM: Clinical evaluation of spinal cord monitoring in scoliosis surgery, Spine 9:636, 1984.

Broadstone T: Consider post-operative immobilization of double-L-rod SSI patients, Orthop Trans 8:171, 1984.

Brown RH and Nash CL Jr: Current status of spinal cord monitoring, Spine 4:466, 1979.

Burrington JD et al: Anterior approach to the thoracolumbar spine: technical considerations, Arch Surg: 111:456, 1976.

Butte FL: Scoliosis treated by the wedging jacket: selection of the area to be fused, J Bone Joint Surg 20:1, 1938.

Cloward RB: The anterior approach for ruptured cervical discs, J Neurosurg 15:602, 1958.

Cobb JR: The treatment of scoliosis, Conn Med J 7:467, 1943.

Cobb JR: Technique, after-treatment, and results of spine fusion for scoliosis. In The American Academy of Orthopaedic Surgeons: Instructional course lectures, vol 9, Ann Arbor, Mich, 1952, JW Edwards Co.

Cobb JR: Spine arthrodesis in the treatment of scoliosis, Bull Hosp J Dis Orthop Inst 19:187, 1958.

Cobb JR: The problem of the primary curve, J Bone Joint Surg 42A:1413, 1960.

Cochran T, Irstam L, and Nachemson A: Long-term anatomic and function changes in patients with adolescent idiopathic scoliosis treated by Harrington rod fusions, Spine 8:576, 1983.

Cook CD et al: Pulmonary physiology in children. III. Lung volumes, mechanics of respiration and respiratory muscle strength in scoliosis, J Pediatr 25:766, 1960.

Cook WA: Transthoracic vertebral surgery, Ann Thorac Surg 12:54, 1971.

Cotrel Y and Dubousset J: New segmental posterior instrumentation of the spine, Orthop Trans 9:118, 1985.

Cotrel Y, Dubousset J, and Guillaumat M: New universal instrumentation and spinal surgery, Clin Orthop 227:10, 1988.

Cowell HR and Swickard JW: Autotransfusion in children's orthopaedics, J Bone Joint Surg 56A:908, 1974.

Dawson EG, Moe JH, and Caron A: Surgical measurement of scoliosis in the adult: Scoliosis Research Society–1972, J Bone Joint Surg 55A:437, 1973.

Denis F: Cotrel-Dubousset instrumentation in the treatment of idiopathic scoliosis, Orthop Clin North Am 19:291, 1988.

DeWald RL: New trends in the operative treatment of scoliosis. In Ahstrom JP Jr, editor: Current practices in orthopaedic surgery, vol 5, St Louis, 1973, The CV Mosby Co.

Dickson JH: Spinal instrumentation and fusion in adolescent idiopathic scoliosis: indications and surgical techniques, Contemp Orthop 4:397, 1982.

Dickson JH and Harrington PR: The evolution of the Harrington instrumentation technique in scoliosis, J Bone Joint Surg 55A:993, 1973.

Dolan JA and MacEwen GD: Surgical treatment of scoliosis, Clin Orthop 76:125, 1971.

Dommisse GG: The blood supply of the spinal cord, J Bone Joint Surg 56B:225, 1974.

Donaldson WF Jr and Wissinger HA: The results of surgical exploration of spine fusion performed for scoliosis, West J Surg Obstet Gynecol 72:195, 1964.

Dorang LA, Klebanoff G, and Kemmerer WT: Autotransfusion in long-segment spinal fusion: an experimental model to demonstrate the efficacy of salvaging blood contaminated with bone fragments and marrow, Am J Surg 123:686, 1972.

Dove J et al: Aortic aneurysm complicating spinal fixation with Dwyer's apparatus: report of a case, Spine 6:524, 1981.

Drummond DS: Harrington instrumentation with spinous process wiring for idiopathic scoliosis, Orthop Clin North Am 19:281, 1988.

Drummond DS, Keene JS, and Breed A: The Wisconsin system: a technique of interspinous segmental spinal instrumentation, Contemp Orthop 8:29, 1984.

Drummond D et al: Wisconsin segmental spinal instrumentation, Orthop Trans 6:22, 1982.

Drummond D et al: Interspinous process segmental spinal instrumentation, J Pediatr Orthop 4:397, 1984.

Dunn HK: Spinal instrumentation. I. Principles of posterior and anterior instrumentation. In The American Academy of Orthopaedic Surgeons: Instructional course lectures, vol 32, St Louis, 1983, The CV Mosby Co.

Dunn HK and Bolstad KE: Fixation of Dwyer screws for the treatment of scoliosis: a postmortem study, J Bone Joint Surg 59A:54, 1977.

Dwyer AF: Experience of anterior correction of scoliosis, Clin Orthop 93:191, 1973.

Dwyer AF, Newton NC, and Sherwood AA: An anterior approach to scoliosis: a preliminary report, Clin Orthop 62:192, 1969.

Dwyer AP et al: The late complications after the Dwyer anterior spinal instrumentation for scoliosis, J Bone Joint Surg 59B:117, 1977.

Engler GL et al: Somatosensory evoked potentials during Harrington instrumentation for scoliosis, J Bone Joint Surg 60A:528, 1978.

Erwin WD, Dickson JH, and Gaines JH III: Utilization of Harrington spinal instrumentation and fusion for scoliosis, Surgical technique, Zimmer, 1986.

Erwin WD, Dickson JH, and Harrington PR: The postoperative management of scoliosis patients treated with Harrington instrumentation and fusion, J Bone Joint Surg 58A:479, 1976.

Evarts CM, Winter RB, and Hall JE: Vascular compression of the duodeum associated with the treatment of scoliosis, J Bone Joint Surg 53A:431, 1971.

Farcy J, Weidenbaum M, and Roye DP Jr: Correction of thoracic scoliosis using the Cotrel-Dubousset technique, Surg Rounds Orthop 1:11, 1987.

Ferguson RL and Allen BL Jr: Segmental spinal instrumentation for routine scoliotic curve, Contemp Orthop 2:450, 1980.

Flynn JC and Hoque A: Anterior fusion of the lumbar spine: end-results study with long-term follow-up, J Bone Joint Surg 61A:143, 1979.

Fraser RD: A wide muscle-splitting approach to the lumbosacral spine, J Bone Joint Surg 64B:44, 1982.

Freebody D, Bendall R, and Taylor RD: Anterior transperitoneal lumbar fusion, J Bone Joint Surg 53B:617, 1971.

Gaines RW Jr and Abernathie DL: Mersilene tapes as a substitute for wire in segmental spinal instrumentation for children, Spine 11:907, 1986.

Gaines RW, McKinley LM, and Leatherman KD: Effect of the Harrington compression system on the correction of the rib hump in spinal instrumentation for idiopathic scoliosis, Spine 6:489, 1981.

Gaines RW Jr, York DH, and Watts C: Identification of spinal cord pathways responsible for the peroneal-evoked response in the dog, Spine 9:810, 1984.

Galeazzi R: The treatment of scoliosis, J Bone Joint Surg 11:81, 1929.

Gardner RC: Blood loss after spinal instrumentation and fusion in scoliosis (Harrington procedure): results using a radioactive tracer and an electronic blood volume computer: preliminary report, Clin Orthop 71:182, 1970.

Gazioglu K et al: Pulmonary function in idiopathic scoliosis: comparative evaluation before and after orthopaedic correction, J Bone Joint Surg 50A:1391, 1968.

Goldstein LA: Results in the treatment of scoliosis with turnbuckle plaster cast correction and fusion, J Bone Joint Surg 41A:321, 1959.

Goldstein LA: The surgical management of scoliosis, Clin Orthop 35:95, 1964.

Goldstein LA: Surgical management of scoliosis, J Bone Joint Surg 48A:167, 1966.

Goldstein LA: Treatment of idiopathic scoliosis by Harrington instrumentation and fusion with fresh autogenous iliac bone grafts: results in eighty patients, J Bone Joint Surg 51A:209, 1969.

Goldstein LA: The surgical management of scoliosis, Clin Orthop 77:32, 1971.

Goldstein LA: The surgical treatment of idiopathic scoliosis, Clin Orthop 93:131, 1973.

Goldstein LA and Everts CM: Further experiences with the treatment of scoliosis by cast correction and spine fusion with fresh autogenous iliac-bone grafts, J Bone Joint Surg 48A:962, 1966.

Gollehon D, Kahanovitz N, and Happel LT: Temperature effects on the feline cortical and spinal evoked potentials, Spine 8:443, 1983.

Guadagni J, Drummond D, and Breed A: Improved post-operative course following modified segmental instrumentation and posterior spinal fusion for idiopathic scoliosis, J Pediatr Orthop 4:405, 1984.

Hall JE: The anterior approach to spinal deformities, Orthop Clin North Am 3:81, 1972.

Hall JE: Pre-operative assessment of the patient with a spinal deformity. In The American Academy of Orthopaedic Surgeons: Instructional course lectures, vol 34, St Louis, 1985, The CV Mosby Co.

Hall JE, Levine CR, and Sudhir KG: Intraoperative awakening to monitor spinal cord function during Harrington instrumentation and spine fusion: descriptions of procedure and report of three cases, J Bone Joint Surg 60A:533, 1978.

Hallock H, Francis KC, and Jones JB: Spine fusion in young children, J Bone Joint Surg 39A:41, 1957.

Harmon PC: Results from the treatment of sciatica due to lumbar disc protrusion, Am J Surg 80:829, 1950.

Harrington PR: Surgical instrumentation for management of scoliosis, J Bone Joint Surg 42A:1448, 1960.

Harrington PR: Treatment of scoliosis: correction and internal fixation by spine instrumentation, J Bone Joint Surg 44A:591, 1962.

Harrington PR: The management of scoliosis by spine instrumentation: an evaluation of more than two hundred cases, South Med J 56:1367, 1963.

Harrington PR: Technical details in relation to the successful use of instrumentation in scoliosis, Orthop Clin North Am 3:49, 1972.

Harrington PR: The history and development of Harrington instrumentation, Clin Orthop 93:110, 1973.

Harrington PR and Dickson JH: An eleven-year clinical investigation of Harrington instrumentation: a preliminary report of 578 cases, Clin Orthop 93:113, 1973.

Heilbronner DM and Sussman MD: Early mobilization of adolescent scoliosis patients following Wisconsin interspinous segmental instrumentation as an adjunct to Harrington distraction instrumentation, Clin Orthop 229:52, 1988.

Herndon WA et al: Segmental spinal instrumentation with sublamina wires: a critical appraisal, J Bone Joint Surg 69A:851, 1987.

Herring JA and Wenger DR: Early complications of segmental spinal instrumentation, Orthop Trans 6:22, 1982.

Herring JA and Wenger DR: Segmental spinal instrumentation: a preliminary report of 40 consecutive cases, Spine 7:285, 1982.

Hibbs RA: An operation for progressive spinal deformities, NY Med J 93:1013, 1911.

Hibbs RA: A report of 59 cases of scoliosis treated by the fusion operation, J Bone Joint Surg 6:3, 1924.

Hibbs RA, Risser JC, and Ferguson AB: Scoliosis treated by the fusion operation, J Bone Joint Surg 13:91, 1931.

Hodgson AR and Stock FE: Anterior spine fusion, Br J Surg 44:266, 1956.

Hodgson AR et al: Anterior spine fusion, Br J Surg 48:172, 1960.

Hsu LCS et al: Dwyer instrumentation in the treatment of adolescent idiopathic scoliosis, J Bone Joint Surg 64B:536, 1982.

Jackson JW: Surgical approaches to the anterior aspect of the spinal column, Ann R Coll Surg Engl 48:83, 1971.

James JIP: Two curve patterns in idiopathic structural scoliosis, J Bone Joint Surg 33B:399, 1951.

Johnson BE and Westgate HD: Methods of predicting vital capacity in patients with thoracic scoliosis, J Bone Joint Surg 52A:1433, 1970.

Johnson RM and McGuire EJ: Urogenital complications of anterior approaches to the lumbar spine, Clin Orthop 154:114, 1981.

Johnston CE, Ashman RB, and Sherman MC: Mechanical consequences of rod contouring and residual scoliosis in sublamina pelvic SSI, Orthop Trans 10:5, 1986.

Johnston CE et al: Delayed paraplegia complicating sublamina segmental spinal instrumentation, J Bone Joint Surg 68A:556, 1986.

Jones SJ et al: A system for the electrophysiological monitoring of the spinal cord during operations for scoliosis, J Bone Joint Surg 65B:134, 1983.

Kaneda K, Fujiya N, and Satoh S: Results with Zielke instrumentation for idiopathic thoracolumbar and lumbar scoliosis, Clin Orthop 205:195, 1986.

King HA: Selection of fusion levels for posterior instrumentation and fusion in idiopathic scoliosis, Orthop Clin North Am 19:247, 1988.

King HA et al: The selection of the fusion levels in thoracic idiopathic scoliosis, J Bone Joint Surg 65A:1302, 1983.

Kleinberg S: A survey of structural scoliosis: the principles of treatment and their application. In The American Academy of Orthopaedic Surgeons: Instructional course lectures, vol 7, Ann Arbor, Mich, 1950, JW Edwards Co.

Knapp DR and Jones ET: Use of cortical allograft for posterior spinal fusion, Clin Orthop 229:99, 1988.

Kojima Y et al: Evoked spinal potentials as a monitor of spinal cord viability, Spine 4:471, 1979.

Korovessis P: Combined VDS and Harrington instrumentation for treatment of idiopathic double major curves, Spine 12:244, 1987.

Lagrone MO: Loss of lumbar lordosis: a complication of spinal fusion for scoliosis, Orthop Clin North Am 19:393, 1988.

Lagrone MO et al: Treatment of symptomatic flatback after spinal fusion, J Bone Joint Surg 70A:569, 1988.

Larson SJ et al: Evoked potentials in experimental myelopathy, Spine 5:299, 1980.

Leatherman KD: The management of rigid spinal curves, Clin Orthop 93:215, 1973.

Letts RM and Bobechko WP: Fusion of the scoliotic spine in young children: effect on prognosis and growth, Clin Orthop 101:136, 1974.

Letts RM and Hollenberg C: Delayed paresis following spinal fusion with Harrington instrumentation, Clin Orthop 125:45, 1977.

Lieponis JV et al: Spinal cord injury during segmental sublamina spinal instrumentation: an animal model, Orthop Trans 8:173, 1984.

Lowe TG: Morbidity and mortality committee report. Paper presented at 22nd annual meeting of the Scoliosis Research Society, Vancouver, British Columbia, 1987.

Lueders H et al: A new technique for intraoperative monitoring of spinal cord function: multichannel recording of spinal cord and subcortical evoked potentials, Spine 7:110, 1982.

Luque ER: Anatomy of scoliosis and its correction, Clin Orthop 105:298, 1974.

Luque ER: Segmental spinal instrumentation: a method of rigid internal fixation of the spine to induce arthrodesis, Orthop Trans 4:391, 1980.

Luque ER: The anatomic basis and development of segmental spinal instrumentation, Spine 7:256, 1982.

Luque ER: Segmental spinal instrumentation for correction of scoliosis, Clin Orthop 163:192, 1982.

Luque ER and Cardoso A: Segmental correction of scoliosis with rigid internal fixation, Orthop Trans 1:136, 1977.

MacEwen GD, Bunnell WP, and Sriram K: Acute neurological complications in the treatment of scoliosis: a report of the Scoliosis Research Society, J Bone Joint Surg 57A:404, 1975.

Machida M et al: Spinal cord monitoring: electrophysiological measures of sensory and motor function during spinal surgery, Spine 10:407, 1985.

Mankin HJ, Graham JJ, and Schack J: Cardiopulmonary function in mild and moderate idiopathic scoliosis, J Bone Joint Surg 46A:53, 1964.

Manning EW, Prime FJ, and Zorab PA: Partial costectomy as a cosmetic operation in scoliosis, J Bone Joint Surg 55B:521, 1973.

May VR Jr and Mauck WR: Exploration of the spine for pseudarthrosis following spinal fusion in the treatment of scoliosis, Clin Orthop 53:115, 1967.

McCarroll HR and Costen W: Attempted treatment of scoliosis by unilateral vertebral epiphyseal arrest, J Bone Joint Surg 42A:965, 1960.

McKittrick JE: Banked autologous blood in elective surgery, Am J Surg 128:137, 1974.

McMaster MJ and James JIP: Pseudarthrosis after spinal fusion for scoliosis, J Bone Joint Surg 58B:305, 1976.

Michel CR and Lalain JJ: Late results of Harrington's operation: long-term evolution of the lumbar spine below the fused segments, Spine 10:414, 1985.

Michele AA and Krueger FJ: Surgical approach to the vertebral body, J Bone Joint Surg 31A:873, 1949.

Mir SR et al: Early ambulation following spinal fusion and Harrington instrumentation in idiopathic scoliosis, Clin Orthop 110:54, 1975.

Mirbaha MM: Anterior approach to the thoraco-lumbar junction of the spine by retroperitoneal–extra pleural technique, Clin Orthop 91:41, 1973.

Moe JH: A critical analysis of methods of fusion for scoliosis: an evaluation in 266 patients, J Bone Joint Surg 40A:529, 1958.

Moe JH: Methods of correction and surgical techniques in scoliosis, Orthop Clin North Am 3:17, 1972.

Moe JH and Gustilo RB: Treatment of scoliosis: results in 196 patients treated with cast correction and fusion, J Bone Joint Surg 46A:293, 1964.

Moe JH, Purcel GA, and Bradford DS: Zielke instrumentation (VDS) for the correction of spinal curvature, Clin Orthop 180:133, 1983.

Moore SV: Segmental spinal instrumentation: complications, correction, and indications, Orthop Trans 7:413, 1983.

Moskowitz A et al: Long-term follow-up of scoliosis fusion, J Bone Joint Surg 62A:364, 1980.

Mouradian WH and Simmons EH: A frame for spinal surgery to reduce intra-abdominal pressure while continuous traction is applied, J Bone Joint Surg 59A:1098, 1977.

Mubarak SJ, Wenger DR, and Leach J: Evaluation of Cotrel-Dubousset instrumentation for treatment of idiopathic scoliosis, Update Spinal Disorders 2:3, 1987.

Nach CD and Keim HA: Prophylactic antibiotics in spinal surgery, Orthop Rev 2:27, 1973.

Nachemson AL and Elfstrom G: Intravital wireless telemetry of axial forces in Harrington distraction rods in patients with idiopathic scoliosis, J Bone Joint Surg 53A:445, 1971.

Nachlas IW and Borden JN: The cure of experimental scoliosis by directed growth control, J Bone Joint Surg 33A:24, 1951.

Nasca RJ: Segmental spinal instrumentation, South Med J 78:303, 1985.

Nash CL Jr, Schatzinger L, and Lorig R: Intraoperative monitoring of spinal cord function during scoliosis spine surgery, J Bone Joint Surg 56A:1765, 1974 (abstract).

Nash CL Jr et al: Spinal cord monitoring during operative treatment of the spine, Clin Orthop 126:100, 1977.

Nicastro JF et al: Sublaminar segmental wire fixation: anatomic pathways during their removal, Orthop Trans 8:172, 1984.

Nordwall A et al: Spinal cord monitoring using evoked potentials recorded from feline vertebral bone, Spine 4:486, 1979.

Ogilvie JW: Anterior spine fusion with Zielke instrumentation for idiopathic scoliosis in adolescents, Orthop Clin North Am 19:313, 1988.

Ogilve JW and Millar EA: Comparison of segmental spinal instrumentation devices in the correction of scoliosis. Spine, 8:416, 1983.

Perry J: Surgical approaches to the spine. In Pierce DS and Nickel VH, editors: The total care of spinal cord injuries, Boston, 1977, Little, Brown & Co.

Phillips WA and Hensinger RN: Wisconsin and other instrumentation for posterior spinal fusion, Clin Orthop 229:44, 1988.

Piggott H: Posterior rib resection in scoliosis, J Bone Joint Surg 53B:663, 1971.

Piggott H: Treatment of scoliosis by posterior fusion, Harrington instrumentation and early walking, J Bone Joint Surg 58B:58, 1976.

Ponseti IV and Friedman B: Changes in the scoliotic spine after fusion, J Bone Joint Surg 32A:751, 1950.

Rappaport M et al: Effects of corrective scoliosis surgery on somatosensory evoked potentials, Spine 7:404, 1982.

Relton JES and Hall JE: An operation frame for spinal fusion: a new apparatus designed to reduce haemorrhage during operation, J Bone Joint Surg 49B:327, 1967.

Renshaw TS: Spinal fusion with segmental instrumentation, Contemp Orthop 4:413, 1982.

Renshaw TS: The role of Harrington instrumentation and posterior spine fusion in the management of adolescent idiopathic scoliosis, Orthop Clin North Am 19:257, 1988.

Resina J and Alves AF: A technique for correction and internal fixation for scoliosis, J Bone Joint Surg 59B:159, 1977.

Riseborough EJ: The anterior approach to the spine for the correction of deformities of the axial skeleton, Clin Orthop 93:207, 1973.

Risser JC and Norquist DM: A follow-up study of the treatment of scoliosis, J Bone Joint Surg 40A:555, 1958.

Roaf R: Vertebral growth and its mechanical control, J Bone Joint Surg 42B:40, 1960.

Roaf R: The treatment of progressive scoliosis by unilateral growth arrest, J Bone Joint Surg 45B:637, 1963.

Rose GK, Owen R, and Sanderson JM: Transposition of rib with blood supply for the stabilization of spinal kyphosis, J Bone Joint Surg 57B:112, 1975.

Roth A et al: Scoliosis and congenital heart disease, Clin Orthop 93:95, 1973.

Schmidt AC: Fundamental principles and treatment of scoliosis. In The American Academy of Orthopaedic Surgeons: Instructional course lectures, vol 16, St Louis, 1959, The CV Mosby Co.

Schultz AB and Hirsch C: Mechanical analysis of Harrington rod correction of idiopathic scoliosis, J Bone Joint Surg 55A:983, 1973.

Schultz AB and Hirsch C: Mechanical analysis of techniques for improved correction of idiopathic scoliosis, Clin Orthop 100:66, 1974.

Shands AR Jr et al: End-result study of the treatment of idiopathic scoliosis: report of the research committee of the American Orthopaedic Association, J Bone Joint Surg 23:963, 1941.

Shifrin LZ: The lateral position for spine fusion in Harrington instrumentation for scoliosis: a brief report, Clin Orthop 81:48, 1971.

Shufflebarger HL et al: Segmental spinal instrumentation in idiopathic scoliosis: a retrospective analysis of 234 cases, Orthop Trans 9:124, 1985.

Silverman BJ and Greenbarg PE: Idiopathic scoliosis posterior spine fusion with Harrington rod and sublaminar wiring, Orthop Clin North Am 19:269, 1988.

Smith A, Butte FL, and Ferguson AB: Treatment of scoliosis by the wedging jacket and spine fusion: a review of 265 cases, J Bone Joint Surg 20:825, 1938.

Smith AD, von Lackum WH, and Wylie R: An operation for stapling vertebral bodies in congenital scoliosis, J Bone Joint Surg 36A:342, 1954.

Southwick WO and Robinson RA: Surgical approaches to the vertebral bodies in the cervical and lumbar regions, J Bone Joint Surg 39A:631, 1957.

Spielholz NI et al: Somatosensory evoked potentials during decompression and stabilization of the spine: methods and findings, Spine 4:500, 1979.

Steel HH: Rib resection and spine fusion in correction of convex deformity in scoliosis, J Bone Joint Surg 65A:920, 1983.

Taddonio RF, Weller K, and Appel M: A comparison of patients with idiopathic scoliosis managed with and without post operative immobilization following segmental spinal instrumentation with Luque rods, Orthop Trans 8:172, 1984.

Tambornino JM, Armbrust EN, and Moe JH: Harrington instrumentation in correction of scoliosis: a comparison with cast correction, J Bone Joint Surg 46A:313, 1964.

Thompson GH et al: Segmental spinal instrumentation in idiopathic scoliosis: a preliminary report, Spine 10:623, 1985.

Thompson GH et al: Segmental spinal instrumentation in idiopathic spinal deformities, Orthop Trans 9:123, 1985.

Thompson JD et al: Prior deposition of autologous blood in elective orthopaedic surgery, J Bone Joint Surg 69A:320, 1987.

Thompson WAL and Ralston EL: Pseudarthrosis following spine fusion, J Bone Joint Surg 31A:400, 1949.

Thulborne T and Gillespie R: The rib hump in idiopathic scoliosis: measurement, analysis, and response to treatment, J Bone Joint Surg 58B:64, 1976.

Ulrich HF: The operative treatment of scoliosis, Am J Surg 45:235, 1939.

Van Grouw A et al: Long-term follow-up of patients with idiopathic scoliosis treated surgically: a preliminary subjective study, Clin Orthop 117:197, 1976.

Vauzelle C, Stagnara P, and Jouvinroux P: Functional monitoring of spinal activity during spinal surgery, J Bone Joint Surg 55A:441, 1973.

Von Lackum WH: The surgical treatment of scoliosis. In The American Academy of Orthopaedic Surgeons: Instructional course lectures, vol 5, Ann Arbor, Mich, 1948, JW Edwards Co.

Von Lackum WH: Surgical scoliosis, Surg Clin North Am 31:345, 1951.

Von Lackum WH and Miller JP: Critical observation of the results in the operative treatment of scoliosis, J Bone Joint Surg 31A:102, 1949.

von Rokitansky C: Lehrbuch der pathologischen Anatomie, ed 3, vol 3, Wien, 1861, W Braumuller.

Weiler PJ, McNeice GM, and Medley JB: An experimental study of the buckling behavior of L-rod implants used in the surgical treatment of scoliosis, Spine 11:992, 1986.

Wenger D, Miller S, and Wilkerson J: Evaluation of fixation sites for segmental instrumentation of the human vertebra, Orthop Trans 6:23, 1982.

Wenger DR, Carollo JJ, and Wilkerson JA: Biomechanics of scoliosis correction by segmental spinal instrumentation, Spine 7:260, 1982.

Wenger DR et al: Laboratory testing of segmental spinal instrumentation versus traditional Harrington instrumentation for scoliosis treatment, Spine 7:265, 1982.

Wilber RG et al: Postoperative neurologic deficits and segmental spinal instrumentation: a study using spinal cord monitoring, J Bone Joint Surg 66A:1178, 1984.

Wilson RL, Levine DB, and Doherty JH: Surgical treatment of idiopathic scoliosis, Clin Orthop 81:34, 1971.

Winter RB: Posterior spinal fusion in scoliosis: indications, techniques and results, Orthop Clin North Am 10:787, 1979.

Winter RB: Posterior spinal arthrodesis with instrumentation and sublaminar wire: 100 consecutive cases, Orthop Trans 9:124, 1985.

Winter RB, Lovell WW, and Moe JH: Excessive thoracic lordosis and loss of pulmonary function in patients with idiopathic scoliosis, J Bone Joint Surg 57A:972, 1974.

Woolson ST, Marsh JS, and Tanner JB: Transfusion of previously deposited autologous blood for patients undergoing hip-replacement surgery, J Bone Joint Surg 69A:325, 1987.

Wu Z: Posterior vertebral instrumentation for correction of scoliosis, Clin Orthop 215:40, 1987.

Zielke K: Derotation and fusion—anterior spinal instrumentation, Orthop Trans 2:270, 1978.

Zielke K: Ventral derotation spondylodesis: preliminary report on 58 cases, Beitr Orthop Traumatol 25:85, 1978.

Zuege RC, Blount WP, and Dicus WT: Indications for operative treatment of spinal deformities, Wis Med J 74:S33, 1975.

Neuromuscular scoliosis (general)

Allen BL and Ferguson RL: The Galveston technique for L-rod instrumentation of the scoliotic spine, Spine 7:119, 1982.

Allen BL, and Ferguson RL: L-rod instrumentation (LRI) for scoliosis in cerebral palsy, J Pediatr Orthop 2:87, 1982.

Bonnett C et al: The evolution of treatment of paralytic scoliosis at Rancho Los Amigos Hospital, J Bone Joint Surg 57A:206, 1975.

Brown JC et al: Late spinal deformity in quadriplegic children and adolescents, J Pediatr Orthop 4:456, 1984.

Bunch WH: The Milwaukee brace in paralytic scoliosis, Clin Orthop 110:63, 1975.

Bunch WH, Smith D, and Hakala M: Kyphosis in the paralytic spine, Clin Orthop 128:107, 1977.

DeWald RL and Faut MM: Anterior and posterior spinal fusion for paralytic scoliosis, Spine 4:401, 1979.

Ferguson RL and Allen BL: Staged correction of neuromuscular scoliosis, J Pediatr Orthop 3:555, 1983.

Fisk JR and Bunch WH: Scoliosis in neuromuscular disease, Orthop Clin North Am 10:863, 1979.

Garrett AL, Perry J, and Nickel VL: Paralytic scoliosis, Clin Orthop 21:117, 1961.

Garrett AL, Perry J, and Nickel VL: Stabilization of the collapsing spine, J Bone Joint Surg 43A:474, 1961.

Kepes ER et al: Anesthetic problems in hereditary muscular abnormalities, N Y State J Med 72:1051, 1972.

Lonstein JE and Renshaw TS: Neuromuscular spine deformities. In The American Academy of Orthopaedic Surgeons: Instructional course lectures, vol 36, St Louis, 1987, The CV Mosby Co.

Luque ER: Paralytic scoliosis in growing children, Clin Orthop 163:202, 1982.

Luque ER: Segmental spinal instrumentation for correction of scoliosis, Clin Orthop 163:192, 1982.

Makley J et al: Pulmonary function and paralytic and non-paralytic scoliosis: before and after treatment—a study of 63 cases, J Bone Joint Surg 50A:1379, 1968.

McCarthy RE et al: Allograft bone in spinal fusion for paralytic scoliosis, J Bone Joint Surg 68A:370, 1986.

Moe JH: The management of paralytic scoliosis, South Med J 50:67, 1957.

Nash CL: Current concepts review: scoliosis bracing, J Bone Joint Surg 62A:848, 1980.

Nickel Y et al: Elective surgery on patient with respiratory paralysis, J Bone Joint Surg 39A:989, 1957.

O'Brien JP and Yau AC: Anterior and posterior correction and fusion for paralytic scoliosis, Clin Orthop 86:151, 1972.

Sullivan JA and Conner SB: Comparison of Harrington instrumentation and segmental spinal instrumentation in the management of neuromuscular spinal deformity, Spine 7:299, 1982.

Taddonio RF: Segmental spinal instrumentation in the management of neuromuscular spinal deformity, Spine 7:305, 1982.

Winter RB and Carlson JM: Modern orthotics for spinal deformities, Clin Orthop 23:74, 1977.

Cerebral palsy

Allen BL and Ferguson RL: L-rod instrumentation for scoliosis in cerebral palsy, J Pediatr Orthop 2:87, 1982.

Balmer GA and MacEwen GD: The incidence and treatment of scoliosis in cerebral palsy, J Bone Joint Surg 52B:134, 1970.

Bonnett C, Brown J, and Brooks HL: Anterior spine fusion with Dwyer instrumentation for lumbar scoliosis in cerebral palsy, J Bone Joint Surg 55A:425, 1973.

Bonnett CA, Brown JC, and Grow T: Thoracolumbar scoliosis in cerebral palsy: results of surgical treatment, J Bone Joint Surg 58A:328, 1976.

Brown JC, Swank SM, and Specht L: Combined anterior and posterior spine fusion in cerebral palsy, Spine 7:570, 1982.

Bunnell WP and MacEwen GD: Non-operative treatment in scoliosis in cerebral palsy: preliminary report on the use of a plastic jacket, Dev Med Child Neurol 19:45, 1977.

Carlson JM and Winter RB: The "Gillette" sitting support orthothosis for non-ambulatory children with severe cerebral palsy or advanced muscular dystrophy, Minn Med 61:469, 1978.

Ferguson RL and Allen BL: Considerations in the treatment of cerebral palsy patients with spinal deformities, Orthop Clin North Am 19:419, 1988.

Gersoff WK and Renshaw JS: The treatment of scoliosis in cerebral palsy by posterior spinal fusion with Luque-rod segmented instrumentation, J Bone Joint Surg 70A:41, 1988.

Lonstein JE and Akbarnia BA: Operative treatment of spinal deformities in patients with cerebral palsy or mental retardation: an analysis of 107 cases, J Bone Joint Surg 65A:43, 1983.

MacEwen GD: Operative treatment of scoliosis in cerebral palsy, Reconstr Surg Traumatol 13:58, 1972.

Madigan RR and Wallace SL: Scoliosis in the institutionalized cerebral palsy population, Spine 6:583, 1981.

Robson P: The prevalence of scoliosis in adolescents and young adults with cerebral palsy, Dev Med Child Neurol 10:447, 1968.

Rosenthal RK, Levine DB, and McCarver CL: The occurrance of scoliosis in cerebral palsy, Dev Med Child Neurol 16:664, 1974.

Samilson R and Bechard R: Scoliosis in cerebral palsy: incidence, distribution of curve patterns, natural history and thoughts on etiology, Curr Pract Orthop Surg 5:183, 1973.

Stanitski CL et al: Surgical correction of spinal deformity in cerebral palsy, Spine 7:563, 1982.

Taddonio RF: Segmental spinal instrumentation and the management of neuromuscular spinal deformity, Spine 7:305, 1982.

Heritable neurologic disorders

Aprin H et al: Spine fusion in patients with spinal muscle atrophy, J Bone Joint Surg 64A:1179, 1982.

Axelrod FB, Iyer K, and Fish I: Progressive sensory loss and familial dysautonomia, Pediatrics 67:517, 1981.

Benady SG: Spinal muscle atrophy in childhood: review of 50 cases, Dev Med Child Neurol 20:746, 1978.

Bethea JS III and Doherty JH: Scoliosis and dysautonomia, J Bone Joint Surg 52A:409, 1971.

Cady RB and Bobechko WP: Incidence, natural history, and treatment of scoliosis in Friedrich's ataxia, J Pediatr Orthop 4:673, 1984.

Daher YH et al: Spinal surgery in spinal muscle atrophy, J Pediatr Orthop 5:391, 1985.

Daher YH et al: Spinal deformities in patients with Charcot-Marie-Tooth: a review of 12 patients, Clin Orthop 202:219, 1986.

Daher YH et al: Spinal deformities in patients with Friedreich's ataxia: a review of 19 patients, J Pediatr Orthop 5:553, 1985.

Dancis J and Smith AA: Current concepts and familial dysautonomia, N Engl J Med 274:207, 1966.

Dorr J, Brown J, and Perry J: Results of posterior spine fusion in patients with spinal muscle atrophy: a review of 25 cases, J Bone Joint Surg 55A:436, 1973.

Dubowitz Y: Benign infantile spinal muscular atrophy, Dev Med Child Neurol 16:672, 1974.

Evans GA, Drennan JC, and Russman BS: Functional classification and orthopaedic management of spinal muscle atrophy, J Bone Joint Surg 63B:516, 1981.

Geoffrey G et al: Classifical description and roentgenologic evaluation of patients with Friedreich's ataxia, Can J Neurol Sci 3:279, 1976.

Goldstein LA et al: Surgical treatment of thoracic scoliosis in patients with familial dysautonomia, J Bone Joint Surg 51A:205, 1969.

Hensinger RN and MacEwen GD: Spinal deformity associated with heritable neurologic conditions: spinal muscle atrophy, Friedreich's ataxia, familial dysautonomia, and Charcot-Marie-Tooth disease, J Bone Joint Surg 58A:13, 1976.

Labelle H et al: Natural history in scoliosis in Friedreich's ataxia, J Bone Joint Surg 68A:564, 1986.

McKusick YA et al: The Riley-Day syndrome: observations on genetics and survivorship (an interim report), Isr J Med Sci 3:372, 1967.

Namba T, Aberfeld DC, and Grob D: Chronic proximal spinal muscular atrophy, J Neurol Sci 11:401, 1970.

Riddick M, Winter RB, and Lutter L: Spinal deformities in patients with spinal muscle atrophy, Spine 8:476, 1982.

Riley CM et al: Central autonomic dysfunction with defective lachrymation: report of 5 cases, Pediatrics 3:468, 1949.

Robin GC: Scoliosis in familial dysautonomia, Bull Hosp Jt Dis Orthop Inst 44:16, 1984.

Schwentker EP and Gibson DA: The orthopaedic aspects of spinal muscle atrophy, J Bone Joint Surg 58A:32, 1976.

Shapiro F and Bresnan MJ: Current concepts reviewed: management of childhood neuromuscular disease. I. Spinal muscle atrophy, J Bone Joint Surg 64A:785, 1982.

Shapiro F and Bresnan MJ: Current concepts reviewed: orthopaedic management of childhood neuromuscular disease. II. Peripheral neuropathies, Friedreich's ataxia and arthrogryposis multiplex congenita, J Bone Joint Surg 64A:949, 1982.

Stenquist O and Sigurdson J: The anaesthetic management of a patient with familial dysautonomia, Anaesthesia 37:929, 1982.

Yoslow W et al: Orthopaedic defects in familial dysautonomia: a review of 65 cases, J Bone Joint Surg 53A:1541, 1971.

Syringomyelia

Baker AS and Dove J: Progressive scoliosis as the first presenting sign of syringomyelia: report of a case, J Bone Joint Surg 65B:472, 1983.

Bradford DS: Neuromuscular spinal deformity. In Bradford DS et al, editors: Moe's textbook of scoliosis and other spinal deformities, Philadelphia, 1987, WB Saunders Co.

Gardner WJ and Collis JS: Skeletal anomalies associated with syringomyelia, diastematomyelia and myelomeningocele, J Bone Joint Surg 42A:1265, 1960.

Huebert HT and MacKinnon WB: Syringomyelia and scoliosis, J Bone Joint Surg 51B:338, 1969.

McIlroy WJ and Richardson JC: Syringomyelia: a clinical review of 75 cases, Can Med Assoc J 93:731, 1965.

McRae DL and Standen J: Roentgenologic findings in syringomyelia and hydromyelia, Am J Roentg 98:695, 1966.

Nordwall A and Wikkelso C: A late neurologic complication of scoliosis surgery in connection with syringomyelia, Acta Orthop Scand 50:407, 1979.

Weber FA: The association of syringomyelia and scoliosis, J Bone Joint Surg 56B:589, 1974.

Williams B: Orthopaedic features in the presentation of syringomyelia, J Bone Joint Surg 61B:314, 1979.

Woods WW and Pimenta AM: Intramedullary lesions of the spinal cord, Arch Neurol Psych 52:383, 1944.

Spinal cord injuries

Bedbrook GM: Correction of scoliosis due to paraplegia sustained in pediatric age group, Paraplegia 15:90, 1977-78.

Brown HP and Bonnett CC: Spine deformity subsequent to spinal cord injury. In Proceedings of the Scoliosis Research Society, J Bone Joint Surg 55A:441, 1973.

Bonnett CA: The cord injured child. In Lovell WW and Winter RB, editors: Children's Orthopaedics, Philadelphia, 1978, JB Lippincott Co.

Johnston CE II, Hakaka MW, and Rosenberger R: Paralytic spine deformity: orthotic treatment in spinal discontinuity syndromes, J Pediatr Orthop 2:233, 1982.

Kilfoyle RM, Foley JJ, and Norton PL: Spine and pelvic deformity in childhood and adolescent to paraplegia: a study of 104 cases, J Bone Joint Surg 47A:659, 1965.

Kleinberg S: Scoliosis with paraplegia, J Bone Joint Surg 33A:225, 1951.

Lancourt JC, Dickson JH, and Carter RE: Paralytic spinal deformity following traumatic spinal cord injury in children and adolescents, J Bone Joint Surg 63A:47, 1981.

Leidholt JD: Evaluation of late spinal deformities with fracture-dislocations of the dorsal and lumbar spine in paraplegics, Paraplegia 7:16, 1969.

Luque ER: Paralytic scoliosis in growing children, Clin Orthop 163:202, 1982.

Makin M: Spinal problems of childhood to paraplegia, Isr J Med Sci 9:732, 1973.

Mayfield JK, Erkkila JD, and Winter RB: Spine deformity subsequent to acquired childhood spinal cord injury, J Bone Joint Surg 63A:1401, 1981.

McSweeny T: Spinal deformity after spinal cord injury, Paraplegia 6:212, 1969.

Norton PL and Foley JJ: Paraplegia in children, J Bone Joint Surg 41A:1291, 1959.

Odom JA et al: Scoliosis in paraplegia, Paraplegia 11:290, 1974.

Von Bazan UKB and Paeslack V: Scoliotic growth in children with acquired paraplegia, Paraplegia 15:65, 1977-1978.

Wedge JH and Gillespie R: Problems of scoliosis surgery in paraplegic children, J Bone Joint Surg 57B:536, 1975.

Poliomyelitis

Bonnett C et al: The evolution of treatment of paralytic scoliosis at Rancho Los Amigos Hospital, J Bone Joint Surg 57A:206, 1975.

Colonna PC and Vom Saal F: A study of paralytic scoliosis based on 500 cases of poliomyelitis, J Bone Joint Surg 23:335, 1941.

Garrett AL, Perry J, and Nickel VL: Paralytic scoliosis, Clin Orthop 21:117, 1961.

Garrett AL, Perry J, and Nickel VL: Stabilization of the collapsing spine, J Bone Joint Surg 43A:474, 1961.

Gucker T: Experience in poliomyelitis scoliosis after correction and fusion, J Bone Joint Surg 38A:1281, 1956.

Gui L et al: Surgical treatment of poliomyelitic scoliosis, Ital J Orthop Traumat 2:191, 1976.

Irwin CE: The iliotibial band: its role in producing deformity in poliomyelitis, J Bone Joint Surg 31A:141, 1949.

James JIP: Paralytic scoliosis, J Bone Joint Surg 38B:660, 1956.

Leong JCY et al: Surgical treatment of scoliosis following poliomyelitis: a review of 100 cases, J Bone Joint Surg 63A:726, 1981.

Mayer L: Further studies of fixed paralytic pelvic obliquity, J Bone Joint Surg 18:87, 1936.

Mayer PJ et al: Post-poliomyelitis paralytic scoliosis, Spine 6:573, 1981.

O'Brien JP, Dwyer AP, and Hodgson AR: Paralytic pelvic obliquity: its prognosis and management and the development of a technique for full correction of the deformity, J Bone Joint Surg 57A:626, 1975.

O'Brien JP et al: Combined staged, anterior and posterior correction and fusion of the spine in scoliosis following poliomyelitis, Clin Orthop 110:81, 1975.

Pavon SJ and Manning C: Posterior spine fusion for scoliosis due to anterior poliomyelitis, J Bone Joint Surg 52A:420, 1970.

Roaf R: Paralytic scoliosis, J Bone Joint Surg 38B:640, 1956.

Yount CC: Role of the tensor fascia femoris in certain deformities of the lower extremities, J Bone Joint Surg 8:171, 1926.

Arthrogryposis

Brown LM and Robson MJ: The pathophysiology of arthrogryposis multiplex congenita neurologica, J Bone Joint Surg 62B:291, 1980.

Daher YH et al: Spinal deformities in patients with arthrogryposis: a review of 16 patients, Spine 10:609, 1985.

Drummond D and McKenzie DA: Scoliosis in arthrogryposis, multiplex congenita, Spine 3:146, 1978.

Friedlander HL, Westin GW, and Wood WL: Arthrogryposis multiplex congenita: a review of 45 cases, J Bone Joint Surg 50A:89, 1968.

Gibson DA and Urs NDK: Arthrogryposis multiplex congenita, J Bone Joint Surg 52B:483, 1970.

Herron LD, Westin GW, and Dawson EG: Scoliosis in arthrogryposis multiplex congenita, J Bone Joint Surg 60A:293, 1978.

Mead NG, Lithgow WC, and Sweeney HJ: Arthrogryposis multiplex congenita, J Bone Joint Surg 40A:1285, 1958.

Shapiro F and Bresnan MJ: Current concepts review: Orthopaedic management of childhood neuromuscular disease. II. Peripheral neuropathies, Friedreich's ataxia, and arthrogryposis multiplex congenita, J Bone Joint Surg 64A:949, 1982.

Siebold RM, Winter RB, and Moe JH: The treatment of scoliosis in arthrogryposis multiplex congenita, Clin Orthop 103:191, 1974.

Muscular dystrophy

Cambridge W and Drennan JC: Scoliosis associated with Duchenne muscular dystrophy, J Pediatr Orthop 7:436, 1987.

Daher YH et al: Spinal deformities in patients with muscular dystrophy other than Duchenne: review of 11 patients having surgical treatment, Spine 10:614, 1984.

Dubowitz V: Some clinical observations on childhood muscular dystrophy, Br J Clin Pract 17:283, 1963.

Dubowitz V: Progressive muscular dystrophy: prevention of deformities, Clin Pediatr 3:323, 1964.

Gibson DA et al: The management of spinal deformity in Duchenne's muscular dystrophy, Orthop Clin North Am 9:437, 1978.

Hsu JD: The natural history of spine curvature progression in the nonambulator Duchenne muscular dystrophy patient, Spine 8:771, 1983.

Inkley SR, Oldenburg FC, and Vignos PJ Jr: Pulmonary function in Duchenne muscular dystrophy related to stage of disease, Am J Med 56:297, 1974.

Kurz LT et al: Correlation of scoliosis and pulmonary function in Duchenne muscular dystrophy, J Pediatr Orthop 3:347, 1983.

Luque ER: Segmental spinal instrumentation for correction of scoliosis, Clin Orthop 163:192, 1982.

Milne B and Rosales JK: Anesthetic considerations in patients with muscular dystrophy undergoing spinal fusion and Harrington rod insertion, Can Anaesth Soc J 29:250, 1982.

Rideau Y et al: The treatment of scoliosis in Duchenne muscular dystrophy, Muscle Nerve 7:281, 1984.

Robin GC and Brief LP: Scoliosis in childhood muscular dystrophy, J Bone Joint Surg 53A:466, 1971.

Robin GD: Scoliosis in Duchenne muscular dystrophy, Isr J Med Sci 13:203, 1977.

Sakai DN et al: Stabilization of the collapsing spine in Duchenne muscular dystrophy, Clin Orthop 128:256, 1977.

Seeger BR, Sutherland AD, and Clard MS: Orthotic management of scoliosis in Duchenne muscular dystrophy, Arch Phys Med Rehabil 65:83, 1984.

Shapiro F and Bresnan MJ: Orthopaedic management of childhood neuromuscular disease. III. Diseases of muscle, J Bone Joint Surg 64A:1102, 1982.

Siegel IM: Scoliosis in muscular dystrophy, Clin Orthop 93:235, 1973.

Siegel IM: Spinal stabilization in Duchenne muscular dystrophy: rationale and method, Muscle Nerve 5:417, 1982.

Sullivan JA and Conner SB: Comparison of Harrington instrumentation and segmental spinal instrumentation in the management of neuromuscular spinal deformity, Spine 7:299, 1982.

Swank SM, Brown JC, and Perry RE: Spinal fusion in Duchenne's muscular dystrophy, Spine 7:484, 1982.

Taddonio RF: Segmental spinal instrumentation in the management of neuromuscular spinal deformity, Spine 7:305, 1982.

Wilkins KE and Gibson DA: The patterns of spinal deformity in Duchenne muscular dystrophy, J Bone Joint Surg 58A:24, 1976.

Congenital scoliosis

Akbarnia BA, Heydarian K, and Ganjavian MS: Concordant congenital spine deformity in monozygotic twins, J Pediatr Orthop 3:502, 1983.

Akbarnia BA and Moe JH: Familial congenital scoliosis with unilateral unsegmented bar: case report of two siblings, J Bone Joint Surg 60A:259, 1978.

Andrew T and Piggott H: Growth arrest for progressive scoliosis: combined anterior and posterior fusion of the convexity, J Bone Joint Surg 67B:193, 1985.

Bernard TN Jr et al: Congenital spine deformities: a review of 47 cases, Orthopedics 8:777, 1985.

Bradford DS: Partial epiphyseal arrest and supplemental fixation for progressive correction of congenital spine deformity, J Bone Joint Surg 64A:610, 1982.

Compere EL: Excision of hemivertebrae for correction of congenital scoliosis, J Bone Joint Surg 14:555, 1932.

Drvaric DM et al: Congenital scoliosis and urinary tract abnormalities: are intravenous pyelograms necessary? J Pediatr Orthop 7:436, 1987.

Gillespie R et al: Intraspinal anomalies and congenital scoliosis, Clin Orthop 93:103, 1973.

Goldberg C, Fenlon G, and Blacke NS: Diastematomyelia: a critical review of the natural history and treatment, Spine 9:367, 1984.

Hall JE, Herndon WA, and Levine CR: Surgical treatment of congenital scoliosis with or without Harrington instrumentation, J Bone Joint Surg 63A:608, 1981.

Hathaway GL: Congenital scoliosis in one of monozygotic twins: a case report, J Bone Joint Surg 59A:837, 1977.

Hensinger R, Lang JE, and MacEwen GD: Klippel-Feil syndrome: a constellation of associated anomalies, J Bone Joint Surg 56A:1246, 1974.

Hood RW et al: Diastematomyelia and structural spinal deformities, J Bone Joint Surg 62A:520, 1980.

James CCM and Lassman LP: Diastematomyelia and the tight filum terminale, J Neurol Sci 10:193, 1970.

Keim HA and Greene AF: Diastematomyelia and scoliosis, J Bone Joint Surg 55A:1425, 1973.

Kuhns JE and Hormell RS: Management of congenital scoliosis, Arch Surg 65:250, 1952.

Langenskiold A: Correction of congenital scoliosis by excision of one half of a cleft vertebra, Acta Orthop Scand 38:291, 1967.

Leatherman KD and Dickson RA: Two-stage corrective surgery for congenital deformities of the spine, J Bone Joint Surg 61B:324, 1979.

Letts RM and Hollenberg C: Delayed paresis following spinal fusion with Harrington instrumentation, Clin Orthop 125:45, 1977.

Lhowe D et al: Congenital intraspinal lipomas: clinical presentation and response to treatment, J Pediatr Orthop 7:531, 1987.

Lonstein JE et al: Neurologic deficits secondary to spinal deformity: a review of the literature and report of 43 cases, Spine 5:331, 1980.

MacEwen GD, Conway JJ, and Miller WT: Congenital scoliosis with a unilateral bar, Radiology 40:711, 1968.

MacEwen GD, Winter RB, and Hardy JH: Evaluation of kidney anomalies in congenital scoliosis, J Bone Joint Surg 54A:1341, 1972.

McMaster MJ: Occult intraspinal anomalies and congenital scoliosis, J Bone Joint Surg 66A:588, 1984.

McMaster MJ and David CV: Hemivertebra as a cause of scoliosis: a study of 104 patients, J Bone Joint Surg 68B:588, 1986.

McMaster MJ and Ohtsuka K: The natural history of congenital scoliosis: a study of 251 patients, J Bone Joint Surg 64A:1128, 1982.

Nasca RJ, Stelling FH, and Steel HH: Progression of congenital scoliosis due to hemivertebrae and hemivertebrae with bars, J Bone Joint Surg 57A:456, 1975.

Reckles LH et al: The association of scoliosis and congenital heart defects, J Bone Joint Surg 57A:449, 1975.

Roaf R: Vertebral growth and its mechanical control, J Bone Joint Surg 42B:40, 1960.

Royle ND: Operative removal of an accessory vertebra, Med J Aust 1:467, 1928.

Shapiro F and Eyre D: Congenital scolioses: a histopathologic study, Spine 6:107, 1981.

Slabaugh P et al: A review of lumbosacral hemivertebra with excision in eight, Spine 5:234, 1980.

Smith A et al: An operation for stapling vertebral bodies in congenital scoliosis, J Bone Joint Surg 36A:342, 1954.

Stoll J and Bunch W: Segmental spinal instrumentation for congenital scoliosis: a report of two cases, Spine 8:43, 1983.

Tsou P, Yau A, and Hodgson A: Congenital spinal deformities: natural history, classification, and the role of anterior surgery, J Bone Joint Surg 56A:1767, 1974.

Wiles P: Resection of dorsal vertebrae in congenital scoliosis, J Bone Joint Surg 33A:151, 1951.

Winter RB: Congenital scoliosis, Clin Orthop 93:75, 1973.

Winter RB: Congenital spine deformity: natural history and treatment, Isr J Med Sci 9:719, 1973.

Winter RB: Convex anterior and posterior hemiarthrodesis and epiphyseodesis in young children with progressive congenital scoliosis, J Pediatr Orthop 1:361, 1981.

Winter RB: Congenital scoliosis, Orthop Clin North Am 19:395, 1988.

Winter RB and Moe JH: The results of spinal arthrodesis for congenital spine deformity in patients younger than five years old, J Bone Joint Surg 64A:419, 1982.

Winter RB, Moe JH, and Eilers VE: Congenital scoliosis: a study of 234 patients treated and untreated, J Bone Joint Surg 50A:1, 1968.

Winter RB, Moe JH, and Lonstein JE: Posterior spinal arthrodesis for congenital scoliosis: an analysis of the cases of two hundred and ninety patients, five to nineteen years old, J Bone Joint Surg 66A:1188, 1984.

Winter RB et al: Diastematomyelia and congenital spine deformities, J Bone Joint Surg 56A:27, 1974.

Winter RB et al: The Milwaukee brace and the non-operative treatment of congenital scoliosis, Spine 1:85, 1976.

Scheuermann's kyphosis

Adelstein LJ: Spinal extradural cyst associated with kyphosis dorsalis juvenilis, J Bone Joint Surg 23A:93, 1941.

Ascani E, Ippolito E, and Montanaro A: Scheuermann's kyphosis: histological, histochemical and ultrastructural studies, Orthop Trans 7:28, 1982.

Aufdermaur M: Juvenile kyphosis (Scheuermann's disease): radiography, histology and pathogenesis, Clin Orthop 154:166, 1981.

Berg A: Contribution to the technique and fusion operations on the spine, Acta Orthop Scand 17:1, 1948.

Bick EM and Copel JW: Longitudinal growth of the human vertebra: contribution to human osteogeny, J Bone Joint Surg 33A:783, 1951.

Bradford DS: Neurological complications in Scheuermann's disease, J Bone Joint Surg 51A:657, 1969.

Bradford DS: Juvenile kyphosis, Clin Orthop 128:45, 1977.

Bradford DS: Juvenile kyphosis. In Bradford DS et al, editors: Moe's textbook of scoliosis and other spinal deformities, Philadelphia, 1987, WB Saunders Co.

Bradford DS et al: Scheuermann's kyphosis and roundback deformity: results of Milwaukee brace treatment, J Bone Joint Surg 56A:749, 1974.

Bradford DS et al: Scheuermann's kyphosis: results of surgical treatment in 22 patients, J Bone Joint Surg 57A:439, 1975.

Bradford DS et al: Scheuermann's kyphosis: a form of juvenile osteoporosis? Clin Orthop 118:10, 1976.

Bradford DS et al: The surgical management of patients with Scheuermann's disease: a review of 24 cases managed by combined anterior and posterior spine fusion, J Bone Joint Surg 62A:705, 1980.

Bradford DS and Moe JH: Scheuermann's juvenile kyphosis: a histologic study, Clin Orthop 110:45, 1975.

Bradford DS, Moe JH, and Winter RB: Kyphosis and postural roundback deformity in children and adolescence, Minn Med 56:114, 1973.

Cloward RB and Bucy PC: Spinal extradural cyst and kyphosis dorsalis juvenilis, Am J Roentgenology 38:681, 1937.

Coscia MF, Bradford DS, and Ogilvie JW: Scheuermann's kyphosis: treatment with Luque instrumentation—a review of 19 patients. Paper presented at the 55th Annual Meeting of the American Academy of Orthopaedic Surgeons, Atlanta, Feb 4-9, 1988.

Ferguson AB Jr: Etiology of pre-adolescent kyphosis, J Bone Joint Surg 38A:149, 1956.

Fon GT, Pitt MJ, and Thies AC: Thoracic kyphosis: range in normal subjects, Am J Roentgenology 134:979, 1980.

Hafner RH: Localized osteochondritis: Scheuermann's disease, J Bone Joint Surg 34B:38, 1952.

Hensinger RN, Greene TL, and Hunter LY: Back pain and vertebral changes simulating Scheuermann's kyphosis, Spine 6:341, 1982.

Herndon WA et al: Combined anterior and posterior fusion for Scheuermann's kyphosis, Spine 6:125, 1981.

Ippilito E and Ponsetti I: Juvenile kyphosis: histological and histochemical studies, J Bone Joint Surg 63A:175, 1981.

Kehl D, Lovell WW, and MacEwen GD: Scheuermann's disease of the lumbar spine, Orthop Trans 6:342, 1982.

Knutson F: Observations of the growth of the vertebral body in Scheuermann's disease, Acta Radiol 30:97, 1948.

Kostuik J and Lorenz M: Long-term follow-up of surgical management in adult Scheuermann's kyphosis, Orthop Trans 7:28, 1983.

Lopez RA et al: Osteoporosis in Scheuerman's disease, Spine 13:1099, 1988.

Moe JH: Treatment of adolescent kyphosis by non-operative and operative methods, Manitoba Med Rev 45:481, 1965.

Montgomery SP and Erwin WE: Scheuermann's kyphosis: long-term results of Milwaukee brace treatment, Spine 6:5, 1978.

Nathan L and Kuhns JG: Epiphysitis of the spine, J Bone Joint Surg 22:55, 1940.

Neithard FV: Scheuermann's disease and spondylolysis, Orthop Trans 7:103, 1983.

Outland T and Snedden HE: Juvenile dorsal kyphosis, Clin Orthop 5:155, 1955.

Ponte A, Gebbia F, and Eliseo F: Non-operative treatment of adolescent hyperkyphosis, Orthop Trans 9:108, 1985.

Ryan MD and Taylor TKF: Acute spinal cord compression in Scheuermann's disease, J Bone Joint Surg 64B:409, 1982.

Sachs BL et al: Scheuermann's kyphosis: long-term results of Milwaukee brace treatment, Orthop Trans 9:108, 1985.

Scheuermann H: Kyphosis dorsalis juvenile, Ztschr Orthop Chir 41:305, 1921.

Schmorl G: Die Pathogenese der juvenilen Kyphose, Fortschr Geb Roentgenstr Nuklearmed 41:359, 1930.

Simon RS: The diagnosis and treatment of kyphosis dorsalis juvenilis (Scheuermann's kyphosis) in the early stage, J Bone Joint Surg 24:681, 1942.

Sorenson KH: Scheuermann's juvenile kyphosis, Copenhagen, 1964, Munksgaard.

Sturm PF, Dobson JC, and Armstrong GWD: The surgical management of Scheuermann's disease. Paper presented at the 55th Annual Meeting of The American Academy of Orthopaedic Surgeons, Atlanta, Ga, Feb 4-9, 1988.

Taylor TC et al: Surgical management of thoracic kyphosis in adolescents, J Bone Joint Surg 61A:496, 1979.

Congenital kyphosis

Bjekreim I, Magnaes B, and Semb G: Surgical treatment of severe angular kyphosis, Acta Orthop Scand 53:913, 1982.

Bradford DS: Anterior vascular pedicle bone grafting for the treatment of kyphosis, Spine 5:318, 1980.

Bradford DS et al: Anterior strut-grafting for the treatment of kyphosis: a review of experience with 48 patients, J Bone Joint Surg 64A:680, 1982.

James JIP: Paraplegia in congenital kyphoscoliosis, J Bone Joint Surg 57B:261, 1975.

Lonstein JE et al: Neurologic deficit secondary to spinal deformity: a review of the literature and report of 43 cases, Spine 5:331, 1980.

Mayfield JK et al: Congenital kyphosis due to defects of anterior segmentation, J Bone Joint Surg 62A:1291, 1980.

Montgomery SP and Hall JE: Congenital kyphosis, Spine 7:360, 1982.

Winter RB: Congenital kyphoscoliosis with paralysis following hemivertebra excision, Clin Orthop 119:116, 1976.

Winter RB, Moe JH, and Lonstein JE: The surgical treatment of congenital kyphosis: a review of 94 patients age 5 years or older with 2 years or more follow-up in 77 patients, Spine 10:224, 1985.

Winter RB, Moe JH, and Wang JF: Congenital kyphosis, J Bone Joint Surg 55A:223, 1973.

Spondylolisthesis

Adkins EWO: Spondylolisthesis, J Bone Joint Surg 37B:48, 1955.

Amuso SJ et al: The surgical treatment of spondylolisthesis by posterior element resection, J Bone Joint Surg 52A:529, 1970.

Balderston RA and Bradford DS: Technique for achievement and maintenance of reduction for severe spondylolisthesis using spinous process traction wiring and external fixation of the pelvis, Spine 10:376, 1985.

Baker DR and McHollick W: Spondylolysis and spondylolisthesis in children, Proceedings of the American Academy of Orthopaedic Surgeons, J Bone Joint Surg 38A:933, 1956.

Barash HL et al: Spondylolisthesis and tight hamstrings, J Bone Joint Surg 52A:1319, 1970.

Barr JS: Spondylolisthesis (editorial), J Bone Joint Surg 37A:878, 1955.

Beeler JW: Further evidence on the acquired nature of spondylolysis and spondylolisthesis, Am J Roentgenol Radium Ther Nucl Med 108:796, 1970.

Blackburne JS and Velikas EP: Spondylolisthesis in children and adolescents, J Bone Joint Surg 59B:490, 1977.

Bohlman HH and Cook SS: One-stage decompression and posterolateral and interbody fusion for lumbosacral spondyloptosis through a posterior approach: report of two cases, J Bone Joint Surg 64A:415, 1982.

Borokow SE and Kleiger B: Spondylolisthesis in the newborn, Clin Orthop 81:73, 1971.

Bosworth DM: Technique of spinal fusion in the lumbosacral region by the double clothespin graft (distraction graft; H graft) and results. In The American Academy of Orthopaedic Surgeons: Instructional course lectures, vol 9, Ann Arbor, Mich, 1952, JW Edwards.

Bosworth DM et al: Spondylolisthesis: a critical review of a consecutive series of cases treated by arthrodesis, J Bone Joint Surg 37A:767, 1955.

Boxall D et al: Management of severe spondylolisthesis in children and adolescents, J Bone Joint Surg 61A:479, 1979.

Bradford DS: Spondylolysis and spondylolisthesis, Curr Pract Orthop Surg 8:12, 1979.

Bradford DS: Treatment of severe spondylolisthesis: a combined approach for reduction and stabilization, Spine 4:423, 1979.

Bradford DS: Repair of spondylolysis or minimal degrees of spondylolisthesis by segmental wire fixation and bone grafting, Ortho Trans 6:1, 1982.

Bradford DS: Management of spondylolysis and spondylolisthesis. In The American Academy of Orthopaedic Surgeons: Instructional course lectures, vol 32, St Louis, 1983, The CV Mosby Co.

Buck JE: Direct repair of the defect in spondylolisthesis, J Bone Joint Surg 61A:479, 1979.

Burns BH: Two cases of spondylolisthesis, Proc R Soc Med 25:571, 1932.

Burns BH: An operation for spondylolisthesis, Lancet 1:1233, 1933.

Capener N: Spondylolisthesis, Br J Surg 19:374, 1932.

Cedell C and Wiberg G: Long term results of laminectomy in spondylolisthesis, Acta Orthop Scand 40:773, 1970.

Chandler FA: Lesions of the "isthmus" (pars interarticularis) of the laminae of the lower lumbar vertebrae and their relation to spondylolisthesis, Surg Gynecol Obstet 53:273, 1931.

Cleveland M, Bosworth DM, and Thompson FR: Pseudarthrosis in the lumbosacral spine, J Bone Joint Surg 20A:302, 1948.

Cloward RB: Spondylolisthesis: treatment by laminectomy and posterior interbody fusion: review of 100 cases, Clin Orthop 154:74, 1981.

Davis IS and Bailey RW: Spondylolisthesis: long term follow-up study of treatment with total laminectomy, Clin Orthop 88:46, 1972.

Davis IS and Bailey RW: Spondylolisthesis: indications for lumbar nerve root decompression and operative technique, Clin Orthop 117:129, 1976.

Dawson EG, Lotysch M III, and Urist MR: Intertransverse process lumbar arthrodesis with autogenous bone graft, Clin Orthop 154:90, 1981.

Del Torto U: Surgical reduction and stabilization of spondylolisthesis, Clin Orthop 75:281, 1971.

Devas MB: Stress fractures in children, J Bone Joint Surg 45B:528, 1963.

DeWald RL et al: Severe lumbosacral spondylolisthesis in adolescents and children: reduction and staged circumferential fusion, J Bone Joint Surg 63A:619, 1981.

Farfan HF, Osteria V, and Lamy C: The mechanical etiology of spondylolysis and spondylolisthesis, Clin Orthop 117:40, 1976.

Fisk JR, Moe JH, and Winter RB: Scoliosis, spondylolisthesis, and spondylolysis: their relationship as reviewed in 539 patients, Spine 3:234, 1978.

Fredrickson BE et al: The natural history of spondylolysis and spondylolisthesis, J Bone Joint Surg 66A:699, 1984.

Freeman BL and Donati NL: Spinal arthrodesis for severe spondylolisthesis in children and adolescents: a long term follow-up study, J Bone Joint Surg 71A:594, 1989.

Gaines RW and Nichols WK: Treatment of spondyloptosis by two-stage L-5 vertebrectomy and reduction of L-4 onto S-1, Spine 10:680, 1985.

Garfin SR and Amundson GM: Spondylolisthesis, Update Spinal Disorders 1:3, 1986.

Gelfand MJ, Strife JL, and Kereiakes SG: Radionuclide bone imaging in spondylolysis of the lumbar spine in children, Radiology 140:191, 1981.

Gill GG: Treatment of spondylolisthesis and spina bifida, Exhibit, The American Academy of Orthopaedic Surgeons Meeting, Chicago, January 1952.

Gill GG, Manning JG, and White HL: Surgical treatment of spondylolisthesis without spine fusion, J Bone Joint Surg 37A:493, 1955.

Gill GG and White HL: Surgical treatment of spondylolisthesis without spine fusion: a long term follow-up of operated cases. Paper presented at the Western Orthopaedic Association, San Francisco, Nov 1962.

Goldberg MJ: Gymnastic injuries, Orthop Clin North Am 11:717, 1980.

Goldstein LA et al: Guidelines for the management of lumbosacral spondylolisthesis associated with scoliosis, Clin Orthop 117:135, 1976.

Hammond G, Wise RE, and Haggart GE: Review of seventy-three cases of spondylolisthesis treated by arthrodesis, JAMA 163:175, 1957.

Haraldsson S and Willner S: A comparative study of spondylolisthesis in operations on adolescents and adults, Arch Orthop Trauma Surg 101:101, 1983.

Harrington PR and Dickson JH: Spinal instrumentation in the treatment of severe progressive spondylolisthesis, Clin Orthop 117:157, 1976.

Harrington PR and Tullos HS: Spondylolisthesis in children: observations and surgical treatment, Clin Orthop 79:75, 1971.

Harris IE and Weinstein SL: Long-term follow-up of patients with grade III and IV spondylolisthesis: treatment with and without fusion, J Bone Joint Surg 69A:960, 1987.

Harris RI: Spondylolisthesis, Ann R Coll Surg Engl 8:259, 1951.

Henderson ED: Results of the surgical treatment of spondylolisthesis, J Bone Joint Surg 48A:619, 1966.

Hensinger RN: Spondylolysis and spondylolisthesis in children. In The American Academy of Orthopaedic Surgeons: Instructional course lectures, vol 32, St Louis, 1983, The CV Mosby Co.

Hensinger RN, Lang JR, and MacEwen GD: Surgical management of the spondylolisthesis in children and adolescents, Spine 1:207, 1976.

Hitchcock HH: Spondylolisthesis: observations on its development, progression, and genesis, J Bone Joint Surg 22:1, 1940.

Howorth B: Low backache and sciatica: results of surgical treatment. III. Surgical treatment of spondylolisthesis, J Bone Joint Surg 46A:1515, 1964.

Huizenga BA: Reduction of spondyloptosis with two-stage vertebrectomy, Orthop Trans 7:21, 1983.

Jackson DW, Wiltse LL, and Cirincione RJ: Spondylolysis in the female gymnast, Clin Orthop 117:68, 1976.

Jenkins JA: Spondylolisthesis, Br J Surg 24:80, 1936.

Johnson JR and Kirwan EOG: The long-term results of fusion in situ for severe spondylolisthesis, J Bone Joint Surg 65B:43, 1983.

Kaneda K et al: Distraction rod instrumentation with posterolateral fusion in isthmic spondylolisthesis: 53 cases followed for 18-89 months, Spine 10:383, 1985.

Kettlekamp DB and Wright GD: Spondylolysis in the Alaskan Eskimo, J Bone Joint Surg 53A:563, 1971.

King AB, Baker DR, and McHolick WJ: Another approach to the treatment of spondylolisthesis and spondyloschisis, Clin Orthop 10:257, 1957.

Kiviluoto O et al: Postero-lateral spine fusion, a 1-4 year follow-up of 80 consecutive patients, Acta Orthop Scand 56:152, 1985.

Klinghoffer L and Murdock MG: Spondylolysis following trauma: a case report and review of the literature, Clin Orthop 166:72, 1982.

Krenz J and Troup JDG: The structure of the pars interarticularis of the lower lumbar vertebrae and its relation to the etiology of spondylolysis, with a report of the healing fracture in the neural arch of a fourth lumbar vertebra, J Bone Joint Surg 55B:735, 1973.

Lafond G: Surgical treatment of spondylolisthesis, Clin Orthop 22:175, 1962.

Lance EM: Treatment of severe spondylolisthesis with neural involvement: a report of two cases, J Bone Joint Surg 48A:883, 1966.

Laurent LE: Spondylolisthesis: a study of 53 cases treated by spine fusion and 32 cases treated by laminectomy, Acta Orthop Scand 35(suppl):1, 1958.

Laurent LE and Einola S: Spondylolisthesis in children and adolescents, Acta Orthop Scand 31:45, 1961.

Laurent LE and Osterman K: Operative treatment of spondylolisthesis in young patients, Clin Orthop 117:85, 1976.

Lowe RW et al: Standing roentgenograms in spondylolisthesis, Clin Orthop 117:80, 1976.

Lusskin R: Pain patterns in spondylolisthesis: a correlation of symptoms, local pathology, and therapy, Clin Orthop 40:123, 1965.

Macnab I and Dall D: The blood supply of the lumbar spine and its application to the technique of intertransverse lumbar fusion, J Bone Joint Surg 53B:628, 1971.

Marmor L and Bechtol CO: Spondylolisthesis: complete slip following the Gill procedure: a case report, J Bone Joint Surg 43A:1068, 1961.

McKee BW, Alexander WJ, and Dunbar JS: Spondylolysis and spondylolisthesis in children: a review, J Can Assoc Radiol 22:100, 1971.

McPhee IB and O'Brien JP: Reduction of severe spondylolisthesis: a preliminary report, Spine 4:430, 1979.

McPhee IB and O'Brien JP: Scoliosis in symptomatic spondylolisthesis, J Bone Joint Surg 62B:155, 1980.

Mercer W: Spondylolisthesis: with a description of a new method of operative treatment and notes of ten cases, Edinburgh Med J 43:545, 1936.

Meyerding HW: Spondylolisthesis, Surg Gynecol Obstet 54:371, 1932.

Meyerding HW: Low backache and sciatic pain associated with spondylolisthesis and protruded intervertebral disc: incidence, significance and treatment (symposium), J Bone Joint Surg 23:461, 1941.

Micheli LJ: Low back pain in the adolescent: differential diagnosis, Am J Sports Med 7:361, 1979.

Munster JK and Troup JDG: The structure of the pars interarticularis of the lower lumbar vertebrae and its relation to the etiology of spondylolysis, J Bone Joint Surg 55B:735, 1973.

Nachemson A: Repair of the spondylolisthetic defect and intertransverse fusion for young patients, Clin Orthop 117:101, 1976.

Newman PH: A clinical syndrome associated with severe lumbosacral subluxation, J Bone Joint Surg 47B:472, 1965.

Newman PH: Stenosis of the lumbar spine in spondylolisthesis, Clin Orthop 115:116, 1976.

Newman PH and Stone KH: The etiology of spondylolisthesis, J Bone Joint Surg 45B:39, 1963.

Ohki I et al: Reduction and fusion of severe spondylolisthesis using halo-pelvic traction with a wire reduction device, Inter Orthop (SICOT) 4:107, 1980.

Osterman K, Lindholm TS, and Laurent LE: Late results of removal of the loose posterior element (Gill's operation) in the treatment of lytic lumbar spondylolisthesis, Clin Orthop 117:121, 1976.

Phalen GS and Dickson JA: Spondylolisthesis and tight hamstrings, J Bone Joint Surg 43A:505, 1961.

Riley P and Gillespie R: Severe spondylolisthesis: results of posterolateral fusion, Orthop Trans 9:119, 1985.

Rombold C: Treatment of spondylolisthesis by posterolateral fusion, resection of the pars interarticularis, and prompt mobilization of the patient: an end-result study of seventy-three patients, J Bone Joint Surg 48A:1282, 1966.

Rosenberg NJ, Bargar WL, and Friedman B: The incidence of spondylolysis and spondylolisthesis in nonambulatory patients, Spine 6:35, 1981.

Rosomoff HL: Lumbar spondylolisthesis: etiology of radiculopathy and role of the neurosurgeon, Clin Neurosurg 27:577, 1980.

Rowe GG and Roche MB: The etiology of separate neural arch, J Bone Joint Surg 35A:102, 1953.

Scaglietti O, Frontino G, and Bartolozzi P: Technique of anatomical reduction of lumbar spondylolisthesis and its surgical stabilization, Clin Orthop 117:164, 1976.

Sevastikoglou JA, Spangfort E, and Aaro S: Operative treatment of spondylolisthesis in children and adolescents with tight hamstrings syndrome, Clin Orthop 147:192, 1980.

Shahriaree H, Sajadi K, and Rooholamini SA: A family with spondylolisthesis, J Bone Joint Surg 61A:1256, 1979.

Sherman FC, Rosenthal RK, and Hall JE: Spine fusion for spondylolysis and spondylolisthesis in children, Spine 4:59, 1979.

Sijbrandij S: A new technique for the reduction and stabilisation of severe spondylolisthesis: a report of two cases, J Bone Joint Surg 63B:266, 1981.

Sijbrandij S: Reduction and stabilisation of severe spondylolisthesis: a report of three cases, J Bone Joint Surg 65B:40, 1983.

Snijder JGN et al: Therapy of spondylolisthesis by repositioning and fixation of the olisthetic vertebra, Clin Orthop 117:149, 1976.

Speed K: Spondylolisthesis: treatment by anterior bone graft, Arch Surg 37:175, 1938.

Stanton RP, Meehan P, and Lovell WW: Surgical fusion in childhood spondylolisthesis, J Pediatr Orthop 5:411, 1985.

Stewart TD: The age incidence of neural arch defects in Alaskan natives, considered from the standpoint of etiology, J Bone Joint Surg 35A:937, 1953.

Taillard WF: Etiology of spondylolisthesis, Clin Orthop 117:30, 1976.

Takeda M: A newly devised "three-one" method for the surgical treatment of spondylolysis and spondylolisthesis, Clin Orthop 147:228, 1980.

Todd EM Jr and Gardner WJ: Simple excision of the unattached lamina for spondylolysis, Surg Gynecol Obstet 106:724, 1958.

Troup JDG: Mechanical factors in spondylolisthesis and spondylolysis, Clin Orthop 117:59, 1976.

Turner RH and Bianco AJ Jr: Spondylolysis and spondylolisthesis in children and teen-agers, J Bone Joint Surg 53A:1298, 1971.

Velikas EP and Blackburne JS: Surgical treatment of spondylolisthesis in children and adolescents, J Bone Joint Surg 63B:67, 1981.

Verbiest H: The treatment of spondyloptosis or impending lumbar spondyloptosis accompanied by neurologic deficit and/or neurogenic intermittent claudication, Spine 4:68, 1979.

Vidal J et al: Surgical reduction of spondylolisthesis using a posterior approach, Clin Orthop 154:156, 1981.

Watkins MB: Posterolateral fusion in pseudarthrosis and posterior element defects of the lumbosacral spine, Clin Orthop 35:80, 1964.

Wertzberger KL and Peterson HA: Acquired spondylolysis and spondylolisthesis in the young child, Spine 5:437, 1980.

Wiltse LL: Etiology of spondylolisthesis, Clin Orthop 10:48, 1957.

Wiltse LL: Spondylolisthesis in children, Clin Orthop 21:156, 1961.

Wiltse LL and Hutchinson RH: Surgical treatment of spondylolisthesis, Clin Orthop 35:116, 1964.

Wiltse LL and Jackson DW: Treatment of spondylolisthesis and spondylolysis in children, Clin Orthop 117:92, 1976.

Wiltse LL and Winter RB: Terminology and measurement of spondylolisthesis, J Bone Joint Surg 65A:768, 1983.

Wiltse LL, Newman PH, and Macnab I: Classification of spondylolisis and spondylolisthesis, Clin Orthop 117:23, 1976.

Wiltse LL, Widell EH Jr, and Jackson DW: Fatigue fracture: the basic lesion in isthmic spondylolisthesis, J Bone Joint Surg 57A:17, 1975.

Wiltse LL et al: The paraspinal sacrospinalis-splitting approach to the lumbar spine, J Bone Joint Surg 50A:919, 1968.

Woolsey RD: The mechanism of neurological symptoms and signs in spondylolisthesis at the fifth lumbar, first sacral level, J Neurosurg 11:67, 1954.

Kyphoscoliosis in myelomeningocele

Allen B and Ferguson R: Operative treatment of myelomeningocele spinal deformities, Orthop Clin North Am 10:845, 1979.

Banta JV and Hamada JS: Natural history of the kyphotic deformity in myelomeningocele, J Bone Joint Surg 58A:279, 1960.

Banta JV and Park SM: Improvement in pulmonary function in patients having combined anterior and posterior spine fusion for myelomeningocele scoliosis, Spine 8:766, 1983.

Banta JV et al: Fifteen-year review of myelodysplasia, J Bone Joint Surg 58A:726, 1976.

Bodel JG and Stephane JP: Luque rods in the treatment of kyphosis in myelomeningocele, J Bone Joint Surg 65B:98, 1983.

Brown HP: Management of spinal deformity in myelomeningocele, Orthop Clin North Am 9:391, 1978.

Bunch WH: The Milwaukee brace in paralytic scoliosis, Clin Orthop 110:63, 1975.

Christofersen MR and Brooks AL: Excision and wire fixation of rigid myelomeningocele kyphosis, J Pediatr Orthop 5:691, 1985.

Dickens DVR: The surgery of scoliosis and spina bifida, J Bone Joint Surg 61B:386, 1979.

Drennan JC: The role of muscle in the development of human lumbar kyphosis, Dev Med Child Neurol 12:33, 1970.

Drummond DS, Morear M, and Cruess RL: The results and complications of surgery for the paralytic hip and spine in myelomeningocele, J Bone Joint Surg 62B:49, 1980.

Dunn HK: Kyphosis of myelodysplasia: operative treatment based on pathophysiology, Orthop Trans 7:19, 1983.

Eyring EJ, Wanken JJ, and Sayers MP: Spine ostectomy for kyphosis in myelomeningocele, Clin Orthop 88:24, 1972.

Feiwell E: Selection of appropriate treatment for patients with myelomeningocele, Orthop Clin North Am 12:101, 1981.

Gillespie R, Torode I, and van Olm RS Jr: Myelomeningocele kyphosis fixed by kyphectomy and segmental spinal instrumentation, Orthop Trans 8:162, 1984.

Hall JE and Bobechko WP: Advances in the management of spinal deformities and myelodysplasia, Clin Neurosurg 20:164, 1973.

Hall JE and Poitras B: The management of kyphosis in patients with myelomeningocele, Clinic Orthop 128:33, 1977.

Hall PV et al: Myelodysplasia and developmental scoliosis: a manifestation of syringomyelia, Spine 1:48, 1976.

Hall PV et al: Scoliosis and hydrocephalus in myelocele patients: the affect of ventricular shunting, J Neurosurg 50:174, 1979.

Heydemann JS and Gillespie R: Management of myelomeningocele kyphosis in the older child by kyphectomy and segmental spinal instrumentation, Spine 12:37, 1987.

Hoppenfeld S: Congenital kyphosis in myelomeningocele, J Bone Joint Surg 49B:276, 1967.

Hull WJ, Moe JH, and Winter RB: Spinal deformity in myelomeningocele: natural history, evaluation, and treatment, J Bone Joint Surg 56A:1767, 1974.

Johnston CE, Hakala MW, and Rosenberg R: Paralytic spinal deformity: orthotic treatment in spinal discontinuity syndromes, J Pediatr Orthop 2:233, 1982.

Jones ET: Kyphectomy in myelodysplasia, Orthop Trans 7:432, 1983.

Kahanovitz N and Duncan JW: The role of scoliosis and pelvic obliquity on functional disability in myelomeningocele, Spine 6:494, 1981.

Kilfoyle RM, Foley JJ, and Norton PL: Spine and pelvic deformity in childhood and adolescent paraplegia: a study of 104 cases, J Bone Joint Surg 47A:659, 1976.

Leatherman KD and Dickson RA: Congenital kyphosis in myelomeningocele: vertebral body resection and posterior spinal fusion, Spine 3:222, 1978.

Lindseth RE, and Selzer L: Vertebral excision of kyphosis in myelomeningocele, J Bone Joint Surg 61A:699, 1979.

Lowe GP and Menelaus MB: The surgical management in kyphosis in older children with myelomeningocele, J Bone Joint Surg 60B:40, 1978.

Mackel JL and Lindseth RE: Scoliosis in myelodysplasia, J Bone Joint Surg 57A:131, 1975.

Mayfield JK: Severe spine deformity and myelodysplasia and sacral agenesis: an aggressive surgical approach, Spine 6:498, 1981.

McMaster MJ: Anterior and posterior instrumentation and fusion of thoracolumbar scoliosis due to myelomeningocele, J Bone Joint Surg 69B:20, 1987.

Osebold W et al: Surgical treatment of paralytic scoliosis in myelomeningocele, J Bone Joint Surg 64A:841, 1982.

Park WM and Watt I: The pre-operative aortographic assessment of children with spina bifida cystica and severe kyphosis, J Bone Joint Surg 57B:112, 1975.

Piggott H: The natural history of scoliosis in myelodysplasia, J Bone Joint Surg 61B:122, 1979.

Poitras B and Hall JE: The management of kyphosis in patients with myelomeningocele, Clin Orthop 128:33, 1977.

Poitras B et al: Correction of the kyphosis in myelomeningocele patients by both anterior and posterior stabilization procedure, Orthop Trans 7:432, 1983.

Raycroft JF and Curtis BH: Spinal curvature in myelomeningocele. In The American Academy of Orthopaedic Surgeons Symposium on Myelomeningocele, St Louis, 1972, The CV Mosby Co.

Sharrard WJW: Spinal osteotomy for congenital kyphosis in myelomeningocele, J Bone Joint Surg 50B:466, 1968.

Sharrard WJW and Drennan JC: Osteo-excision of the spine for lumbar kyphosis in older children with myelomeningocele, J Bone Joint Surg 54B:50, 1972.

Shurtleff DB et al: Myelodysplasia: the natural history of kyphosis and scoliosis, Dev Med Child Neurol 18 (suppl 37):126, 1976.

Sriram K, Bobechko WP, and Hall JE: Surgical management of spinal deformities in spina bifida, J Bone Joint Surg 54B:666, 1972.

Winston K et al: Acute elevation of intracranial pressure following transection of non-functional spinal cord, Clin Orthop 128:41, 1977.

Sacral agenesis

Abraham E: Lumbosacral coccygeal agenesis: autopsy case report, J Bone Joint Surg 58A:1169, 1976.

Abraham E: Sacral agenesis with associated anomalies (caudal regression syndrome): autopsy case report, Clin Orthop 145:168, 1979.

Andrish J, Kalamchi A, and MacEwen GD: Sacral agenesis: a clinical evaluation of its management, heredity, and associated anomalies, Clin Orthop 139:52, 1979.

Banta JV, and Nichols O: Sacral agenesis, J Bone Joint Surg 51A:693, 1969.

Blumel J, Evans EB, and Eggers GWN: Partial and complete agenesis or malformation of the sacrum with associated anomalies, J Bone Joint Surg 41A:497, 1959.

Cohn J and Bay-Nielsen E: Hereditary defect of the sacrum and coccyx with anterior sacral meningocele, Acta Pediatr Scand 58:268, 1969.

Duraiswami PK: Experimental causation of congenital skeletal defects and its significance in orthopaedic surgery, J Bone Joint Surg 34B:646, 1952.

Elting JJ and Allen JC: Management of the young child with bilateral anomalous and functionless lower extremities, J Bone Joint Surg 54A:1523, 1972.

Frantz CH and Aitken GT: Complete absence of the lumbar spine and sacrum, J Bone Joint Surg 49A:1531, 1967.

Freedman B: Congenital absence of the sacrum and coccyx: report of a case and review of the literature, Brit J Surg 37:299, 1950.

Ignelzi RJ and Lehman RAW: Lumbosacral agenesis: management and embryological implications, J Neurol Neurosurg Psychiatry 37:1273, 1974.

Koff SA and Deridder PA: Patterns of neurogenic bladder dysfunction in sacral agenesis, J Urol 188:87, 1977.

Marsh HO and Tejano NA: Four cases of lumbo-sacral and sacral agenesis, Clin Orthop 92:214, 1973.

Mongeau M and LeClaire R: Complete agenesis of the lumbosacral spine: a case report, J Bone Joint Surg 54A:161, 1972.

Nicol WJ: Lumbosacral agenesis in a 60-year-old man, Br J Surg 59:577, 1972.

Nogami H and Ingalls TH: Pathogenesis of spinal malformations induced in the embryos of mice, J Bone Joint Surg 49A:1551, 1967.

Passarge E and Lenz W: Syndrome of caudal regression in infants of diabetic mothers: observation of further cases, Pediatrics 37:672, 1966.

Perry J, Bonnett CA, and Hoffer MM: Vertebral pelvic fusions in the rehabilitation of patients with sacral agenesis, J Bone Joint Surg 52A:288, 1970.

Phillips WA et al: Orthopaedic management of lumbosacral agenesis: long-term follow-up, J Bone Joint Surg 64A:1282, 1982.

Price DL, Dooling EC, Richardson EP Jr: Caudal dysplasia (caudal regression syndrome), Arch Neurol 23:212, 1970.

Redhead RG, Vitali M, and Trapnell DH: Congenital absence of the lumbar spine, Br Med J 3:595, 1968.

Redman JF: Congenital absence of the lumbosacral spine, South Med J 66:770, 1973.

Reeve AW and Mortimer JG: Lumbosacral agenesis or rumplessness, N Z Med J 73:340, 1971.

Renshaw TS: Sacral agenesis: a classification in review of 23 cases, J Bone Joint Surg 60A:373, 1978.

Rosenthal RK: Congenital absence of the coccyx, sacrum, lumbar vertebrae and the lower two thoracic vertebrae, Bull Hosp J Dis Orthop Inst 29:287, 1968.

Ruderman RJ, Keats P, and Goldner JL: Congenital absence of the lumbo-sacral spine: a report of an unusual case, Clin Orthop 124:177, 1977.

Rusnak SL and Driscoll SG: Congenital spinal anomalies in infants of diabetic mothers, Pediatrics 35:989, 1965.

Russell HE and Aitken GT: Congenital absence of the sacrum and lumbar vertebrae with prosthetic management: a survey of the literature and presentation of five cases, J Bone Joint Surg 45A:501, 1963.

Sinclair JE, Duren N, and Rude JC: Congenital lumbosacral defect, Arch Surg 43:473, 1941.

Smith ED: Congenital sacral anomalies in children, Aust N Z J Surg 29:165, 1959.

White RI and Klauber GT: Sacral agenesis: analysis of 22 cases, Urology 8:521, 1976.

Williams DI and Nixon HH: Agenesis of the sacrum, Surg Gynecol Obstet 105:84, 1957.

Neurofibromatosis

Bradford DS: Anterior vascular pedicle bone grafting for the treatment of kyphosis, Spine 5:318, 1980.

Brooks B and Lehman E: The bone changes in Recklinghausen's neurofibromatosis, Surg Gynecol Obstet 38:587, 1924.

Casselman E and Mandell G: Vertebral scalloping in neurofibromatosis, Radiology 131:89, 1979.

Chaglassian J, Riseborough E, and Hall J: Neurofibromatosis, J Bone Joint Surg 58A:695, 1976.

Crowe F and Schull W: Diagnostic importance of café au lait spot in neurofibromatosis, Arch Intern Med 91:758, 1953.

Curtis B et al: Neurofibromatosis with paraplegia, J Bone Joint Surg 51A:843, 1969.

Fulton J: Robert W Smith's description of generalized neurofibromatosis (1849), N Engl J Med 200:1315, 1929.

Heard G, Holt J, and Naylor B: Cervical vertebral deformity in Von Recklinghausen's disease of the nervous system, J Bone Joint Surg 44B:880, 1962.

Hensinger R: Kyphosis secondary to skeletal dysplasias and metabolic disease, Clin Orthop 128:113, 1977.

Holt J: Neurofibromatosis in children, Am J Roentgenol 130:615, 1978.

Hsu L, Lee P, and Leong J: Dystrophic spinal deformities in neurofibromatosis, J Bone Joint Surg 66B:495, 1984.

Hunt J and Pugh D: Skeletal lesions in neurofibromatosis, Radiology 76:1, 1961.

Lonstein J et al: Neurologic deficits secondary to spinal deformity, Spine 5:331, 1980.

Mandell G: The pedicle in neurofibromatosis, Am J Roentgenol 130:675, 1978.

McCarroll H: Clinical manifestations of congenital neurofibromatosis, J Bone Joint Surg 32A:601, 1950.

Miller A: Neurofibromatosis: with reference to skeletal changes, compression myelitis and malignant degeneration, Arch Surg 32:109, 1936.

Mitchell G, Lourie H, and Berne A: The various causes of scalloped vertebrae with notes on their pathogenesis, Radiology 89:67, 1967.

Nanson E: Thoracic meningocele associated with neurofibromatosis, J Thorac Cardiovasc Surg 33:650, 1967.

Rezaian S: The incidence of scoliosis due to neurofibromatosis, Acta Orthop Scand 47:534, 1976.

Riccardi V: Von Recklinghausen neurofibromatosis, N Engl J Med 305:1617, 1981.

Salerno N and Edigken J: Vertebral scalloping in neurofibromatosis, Radiology 97:509, 1970.

Savini R, et al: Surgical treatment of vertebral deformities in neurofibromatosis, Ital J Orthop Traumatol 9:13, 1983.

von Recklinghausen F: Ueber die multiplen Fibrome der Haut und ihre Beziehung zu den multiplen Neuromen, Festschrift dur Rudolph Virchow, Berlin, 1882, August Hirschwald.

Whitehouse D: Diagnostic value of the café au lait spot in children, Arch Dis Child 41:316, 1966.

Winter RB and Edwards W: Neurofibromatosis with lumbosacral spondylolisthesis, J Pediatr Orthop 1:91, 1981.

Winter RB, Lonstein JE, and Anderson M: Neurofibromatosis kyphosis. Paper presented at the Fifty-fifth Annual Meeting of the American Academy of Orthopaedic Surgeons, Atlanta, Feb 4-9, 1988.

Winter RB et al: Spine deformity in neurofibromatosis, J Bone Joint Surg 61A:677, 1979.

Yong-Hing K, Kalamchi A, and MacEwen GD: Cervical spine abnormalities in neurofibromatosis, J Bone Joint Surg, 61A:695, 1979.

Marfan syndrome

Amis J and Herring J: Iatrogenic kyphosis: complication of Harrington instrumentation in Marfan's syndrome, J Bone Joint Surg 66A:460, 1984.

Birch JG and Herring JA: Spinal deformity in Marfan's syndrome, J Pediatr Orthop 7:546, 1987.

Boucek RJ et al: The Marfan's syndrome: a difficiency in chemically stable collogen cross-links, N Engl J Med 305:988, 1981.

Bowers D: Marfan syndrome: the S family revisited, Can Med Assoc J 89:337, 1963.

Brenton DP and Dow DJ: Homocystinuria and Marfan's syndrome: a comparison, J Bone Joint Surg 54B:277, 1972.

McKusick VA: Heritable disorders of connective tissue, ed 3, St Louis, 1966, The CV Mosby Co.

Murdoch JL et al: Life expectancy and causes of death in Marfan's syndrome, N Engl J Med 286:804, 1972.

Orcutt FV and DeWald RL: The special problems which the Marfan syndrome introduces to scoliosis, J Bone Joint Surg 56A:1763, 1974.

Pyeritz RE and McKusick VA: The Marfan syndrome: diagnosis and management, N Engl J Med 300:772, 1979.

Pyeritz RE and McKusick VA: Basic defects in the Marfan syndrome, N Engl J Med 305:1011, 1981.

Robins PR, Moe JH, and Winter RB: Scoliosis in Marfan syndrome: its characteristics and results of treatment in 35 patients, J Bone Joint Surg 57A:358, 1975.

Savini R, Cerrellati S, and Beroaldo E: Spinal deformities in Marfan's syndrome, Ital J Orthop Traumatol 6:19, 1980.

Wilner HI and Finby J: Skeletal manifestations in the Marfan syndrome, JAMA 197:490, 1975.

Winter RB: Severe spondylolisthesis in Marfan's syndrome: report of two cases, J Pediatr Orthop 2:51, 1982.

Vertebral column tumors

Akbarnia BA, Bradford DS, and Winter RB: Osteoid osteoma of the spine: an analysis of 14 patients, Orthop Trans 6:4, 1982.

Akbarnia BA and Rooholamini SA: Scoliosis caused by benign osteoblastoma of the thoracic or lumbar spine, J Bone Joint Surg 63A:1146, 1981.

Allison DJ: Therapeutic embolization, J Bone Joint Surg 64B:151, 1982.

Barwick KW, Huvos AG, and Smith J: Primary osteogenic sarcoma of the vertebral column, Cancer 46:595, 1980.

Caldicott WJH: Diagnosis of spinal osteoid osteoma, Radiology 92:1192, 1969.

Dick HM et al: Adjuvant arterial embolization in the treatment of benign primary bone tumors in children, Clin Orthop 139:133, 1979.

Dunlop JAY, Morton KS, and Elliott GB: Recurrent osteoid osteoma: report of a case with a review of the literature, J Bone Joint Surg 52B:128, 1970.

Dunn HK: Tumors of the thoracic and lumbar spine. In Evarts CM, editor: Surgery of the musculoskeletal system, New York, 1983, Churchill Livingstone.

Feldman F et al: Selective intra-arterial embolization of bone tumors: a useful adjunct in the management of selected lesions, J Roentgenol 123:130, 1975.

Freiberger RH: Osteoid osteoma of the spine: a cause of backache and scoliosis in children and young adults, Radiology 75:232, 1960.

Golding JSR: The natural history of osteoid osteoma: with a report of 20 cases, J Bone Joint Surg 36B:218, 1954.

Heiman ML, Cooley CJ, and Bradford DS: Osteoid osteoma of a vertebral body, Clin Orthop 118:159, 1976.

Hekster REM, Luyendijk W, and Tan TI: Spinal-cord compression caused by vertebral hemangioma relieved by percutaneous catheter embolization, Neuroradiology 3:160, 1972.

Henderson ED and Dahlin DC: Chondrosarcoma of bone: a study of 280 cases, J Bone Joint Surg 54A:1451, 1972.

Inglis AE et al: Osteochondroma of the cervical spine: case report, Clin Orthop 126:127, 1977.

Israeli A et al: Use of radionuclide method in preoperative and intra-operative diagnosis of osteoid osteoma of the spine: case report, Clin Orthop 175:194, 1983.

Jackson RP, Reckling FW, and Mantz FA: Ostroidosteoma and osteoblastoma: similar histologic lesions with different natural histories, Clin Orthop 128:303, 1977.

Jaffee HL: "Osteoid osteoma": a benign osteoblastic tumor composed of osteoid and atypical bone, Arch Surg 31:709, 1935.

Jelsma RK and Kirsch PT: The treatment of malignancy of a vertebral body, Surg Neurol 13:189, 1980.

Keim HA and Reina EG: Osteoid osteoma as a cause of scoliosis, J Bone Joint Surg 57A:159, 1975.

Larsson SE, Lorentzon R, and Boquist L: Giant-cell tumors of the spine and sacrum, causing neurological symptoms, Clin Orthop 111:201, 1975.

Lichenstein L and Jaffee HL: Eosinophilic granuloma of bone— with report of a case, Am J Pathol 16:595, 1940.

Lichtenstein L and Sawyer WR: Benign osteoblastoma: further observations and report of 20 additional cases, J Bone Joint Surg 46A:755, 1964.

Maclellan DI and Wilson FC Jr: Osteoid osteoma of the spine: a review of the literature and report of 6 new cases, J Bone Joint Surg 49A:111, 1967.

Marsh BW et al: Benign osteoblastoma: range of manifestations, J Bone Joint Surg 57A:1, 1975.

Marsh HO and Choi CB: Primary osteogenic sarcoma of the cervical spine, originally mistaken for benign osteoblastoma, J Bone Joint Surg 52A:1467, 1970.

Mehta MH: Pain provoked scoliosis: observations on the evolution of the deformity, Clin Orthop 135:58, 1978.

Mehta MH and Murray RO: Scoliosis provoked by painful vertebral lesions, Skel Radiol 1:223, 1977.

Merryweather R, Middlemiss JH, and Sanerkin NG: Malignant transformation of osteoblastoma, J Bone Joint Surg 62B:381, 1980.

Michele A and Krueger FJ: A surgical approach to the vertebral body, J Bone Joint Surg 31A:873, 1949.

Moon KL, Genant HK, and Holmes CA: Muscular skeletal applications of nuclear magnetic resonance imaging, Radiology 147:161, 1983.

Nelson OA and Greer RB III: Localization of osteoid osteoma of the spine using computerized tomography, J Bone Joint Surg 65A:263, 1983.

Ottolenghi CE: Aspiration biopsy in the diagnosis of lesion of the vertebral bodies, J Bone Joint Surg 37A:443, 1955.

Pettine KA and Klassen RA: Osteoid-osteoma and osteoblastoma of the spine, J Bone Joint Surg 68A:354, 1986.

Ponseti I and Barta CK: Osteoid osteoma, J Bone Joint Surg 29:767, 1947.

Ransford AO et al: The behavior pattern of the scoliosis associated with osteoid osteoma or osteoblastoma of the spine, J Bone Joint Surg 66B:16, 1984.

Rinsky LA et al: Intraoperative skeletal scintigraphy for localization of osteoid-osteoma in the spine, J Bone Joint Surg 62A:143, 1980.

Rodrigues RJ and Lewis HH: Eosinophilic granuloma of bone, Clin Orthop 77:183, 1971.

Rushton JG, Mulder DW, and Lipscom PR: Neurologic symptoms with osteoid osteoma, Neurology 5:794, 1955.

Schacked I, et al: Aneurysmal bone cyst of a vertebral body with acute paraplegia, Paraplegia 19:294, 1981.

Schajowicz F and Lemos C: Osteoid osteoma and osteoblastoma: closely related entities of osteoblastic derivation, Acta Orthop Scand 41:272, 1970.

Seiman LP: Eosinophilic granuloma of the spine, J Pediatr Orthop 1:371, 1981.

Sherman MS: Osteoid osteoma: review of the literature and report of 30 cases, J Bone Joint Surg 29:918, 1947.

Valls J, Ottolenghi CE, and Schajowicz F: Aspiration biopsy in the diagnosis of lesions of the vertebral bodies, JAMA 136:376, 1948.

Wedge JH, Tchang S, and MacFadyen DJ: Computed tomography and localization of spinal osteoid osteoma, Spine 6:423, 1981.

Osteochondrodystrophies

Bethem D et al: Spinal disorders of dwarfism: review of the literature and report of 80 cases, J Bone Joint Surg 63A:1412, 1981.

Postirradiation—spine deformity

Arkin AM et al: Radiation-induced scoliosis: a case report, J Bone Joint Surg 32A:401, 1950.

Arkin AM and Simon N: Radiation scoliosis: an experimental study, J Bone Joint Surg 32A:396, 1950.

Barr JS, Lingley JR, and Gall EA: The effect of roentgen irradiation on epiphyseal growth, Am J Roentgenol 49:104, 1943.

Bick EM and Copel JW: Longitudinal growth of the human vertebra: a contribution to human osteogeny, J Bone Joint Surg 32A:803, 1950.

Engel D: Experiments on the production of spinal deformities by radium, Am J of Roentgenol 42:217, 1939.

Frantz CH: Extreme retardation of epiphyseal growth from roentgen irradiation, Radiology 55:720, 1950.

Heaston DK, Libshitz HJ, and Chan RC: Skeletal affects of megavoltage irradiation and survivors of Wilms' tumors, Am J Roentgenol 133:389, 1979.

Hinkel CL: The effect of roentgen rays upon the growing long bones of albino rats. II. Histopathological changes involving inchondral growth centers, Am J Roentgenol 49:321, 1943.

Katzman H, Waugh T, and Berdon W: Skeletal changes following irradiation of childhood tumors, J Bone Joint Surg 51A:825, 1969.

King J and Stowe S: Results of spinal fusion for radiation scoliosis, Spine 7:574, 1982.

Mayfield JK et al: Spinal deformity in children treated for neuroblastoma, J Bone Joint Surg 63A:183, 1981.

Murphy FD and Blount WP: Cartilagenous exostoses following irradiation, J Bone Joint Surg 44A:662, 1962.

Neuhauser EB et al: Radiation effects of roentgen therapy on the growing spine, Radiology 59:637, 1952.

Ogilvie JW: Spinal deformity following radiation. In Bradford DS et al: Moe's textbook of scoliosis and other spinal deformities, ed 2, Philadelphia, 1987, WB Saunders Co.

Phemister DB: Radium necrosis of bone, Am J Roentgenol 16:340, 1926.

Reidy JA, et al: The effect of roentgen irradiation on epiphyseal growth, J Bone Joint Surg 29:853, 1947.

Riseborough EJ, et al: Skeletal alterations following irradiation for Wilm's tumor, J Bone Joint Surg 58A:526, 1976.

Rubin P, et al: Radiation induced dysplasias of bone, Am J Roentgenol 82:206, 1959.

Whitehouse, WM and Lampe I: Osseous damage in irradiation of renal tumors in infancy and childhood, Am J Roentgenol 70:721, 1953.

Osteogenesis imperfecta

Albright JA: Management overview of osteogenesis imperfecta, Clin Orthop 159:80, 1981.

Albright JA and Grunt JA: Studies of patients with osteogenesis imperfecta, J Bone Joint Surg 53A:1415, 1971.

Benson DR and Donaldson DH: The spine in osteogenesis imperfecta, J Bone Joint Surg 60A:925, 1978.

Benson DR and Newman DC: The spine and surgical treatment in osteogenesis imperfecta, Clin Orthop 159:147, 1981.

Bradford DS: Osteogenesis imperfecta. In Bradford DS et al, editors: Moe's textbook of scoliosis and other spinal deformities, Philadelphia, 1987, WB Saunders Co.

Cristofaro RL et al: Operative treatment of spine deformity in osteogenesis imperfecta, Clin Orthop 139:40, 1979.

Falvo KA, Root L, and Bullough PG: Osteogenesis imperfecta: clinical evaluation and management, J Bone Joint Surg 56A:783, 1974.

Gitelis S, Whiffen J, and DeWald RL: The treatment of severe scoliosis in osteogenesis imperfecta, Clin Orthop 175:56, 1983.

Hanscom DA and Bloom BA: The spine in osteogenesis imperfecta, Orthop Clin North Am 19:449, 1988.

Herndon CN: Osteogenesis imperfecta: some clinical and genetic considerations, Clin Orthop 8:132, 1956.

King JD and Bobechko WP: Osteogenesis imperfecta, J Bone Joint Surg 53B:72, 1971.

Moorefield WG and Miller GR: Aftermath of osteogenesis imperfecta: the disease of adulthood, J Bone Joint Surg 62A:113, 1980.

Norimatsu H, Mayuzumi T, and Takahashi T: The development of the spinal deformities in osteogenesis imperfecta, Clin Orthop 162:20, 1982.

Rask MR: Spondylolisthesis resulting from osteogenesis imperfecta: report of a case, Clin Orthop 139, 164, 1979.

Renshaw TS, Cook RS, and Albright JA: Scoliosis in osteogenesis imperfecta, Clin Orthop 145:163, 1979.

Waugh TR: The biomechanical basis for the utilization of methyl methacrylate in the treatment of scoliosis, J Bone Joint Surg 53A:194, 1971.

Yong-Hing K and MacEwen GD: Scoliosis associated with osteogenesis imperfecta: results of treatment, J Bone Joint Surg 64B:36, 1982.

Postlaminectomy spine deformity

Brown HP and Bonnett CC: Spine deformity subsequent to spinal cord injury, J Bone Joint Surg 55A:441, 1973.

Cattell HE and Clark LG: Cervical kyphosis and instability following multiple laminectomies in children, J Bone Joint Surg 49A:713, 1967.

Fraser RD, Patterson DC, and Simpson DA: Orthopaedic aspects of spinal tumors in children, J Bone Joint Surg 59B:143, 1977.

Haft H, Ransohoff J, and Carter S: Spinal cord tumors in children, Pediatrics 23:1152, 1959.

Jenkins DHR: Extensive cervical laminectomy: long-term results, Br J Surg 60:852, 1973.

Johnston CE II: Post-laminectomy kyphoscoliosis following surgical treatment for spinal cord astrocytoma, Orthopaedics 9:587, 1986.

Kilfoyle RM, Foley JJ, and Norton PL: Spine and pelvic deformity in childhood and adolescent paraplegia: a study of 104 cases, J Bone Joint Surg 47A:659, 1965.

Lonstein JE: Post-laminectomy kyphosis, Clin Orthop 128:93, 1977.

Lonstein JE et al: Post-laminectomy spine deformity, J Bone Joint Surg 58A:727, 1976.

Munechika Y: Influence of laminectomy on the stability of the spine: an experimental study with special reference to the extent of the laminectomy and resection of the intervertebral joint, J Jpn Orthop Assoc 47:111, 1973.

Panjabi MM, White AA, and Johnson RM: Cervical spine mechanics as a function of transection on components, J Biomech J 8:327, 1975.

Pachdjian MO and Matson DD: Orthopaedic aspects of intraspinal tumors in infants and children, J Bone Joint Surg 47A:223, 1965.

Yasuoka S, Peterson HA, and MacCarty CS: Incidence of spinal column deformity after multilevel laminectomy in children and adults, J Neurosurgery 57:441, 1982.

Yasuoka S et al: Pathogenesis and prophylaxis of post-laminectomy deformity of the spine after multiple level laminectomy: difference between children and adults, Neurosurgery 9:145, 1981.

Skeletal dysplasias

Amuso ST: Diastrophic dwarfism, J Bone Joint Surg 50A:113, 1963.

Bailey JA: Orthopaedic aspects of achondroplasia, J Bone Joint Surg 52A:1285, 1970.

Beals RK: Hypochondroplasia, J Bone Joint Surg 51A:728, 1969.

Beighton P: Orthopaedic problems in dwarfism, J Bone Joint Surg 62B:116, 1980.

Bethem D, Winter RB, and Lutter L: Disorders of the spine in diastrophic dwarfism: a discussion of 9 patients and review of the literature, J Bone Joint Surg 62A:529, 1980.

Bethem D et al: Spinal disorders of dwarfism: review of the literature and report of 80 cases, J Bone Joint Surg 63A:1412, 1981.

Blaw MD and Langer LO: Spinal cord compression in Morquio-Brailsford disease, J Pediatr 74:593, 1969.

Caffey J: Achondroplasia of pelvis and lumbosacral spine, Am J Roentgenol 80:449, 1958.

Diamond LS: A family study of spondyloepiphyseal dysplasia, J Bone Joint Surg 52A:1587, 1970.

Duvisin RC and Yahr MD: Compression spinal cord and root syndromes in achondroplastic dwarfs, Neurology 12:202, 1962.

Eulert J: Scoliosis and kyphosis in dwarfing conditions, Arch Orthop Traum Surg 102:45, 1983.

Fairbank HAT: Dysplasia epiphysealis punctata: synonyms—stippled epiphysis, chondrodystrophia calcificans congenita (Hunermann), J Bone Joint Surg 31B:114, 1949.

Hensinger RN: Kyphosis secondary to skeletal dysplasias and metabolic disease, Clin Orthop 128:113, 1977.

Herring JA: Rapidly progressive scoliosis in multiple epiphyseal dysplasia: a case report, J Bone Joint Surg 58A:703, 1976.

Herring JA: The spinal disorders in diastrophic dwarfism, J Bone Joint Surg 60A:177, 1978.

Herring JA and Winter RB: Kyphosis in an achondroplastic dwarf, J Pediatr Orthop 3:250, 1983.

Hollister DW and Lachman RS: Diastrophic dwarfism, Clin Orthop 114:61, 1976.

Johnston CE II: Scoliosis in metatrophic dwarfism, Orthopaedics 6:491, 1983.

Jones E and Hensinger RN: Spinal deformity in individuals with short stature, Orthop Clin North Am 10:877, 1979.

Kash IJ et al: Cervical cord compression in diastrophic dwarfism, J Pediatr 84:862, 1974.

Kopits SE: Orthopaedic complications of dwarfism, Clin Orthop 114:153, 1976.

Kopits SE: Cervical myelopathy and dwarfism, Orthop Trans 3:119, 1979.

Kopits SE et al: Congenital atlantoaxial dislocations in various forms of dwarfism, J Bone Joint Surg 54A:1349, 1972.

Kozlowski K and Beighton P: Radiographic features of spondyloepimetaphyseal dysplasia with joint laxity and progressive kyphoscoliosis, Fortschr Roentgenstr 141:337, 1984.

Lamy M and Maroteaux P: Le nanisme diastrophique, Presse Med 68:1977, 1960.

Langer LO: Diastrophic dwarfism in early infancy, Am J Roentgenol 93:399, 1965.

Langer LO, Bauman PA, and Gorlin RJ: Achondroplasia, Am J Roentgenol 100:12, 1967.

Langer LO, Bauman PA, and Gorlin RJ: Achondroplasia: clinical radiologic features with comment on genetic implications, Clin Pediatr 7:474, 1968.

Langer LO and Carey LS: The roentgenographic features of the KS mucopolysaccharidosis of Morquio, Am J Roentgenol 97:1, 1966.

Lipson SJ: Dysplasia of the odontoid process in Morquio's syndrome causing quadriparesis, J Bone Joint Surg 59A:340, 1977.

Lutter LD and Langer LO: Neurological symptoms in achondroplastic dwarfs—surgical treatment, J Bone Joint Surg 59A:87, 1977.

Lutter LD et al: Anatomy of the achondroplastic lumbar canal, Clin Orthop 126:139, 1977.

Maroteaux P: Spondyloepiphyseal dysplasias and metatropic dwarfism, Birth Defects 5:35, 1969.

Maroteaux P and Lamy M: Achondroplasia in man and animals, Clin Orthop 33:91, 1964.

Medlar RC and Crawford AH: Frontometaphyseal dysplasia presenting as scoliosis, J Bone Joint Surg 60A:392, 1978.

Morquio L: Sur une forme de dystrophie osseuse familiale, Arch Med Enf 32:129, 1929.

Nelson MA: Spinal stenosis in achondroplasia, Proc R Soc Med 65:1028, 1972.

Ponseti IV: Skeletal growth in achondroplasia, J Bone Joint Surg 52A:701, 1970.

Rimoin DS et al: Metatrophic dwarfism, the Kneist syndrome and the pseudoachondroplastic dysplasias, Clin Orthop 114:70, 1976.

Selakovich WG and White JW: Chondrodystropia calcificans congenita, J Bone Joint Surg 37A:1271, 1955.

Spranger JW and Langer LO: Spondyloepiphyseal dysplasia congenita, Radiology 94:313, 1970.

Stanescu V, Stanescu R, and Maroteaux P: Pathogenic mechanisms in osteochondrodysplasias, J Bone Joint Surg 66A:817, 1984.

Stover C, Hayes JY, and Holt JF: Diastrophic dwarfism, Am J Roentgenol 89:914, 1963.

Tolo VT: Surgical treatment of thoracolumbar kyphosis in achondroplasia. Paper presented at the Fifty-fifth Annual Meeting of the American Academy of Orthopaedic Surgeons, Atlanta, Feb 4-9, 1988.

Infections of the spine

Ahn BH: Treatment of Pott's paraplegia, Acta Orthop Scand 39:145, 1968.

Albee FH: Orthopedic and reconstruction surgery, Philadelphia, 1919, WB Saunders Co.

Albee FH, Powers EJ, and McDowell HC: Surgery of the spinal column, Philadelphia, 1945, FA Davis Co.

Alexander GL: Neurological complications of spinal tuberculosis, Proc R Soc Med 39:730, 1945-1946.

Allen AR and Stevenson AW: The results of combined drug therapy and early fusion in bone tuberculosis, J Bone Joint Surg 39A:32, 1957.

Allen AR and Stevenson AW: A ten-year follow-up of combined drug therapy and early fusion in bone tuberculosis, J Bone Joint Surg 49A:1001, 1967.

Altemeier WA, and Largen T: Antibiotic and chemotherapeutic agents in infections of the skeletal system, JAMA 150:1462, 1952.

Ambrose GB, Alpert M, and Neer CS: Vertebral osteomyelitis: a diagnostic problem, JAMA 197:619, 1966.

Arct W: Operative treatment of tuberculosis of the spine in old people, J Bone Joint Surg 50A:255, 1968.

Avila L Jr: Primary pyogenic infections of the sacro-iliac articulation: a new approach to the joint, J Bone Joint Surg 23:922, 1941.

Badgley CE: Osteomyelitis of the ilium, Arch Surg 28:83, 1934.

Bailey HL et al: Tuberculosis of the spine in children: operative findings and results in one hundred consecutive patients treated by removal of the lesion and anterior grafting, J Bone Joint Surg 54A:1633, 1972.

Bakalim G: Tuberculosis spondylitis: a clinical study with special reference to the significance of spinal fusion and chemotherapy, Acta Orthop Scand (suppl) 47, 1960.

Bakalim G: Results of radical evacuation and arthrodesis in sacro-iliac tuberculosis, Acta Orthop Scand 37:375, 1966.

Batson OV: The vertebral vein system as a mechanism for the spread of metastases, Am J Roentgenol Radium Ther 48:715, 1942.

Bickel WH: Tuberculosis of bones and joints, Mayo Clin Proc 28:370, 1953.

Bickham WS: Operative surgery, vol 2, Philadelphia, 1924, WB Saunders Co.

Blanche DW: Osteomyelitis in infants, J Bone Joint Surg 34A:71, 1952.

Bonfiglio M, Lange TA, and Kim YM: Pyogenic vertebral osteomyelitis: disk space infections, Clin Orthop 96:234, 1973.

Boston HC Jr, Bianco AJ Jr, and Rhodes KH: Disk space infections in children, Orthop Clin North Am 6:953, 1975.

Bosworth D: Tuberculosis of the osseous system. VI. Operative methods, Quart Bull Sea View Hosp 5:441, 1940.

Bosworth DM: The treatment of tuberculous lesions of bones and joints with iproniazid (Marsilid), NY State J Med 56:1281, 1956.

Bosworth DM: Surgery of the spine. In The American Academy of Orthopaedic Surgeons: Instructional course lectures, vol 14, Ann Arbor, Mich, 1957, JW Edwards Co.

Bosworth DM: Treatment of bone and joint tuberculosis in children, J Bone Joint Surg 41A:1255, 1959.

Bosworth DM: Treatment of tuberculosis of bone and joint, Bull NY Acad Med 35:167, 1959.

Bosworth DM, Della Pietra A, and Rahilly G: Paraplegia resulting from tuberculosis of the spine, J Bone Joint Surg 35A:735, 1953.

Bosworth DM and Wright HA: Streptomycin in bone and joint tuberculosis, J Bone Joint Surg 34A:255, 1952.

Bosworth DM et al: The use of iproniazid in the treatment of bone and joint tuberculosis, J Bone Joint Surg 35A:577, 1953.

Brant-Zawadzki M, Burke VD, and Jeffrey RB: CT in the evaluation of spine infection, Spine 8:358, 1983.

Brashear HR Jr, and Rendleman DA: Pott's paraplegia, South Med J 71:1379, 1978.

Butler RW: Paraplegia in Pott's disease with special reference to the pathology and etiology, Br J Surg 22:738, 1934-1935.

Campos OP: Bone and joint tuberculosis and its treatment, J Bone Joint Surg 37A:937, 1955.

Capener N: Personal communication to Girdlestone GR, 1934, Cited in Platt H, editor: Modern trends in orthopaedics, New York, 1950, Paul B Hoeber, Inc.

Capener N: The evolution of lateral rhachotomy, J Bone Joint Surg 36B:173, 1954.

Cardoso A, Flores A, and Galvan R: Segmental instrumentation in Pott's Disease, Orthop Trans 9:125, 1985.

Chahal AS and Jyoti SP: The radical treatment of tuberculosis of the spine, Intern Orthop 4:93, 1980.

Chu C-B: Treatment of spinal tuberculosis in Korea, using focal debridement and interbody fusion, Clin Orthop 50:235, 1967.

Conrad SE, Breivis J, and Fried MA: Vertebral osteomyelitis, caused by *Arachni propionica* and resembling actinomycosis, J Bone Joint Surg 60A:549, 1978.

Coventry MB, Ghormley RK, and Kernohan JW: The intervertebral disc: its microscopic anatomy and pathology. I. Anatomy, development, and physiology, J Bone Joint Surg 27A:105, 1945.

Crock HV and Yoshizawa H: The blood supply of the lumbar vertebral column, Clin Orthop 115:6, 1976.

Davies PDO et al: Bone and joint tuberculosis: a survey of notifications in England and Wales, J Bone Joint Surg 66B:326, 1984.

Dickson JA: Spinal tuberculosis in Nigerian children: a review of ambulant treatment, J Bone Joint Surg 49B:682, 1967.

Digby JM and Kersley JB: Pyogenic non-tuberculous spinal infection, J Bone Joint Surg 61B:47, 1979.

Dott NM: Skeletal traction and anterior decompression in the management of Pott's paraplegia, Edinburgh Med J 54:620, 1947.

Dove J, Hsu LCS, and Yau ACMC: The cervical spine after halopelvic traction: an analysis of the complications in 83 patients, J Bone Joint Surg 62B:158, 1980.

Du Toit G: Anterior spinal cord decompression in kyphosis with particular reference to healed tuberculosis, J Bone Joint Surg 66B:455, 1984.

Editorial: Chemotherapy in orthopaedic tuberculosis, Lancet 1:1227, 1954.

Eismont FJ et al: Pyogenic and fungal vertebral osteomyelitis with paralysis, J Bone Joint Surg 65A:19, 1983.

El-Gindi S et al: Infection of intervertebral discs after operation, J Bone Joint Surg 58B:114, 1976.

Erlacher PJ: The radical operative treatment of bone and joint tuberculosis, J Bone Joint Surg 17:536, 1935.

Evans ET: Tuberculosis of the bones and joints, J Bone Joint Surg 34A:267, 1952.

Fang D, Leong JCY, and Fang HSY: Tuberculosis of the upper cervical spine, J Bone Joint Surg 65B:47, 1983.

Fang HSY, Ong GB, and Hodgson AR: Anterior spinal fusion, the operative approaches, Clin Orthop 35:16, 1964.

Felländer M: Radical operation in tuberculosis of the spine, Acta Orthop Scand (suppl) 19, 1955.

Fifth report of the Medical Research Council Working Party on Tuberculosis of the Spine, Brompton Hospital, London, England: A five-year assessment of controlled trials of in-patient and out-patient treatment and of plaster-of-Paris jackets for tuberculosis of the spine in children on standard chemotherapy: studies in Masan and Pusan, Korea, J Bone Joint Surg 58B:399, 1976.

First report of the Medical Research Council Working Party on Tuberculosis of the Spine: A controlled trial of ambulant outpatient treatment and in-patient rest in bed in management of tuberculosis of the spine in young Korean patients on standard chemotherapy: a study in Masan, Korea, J Bone Joint Surg 55B:678, 1973.

Ford LT: Postoperative infection of lumbar intervertebral disk space, South Med J 69:1477, 1977.

Fountain SS et al: Progressive kyphosis following solid anterior spine fusion in children with tuberculosis of the spine: a long term study, J Bone Joint Surg 57A:1104, 1975.

Fourth report of the Medical Research Council Working Party on Tuberculosis of the Spine: A controlled trial of anterior spinal fusion and debridement in the surgical management of tuberculosis of the spine in patients on standard chemotherapy: a study in Hong Kong, Br J Surg 61:853, 1974.

Freehafer AA, Heiser DP, and Saunders AP: Infection of the lower lumbar spine with Neisseria meningitidis, J Bone Joint Surg 60A:1001, 1978.

Friedman B: Chemotherapy of tuberculosis of the spine, J Bone Joint Surg 48A:451, 1966.

Friedman B and Kapur VN: Newer knowledge of chemotherapy in the treatment of tuberculosis of bones and joints, Clin Orthop 97:5, 1973.

Garceau GJ and Brady TA: Pott's paraplegia, J Bone Joint Surg 32A:87, 1950.

Garcia A Jr and Grantham SA: Hematogenous pyogenic vertebral osteomyelitis, J Bone Joint Surg 42A:429, 1960.

Ghormley RK, Bickel WH, and Dickson DD: A study of acute infectious lesions of the intervertebral disks, South Med J 33:347, 1940.

Girdlestone GR: The operative treatment of Pott's paraplegia, Br J Surg 19:121, 1931.

Girdlestone GR: Tuberculosis of bones and joints. In Platt H, editor: Modern trends in orthopaedics, New York, 1950, Paul B Hoeber, Inc.

Girdlestone GR and Somerville EW: Tuberculosis of bone and joint, ed 2, New York, 1952, Oxford University Press.

Goel MK: Treatment of Pott's paraplegia by operation, J Bone Joint Surg 49B:674, 1967.

Golimbu C, Firooznia H, and Rafii M: CT of osteomyelitis of the spine, AJR 142:159, 1984.

Griffiths DL: Pott's paraplegia and its operative treatment, J Bone Joint Surg 35B:487, 1953.

Griffiths HED and Jones DM: Pyogenic infection of the spine: a review of twenty-eight cases, J Bone Joint Surg 53B:383, 1971.

Guirguis AR: Pott's paraplegia, J Bone Joint Surg 49B:658, 1967.

Hale JE and Aichroth P: Vertebral osteomyelitis: a complication of urological surgery, Br J Surg 61:867, 1974.

Hallock H and Jones JB: Tuberculosis of the spine, J Bone Joint Surg 36A:219, 1954.

Halpern AA et al: Coccidioidomycosis of the spine: unusual roentgenographic presentation, Clin Orthop 140:78, 1979.

Harris RI, Coulthard HS, and Dewar FP: Streptomycin in the treatment of bone and joint tuberculosis, J Bone Joint Surg 34A:279, 1952.

Harris HN and Kirkaldy-Willis WH: Primary subacute pyogenic osteomyelitis, J Bone Joint Surg 47B:526, 1965.

Hartman JT and Phalen GS: Needle biopsy of bone: report of three representative cases, JAMA 200:201, 1967.

Hassler O: The human intervertebral disc: a microangiographical study on its vascular supply at various ages, Acta Orthop Scand 40:765, 1969.

Hazlett JW: Pyogenic osteomyelitis of the spine, Can J Surg 1:243, 1958.

Henson SW Jr and Coventry MB: Osteomyelitis of the vertebrae as the result of infection of the urinary tract, Surg Gynecol Obstet 102:207, 1956.

Hodgson AR, Skinsnes OK, and Leong CY: The pathogenesis of Pott's paraplegia, J Bone Joint Surg 49A:1147, 1967.

Hodgson AR and Stock FE: Anterior spinal fusion: a preliminary communication on the radical treatment of Pott's disease and Pott's paraplegia, Br J Surg 44:266, 1956.

Hodgson AR and Stock FE: Anterior fusion. In Rob C and Smith R, editors: Operative surgery service, vol 9, London, 1960, Butterworth & Co, Ltd.

Hodgson AR and Stock FE: Anterior spine fusion for the treatment of tuberculosis of the spine: the operative findings and results of treatment of the first one hundred cases, J Bone Joint Surg 42A:295, 1960.

Hodgson AR et al: Anterior spinal fusion: the operative approach and pathological findings in 412 patients with Pott's disease of the spine, Br J Surg 48:172, 1960.

Hodgson AR et al: A clinical study of 100 consecutive cases of Pott's paraplegia, Clin Orthop 36:128, 1964.

Hoover MJ Jr: The treatment of the tuberculous psoas abscess, South Surg 16:729, 1950.

Hoover NW: Methods of lumbar fusion, J Bone Joint Surg 50A:194, 1968.

Hsieh CK, Miltner LJ, and Chang CP: Tuberculosis of the shaft of the large bones of the extremities, J Bone Joint Surg 16:545, 1934.

Hsu LCS and Leong JCY: Tuberculosis of the lower cervical spine (C-2-C-7): report on forty cases, J Bone Joint Surg 66B:1, 1984.

Ito H, Tsuchiya J, and Asami G: A new radical operation for Pott's disease, J Bone Joint Surg 16:499, 1934.

James JIP: Pott's paraplegia, Med Pregl 13:9, 1960.

Janeway T and Moseberg WH Jr: Tuberculous paraplegia with lateral vertebral dislocation: a case report, J Bone Joint Surg 59A:554, 1977.

Jenkins DHR et al: Stabilization of the spine in the surgical treatment of severe spinal tuberculosis in children, Clin Orthop 110:69, 1975.

Johnson RW Jr, Hillman JW, and Southwick WO: The importance of direct surgical attack upon lesions of the vertebral bodies, particularly in Pott's disease, J Bone Joint Surg 35A:17, 1953.

Jones AR: The influence of Hugh Owen Thomas on the evolution of treatment of skeletal tuberculosis, J Bone Joint Surg 35B:309, 1958.

Jones BS: Pott's paraplegia in the Nigerian, J Bone Joint Surg 40B:16, 1958.

Kaplan CJ: Conservative therapy in skeletal tuberculosis: an appraisal based on experience in South Africa, Tubercle 40:355, 1959.

Karlén A: Early drainage of paraspinal tuberculous abscesses in children: a preliminary report, J Bone Joint Surg 41B:491, 1959.

Kattapuram SV, Phillips WC, and Boyd R: Computed tomography in pyogenic osteomyelitis of the spine, AJR 140:1199, 1983.

Kemp HBS et al: Anterior fusion of the spine for infective lesions in adults, J Bone Joint Surg 55B:715, 1973.

Kemp HBS et al: Pyogenic infections occurring primarily in intervertebral discs, J Bone Joint Surg 55B:698, 1973.

Kemp HBS, Jackson JW, and Shaw NC: Laminectomy in paraplegia due to infective spondylosis, Br J Surg 61:66, 1974.

King DM and Mayo KM: Infective lesions of the vertebral column, Clin Orthop 96:248, 1973.

Kirkaldy-Willis WH and Thomas TG: Anterior approaches in the diagnosis and treatment of infections of the vertebral bodies, J Bone Joint Surg 47A:87, 1965.

Kite JH: Tuberculosis of the spine with paraplegia, South Med J 29:883, 1936.

Kocher T: Textbook of operative surgery, London, 1911, A & C Black, Ltd.

Kohli SB: Radical surgical approach to spinal tuberculosis, J Bone Joint Surg 49B:668, 1967.

Kondo E and Yamada K: End results of focal débridement in bone and joint tuberculosis and its indications, J Bone Joint Surg 39A:27, 1957.

Konstam PG and Blesovsky A: The ambulant treatment of spinal tuberculosis, Br J Surg 50:26, 1962-1963.

Kulowski J: Pyogenic osteomyelitis of the spine: an analysis and discussion of 102 cases, J Bone Joint Surg 18:343, 1936.

Lame EL: Vertebral osteomyelitis following operation on the urinary tract or sigmoid: the third lesion of an uncommon syndrome, Am J Roentgenol Radium Ther Nucl Med 75:938, 1956.

Langenskiöld A and Riska EB: Pott's paraplegia treated by anterolateral decompression in the thoracic and lumbar spine: a report of twenty-seven cases, Acta Orthop Scand 38:181, 1967.

Lindholm TS and Pylkkänen P: Discitis following removal of intervertebral disc, Spine 7:618, 1982.

Ling CM: Pyogenic osteomyelitis of the spine, Orthop Rev 4:23, September 1975.

Lougheed JC and White WG: Anterior dependent drainage for tuberculous lumbosacral spinal lesions: coccygectomy and dependent drainage in treatment of tuberculous lesions of the lower spine with associated soft-tissue abscesses, Arch Surg 81:961, 1960.

Malawski SK: Pyogenic infection of the spine, Inter Orthop 1:125, 1977.

Martin NS: Tuberculosis of the spine: a study of the results of treatment during the last twenty-five years, J Bone Joint Surg 52B:613, 1970.

Martin NS: Pott's paraplegia: a report of 120 cases, J Bone Joint Surg 53B:596, 1970.

Matsushita T and Suzuki K: Spastic paraparesis due to cryptococcal osteomyelitis: a case report, Clin Orthop 196:279, 1985.

Mawk JR et al: *Aspergillus* infections of the lumbar disc spaces: report of three cases, J Neurosurg 58:270, 1983.

Mazet R Jr: Skeletal lesions of coccidioidomycosis, Arch Surg 70:633, 1955.

Medical Resource Council Working Party on Tuberculosis of the Spine: Five-year assessments of controlled trials of ambulatory treatment, debridement and anterior spinal fusion in the management of tuberculosis of the spine—studies in Bulawayo (Rhodesia) and in Hong Kong, J Bone Joint Surg 60B:163, 1978.

Menelaus MB: Discitis: an inflammation affecting the intervertebral discs in children, J Bone Joint Surg 46B:16, 1964.

Ménard V: Étude pratique sur le mal du Pott, Paris, 1900, Masson et Cie.

Morrey BF, Kelly PJ, and Nichols DR: Viridans streptococcal osteomyelitis of the spine, J Bone Joint Surg 62A:1009, 1980.

Nagel DA et al: Closer look at spinal lesions: open biopsy of vertebral lesions, JAMA 191:975, 1965.

Naim-Ur-Rahman: Atypical forms of spinal tuberculosis, J Bone Joint Surg 62B:162, 1980.

Neville CH Jr and Davis WL: Is surgical fusion still desirable in spinal tuberculosis? Clin Orthop 75:179, 1971.

Norris SH et al: The radioisotopic study of an experimental model of disc space, J Bone Joint Surg 60B:281, 1978.

O'Connor BT, Steel WM, and Sanders R: Disseminated bone tuberculosis, J Bone Joint Surg 57A:537, 1970.

Otani K et al: Spinal osteotomy to correct kyphosis in spinal tuberculosis, Intern Orthop 3:299, 1979.

Puig-Guri J: Pyogenic osteomyelitis of the spine: differential diagnosis through clinical and roentgenographic observations, J Bone Joint Surg 28:29, 1946.

Puranen J, Mäkelä J, and Lähde S: Postoperative intervertebral discitis, Acta Orthop Scand 55:461, 1984.

Ray MJ and Bassett RL: Pyogenic vertebral osteomyelitis, Orthopedics 8:506, 1985.

Risko T and Novoszel T: Experiences with radical operations in tuberculosis of the spine, J Bone Joint Surg 45A:53, 1963.

Roaf R: Tuberculosis of the spine, J Bone Joint Surg 40B:3, 1958 (editorial).

Roaf R, Kirkaldy-Willis WH, and Cathro AJM: Surgical treatment of bone and joint tuberculosis, Edinburgh, 1959, E & S Livingstone, Ltd.

Robertson RC and Ball RP: Destructive spine lesions: diagnosis by needle biopsy, J Bone Joint Surg 17:749, 1935.

Ross PM and Fleming JL: Vertebral body osteomyelitis: spectrum and natural history: a retrospective analysis of 37 cases, Clin Orthop 118:190, 1976.

Ryan LM et al: The radiographic diagnosis of sacroiliitis: a comparison of different views with computed tomograms of the sacroiliac joint, Arthritis Rheum 26:760, 1983.

Saenger EL: Spondylarthritis in children, Am J Roentgenol Radium Ther 64:20, 1950.

Scoles PV and Quinn TP: Intervertebral discitis in children and adolescents, Clin Orthop 162:31, 1982.

Seddon HJ: Pott's paraplegia, Br J Surg 22:769, 1935.

Seddon HJ: The pathology of Pott's paraplegia, Proc R Soc Med 39:723, 1945-1946.

Seddon HJ: Antero-lateral decompression of Pott's paraplegia, J Bone Joint Surg 33B:461, 1951.

Seddon HJ: Treatment of Pott's paraplegia by anterolateral decompression, Mem Acad Chir 79:281, 1952.

Seddon HJ: Pott's paraplegia and its operative treatment, J Bone Joint Surg 35B:487, 1953.

Seddon HJ: Pott's paraplegia. In Platt H, editor: Modern trends in orthopaedics (second series), London, 1956, Butterworth & Co, Ltd.

Seddon HJ and Alexander GL: Discussion of spinal caries with paraplegia, Proc R Soc Med 39:723, 1946.

Shaw NE and Thomas TG: Surgical treatment of chronic infective lesions of the spine, Br Med J 1:162, 1963.

Sherman M and Schneider GT: Vertebral osteomyelitis complicating postabortal and postpartum infection, South Med J 48:333, 1955.

Siebert WT, Moreland N, and Williams TW Jr: Methicillin-resistant Staphylococcus epidermidis, South Med J 7:1353, 1978.

Smith AD: The treatment of bone and joint tuberculosis, J Bone Joint Surg 37A:1214, 1955.

Smith AD: Tuberculosis of the spine: results in 70 cases treated at the New York Orthopaedic Hospital from 1945 to 1960, Clin Orthop 58:171, 1968.

Speed JS and Boyd HB: Bone syphilis, South Med J 29:371, 1936.

Spiegel PG et al: Intervertebral disc-space inflammation in children, J Bone Joint Surg 54A:284, 1972.

Stauffer RN: Pyogenic vertebral osteomyelitis, Orthop Clin North Am 6:1015, 1975.

Steindler A: Posterior mediastinal abscess in tuberculosis of the dorsal spine, Illinois Med J 50:201, 1926.

Steindler A: Diseases and deformities of the spine and thorax, St. Louis, 1929, The CV Mosby Co.

Steindler A: On paraplegia in Pott's disease, Lancet 54:281, 1934.

Stern WE and Balch RE: Surgical aspects of nonspecific inflammatory and suppurative disease of the vertebral column, Am J Surg 122:314, 1966.

Stevenson FH: The chemotherapy of orthopaedic tuberculosis, J Bone Joint Surg 36B:5, 1954.

Surgarman B: Osteomyelitis in spinal cord injury, Arch Phys Med Rehabil 65:132, 1984.

Torres-Rojas J, Taddonio RF, and Sanders CV: Spondylitis caused by *Brucella abortus,* South Med J 72:1166, 1979.

Tuli SM: Tuberculosis of the craniovertebral region, Clin Orthop 104:209, 1974.

Tuli SM: Results of treatment of spinal tuberculosis by "middle-path" regime, J Bone Joint Surg 57B:13, 1975.

Tuli SM and Kumar S: Early results of treatment of spinal tuberculosis of triple drug therapy, Clin Orthop 81:56, 1971.

Tuli SM et al: Tuberculosis of spine, Acta Orthop Scand 38:445, 1967.

Waldvogel FA, Medoff G, and Swartz MN: Osteomyelitis: a review of clinical features, therapeutic considerations and unusual aspects (first of three parts), N Engl J Med 282:198, 1976.

Wedge JH et al: Atypical manifestations of spinal infections. Clin Orthop 123:155, 1977.

Weinberg JA: The surgical excision of psoas abscesses resulting from spinal tuberculosis, J Bone Joint Surg 39A:17, 1957.

Wenger DR, Bobechko WP, and Gilday DL: The spectrum of intervertebral disc-space infection in children, J Bone Joint Surg 60A:100, 1978.

Whalen JL et al: The intrinsic vasculature of developing vertebral end plates and its nutritive significance to the intervertebral discs, J Ped Ortho 5:403, 1985.

Wiley AM and Trueta J: The vascular anatomy of the spine and its relationship to pyogenic vertebral osteomyelitis, J Bone Joint Surg 41B:796, 1959.

Wilkinson MC: The treatment of tuberculosis of the spine by evacuation of the paravertebral abscess and curettage of the vertebral bodies, J Bone Joint Surg 37B:382, 1955.

Wiltberger BR: Resection of the vertebral bodies and bone-grafting for chronic osteomyelitis of the spine, J Bone Joint Surg 34A:215, 1952.

Winter WG Jr et al: Coccidioidal spondylitis, J Bone Joint Surg 60A:240, 1978.

Yau ACMC and Hodgson AR: Penetration of the lung by the paravertebral abscess in tuberculosis of the spine, J Bone Joint Surg 50A:243, 1968.

Yau ACMC et al: Tuberculous kyphosis: correction with spinal osteotomy, halo-pelvic distraction, and anterior and posterior fusion, J Bone Joint Surg 56A:1419, 1974.

Neil E. Green

Cerebral palsy is a nonprogressive disease of the central nervous system that results from a prenatal, neonatal, or postnatal injury to the brain from various causes. It is important to remember that this disease is the result of an isolated etiologic factor. The cerebral lesion itself does not progress, and the resulting signs and symptoms lessen with growth and with the maturation of the nervous system. The cerebral lesion produces abnormalities of motor function that are manifested by movement disorders.

CLASSIFICATION OF MOVEMENT DISORDERS

The movement disorders associated with cerebral palsy are spasticity, athetosis, ataxia, and mixed types. Spasticity is manifested by increased muscle tone and increased stretch reflexes of the skeletal muscles. The increased muscle tone can be felt clinically as resistance to passive movement of an extremity. Hyperreflexia and clonus of the involved muscles are evident on examination, as well as the clasped-knife type of muscle tightness seen in spasticity. Attempts at passive movement of a joint (especially a large joint) through a range of motion meet with constant resistance throughout the range of motion until the muscle tone finally gives way and the joint then flexes easily, producing a feeling similar to that of closing an opened jack knife.

Athetosis is characterized by abnormal involuntary movements of the muscles of the involved extremity. Different types of athetosis (dyskinesias) produce different clinical movement abnormalities. The form most commonly associated with cerebral palsy includes dystonia, chorea, and ballismus and is characterized by abnormal, involuntary movements of muscles anywhere in the body. Children with this form of cerebral palsy rarely have joint contractures because the athetoid extremities usually move through a full range of motion. It is important to distinguish between tension athetosis and spasticity. This can be accomplished by shaking the involved extremity; the spastic extremity will remain spastic, whereas the extremity with tension athetosis will loosen. Another type of dyskinesia is rigidity, either of the "lead pipe" or the "cogwheel" type, that resists all attempts at movement. The lead pipe type of rigidity is a continuous muscle resistance, whereas the cogwheel type is characterized by intermittent resistance to passive movement.

Ataxia is typified by a loss of the sense of balance and position in space. Infants with ataxia have hypotonia of the peripheral muscles and typical findings of the abnormal cerebellum: abnormal finger-to-nose and heel-to-shin tests. Ataxia usually is the result of congenital or hereditary cerebellar abnormalities.

The mixed type of cerebral palsy usually combines spasticity and athetosis. It is important, although sometimes difficult, to recognize the mixture of spasticity and athetosis because pure athetosis does not respond well to muscle surgery. Although mixed cerebral palsy with spasticity as the major component responds to muscle procedures, if the athetosis predominates, muscle surgery may worsen the deformity.

INCIDENCE AND ETIOLOGY

The incidence of cerebral palsy averages two per 1000 live births in Western nations. Because it is the result of a cerebral injury, cerebral palsy is not a hereditary disease and is not progressive; it must be differentiated from hereditary spastic paraplegia, which usually is transmitted by an autosomal dominant mode of inheritance and is slowly progressive. Hereditary spastic paraplegia should be suspected when more than one child in a family has a spastic diplegia–like condition or when there is no history of a possible neonatal cause for symptoms of spastic diplegia.

Cerebral palsy results from a variety of cerebral insults. The type of insult, the development of the fetus or infant at the time of the insult, and the localization of the lesion in the brain determine the motor manifestations. The most common causes of cerebral palsy are prematurity and low birth weight. The immature neurons of the premature infant's brain may not be able to withstand the trauma of birth, and there is a higher than average incidence of intracerebral hemorrhage in very premature infants of low birth weight. Intrauterine environmental problems that cause premature birth also may result in brain injury. Certain intrauterine abnormalities such as placenta previa and abruptio placentae increase the incidence of cerebral palsy, and intrauterine infections such as rubella and cytomegalovirus are known causes of cerebral damage. Neonatal asphyxia has been associated with an increased incidence of cerebral palsy. There is a higher probability that cerebral palsy will develop in children with low Apgar scores; however, in a study of 99 children with Apgar scores of 3 or less at 20 minutes, cerebral palsy developed in only 12%, which indicates that neonatal asphyxia is not a certain precursor of cerebral palsy. The most common postnatal cause of cerebral palsy is infection of the immature brain, either viral or bacterial. Direct trauma to the brain in the neonate or infant may result in cerebral palsy. One cause of postnatal cerebral trauma is child abuse; shaking the child may result in permanent brain damage from intracranial or intracerebral bleeding. A nontraumatic, idiopathic, or thrombotic cerebral vascular accident is another frequent cause of cerebral palsy, as manifested by hemiplegia. The middle cerebral artery is the usual site of the lesion, and the extent of the vascular occlusion determines the severity of the clinical condition.

CLINICAL DESCRIPTION OF MOTOR DEFICITS

Because the lesion in the brain is localized, the motor deficit in patients with cerebral palsy may be classified according to the area of the body involved.

Monoplegia

The term *monoplegia* should be restricted to the true paralysis of only one extremity and is extremely uncommon in cerebral palsy. Monoplegia is most commonly the result of a peripheral nerve lesion rather than a brain lesion. Monoplegia in a child with cerebral palsy may result from a stretch injury to the brachial plexus at birth. Monoplegia may be mistaken for hemiplegia, but a careful examination of the more normal extremity, including reflex evaluation, usually provides the correct diagnosis.

Hemiplegia

Hemiplegia involves the ipsilateral upper and lower extremity, most commonly with spasticity. The upper extremity involvement usually is greater than the involvement of the lower extremity. The upper extremity tends to be adducted and internally rotated at the shoulder; the elbow, wrist, and fingers are flexed with pronation of the forearm. The severity of the deformity varies from very mild to severe and depends on the extent of the cerebral damage.

Paraplegia

True paraplegia does not exist in cerebral palsy. Diplegia with very mild involvement of the upper extremities may be mistaken for paraplegia, but careful examination usually reveals decreased fine motor function in the upper extremities. When children with mild diplegia run, they usually pronate the forearm and flex the elbow and wrist.

Diplegia

Diplegia resembles paraplegia in that there is greater involvement of the lower extremities; upper extremity involvement may be extremely mild, manifested only by a decrease in fine motor movement.

Tetraplegia, Quadriplegia, or Total Body Involvement

These children may have spasticity, athetosis, or a mixed type of movement disorder. They usually have the most profound motor deficit, which often includes those muscles responsible for speech and swallowing in addition to extremity involvement. Although children with cerebral palsy may be mentally retarded, most of the noninstitutionalized children are of normal intellect. This may be very frustrating for the child with severe motor deficits that preclude self-care and communication with comprehensible speech. Fortunately, computers designed to allow the aphonic, intelligent child or adult to communicate may be adapted to almost any functional level.

CLINICAL PRESENTATION

Most, although not all, children with cerebral palsy have a clear history of neonatal difficulties; in those who do not, a definite cause may be difficult to establish. Awareness of normal developmental milestones is important inasmuch as the hallmark of cerebral palsy in the infant is developmental delay. The average child pulls to standing by the age of 9 to 10 months and begins to walk independently by age 12 to 18 months. If a child is not even standing at age 16 months, a cause for the delay in development should be sought. Most developmentally delayed infants should be evaluated by a pediatric neurologist and perhaps by a physical or occupational therapist. Two of the tests most commonly used are the Denver Developmental Screening Test and that of Paine and Oppé for the older child (Table 11-1).

Cerebral palsy is diagnosed in some children later in childhood because of gait abnormalities, usually caused by very mild hemiplegia or diplegia. A child with mild hemiplegia may have normal developmental milestones; however, when asked, the parents may relate that the child has preferred one hand over the other since birth. It is decidedly uncommon for the normal child to develop handedness before the age of 3 years, and children often remain ambidextrous until the age of 5 or 6 years. If parents report that their child has long preferred one hand or the other, this may indicate that the hand not used as often or as well actually is weaker or less well-coordinated than the other. Watching the child walk and, especially, run aids in diagnosis because the abnormal upper extremity may be held in a somewhat flexed position at the elbow, with pronation of the forearm and flexion of the wrist, or it simply may not swing normally.

Table 11-1   Check-list for assessment by observation of developmental level of preschool children

Age (yr)	Historical (or observed) items	Items to be tested
2	Runs well	Builds tower of six cubes
	Walks up and down stairs—one step at a time	Circular scribbling
		Copies horizontal stroke with pencil
	Opens doors	Folds paper once
	Climbs on furniture	
	Puts three words together	
	Handles spoon well	
	Helps to undress	
	Listens to stories with pictures	
2½	Jumps	Builds tower to eight cubes
	Knows full name	Copies horizontal and vertical strokes (not a cross)
	Refers to self by pronoun "I"	
	Helps put things away	
3	Goes upstairs, alternating feet	Builds tower of nine cubes
	Rides tricycle	Imitates construction of bridge with three cubes
	Stands momentarily on one foot	Imitates a cross and circle
	Knows age and sex	
	Plays simple games	
	Helps in dressing	
	Washes hands	
4	Hops on one foot	Copies bridges from a model
	Throws a ball overhand	Imitates construction of a gate with five cubes
	Climbs well	Copies a cross and circle
	Uses scissors to cut out pictures	Draws a man with two to four parts—other than head
	Counts four pennies accurately	Names longer of two lines
	Tells a story	
	Plays with several children	
	Goes to toilet alone	
5	Skips	Copies a square and triangle
	Names four colors	Names four colors
	Counts 10 pennies correctly	Names heavier of two weights
	Dresses and undresses	
	Asks questions about meaning of words	

From Paine RS and Oppé TE: Neurological examination of children, Clin Dev Med 20/21, London, 1966, SIMP with Heinemann Publishers.

PHYSICAL EXAMINATION

The physical examination should include a thorough neurologic examination in addition to evaluation of the developmental milestones.

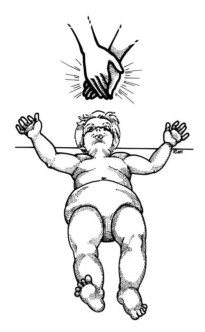

Fig. 11-1 Moro's reflex, which is elicited by placing infant supine and making loud noise or jarring bed. Child responds with abduction and extension of arms at shoulders; circumduction and flexion of arms then occurs. (Redrawn from Bleck EE: Orthopaedic management of cerebral palsy, Philadelphia, 1979, WB Saunders Co.)

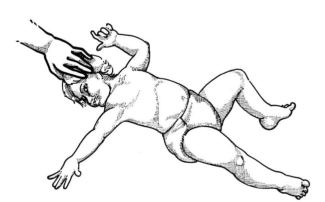

Fig. 11-2 Asymmetric tonic neck reflex. Patient is placed supine with head turned to one side. Arm and leg on mental (chin) side will extend while arm and leg on occipital side will flex at elbow and knee. (Redrawn from Bleck EE: Orthopaedic management of cerebral palsy, Philadelphia, 1979, WB Saunders Co.)

Neurologic Examination
Primitive Reflexes and Postural Responses

Certain primitive reflexes and postural responses should be evaluated because they tell much about the prognosis of the child with delayed development. The Moro reflex that is present in the newborn should disappear in the normal child by the age of 6 months. The Moro reflex is elicited by startling the child with a loud noise or by slapping the examining table. The infant responds by abducting and extending the arms, which then are brought into the position of an embrace (Fig. 11-1). In the child with hemiplegia or brachial plexus palsy, the involved arm will not respond in the same manner as the normal arm.

The asymmetric tonic neck reflex is tested with the child supine. As the head is turned to one side, the upper and lower extremities on the mental (face) side are extended and the extremities on the occipital side are flexed (the "fencing position") (Fig. 11-2). Although mild manifestations of this reflex may be present up to the age of 7 months, after this it is definitely abnormal.

The symmetric tonic neck reflex is demonstrated with the child placed on all fours. As the neck and

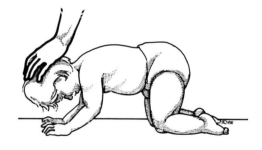

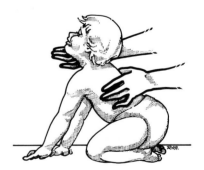

Fig. 11-3 Symmetric tonic neck reflex, which is present in crawling. Patient is placed on all fours in crawling position. If head is flexed, elbows flex; if head is extended, elbows extend and knees and hips flex fully. (Redrawn from Bleck EE: Orthopaedic management of cerebral palsy, Philadelphia, 1979, WB Saunders Co.)

head are flexed ventrally, the arms flex and the legs extend; if the head and neck are extended, the arms extend and the legs flex (Fig. 11-3). If this reflex is present, crawling is impossible. It is normal for this reflex to be present up to the age of 6 months.

The neck-righting reflex is tested with the child supine. As the head is turned to one side, the body follows the turned head (log rolling) (Fig. 11-4); it is normal for this reflex to be present between birth and 6 months of age.

The foot placement reaction is demonstrated by holding the child upright by the chest and body. When the dorsa of the feet are brought upward against the edge of a table top, the child normally will lift the leg that has been stimulated and bring it upward and forward onto the table top (Fig. 11-5). This response is normal in all infants and usually disappears by the age of 3 or 4 years.

The extensor thrust is an abnormal response seen in infants and children with spasticity but never in normal children. To demonstrate this response, the child is lifted by the body in the upright position and lowered so that the feet touch the floor or the top of a table. The normal infant will flex the legs, but the child with spasticity will stiffen the lower extremities and trunk into forced extension (Fig. 11-6).

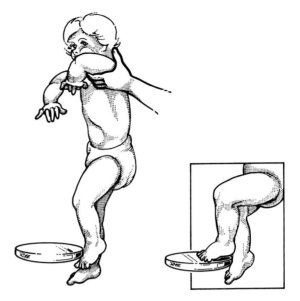

Fig. 11-5   Foot placement. Child is suspended by examiner holding child's thorax. Dorsum of child's foot is placed against stable object such as table top or chair. Child then will lift foot to place it on top of table or chair *(inset)*.

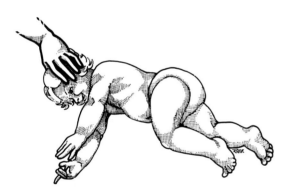

Fig. 11-4   Neck-righting reflex. As head is turned to one side, child rolls to that same side and will continue to follow the head as it is turned. (Redrawn from Bleck EE: Orthopaedic management of cerebral palsy, Philadelphia, 1979, WB Saunders Co.)

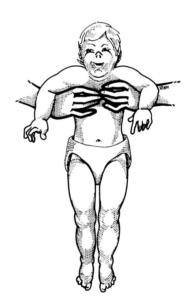

Fig. 11-6   Extensor thrust. Child is held upright and vertical by thorax. In this position child's hips and knees will extend fully and rigidly with feet in forced equinus. (Redrawn from Bleck EE: Orthopaedic management of cerebral palsy, Philadelphia, 1979, WB Saunders Co.)

The parachute response is not present in the newborn but develops in normal infants before the age of 12 months. The response is demonstrated by holding the child by the body in the prone position. As the child is lifted into the air and then quickly tilted head down toward the table top, both arms will extend to protect the head and body (Fig. 11-7). The response, which may be present unilaterally in the child with hemiplegia or brachial plexus palsy, still is considered normal if the unaffected extremity responds appropriately.

Although it is not always possible to predict the ability of a given child, Bleck (1988) has been able to determine walking prognosis fairly accurately by means of an examination based on retained infantile automatisms and postural reflexes in the 1-year-old child. He assigns one point for each persistent infantile automatism (asymmetric tonic neck reflex, neck-righting reflex, Moro's reflex, symmetric neck reflex, and extensor thrust) and for each absent postural reflex (parachute reaction and foot placement reaction). On the basis of this scale a score of two points or more indicates a poor prognosis for walking; a score of one point a guarded prognosis (undetermined); and a score of zero a good prognosis.

Bleck also determined that most children with hemiplegia walk between the ages of 18 and 21 months. Children with diplegia usually walk sometime between the ages of 2 and 4 years. Children with quadriplegia have a much more variable walking prognosis.

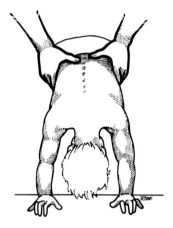

Fig. 11-7 Parachute response. When suspended by thorax and quickly tilted forward toward table, chair, or bed, child reaches forward for protection. (Redrawn from Bleck EE: Orthopaedic management of cerebral palsy, Philadelphia, 1979, WB Saunders Co.)

Reflexes

The neurologic examination should include a thorough search for other pathologic reflexes, including deep tendon reflexes, to determine the presence of an increased response. An increased response may not be obtained if the child has severe spasticity or rigidity. The child with athetosis or ataxia will not show an increase in these reflexes.

The Babinski sign is demonstrated by stroking the bottom of the child's foot along the lateral side of the sole beginning at the heel and proceeding toward the forefoot. Extension and spreading of the toes are normally present in the infant but should disappear by 1 to 2 years of age.

Muscle Examination

The muscle control of the upper and lower extremities is tested to establish the strength of each individual muscle. Muscle testing in the child with spasticity is more difficult than in the normal child; however, by palpating the muscle and tendon while testing strength against gravity and resistance, a relatively accurate assessment of the strength of each individual muscle can be made. For example, to examine the flexor carpi ulnaris muscle, the examiner palpates the muscle belly and the tendon to feel the amount of contraction of the muscle (as the child flexes the wrist against the resistance of one of the examiner's hands).

Joint Motion

Although there is increased muscle tone in the extremities, a careful assessment of joint range of motion is possible; the child should be relaxed to decrease spasticity. In the upper extremity the ranges of motion of the shoulder, elbow, wrist, and fingers are tested in the routine manner; evaluation of the lower extremity is more complicated. The hip must be tested for abduction in both flexion and in extension. Abduction is greater if the test is performed slowly; if the hips are abducted quickly, the adductor muscles contract forcibly, restricting abduction of the hip.

Flexion of the hip is tested in the normal manner. The amount of extension of the hip (flexion contracture) may be tested in two ways. The most familiar is the standard Thomas test, which is performed with the child supine. The opposite hip is flexed enough to flatten the lumbar spine and to eliminate lordosis. The hip being tested is flexed maximally and then adducted to neutral and finally extended to the point of resistance, which marks the amount of flexion contracture. This test may not be accurately reproducible in some patients with spasticity. Staheli has described a test that he believes is more accurate in children with spasticity. To perform this test the child is placed

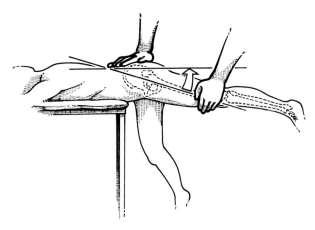

Fig. 11-8 Prone measure of hip flexion contracture. Child is placed prone with abdomen, thorax, and chest on table but pelvis and legs suspended over edge of table, with hips flexed fully. Examiner places one hand on back of sacrum and pelvis; other hand extends one leg. Hip is extended until pelvis begins to move, which is maximum amount of flexion contracture of hips; angle that thigh and femur makes with horizontal provides measure of hip flexion contracture. (Redrawn from Bleck EE: Orthopaedic management of cerebral palsy, Philadelphia, 1979, WB Saunders Co.)

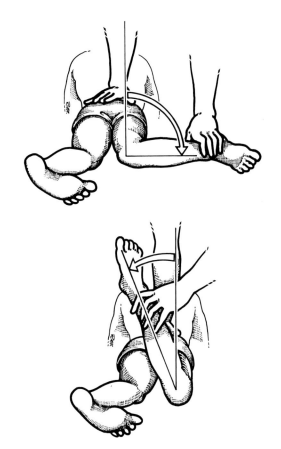

Fig. 11-9 Measurement of internal and external rotation of hips. Patient is placed prone with hips extended and knees flexed to 90 degrees; hips then are internally and externally rotated to maximum hips will allow without motion of pelvis. (Redrawn from Bleck EE: Orthopaedic management of cerebral palsy, Philadelphia, 1979, WB Saunders Co.)

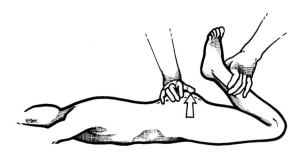

Fig. 11-10 Rectus femoris (Ely) test. Patient is placed prone with hip and knee extended; as knee is flexed quickly, examiner's opposite hand holds pelvis on ipsilateral side. If rectus femoris is tight, pelvis elevates on that side. (Redrawn from Bleck EE: Orthopaedic management of cerebral palsy, Philadelphia, 1979, WB Saunders Co.)

in the prone position with the anterior iliac spines of the pelvis at the edge of the table and the legs hanging suspended over the edge of the table. The examiner holds the leg to be tested with one hand while placing the other hand on the pelvis. The leg being tested is gently extended until the hand on the pelvis detects movement, which indicates the maximum amount of hip extension. The angle that the leg makes with the body at the point that the pelvis begins to move is the measure of the hip flexion contracture (Fig. 11-8).

Rotation of the hip is tested with the hip in both flexion and extension; the extension measurement is the more important because it indicates the functional rotation of the hip in the standing position. This may be performed with the patient supine but is more accurate with the patient prone. The knees are flexed to 90 degrees, and the hips are rotated internally and then externally rotated to test the range of their rotation (Fig. 11-9).

The range of motion of the knee first is tested in the routine fashion. The amount of flexion contracture is estimated by extending the knee with the hip fully extended and the patient supine. The spasticity of the rectus femoris muscle is tested with the Ely test; the patient is placed prone with the knee extended, and the knee then is flexed to the point that the pelvis lifts off the table (Fig. 11-10). Perry has shown that when this test is performed, the iliopsoas muscle also contracts; thus spasticity of the rectus femoris alone is not determined.

The tightness of the hamstring muscles may be tested in two ways. The straight leg-raising test stresses the hamstring muscles, enabling the examiner to determine their relative tightness. A more reproducible method is the measure of the popliteal angle. With the patient supine on the examining table the leg to be tested is lifted from the table and the knee is flexed maximally; then the hip is flexed to 90 degrees and held in that position. The knee is slowly extended, and the point at which resistance is met is noted. The angle that the knee makes determines the amount of hamstring tightness (Fig. 11-11). Ninety degrees of hip flexion must be maintained throughout the examination because if the hip is extended, the hamstrings will be less tight and a false impression will be recorded.

The examination of the foot and ankle in the spastic child is performed in much the same manner as in a child without spasticity. It is important to examine the ankle for tendo Achilles contracture, with the foot held in inversion to lock the midfoot and the hindfoot. If the foot is held in a neutral position, the foot and ankle tend to go into valgus and there is dorsiflexion in the midfoot rather than at the ankle. With the foot held in inversion the lateral rather than the medial border of the foot should be observed to determine the amount of dorsiflexion possible (Fig. 11-12).

Ankle dorsiflexion should be evaluated with the knee in both flexion and extension. Silfverskiöld developed a test to determine which muscles were responsible for tendo Achilles contracture, postulating that if the tendo Achilles was tight only with the knee extended, the gastrocnemius muscle alone was responsible, whereas if it were tight with the knee both flexed and extended, both the soleus and gastrocnemius muscles were responsible (Fig. 11-13). Using electromyography, Perry demonstrated that both the gastrocnemius and the soleus muscles were active electrically when this test was performed; thus he questioned the accuracy of the Silfverskiöld test.

Hindfoot varus or valgus should be evaluated by testing the position of the calcaneus in the resting position both on standing and with the foot suspended. The heel also should be tested to ascertain if it is mobile or fixed. This is done by grasping the heel with one hand and holding the tibia with the other, then inverting and everting the heel to determine passive motion of the hindfoot. If there is a varus deformity of the foot, the posterior tibial tendon should be checked for contracture. Tenting of the skin behind the medial malleolus usually occurs when eversion of the foot is attempted. Hindfoot varus is more common in children with hemiplegia, and valgus occurs more frequently in children with diplegia or tetraplegia.

A cavus deformity of the foot may be present, especially in children with hemiplegia. Recognition of the cavus deformity is important because some children walk on their toes as a result of pes cavus rather than

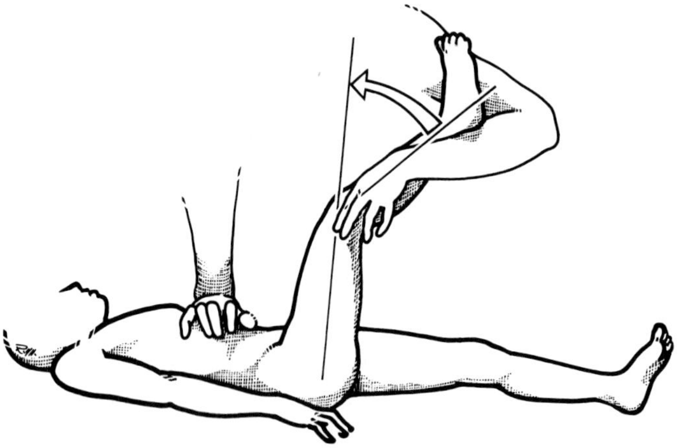

Fig. 11-11 Test of hamstring tightness. Patient is placed prone, and hip is flexed and held in 90 degrees of flexion. Knee is allowed to flex fully and is extended to a point where resistance is felt. Popliteal angle at that point is measured, which provides amount of hamstring tightness. (Redrawn from Bleck EE: Orthopaedic management of cerebral palsy, Philadelphia, 1979, WB Saunders Co.)

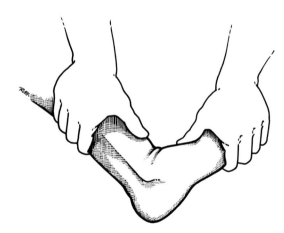

Fig. 11-12 Measurement of equinus deformity. Foot is inverted to lock subtalar joint and is placed in dorsiflexion with subtalar joint held in position of stability; lateral border of foot is observed. Angle of lateral border of heel and longitudinal axis of fibula provides degree of deformity.

tendo Achilles contracture. If pes cavus is responsible for the toe walking, tendo Achilles lengthening will not correct the problem and may actually worsen it inasmuch as the cavus remains and the triceps surae muscle is weakened.

Hallux valgus is seen in children with spastic diplegia and quadriplegia. There are several possible causes of this deformity. The adductor of the great toe should be tested for tightness and spasticity. In addition, the position of the hindfoot should be evaluated because spastic children with hallux valgus usually have a tendo Achilles contracture combined with a valgus heel. This pronation of the foot, combined with equinus of the ankle and tendo Achillis contracture, results in increased weight bearing on the medial border of the great toe, producing the valgus deformity.

Sensory Examination

Although it may be difficult to perform, a sensory examination of the upper and lower extremities is important. The function of the hand after any surgical procedures depends in part on the degree of sensory deficit. Of the different methods of determining sensory status the one most useful for the young or retarded patient is testing stereognosis, which involves the identification of objects placed in the child's hand with the patient either blindfolded or with closed eyes. Any available objects that are easily recognizable such as a pen or a coin may be used. Another method is dermographics, in which a number under 10 is drawn on the patient's palm and the child is asked to identify it. Sensation of the hand also may be determined with the Moberg two-point discrimination test.

DIAGNOSTIC TOOLS
Gait Analysis

Gait analysis is the most useful laboratory test in the treatment of the child with cerebral palsy. In modern gait analysis laboratories several types of analyses are performed simultaneously. Gait electromyography (EMG) allows determination of the action of a given muscle during a known period in the gait cycle. The gait laboratory is equipped with a walkway where the patient may walk unimpeded. In the middle of the walkway there usually is a force plate, and either video cameras or motion picture cameras are used to record the actual gait cycle. In addition, the patient usually is connected to an EMG analyzer through electrodes placed over the muscles to be tested. Some muscles, such as the posterior tibial and the iliopsoas, require needle electrodes. The information from the electrodes is transmitted to a com-

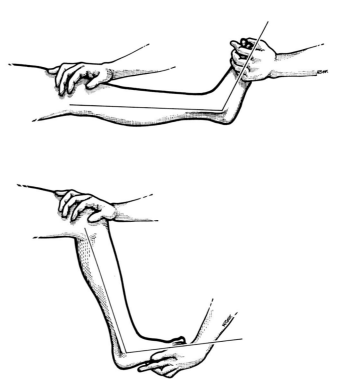

Fig. 11-13 Silfverskiöld test, which is performed by testing equinus deformity with knee in extension and in flexion. If amount of equinus deformity is less with knee in flexion than in extension, gastrocnemius muscle is major cause of equinus deformity.

puter through telemetry equipment. Force-sensitive switches attached to the foot of the patient also record the swing and stance phases of gait, and this information is recorded and analyzed by a computer that provides insight into the action of the recorded muscles during the different phases of gait, for example, the action of the posterior tibial muscle, which frequently is responsible for hindfoot varus in the child with hemiplegia.

Motion Analysis

Motion analysis, which is another diagnostic tool in the gait analysis laboratory, is used to determine active ranges of motion of the joints of the body. Light-sensitive or light-emitting objects are placed strategically on the patient and recorded by a computer as the patient walks along a walkway. This is compared with normal data and provides information regarding the motion of the various joints during the gait cycle. Because of the speed of the gait cycle, it is difficult to determine how much the hip and knee flex during gait, but with motion analysis, the exact motion of these joints can be determined quickly and compared with normal function. This information aids decision making about surgical treatment and provides excellent documentation of the results of treatment.

Myoneural Blocks

The use of muscle blocks to determine the effect of paralysis or weakening of a certain muscle occasionally is helpful in decision making. The muscle may be temporarily paralyzed with a local anesthetic such as lidocaine, after which the effect of the muscle paralysis or weakening is tested clinically and in the gait laboratory. This procedure is of potential benefit only if the muscle in question is dynamically tight and there is no fixed contracture of the muscle. Alcohol has been used for the same effect; this block lasts for several weeks, allowing more time for analysis.

NONSURGICAL MANAGEMENT
Neurodevelopmental Therapy

Many different forms of physical therapy have been developed for the child with cerebral palsy, the most current being neurodevelopmental therapy (NDT). This form of therapy is based on the work of Bobath and attempts to follow and implement normal development in the child with cerebral palsy. The therapist may require the child to achieve each normal stage of development before continuing to the next; for example, if a child is ready to walk but has not yet crawled, walking is restricted until crawling had been accomplished. Therapists who adhere to this philosophy also advocate early intervention in the neonatal unit. Controversy exists as to whether this form of therapy is effective in accomplishing its stated goals: to allow the child to achieve milestones that would have been unattainable without therapy. Several studies have shown no positive effect of NDT therapy, and Sullivan and Conner found no difference between children who underwent early intervention therapy and those who did not. Whatever the form of therapy the physical therapist is important in the overall care of the child with cerebral palsy and is usually the person with whom the family has the most contact during the early years of the child's life. The therapist can assist the family in the care of the handicapped child, can play an important role in the clinical evaluation, can assist in attempts at ambulation with walkers and crutches, and can provide exercises that may help to decrease the severity of contractures. A clinic that specializes in seating, staffed by persons knowledgeable about seating devices and the special needs of the handicapped child, also is important for children with special seating needs. The child may need only a standard chair or may require custom fitting of a specialized chair or insert.

Orthoses

Full-control hip-knee-ankle-foot orthoses (HKAFO) once were popular as a means of standing the child who could not stand unaided, but this practice has been almost completely abandoned because, in addition to being ineffective, the braces were a hindrance to normal development.

Knee-ankle-foot orthoses (KAFO) also are usually unnecessary for the child with cerebral palsy. These orthoses, like the HKAFOs, inhibit function rather than assist it and are not recommended for the child with spasticity. This type of bracing is only very occasionally needed for the child with an unusual athetosis or dystonia that is supple but that the patient cannot control. In this instance the orthosis may control abnormal movement and allow the child to ambulate. This type of orthosis also may be used to prevent hyperextension of the knee during gait in the child with genu recurvatum. Another less cumbersome method of preventing knee hyperextension is an ankle-foot-orthosis (AFO) with the ankle in 5 degrees of dorsiflexion. Putting the foot in a mild calcaneus position causes the child to assume a very slight crouched posture that prevents genu recurvatum.

The AFO is the most commonly used orthosis for children with cerebral palsy. The metal upright attached to a high-topped "orthopaedic shoe" has been, for the most part, replaced by the rigid plastic custom-molded AFO. Although an orthosis may help control a mild dynamic equinus deformity or prevent a recurrence of an equinus deformity after surgery, no orthosis can overcome a fixed contracture or control the very spastic dynamic deformity. The AFO for a child with spasticity must be different from that for a patient with flaccid paralysis of the foot. The flaccid foot and ankle require an AFO with some spring in its design to provide some dorsiflexion assistance during ambulation. This orthosis usually is very lightweight and made of thin plastic. The AFO for the child with spasticity, on the other hand, must be rigid to help control the spasticity of the triceps surae muscle.

The use of short-leg casts to reduce the spasticity of the muscles of the lower portion of the leg has gained some popularity. The object, according to proponents, is to inhibit the plantar grasp response, to extend the toes, and to provide a stable base for support. Maintaining the muscles that are stretched is believed to reduce the spastic muscle's response to stretch.

Seating Devices

Children with quadriplegia frequently require a wheelchair for longer distances. Children who walk as youngsters may find their ability to ambulate decreased with age, and other children never develop the ability to ambulate; therefore the proper fitting of a wheelchair is important. Many different types of chairs are available to fit the varied needs of those with cerebral palsy. The infant who is unable to sit without support will need a stroller for transportation. A simple, unmodified wheelchair is appropriate for the child with normal head and trunk control who simply lacks the lower extremity strength and control to walk. The standard wheelchair frequently is replaced by a lightweight and sturdy "sport wheelchair" that is easier to maneuver. Children who lack good trunk control or who have deformities of the spine or pelvis require some modification of the chair to provide trunk support to allow sitting. These supports vary from pads attached to a standard wheelchair to custom-molded seating systems that fit into a wheelchair. If a child is unable to propel the wheelchair, an electric wheelchair is of great benefit in increasing independence and improving the quality of life. The control switches for these chairs are quite sophisticated and can be modified to enable even the child with minimal voluntary control of only one extremity to operate the chair.

Communication Devices

Some children with cerebral palsy lack the motor control necessary for intelligible communication. Through the use of communication devices a nonverbal but intelligent child may be able to communicate. Some of these devices are simple, such as a communication board that contains pictures of persons or objects to which the child points. This type of device is used for the young child as a first means of nonverbal communication. As the child grows, more sophisticated devices, such as computers that speak for the child, are used to allow communication.

SURGICAL MANAGEMENT
Nonorthopaedic Surgical Management

There was a brief wave of enthusiasm for cerebellar stimulation among families of children with cerebral palsy, but that enthusiasm has waned. This treatment method, which consists of a "cerebellar stimulator" implanted on the surface of the cerebellum, remains controversial. A newer neurologic procedure that currently is popular is selective posterior rhizotomy. This involves severing some of the dorsal rootlets of the lumbar nerve roots. The early reports by the advocates of this procedure are favorable; however, several more years of study are required before its final value is known. At the present time it remains experimental.

Principles of Orthopaedic Surgical Management

It is important to remember that any treatment of a patient with cerebral palsy affects the symptoms of the disease but does not affect the cause, which is brain damage. Therefore, although the function of an individual can be improved, function never will be totally normal. Surgical lengthening of a spastic muscle weakens that muscle, thereby decreasing its stretch reflex, which reduces its spasticity. This may allow the antagonist muscles that were inhibited by the overpull of a spastic muscle to function better.

Spastic muscles usually should not be transferred to another location if they are producing a deformity where they are because they invariably will produce a deformity in their transferred location. To effectively transfer a muscle in a child with spasticity, the muscle should be under good volitional control. Spastic muscles may, however, be split and then half the tendon transferred to an antagonist muscle. This leaves a portion of the tendon of the transferred muscle intact but balances its spasticity, thus correcting the deformity from muscle spasticity and preventing the overcorrection from transfer of the entire muscle. Athetoid muscles should not be transferred or lengthened because of the almost certain development of an opposite deformity.

It is important to remember that muscle transfers cannot overcome fixed bony deformity. A tendon transfer may be performed in the presence of a fixed bony deformity if the bony deformity is corrected at the same time.

Abnormal sensation is not a problem in the lower extremity, but abnormal sensation in the hand precludes normal function even after surgery. Decreased sensation requires the child to visually control any use of the affected hand, thereby making that hand dependent rather than independent. This does not mean that surgery is not worthwhile, but realistic goals must be set and results graded accordingly. Most often the affected hand will be a "helper" rather than an independent hand.

The age of the child when surgical treatment is performed differs, depending on the planned procedures and the functional level of the child. Surgery on the lower extremities usually is appropriate between the ages of 3 and 7 years. Some authors recommend waiting until the child is 6 or 7 years of age before considering surgical treatment because they believe that before this age the child's nervous system has not sufficiently matured. Bleck (1988) believes that recurrence of deformity, such as an equinus deformity after tendo Achilles lengthening, is greater if the child is younger than 7 years old at the time of surgery. On the other hand, children who can pull to standing but have too much spasticity to walk, frequently are able to walk after appropriate lengthening of the muscles of the lower extremity. The appropriate age for surgical treatment of all children with cerebral palsy cannot be determined exactly; each child must be evaluated individually and the timing of surgery determined by the needs of that particular patient. The best time for surgical treatment is when the child is being hindered by the spasticity and/or contractures of the lower extremities. The timing of surgical treatment of the upper extremity differs from that of the lower extremity. To adequately evaluate the spastic upper extremity, the child's complete cooperation is required and postoperative care requires patient cooperation. Surgery should not be delayed too long, however, because of the possibility that contractures will develop. The ideal age varies between 4 and 8 years.

UPPER EXTREMITY

Surgery in the upper extremity usually is beneficial to children with hemiplegia. Children with spastic diplegia do not have severe enough involvement of the upper extremities to warrant surgical correction, and those with total body involvement usually have too much spasticity and too little voluntary control for surgery on the hand to be of benefit; however, these children may benefit from releases to prevent fixed deformity or for cosmesis.

Shoulder, Elbow, and Forearm

Release of adduction and internal rotation contracture of the shoulder. The spastic shoulder occasionally develops a severe adduction and internal rotation deformity that may require correction if it limits the patient's ability to reach for objects, thus limiting the function of the upper portion of the limb. Children with severe spasticity and minimal function may benefit from correction of this contracture to improve hygiene. Generally, the muscles responsible for this contracture are the pectoralis major and the subscapularis.

▲ *Technique.* Approach the shoulder through a deltopectoral incision. Identify the subscapularis muscle, and separate it from the underlying capsule of the shoulder joint. Pass a probe or clamp under the subscapularis, and release the tendon of the muscle from the lesser tuberosity. Identify the pectoralis major and perform a Z-plasty lengthening of its tendon.

▲ *Postoperative management.* After surgery the shoulder is splinted for comfort, and range of motion exercises are begun as soon as comfort allows.

Occasionally a fixed abduction contracture of the shoulder may develop. If the neurologic injury is very severe, the child may assume a chronic posture with the head directed toward one side. Because of the persistent asymmetric tonic neck reflex, the involved arm is maintained in constant abduction and external rotation. A high degree of spasticity may cause dislocation of the humeral head inferiorly, which requires open reduction of the shoulder with release of the deltoid muscle and lengthening of the teres major and infraspinatus muscles.

Lengthening of the biceps and brachialis muscles.
Elbow flexion contracture is a common problem in the child with hemiplegia. The contracture limits the use of the hand and also may limit the child's use of crutches. In severely spastic children with total body involvement a flexion deformity of the elbow may be severe enough to cause maceration of the skin in the flexion crease of the elbow. Posterior dislocation of the head of the radius develops in some children with elbow flexion contractures and pronation deformities of the forearm. Lengthening of the biceps and brachialis muscles is indicated if the contracture is severe or if it limits hand function.

▲ *Technique.* Approach the elbow through an S-shaped incision, beginning the proximal limb of the incision on the anterolateral aspect of the upper portion of the arm and crossing the elbow flexion crease at a 45-degree angle. Continue the distal limb of the incision on the anteromedial aspect of the proximal forearm (Fig. 11-14, *A*). Preserve the veins on the volar side of the elbow if possible. Identify the muscle of the biceps brachii, and trace it distally to its main tendon and to the lacertus fibrosus, which usually is thick and tight. Isolate the lacertus fibrosus, and completely divide it (Fig. 11-14, *B*).

The lateral antebrachial cutaneous nerve, which is the distal continuation of the musculocutaneous nerve, enters the cubital fossa between the biceps and the brachialis muscles lateral to the tendon of the biceps. Identify and protect this nerve by gently retracting it laterally. Identify the biceps tendon, and trace it distally to the insertion on the bicipital tuberosity of the radius. Once the tendon is completely freed, perform a Z-plasty lengthening of the tendon (Fig. 11-14, *C*). Directly posterior to the biceps tendon is the muscle belly of the brachialis muscle. Isolate the tendon almost to the point where the brachialis muscle inserts on the coronoid process of the proximal ulna. The distal portion of the brachialis is covered with a strong aponeurosis that extends proximally for more than 3 cm. Lateral to the tendon and partially covered by the brachioradialis muscle is the radial nerve; identify and protect the radial nerve throughout the surgical procedure. Also identify and

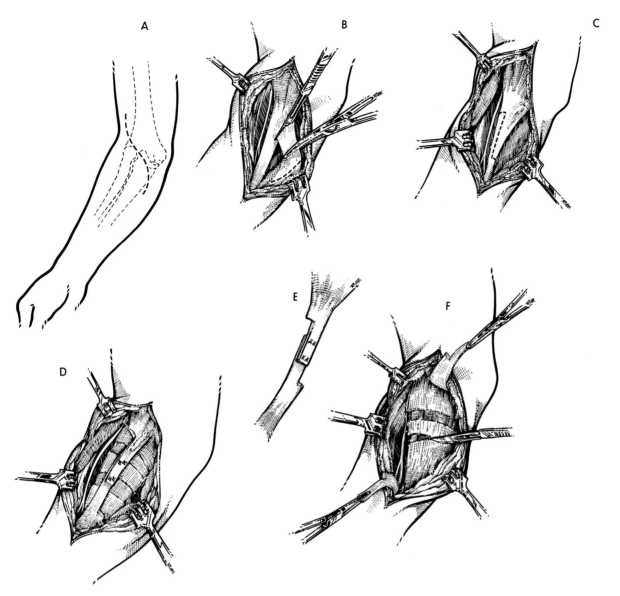

Fig. 11-14 Lengthening of elbow flexion contracture (see text). **A,** S-shaped incision. **B,** Biceps femoris muscle and tendon are identified; lacertus fibrosus is identified and divided. **C** to **E,** Z-plasty lengthening of biceps tendon, which then is repaired. **F,** Fractional lengthening of brachialis muscle is performed by making one or two transverse cuts through aponeurosis of the muscle tendon unit proximal to musculotendinous junction. (Redrawn from Mital MA: J Bone Joint Surg 61A:515, 1979.)

protect the median nerve and brachial artery on the medial side of the brachialis muscle. Once all the vital structures are protected, cut the aponeurosis transversely in one or two places, making certain that the aponeurosis is completely cut from medial to lateral but that the fibers of the muscle are left undisturbed (Fig. 11-14, *F*). If a significant flexion deformity of the elbow remains, an anterior capsulotomy of the elbow joint may be performed.

With the elbow in the position of splinting, release the tourniquet and evaluate the circulation to the arm. If the pulse in the radial artery is not strong, position the arm in less extension to reduce the stretch on the brachial artery. Repair the tendon of the biceps with the elbow in moderate extension (Fig. 11-14, *D* and *E*). Close the incision in layers over a suction drain. The skin may be closed with a subcuticular absorbable suture.

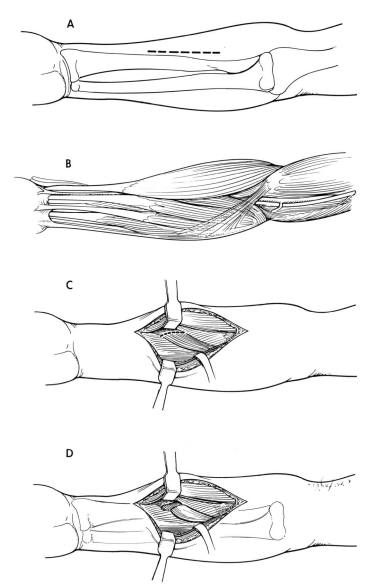

Fig. 11-15 Release of pronator teres (see text). **A,** Longitudinal incision on volar aspect of forearm. **B,** Brachioradialis is retracted radially with neurovascular bundle; pronator teres muscle and tendon are identified by oblique direction. **C,** Distal insertion of pronator teres on radius is released. Note dotted line, which identifies insertion of pronator teres on radius. **D,** Release has been completed; muscle separates from its insertion by about 1 cm. (After Hoppenfeld S and deBoer P: Surgical exposures in orthopaedics: the anatomic approach, Philadelphia, 1984, JB Lippincott Co.)

▲ *Postoperative management.* The arm is placed in a long-arm cast with the forearm in supination and the elbow in moderate extension, but it is important to limit the extension to the degree that the circulation in the brachial artery is able to tolerate. If the procedure was performed for hygiene, the cast is left in place for 4 to 6 weeks. If the procedure was performed to improve function in a child with an extremity capable of independent functioning, then as soon as the patient is comfortable, the cast is bivalved (usually in 1 to 2 weeks) and active range-of-motion exercises are begun. The cast is continued full-time, except for periods of exercise, for 6 weeks. At that time the cast is removed during the day, but night splinting is continued for 6 months.

Release of the pronator teres muscle in pronation contracture of the forearm. Pronation contracture of the forearm is common in children with hemiplegia and frequently is associated with other deformities of the hand and wrist that may require simultaneous surgical procedures. The pronation contracture limits function of the hand and wrist and may contribute to posterior dislocation of the radial head. The forearm is pronated because of the spasticity of the pronator teres muscle and weakness of the supinator muscle. Correction of this deformity may be directed toward the spastic pronator or the weak supinator, or both. To reduce the pronator spasticity and overpull of this muscle, the pronator may be released or transferred around the radius, creating a supination force. Simple release of the insertion of the pronator teres has been very successful in patients with spasticity. Sakellarides et al prefer transfer of the pronator teres around the anterolateral border of the radius, converting it into a supinator. If the pronator is spastic, a supination deformity might be produced with this transfer, and simple release is preferred.

Another method of reducing the pronation deformity is creation of a new supinator of the forearm by rerouting the flexor carpi ulnaris muscle around the ulnar side of the forearm and transferring it either to the wrist extensors or to the finger extensors. Transfer of the flexor carpi ulnaris is discussed in the section on treatment of the hand and wrist.

▲ *Technique.* The approach for both simple release of the pronator teres and transfer of the pronator to the anterolateral border of the radius is the same: either a straight or a curved incision on the anterolateral aspect of the mid to proximal part of the forearm (Fig. 11-15). Identify and protect the lateral cutaneous nerve of the forearm and the superficial radial nerve. Identify the edge of the brachioradialis muscle, then mobilize and lift the muscle from the underlying soft tissues. Identify the muscle and tendon of the prona-tor teres by the oblique direction of the muscle fibers and the attachment of the tendon to the radius at this level (Fig. 11-15). Release the attachment of the pro-nator teres onto the radius, and supinate the forearm. Release the tourniquet and control bleeding; then close the wound and apply a long-arm cast with the forearm in supination.

▲ *Postoperative management.* The cast is left intact for 2 weeks, at which time it is bivalved and active range-of-motion, supination, and pronation exercises are begun. The cast is worn when the patient is not exer-cising. At the end of 6 weeks the cast may be discon-tinued during the day but is worn at night for at least 3 months to prevent recurrence of the supination contracture.

Transfer of the pronator teres muscle in pronation contracture of the forearm

▲ *Technique.* Make a straight or curved incision on the anterolateral aspect of the mid to proximal part of the forearm. Isolate the tendon of the pronator teres muscle by sharp dissection, and lengthen the tendon as much as possible by removing a strip of perios-teum from the radius, leaving it attached to the end of the tendon. Insert a nonabsorbable suture into the end of the tendon and periosteum with a Bunnell stitch (Fig. 11-16, *A*). Then mobilize the tendon as far proximally as possible. Free all soft tissue attach-ments subperiosteally from the radius posteriorly and laterally. Also free the interosseous membrane from the radius as far distally and proximally as possible to gain maximum passive supination. Do not disturb the pronator quadratus attachment distally in the fore-arm.

Pass the pronator teres posterior and lateral to the radius toward its anterolateral border. Using a 1.6-mm Kirschner wire, make a small hole through the radius at the same level as the original attachment of the tendon, but direct it from the anterolateral cortex posteromedially. Enlarge the hole in the anterolateral cortex with a 2.8-mm (⁷⁄₆₄-inch) drill bit (Fig. 11-16, *B*). Pass the suture attached to the tendon through the drill hole from anterolateral to posteromedial (Fig. 11-16, *C*). Pull the tendon tightly into the hole created in the radius, and attach the suture to the portion of the tendon that did not pass through the hole (Fig. 11-16, *D*). Use additional sutures from the tendon to the surrounding soft tissues to secure the transferred tendon.

▲ *Postoperative management.* After wound closure the arm is immobilized in a long-arm cast, with the

forearm held in a position of 60 degrees of supina-tion and the elbow flexed to 90 degrees, which will decrease the tension on the transferred tendon. The cast is left in place for 5 weeks, at which time it is bi-valved and then removed during the day for active range-of-motion exercises that include supination, pr-onation, and elbow flexion and extension. After 4 weeks the bivalved cast is removed during the day but is continued at night for 6 months.

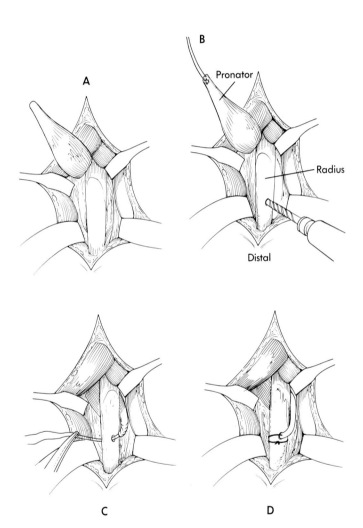

Fig. 11-16 Transfer of pronator teres (see text). **A,** Pro-nator teres muscle is released from attachment to radius with strip of periosteum. **B,** Drill hole is made through ra-dius. **C,** Pronator teres is passed underneath and poste-rior to radius, and with a suture the tendon itself is pulled into drill hole in radius. **D,** Tendon then is sutured to it-self and to surrounding structures. (Redrawn from Sakel-larides MT, Mital MA, and Lenzi WD: J Bone Joint Surg 63A:645, 1981.)

Hand and Wrist
Evaluation

The ease of the evaluation of the hand of a child with spastic cerebral palsy depends on the age and intelligence of the patient. Control of the hand is difficult for these children because of the spasticity of the muscles to be tested, in addition to the spasticity of the antagonist muscles. Palpation of the tendon of the muscle being tested may be necessary to determine if it is functioning inasmuch as there may be little movement of the joint in question. Patience and persistence are required in the evaluation of these children.

Because athetosis is a contraindication to muscle surgery, it is extremely important to determine the type of neurologic damage. A thorough sensory examination is helpful to predict the postoperative level of use of the hand; the better the sensation the better will be the independent use of the hand. Although few children with spastic hemiplegia have good sensation, surgical treatment may improve the function of the hand. It must be remembered that after surgery the hand may be used only as a helper, and if the sensation of the hand is not good, the child will require visual assistance in using the hand.

Although multiple problems exist in the spastic upper extremity, it is impossible to cover all possible combinations of deformities; therefore in this chapter individual problems are discussed separately, and the reader must keep in mind that many occur in combination. The treatment of multiple deformities should be undertaken at one time even though they are described separately in this chapter.

Zancolli et al classified spastic deformity of the upper extremity into three patterns.

Group I. Flexion spasticity is minimal and occurs only in the flexor carpi ulnaris muscle. These patients can completely extend their fingers with the wrist in neutral position or in less than 20 degrees of flexion. The main characteristic is the inability to hyperextend the wrist with the fingers fully extended.

Group II. The fingers can be fully extended but only with the wrist flexed more than 20 degrees. The spasticity is believed to be located in the wrist and finger flexor muscles. This group can be further subdivided according to the severity of the spasticity and the strength of the wrist extensor muscles.

In subgroup IIa the patient can actively extend the wrist with the fingers flexed, indicating that the extensor muscles of the wrist are active and the flexor muscles of the wrist are not very spastic. Most spasticity is located in the finger flexor muscles. The goal of treatment is to reduce the spasticity of the finger flexors.

In subgroup IIb the patient cannot extend the wrist with the fingers flexed because of the paralysis of the wrist extensor muscles, and the strength of the wrist extensor muscles must be increased to improve function.

Group III. The spasticity of the flexor-pronator muscles and the paralysis of the extensor-supinator muscles are so marked that finger or wrist extension is not possible, even with maximum flexion of the wrist. This is the most difficult group to treat, and the functional results of treatment may be limited simply to reducing the contracture without improving the function of the hand and wrist.

Wrist Flexion Deformity

Flexion deformity of the wrist is due to spasticity with or without a fixed contracture of the wrist flexor muscles. Weakness of the wrist dorsiflexors also may contribute to the inability to achieve dorsiflexion of the wrist. Although the flexor carpi ulnaris muscle may be the cause of the wrist flexion posture, the most common cause is spasticity of the flexor carpi radialis muscle, which Goldner terms the *heel cord of the upper extremity*. The wrist extensors usually are weak, with little active function. The extensor carpi ulnaris, although weak, frequently is functioning, but because of the persistent flexed posture of the wrist, this tendon becomes subluxated volarly. It then functions as an ulnar deviator and a flexor of the wrist, which increases the deformity.

Multiple procedures have been described to help reduce the wrist flexion deformity. Some of the more commonly used are described.

Transfer of the flexor carpi ulnaris to the extensor carpi radialis brevis or extensor digitorum communis. According to Zancolli et al, for patients with class I involvement who have full finger extension with the wrist flexed less than 30 degrees, simple lengthening of the spastic wrist flexor usually is sufficient to improve function. They recommend lengthening the flexor carpi ulnaris muscle, but the flexor carpi radialis muscle seems to be a more common cause of the flexion deformity of the wrist in children with spastic hemiplegia. With a group II deformity Zancolli et al recommend transfer of the flexor carpi ulnaris around the ulnar border of the wrist as described by Green and Banks. This theoretically decreases the flexion deformity of the wrist and increases the dorsiflexion power of the wrist. In addition, because of the new route of the flexor carpi ulnaris around the ulna, the pull of the muscle tends to supinate the forearm, which helps reduce the pronation deformity.

Although this procedure produces the desired effect in many patients, results are not always predictable. Some patients are left with a dorsiflexion deformity after transfer of the flexor carpi ulnaris. This transfer never should be combined with lengthening of the flexor carpi radialis because there may be too little flexion strength remaining to oppose the transferred flexor carpi ulnaris.

Using EMG analysis of children with spastic cerebral palsy, Hoffer et al (1986) found the flexor carpi ulnaris to be sometimes active during grasp and at other times in release. Because muscles in cerebral palsy are phase-dependent and will not change phase, the authors believe it is important to transfer a muscle that will operate in the same phase as the muscle to which it is transferred. If the flexor carpi ulnaris is active in grasp, its transfer to the extensor carpi radialis brevis should be in phase because the extensor carpi radialis brevis and longus contract during grasp. On the other hand, if the flexor carpi ulnaris is active during release, its transfer to the extensor carpi radialis brevis will not function as desired. Hoffer et al recommend EMG to determine the phase of the flexor carpi ulnaris before transfer. They transfer the flexor carpi ulnaris to the extensor carpi radialis brevis if the flexor carpi ulnaris is active in grasp, but they believe the transfer should be to the extensor digitorum comminus muscle if the flexor carpi ulnaris is active in release.

Clinical evaluation also may help to determine the appropriate transfer of the flexor carpi ulnaris. If a child lacks wrist extension and has a poor grasp, then transfer to the extensor carpi radialis brevis is indicated. If the child has poor release but adequate grasp, then transfer to the finger extensors will improve the finger release.

◣ *Technique.* Make an anterior longitudinal incision about 10 to 12 cm long from the flexor crease of the wrist proximally (Fig. 11-17, *A*). Expose the tendon of the flexor carpi ulnaris from its insertion on the pisiform. Sever this attachment to the pisiform, and free the muscle completely from its attachment on the ulna as far proximally as possible. Identify the lateral margin of the muscle, and make an incision in the deep fascia to expose this margin and the posterior surface of the muscle. Then dissect the muscle free from its origin on the ulna distally and from the fascia. Once the muscle is completely freed, release as much of the muscle as necessary to be certain that the pull of the tendon will be in a straight line in its transferred position (Fig. 11-17, *B*). Identify and protect the nerve supply to the muscle from the ulnar nerve inasmuch as it usually limits the proximal extent of the dissection. Open the intermuscular septum that separates the volar and dorsal compartments at the lateral margin of the ulna to allow entry into the dorsal compartment of the forearm.

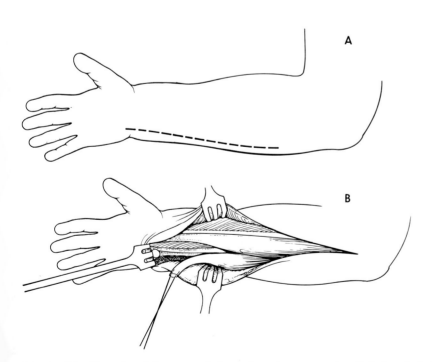

Fig. 11-17 Transfer of flexor carpi ulnaris to extensor carpi radialis brevis (see text). **A,** Anterior longitudinal incision. **B,** Flexor carpi ulnaris muscle is detached from insertion on pisiform. *Continued.*

Make a third incision over the extensor carpi radialis brevis and longus tendons, beginning just proximal to the dorsal wrist crease and extending proximally for about 3 cm (Fig. 11-17, *C*). Pull the tendon of the flexor carpi ulnaris into this wound, and insert the tendon into the extensor carpi radialis brevis through a buttonhole in its tendon. Suture the transfer under tension with the forearm supinated fully and the wrist in dorsiflexion 45 degrees (Fig. 11-17, *D*).

Transfer the flexor carpi ulnaris to the finger extensors in the same manner; however, insert it into the tendon of the extensor digitorum comminus under sufficient tension so that the metacarpophalangeal joints will hyperextend with the wrist in neutral position.

▲ *Postoperative management.* The arm is placed in a long-arm cast that may be bivalved in 3 to 4 weeks to begin active range-of-motion exercises. The cast usually is discontinued during the day 6 weeks after the operation, but it is continued at night for 6 months or more.

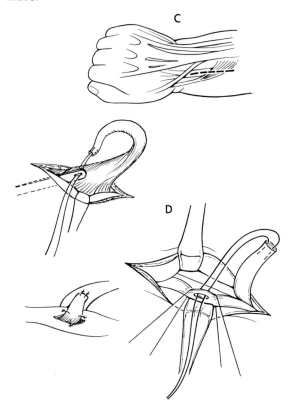

Fig. 11-17, cont'd   C, Small longitudinal incision on dorsum of wrist over extensor carpi radialis brevis. **D,** Tendon of flexor carpi ulnaris is passed subcutaneously around ulnar border of forearm and sutured to extensor carpi radialis brevis under moderate tension. Tension should be adjusted to hold wrist in flight dorsiflexion.

Lengthening of the flexor carpi radialis muscle and finger flexors. Not all children with spastic hemiplegia will benefit from selective lengthening of the wrist and finger flexors. Those children who are unable to fully extend the wrist because of spasticity of the wrist flexors or finger flexors, or both, will have improved function of the hand after lengthening of these muscles.

▲ *Technique.* Make a curved volar incision over the forearm from about 3 cm proximal to the volar wrist crease, and continue it proximally for 6 cm. Identify the flexor carpi radialis muscle, and follow it proximally to the musculotendinous junction and then proximally until the muscle belly is identified. The distal portion of the muscle belly is surrounded by an aponeurosis that thickens distally and forms the tendon of the muscle itself. Lengthen the muscle-tendon unit, and leave it in continuity by making transverse cuts in the aponeurosis proximal to the musculotendinous junction. Completely identify the muscle circumferentially, and make a transverse cut through the aponeurosis but not the muscle (Fig. 11-18). It is important to completely cut the aponeurosis transversely and not leave any of the tendon intact or the muscle-tendon unit will not lengthen. After the cut in the aponeurosis is made, place the wrist in dorsiflexion. The transverse cut in the aponeurosis will widen as the muscle lengthens, but the entire muscle tendon unit will remain intact. A second cut for recession may be made if necessary.

Other musculotendinous units may be contracted in addition to the flexor carpi radialis muscle. Frequently the palmaris longus muscle also is spastic and contracted and also may require lengthening in the same manner as the flexor carpi radialis.

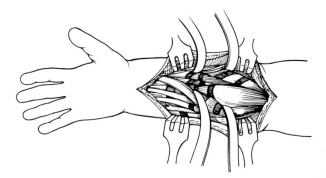

Fig. 11-18   Lengthening of flexor carpi radialis and finger flexors (see text). Each muscle to be lengthened is identified circumferentially, and transverse incision is made through tendon of muscle tendon unit proximal to musculotendinous junction. Incision is carried only through tendinous portion and not through muscle, which allows tendon unit to slide on itself but maintains continuity in musculotendinous unit.

Through this same incision the finger flexors may be lengthened in a similar manner. First lengthen the flexor digitorum superficialis muscles and then the flexor digitorum profundus if they contribute to the contracture.

▶ *Postoperative management.* A palmar (volar) short-arm splint with the wrist in neutral or slightly extended position is worn for 3 to 4 weeks. Then mobilization of the wrist is begun, and a removable splint is used for protection. A volar short-arm night splint is used for an additional 4 to 6 months.

Flexor slide. Another method of decreasing the spastic contracture of the wrist and fingers is by releasing the origin of the common flexors and pronator from the medial epicondyle of the distal humerus as proposed by Inglis and Cooper. This is a nonselective surgical procedure that lengthens all the muscles that originate from the medial epicondyle whether or not they are contracted. Because this requires an extensive dissection, selective fractional lengthenings usually are preferable.

▶ *Technique.* Approach the proximal half of the forearm and the medial epicondyle through a 10-cm incision centered over the medial aspect of the elbow. Begin the incision 5 cm proximal to the medial epicondyle, and continue it distally to the midpoint of the forearm over the ulna (Fig. 11-19). The medial antebrachial cutaneous nerve frequently is observed in the distal limb of the incision, and the medial brachial cutaneous nerve may be observed posterior to the medial part of the epicondyle. Identify the ulnar nerve proximal to the epicondyle, and gently lift it out of its groove behind the medial epicondyle. Free the ulnar nerve distally, and identify the nerves to the flexor carpi ulnaris and to the two heads of the flexor digitorum profundus muscles.

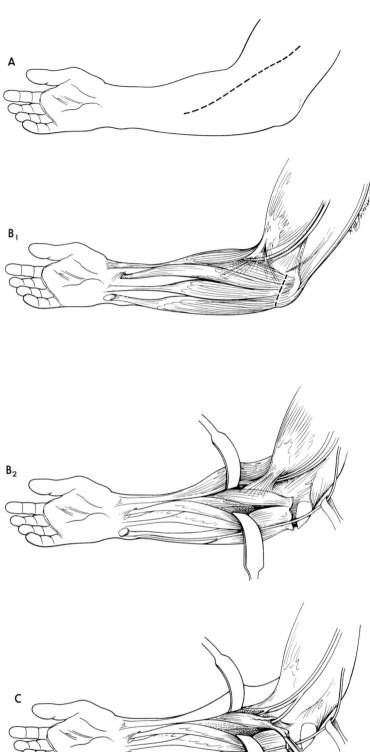

Fig. 11-19 **A,** Incision of 10 cm is made on medial aspect of volar side of arm, beginning approximately 5 cm proximal to medial epicondyle and continuing distally to midpoint of forearm over ulna. **B₁,** Wrist and finger flexor muscles are attached to medial epicondyle and are to be released from their origin on medial epicondyle. **B₂,** Ulnar nerve is identified, protected, and released from ulnar groove. Attachment of muscles to medial epicondyle is cut, and flexor carpi ulnaris and flexor digitorum profundus muscles are completely released. Both are from medial epicondyle and from ulna. **C,** Lacertus fibrosus is divided along with any remaining portions of flexor muscle origin.

Once the ulnar nerve has been released from the ulnar groove and completely identified, release the flexor carpi ulnaris and flexor digitorum profundus muscle origins. Begin the release distally at about the midpoint of the ulna. Elevate both muscles from the ulna at the subcutaneous border, and expose the interosseous membrane around the volar surface. Continue the dissection proximally along the ulna as far as the ulnar groove in the medial part of the epicondyle. During this dissection the interosseous membrane and the fascia of the brachialis muscle can be seen in the bottom of the wound. Replace the ulnar nerve in its groove, and divide the entire flexor-pronator muscle mass at its origin from the medial part of the epicondyle of the humerus. At the completion of this dissection the median nerve can be seen as it passes through the pronator teres muscle. Identify the lacertus fibrosus anteriorly, and divide it and any remaining portions of the flexor muscle origin. Remove the ulnar nerve from its groove, and transplant it anteriorly (Fig. 11-19). At the end of the procedure the wrist should extend 45 to 60 degrees with the fingers extended. The flexor muscle mass should be displaced 3 to 4 cm distal to its origin. Leave the fascia open, and release the remainder of the forearm fascia to prevent compartment ischemia. Close the wound over a suction drain, and splint the arm with the elbow flexed to 90 degrees and the forearm supinated, keeping the fingers and wrist in neutral position.

▶ *Postoperative management.* The splint is worn for 3 weeks, at which time a splint that keeps the wrist in neutral position is applied. This splint is worn for a minimum of 3 months full time and then at night.

Wrist arthrodesis. Arthrodesis of the wrist rarely is indicated in children with cerebral palsy. The function of the fingers in the spastic hand depends on the grasp-release function of the wrist, which is lost if wrist movement is lost. Some children with severe spasticity are able to open their fingers only when the wrist is flexed, relaxing the tight finger flexors, and conversely they are able to close their fingers when the wrist is in dorsiflexion. Wrist arthrodesis eliminates this important function of the wrist (Fig. 11-20).

Arthrodesis of the wrist should not be considered if any other procedures will improve function. Wrist arthrodesis may be performed for cosmetic improvement of the wrist. Although it will not improve function, it may allow the child to put the hand in a pocket or glove.

▶ *Technique.* Perform the fusion through a dorsal incision, exposing the carpal bones, the distal radius, and the second and third metacarpals. Remove the articular surfaces of these bones, and use iliac crest

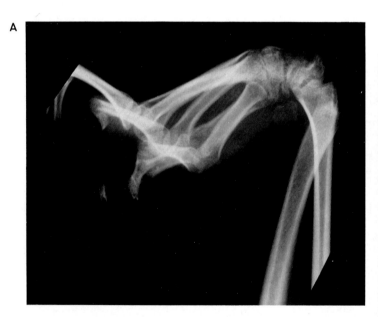
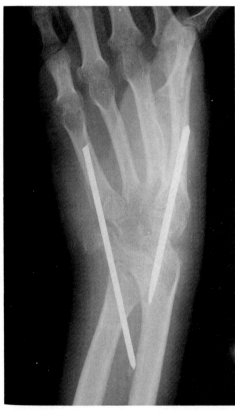

Fig. 11-20 Wrist arthrodesis. **A,** Position of wrist shows fixed deformity before wrist fusion. **B,** Improvement in wrist position after fusion.

bone graft to supplement the fusion. Insert intramedullary fixation through the third metacarpal and into the distal radius, and apply a plaster cast with the wrist in neutral alignment. Occasionally a proximal row carpectomy may be required to allow dorsiflexion of the wrist to neutral.

▶ *Postoperative management.* A long-arm cast is applied with the elbow at a right angle, the forearm in a neutral position, and the wrist in the position of fusion. Active extension and flexion of the fingers are encouraged. Three weeks after surgery, this may be converted to a short cast (below the elbow to just proximal to the metacarpophalangal joints). Support

is continued until firm fusion is present, usually 10 weeks. Internal fixation may be removed when fusion is solid.

Thumb-in-Palm Deformity

Multiple thumb positions are referred to collectively as a *thumb-in-palm deformity.* The thumb simply may be held adducted with the metacarpophalangeal and interphalangeal joints extended but the metacarpal joint adducted. In this instance the adductor of the thumb is spastic and responsible for the deformity. The first dorsal interosseous muscle also may be contributing to the deformity (Fig. 11-21). A second deformity that is truly a thumb-in-palm deformity is adduction and flexion of the thumb. The adductor of the thumb and the first dorsal interosseus muscles are responsible for the adduction posture of the thumb. The spasticity of the flexor pollicis longus muscle usually is responsible for the flexion of the interphalangeal joint of the thumb (Fig. 11-22). A third deformity is identical to the second except that the thumb metacarpal joint also is flexed and adducted into the palm, and the joint of the thumb may be hyperextended. In this instance the adductor and the first dorsal interosseus are spastic and tight. If the interphalangeal joint of the thumb is flexed, the flexor pollicis longus is spastic and tight. Spasticity of the flexor pollicis brevis, abductor pollicis brevis, or opponens pollicis muscles (or all three) is responsible for the flexion and apposition of the metacarpal (Fig. 11-23).

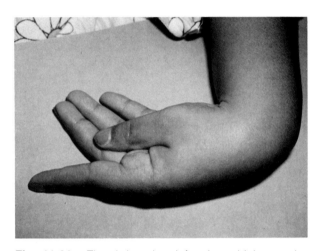

Fig. 11-21 Thumb-in-palm deformity, which may be caused by different muscle contractures. Here abductor of thumb is spastic and contracted and mainly responsible for deformity.

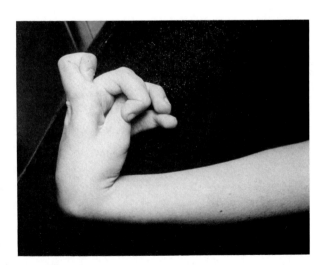

Fig. 11-22 Thumb-in-palm deformity with multiple causes. Adductor of thumb is spastic and flexor pollicis longus is very tight, producing flexion deformity of interphalangeal joint.

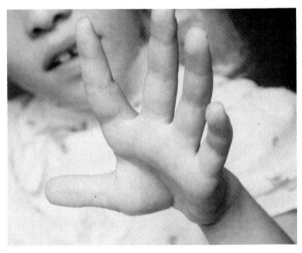

Fig. 11-23 Thumb-in-palm deformity produced by both adductor and short flexor of thumb. Note flexion and adduction posture of thumb metacarpal. Simple release of thumb adductor would not solve this child's deformity and would produce hypertension deformity of metacarpophalangeal joint.

In addition to the spastic musculature there is weakness or absence of the antagonist muscles, which allows the spastic muscles to produce the thumb deformities. The abductor pollicis longus and the extensor pollicis brevis muscles usually are weak or nonfunctioning and are overpowered by the spastic adductor pollicis and first dorsal interosseus muscles. In addition, the extensor pollicis longus may be weak, but if it functions, it usually is overpowered by the spasticity of the flexors, producing hyperextension and instability of the metacarpophalangeal joint.

Many procedures have been described to correct the thumb deformities in the child with spastic cerebral palsy. Because each child has different problems, each must be critically evaluated before any treatment decisions are made. The thumb deformities are complex, with multiple causes for the poor function; although surgical procedures are described individually, frequently multiple procedures are indicated for an individual child and can be performed in one operation combined with other procedures on the upper extremity.

Release of thumb web contracture. Occasionally the skin in the thumb web becomes contracted and requires Z-plasty to increase the width of the thumb web. Goldner recommends correction through an incision in the thumb web for the release of the contracted musculature.

▶ *Technique (Goldner).* Make a straight incision along the tight skin in the thumb web in a line directly from the base of the index finger to the base of the thumb. To define this skin contracture, distract the index finger and the thumb as much as possible. Then make the incision along this skin fold. Make two oblique cuts at angles of 45 to 60 degrees on opposite sides so that they can be rotated at the time of skin closure to increase the amount of skin in the web and thereby release the contracture (Fig. 11-24).

▶ *Postoperative management.* The hand is immobilized for 6 weeks with the thumb in abduction and

the wrist in 30 degrees of flexion. The thumb is splinted with a C-splint in the web for an additional 6 weeks.

• • •

Goldner also recommends this incision for release of the adductor pollicis muscle from the proximal phalanx of the thumb as the tendon is lengthened and then reattached to the neck of the thumb metacarpal. The first dorsal interosseous muscle also is released from the thumb and index matecarpals. This procedure is easily accomplished and usually produces a good result; however, occasionally a fixed abduction contracture may occur if the abductor pollicis longus is lengthened at the same time. If it is spastic, the short flexor of the thumb cannot be lengthened through this approach. Many authors recommend that the adductor pollicis be approached through an incision in the palm and the origin from the third metacarpal be released, because this will preserve its attachment on the thumb and will prevent an abduction deformity.

Matev release of the thumb-in-palm deformity. Matev found that a simple release of the adductor pollicis muscle increased the hyperextension deformity of the metacarpophalangeal joint of the thumb (Fig. 11-25); this deformity traditionally was treated with arthrodesis of the metacarpophalangeal joint, which reduced mobility of the thumb. If the abductor pollicis brevis and the flexor pollicis brevis muscles are spastic, they produce a fixed flexion position of the thumb metacarpal after simple adductor release. To avoid both problems Matev recommended that release of the thenar muscles be performed in addition

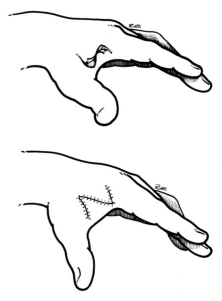

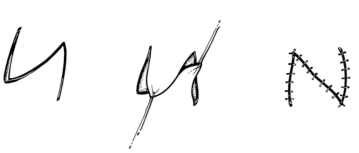

Fig. 11-24 Release of thumb web contracture by straight incision and two Z-plasty procedures. Alternative is to begin with Z-plasty; then flaps rotate to increase depth of thumb web as demonstrated here.

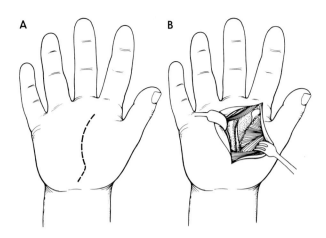

Fig. 11-25 Matev technique for release of thumb-in-palm deformity (see text). **A,** Incision in palmar crease at base of thenar eminence. **B,** Retraction of flexor tendons of index and long fingers along with neurovascular bundle and interosseus muscles toward ulnar side, exposing adductor pollicis muscle and short flexor and opponens of thumb. (Redrawn from Matev I: J Bone Joint Surg 45B:703, 1963.)

to release of the adductor pollicis from the third metacarpal. Some authors maintain that only release of the adductor pollicis longus is necessary, but they still prefer the palmar incision because it affords a direct approach to the origin of the muscle. The choice between complete release or simple release of the adductor depends on the individual patient. If the thumb metacarpal is flexed and even slightly opposed in addition to being adducted, then release of the short flexor, abductor, and opponens, in addition to a release of the origin of the adductor pollicis, is recommended (Fig. 11-25).

▲ *Technique (Matev).* Make an incision in the palmar crease at the base of the thenar eminence (Fig. 11-25, *A*). Retract the flexor tendons of the fingers toward the ulnar side along with the neurovascular bundles, exposing the adductor pollicis (Fig. 11-25, *B*). Avoid the motor branch of the ulnar nerve, and release the transverse and oblique heads of the adductor pollicis from the third metacarpal and from the carpus. Release the origins of the flexor pollicis brevis, opponens pollicis, and two thirds of the abductor pollicis brevis muscles from their origins from the volar carpal ligament, and recess them distally. If required, the first dorsal interosseous muscle also may be released from the second metacarpal through the same incision.

▲ *Postoperative management.* The hand is splinted with the thumb metacarpal abducted. It is important not to hyperextend the metacarpophalangeal joint. Active motion is begun within 2 weeks if no other procedures have been performed; however, usually

tendon transfers are performed at the same time and the postoperative care depends on the extent of those procedures.

Lengthening of the flexor pollicis longus muscle. If the flexor pollicis longus muscle is spastic, it will contribute to the thumb-in-palm deformity. Contracture of the flexor pollicis longus can be tested by holding the wrist in neutral position and extending the thumb. The distal phalanx of the thumb should extend to neutral with the metacarpal extended. If this is not possible, the flexor pollicis longus probably is contracted and release of the adductor of the thumb alone will not correct the thumb-in-palm deformity; lengthening of the flexor pollicis longus in addition to a release of the adductor pollicis should be performed. If the flexor pollicis longus is contracted, it may be weak or nonfunctional, and lengthening alone may result in a nonfunctioning interphalangeal joint of the thumb. If the flexor pollicis longus is weak but must be lengthened, then it should be reinforced with a functioning tendon if one is available, but if none exists, tenodesis to the radius will prevent hyperextension and strengthen the grasp when the wrist is in dorsiflexion.

The two muscles usually used for transfer to the weak flexor pollicis longus are the brachioradialis and flexor digitorum superficialis. The brachioradialis usually is functional in the spastic upper extremity, but its excursion is not as long as other muscles. Its excursion can be lengthened from 1.5 to 3 cm with complete mobilization of the muscle. The brachioradialis generally is preferred for transfer. If the flexor digitorum superficialis is to be transferred, it must function independently as must the flexor digitorum profundus to the same finger.

▲ *Technique.* Make a curved volar incision over the forearm from about 3 cm proximal to the volar crease, and continue it proximally for 5 to 6 cm. Perform an aponeurotic lengthening of the muscle with one or two cuts in the aponeurosis. After the muscle is lengthened, the interphalangeal joint of the thumb should extend to neutral with the thumb abducted. If the flexor pollicis longus is to be reinforced with the flexor digitorum superficialis, it is obtained through the same incision. It is not necessary to release the tendon from the palm inasmuch as more length is not required. With the wrist flexed maximally, incise the flexor digitorum superficialis transversely as far distally as possible and then transfer it to the flexor pollicis longus, passing it through a buttonhole in the tendon under moderate tension with the thumb and wrist in neutral position.

Another choice for reinforcement of the lengthened flexor pollicis longus is the brachioradialis; however, it is used more frequently to strengthen the abductor pollicis longus after plication. In either transfer the brachioradialis must be mobilized extensively to increase the excursion of the muscle.

◣ *Postoperative management.* After surgery both the hand and wrist should be immobilized in neutral position for 6 weeks, after which active range-of-motion exercises are begun.

Flexor pollicis longus abductor–plasty. This is another method of reducing the spasticity of the flexor pollicis longus muscle and improving its pull. The procedure is technically more demanding, but it seems to be effective.

◣ *Technique (Smith).* Make a radial incision from the middle of the distal phalanx of the thumb to the neck of the first metacarpal. Elevate a volar skin flap, and transect the flexor pollicis longus opposite the proximal phalanx (Fig. 11-26, *A*). Tenodesis of the distal stump of the cut tendon may be performed across the interphalangeal joint to prevent hyperextension

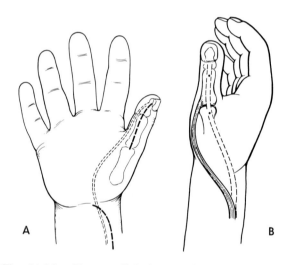

Fig. 11-26 Flexor pollicis longus abductor–plasty. **A,** Medial radial incision on distal phalanx of thumb and second incision over volar aspect of wrist, either longitudinal or slightly curved. **B,** Flexor pollicis longus tendon is passed subcutaneously on radial side of thumb and sutured to base of proximal phalanx of thumb on its radial side. (After Smith RJ: J Hand Surg 7:327, 1982.)

of the joint, or the joint may be fused. In either instance the joint should be placed in 15 degrees of flexion. Make a longitudinal incision in the forearm just radial to the tendon of the flexor carpi radialis, curving ulnarly proximal to the wrist crease. Identify the flexor pollicis longus, and draw its distal end into the wrist wound. Develop a subcutaneous tunnel from the lateral side of the metacarpophalangeal joint of the thumb to the apex of the wrist wound, and pass the distal end of the flexor pollicis longus through this tunnel. With the wrist in neutral position and the thumb in 50 degrees of abduction, suture the transferred tendon to the dorsoradial aspect of the base of the proximal phalanx of the thumb without tension (Fig. 11-26, *B*).

◣ *Postoperative management.* A plaster splint is worn for 6 weeks with the thumb abducted and the wrist slightly flexed if no other procedures have been performed at the same time.

Plication and reinforcement of the abductor pollicis longus muscle. The thumb-in-palm deformity of the spastic hand is a complex deformity that results not only from spasticity and contracture of the muscles that adduct and flex the thumb but also from weakness of the abductor and extensor muscles. These muscles may be strengthened by plication of their tendons or by reinforcing them with tendon transfer, or both.

Plication of the abductor pollicis longus muscle

◣ *Technique.* Approach the abductor pollicis longus tendon through an incision over the tendon itself on the radial side of the distal forearm. Take care to preserve the superficial branch of the radial nerve. The tendon of the abductor usually is composed of multiple slips, and once the adduction and web contractures have been released, the abductor tendons are redundant. Plicate them by transecting and then resuturing with the ends overlapped. Adjust the tension so that the thumb rests in 30 degrees of abduction with the wrist in neutral position.

◣ *Postoperative management.* The thumb is splinted in abduction with the wrist in neutral for 6 weeks, and then range-of-motion exercises are begun.

Reinforcement of abductor pollicis longus muscle

Plication of the abductor pollicis longus muscle alone may not be sufficient to provide active abduction of the thumb because of weakness of the muscle, and reinforcement frequently is necessary. This can be accomplished by transfer of the brachioradialis, the palmaris longus, or flexor digitorum superficialis muscle, or by rerouting the extensor pollicis longus muscle. Which muscle is used depends on what other procedures are to be performed and which muscles are strong and available for transfer.

▶ *Technique.* If the brachioradialis is to be used for reinforcement of the abductor pollicis longus, the incision should be placed slightly more toward the radial side of the forearm and must extend much further proximally to allow full mobilization of the brachioradialis (Fig. 11-27, *A*).

Expose the brachioradialis insertion into the radial styloid, and identify the flexor carpi radialis anterior to the brachioradialis. Protect the radial artery between these two muscles and the superficial branch of the radial nerve beneath the brachioradialis. Mobilize the brachioradialis proximally as completely as possible to obtain sufficient excursion of the muscle; otherwise the muscle transfer will function only as a tenodesis. Dissect the brachioradialis free of the antebrachial fascia, from the extensor carpi radialis longus posteriorly and from the flexor carpi radialis anteriorly. Free the vertical septa because they not only restrict the amplitude of the transferred muscle but also prevent it from following a straight course to its transferred position. Identify and protect the neurovascular supply of the brachioradialis that enters the muscle proximally.

Remove the abductor pollicis longus from the first dorsal compartment, and allow it to slide volarly. Suture the transferred tendon into the abductor pollicis longus through a buttonhole in the tendon, or pass it through the slips of the tendon and suture it to them and then to itself (Fig. 11-27, *B*). Adjust the tension so that with the elbow flexed to 90 degrees and the wrist in neutral the thumb is in 30 degrees of flexion.

If the palmaris longus muscle is to be used for reinforcement of the abductor pollicis longus, detach it from its insertion in the palmar fascia and transfer it to the abductor pollicis longus after that tendon has been removed from the first dorsal compartment. Adjust the tension in a fashion similar to that for transfer of the brachioradialis.

▶ *Postoperative management.* A pressure dressing and cast are applied while the first metacarpal (not phalanx) is held in wide abduction and opposition. At 3 weeks the cast and sutures are removed and a splint is applied to hold the thumb in this same position. Splinting is continued for 4 to 6 weeks; then splinting at night may be used.

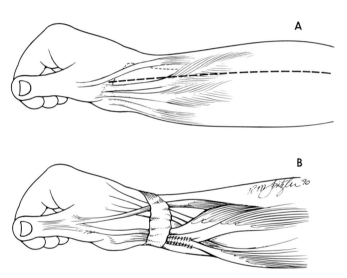

Fig. 11-27   Transfer of brachioradialis to abductor pollicis longus. **A,** Straight incision on radial aspect of forearm from radial styloid, extending proximally for 10 to 12 cm. **B,** Brachioradialis has been mobilized. Abductor pollicis longus has been plicated; brachioradialis is sutured to plicated abductor pollicis longus.

Rerouting of the extensor pollicis longus muscle.
The extensor pollicis longus frequently is functional
in children with spasticity, but it is overpowered by
the spastic flexor pollicis longus, flexor pollicis brevis,
and adductor of the thumb. To test the function of
the extensor pollicis longus the wrist should be
slightly flexed to relax the flexor pollicis longus and
the thumb should be adducted slightly. The extensor
pollicis longus then is tested to determine if it is able
to extend the interphalangeal joint of the thumb. If it
does function, its action can be improved by redirect-
ing its pull toward the radial side of the wrist to help
increase the abduction of the thumb. Moving the extensor pollicis longus to the abductor pollicis longus
will increase the abduction strength of the thumb and
improve its function.

▲ *Technique.* Make a straight dorsoradial incision between the abductor pollicis longus and the extensor
pollicis longus, beginning just distal to the radial styloid and continuing proximally for a distance of 4 cm
(Fig. 11-28, *A*). Take care to preserve the superficial
branch of the radial nerve. Identify and remove the
extensor pollicis longus from the third dorsal compartment. Identify the abductor pollicis longus, but
leave it in its first dorsal compartment. Usually its tendon consists of multiple slips. Cut one or two of
these slips transversely and bring the extensor pollicis longus to lie underneath the cut ends of the abductor pollicis longus. Plicate these cut ends, and suture them overlapped to tighten the tendon (Fig. 11-
28, *B*).

▲ *Postoperative management.* A pressure dressing and
cast are applied while the first metacarpal (not phalanx) is held in wide abduction and opposition. At 3
weeks the cast and sutures are removed. Splinting at
night may be necessary.

***Fusion of the metacarpophalangeal joint of the
thumb.*** Because hyperextension deformity of the
metacarpophalangeal joint of the thumb is common
in spastic cerebral palsy in spite of appropriate releases and transfers, stabilization of the joint is necessary for function of the thumb. This can be accomplished by either arthrodesis or capsulodesis. Joint
fusion can be performed even with open physes
without damage.

▲ *Technique.* Approach the metacarpophalangeal
joint of the thumb through a midlateral ulnar incision, and displace the lateral band dorsally. Incise the
ulnar collateral ligament and the capsule to open the
joint. Remove the articular surfaces of both the proximal phalanx and the metacarpal, taking care not to
injure the physis. Approximate the joint in 5 degrees
of flexion, and hold it in position with crossed
smooth Kirschner wires.

▲ *Postoperative management.* The thumb is immobilized in a plaster cast for 6 weeks or longer until the
arthrodesis is solid, at which time the pins are removed.

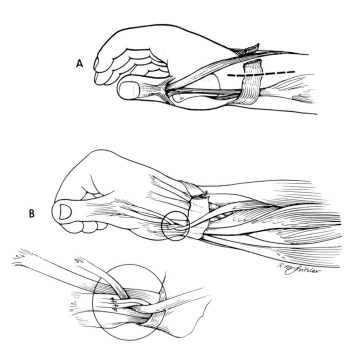

Fig. 11-28   Rerouting of extensor pollicis longus. **A,**
Straight dorsoradial incision between abductor pollicis
longus and extensor pollicis longus. **B,** Extensor pollicis longus is removed from third dorsal compartment. One or two slips of abductor pollicis longus
are cut, and extensor pollicis longus is rerouted between cut slips of abductor pollicis longus, which then
are repaired over top of extensor pollicis longus, forming
sling for extensor pollicis longus.

Capsulodesis of the metacarpophalangeal joint of the thumb

▶ *Technique.* Use a transverse incision parallel to the proximal flexor crease of the thumb. Expose the flexor pollicis longus muscle, and remove a portion of the sheath, including the thickened transverse pulley fibers between the two sesamoid bones. Carefully protect the neurovascular bundles, and retract the tendon to expose the volar plate. Incise this plate at its proximal attachment and along each side, leaving only the strong distal attachment intact (Fig. 11-29, *A*). This can be done easily by making two incisions, one on either side of the volar plate just outside the sesamoid bone, which divides the fibers of the intrinsic muscles that insert into the volar plate. Leave intact the fibers that insert into the extensor wing and base of the proximal phalanx of the thumb. Once the volar plate has been freed, it can be hinged distally.

Place the metacarpophalangeal joint in 30 to 35 degrees of flexion, and insert the proximal margin of the volar plate into a slot in the metacarpal neck. Make two small drill holes through the neck of the metacarpal from volar to dorsal. Pass a suture through the volar plate, and then pass each end of the suture through one of the drill holes exiting the skin on the dorsum of the thumb (Fig. 11-29, *B*). Then pass the suture through a piece of sterile felt and then through a button, and secure it.

▶ *Postoperative management.* The thumb is immobilized in abduction, with the metacarpophalangeal joint flexed 35 degrees, for 8 weeks, at which time the pull-out suture is removed. Active range-of-motion exercises are then begun.

Swan-Neck Deformity

Swan-neck deformity of the digits is relatively common in spastic cerebral palsy because of muscle imbalance combined with ligamentous laxity. The common extensor band becomes short relative to the lateral band as a result of persistent flexion posture of the wrist with constant pull on the central slip from the extensor and the intrinsic muscles. In addition, ligamentous laxity allows severe stretch of the joints. The deformity may be so severe that the proximal interphalangeal joints become subluxated and lock in this extended position. Sublimis tenodesis has been successful in correcting the deformity.

Sublimis tenodesis

▶ *Technique.* Through a midlateral incision expose the flexor sheath at the proximal interphalangeal joint and incise it longitudinally to give access to the flexor tendons. Resect the palmar capsule, the volar plate, the vincula brevae, and the periosteum proximal to the joint. Make two small drill holes approximately 0.6 cm apart through the neck of the proximal phalanx from the palmar to the dorsal side. Connect the two holes on the volar side with a small curet to give a broad exposure of bone for the attachment of the tendon. Then pass a suture through the superficialis tendon, with the proximal interphalangeal joint held in 30 to 40 degrees of flexion (Fig. 11-30); the further distal the suture in the superficialis tendon, the greater the amount of flexion of the proximal interphalangeal joint. Then pass the suture through the two drill holes and out through the skin on the dorsum of the finger. Pass the suture through a piece of sterile felt, and then tie it over a button. Insert a small Kirschner wire across the joint to hold it in about 30 degrees of flexion.

▶ *Postoperative management.* The hand is splinted for 8 weeks, at which time the suture and wire are removed.

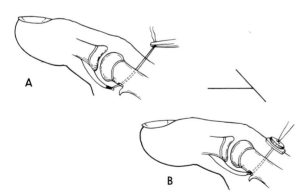

Fig. 11-29 Capsulodesis of metacarpophalangeal joint of thumb. **A,** Volar plate of metaphalangeal joint of thumb is incised transversely at its proximal attachment and then medially and laterally, leaving distal attachment intact. **B,** Thumb metaphalangeal joint is flexed 35 degrees, and metacarpal neck is roughened. Volar plate is pulled into roughened area through drill hole and sutured over button on dorsum of thumb.

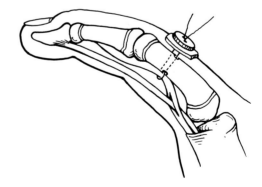

Fig. 11-30 Sublimis tenodesis of superficialis tendon to proximal phalanx after roughening of bone, with tendon attached by means of pull-out suture.

Spine

The incidence of scoliosis in patients with cerebral palsy varies according to the age of the patient and the severity of the neurologic involvement. The child with spasticity is at greater risk of development of scoliosis than are those with other movement disorders. In addition, children with total body involvement are at greatest risk of scoliosis development. Samilson reported that scoliosis occurs in 7% of ambulatory children with spasticity and in 39% of those who are nonambulatory. Madigan and Wallace found that 64% of institutionalized patients had a scoliosis of greater than 10 degrees.

Scoliosis is much more likely to progress in the patient who has cerebral palsy and spastic quadriplegia than in children with adolescent idiopathic scoliosis. The more severe the neurologic involvement the more likely and the more significant the progression of the scoliosis.

Problems that result from scoliosis in patients with cerebral palsy are similar to those in patients with other neurologic diseases. Severe scoliosis may prevent the patient from sitting even if supported, thus limiting the patient's ability to function and making caretaking more difficult. Progression of scoliosis may decrease pulmonary function, increasing the pa-

tient's susceptibility to respiratory infections. Pressure sores are much more likely to occur in patients with severe scoliosis.

Curve Types

The long C-type curve usually associated with neuromuscular scoliosis is seen in the most severely impaired patients with cerebral palsy. According to Madigan and Wallace the most common C curves are the right thoracic curve and the right thoracolumbar curve. The lumbar curves are the least common and usually have an apex to the left. Lumbar curves were found to be less severe and more flexible than other curves. The most common S-curve pattern is the double major, with the thoracic curve usually convex to the right and the lumbar curve convex to the left. The single right thoracic curve is the most severe of all curve types.

Lonstein and Akbarnia described two main curve types in spastic cerebral palsy. Type I is a double major curve with the lumbar and thoracic curves about equal. These curves are either well balanced and compensated, or the thoracic curve is larger, with a fractional and poorly compensated lumbar curve. This type is seen most commonly in patients with mental retardation and in patients who are ambula-

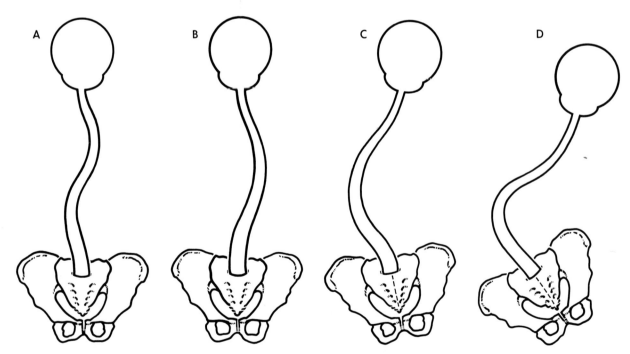

Fig. 11-31 Curve patterns in patients with neuromuscular scoliosis resulting from cerebral palsy. **A** and **B,** Group 1, double curves with thoracic and lumbar components; **C** and **D,** group 2, large lumbar or thoracolumbar curves with marked pelvic obliquity. (Redrawn from Lonstein JE and Akbarnia BA: J Bone Joint Surg 65A:43, 1983.)

tory and live at home. These patients have fewer problems with hip subluxation and dislocation. Type II curves include more severe lumbar or thoracolumbar curves, with marked pelvic obliquity. Many patients with type II curves have a short fractional curve between the end of the curve and the sacrum, and in many the curve continues into the sacrum (Fig. 11-31).

The treatment of scoliosis depends on many factors, including the severity of the curve and the age, functional ability, and intellectual level of the patient. The patient's caregivers are extremely important in assisting the orthopaedic surgeon in deciding on a course of treatment because they know the functional abilities of the patient. Treatment options include observation, bracing and adaptive seating devices to improve sitting posture, and spinal fusion to correct the deformity and stabilize the spine.

Bracing and Adaptive Seating

Bracing helps support the child who is unable to sit because of a severe spinal deformity or collapsing spine. Bracing may slow the progression of the curve, but most curves will continue to worsen. Bunnell and MacEwen reported successful bracing in 48 patients, and several authors have reported success in slowing the progression of curves until spinal growth has matured sufficiently for spinal fusion.

Bracing may consist of a custom-molded plastic orthosis or a custom seat molded to body contours. Various types of seating systems are available. Some are modular and can be modified for the individual needs of each patient. Other systems are constructed from a mold of the patient, allowing the chair to act as a brace to support the child in the appropriate manner. These seating systems increase the pulmonary capacity of the child and free the hands for play or other activities. Custom seating usually can relieve the discomfort of severe scoliosis and allow the child to sit for long periods of time, as well as allow for easier transportation.

Spinal Fusion

Spinal fusion is indicated for progressive scoliosis that may result in deterioration of function. The decision to correct scoliosis surgically in a patient with a severe neuromuscular deformity frequently is difficult. If the patient is functional and able to communicate, the decision may be relatively straightforward. On the other hand, if the child is institutionalized, the decision is more difficult. For children who are aware of their surroundings and respond to those around them, careful consideration should be given to preventing curve progression that would inhibit sitting. Spinal fusion also may be appropriate for a nonambulatory child whose care would be made more difficult by the loss of sitting ability.

Early results of spinal fusion in children with cerebral palsy were not good, with a high incidence of pseudarthrosis after posterior fusion with nonsegmental fixation. Bonnett et al reported more than 50% pseudarthroses in patients with cerebral palsy who underwent spinal fusion with various forms of internal fixation, including Harrington posterior instrumentation and Dwyer anterior instrumentation alone. Other authors also have reported a higher risk of pseudarthrosis with posterior Harrington instrumentation in patients with spasticity. All found that combined anterior and posterior instrumentation and fusion gave better results in these patients (Fig. 11-32).

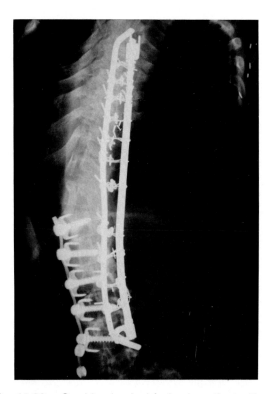

Fig. 11-32 Combined spinal fusion in patient with cerebral palsy by means of both anterior and posterior instrumentation.

Lonstein and Akbarnia reported a 17% overall incidence of pseudarthrosis in patients with cerebral palsy undergoing spinal fusion; however, those with type I curves (balanced double curves) had a much lower incidence of pseudarthrosis than those with type II curves (large unbalanced lumbar and thoracolumbar curves). They also found that patients with type II curves who underwent combined anterior and posterior spinal fusion had a much lower incidence of pseudarthrosis: 5.9% with a combined approach compared with 22% with posterior fusion and instrumentation alone. Thus they recommended that patients with type I curves be treated with a posterior approach alone, but those with type II curves should be treated with combined anterior and posterior fusion.

More recently segmental spinal instrumentation has been used for correction and stabilization of spastic spinal curves. Reports of this technique have indicated a very low incidence of pseudarthrosis. Allen and Ferguson found that the combined anterior and posterior approach was required for some patients but only posterior fusion was needed for others. Gersoff and Renshaw, using the same posterior segmental technique with Luque rods and segmental sublaminar wiring, reported good results with posterior fusion alone. According to Allen and Ferguson the choice of one-stage posterior fusion or two-stage anterior and posterior fusion depends on the correctability of the curve as shown on bending roentgenograms. If the trunk can be aligned over the pelvis on bending roentgenograms, they recommend a one-stage posterior fusion with Luque rods and sublaminar segmental fixation. If compensation of the trunk over the pelvis cannot be obtained on bending roentgenograms, they recommend a two-stage procedure of anterior fusion and release without instrumentation, followed by posterior fusion and instrumentation with Luque rods and sublaminar segmental fixation. They obtained greater than 25% more correction of the scoliosis with the two-stage procedure than with posterior fusion alone. They believe this increased correction is important in patients whose curves cannot be compensated inasmuch as it decreases the strain placed on the instrumentation and leads to an improved rate of arthrodesis (Fig. 11-33).

Sponseller et al reported that segmental fixation by means of Harrington rods and button-wire implants that pass through the base of the spinous process affords excellent correction of the scoliosis and results in an acceptable rate of pseudarthrosis. The advantage of this technique is that the wires used for the segmental fixation do not pass through the spinal canal, thereby reducing the risk of neurologic injury from the passage of the sublaminar wires (Fig. 11-34).

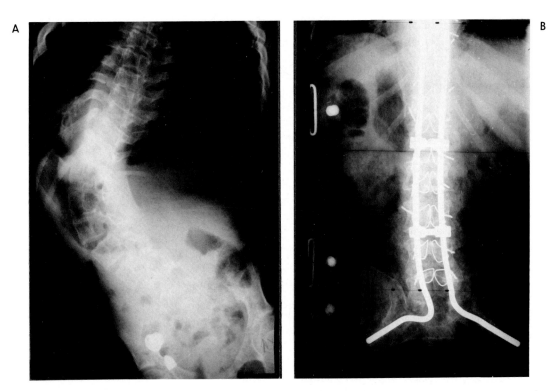

Fig. 11-33 Large thoracolumbar curve in patient with cerebral palsy. **A,** Large group 2 curve with pelvic obliquity. **B,** Postoperative roentgenogram of spine showing sublaminar segmental and Luque-rod instrumentation to pelvis, with rods stabilized by cross-links.

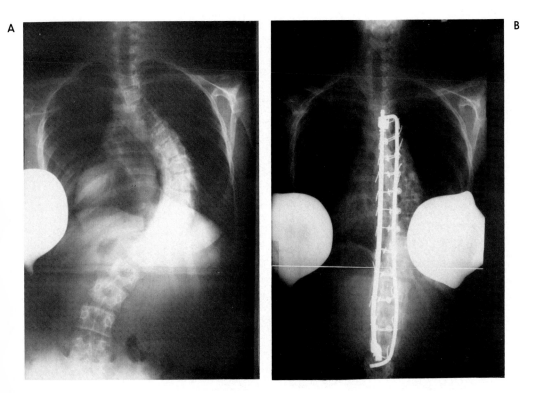

Fig. 11-34 Teenager with severe scoliosis of right side of thorax and cerebral palsy. **A,** Preoperative anteroposterior roentgenogram. **B,** Postoperative anteroposterior view demonstrating significant scoliosis correction and spinal stabilization with intersegmental spinal instrumentation.

The fusion levels depend on the extent and location of the curve. The paralytic curve that is collapsing should be fused throughout the extent of the spine to prevent progression of the deformity above and below the fusion area. Structural scoliosis, on the other hand, does not require fusion of the entire spine. In general the levels appropriate for a nonparalytic curve are selected for the child with cerebral palsy. The exception is the child with pelvic obliquity as a part of the scoliosis. For such children the fusion should extend to the sacrum to prevent progression of the curve below the fusion area and to balance the spine and improve sitting balance. The current method of instrumentation to the sacrum that provides the best security is the Galveston technique of fixation to the pelvis (Fig. 11-33). This technique, when combined with segmental fixation, usually does not require postoperative cast immobilization. Cotrel-Dubousset instrumentation may be used for scoliosis in patients with cerebral palsy; however, there have been no studies documenting its efficacy (Fig. 11-35). The nutritional level of the patient, especially if a

combined anterior and posterior fusion is to be performed, must be considered. Frequently patients with severe neurologic deficits are poorly nourished and much more susceptible to complications. This is especially true if an interval of a week is planned between stages of the fusion. During this time even the neurologically normal person does not consume enough calories to prevent a negative nitrogen balance. Therefore it may be advisable to improve the nutritional level of the patient with parenteral hyperalimentation preoperatively and between the two stages of spinal fusion.

Techniques of spinal fusion using the Luque or Cotrel-Dubousset instrumentation or interspinous segmental spinal instrumentation, as well as the Galveston technique for fixation to the pelvis, are described in Chapter 10. Special considerations for cerebral palsy patients include the use of the larger (0.25 inch) Luque rods for very spastic patients to provide more postoperative control and the occasional need for a postoperative cast or brace in athetoid or very spastic patients.

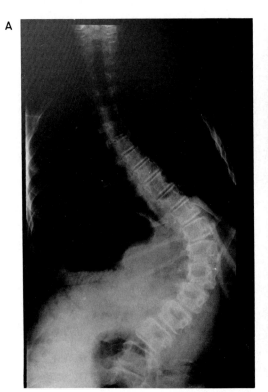 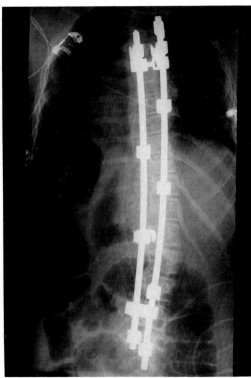

Fig. 11-35 Large thoracolumbar curve on right side in patient with spasticity that was corrected and stabilized by Cotrel-Dubousset instrumentation. Preoperative **(A)** and postoperative **(B)** roentgenograms.

LOWER EXTREMITY
Hip
Adduction Deformity

The adductor muscles originate from the pubis anteriorly and insert on the femur medially. They are innervated by the obturator nerve except for the medial half of the adductor magnus muscle, which may be innervated by the sciatic nerve. The obturator nerve divides into anterior and posterior branches. The anterior branch supplies the adductor longus, the adductor brevis, and the gracilis muscles; the posterior branch supplies the adductor magnus and occasionally a portion of the adductor brevis. These muscles contract at the end of the stance phase of gait to prevent excessive lateral shift of the trunk. In the child with spasticity, however, the adductor muscles may contract during the swing phase of gait, which causes scissoring (crossing over of the swing leg in front of the stance leg) of the lower extremities (Fig. 11-36). The legs thus remain together during stance and cross in front of one another as one leg is raised from the ground to begin the swing phase of gait. When the child walks, adductor spasticity is obvious and is characterized by close approximation of the knees and thighs and a short stride length.

The measurement of adduction contracture is made with the child supine and the pelvis level. Hip abduction is assessed with the hips in both flexion and extension. Scissoring is corrected by lengthening the adductor longus and sometimes the adductor brevis also. The adductor longus may be released percutaneously; however, an open procedure is required if both muscles are to be sectioned.

Hip Subluxation and Dislocation

Untreated adductor contractures may decrease ambulatory ability in those children who are ambulators and may produce hip subluxation and dislocation in nonambulatory patients. Although roentgenographic evidence of hip instability may develop in ambulatory children, it is much more common in the nonambulatory child. Because the adductor muscles are spastic, they adduct the legs, which tends to "uncover" the femoral head (Fig. 11-37). If this is allowed to continue, the acetabulum, which develops along lines of stress, will become dysplastic as a result of abnormal forces (a concentric placement of the femoral head in the acetabulum will stimulate normal acetabular growth). Another factor that contributes to subluxation and dislocation of the hip is the valgus angulation and anteverted posture of the femoral neck. In the newborn femoral anteversion may be as great as 50 to 60 degrees, but in the normal child it decreases with growth to the adult average of 15 degrees. In the child with spasticity this normal derotation of the up-

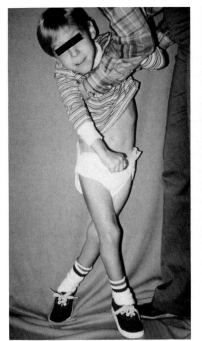 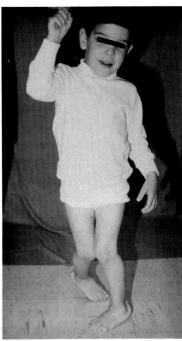

A   B

Fig. 11-36 Two children with adductor spasticity producing scissoring. **A,** Severe spasticity in nonambulatory child who has adduction deformity and severe scissoring. **B,** Ambulatory child with spastic diplegia whose legs scissor during walking. Note crossing of one foot over path of other and position of forward knee in front of and crossed over knee behind.

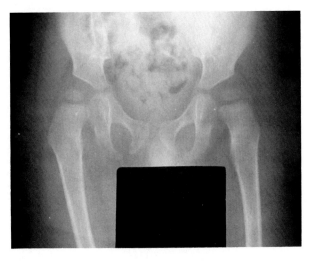

Fig. 11-37 Anteroposterior roentgenogram of hips and pelvis of child with spastic quadriparesis. Shenton's line is broken on right hip, which is dysplastic.

per end of the femur does not occur. The abnormal pull of the iliopsoas muscle that flexes and externally rotates the hip also contributes to hip subluxation. If the iliopsoas muscle is spastic, the hip develops a flexion contracture with a tendency toward external rotation. When this is combined with an anteverted, valgus femoral neck, the acetabulum and the femoral head do not remain in their normal relationship and the acetabulum becomes dysplastic, with subsequent subluxation and possibly dislocation of the hip.

This tendency of the hip to become subluxated and eventually dislocated has been shown to be a progressive change in the femoral head–acetabulum relationship; therefore frequent evaluations with clinical examination and roentgenograms are necessary. Reimers, using the migration percentage, which is defined as the width of the femoral head lateral to Perkins' line divided by the width of that entire femoral head (Fig. 11-38), stated that a stable hip has more than two thirds of the femoral head covered by the acetabulum and a subluxated femoral head has a migration percentage of less than 33%. Sharrard et al defined hip stability in patients with spasticity by comparison with the normal hip that has no break in Shenton's line and in which the head of the femur is completely covered by the acetabulum. According to their classification a dysplastic hip has more than two thirds of the femoral head covered by the acetabulum, there is a break in Shenton's line, and/or there is an abnormality of the roof of the acetabulum as measured on roentgenogram; a subluxated hip is less

than two thirds covered by the acetabulum, and a dislocated hip represents complete loss of contact between the femoral head and the acetabulum.

Because a dislocated hip most likely will become painful, subluxation of the hip should be treated and dislocation should be prevented, even in children who never will ambulate. Even a nonpainful dislocated hip in the nonambulatory child will produce marked limitation of hip abduction, which results in difficulty in perineal care and a marked pelvic obliquity. Hip reduction should be maintained, with no hip dysplasia if possible, even in the nonambulatory child.

Indications for treatment. The techniques for treatment of the spastic hip vary according to the stage and severity of the hip deformity. In the ambulatory child with less than 30 degrees of hip abduction with the hips extended or with scissoring of the legs during gait, or both, an adductor tenotomy is indicated. Usually the adductor longus and brevis muscles are sectioned at their origin, along with the gracilis muscle. Some advocate a neurectomy of the anterior branch of the obturator nerve; however, this procedure usually is not performed. Lengthening of the adductor muscles provided by the tenotomy decreases the stretch reflex and reduces the contracture, enabling the child to walk without scissoring, and increases the length of the stride. Another method of decreasing the stretch reflex of the adductor muscles and reducing the adduction contracture is transfer of the adductor muscles to the ischium. Those who favor this procedure believe that it does not weaken the hip as much as does tenotomy of the adductors. In addition, Root and Spero believe that the transfer to the ischium increases the strength of hip extension, thereby controlling the flexion contracture. Although there was a wave of popularity for this procedure, most authors at this time simply perform tenotomy of the adductors. This procedure is much simpler, and rather than undergoing postoperative immobilization, the children are allowed to return to full ambulation as soon as postoperative pain diminishes.

Indications for surgery on the hip of the nonambulatory child depend on the roentgenographic appearance of the hips. Children with severe spasticity should have frequent roentgenograms to determine the status of the hips. If the migration percentage is greater than 50%, simple adductor surgery alone will not prevent hip subluxation, and proximal femoral osteotomy is indicated. This is especially true because there is less potential for acetabular remodeling in the child older than 4 years. The femoral osteotomy usually is designed to decrease the femoral neck-shaft angle and reduce femoral anteversion.

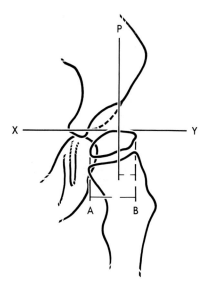

Fig. 11-38 Migration percentage: width of femoral head lateral to Perkins' line divided by the width of the entire femoral head. (Redrawn from Reimers J and Poulsen S: J Pediatr Orthop 4:52, 1984.)

In the child with severe spasticity older than 4 years, there frequently is a variable degree of acetabular dysplasia. Although this abnormality in the contour of the acetabulum has been shown to remodel with treatment, the likelihood of this occurring is small after the age of 5 or 6 years, even with femoral osteotomy and adductor tenotomy. In older children with significant acetabular dysplasia, surgical correction of the acetabular dysplasia at the same time as the femoral osteotomy is indicated. The standard technique for acetabular redirection has been the innominate osteotomy of Salter or triple osteotomy in the older child, as described by Steel (1977). These osteotomies, however, rotate the acetabulum anteriorly to increase the anterior coverage of the femoral head. In the child with neurologic abnormality the acetabular dysplasia usually is the result of deficient posterior coverage of the femoral head. Rotation of the acetabulum anteriorly, especially when combined with derotation of the proximal femur to reduce anteversion, may result in posterior dislocation of the hip in children with posterior deficiency (Fig. 11-39).

The Pemberton osteotomy increases the coverage of the femoral head by the lateral roof of the acetabulum, without decreasing the coverage of the femoral head anteriorly. It also reduces the size of the acetabulum, which usually is large in the child with cerebral palsy. It is therefore the preferred method of increasing the acetabular coverage of the femoral head (Fig. 11-40).

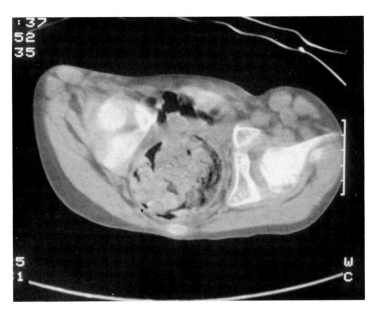

Fig. 11-39 CT scan of hips demonstrates poor acetabular coverage posteriorly. Note posteriorly pointing femoral head; derotational osteotomy likely would produce posterior dislocation of femoral head.

A 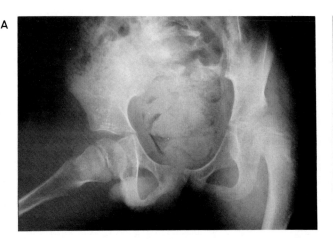 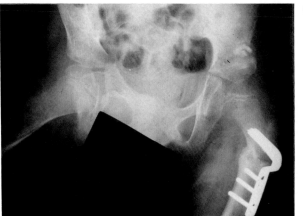 B

Fig. 11-40 Subluxation of left hip in child with spastic quadriparesis. **A,** Anteroposterior roentgenogram of pelvis and hips showing subluxation of left femoral head with marked dysplasia of acetabulum. **B,** Improved coverage of left femoral head after varus osteotomy of proximal femur and Pemberton osteotomy of acetabulum.

The Chiari osteotomy affords coverage of the femoral head in the patient with acetabular dysplasia by increasing the lateral and both anterior and posterior coverage of the femoral head without reducing one or the other inasmuch as the acetabulum is not rotated. Although this osteotomy is effective in "covering" an uncovered femoral head, it is at best a capsular interposition arthroplasty and therefore is best used to "salvage" the hip in the older child. Another procedure that provides coverage of the spastic dysplastic hip is the shelf procedure. These techniques are described in Chapter 2.

Percutaneous adductor longus tenotomy. For the ambulatory child with very mild spastic diplegia, percutaneous adductor longus tenotomy may be performed. These children ambulate well, but scissoring occurs when they walk. The spastic, contracted adductor longus muscle usually is the cause, and tenotomy of this muscle improves gait. Although this technique may be performed as an open surgical procedure, percutaneous tenotomy is easier and results in less postoperative pain with quicker return to normal function.

▶ *Technique.* Exclude the perineum from the operative field with the use of an adhesive drape, but include the pelvis and both hips and legs in the operative field. Flex both hips and abduct them maximally, placing the adductor longus muscles under tension. The tendon is easily palpated because it originates from the pubis. With the hips held flexed to 80 to 90 degrees and maximally abducted, insert a No. 15 knife blade longitudinally next to the tendon of the adductor longus 2 cm distal to the pubis. Then turn the scalpel horizontally with the blade toward the tendon of the adductor longus. This tendon is easily felt and offers resistance to the scalpel. Keeping the tendon under maximum tension with both hips abducted, incise the entire tendon of the adductor longus. As this occurs, the assistant can feel the release of the adduction contracture. Close the small wound with one or two absorbable sutures or with skin strips.

▶ *Postoperative management.* This procedure frequently is performed in conjunction with other operations on the lower extremities such as hamstring and tendo Achilles lengthenings, and the postoperative care depends on the extent of other surgery. Diazepam can be used postoperatively for 1 to 2 days to decrease muscle spasms. These children are mobilized as quickly as possible so that they may return to normal function. Immobilization is not required after adductor tenotomy alone.

Open adductor tenotomy with or without obturator neurectomy. Open tenotomy is indicated if proximal lengthening of the gracilis muscle is required or if the child has moderate or severe contractures and requires more extensive muscle releases. This operation usually is performed in patients with total body involvement.

▶ *Technique.* Make a transverse incision 1.5 to 2 cm distal to the origin of the adductor longus muscle on the pubis (Fig. 11-41, *A*), beginning 1 cm anterior to the tendon of the adductor longus and continuing posteriorly for 3 to 4 cm. Identify and protect the saphenous vein, and incise the deep fascia to expose the tendon of the adductor longus, detectable when the hip is abducted (Fig. 11-41, *B*). Identify the anterior and posterior margins of this tendon, and place a finger around the tendon close to the pubis. Perform this gently to avoid injury to the anterior branch of the obturator nerve that lies posterior to the adductor longus and anterior to the adductor brevis muscle. Once the tendon of the adductor longus muscle is completely freed from the adductor brevis (Fig. 11-41, *C*), section it through the tendinous portion close to its origin, which reduces muscle bleeding. The muscle retracts distally, and hip abduction will increase significantly.

The anterior branch of the obturator nerve may be seen on the muscle belly of the adductor brevis (Fig. 11-41, *D*). The gracilis muscle is a thin but wide muscle that lies subcutaneous and posterior to the adductor longus and extends from the origin of the adductor longus to the ischium. Identify the entire extent of the muscle with blunt dissection both anterior and posterior to the muscle. Because there is very little identifiable tendon, release the muscle from its bony attachment beginning anteriorly on the pubis and continuing posterior to the ischium until it is completely free.

The anterior branch of the obturator nerve now can be easily sectioned if desired (Fig. 11-41, *E*). Even after release of the adductor longus and the gracilis, the hip still may have a significant adduction contracture, especially in the child with total body involvement. In these children a portion of the adductor brevis muscle may be released by sectioning the muscle belly with electrocautery as close to the origin from the pubis as possible (Fig. 11-41, *F*). It usually is not necessary to section all the fibers of the adductor brevis, but only the anterior fibers.

▶ *Postoperative management.* Although the wound is small after release of these muscles, a large dead space is created that will fill with hematoma. A suction drain should be used for 24 to 48 hours until the drainage slows or ceases. No postoperative immobilization, splinting, or bracing is used, and these children are returned to their normal level of function as quickly as possible.

Splinting may benefit children with severe involvement, and nonambulatory children are maintained in an abduction orthosis at night. If there is a tendency toward "windblown" deformity (abduction of one hip with adduction of the other), the pelvis is included in the orthosis.

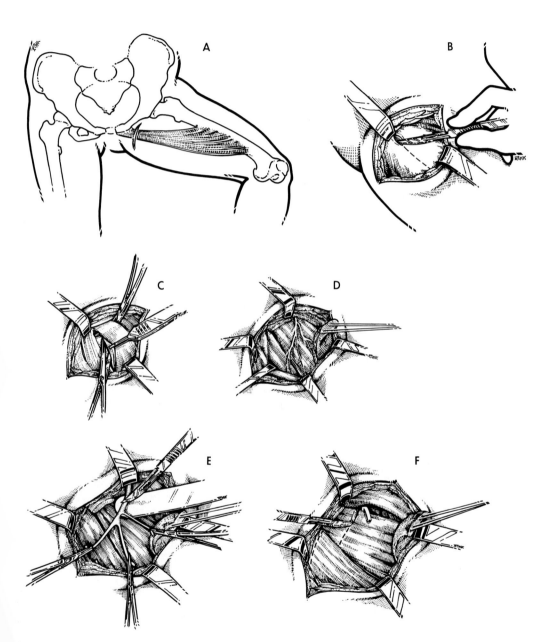

Fig. 11-41 Open adductor tenotomy. **A,** Transverse incision distal to origin of adductor longus. **B,** Fascia is incised longitudinally. **C,** Hemostat is placed around tendon of adductor longus as far proximally as possible; tendon then is sectioned. **D,** Adductor longus muscle is reflected distally exposing anterior branch of obturator nerve. **E,** Anterior branch of obturator nerve may be sectioned if desired. **F,** Adductor brevis muscle is being sectioned; gracilis muscle should be sectioned as well. (Redrawn from Tachdjian MO: Pediatric orthopedics, Philadelphia, 1972, WB Saunders Co.)

Adductor muscle transfer to ischium

▶ *Technique.* Drape both hips and legs in the same manner as for the adductor tenotomy. Make a transverse incision parallel to and 1 to 2 cm distal to the inguinal crease, beginning 1 cm anterior to the adductor longus and continuing posteriorly for 5 to 6 cm. Incise the fascia over the adductor muscles, exposing the muscle bellies and the tendons. Carefully define the interval between the adductor longus and the pectineus muscles, and protect the anterior branch of the obturator nerve. Expose the entire origin of the gracilis from the pubis posteriorly to the ischium. Remove the origins of the adductor longus, adductor brevis, and the gracilis en bloc from the pubic ramus by incising the periosteum of the pubis and stripping the periosteum off the pubis with the muscle attachments in order to provide more tendon to suture to the ischium. Suture this fibrous muscle origin to the anteroinferior aspect of the ischium with heavy nonabsorbable sutures (Fig. 11-42). Close the wound over a suction drain, and apply a bilateral hip spica cast.

▶ *Postoperative management.* The cast is worn for 3 to 6 weeks, and then mobilization of the child is begun. No postoperative splinting is used once the cast has been removed.

Flexion Deformity

In patients with spastic involvement of both lower extremities, flexion deformity of the hip is frequent, usually caused by the psoas muscle. Increased lumbar lordosis is present when the patient is standing, and if hip flexion contracture is greater than the degree compensated by the increased lordosis, the child walks with hips flexed, producing an anterior inclination of the pelvis. The child thus walks with the body tilted forward or in a crouched posture. It must be remembered that the crouched posture of patients with cerebral palsy is due not only to hamstring tightness but also to hip flexion deformity and a calcaneus deformity of the feet (Fig. 11-43).

The amount of hip flexion deformity is tested clinically by the prone measurement as described by Staheli or by the Thomas test, which may be unreliable in the patient with spasticity (see Fig. 11-8). The flexion posture may be estimated by measurement of the sacrofemoral angle on a standing lateral roentgenogram of the lumbar spine that includes the upper femora. A line is drawn along the top of the sacrum to locate the sacral inclination, and a second line is drawn along the shaft of the femur (Fig. 11-44). The angle formed by the intersection of these two lines is the sacrofemoral angle. In normal children and adolescents this angle measures between 50 and 65 degrees. The smaller the angle the worse the hip flexion deformity. Lengthening of the iliopsoas tendon

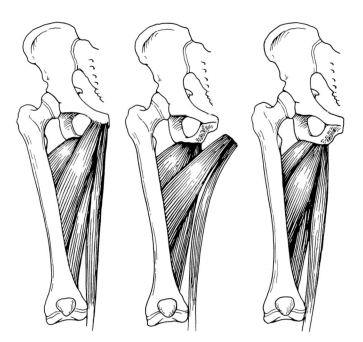

Fig. 11-42 Adductor muscle transfer to ischium. Origins of adductor longus, adductor brevis, and gracilis muscles are exposed through transverse incision distal to pubis. Origins are removed with small amount of periosteum and then transferred to ischium as far posteriorly as possible.

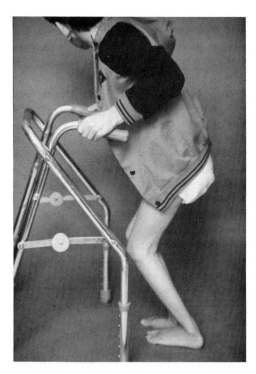

Fig. 11-43 Child with crouched gait; note hip flexion, knee flexion, and calcaneus deformity.

decreases the hip flexion deformity and increases the sacrofemoral angle. The psoas muscle may be lengthened by distal release of the psoas tendon, but this may result in excessive weakness of the psoas. The psoas muscle is important for hip flexion and should be maintained; therefore lengthening of the psoas by either recession or intramuscular lengthening is preferable to complete release in the ambulatory child.

Iliopsoas recession

▶ *Technique.* Position the patient supine, and exclude the perineum with an adhesive transparent drape. Include both hips and legs in the operative field. Make a transverse incision that parallels the inguinal crease, beginning about 1.5 cm distal to the anterosuperior iliac spine and continuing distally and medially for 10 to 15 cm, depending on the size of the patient.

Identify the medial border of the sartorius muscle, and retract it laterally along with the lateral femoral cutaneous nerve. The straight head of the rectus femoris muscle originates from the anteroinferior iliac spine; partially overlying it and medial is the iliacus muscle. Free this from the anterior capsule of the hip. When freeing the iliopsoas from the hip capsule,

flex and externally rotate the hip to relax the iliopsoas muscle. Using a periosteal elevator free the iliacus muscle fibers from the capsule. Pushing a gauze sponge with the elevator facilitates this maneuver. Identify and gently retract the femoral nerve on the anterior surface of the iliacus. Retract the bulky iliacus fibers laterally to expose the broad tendon of the psoas that lies on the anterior capsule of the hip. Remove the sheath and fibrous tissue from the psoas tendon.

Then cut the distal iliacus muscle fibers from lateral to medial in an oblique line as far as the psoas tendon. Incise the tendon close to its insertion on the lesser trochanter, deliver it into the wound, and suture it to the anterior capsule of the hip joint at the base of the femoral neck. Then suture the iliacus fibers over the psoas tendon. Adductor tenotomies may be performed through this same incision. Close the wound over a suction drain (Fig. 11-45).

▶ *Postoperative management.* No cast is applied unless other procedures were performed simultaneously; however, Bleck (1987) recommends that the patient be kept in bed for 3 weeks and not allowed to sit upright. Gentle exercises are performed to maintain hip extension, abduction, and external rotation. Strength in the upper extremities is maintained with regular exercises. At the end of 3 weeks of bed rest, gait training is begun, first in the parallel bars, then with a walker or crutches, and finally independent ambulation if possible.

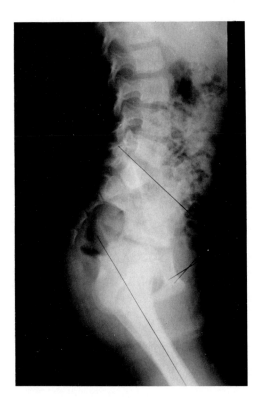

Fig. 11-44 Lateral roentgenogram of spine and femur demonstrating measurement of sacrofemoral angle. Line is drawn parallel to upper border of sacrum, and second line is drawn parallel to shaft of femur; intersection of right angles to these two lines measures sacrofemoral angle.

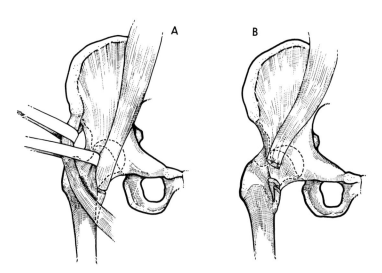

Fig. 11-45 Iliopsoas recession. **A,** Iliopsoas muscle and tendon are freed from attachment to lesser trochanter. **B,** Tendon and muscle then are sutured to anterior aspect of hip capsule. (Redrawn from Bleck EE: Orthopaedic management of cerebral palsy, Philadelphia, 1979, WB Saunders Co.)

Iliopsoas lengthening

▶ *Technique.* Make an incision beginning in the inguinal crease 2 cm medial to the anterosuperior iliac spine and continuing lateral for 4 cm just inferior to the crest of the ilium. Dissect the iliacus muscle free from the hip capsule, and identify the psoas tendon. Protect the femoral nerve. Perform a Z-plasty lengthening of the tendon, and suture the ends.

Intramuscular lengthening of the psoas also may be performed through the same approach. Once the femoral nerve is protected and the psoas tendon is identified on the posterior surface of the iliacus muscle, the muscle fibers of the iliacus muscle are visible extending distally well beyond the proximal extent of the psoas tendon. Intramuscular lengthening of the psoas maintains continuity of the muscle-tendon unit and prevents overlengthening. Retract the muscle belly of the iliacus medially along with the femoral nerve. Maintain the hip in a flexed and externally rotated position to relax the psoas tendon. Invert the iliacus muscle and find the tendon of the psoas muscle, which lies in a sheath on the posterior surface of the iliacus. Make a transverse cut in the tendinous portion of the psoas tendon, being careful to maintain continuity of the iliacus muscle (Fig. 11-46).

▶ *Postoperative management.* After surgery the child is allowed to ambulate and return to normal function as soon as comfort allows.

Iliopsoas tenotomy. Simple release of the psoas tendon at the time of the adductor tenotomy is indicated for the child with total body involvement and hip subluxation who is not going to be an upright ambulator.

▶ *Technique.* Include the hips and legs in the operative field. Make a transverse incision 2 cm distal to the inguinal crease beginning just anterior to the adductor longus tendon and continuing posterior for about 5 cm. Perform the adductor tenotomy, and, with finger dissection, identify the interval between the pectineus and the adductor brevis muscles. Palpate the lesser trochanter in the depths of the wound. Place retractors around the femur, and then identify the psoas tendon by removing the connective tissue that envelops the tendon. Pass a right-angle clamp around the tendon adjacent to the lesser trochanter, and divide the tendon.

▶ *Postoperative management.* Postoperative care is the same as for other surgical procedures on the adductor and psoas muscles.

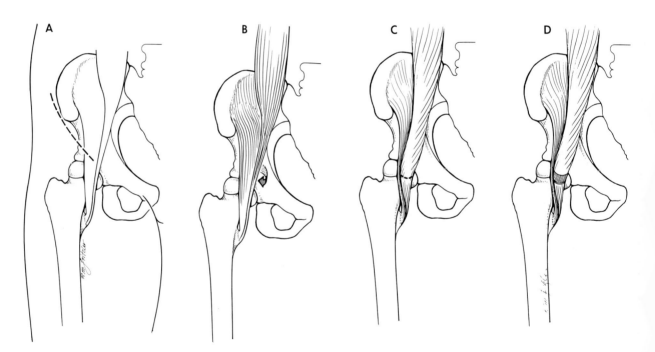

Fig. 11-46 Iliopsoas lengthening. **A,** Anterior incision lateral to anterosuperior iliac spine and along inguinal crease. **B,** Tendon of psoas muscle is identified on posterior surface of iliacus muscle. This is accomplished by elevation of iliacus muscle. To do this, hip must be flexed as much as possible and placed in external rotation. Iliacus muscle may then be elevated and externally rotated itself, revealing psoas tendon on undersurface of iliacus. **C,** Tendon of psoas is cut well proximal to musculotendinous junction. Location of this incision is identified by dotted line on psoas tendon. Note that iliacus muscle has been inverted to reveal psoas tendon on posterior surface. **D,** Tendon of psoas muscle has been cut and the tendon ends separated by about 1 to 1½ cm, but muscle tendon unit remains in continuity.

Proximal femoral osteotomy. The primary indication for proximal femoral varus osteotomy is subluxation of the hip or progressive hip dysplasia after adductor tenotomy and psoas lengthening. This is especially true in the child older than 4 years of age.

The technique of proximal femoral osteotomy is described elsewhere (Chapter 1). There are, however, some pertinent technical details unique to the child with spasticity. Because the child with spasticity has more valgus of the femoral neck than the child with normal neurologic function, more reduction in the femoral neck-shaft angle is necessary. In addition, because of the muscle imbalance, the valgus deformity of the proximal femur tends to recur if there is sufficient time for remodeling after osteotomy. Thus a greater varus inclination in the femoral neck-shaft angle than normal is required.

The neck-shaft angle obtained by osteotomy depends on the neurologic status of the child. If the child is an ambulator, then to avoid excessive weakening of the hip abductor muscles, which will lead to a Trendelenburg gait, the femoral neck-shaft angle should not be reduced to less than 115 degrees. An osteotomy in the nonambulatory child does not carry this risk, and a more varus femoral neck-shaft angle may be produced. Frequently, derotation of the femur is needed to reduce femoral anteversion, and this may be performed at the same time as the varus osteotomy.

Internal fixation of the osteotomy is mandatory to maintain correction. A spica cast should be used postoperatively to prevent loss of the correction in the child with spasticity (Fig. 11-47).

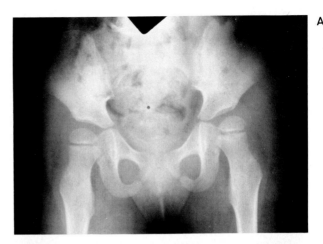

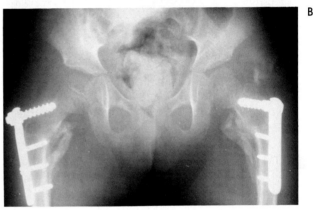

Fig. 11-47 Patient with spastic quadriparesis. **A,** Anteroposterior view of pelvis and hips demonstrating increasing migration percentage and valgus femoral neck. **B,** Reduction of femoral neck-shaft angle after proximal femoral osteotomy, adductor tenotomy, and psoas lengthening.

Acetabular Dysplasia

In long-standing hip subluxation the acetabulum becomes dysplastic because of the incongruous reduction of the femoral head. The acetabulum may remodel after redirection of the femoral head if sufficient growth remains. After varus derotational osteotomy in the child younger than 5 years, 1 to 2 years may be allowed for correction of the acetabular dysplasia; in children older than 5 or 6 years, correction of the acetabular dysplasia is indicated.

The Salter innominate osteotomy (Chapter 2) is not recommended for correction of acetabular dysplasia in children with spasticity because it increases the posterior deficiency. The Pemberton osteotomy (Chapter 2) is preferred (see Fig. 11-40) because it does not reduce the amount of posterior acetabular coverage. Because it hinges the acetabulum at the triradiate cartilage rather than at the symphysis pubis, the Pemberton osteotomy can be performed only in the young child with an open triradiate cartilage.

In the child older than 9 years the triple innominate described by Steel (1977) (Chapter 2) can be used. This rotates the acetabulum anteriorly and may decrease posterior coverage of the femoral head. Rotating the acetabulum only laterally and not anteriorly will avoid this. Procedures that do not depend on acetabular rotation include the Chiari osteotomy (Chapter 2) and the "shelf" procedure (Fig. 11-48) (Chapter 2). These two procedures increase the size of the acetabulum without decreasing the posterior acetabular coverage as do the rotational osteotomies. The major objection to these surgical procedures is that bone without cartilage is placed over the femoral head. Both leave the capsule of the hip joint as an interposition, but a normal articular surface is not created.

For painful, severe hip dysplasia in adolescents and young adults the choice of treatment depends on the severity of the dysplasia and the functional status of the patient and may include proximal femoral resection, hip fusion, or total hip replacement. Hip fusion relieves pain but, if the hip is flexed enough to allow sitting, severely limits the ability to lie supine. It rarely is indicated. Total hip replacement is appropriate only for the ambulatory adult with mild neurologic involvement and severe degenerative hip disease. Proximal femoral resection has been associated with recurrence of deformities, stiffness, and periarticular ossification. Castle and Schneider reported that resection of the proximal femur with muscle interposition is more successful than simple resection of the femoral head and neck. This procedure is indicated for the patient with a painful hip who has very severe involvement that cannot be improved by osteotomy and for the patient with a dislocated hip that is either painful or produces difficulty in sitting.

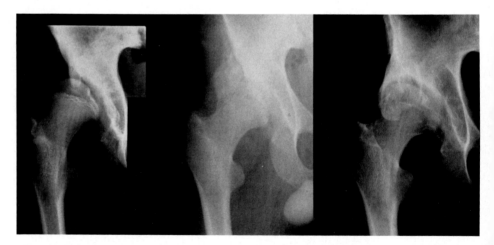

Fig. 11-48 Shelf procedure to increase coverage of very dysplastic hip in child with spasticity. (Courtesy Dr. Lynn Staheli.)

Hip Dislocation

Dislocation of the hip is most common in the child with total body involvement. Prevention of the dislocation is the best treatment but is not always possible. The choice of treatment depends on the age, function, and intellectual status of the patient. Open reduction combined with femoral shortening (Chapter 2) is appropriate in children younger than 6 years to prevent painful, severely contracted hips later in life. The treatment of the dislocated hip in the older child depends on the symptoms. If the child is symptom-free, no treatment is necessary. If the hip becomes painful, then resection of the proximal femur probably is the best procedure.

Proximal femoral resection—interposition arthroplasty

▶ *Technique.* Position the patient supine with a sandbag under the hip. Make a straight lateral incision beginning 10 cm proximal to the greater trochanter and extending distally along the shaft of the femur to provide sufficient exposure of the proximal femur (Fig. 11-49, *A*). Split the fascia lata, and detach the vastus lateralis and the gluteus maximus muscles from their insertions on the femur. Also detach the gluteus medius and minimus from their attachment on the greater trochanter. Then detach the rectus femoris and sartorius muscles from the anteroinferior and superior iliac spines, and cut the tensor fasciae latae muscle transversely. Expose the femur extraperiosteally, and incise the periosteum circumferentially just distal to the gluteus maximus insertion. Cut the bone transversely at this level, leaving the lesser and greater trochanters as part of the proximal fragment. Cut the iliopsoas tendon from its attachment on the lesser trochanter. Divide the short external rotators

of the hip, and cut the hip capsule circumferentially. Cut the ligamentum teres, and remove the proximal end of the femur.

Cover the acetabulum by oversewing the edges of the hip capsule. Suture the vastus lateralis and the rectus femoris over the proximal end of the femur. Suture the gluteal muscles to the depths of the acetabulum so that they are interposed between the cut end of the femur and the acetabulum. Close the wound over suction drainage (Fig. 11-49, *B* and *C*).

▶ *Postoperative management.* The patient is placed in split Russell's traction until comfortable and then in a cast or brace to limit hip adduction while the soft tissues heal. Postoperative skeletal traction is not necessary.

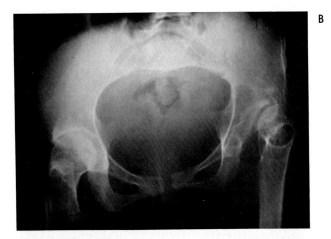

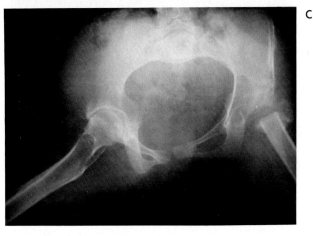

Fig. 11-49 Proximal femoral resertion—interposition arthroplasty. **A,** Incision for lateral approach to hip. **B,** Pelvis and hips of patient with painful dysplastic left hip. **C,** After resection of proximal femur; note level of resection well below lesser trochanter and formation of heterotopic ossification.

Extension and Abduction Contracture of the Hip

Extension-abduction contracture of the hip most commonly occurs after release of the adductors and flexors of the hips and neurectomy of the obturator nerve in patients with rigidity and severe spasticity of the hip extensors and abductors. It also may occur in patients with athetosis after release of the hip flexor and adductor muscles. Treatment depends on the severity of the deformity. For mild contractures, simple positioning of the patient usually allows sitting. With very severe deformity, sitting is not possible, and, if the hips are rigidly positioned in extension, anterior dislocation may occur. Severe deformity requires release of all tight structures, most commonly the hamstrings, and in more severe contractures the gluteus maximus insertion into both the iliotibial band and the femur also must be released. The external rotators of the hip and the hip capsule may have to be cut to correct the deformity. For the most severe contractures, femoral shortening must be performed to reduce the stretch on the sciatic nerve.

◤ *Technique.* Position the patient in the lateral decubitus position, and exclude the perineum from the operative field. Include the entire hip, flank, and leg in the operative field. Make a straight incision 1 to 1.5 cm posterior to the greater trochanter, beginning 2 to 3 cm proximal to the tip of the greater trochanter and continuing distally for at least 6 cm (Fig. 11-50). The length of the incision is determined by the necessity of a femoral shortening. Identify the superior border of the gluteus maximus, and isolate it from the gluteus medius. Release the insertion of the gluteus maximus first from the iliotibial tract and then from the posterior femur (Fig. 11-50). Then retract this muscle medially, exposing the sciatic nerve, which must be protected. Identify the piriformis and the gluteus medius muscles, and release completely their insertion on the greater trochanter. The gluteus minimus, which lies below the gluteus medius, usually requires release as well. If the obturator internus and the gemelli muscles are tight, release them also. Carefully retract the sciatic nerve laterally, and identify the origin of the hamstring muscles. Release these as described in the technique for proximal hamstring lengthening (p. 659).

Once all the muscles have been released, the hip should flex and adduct. While flexing the hip, carefully observe the sciatic nerve for tension. If it is tight and prevents hip flexion, shorten the femur. To resect a portion of the femur, extend the incision distally to expose the subtrochanteric portion of the femur at least 6 cm below the greater trochanter. Expose the femur subperiosteally, and perform an osteotomy sufficiently distal to the greater trochanter to allow application of a 4- or 6-hole plate to secure the osteotomy. Remove sufficient bone so that the hip may be flexed without tension on the sciatic nerve.

Repeat the procedure on the opposite hip, and apply a hip spica cast with the hips flexed to at least 60 degrees and 30 degrees of abduction of each hip.

◤ *Postoperative management.* The cast is worn for 6 to 8 weeks until the femoral osteotomy has united. Postoperative bracing usually is unnecessary.

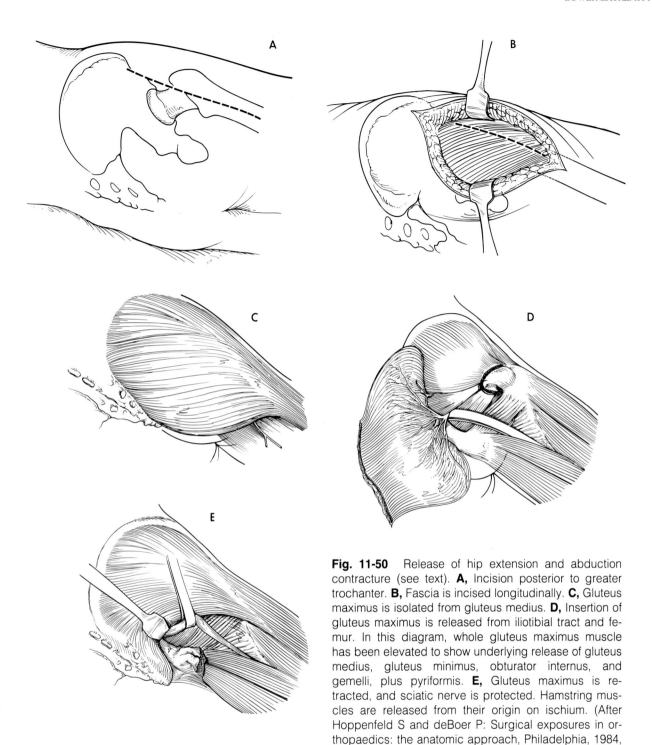

Fig. 11-50 Release of hip extension and abduction contracture (see text). **A,** Incision posterior to greater trochanter. **B,** Fascia is incised longitudinally. **C,** Gluteus maximus is isolated from gluteus medius. **D,** Insertion of gluteus maximus is released from iliotibial tract and femur. In this diagram, whole gluteus maximus muscle has been elevated to show underlying release of gluteus medius, gluteus minimus, obturator internus, and gemelli, plus pyriformis. **E,** Gluteus maximus is retracted, and sciatic nerve is protected. Hamstring muscles are released from their origin on ischium. (After Hoppenfeld S and deBoer P: Surgical exposures in orthopaedics: the anatomic approach, Philadelphia, 1984, JB Lippincott Co.)

In-Toed Gait

Children with cerebral palsy are born with a normal amount of femoral anteversion (average, 35 to 40 degrees), but in the child with spasticity this femoral anteversion does not decrease with growth as in the normal child. This persistent femoral anteversion causes children with spastic diplegia and quadriplegia to walk with an in-toed gait (Fig. 11-51). Although several procedures have been described to reduce the in-toeing, the mainstay of treatment is derotational osteotomy of the femur. Neither adductor tenotomy nor iliopsoas lengthening significantly reduces the amount of in-toeing, although Bleck (1987) reported that iliopsoas recession resulted in a decrease in in-toeing over 3 to 5 years and reduced the need for derotational osteotomy. Semitendinosus muscle

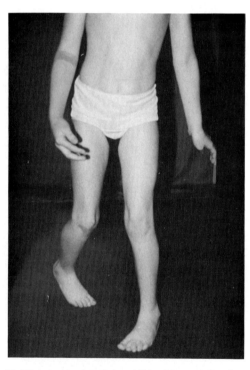

Fig. 11-51 In-toed gait in child with spastic diplegia. Note that legs internally rotate from hip down because of femoral anteversion.

transfer to the lateral aspect of the femur has not produced predictable results. Steel (1977) described transfer of the insertion of the gluteus medius and minimus muscles to decrease in-toeing, but he noted that the procedure may produce a Trendelenburg gait in some patients, especially if the transfer is not secure.

Femoral derotational osteotomy, either proximal or distal, will decrease the in-toed gait. The proximal osteotomy is a more extensive operation that requires internal fixation and a postoperative hip spica cast. Supracondylar femoral osteotomy produces the desired amount of derotation with a less extensive surgical procedure. Implant fixation is unnecessary with the supracondylar osteotomy; a cylinder cast that incorporates pins above and below the osteotomy is all that is required. If varus correction of the proximal femur is desired, femoral anteversion also may be corrected with the proximal osteotomy. If only femoral derotation is desired, then osteotomy in the supracondylar region of the femur is preferable.

Advancement of insertion of gluteus medius and minimus

▶ *Technique.* Position the patient supine on the operating table, and include the flank, hip, and lower extremity in the operative field. Abduct the leg to relax the fascia lata and facilitate the approach to the gluteus medius and minimus muscles.

Begin the incision at the junction of the anterior border of the gluteus maximus and the posterior border of the gluteus medius. Extend it far enough superiorly to allow exposure of the distal muscle bellies of the gluteus medius and minimus and their tendons. Then curve the incision anteriorly to the greater trochanter and then posteriorly and distally to the posterior margin of the femur 5 cm distal to the greater trochanter (Fig. 11-52, *A*). Incise the fascia lata overlying the gluteus medius and minimus in the bloodless interval between the gluteus maximus and the tensor fasciae latae. Then continue this fascial incision distally along the shaft of the femur to 5 cm below the greater trochanter. The fascia lata remains lax if the hip is kept abducted, allowing it to be retracted anteriorly along with the tensor fasciae latae muscle.

Also retract the fascia lata posteriorly to expose the posterior margin of the greater trochanter. Expose the gluteus medius and minimus muscles by retracting the fascia lata, and free them for mobilization. Free the gluteus minimus from the hip capsule so that both muscles may be transposed as a single unit.

With an osteotome, excise the conjoined tendon of these muscles along with a piece of bone from the greater trochanter distal to the physis (Fig. 11-52, *B*). Expose the origin of the vastus intermedius, just distal to the intertrochanteric line anteriorly on the femur, and reflect it far enough distally to allow the transferred bony insertion of the gluteal muscles to be reattached anterior to the greater trochanter. Roughen the surface of the femur underlying the vastus intermedius (Fig. 11-52, *C*). Establish the maximum range of hip abduction and external rotation, and position the hip at 10 degrees less than these two measurements. Attach the bony attachment of the gluteus medius and minimus to the roughened surface of the femur under maximum tension, and hold it in place with crossed pins, a staple, or a screw (Fig. 11-52, *D*). Secure the origin of the vastus intermedius over the transferred gluteal muscles. Repair the fascia lata, and close the wound in layers over a suction drain. Apply a 1½ hip spica cast that includes the foot on the operated leg. This cast is worn for 6 weeks.

Derotational proximal femoral osteotomy. This procedure is performed in the same manner as a varus derotation femoral osteotomy (p. 146), including external rotation of the distal femoral fragment. It is not necessary to measure the exact amount of femoral anteversion roentgengraphically inasmuch as the goal is simply to reduce the amount of in-toeing. Thus the amount of excessive internal rotation is determined clinically, and the distal fragment of the femur is externally rotated enough to allow the foot to be directed straight ahead or in 5 to 10 degrees of external rotation during gait.

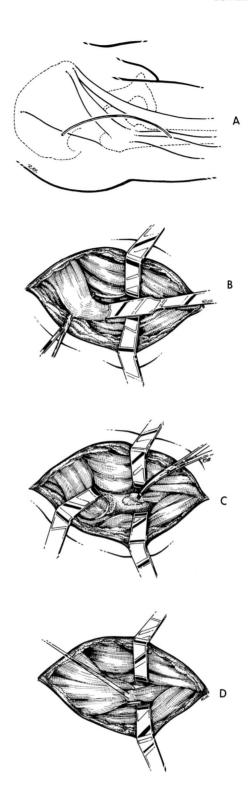

Fig. 11-52 Advancement of gluteus medius (see text). **A,** Incision. **B,** Gluteus medius and minimus muscles are freed. Conjoined tendon of these muscles is detached with small piece of bone. **C,** Surface of femur anterior and distal to original insertion is exposed. **D,** Conjoined tendon is then reattached to femur in new position. (Redrawn from Steel HH: J Bone Joint Surg 62A:919, 1980.)

Supracondylar derotational osteotomy of the femur

▶ *Technique.* Place the patient supine, and include the entirety of the hip and lower extremity in the operative field. Approach the distal femur through a longitudinal midlateral incision beginning at the level of the superior pole of the patella and continuing proximally for 5 cm (Fig. 11-53). Split the fascia lata longitudinally, and expose the femur subperiosteally. Determine the level of the osteotomy and mark the femur, being certain the osteotomy is above the superior pole of the patella to avoid producing an irregular gliding surface for the patella. Using an oscillating saw, perform a transverse osteotomy three fourths of the way through the femur. Then insert two large (4 or 5 mm) Steinmann pins in the lateral surface of the proximal fragment of the femur, with the femur rotated directly anteriorly (the patella should point anteriorly). Insert these two pins parallel to each other. Then insert two parallel pins distal to the osteotomy at an angle to the proximal pins equal to the desired amount of derotation of the femur. Complete the osteotomy, and externally rotate the distal fragment of the femur so that the four pins become parallel. An external fixation device may be applied to secure the osteotomy. Once the osteotomy is stabilized, assess the rotation of the leg to be certain that the desired amount of correction has been obtained. Close the wound over a suction drain. Apply a cylinder cast that incorporates the four pins, and remove the external fixation device if used (Fig. 11-54).

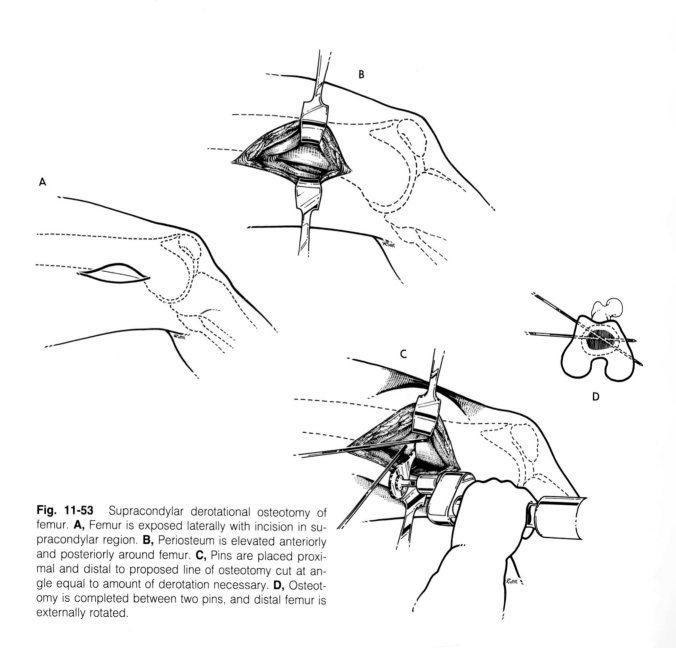

Fig. 11-53 Supracondylar derotational osteotomy of femur. **A,** Femur is exposed laterally with incision in supracondylar region. **B,** Periosteum is elevated anteriorly and posteriorly around femur. **C,** Pins are placed proximal and distal to proposed line of osteotomy cut at angle equal to amount of derotation necessary. **D,** Osteotomy is completed between two pins, and distal femur is externally rotated.

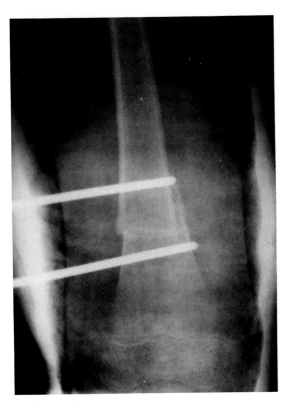

Fig. 11-54 Supracondylar osteotomy of femur secured with one or two pins above and below osteotomy.

▶ *Postoperative management.* The child is kept non-weight bearing for 4 to 6 weeks, at which time the osteotomy usually is sufficiently healed to permit removal of the pins. A new cylinder cast is applied, and ambulation is begun. This cast is worn for approximately 4 more weeks or until there is adequate healing of the osteotomy to allow unprotected weight bearing.

Crouched Gait

The most common causes of a crouched gait are hamstring contracture and spasticity, but other causes also may be implicated. Hip flexion deformity may be the cause of the crouched posture. If a hip flexion contracture exceeds the ability to compensate by increasing lumbar lordosis, the child must bend forward at the hips or walk with the hips and knees flexed (see Fig. 11-43). Another cause of the crouched gait is a calcaneus deformity, which forces the child to stand on the heels when the knees are extended. The feet may be kept flat on the floor only by flexing the knees, which accommodates the calcaneus deformity but produces a crouched gait. The most common cause of this calcaneus deformity is not overlengthening of the heel cord but rather neglecting to lengthen the hamstrings along with tendo Achilles when indicated. In this instance the hamstring contracture forces the child to walk with the knees flexed, but tendo Achilles lengthening causes the feet to remain flat on the floor, which results in further crouching.

It is therefore important to accurately evaluate the child with a crouched gait to determine the exact cause. Frequently more than one cause exists. Treatment depends on the deformities that are present. Correction may be required at the level of the hip, knee, and ankle. Hip flexion deformity is discussed on p. 648. Hamstring contracture and calcaneus deformity are discussed here.

Hamstring lengthening. Because the hamstring muscles originate from the ischium and then insert on the proximal portion of the tibia, crossing the hip and knee, hamstring contracture may produce deformity of both joints. Contracture of the hamstring muscles produces extension of the pelvis, resulting in a decrease in the normal lumbar lordosis, loss of knee extension, and decreased stride length.

Any child for whom tendo Achilles lengthening is planned should be carefully assessed for hamstring spasticity. If there is limited knee extension with the hips flexed to 90 degrees, the hamstring muscles should be lengthened simultaneously with the tendo Achilles.

Various procedures have been described for the correction of hamstring overactivity; however, not all are described here because their effectiveness has not been proved. Tenotomy of the hamstrings results in knee hyperextension, and the Eggers transfer of the hamstrings to the femur has been reported to increase the risk of knee hyperextension deformity; neither procedure is recommended. Lengthening of the hamstring muscles either proximally or distally is the most common procedure.

Proximal hamstring lengthening has been reported to be effective without development of knee extension deformity, as may occur after distal hamstring lengthening. Knee extension deformity after distal hamstring lengthening usually is caused by hamstring tenotomy or failure to lengthen the tendo Achilles when indicated. Failure to lengthen a tight tendo Achilles causes hyperextension of the knee during the stance phase of gait as a result of the equinus posture of the foot. Drummond et al found marked increase in lumbar lordosis after proximal hamstring release and no longer recommend the procedure. Distal hamstring lengthening is the procedure of choice, but occasionally release of the hamstring muscles proximally is appropriate in a nonambulatory child who has difficulty sitting because of extension of the pelvis or in the child with extension and abduction contracture of the hip.

Proximal hamstring release

▶ *Technique*. Position the patient supine with a sandbag or folded towels under the sacrum. Drape the buttocks, the hips, and both lower extremities free. Exclude the perineum with an adhesive drape. Make a 7- to 10-cm transverse incision in the subgluteal crease (Fig. 11-55, *A*), with the hip and knee both flexed to 90 degrees. Identify the gluteus maximus, and retract it laterally. Take care not to injure the sciatic nerve beneath the muscle, and gently retract it laterally. Identify the origin of the hamstring muscles on the ischium and 2 cm distally. Place a finger around this muscle mass, and section with electrocautery (Fig. 11-50, *E,* and 11-55, *B*). It is not always necessary to release the entire muscle mass of the hamstrings; only a portion of the origin is released if sufficient release of the muscle tightness can be accomplished. Once the muscle is released, knee extension should be 45 degrees or less. Close the wound over a suction drain.

▶ *Postoperative management*. Sharps et al recommend bilateral long-leg casts after surgery, with the patient alternating between sitting with the hips flexed and reclining. Residual knee flexion contracture is corrected with repeated cast changes.

Fractional lengthening of the hamstrings distally

▶ *Technique*. This procedure may be performed with the patient prone or supine. It is technically easier with the patient prone, but because as other procedures often are performed concurrently, the patient usually is placed supine.

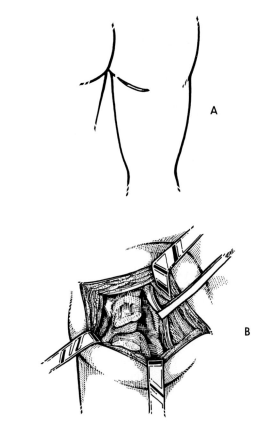

Fig. 11-55 Proximal hamstring release (see text). (Redrawn from Drummond DS, Rogala E, and Templeton J: J Bone Joint Surg 56A:1598, 1974.)

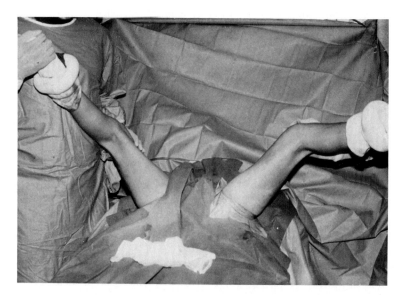

Fig. 11-56 Patient positioned supine for distal hamstring lengthenings; hips are abducted and externally rotated flexed maximally. Surgeon stands between patient's abducted leg and operating table. Note that assistant holds patient's leg in this position.

With the patient supine, prepare and drape both hips, groin, and the lower extremities. Do not use a tourniquet. If adductor tenotomy is planned, perform it first to allow sufficient hip abduction. Flex the hip to more than 90 degrees, and have an assistant hold the leg. Abduct the hip maximally, and extend the knee maximally (Fig. 11-56).

Make an 8 to 10 cm incision in the midline posteriorly beginning approximately 3 to 4 cm proximal to the popliteal crease (Fig. 11-57, *A*). Divide the subcutaneous tissue and the deep fascia. Reflect the subcutaneous tissue from the fascia medially to expose the medial hamstrings. The semitendinosus muscle is the most medial and has the thinnest tendon. Its muscle belly does not extend as far distally as the other hamstring muscles. The semimembranosus is just medial to the semitendinosus and has a broad tendon that envelops its muscle belly, which extends far distally. The most medial tendon is the gracilis. Divide the fascia overlying these muscles, and expose the muscles completely (Fig. 11-57, *B*). It is very important to expose each muscle from the medial to lateral extent to perform a complete fractional lengthening (Fig. 11-57, *C*). Identify the semitendinosus muscle belly at the proximal extent of the wound, and make one or two transverse incisions, approximately 1 to 2 cm apart, in the aponeurosis overlying the muscle. These cuts must go from the medial to lateral extent of the aponeurosis to allow for separation of the tendon ends. Make the cuts all the way through the very thin aponeurosis, but do not cut into the muscle belly (Fig. 11-57, *D*). Extend the knee to separate the incisions in the aponeurosis. If the musculotendinosus junction of the semitendinosus is too far proximal to reach, a Z-plasty lengthening may be performed.

Next identify the semimembranosus just medial to the semitendinosus, outlining it completely from the medial to the lateral extent of the muscle. Make one or two cuts, 1 to 2 cm apart, in the aponeurosis of the muscle, but do not go through the underlying muscle fibers. Again gently extend the knee to separate the cuts in the aponeurosis. Finally identify the gracilis muscle medial to the semitendinosus muscle if this muscle has not been lengthened proximally. Perform a fractional lengthening in the same manner by making two cuts in the aponeurosis of the muscle.

Next dissect the subcutaneous tissue away from the lateral fascia to expose the underlying biceps femoris muscle. Do not disturb the neurovascular bundle lying between the medial and lateral hamstrings. Identify the biceps from medial to lateral extent. Take care not to injure the peroneal nerve. Make two transverse incisions 1 to 2 cm apart in the aponeurosis of the biceps muscle, and gently extend the knee. Close the wounds (drainage usually is not re-

quired), and apply cylinder casts with the knees in neutral extension if this is the only procedure that has been performed. Long-leg casts will be required if tendo Achilles lengthening also has been performed.

▶ *Postoperative management.* As soon as the patient is comfortable, ambulation is allowed with crutches or walker if required. The casts are bivalved in 2 to 3 weeks and worn at night for 2 to 6 months. The length of splinting depends on the amount of preoperative contracture and the propensity for recurrence of the contracture.

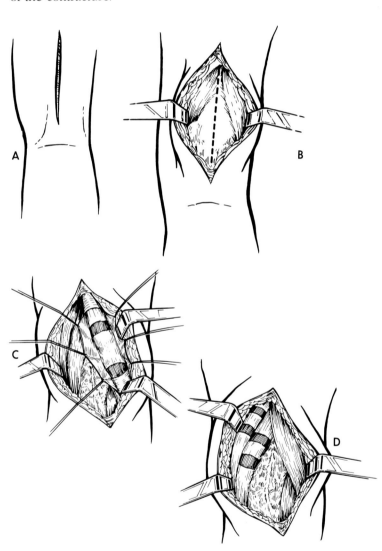

Fig. 11-57 Fractional lengthening of hamstring muscles distally. **A,** Incision proximal to popliteal crease on posterior surface of thigh. **B,** Fascia is incised longitudinally, exposing medial and lateral hamstrings. **C,** Biceps femoris muscle is identified; fractional lengthening of muscle is performed by cutting fascia proximal to musculotendinous junction but leaving muscle fibers intact. **D,** Same procedure is performed on semitendinosus, semimembranosus, and gracilis muscles.

Stiff-Legged Gait

A stiff-legged gait is less common than a crouched gait but may be seen in ambulatory patients with spastic diplegia and spastic quadriplegia. Children with a stiff-legged gait show a relative loss of sagittal plane knee motion (flexion), which interferes with foot clearance during the swing phase of gait. It has been shown that frequently both the hamstrings and the quadriceps are spastic at the midswing phase. In the spastic gait the rectus femoris muscle assumes the role of a primary hip flexor, contracting during the swing phase of gait, which keeps the knee extended. As a result the foot does not clear the floor during swing but drags as the leg moves forward. Spasticity of the rectus femoris muscle usually accompanies hamstring tightness. Simple lengthening of the hamstrings alone will allow more knee extension during stance but will not increase knee flexion during swing. Proximal release of the rectus femoris does not improve knee flexion. Both Gage et al and Perry recommend release of the rectus femoris distally and transfer of the tendon posterior to the knee axis to allow knee extension in stance and preserve or augment knee flexion in swing. They also recommend transfer of the tendon to the sartorius muscle in children with an internal rotation gait and to the iliotibial band in patients with an external rotation gait.

Distal release or transfer of rectus femoris muscle

▲ *Technique.* Make a 4-cm transverse incision 4 cm proximal to the superior pole of the patella (Fig. 11-58, *A*). Make the incision toward the anteromedial aspect of the distal thigh if the rectus tendon is to be transferred to the sartorius and on the anterolateral side of the anterior distal thigh if transfer is to the iliotibial band. Isolate the rectus femoris tendon at its point of insertion into the quadriceps tendon. The tendon of the rectus frequently is partially covered with muscle fibers of the vastus lateralis and the vastus medialis muscles. Reflect these laterally and medially to reveal the rectus tendon. Separate the tendon of the rectus femoris from the vastus intermedius (Fig. 11-58, *B*). Then follow the tendon of the rectus femoris to its insertion into the quadriceps tendon and divide the attachment, taking care not to divide the entire quadriceps tendon but only that of the rectus femoris. Mobilize the rectus femoris muscle from the rest of the quadriceps sufficiently to allow transfer to the sartorius. Place a heavy nonabsorbable suture in the tendon of the rectus, and outline the course of the transfer through the medial intermuscular septum as the septum is opened for a distance of about 10 cm. Palpate the sartorius through the opening in the septum, and bring it into the wound. Place the knee in 20 degrees of flexion, pass the rec-

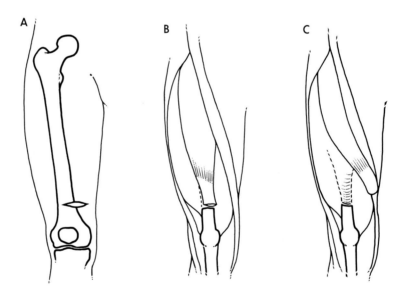

Fig. 11-58 Distal release or transfer of rectus femoris. **A,** Transverse incision. **B,** Rectus femoris is separated from vastus medialis, vastus lateralis, and vastus intermedius. **C,** Rectus femoris may be transferred through medial intermuscular septum to sartorius if desired.

tus tendon through the tendon of the sartorius, and then suture it to itself and to the sartorius under moderate tension (Fig. 11-58, *C*). If the tendon is to be transferred to the iliotibial band, suture it into the posterior portion of the iliotibial band posterior to the axis of knee flexion.

▶ *Postoperative management.* A knee immobilizer is applied, and ambulation is begun as soon as possible, usually by the fourth postoperative day. On the third postoperative day, gentle range of knee motion is begun. The knee immobilizer is discontinued when the patient has good active control of the knee and can extend the knee against gravity.

Ankle and Foot
Equinus

Equinus is the most common deformity in patients with cerebral palsy. The cause of the deformity is a combination of increased strength and spasticity of the triceps surae muscles combined with weakness of the ankle dorsiflexors. The presence of an equinus deformity is not an absolute indication for treatment of that deformity, but the equinus posture of the foot and ankle increase the instability of already compromised balance. If the child has hemiplegia, the leg with the equinus ankle appears longer than the other, and the child has difficulty clearing the ground with the foot during the swing phase of gait. This causes an increase in knee and hip flexion during swing or circumduction of the leg if knee flexion cannot be increased.

Surgical lengthening is indicated if there is a true contracture of the tendo Achilles or if there is significant equinus during gait and other means such as bracing are not successful. Westin and Dye, who advocate casting for spastic equinus, found tendo Achilles surgery was needed less frequently with the use of this approach. They believe that spasticity of the hamstring muscles is one cause of the equinus position of the ankle. Spastic hamstring muscles tend to pull the child backward, making the center of gravity posterior to the base of support with the feet flat on the ground. The equinus position places the weight-bearing line anterior to the center of gravity, thereby increasing stability.

Although many different surgical procedures have been described for lengthening of the tendo Achilles, there are three basic types: lengthening of the gastrocnemius alone, anterior translocation of the tendo Achilles, and lengthening of the tendo Achilles.

Lengthening of the gastrocnemius was first described by Vulpius and Stoffel and later by Strayer (1950) and Baker (1954). The basis for gastrocnemius lengthening alone is the Silfverskiöld test, which evaluates the amount of ankle dorsiflexion with the knee in both flexion and extension. Although this test probably is accurate for nonspasticity, Perry et al showed that it was not reliable for the child with spasticity. They found that when the ankle was in dorsiflexion, electrical activity was recorded in both muscles, accounting for the high recurrence rate in patients after gastrocnemius lengthening.

Anterior translocation of the tendo Achilles, as described by Throop et al, involves detachment of the tendo Achilles from the posterior aspect of the calcaneus and transfer anterior to a new location on the calcaneus. Results of this have not been superior to other means of tendo Achilles lengthening, and because this procedure is much more complicated than a simple tendo Achilles lengthening, generally it is not recommended.

The most commonly performed procedure to decrease the tendo Achilles contracture in patients with cerebral palsy is tendo Achilles lengthening, by either Z-plasty lengthening or sliding lengthening.

Two types of sliding lengthening lengthen the tendo Achilles while maintaining continuity. The double-cut technique takes into account the 90-degree rotation of the fibers of the tendo Achilles. The Hoke or triple-cut technique disregards the rotation of the tendo Achilles fibers by making three cuts midway through the tendon. Both sliding lengthenings maintain continuity in the tendon, which reduces the risk of overlengthening and promotes more rapid healing than the Z-plasty lengthening, which completely separates the tendon ends. Percutaneous sliding lengthening may be performed, but there is a risk of completely severing the tendo Achilles.

Complications of tendo Achilles lengthening are rare, but a calcaneus deformity may occur. Although overlengthening of the tendo Achilles is possible, a calcaneus deformity is more commonly caused by failure to lengthen the hamstrings or transfer of a spastic posterior tibial tendon to the dorsum of the foot at the time of tendo Achilles lengthening. Lengthening of the tendo Achilles in patients with athetosis may result in a calcaneus deformity because the balance between the plantarflexion and dorsiflexion musculature has been changed.

Vulpius lengthening

▶ *Technique.* Place the patient in the prone position, with the lower extremity in the operative field. Apply a tourniquet. Make an 8 to 10 cm longitudinal incision over the posterior aspect of the lower third of the calf (Fig. 11-59, *A*). Split the fascia overlying the triceps surae in line with the skin incision. Identify the aponeurosis of the gastrocnemius, and make an inverted V-shaped cut through the aponeurosis only from the medial edge of the tendon to the lateral edge (Fig. 11-59, *B*). Then place the foot in dorsiflexion to separate the cut edges of the aponeurosis (Fig. 11-59, *C*). Using fine-pointed scissors separate the fibers of the soleus muscle in the midline. Divide the median raphe (septum) of the soleus muscle. Occasionally two of these septae will be encountered, and both should be divided. Close the fascia, and then suture the skin with an absorbable suture or with a subcuticular suture plus skin strips.

▶ *Postoperative management.* A long-leg cast is applied initially and then changed to a short-leg cast as soon as the child is comfortable, usually in about a week. Postoperative full-time bracing is required if the child does not have control of the anterior tibial muscle, usually with a plastic ankle-foot orthosis. If the anterior tibial muscle functions with flexion of the hip and knee (withdrawal), then only night bracing is required.

Z-plasty lengthening of tendo Achilles

▶ *Technique.* The child may be positioned either prone or supine. Make a posteromedial incision midway between the tendo Achilles and the posterior aspect of the medial malleolus. The lower extent of the incision is at the superior border of the calcaneus, and it then continues cephalad for 4 to 5 cm (Fig. 11-60, *A*). Expose the tendo Achilles with sharp dissection directed posterior toward it. Incise the sheath of the tendo Achilles longitudinally from the superior to the inferior extent of the incision. Free the tendo Achilles from the surrounding tissues. Make a longitudinal incision in the center of the tendo Achilles from proximal to distal. Turn the scalpel either medially or laterally distally, and divide that half of the tendon transversely. Make the distal cut toward the medial side for a varus deformity and lateral for a valgus deformity. Hold this cut portion of the tendo Achilles with forceps, and bring the scalpel to the proximal portion of the longitudinal incision in the tendo Achilles. Then turn the scalpel opposite the distal cut, and divide that half of the tendon transversely to completely free the tendo Achilles. Divide the plantaris tendon on the medial aspect of the tendo Achilles transversely.

Evaluate the passive excursion of the triceps surae muscle using a Kocher clamp to pull the proximal stump of the tendon to its maximally stretched

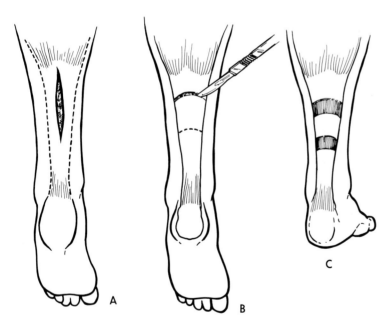

Fig. 11-59 Vulpius technique of gastrocnemius lengthening. **A,** Incision over posterior aspect of lower third of calf. **B,** Two transverse cuts through tendon of gastrocnemius are performed well above musculotendinous junction, leaving muscle fibers intact. **C,** Foot is placed in dorsiflexion to neutral, which separates tendon ends but maintains continuity in muscle fibers.

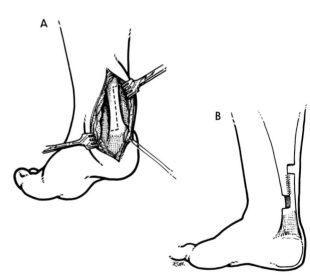

Fig. 11-60 Z-plasty lengthening of tendo Achilles. **A,** Longitudinal incision, halfway between posterior aspect of medial malleolus and tendo Achilles. Longitudinal cut in tendon is brought out proximally in one direction and distally in opposite direction. **B,** Ends are sutured to repair tendon.

length. Allow the tendon to retract halfway back to its resting length, and then suture it to the distal tendon end at that point (Fig. 11-60, *B*). Further control tension by adjusting the foot position. According to Gaines and Ford the ankle is placed in neutral position for mild spasiticity, in 10 degrees of dorsiflexion for moderate involvement, and in 20 degrees of dorsiflexion for the most severe involvement. Perform the repair in a side-to-side manner with a heavy absorbable suture. Close the wound with absorbable sutures or subcuticular sutures and skin strips. Apply a long-leg cast.

▶ *Postoperative management.* Ambulation is allowed as soon as the patient is comfortable. When pain is gone (usually 5 to 10 days), the cast is changed to a short-leg cast and walking is continued. Cast immobilization is continued for a total of 6 weeks. Bracing is used if the anterior tibial muscle is not strong or is not under volitional control. If there is no function in the anterior tibial muscle, full-time bracing is required. If the anterior tibial muscle functions only with withdrawal, full-time bracing is required for several months and then at night only to prevent recurrence of the tendo Achilles contracture.

White (double-cut) sliding lengthening of tendo Achilles

▶ *Technique.* Position the patient either prone or supine. Make a longitudinal incision on the posteromedial aspect of the ankle midway between the posterior aspect of the medial malleolus and the tendo Achilles (Fig. 11-61, *A*). The incision should not be placed directly over the tendon because of irritation of the scar from the counter of the shoe and the possibility of skin slough. Begin the incision distally at the superoposterior border of the calcaneus, and continue it proximally for 4 to 8 cm. Sharply divide the subcutaneous tissue and the tendon sheath in one plane so that the sheath remains attached to the subcutaneous tissue and can be closed after lengthening. It is not necessary to dissect completely around the tendo Achilles as in the Z-plasty lengthening.

Determine the rotation of the fibers of the tendon. The tendon usually rotates 90 degrees so that the fibers that are medial in the proximal portion of the heel cord are posterolateral in the distal end at the insertion into the calcaneus.

Use a scalpel with a No. 15 blade to divide the tendo Achilles transversely proximally and distally, making each cut halfway through the tendon. The placement of the two cuts depends on the rotation of the fibers; usually the anteromedial half of the tendon is divided distally and the posteromedial half proximally (Fig. 11-61, *B*).

Then place the foot in dorsiflexion, causing the fibers of the tendon to slide on each other and lengthen the tendon. If sliding does not occur, make a third incision halfway between the proximal and the distal incisions. Close the tendon sheath and the subcutaneous tissues with absorbable sutures. Close the skin with either subcuticular absorbable sutures or with absorbable skin sutures.

▶ *Postoperative management.* The leg is immobilized in a long-leg plaster cast with the knee in full extension. Ambulation is encouraged immediately, and once the child is comfortable, usually about 1 week after surgery, the cast is trimmed to a short-leg cast. Immobilization is continued for a total of 6 weeks. If the anterior tibial muscle can produce active dorsiflexion of the foot to a right angle, no postoperative bracing is necessary. If the foot cannot be actively dorsiflexed or if dorsiflexion occurs only with a withdrawal response, then bracing usually is required to improve gait and help prevent recurrence of the contracture. A plastic ankle-foot orthosis is worn full-time by the child with no function in the anterior tibial muscle and at night by the child with an anterior tibial muscle that functions only with withdrawal.

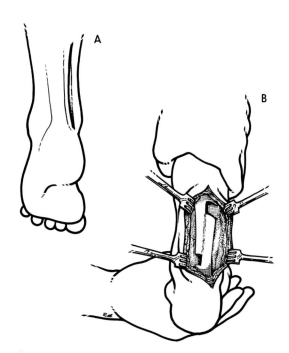

Fig. 11-61 Sliding lengthening of tendo Achilles. **A,** Posteromedial incision. **B,** Two cuts are made through one half of tendon in opposite directions. Rotation of fibers must be followed accurately; as foot is placed in dorsiflexion, tendon fibers separate.

Continued.

Hoke sliding lengthening of the tendo Achilles

▲ *Technique.* Use the same incision as for the White sliding lengthening. Split the sheath with the subcutaneous tissues to allow for easy closure of the sheath at the end of the procedure. Make three transverse half-cuts in the tendon, the most proximal and most distal cuts medially and the middle cut laterally (Fig. 11-61, *C*). Insert a No. 15 scalpel blade longitudinally into the tendo Achilles in the exact midportion of the tendon. Place the first proximal cut just above the musculotendinous junction. Turn the knife medially to completely sever the medial half of the tendon. Repeat this procedure distally in the tendon. Make the final cut midway between these two cuts, directing it laterally. Once these cuts have been made, place the foot in dorsiflexion just to neutral, allowing the tendon ends to slide on themselves (Fig. 11-61, *D*). The tendon remains in continuity, and no suturing is necessary.

▲ *Postoperative management.* Treatment after surgery is the same as after the White sliding lengthening.

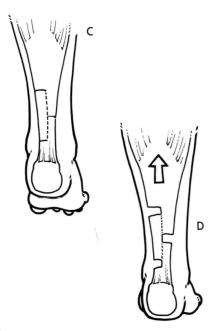

Fig. 11-61, cont'd   C, Three cuts may be made in tendon: proximal and distal cuts in same direction and middle cut in opposite direction. **D,** Tendon cuts then separate as foot is placed in dorsiflexion, maintaining continuity in tendon.

Varus Deformity of Hindfoot

Varus deformity of the hindfoot occurs most commonly in patients with spastic hemiplegia, although occasionally it may occur in those with bilateral involvement. The varus deformity usually is associated with equinus of the ankle. The varus deformity has been attributed to spasticity of either the anterior or the posterior tibial muscle. Although spasticity of either muscle may produce a varus deformity of the foot, the posterior tibial muscle is the more common cause of a varus deformity of the hindfoot, and the anterior tibial muscle, a varus deformity of the midfoot with supination of the forefoot. A gait study helps to determine the cause of the varus deformity. In children with spastic hemiplegia from perinatal causes, the varus deformity usually is caused by spasticity of the posterior tibial muscle and the anterior tibial muscle is weak or nonfunctional. Hemiplegia that occurs later in life may result in overactivity of the anterior tibial muscle with resultant varus of the midfoot. It is important to determine the cause of the deformity because treatment depends on etiologic factors.

If the posterior tibial muscle is the cause of the hindfoot varus, it should be either lengthened or transferred. Lengthening the posterior tibial muscle decreases its stretch reflex, reduces its spasticity, and weakens it. The posterior tibial muscle may be lengthened either with a Z-plasty lengthening in the supramalleolar region or with an intramuscular sliding lengthening, which maintains continuity of the muscle-tendon unit. These procedures usually are effective, but the varus deformity may recur or a calcaneus deformity may be produced if the tendon is lengthened too much. Tenotomy of the posterior tibial tendon, which may result in a valgus deformity of the foot with breakdown of the longitudinal arch, is not recommended.

Anterior transposition of the posterior tibial tendon, as described by Baker and Hill, involves rerouting the tendon anterior to the medial malleolus, thus decreasing its plantar flexion drive. Although the posterior tibial muscle is effectively lengthened by this technique, the deformity may not be corrected because the muscle retains its varus pull. In addition, if the muscle is continuously spastic, a calcaneus deformity may result because the posterior tibial muscle is converted to an ankle dorsiflexor by the transposition. Anterior transfer of the posterior tibial muscle through the interosseous membrane removes the actual deforming force and balances the absent or weak anterior tibial and peroneal muscles. If the posterior tibial muscle is phasic, the muscle fires appropriately, and transfer is not likely to cause a calcaneus deformity. If, however, the posterior tibial muscle is continuously spastic and if a tendo Achilles lengthening accompanies transfer, a calcaneus deformity is likely to result. A gait study determines whether the posterior tibial muscle is continuously firing or phasic. Because the results of this transfer are so variable in spastic feet, it rarely is recommended for the treatment of the varus hindfoot.

Split posterior tibial tendon transfer may be performed in the flexible spastic varus foot as an alternative to lengthening. The plantar flexion power of the posterior tibial muscle is retained, thereby decreasing the chance of a calcaneus deformity, and because half the tendon is transferred to the lateral side of the foot, the weak peroneal muscles are balanced.

If the varus deformity is caused by overactivity of the anterior tibial muscle, a split transfer of this muscle is indicated. This procedure balances the spastic deforming anterior tibial muscle while maintaining the normal pull of the muscle, thus preventing overcorrection. It must be remembered that this procedure is effective in correcting a dynamic varus deformity of the hindfoot. Regardless of the procedure chosen, a soft tissue procedure corrects only a dynamic deformity. For a fixed bony deformity the structural deformity must be corrected in addition to the soft tissue balancing procedure. If the hindfoot deformity is fixed, a lateral-based wedge osteotomy of the calcaneus (p. 90) must be performed in addition to the split posterior tibial tendon transfer.

Intramuscular lengthening of the posterior tibial tendon

▶ *Technique.* Place the patient in the supine position, and include the entire foot and leg in the operative field. Apply a pneumatic tourniquet around the thigh. Make a 3- to 5-cm incision posterior to the medial border of the tibia at the junction of its mid and distal thirds (Fig. 11-62, *A*). Incise the fascia in line with the skin incision, which opens into the deep posterior compartment of the lower leg. Retract the flexor digitorum longus muscle medially to expose the posterior tibial tendon.

The musculotendinous portion of the posterior tibial muscle now should be exposed by this maneuver. Place a small hemostat around the tendinous portion of the tibialis posterior to isolate it from the muscle fibers that envelop it. Divide the tendon transversely well proximal to the musculotendinous junction so as to leave the muscle fibers intact (Fig. 11-62, *B*). Then place the foot in dorsiflexion, and stretch it into valgus to separate the cut ends of the tendon while maintaining continuity of the muscle-tendon unit (Fig. 11-62, *C*). If the posterior tibial muscle is still tight after one cut has been made, make a second cut in the tendon 1 to 2 cm from the first.

▶ *Postoperative management.* Postoperative immobilization is not required, and the patient is allowed to ambulate immediately. This procedure usually is performed along with other procedures on the lower extremity, such as a tendo Achilles lengthening, and plaster immobilization for that procedure is indicated.

Z-plasty lengthening of the posterior tibial tendon

▶ *Technique.* Include the foot and leg in the operative field, and apply a pneumatic tourniquet. Make a posteromedial incision as for tendo Achilles lengthening (p. 664). Expose the flexor digitorum communus and the tibialis posterior muscles. Isolate the tendon of the posterior tibia, and lengthen it by Z-plasty. Adjust the amount of lengthening so that the foot can be brought into a slight valgus position.

▶ *Postoperative management.* The leg is immobilized in a short-leg cast for 6 weeks. Bracing is not necessary unless other procedures performed at the same time require postoperative bracing.

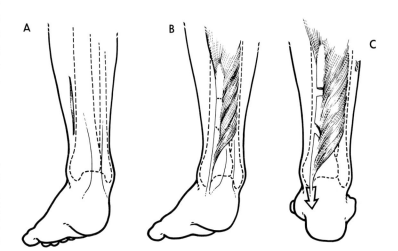

Fig. 11-62   Sliding lengthening of posterior tibial tendon. **A,** Longitudinal incision posterior to tibia. **B,** One or two cuts are made through posterior tibial tendon proximal to musculotendinous junction. **C,** As foot is placed in dorsiflexion, tendon cuts separate.

Split posterior tibial tendon transfer

▶ *Technique.* Three or four incisions are required for the split posterior tibial tendon transfer: two medial and one or two lateral. Make the first medial incision over the insertion of the posterior tibial tendon in the navicular, extending proximally for about 3 cm. Split the posterior tibial tendon longitudinally, and detach the plantar half of the tendon from its insertion in the navicular, leaving the dorsal half intact.

Continue the longitudinal split as far proximally as the wound permits. Make a second incision posterior to the medial malleolus. Pass the tendon into this wound beneath the tendon sheath of the posterior tibial tendon. Continue the longitudinal split proximally to the musculotendinous junction. Pass the split portion of the posterior tibial tendon posterior to the tibia and fibula but anterior to the neurovascular structures.

Make a third incision on the lateral side of the foot just posterior to the lateral malleolus. This incision may curve distally, following the peroneal muscles, or it may be separated into two incisions. Pass the split tendon into the lateral wound into the sheath of the peroneus brevis tendon. Then pass the split tendon in and out of two small slits made in the peroneus brevis tendon, and suture it to this tendon under maximal tension (Fig. 11-63). At the end of the procedure the foot should lie in a neutral to slightly valgus position because the split tendon serves as a dynamic sling to balance the spasticity of the posterior tibial muscle.

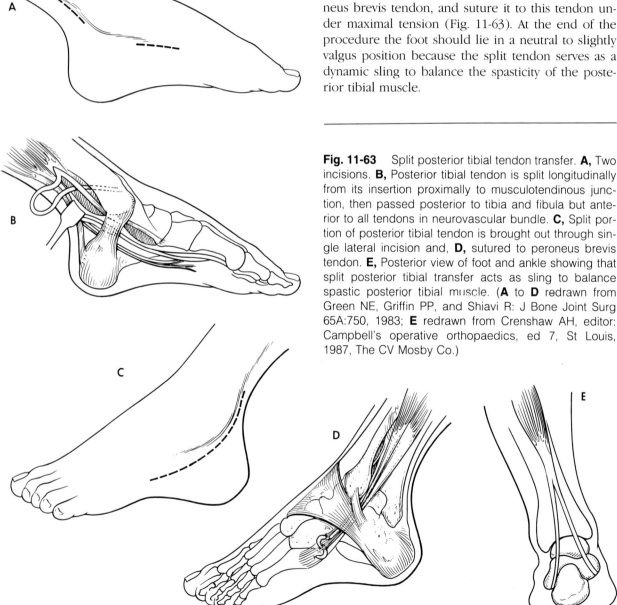

Fig. 11-63 Split posterior tibial tendon transfer. **A,** Two incisions. **B,** Posterior tibial tendon is split longitudinally from its insertion proximally to musculotendinous junction, then passed posterior to tibia and fibula but anterior to all tendons in neurovascular bundle. **C,** Split portion of posterior tibial tendon is brought out through single lateral incision and, **D,** sutured to peroneus brevis tendon. **E,** Posterior view of foot and ankle showing that split posterior tibial transfer acts as sling to balance spastic posterior tibial muscle. (**A** to **D** redrawn from Green NE, Griffin PP, and Shiavi R: J Bone Joint Surg 65A:750, 1983; **E** redrawn from Crenshaw AH, editor: Campbell's operative orthopaedics, ed 7, St Louis, 1987, The CV Mosby Co.)

▶ *Postoperative management.* The foot is maintained in a short-leg cast for 6 weeks. The child is allowed to ambulate, bearing full weight in the cast. No postoperative bracing is required.

Split anterior tibial tendon transfer

▶ *Technique.* Include the entire foot and leg in the operative field, and apply a pneumatic tourniquet. Make a 2- to 3-cm longitudinal incision dorsomedial over the medial cuneiform. Identify the anterior tibial tendon, and split it longitudinally in the midportion. Detach the lateral half of the tendon from its insertion, preserving as much length as possible, and continue the split proximally to the extent of the incision.

Make a second 2- to 3-cm incision anteriorly over the distal tibia, identify the anterior tibial tendon sheath, and split it longitudinally. Continue the split in the anterior tibial tendon proximally into this incision proximal to the musculotendinous junction. Umbilical tape may be used to continue the split in the tendon. Place the tape into the split, and bring the two ends of the tape into the proximal incision. Before the lateral half of the tendon is detached, continue the split to the musculotendinous junction by pulling on the tape. Once the split in the tendon is complete, detach the lateral half of the anterior tibial tendon and bring this half of the tendon into the proximal wound.

Make a third 2- to 3-cm longitudinal incision over the cuboid on the dorsolateral aspect of the foot. Make two drill holes in the cuboid. Place the holes as far away from each other as possible so that they meet well within the body of the cuboid. Enlarge the holes with a curet if necessary, but be certain to leave a bridge of bone between the two holes. Pass the split portion of the anterior tibial tendon distally through the subcutaneous tunnel from the proximal incision to the dorsolateral incision over the cuboid. Attach a nonabsorbable suture to the end of the tendon, and then pass it into one hole in the cuboid and out the other (Fig. 11-64). Hold the foot in dorsiflexion, pull the tendon tight, and suture the free end to the proximal portion of the tendon under moderate tension.

As an alternative, make a drill hole in the cuneiform through the plantar cortex; pass the tendon through this hole and anchor it on the plantar aspect of the foot with a suture over felt and a button.

▶ *Postoperative management.* A short-leg cast is worn for about 6 weeks. Hoffer et al recommend the use of a brace for 6 months, after which it is discontinued if possible.

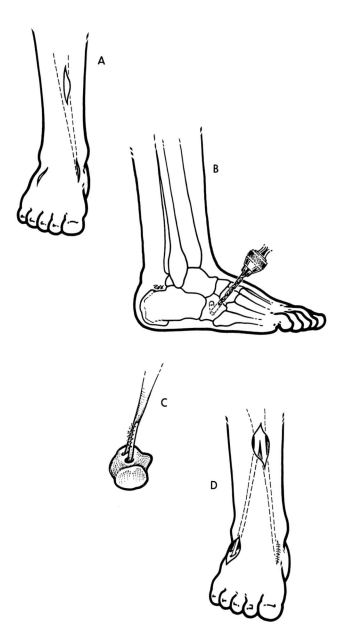

Fig. 11-64 Split anterior tibial tendon transfer. **A,** Three incisions: longitudinal over insertion of anterior tibial tendon, longitudinally over distal leg, and over cuboid. **B,** Two drill holes are made in cuboid. **C,** Split portion of anterior tibial tendon is pulled into one hole in cuboid and out the other and then sutured to itself. **D,** New split portion of tendon in its redirected position. (Redrawn from Hoffer MM et al: Orthop Clin North Am 5:31, 1974.)

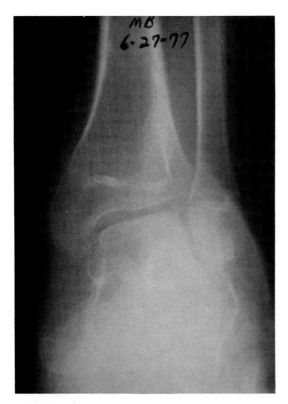

Fig. 11-65   Valgus deformity of distal tibia.

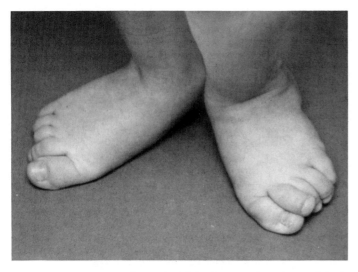

Fig. 11-66   Feet of child with spastic valgus of both feet; dorsiflexion in midfoot produces valgus of midfoot and forefoot.

Pes Valgus

Valgus deformity of the foot is common in patients with spastic diplegia and spastic quadriplegia; however, standing anteroposterior roentgenograms are mandatory to determine whether the valgus deformity is truly in the foot or in the distal tibia, as evidenced by valgus angulation of the distal tibial epiphysis (Fig. 11-65). Valgus angulation of the distal tibial epiphysis frequently results from undergrowth of the distal fibula, which may produce a tether that inhibits growth of the lateral portion of the distal tibial physis. Angular deformity of the distal tibia in children with spastic diplegia or quadriplegia may be corrected either by stapling of the medial side of the distal tibial physis (Chapter 1) or by corrective osteotomy of the distal tibia and fibula (Chapter 1).

Children with spasticity of both lower extremities usually have an associated equinus deformity, either dynamic or fixed, because of inherent ligamentous laxity. Although the hindfoot remains in equinus, the midfoot and the hindfoot deviate into valgus with the midfoot in dorsiflexion, allowing the foot to be plantigrade but causing breakdown of the midfoot. Spasticity of the peroneal muscles also tends to pull the foot into valgus (Fig. 11-66). Bennet et al reported that gait analyses of patients with spastic diplegia showed the posterior tibial muscle to be weak or nonfunctional in patients with pes valgus.

The physical consequences of a valgus deformity usually are less severe than those of a comparable varus deformity inasmuch as the valgus position of the foot does not make it unstable. If the deformity is severe, a painful callus may develop over the prominent head of the talus in the middle of the depressed longitudinal arch; in addition weight bearing on the medial border of the great toe may produce hallux valgus (Fig. 11-67). The medial side of the head of the first metatarsal or the medial side of the interphalangeal joint of the great toe may become painful.

The treatment of pes valgus depends on the severity of the deformity and the symptoms it produces. Tendo Achilles lengthening alone generally will not correct pes valgus. Peroneus brevis tendon lengthening has been reported to provide correction of the valgus deformity if performed before adaptive changes in the bones of the hindfoot have become severe. Intramuscular fractional lengthening should be performed to prevent overlengthening of the peroneus brevis. Lengthening of both peroneal muscles or anterior transfer of the peroneal tendons have not yielded good results and are not recommended.

Bennet et al reported transfer of the peroneus brevis to the posterior tibial muscle in patients with spastic pes valgus, believing the valgus deformity to be caused, at least in part, by the paralysis of the pos-

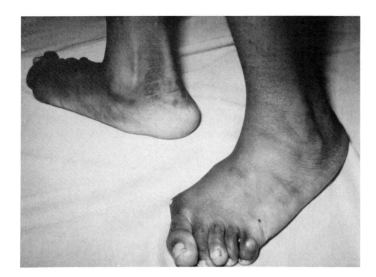

Fig. 11-67 Persistent valgus of midfoot and forefoot and equinus of hindfoot are predisposing factors in development of hallux valgus.

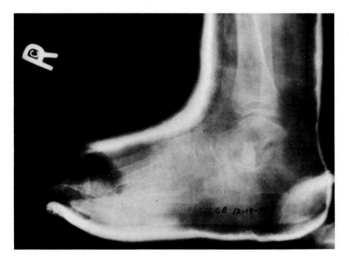

Fig. 11-68 Correct position of graft in sinus tarsi for traditional Grice arthrodesis. Graft is parallel to longitudinal axis of tibia.

terior tibial muscle. Their results have not been adequately evaluated through long-term follow-up, nor have they been confirmed by others.

Grice subtalar extraarticular arthrodesis (Chapter 2) has yielded the most consistent correction of the valgus foot in the child with spasticity, but proper patient selection and careful attention to the surgical technique are of utmost importance. The valgus deformity must be flexible; if the foot is rigid, a triple arthrodesis (Chapter 2) is the best means of correction. The technique as first described by Grice involved the use of a bone graft from the anterior cortex of the proximal tibia, although others have used fibular or bank bone. The bone graft must be inserted into the sinus tarsi perfectly parallel with the longitudinal axis of the tibia (Fig. 11-68). Because the graft also serves as internal fixation, if it is not parallel it may dislodge, resulting in loss of correction (Fig. 11-69). Another complication of this procedure is the

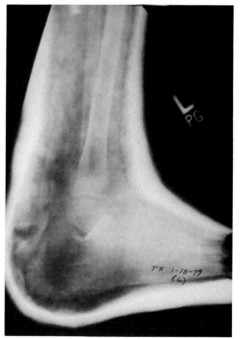

Fig. 11-69 Incorrect position of graft, which is not parallel to tibia and is not supporting subtalar joint.

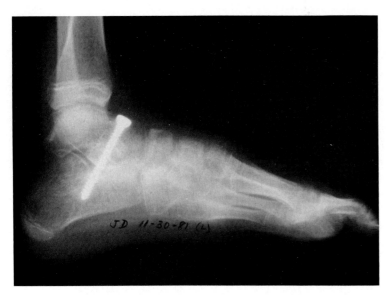

Fig. 11-70 Internal fixation of subtalar arthrodesis with screw inserted into neck of talus and crossing subtalar joint into calcaneus; bone has been placed in sinus tarsi.

development of a varus hindfoot, which tends to be less satisfactory than the original valgus deformity. This can be avoided by inserting a graft of adequate length to maintain the hindfoot in a neutral or slightly valgus position. Too much valgus is preferable to attempting a perfectly neutral heel and risking the development of a varus hindfoot.

Another method of subtalar arthrodesis, reported by Dennyson and Fulford, combines a screw across the subtalar joint for internal fixation with an iliac crest graft placed in the sinus tarsi. Because the screw provides the internal fixation, maintainance of the correct position does not depend on a piece of bone wedged into the sinus tarsi. In addition, the iliac crest bone provides graft material that is superior to a cortical tibial graft (Fig. 11-70).

If the valgus deformity of the foot is rigid, correction is possible only with a triple arthrodesis. The object of this operation is a solid arthrodesis of the hindfoot in a corrected position. Because growth is retarded if the procedure is performed in the young foot, triple arthrodesis usually is performed in the mature or near-mature foot. In addition, much of the surface area of the skeletally immature tarsal bone is cartilage; thus less bone surface is available for fusion, resulting in a higher rate of nonunion than in the older child.

Intramuscular lengthening of the peroneus brevis muscle

▶ *Technique.* Include the foot and leg in the operative field, and apply a pneumatic tourniquet. Make a 4-cm longitudinal incision just posterior to the fibula, beginning 2 to 3 cm proximal to the lateral malleolus and continuing proximally for 4 cm. Expose the two peroneal tendons at their musculotendinous junction. Make one or two transverse cuts through only the tendinous portion of the peroneus brevis well proximal to the distal end of the muscle fibers of the peroneus brevis. Stretch the foot into varus to separate the cut ends of the peroneus brevis tendon (Fig. 11-71).

▶ *Postoperative management.* A short-leg walking cast is worn for 6 weeks.

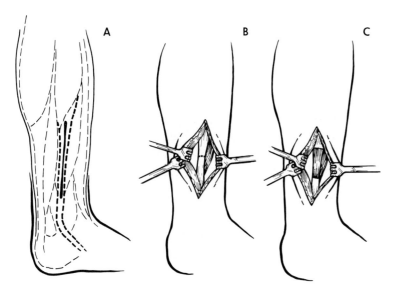

Fig. 11-71 Fractional lengthening of peroneus brevis. **A,** Incision over distal fibula. **B,** Peroneus brevis is exposed, and one or two transverse cuts are made through tendon proximal to musculotendinous junction. **C,** Foot is placed in dorsiflexion and into varus, allowing tendon ends to separate but maintaining continuity in tendon.

Subtalar arthrodesis with internal fixation

▲ *Technique.* Include the foot and leg in the operative field, and apply a pneumatic tourniquet. Make an oblique incision in line with the skin creases centered over the sinus tarsi. Extend the incision from the middle of the front of the ankle downward and laterally to the peroneal tendons. Raise the origin of the extensor digitorum brevis muscle, together with a pad of subcutaneous fat, proximally, and reflect it distally to expose the sinus tarsi. Remove the fat of the sinus tarsi in one piece by sharp dissection close to the bone. With either a gouge or a curved osteotome, remove cortical bone from the apex of the sinus tarsi to expose cancellous bone on both the undersurface of the neck of the talus and on the nonarticular area on the upper surface of the calcaneus. Expose the depression on the upper surface of the neck of the talus by blunt dissection between the tendons of the extensor digitorum longus muscle and the neurovascular bundle.

With the heel held in the corrected position, advance a Kirschner wire from the neck of the talus into the calcaneus across the subtalar joint. Insert this Kirschner wire as close as possible to the talonavicular joint to allow insertion of the transfixing screw. At this point, be certain that the position of the hindfoot is acceptable and not in varus. Reposition the Kirschner wire if the foot is not in the correct position. Then place a 4.5-mm cortical screw posterior to the Kirschner wire through the neck of the talus and across the talocalcaneal joint into the calcaneus. Do not allow the screw to protrude through the inferior cortex of the calcaneus. Obtain iliac crest graft from the ipsilateral anterior portion of the ilium, and pack it into the sinus tarsi, filling it with the graft (Fig. 11-72).

Close the wound with absorbable sutures or a subcuticular suture with skin strips. Insert suction drains in the foot and iliac crest incisions. Apply a short-leg, nonweight-bearing cast.

▲ *Postoperative management.* The cast is worn for 6 weeks, and then a weight-bearing cast is applied and worn for another 4 to 6 weeks. An ankle-foot orthosis may be worn for 6 months after cast removal to allow for maturation of the fusion.

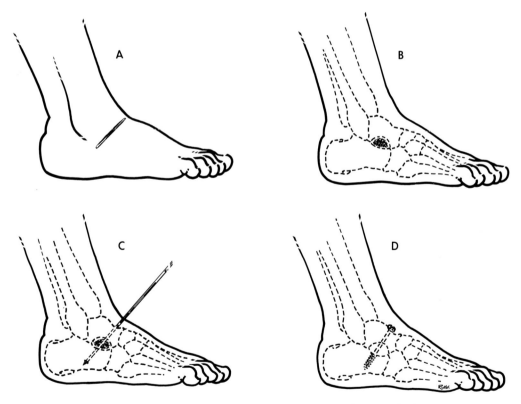

Fig. 11-72   Technique of subtalar arthrodesis with internal fixation. **A,** Oblique incision over sinus tarsi dorsal. **B,** Exposure of sinus tarsi, cancellous bone of the calcaneus, and talus. **C,** Steinmann pin is placed across subtalar joint entering talus as far distal as possible, with foot held in correct position. **D,** Placement of screw across subtalar joint from talar neck into calcaneus; sinus tarsi is filled with iliac crest bone. (Redrawn from Dennyson WG and Fulford GE: J Bone Joint Surg 58B:507, 1976.)

Triple arthrodesis. Triple arthrodesis requires exactness and precision and an intimate knowledge of the normal anatomy and function of the foot. Depending on the severity and rigidity of the deformity of the foot, bony wedges are removed to restore the normal anatomy. According to Hoke a satisfactorily stabilized foot looks natural in shoes, does not turn laterally on its longitudinal axis when the patient is standing or walking, does not require a brace to maintain a natural or nearly natural position, or, when a brace is used, does not look grossly deformed. Thompson recommended that weight be distributed evenly over the plantar surface during stance with the axis of the ankle joint well forward and at a right angle to the long axis of the foot; the patient should be able to control ankle motion and have no pain.

▶ *Technique.* Place the patient in the supine position, and apply a pneumatic tourniquet on the thigh. Place a sandbag or folded towels or sheets under the ipsilateral buttock to tilt the pelvis upward on the side to be operated and facilitate exposure of the lateral side of the foot. Include the foot and leg below the tourniquet in the operative field. Make an oblique incision centered over the sinus tarsi in one of the skin creases on the lateral side of the foot, beginning dorsolaterally at the lateral border of the tendons of the long toe extensors at the level of the talonavicular joint. Continue the incision posteriorly, angling plantarward and ending at the level of the peroneal tendons. Carefully protect the extensor and peroneal tendons, and carry the incision sharply down through the sinus tarsi to the bones at the floor of the sinus tarsi. Reflect the origin of the extensor digitorum brevis muscle distally along with the fat in the sinus tarsi. Clean the remainder of the sinus tarsi of all tissue to expose the subtalar and calcaneocuboid joints, and the lateral portions of the talonavicular joint.

Cut the capsules of the talonavicular, calcaneocuboid, and subtalar joints circumferentially to obtain as much mobilization as possible. If this release allows the foot to be placed in a normal position, bony wedges are not required. If the normal anatomy is not restored with the soft tissue release, appropriate bony wedges must be taken to correct the deformity.

Identify the anterior articular process of the calcaneus, and excise it at the level of the floor of the sinus tarsi for better exposure of the talonavicular joint. Perform this osteotomy with an osteotome placed parallel to the plantar surface of the foot, and preserve the bone for the graft. Next remove the articular surfaces of the calcaneocuboid joint with an osteotome to expose cancellous bone. Remove an equal amount of bone from both bones unless correction of a bony deformity is required. Next remove the distal portion of the head of the talus perpendicular to the long axis of the talus. Remove only enough bone to expose the cancellous bone of the head of the talus unless a wedge is required to correct a fixed deformity. A second medial incision may be required to expose the most medial portion of the talonavicular joint. Remove the proximal articular surface and subchondral bone of the navicular, and shape and roughen the surfaces for a snug fit with the talus. Next excise the articular surfaces of the sustentaculum tali and the anterior facet of the subtalar joint.

Now approach the subtalar joint, and completely remove the articular surfaces of this joint. For better exposure of the most posterior portion, use a small laminar spreader to expose the subtalar joint. Remove appropriate wedges from this joint if necessary; otherwise make the bony cuts parallel. Cut the removed bone into small pieces, and use for bone graft. Place most of the graft material around the talonavicular joint inasmuch as this joint is at highest risk for nonunion (Fig. 11-73).

In spastic feet it is wise to provide internal fixation of the fused joints with either staples or Steinmann pins. Close the muscle pedicle of the extensor digitorum brevis over the sinus tarsi to obliterate the dead space. Close the wound over suction drains, and apply a well-padded, long-leg cast with the knee flexed.

▶ *Postoperative management.* Considerable bleeding from the drain and through the wound itself can be expected. The foot should be elevated to minimize swelling. The patient is allowed to walk with crutches or a walker if able; however, no weight bearing is allowed on the operated foot. Six weeks after surgery the cast and pins are removed, and a short-leg walking cast is worn until union is complete, which usually occurs at about 12 weeks.

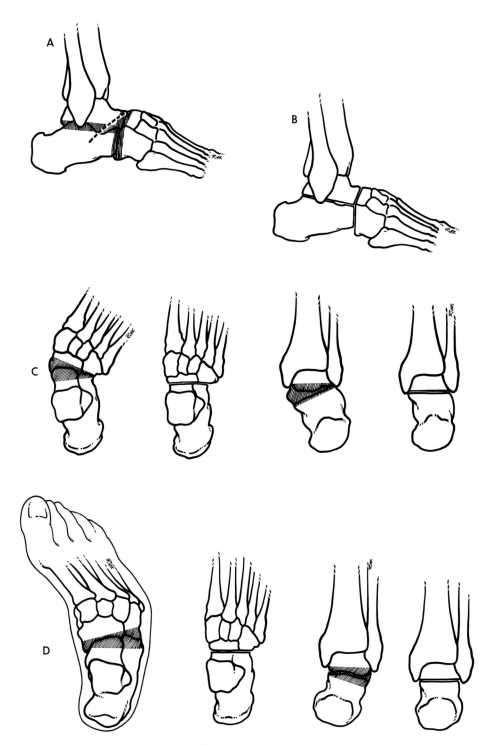

Fig. 11-73 Triple arthrodesis. **A,** Oblique incision in sinus tarsi; subtalar, talonavicular, and calcaneocuboid joints completely exposed. **B,** Cartilage and cortical bone removed from all joint surfaces; appropriate wedges are removed if necessary. **C,** Wedges necessary for correction of valgus foot. **D,** Removal of wedges necessary to correct varus foot. (Redrawn from Ingram AJ: Paralytic disorders. In Crenshaw AH, editor: Campbell's operative orthopaedics, ed 7, St Louis, 1987, The CV Mosby Co.)

Hallux Valgus

In the spastic foot, as in the nonspastic foot, a metatarsus primus varus may be the primary deformity, but even in the absence of this deformity the child with spastic diplegia or quadriplegia is at risk for the development of hallux valgus because of two mechanisms. The first is the equinovalgus posture of the foot, which forces the medial border of the great toe against the floor, producing a lateral thrust on the proximal phalanx. In time the proximal phalanx of the great toe deviates laterally, producing the valgus deformity of the metatarsophalangeal joint (see Fig. 11-67). The second cause unique to patients with spasticity is the spasticity of the adductor hallucis muscle, which pulls the proximal phalanx into valgus.

Treatment of the hallux valgus depends on the symptoms. Most procedures described for correction of hallux valgus are directed to the correction of the metatarsus primus varus, which may not exist in the spastic foot. If the adductor hallucis muscle is spastic, it must be released from the proximal phalanx of great toe; however, it should not be transferred to the neck of the first metatarsal.

If metatarsus primus varus exists, then correction of the varus angle of the first metatarsal is necessary, usually by opening wedge osteotomy of the base of the first metatarsal (Chapter 2).

Recurrence of the hallux valgus is a definite possibility in patients with spasticity, most commonly because of an uncorrected equinovalgus deformity of the foot. This deformity must be corrected before or at the time of correction of the hallux valgus. The second most common cause for recurrence of the deformity is failure to lengthen the adductor hallucis at the time of correction of the hallux valgus. Renshaw et al reported that the McKeever arthrodesis of the metatarsophalangeal joint of the great toe provided better results in the correction of severe or recurrent spastic hallux valgus than did other procedures.

McKeever arthrodesis of the metatarsophalangeal joint

▶ *Technique.* Apply a pneumatic tourniquet, and include the foot and leg in the operative field. Make a straight incision on the medial aspect of the bunion, beginning at the interphalangeal joint and then continuing proximally to about the central portion of the first metatarsal. As an alternative a shorter incision may be made here and a separate incision made on the plantar aspect of the metatarsophalangeal joint. Denude the proximal 0.75 cm of the proximal phalanx on the medial side and the distal 2 cm of the first metatarsal of periosteum and ligaments, and dislocate the joint.

Trim the distal end of the metatarsal to a blunt point about 1 cm in diameter. Remove most of the bone from the medial side of the metatarsal head to reduce the prominence. Then drill a 0.6-cm hole in the proximal phalanx, beginning at the articular surface and continuing within the canal of the bone for a depth of about 1 cm. Using curets or a power burr, enlarge this hole so that it will accept the head of the metatarsal.

Expose the plantar surface of the proximal phalanx, either by extending the incision in a plantar direction or by making a small incision on the plantar surface. Appose the metatarsal and the proximal phalanx with the joint in 10 to 15 degrees of dorsiflexion. With the joint held in this position, drill a hole from the plantar aspect of the midportion of the proximal phalanx, across the joint, and into the medullary canal of the metatarsal. Fix the osteotomy with an intramedullary screw that follows this tract (Fig. 11-74). Close the wound, and apply a short-leg cast. The cast is worn for 8 to 12 weeks until union is complete.

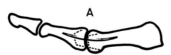
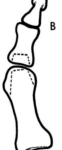
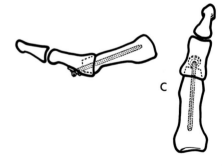

Fig. 11-74 McKeever arthrodesis of metatarsophalangeal joint. **A,** Lateral incision over metatarsophalangeal joint. **B,** Metatarsal is trimmed, and hole is made in base of proximal phalanx to accept head of metatarsal. **C,** Screw is placed from plantar aspect of base of proximal phalanx into metatarsal, with metatarsophalangeal joint in about 5 degrees of dorsiflexion. (Redrawn from McKeever DC: J Bone Joint Surg 34A:129, 1952.)

REFERENCES

General

Amiel-Tinson C: Neurological assessment from birth to 7 years of age. In Harel S, editor: The at risk infant, Baltimore, 1985, Paul H Brookes.

Baker LD: A rational approach to the surgical needs of the cerebral palsy patient, J Bone Joint Surg 38A:313, 1956.

Bax M: Controlled trial of physical therapy at Johns Hopkins, Dev Med 30:285, 1988.

Bleck EE: Severe orthopaedic disability in childhood: solutions provided by rehabilitation engineering, Orthop Clin 9:509, 1977.

Bleck EE: Orthopaedic management in cerebral palsy, Oxford, 1987, MacKeith Press.

Bleck EE: Locomotor prognosis in cerebral palsy, Dev Med Child Neurol 17:18, 1988.

Bobath K: The very early treatment of cerebral palsy, Dev Med Child Neurol 9:373, 1967.

Bobath K: A neurophysiological basis for the treatment of cerebral palsy. In Clinics in Developmental Medicine, Philadelphia, 1980, JB Lippincott Co.

Carlson JM and Winter R: The Gillette sitting support orthosis, Orthotics Prosthetics 4:35, 1978.

Cooper IS et al: Chronic cerebellar stimulation in cerebral palsy, Neurology 26:744, 1976.

Dahlback GO and Norlin R: The effect of corrective surgery on energy expenditure during ambulation in children with cerebral palsy, Eur J Appl Physiol 54:67, 1985.

Davis R, Barolat-Romana G, and Engle H: Chronic cerebellar stimulation for cerebral palsy, Acta Neurochir (Wien) 30:317, 1980.

Drvaric DM et al: Gastroesophageal evaluation in totally involved cerebral palsy patients, J Pediatr Orthop 7:187, 1987.

Ferry PC: On growing new neurons: are early intervention programs effective? Pediatrics 67:38, 1981.

Gage JR: Gait analysis for decision-making in cerebral palsy, Bull Hosp Jt Dis Orthop Inst 43:147, 1983.

Hayes NK and Burns YR: Discussion on use of weight-bearing plasters in reduction of hypertonicity, Am J Physioth 16:108, 1970.

Herndon WA et al: Effects of neurodevelopmental treatment on movement patterns of children with cerebral palsy, J Pediatr Orthop 7:395, 1987.

Highland TR and LaMont RL: Deep, late infections associated with internal fixation in children, J Pediatr Orthop 5:59, 1985.

Hoffer MM: Basic considerations and classification of cerebral palsy. In The American Academy of Orthopaedic Surgeons: Instructional course lectures, vol 25, St Louis, 1976, The CV Mosby Co.

Ireland ML and Hoffer M: Triple arthrodesis for children with spastic cerebral palsy, Dev Med Child Neurol 27:623, 1985.

Morrissy RT, editor: Lovell and Winter's pediatric orthopaedics, ed 3, Philadelphia, 1990, JB Lippincott.

Nelson KB and Ellenberg JH: Apgar scores as a predictor of chronic neurologic disability, Pediatrics 68:36, 1981.

Nwaobi OM and Smith PD: Effect of adaptive seating on pulmonary function of children with cerebral palsy, Dev Med Child Neurol 28:351, 1986.

Paine RS and Oppe TE: Neurological examination of children. In Clinics in Developmental Medicine, vol 20/21, London, 1966, SIMP with Heinemann.

Palmer FB et al: The effects of physical therapy on cerebral palsy: a controlled trial in infants with spastic diplegia, N Engl J Med 318:803, 1988.

Peterson HA and Coventry MB: Long-term results of surgery of adults with cerebral palsy, Dev Med Child Neurol 10:253, 1968.

Phelps WM: Complications of orthopaedic surgery in the treatment of cerebral palsy, Clin Orthop 53:39, 1967.

Pollock GA and Sharrard WJW: Orthopaedic surgery in the treatment of cerebral palsy. In Illingworth RS, editor: Recent advances in cerebral palsy, London, 1958, Churchill.

Rang M: The Easter Seal guide to children's orthopaedics, Ontario, Canada, 1982, The Easter Seal Society.

Reimers J: Static and dynamic problems in spastic cerebral palsy, J Bone Joint Surg 55B:822, 1973.

Sharrard WJW: Indications for bracing in cerebral palsy. In Murdoch G, editor: The advance in orthotics, London, 1976, Edward Arnold.

Silver CM, Simon SD, and Lichtman HM: The use and abuse of obturator neurectomy, Dev Med Child Neurol 8:203, 1966.

Sussman MD: Casting as an adjunct to neurodevelopmental therapy in cerebral palsy, Dev Med Child Neurol 25:804, 1983.

Tachdjian MO: Pediatric orthopedics, ed 2, Philadelphia, 1990, WB Saunders Co.

Trefler JP et al: A modular seating system for cerebral palsied children, Dev Med Child Neurol 20:199, 1978.

Watt J et al: A prospective study of inhibitive casting as an adjunct to physiotherapy in the cerebral palsied child, Orthop Trans 8:110, 1984 (abstract).

Wheeler ME and Weinstein SL: Adductor tenotomy—obturator neurectomy, J Pediatr Orthop 4:48, 1984.

Winters TF Jr, Gage JR, and Hicks R: Gait patterns in spastic hemiplegia in children and young adults, J Bone Joint Surg 69A:437, 1987.

Zachazewski JE, Eberle ED, and Jefferies M: Effect of tone-inhibiting casts and orthoses on gait, Phys Ther 62:453, 1982.

Upper extremity

Goldner JL: Upper extremity reconstructive surgery in cerebral palsy or similar conditions. In The American Academy of Orthopaedic Surgeons: Instructional course lectures, vol 18, St Louis, 1961, The CV Mosby Co.

Goldner JL: Reconstructive surgery of the upper extremity affected by cerebral palsy or brain or spinal cord trauma, Curr Pract Orthop Surg 3:125, 1966.

Inglis AE and Cooper W: Release of flexor pronator origin for flexion deformities of the hand and wrist in spastic paralysis: a study of eighteen cases, J Bone Joint Surg 48A:847, 1966.

Sakellarides HT, Mital MA, and Lenzi MD: Treatment of pronation contractures of the forearm in cerebral palsy by changing the insertion of the pronator radii teres, J Bone Joint Surg 63A:645, 1981.

Samilson RL: Surgery of the upper limbs in cerebral palsy, Dev Med Child Neurol 9:109, 1967.

Samilson RL and Green WL: Long-term results of upper limb surgery in cerebral palsy, Reconstr Surg Traumatol 13:43, 1972.

Skoff H and Woodbury DF: Management of the upper extremity in cerebral palsy, J Bone Joint Surg 67A:500, 1985.

Zancolli EA, Goldner LJ, and Swanson AB: Surgery of the spastic hand in cerebral palsy: report of the Committee on Spastic Hand Evaluation (International Federation of Societies for Surgery of the Hand), J Hand Surg 8A:766, 1983.

Shoulder, elbow, and forearm

Fuji T Y et al: Cervical radiculopathy or myelopathy secondary to athetoid cerebral palsy, J Bone Joint Surg 69A:815, 1987.

Pernet A et al: Management of forearm pronator teres contractures, Int Surg 69:341, 1984.

Hand and wrist

Ferlic DC, Turner BD, and Clayton ML: Compression arthrodesis of the thumb, J Hand Surg 8A:207, 1983.

Goldner JL and Ferlic DC: Sensory status of the hand as related to reconstructive surgery of the upper extremity in cerebral palsy, Clin Orthop 46:87, 1966.

Green WT and Banks HH: Flexor carpi ulnaris transplant and its use in cerebral palsy, J Bone Joint Surg 44A:1343, 1962.

Hoffer MM, Lehman M, and Mitani M: Long-term follow-up on tendon transfers to the extensors of the wrist and fingers in patients with cerebral palsy, J Hand Surg 11A:836, 1986.

Hoffer MM et al: Adduction contracture of the thumb in cerebral palsy: a preoperative electromyographic study, J Bone Joint Surg 65A:755, 1983.

Inglis AE, Cooper W, and Bruton W: Surgical correction of thumb deformities in spastic paralysis, J Bone Joint Surg 52A:253, 1970.

Kessler I: Etiology and management of adduction contracture of the thumb, Bull Hosp Jt Dis Orthop Inst 44:260, 1984.

Manske PR: Redirection of extensor pollicis longus in the treatment of spastic thumb-in-palm deformity, J Hand Surg 10A:553, 1985.

Matev I: Surgical treatment of spastic "thumb-in-palm" deformity, J Bone Joint Surg 45B:703, 1963.

McCue FC et al: Transfer of the brachioradialis for the hands deformed by cerebral palsy, J Bone Joint Surg 52A:1171, 1970.

Sarkin TL: Surgery of the hand in infants with cerebral palsy, S Afr Med J 45:655, 1972.

Smith RJ: Flexor pollicis longus abductor–plasty for spastic thumb-in-palm deformity, J Hand Surg 7A:327, 1982.

Swanson AB: Surgery of the hand in cerebral palsy and muscle origin release procedures, Surg Clin North Am 48:1129, 1968.

Spine

Allen BL Jr and Ferguson RL: The Galveston technique for L rod instrumentation of the scoliotic spine, Spine 7:276, 1982.

Allen BL Jr and Ferguson RL: L-rod instrumentation for scoliosis in cerebral palsy, J Pediatr Orthop 2:87, 1982.

Allen BL Jr and Ferguson RL: Technique: L-rod instrumentation for scoliosis in cerebral palsy, J Pediatr Orthop 2:87, 1982.

Balmer GA and MacEwen GD: The incidence of scoliosis in cerebral palsy, J Bone Joint Surg 52B:134, 1970.

Bonnett C, Brown JC, and Grow T: Thoracolumbar scoliosis in cerebral palsy: results of surgical treatment, J Bone Joint Surg 58A:328, 1976.

Brown JC, Swank S, and Specht L: Combined anterior and posterior spine fusion in cerebral palsy, Spine 7:570, 1982.

Bunnell WP and MacEwen GD: Non-operative treatment of scoliosis in cerebral palsy: a preliminary report on the use of a plastic jacket, Dev Med Child Neurol 19:45, 1977.

Drummond DS Keene JS, and Breed A: The Wisconsin system: a technique of interspinous segmental spinal instrumentation, Contemp Orthop 8:29, 1984.

Drummond DS et al: Interspinous process segmental spinal instrumentation, J Pediatr Orthop 4:397, 1984.

Gersoff WK and Renshaw TS: The treatment of scoliosis in cerebral palsy by posterior spinal fusion with Luque-rod segmental instrumentation, J Bone Joint Surg 70A:41, 1988.

Lonstein JE and Akbarnia A: Operative treatment of spinal deformities in patients with cerebral palsy or mental retardation: an analysis of one hundred and seven cases, J Bone Joint Surg 65A:43, 1983.

Madigan RR and Wallace SL: Scoliosis in the institutionalized cerebral palsy population, Spine 6:583, 1981.

Peacock WJ and Arens LJ: Selective posterior rhizotomy for relief of spasticity in cerebral palsy, S Afr Med J 62:119, 1982.

Robson P: The prevalence of scoliosis in adolescents and young adults with cerebral palsy, Dev Med Child Neurol 10:447, 1968.

Rosenthal RK, Levine DB, and McCarver CL: The occurrence of scoliosis in cerebral palsy, Dev Med Child Neurol 16:664, 1974.

Samilson RL: Orthopedic surgery of the hips and spine in retarded cerebral palsy patients, Orthop Clin North Am 12:83, 1981.

Samilson RL and Bechard R: Scoliosis in cerebral palsy: incidence, distribution of curve paterns, natural history, and thoughts on etiology, Curr Pract Orthop Surg 5:183, 1973.

Sponseller PD, Whiffen JR, and Drummond DS: Interspinous process segmental spinal instrumentation for scoliosis in cerebral palsy, J Pediatr Orthop 6:559, 1986.

Stanitski CL et al: Surgical correction of spinal deformity in cerebral palsy, Spine 7:563, 1982.

Sullivan JA and Conner SB: Comparison of Harrington instrumentation and segmental spinal instrumentation in the management of neuromuscular spinal deformities, Spine 7:299, 1982.

Taddonio RF: Segmental spinal instrumentation in the management of neuromuscular spinal deformities, Spine 7:305, 1982.

Lower extremity

Banks HH and Panagakos P: Orthopaedic evaluation in the lower extremity in cerebral palsy, Clin Orthop 47:117, 1966.

Browne AO and McManus F: One-session surgery for bilateral correction of lower limb deformities in spastic diplegia, J Pediatr Orthop 7:259, 1987.

Evans EB: The status of surgery of the lower extremities in cerebral palsy, Clin Orthop 47:127, 1966.

Grogan DP, Lundy MS, and Ogden JA: A method for early postoperative mobilization of the cerebral palsy patient using a removable abduction bar, J Pediatr Orthop 7:338, 1987.

Harris S et al: Effects of tone rescuing and standard short leg casts: a single subject study design, Proc Am Acad Cereb Palsy Dev Med, 1985 (abstract).

Mullaferoze P and Vora PH: Surgery in lower limbs in cerebral palsy, Dev Med Child Neurol 14:45, 1972.

Norlin R and Tkaczuk H: One-session surgery for correction of lower extremity deformities in children with cerebral palsy, J Pediatr Orthop 5:208, 1985.

Silfverskiöld N: Reduction of the uncrossed two-joint muscles of the leg to one-joint muscles in spastic conditions, Acta Chir Scand 56:315, 1923.

Hip

Allen BL: Basic considerations in pelvic fixation cases. In Luque ER, editor: Segmental spinal instrumentation, Thorofare, NJ, Charles B Slack, Inc.

Bailey TE and Hall JE: Ciari medial displacement osteotomy, J Pediatr Orthop 5:635, 1985.

Baker LD, Dodelin R, and Bassett FH: Pathological changes in the hip in cerebral palsy: incidence, pathogenesis, and treatment, J Bone Joint Surg 44A:1331, 1962.

Banks HH and Green WT: Adductor myotomy and obturator neurectomy for the correction of adduction contracture of the hip in cerebral palsy, J Bone Joint Surg 42A:111, 1960.

Baxter MP and D'Astous JL: Proximal femoral resection—interposition arthroplasty: salvage hip surgery for the severely disabled child with cerebral palsy, J Pediatr Orthop 6:681, 1986.

Bleck EE: The hip in cerebral palsy. In vol 20, The American Academy of Orthopaedic Surgeons, Instructional course lectures, St Louis, 1971, The CV Mosby Co.

Bleck EE: Postural and gait abnormalities caused by hip flexion contractures in spastic cerebral palsy, J Bone Joint Surg 53A:1468, 1971.

Bleck EE: The hip in cerebral palsy, Orthop Clin North Am 11:79, 1980.

Bowen JR, MacEwen GD, and Mathews PA: Treatment of extension contracture of the hip in cerebral palsy, Dev Med Child Neurol 23:23, 1981.

Carr C and Gage JR: The fate of the nonoperated hip in cerebral palsy, J Pediatr Orthop 7:262, 1987.

Castle ME and Schneider C: Proximal femoral resection—interposition arthroplasty, J Bone Joint Surg 60A:1051, 1978.

Chiari K: Medial displacement osteotomy of the pelvis, Clin Orthop 98:55, 1974.

Drummond DS, Rogala E, and Templeton J: Proximal hamstring release for knee flexion and crouched posture in cerebral palsy, J Bone Joint Surg 56A:1598, 1974.

Eyre-Brook AL, Jones DA, and Harris FC: Pemberton's iliac acetabuloplasty for congenital dislocation or subluxation of the hip, J Bone Joint Surg 60B:18, 1978.

Feldkamp M: Late results of hip and knee surgery in severely handicapped cerebral palsy patients, Arch Orthop Trauma Surg 100:217, 1982.

Girdlestone GR: Arthrodesis and other operations for tuberculosis of the hip. In The Robert Jones birthday volume, Cambridge, 1928, Oxford University Press.

Graham S et al: The Chiari osteotomy: a review of 58 cases, Clin Orthop 208:249, 1986.

Gugenheim JJ et al: Pathologic morphology of the acetabulum in paralytic and congenital hip instability, J Pediatr Orthop 2:397, 1982.

Haas SS, Epps CH, and Adams CH: Normal ranges of hip motion in the newborn, Clin Orthop 91:114, 1973.

Harris NH, Lloyd-Roberts GC, and Gallien R: Acetabular development in congenital dislocation of the hip, J Bone Joint Surg 57B:46, 1975.

Hoffer MM: Management of the hip in cerebral palsy, J Bone Joint Surg 68A:629, 1986.

Hoffer MM, Abraham E, and Nickel VL: Salvage surgery at the hip to improve sitting posture of mentally retarded, severely disabled children with cerebral palsy, Dev Med Child Neurol 14:51, 1972.

Houkom JA et al: Treatment of hip subluxation in cerebral palsy, J Pediatr Orthop 6:285, 1986.

Howard CB et al: Factors affecting the incidence of hip dislocation in cerebral palsy, J Bone Joint Surg 67B:530, 1985.

Howard CB and Williams LA: A new radiological sign in the hips of cerebral palsy patients, Clin Radiol 35:317, 1984.

Kalen V and Bleck EE: Prevention of spastic paralytic dislocation of the hip, Dev Med Child Neurol 27:17, 1985.

Keats S: Combined adductor-gracilis tenotomy and selected obturator nerve resection for the correction of adduction deformity of the hip in children with cerebral palsy, J Bone Joint Surg 39A:1087, 1957.

Lonstein JE and Beck K: Hip dislocation and subluxation in cerebral palsy, J Pediatr Orthop 6:521, 1986.

Mitchell GP: Chiari medial displacement osteotomy, Clin Orthop 98:146, 1974.

Mowery CA et al: A simple method of hip arthrodesis, J Pediatr Orthop 6:7, 1986.

Pemberton PA: Pericapsular osteotomy for congenital dislocation of the hip, J Bone Joint Surg 47A:65, 1965.

Perry J et al: Electromyography before and after surgery for hip deformity in children with cerebral palsy: a comparison of clinical and electromyographic findings, J Bone Joint Surg 58A:201, 1976.

Phelps WM: Prevention of acquired dislocation of the hip in cerebral palsy, J Bone Joint Surg 41A:440, 1959.

Reimers J: The stability of the hip in children: a radiological study of the results of muscle surgery in cerebral palsy, Acta Orthop Scand 184:1, 1980.

Reimers J and Poulsen S: Adductor transfer versus tenotomy for stability of the hip in spastic cerebral palsy, J Pediatr Orthop 4:52, 1984.

Root L, Goss JR, and Mendes J: The treatment of the painful hip in cerebral palsy by total hip replacement or hip arthrodesis, J Bone Joint Surg 68A:590, 1986.

Root L and Spero CR: Hip adductor transfer compared with adductor tenotomy in cerebral palsy, J Bone Joint Surg 63A:767, 1981.

Samilson RL: Orthopedic surgery of the hips and spine in retarded cerebral palsy patients, Orthop Clin North Am 12:83, 1981.

Schultz RS, Chamberlain SE, and Stevens PM: Radiographic comparison of adductor procedures in cerebral palsied hips, J Pediatr Orthop 4:741, 1984.

Sharrard WJW et al: Surgical prophylaxis of subluxation and dislocation of the hip in cerebral palsy, J Bone Joint Surg 57B:160, 1975.

Sherk HH, Pasquariello PD, and Doherty J: Hip dislocation in cerebral palsy: selection for treatment, Dev Med Child Neurol 25:738, 1983.

Staheli LT: Slotted acetabular augmentation, J Pediatr Orthop 1:321, 1981.

Steel HH: Triple osteotomy of the innominate bone, Clin Orthop 122:116, 1977.

Steel HH: Gluteus medius and minimus insertion advancement for correction of internal rotation gait in cerebral palsy, J Bone Joint Surg 62A:919, 1980.

Sutherland DH and Greenfield R: Double innominate osteotomy, J Bone Joint Surg 59A:1082, 1977.

Szalay EA et al: Extension abduction contracture of the spastic hip, J Pediatr Orthop 6:1, 1986.

Westin GW: Tendon transfers about the foot, ankle, and hip in the paralyzed lower extremity, J Bone Joint Surg 47A:1430, 1965.

Zuckerman JD, Staheli LT, and McLaughlin JF: Acetabular augmentation for progressive hip subluxation in cerebral palsy, J Pediatr Orthop 4:436, 1984.

Femur/thigh

Brookes M and Wardle EN: Muscle action and the shape of the femur, J Bone Joint Surg 44B:398, 1962.

Couch WH, DeRosa GP, and Throop FB: Thigh adductor transfer for spastic cerebral palsy, Dev Med Child Neurol 19:343, 1977.

Crane A: Femoral torsion and its relation to toeing-in and toeing-out, J Bone Joint Surg 41A:421, 1959.

Eilert RE and MacEwen GD: Varus derotational osteotomy of the femur in cerebral palsy, Clin Orthop 125:168, 1977.

Fabry G, MacEwen GD, and Shands AR: Torsion of the femur: a study in normal and abnormal conditions, J Bone Joint Surg 55A:1726, 1973.

Griffin PP, Wheelhouse WW, and Shiavi R: Adductor transfer for adductor spasticity: clinical and electromyographic gait analysis, Dev Med Child Neurol 19:783, 1977.

Hoffer MM: Supracondylar derotation osteotomy of the femur for internal rotation of the thigh in the cerebral palsied child, J Bone Joint Surg 63A:389, 1981.

Hoffer MM et al: Femoral varus-derotation osteotomy in spastic cerebral palsy, J Bone Joint Surg 67A:1229, 1985.

Michele AA: Iliopsoas. In Michele AA, editor: Development of anomalies of man, Springfield, Ill, 1962, Charles C Thomas, Publisher.

Perry J: Distal rectus femoris transfer, Dev Med Child Neurol 29:153, 1987.

Reimers J: Contracture of the hamstrings in spastic cerebral palsy, J Bone Joint Surg 65B:102, 1974.

Samilson RL et al: Results and complications of adductor tenotomy and obturator neurectomy in cerebral palsy, Clin Orthop 54:61, 1967.

Seymour N and Sharrard WJW: Bilateral proximal release of the hamstrings in cerebral palsy, J Bone Joint Surg 50B:274, 1968.

Shands AR and Steele MK: Torsion of the femur, J Bone Joint Surg 40A:803, 1958.

Sharps CH, Clancy M, and Steel HH: A long-term retrospective study of proximal hamstring release for hamstring contracture in cerebral palsy, J Pediatr Orthop 4:443, 1984.

Silver RL et al: Adductor release in nonambulant children with cerebral palsy, J Pediatr Orthop 5:672, 1985.

Tylkowski CM, Rosenthal RK, and Simon SR: Proximal femoral osteotomy in cerebral palsy, Clin Orthop 151:183, 1980.

Knee

Banks HH: The knee and cerebral palsy, Orthop Clin 3:113, 1972.

Evans EB: The knee in cerebral palsy. In Samilson RL, editor: Orthopaedic aspects of cerebral palsy, London, 1975, Heinemann.

Feldkamp M: Late results of hip and knee surgery in severely handicapped cerebral palsy patients, Arch Orthop Trauma Surg 100:217, 1982.

Gage JR et al: Rectus femoris transfer to improve knee function of children with cerebral palsy, Dev Med Child Neurol 29:159, 1987.

Green NE: The orthopaedic management of the ankle, foot, and knee in patients with cerebral palsy. In The American Academy of Orthopaedic Surgeons: instructional course lectures, vol 36, St Louis, 1987, The CV Mosby Co.

Grujic H and Aparisi T: Distal hamstring tendon release in knee flexion deformity, Int Orthop 6:103, 1982.

Kaye JJ and Freiberger BH: Fragmentation of the lower pole of the patella in spastic lower extremities, Radiology 101:972, 1971.

Lloyd Roberts GC, Jackson AM, and Albert JS: Avulsion of the distal pole of the patella in cerebral palsy: a cause of deteriorating gait, J Bone Joint Surg 67B:252, 1985.

Perry J, Antonelli D, and Ford W: Analysis of knee-joint forces during flexed-knee stance, J Bone Joint Surg 57A:961, 1975.

Rosenthal RK and Levine DB: Fragmentation of the distal pole of the patella in spastic cerebral palsy, J Bone Joint Surg 59A:934, 1977.

Strayer LM: Recession of the gastrocnemius, J Bone Joint Surg 32A:671, 1950.

Strayer LM: Gastrocnemius recession: five year report of cases, J Bone Joint Surg 40A:1019, 1958.

Ankle and foot

Baker LD: Triceps surae syndrome in cerebral palsy, Arch Surg 68:216, 1954.

Baker LD and Dodelin RA: Extra-articular arthrodesis of the subtalar joint (Grice procedure), JAMA 168:1005, 1958.

Baker LD and Hill LM: Foot alignment in the cerebral palsy patient, J Bone Joint Surg 46A:1, 1964.

Banks HH: The management of spastic deformities of the foot and ankle, Clin Orthop 122:70, 1977.

Banks HH: Equinus and cerebral palsy, Foot Ankle 4:149, 1983.

Banks HH and Green WT: The correction of equinus deformity in cerebral palsy, J Bone Joint Surg 40A:1359, 1958.

Barrasso JA, Wile PB, and Gage JR: Extraarticular subtalar arthrodesis with internal fixation, J Pediatr Orthop 4:555, 1984.

Bassett FH and Baker LD: Equinus deformity in cerebral palsy, Curr Pract Orthop Surg 3:59, 1966.

Bennet GC, Rang M, and Jones D: Varus and valgus deformities of the foot in cerebral palsy, Dev Med Child Neurol 24:499, 1982.

Bleck EE: The shoeing of children: sham or science? Dev Med Child Neurol 13:188, 1971.

Bleck EE: Forefoot problems in cerebral palsy—diagnosis and management, Foot Ankle 4:188, 1984.

Bleck EE and Berzins UJ: Conservative management of pes valgus with plantar flexed talus flexible, Clin Orthop 122:85, 1977.

Carpenter EB: Role of nerve blocks in the foot and ankle in cerebral palsy: therapeutic and diagnostic, Foot Ankle 4:164, 1983.

Dennyson WG and Fulford R: Subtalar arthrodesis by cancellous grafts and metallic fixation, J Bone Joint Surg 58B:507, 1976.

Dias LS: Valgus deformity of the ankle joint: pathogenesis of fibular shortening, J Pediatr Orthop 5:176, 1985.

Dillin W and Samilson RL: Calcaneus deformity in cerebral palsy, Foot Ankle 4:167, 1983.

Duncan WR and Mott DH: Foot reflexes and the use of the inhibitive cast, Foot Ankle 4:145, 1984.

Eilert RE: Cavus foot in cerebral palsy, Foot Ankle 4:185, 1984.

Gaines RW and Ford TB: A systematic approach to the amount of Achilles tendon lengthening in cerebral palsy, J Pediatr Orthop 4:448, 1984.

Garbarino JL and Clancy M: A geometric method of calculating tendo Achillis lengthening, J Pediatr Orthop 5:573, 1985.

Grant AD, Feldman R, and Lehman WB: Equinus deformity in cerebral palsy: a retrospective analysis of treatment and function in 39 cases, J Pediatr Orthop 5:678, 1985.

Green NE: The orthopaedic management of the ankle, foot, and knee in patients with cerebral palsy. In The American Academy of Orthopaedic Surgeons: instructional course lectures, vol 36, St Louis, 1987, The CV Mosby Co.

Green NE, Griffin PP, and Shiavi R: Split posterior tibial tendon transfer in spastic cerebral palsy, J Bone Joint Surg 65A:748, 1983.

Greene WB: Achilles tendon lengthening in cerebral palsy: comparison of inpatient versus ambulatory surgery, J Pediatr Orthop 7:256, 1987.

Grice DS: An extra-articular arthrodesis of the subastragalar joint for correction of paralytic feet in children, J Bone Joint Surg 34A:927, 1952.

Hoffer MM et al: The split anterior tibial tendon transfer in treatment of spastic varus of the hindfoot in childhood, Orthop Clin North Am 5:31, 1974.

Hoke M: An operation for stabilizing paralytic feet, J Orthop Surg 3:494, 1921.

Javors JR and Klaaren HE: The Vulpius procedure for correction of equinus deformity in cerebral palsy, J Pediatr Orthop 7:191, 1987.

Keats S and Kouten J: Early surgical correction of the planovalgus foot in cerebral palsy, Clin Orthop 61:223, 1968.

Kling TF, Kaufer H, and Hensinger RN: Split posterior tibial tendon transfers in children with cerebral spastic paralysis and equinovarus deformity, J Bone Joint Surg 67A:186, 1985.

Lee CL and Bleck EE: Surgical correction of equinus deformity in cerebral palsy, Dev Med Child Neurol 22:287, 1980.

Majestro TC, Ruda R, and Frost HM: Intramuscular lengthening of the posterior tibialis tendon, Clin Orthop 79:59, 1971.

Mann R: Biomechanics in cerebral palsy, Foot Ankle 4:114, 1983.

Moreau MJ and Lake DM: Outpatient percutaneous heel cord lengthening in children, J Pediatr Orthop 7:253, 1987.

Moreland JR and Westin GW: Further experience with Grice subtalar arthrodesis, Clin Orthop 207:113, 1986.

Nather A, Fulford GE, and Stewart K: Treatment of valgus hindfoot in cerebral palsy by peroneus brevis lengthening, Dev Med Child Neurol 26:335, 1984.

Otis JC, Root L, and Kroll MA: Measurement of plantar flexor spasticity during treatment with tone-reducing casts, J Pediatr Orthop 5:682, 1985.

Otis JC et al: Biomechanical measurement of spastic plantarflexors, Dev Med Child Neurol 25:60, 1983.

Perry J, Hoffer M, and Giovan P: Gait analysis of the triceps surae in cerebral palsy, Orthop Clin 5:31, 1974.

Perry J et al: Gait analysis of the triceps surae in cerebral palsy: a preoperative clinical and electromyographic study, J Bone Joint Surg 56A:511, 1974.

Renshaw T, Sirkin R, and Drennan J: The management of hallux valgus in cerebral palsy, Dev Med Child Neurol 21:202, 1979.

Root L: Tendon surgery on the feet of children with cerebral palsy, Dev Med Child Neurol 18:671, 1976.

Root L: Varus and valgus foot in cerebral palsy and its management, Foot Ankle 4:174, 1984.

Root L and Kirz P: The result of posterior tibial tendon surgery in 83 patients with cerebral palsy, Dev Med Child Neurol 24:241, 1982.

Rosenthal RK: The use of orthotics in foot and ankle problems in cerebral palsy, Foot Ankle 195, 1984.

Ross PM and Lyne ED: The Grice procedure: indications and evaluations of long-term results, Clin Orthop 153:194, 1980.

Schneider M and Balon K: Deformity of the foot following anterior transfer of the posterior tibial and lengthening of the Achilles tendon for spastic equinovarus, Clin Orthop 125:113, 1977.

Schwartz JR et al: Lessons learned in the treatment of equinus deformity in ambulatory spastic children, Orthop Trans 1:84, 1977.

Skinner SR and Lester DK: Gait electromyographic evaluation of the long-toe flexors in children with spastic cerebral palsy, Clin Orthop p 70, 1986.

Strayer LM: Recession of the gastrocnemius, J Bone Joint Surg 32A:671, 1950.

Strayer LM: Gastrocnemius recession: five year report of cases, J Bone Joint Surg 40A:1019, 1958.

Thompson TC: Astragalectomy and the treatment of calcaneovalgus, J Bone Joint Surg 21:627, 1939.

Throop FB et al: Correction of equinus in cerebral palsy by the Murphy procedure of tendocalcaneus advancement: a preliminary communication, Dev Med Child Neurol 17:182, 1975.

Turner JW and Cooper RR: Anterior transfer of the tibialis posterior through the interosseous membrane, Clin Orthop 83:241, 1972.

Vulpius O and Stoffel A: Orthopadische Operationslehre, Stuttgart, 1913, Ferdinand Enke.

Westin GW: Tendon transfers about the foot, ankle, and hip in the paralyzed lower extremity, J Bone Joint Surg 47A:1430, 1965.

Westin GW and Dye S: Conservative management of cerebral palsy in the growing child, Foot Ankle 4:160, 1983.

12 Myelomeningocele

LUCIANO S. DIAS

OVERVIEW

Myelomeningocele is a hernial protrusion of the spinal cord and its meninges through a defect in the vertebral canal. The nervous system develops by neurulation, the formation of a tubular structure. Closure of the neural tube is completed by closure of the cranial and caudal neuropores (at about days 24 to 26 of gestation). Much of the caudal extremity of the neural tube undergoes regression and finally is represented by the filum terminale. True myelomeningocele is believed to result from failure of fusion of the neural folds during neurulation. The myelomeningocele is a fluid-filled cystic swelling, formed by dura and arachnoid, protruding through a deficit in the vertebral arches under the skin, and the spinal cord nerve roots are carried out into the fundus of the sac (Fig. 12-1). In the United States the incidence of myelomeningocele is from 0.6 to 0.9:1,000 births. Recent studies suggest that the sibling recurrence is approximately 2% to 7%. Prenatal diagnosis can be made by biochemical and enzyme evaluation, as well as by

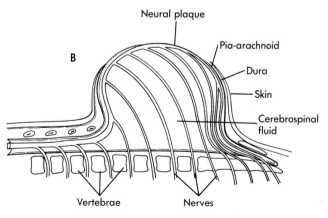

Fig. 12-1 Myelomeningocele lesion **(A)** may be small extension or may assume a large sessile protrusion **(B).**

Many figures in this chapter were taken from Schafer MF and Dias LS: Myelomeningocele: orthopaedic treatment, Baltimore, 1983, The Williams & Wilkins Co.

roentgenographic or ultrasound examination. The least invasive method is maternal serum alpha fetal protein screening, which has an accuracy rate of 60% to 95%. Prenatal diagnosis by serum screen or ultrasonography permits delivery by cesarean section, which avoids trauma to a large myelomeningocele sac. Other abnormalities of the spinal cord often are associated with myelomeningocele, including duplication of the cord, diastematomyelia, and severe vertebral bony anomalies such as defects in segmentation and failure of fusion of vertebral bodies, which causes congenital scoliosis, kyphosis, and kyphoscoliosis (Chapter 10).

The orthopaedist is only one of a multidisciplinary team of physicians involved in the care of children with myelomeningocele, and often medical, neurosurgical, or urologic treatment is of primary concern. The goal of orthopaedic treatment is to make the musculoskeletal system as functional as possible; ambulation is not the goal for every child with myelomeningocele. Quite often the child or adult with myelomeningocele can perform activities of daily living without lower extremity muscle function or the ability to walk. Often surgery is more detrimental than helpful, resulting in long-term disability. Before aggressive orthopaedic treatment is initiated, consideration must be given to the lifetime prognosis for these patients. Only 30% of all patients with myelomeningocele are functionally independent, and only 30% of adults with myelomeningocele are employed full- or part-time. Wheelchair use is common. Almost all patients with L2 to L3 and higher lesions are wheelchair users; of those with lower-level lesions (from L3 to L5), more than two thirds use a wheelchair at least part of the time. Statistically, if a child with myelomeningocele is not standing independently by the age of about 6 years, walking is unlikely. The pattern of mobility established by the age of 10 years will continue into adulthood. More important than the use of the lower extremities, however, is the child's total development. Recent emphasis on the intellectual and personality development of children with myelomeningocele, including emphasis on wheelchair mobility, aggressive wheelchair-sports programs beginning in preschool, and educational mainstreaming, has dramatically increased the independence of these patients.

Associated Neurologic Conditions

Hydrocephalus. Of the children with myelomeningocele 80% to 90% have hydrocephalus that requires cerebrospinal shunting. The incidence of hydrocephalus is related to the neurologic level of the lesion: 83% in high lesions and 60% in low lesions. Infection and obstruction are the most serious late complications of cerebrospinal fluid shunts because they affect the child's motor and intellectual development. In terms of upper extremity function and trunk balance, as well as lower incidences of hydromelia and tethered cord, children who do not require shunting may have a better prognosis than children who require shunting.

Arnold-Chiari malformation. The Arnold-Chiari malformation (Chiari II) is a consistent clinical and pathologic finding in patients with myelomeningocele. The basic lesion is caudal displacement of the posterior lobe of the cerebellum. The clinical manifestation of Arnold-Chiari malformation is dysfunction of the lower cranial nerves, causing weakness or paralysis of vocal cords and difficulty in feeding, crying, and breathing. Respiratory difficulties, such as apnea, cyanotic attacks, and associated brachycardia, are not uncommon. Ocular manifestations also are typical of this condition.

Tethered spinal cord. The spinal cord ascends during fetal development until at birth it is at the L3 level and by the second month of life has reached the adult L1-2 level. Most children with myelomeningocele show signs of tethering on magnetic resonance imaging (MRI), but the clinical manifestations of tethered cord are present in only approximately 20% of children. The clinical signs of tethering are variable, but the most consistent are (1) loss of motor function, (2) development of spasticity in the lower extremity, mainly the medial hamstrings and ankle dorsiflexors and evertors (rarely, spastic paralysis is present at birth), (3) development of scoliosis (before the age of 6 years) in the absence of congenital anomalies of the vertebral bodies, (4) back pain and increased lumbar lordosis in the older child, and (5) changes in urologic function. All children with suspected tethered cord syndrome should be evaluated by MRI (Fig. 12-2, *A*) and, if necessary, computed tomography–myelography scan. Surgical treatment is indicated to prevent further deterioration of the motor function and to decrease the progress of spasticity and scoliosis when clinical signs are documented.

Hydromelia. Hydromelia is an accumulation of fluid in the enlarged central canal of the spinal cord. It is frequent in children with myelomeningocele and may manifest as scoliosis. Hall et al reported progressive scoliosis ranging from 30 to 85 degrees and hydromelia in 12 patients. After surgical treatment of the hydromelia there may be some scoliosis regression. Evaluation of hydromelia should include CT scanning of the head and MRI of the entire spine (Fig. 12-2, *B*).

Types of Paralysis

Mazur et al reported that only 54% of their patients with myelomeningocele whose upper extremities were normal demonstrated the classic flaccid paralysis in the lower extremities; 9% had flaccid lower extremity paralysis with spastic upper extremities, 24% had spastic lower limbs, and 13% had spastic upper and lower limbs. The spasticity in the upper extremities was directly related to the number of shunt revisions. In the authors' series 86% of children with normal upper extremities and flaccid lower extremities were community ambulators, but only 1 of 14 patients with spastic upper and lower extremities was a community ambulator.

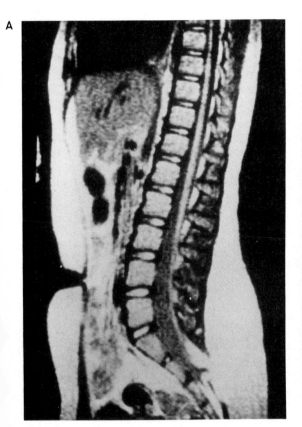
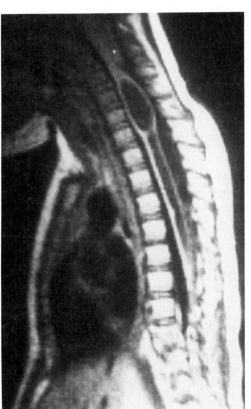

Fig. 12-2 **A,** MRI clearly shows evidence of tethered spinal cord. **B,** MRI shows large hydrocele at cervicothoracic junction.

Classification

The best known classification of myelomeningocele is based on the neurologic level of the lesion (Fig. 12-3): group I, children with thoracic and high lumbar level lesions and no quadriceps function; group II, children with low lumbar level lesions and quadriceps and medial hamstring function, but no gluteus medius function; and group III, children with sacral level lesions and quadriceps and gluteus medius function. Children in group I rarely become community ambulators as adults unless they have excellent trunk balance and upper extremity function and are not obese. Most children in group II require ankle-foot orthoses for support and crutches for trunk stability. Children in group III should walk with no external support and may or may not require ankle-foot orthoses. According to Asher and Olson there is a significant difference in the ability to walk between children with L4 level lesions and those with L3 level lesions. They stress that knee extensor power also is necessary for community ambulation. Children with L3 or L4 level lesions have the most to gain from proper care of musculoskeletal deformities.

ORTHOPAEDIC EVALUATION

Orthopaedic evaluation of the child with myelomeningocele should always include the following:

1. Serial sensory and motor examinations to evaluate neurologic level of function. Children may be 3 to 4 years old before a neurologic level is absolutely defined. The loss of prior motor function and increased spasticity is associated with tethered cord.

2. Sitting balance. The ability to sit without hand support is a good indication of more nearly normal central nervous sytem function. If one- or two-hand support is required for sitting, walking ability with an orthosis and external support is severely impaired.

3. Upper extremity function. Grip strength and atrophy of the thenar musculature are reliable signs of hydromelia. Impaired hand function is found in 82% of children with myelomeningocele, with differences in hand function between children with high level lesions and those with low level lesions.

4. Spine curvature. Spinal roentgenograms should be obtained once a year to evaluate any abnormal curvature such as scoliosis, kyphosis, and increased lumbar lordosis.

5. Hip range of motion and stability. Hip flexion contractures should be evaluated by the Thomas test. Either adduction or abduction contractures of the hip can cause infrapelvic obliquity that interferes with bracing and ambulation.

6. Knee alignment and range of motion. Knee flexion contractures and spasticity should be accurately measured and recorded.

7. Rotational deformities. External tibial torsion is frequent in children with low lumbar level lesions and often is associated with valgus deformity of the ankle joint and calcaneus or calcaneovalgus deformity of the foot.

8. Ankle valgus deformity. Valgus deformity at the ankle may hinder orthotic wear or cause pressure sores at the medial malleolus.

9. Foot deformities. Congenital vertical talus is present in approximately 80% of children with sacral level lesions. A varus foot deformity is an indication of an active posterior tibial muscle, and supination deformity is indicative of an active anterior tibial muscle. Spasticity may indicate a tethered cord. Involvement of the peroneus brevis, longus, and tertius muscles may cause a calcaneovalgus deformity.

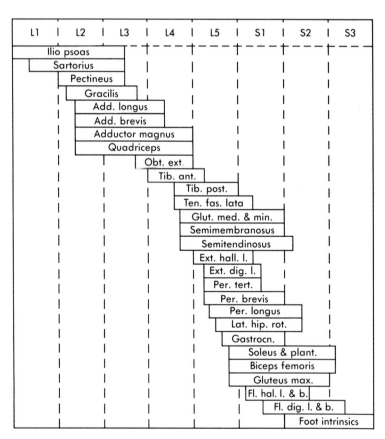

Fig. 12-3 Neurosegmental innervation of lower limb muscles. (From Sharrard WJW: J Bone Joint Surg 46B:427, 1964.)

Principles of Orthopaedic Management

Orthopaedic deformities in children with myelomeningocele are caused by (1) muscle imbalance as a result of the neurologic abnormality, (2) habitually assumed posture after birth, and (3) associated congenital malformations.

The aim of treatment of children with myelomeningocele is to establish a pattern of development that is as near normal as the levels of paraplegia and central nervous system involvement allow. Orthopaedic management should be tailored to meet specific goals during childhood, taking into account the expected adult function. In spite of the best medical and surgical care about 40% of children with myelomeningocele will be nonambulators as adults; thus care must be taken to prevent pelvic obliquity and correct spinal deformities. The goal of orthopaedic treatment is to establish a stable posture.

Most children achieve their maximum level of ambulation around the age of 4 years. A child who is not walking outdoors by the age of 6 years probably will not walk as an adolescent, and increased walking therapy beyond the age of 6 years is not likely to be effective. Walking requires the spine to be balanced over the pelvis, allows only small degrees of hip flexion contractures and knee contractures, and mandates a plantigrade, supple, braceable foot with the center of gravity over the feet. At least 80% of children with myelomeningocele have some impairment of the upper extremities, making effective ambulation with low energy consumption and minimal bracing possible in only about 50% of adult patients. The orthopaedic surgeon should aim for effective mobility by any efficient and effective means of moving about in space that allows the patient to go easily from place to place, explore the environment, and grow and develop. Recently Mazur et al have shown that children with high level lesions, in spite of the low percentage who are effective ambulators as adults, can benefit from walking in the first 10 years of life. Those who walk tend to be more mobile than children who never walk, and they have fewer fractures and skin pressure sores. If the child has quadriceps and medial hamstring function with good sitting balance and upper extremity function, all efforts, both conservative and surgical, should be made to achieve effective ambulation. If quadriceps function is absent, effective ambulation can be achieved only in a small percentage of patients (25% between the ages of 5 and 10 years) even when sitting balance and upper extremity function are normal. All others will be either exercise ambulators or nonambulators and will require a wheelchair for effective mobility.

ORTHOTIC MANAGEMENT

The goal of orthotic treatment is to achieve effective mobility with minimal restriction. Because immobilization of any lower limb segment or joint increases energy consumption by 10%, orthoses should be kept to a minimum. Bracing and splinting vary with the degree of motor deficit and trunk balance, and each child should be carefully assessed by the orthopaedic surgeon, orthotist, and physical therapist.

The A-frame (Fig. 12-4) is recommended for children aged 12 to 18 months, unless there is marked lack of head control. The A-frame is a prefabricated device, is fitted easily, and does not require adjustment for at least 6 to 8 months. It allows the child to stand without hand support and should be used up to 2.5 hours a day divided into periods of 20 to 30 minutes.

A parapodium is indicated for older children (over 2 years) with poor trunk balance and/or spastic upper extremities when walking with an orthosis is impossible. The parapodium supports the spine in both sitting and standing positions. It is aligned so that the child can stand without crutches, and a swing-to or swing-through gait is possible with crutches or walker. The parapodium allows the paralyzed child to stand and engage in activities at regular work benches. Minor foot deformities can be accommo-

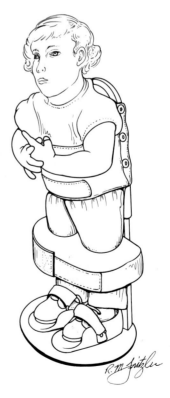

Fig. 12-4   A-frame permits standing without hand support.

dated without special modifications. The Orlau parapodium is recommended for severe neurologic involvement in a child with poor trunk balance and upper extremity function. The child is held upright in a rigid stable frame, the base plate of which is mounted on swiveling foot plates. The user rocks from side to side with movement of the upper portion of the trunk, and as one foot plate clears the ground, the whole device swivels forward automatically on the other foot plate. Ambulation is achieved without the use of crutches, and free use of the hands is achieved. Rose et al advise the use of the Orlau parapodium in all children with lesions at the level of L3 and above because of its lower energy consumption. Those with severe impairment involving the upper limbs, obesity, or other problems that have precluded walking can continue using the device into adulthood.

An ankle-foot orthosis (AFO) is used in children with low lumbar or sacral level lesions who have fair quadriceps function. The AFO should be rigid enough to provide ankle and foot stabilization and maintain the ankle at 90 degrees. Some special padding may be required over the medial malleolus, the head of the talus, and the navicular. In patients with pronation and abnormal hindfoot valgus, the orthosis should maintain the forefoot in slight supination to help control the hindfoot valgus. Rotational problems in children with low lumbar level lesions may be controlled by a twister cable attached to a pelvic band.

The indications for a knee-ankle-foot orthosis (KAFO) are less clear. It is used for a child with weak quadriceps (L1-3 level lesion) or with a low lumbar lesion to protect the knee from abnormal valgus or varus stress during the stance phase of gait. Children with high level lesions often have excessive anterior pelvic tilt and lumbar lordosis and require a pelvic band, either as a conventional hip-knee-ankle-foot orthosis (HKAFO) or a reciprocating gait orthosis.

The conventional HKAFO is most appropriate for children with high lumbar–thoracic level lesions in whom the hip and knee joints are locked. A butterfly pelvic band is recommended to provide better control of anterior pelvic tilt.

The reciprocating gait orthosis (RGO) is a modification of the HKAFO first proposed by Carroll and subsequently refined by Douglas. Through a special cable system, flexion of the hip assists extension of the opposite hip, leading to a reciprocal gait with crutches or walker (Fig. 12-5). A cable release allows bilateral hip flexion for sitting. Light-weight, thermoplastic, and aluminum components have decreased the weight of the orthosis to the range of 2.5 to 7 pounds depending on size. Yngve et al, in a review of their initial experience with the RGO, found the most striking feature of ambulation was the smoothness of the gait pattern and a higher ambulatory speed compared with the HKAFO. Dias et al in 1986 reported initial experience with the RGO and found a direct relationship between normal sitting balance with no hand support and the effectiveness of the orthosis. When trunk balance was normal, 35% were community ambulators and 50% were household ambulators. The RGO can be used as soon as the child has shown good sitting balance, usually around the age of 2 years. Other factors, such as obesity and motivation, can adversely affect the walking ability of the adolescent with myelomeningocele.

Contraindications for the RGO include (1) poor trunk balance that requires hand support, (2) severe upper extremity involvement, (3) mental retardation, (4) severe visual defects, (5) severe scoliosis (more than 50 degrees), and (6) hip flexion contracture (more than 20 to 30 degrees). Accurate fitting of the orthosis is mandatory. Any leg-length discrepancy must be compensated by adequate shoe lift.

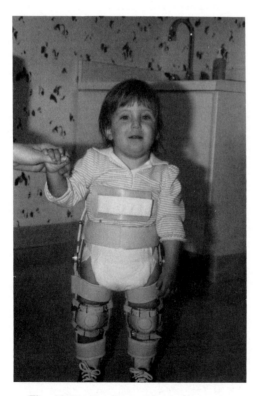

Fig. 12-5   Reciprocating gait orthosis.

SURGICAL TREATMENT

Surgical procedures frequently are required for correction of deformities in children with myelomeningocele, the majority of which are performed during the first 15 years of life. Deformity should be completely and permanently corrected, which often requires radical soft tissue release. Menelaus noted the necessity of overcoming the physician's natural reluctance to sacrifice motor function, as there are few reliable tendon transfers for children with myelomeningocele. Tendon lengthening rarely is done; the tendon is divided and a portion is excised. All deformities, if possible, should be treated during one period of anesthesia. When this is not possible, operations should be performed a short time apart so that only one period of plaster immobilization is necessary. Early weight bearing is encouraged to minimize osteoporosis and pathologic fractures after cast removal. When the period of immobilization in a hip spica cast exceeds 3 to 4 weeks, the cast should be removed while the child is hospitalized to allow a well-controlled physical therapy program for regaining range of motion and ambulation. Pathologic fractures around the knee occur in about 20% of patients after surgery. Pathologic fractures should be treated with brace immobilization rather than casting when possible. After radical soft tissue release, prolonged night splinting is recommended to decrease the recurrence of the deformity. Muscle imbalance should be corrected before, or at the same time as, correction of the structural bony deformities.

Foot

Approximately three fourths of children with myelomeningocele have deformities of the foot, and because ambulation is possible only with a plantigrade foot, these deformities can seriously limit function. Repeated operations frequently are necessary for correction of foot deformities, either because of

Table 12-1 Foot deformities in patients with myelomeningocele*

Level	Clubfoot	Calcaneovalgus deformity	Vertical talus	No deformity
Thoracic	40	8	0	38
L1, L2	22	4	1	13
L3	24	2	1	9
L4	50	4	0	14
L5	11	38	5	20
Sacral	19	4	0	41
TOTAL	166	60	7	135

From Schafer MF and Dias LS: Myelomeningocele: orthopaedic treatment, Baltimore, 1983, Williams & Wilkins Co.
*In patients with asymmetric paralysis, each foot was counted separately.

inadequate correction or unrecognized muscle imbalance and spasticity. Sharrard and Grossfield reported that 14% of children with foot deformities required repeated procedures and that 19% had persistent deformity despite multiple surgeries. A mobile, braceable foot is the goal of orthopaedic treatment, and muscle-balancing procedures that remove motors are more reliable than tendon-transfer procedures. Arthrodesis should be avoided whenever possible, and correction of bony deformities can be obtained by appropriate osteotomies that preserve joint motion.

Foot deformities can be classified (Table 12-1) as (1) clubfoot, (2) acquired equinovarus, (3) varus, (4) metatarsus adductus, (5) equinus, (6) equinovalgus, (7) congenital vertical talus, (8) developmental vertical talus, (9) calcaneus, (10) calcaneovalgus, (11) calcaneovarus, (12) calcaneocavus, (13) cavus, (14) cavovarus, (15) supination, (16) pes planovalgus, and (17) toe deformities.

Clubfoot

Approximately 30% of children with myelomeningocele have clubfoot at birth. There is a marked difference between idiopathic clubfoot and the equinovarus deformity in children with myelomeningocele, which resembles the deformity in arthrogryposis multiplex congenita. The clubfoot deformity is characterized by a severely rigid foot. Supination-varus deformity may be caused by the unopposed action of an active anterior tibial muscle. Rotational malalignment of the calcaneus and talus and calcaneocuboid and talonavicular subluxation are always present, and a cavus component may occur. Menelaus emphasizes that severe internal tibial torsion often is associated with equinovarus foot deformity.

Equinovarus deformities have a high incidence of recurrence despite adequate initial surgical correction. Correction rarely, if ever, is achieved by only serial casting, but serial casting may be used initially to achieve partial correction and to stretch the soft tissues. Surgery should be performed when the child is 10 to 18 months of age. Radical posteromedial-lateral release by means of the Cincinnati incision (p. 82) is recommended. All tendons should be excised rather than lengthened.

If the anterior tibial tendon is active, simple tenotomy should be performed to prevent supination adduction deformity. In the older child (older than the age of 2 to 3 years), the imbalance between the medial and lateral column lengths may be so severe that soft tissue release alone will not fully correct the adduction deformity. Shortening of the lateral column should be performed either by closing wedge osteotomy of the cuboid, lateral wedge resection of the distal end of the calcaneus, preserving the joint surface as described by Lichtblau (p. 93), or calcaneocuboid fusion as described by Evans (p. 90).

Talectomy is indicated for the severely deformed, rigid clubfoot in the older child mainly as a salvage procedure when, because of previous surgeries, the foot has inadequate skin on the medial side. Because of the fibrosis caused by previous operations, dissection around the neurovascular bundle for a complete radical posteromedial release is difficult. Talectomy is done through a curved lateral incision that follows the line of the subtalar and talonavicular joints (p. 94). The talus should be completely removed, because any fragment left behind will resume its growth and cause recurrence of the deformity. The talectomy will correct the hindfoot deformity, but any adduction deformity should be corrected by shortening of the lateral column through the same surgical incision. Reports in the literature indicate that talectomy corrects the hindfoot deformity in most patients, but severe forefoot deformities require midtarsal or metatarsal osteotomies.

Varus Deformity

Isolated varus deformity of the hindfoot is rare. Usually it is associated with adduction deformity of the forefoot, cavus deformity, or supination deformity. Careful examination is required to detect any imbalance between the invertors and evertors. When the rigid hindfoot varus is an isolated deformity, a closing wedge osteotomy (p. 90) is indicated. After removal of the lateral wedge (Fig. 12-6, *A*), an attempt should be made to shift the calcaneus laterally to increase the correction of the hindfoot varus.

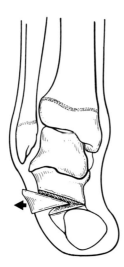

Fig. 12-6 Lateral closing wedge osteotomy of calcaneus for isolated varus deformity of hindfoot.

Cavovarus Deformity

Cavovarus deformities occur mainly in children with sacral-level lesions. Cavus is the primary deformity, and the varus is caused by the cavus. The Coleman test (p. 725) should be used to judge the degree of rigidity of the varus deformity. If the varus is supple, radical plantar release (p. 727) should be performed for the cavus deformity without hindfoot surgery. If the varus is rigid, in spite of plantar release with or without midtarsal osteotomy, the varus deformity of the hindfoot should be corrected by closing wedge osteotomy of the calcaneus (p. 93). Any muscle imbalance must be corrected either before the bony procedures or at the same time. Triple arthrodesis (p. 94) occasionally is performed in patients with myelomeningocele. Hayes and Gross in 1964 reported that triple arthrodesis failed in 13 of 45 feet (28%) in their patients with myelomeningocele. Olney and Menelaus reported 83% satisfactory results in 18 feet. They concluded that triple arthrodesis in patients with myelomeningocele is a demanding operation that may require revision, but once the deformity is corrected and a solid fusion obtained, the results do not deteriorate with time.

Supination Deformity

Supination deformity of the forefoot may be associated with adduction deformity and is produced by the unopposed action of the tibialis anterior when the peroneus brevis and longus are inactive. This deformity occurs most often in children with L5-S1–level lesions. If muscle imbalance is not corrected, the deformity will become fixed. If the foot is supple, simple tenotomy of the anterior tibial tendon is adequate. If there is some gastrocsoleus activity and no spasticity, the anterior tibial tendon can be transferred to the midfoot in line with the third metatarsal. Occasionally, split transfer of the anterior tibial tendon (p. 669) can be used with the lateral half of the tendon inserted in the cuboid. When bony deformity is present, in addition to the transfer of the anterior tibial tendon, osteotomy of the first cuneiform or at the base of the first metatarsal may be required.

Equinus Deformity

Equinus foot deformity occurs most frequently in children with high lumbar– and thoracic-level lesions. It usually is an acquired deformity that can be prevented by bracing and splinting, but when it occurs, it requires surgical treatment because of difficulties with orthotic fitting. Simple tendo Achilles excision corrects mild deformities. The tendo Achilles is exposed through a tranverse incision, and about 2 cm of the tendon is excised. A short-leg cast is applied with the foot in neutral rotation and is worn for 10 days; then an AFO is used at night. For more severe equinus deformity, radical posterior release is necessary. Through a Cincinnati incision (p. 84), all tendons are excised, and extensive capsulotomies of the ankle and subtalar joints are performed. A short-leg cast with the foot in a neutral position is worn for 6 weeks, followed by an AFO worn at night. Rarely, osteotomy or talectomy may be necessary to correct symptomatic equinus deformity.

Calcaneus Deformity

Calcaneus deformity occurs in approximately one third of children with myelomeningocele, most often those with lesions of the L5-S1 level. Calcaneovalgus deformity is the most common because of active muscles in the anterior compartment of the leg and inactive muscles in the posterior compartment. In children with high-level lesions, spasticity of the evertors and dorsiflexors may cause the deformity. The valgus may be either at the subtalar joint or associated with valgus deformity at the ankle joint. When the deformity is present at birth, the foot appears to be in acute dorsiflexion because of the active dorsiflexors. Usually the deformity is not rigid, and the foot can be brought to a neutral position by simple manipulation and held in this position by splinting. If the deformity is quite rigid, serial casting may be used, followed by splinting. If untreated, calcaneus deformity produces a bulky, prominent heel that is prone to pressure sores and that makes shoe wear difficult. External tibial torsion frequently is associated with calcaneovalgus deformity. Early correction of muscle imbalance can be achieved by simple tenotomy of all ankle dorsiflexors and tenotomy of the peroneus brevis and longus.

Anterolateral release

▶ *Technique.* With the patient supine on the operating table, apply and inflate a pneumatic tourniquet. Make a transverse incision about 2.5 cm in length 2 to 3 cm above the ankle joint (Fig. 12-7, *A*). With sharp dissection, divide the superficial fascia to expose the tendons of the extensor hallucis longus, extensor digitorum communis, and anterior tibial tendons. Divide each tendon, and excise at least 2 cm of each (Fig. 12-7, *B*). Locate the peroneus tertius tendon in the most lateral part of the wound and divide it. Make a second incision longitudinally above the ankle joint laterally and posterior to the fibula (Fig. 12-7, *A*). Identify and divide the peroneus brevis and longus tendons, and excise a section of each (Fig. 12-7, *C*). Close the wound, and apply a short-leg walking cast.

▶ *Postoperative management.* The cast is worn for 10 days, and then an AFO is fabricated for night wear.

• • •

After anterolateral release, in some patients spasticity may develop in the gastrocsoleus muscle, causing an equinus deformity that requires tenotomy of the tendo Achilles or posterior release.

Although transfer of the anterior tibial tendon through the interosseous membrane to the calcaneus has been used successfully for calcaneus deformity in poliomyelitis, the results of this procedure are not as good in children with myelomeningocele. The frequent spastic component in these children often causes an equinus deformity. Banta et al added tendo Achilles tibial tenodesis to the tendon transfer in seven patients with bilateral deformities and reported improvement of hindfoot and midfoot support, as well as control over ankle and knee motion and walking velocity with an orthosis. Menelaus reported that the best results in 51 feet were obtained when the tibialis anterior alone was transferred. The transfer of several tendons was complicated by the development of equinus deformity that required division of the transferred tendons in four feet. Valgus deformities developed in 35 feet and required subtalar fusion in 18 and triple arthrodesis in 10.

Anterior tibial transfer to calcaneus

▶ *Technique.* With the patient supine on the operating table, make an incision in the dorsal aspect of the foot at the level of the insertion of the anterior tibial tendon at the base of the first metatarsal. Carefully detach the tendon from its insertion, and free it as far proximally as possible. Make a second incision on the anterolateral aspect of the leg, just lateral to the tibial crest, about 3 to 4 cm above the ankle joint. Free the tendon as far distally as possible, and bring it up into the proximal wound. Expose the interosseous membrane, and make a wide opening. Then make a third transverse incision posteriorly at the level of the insertion of the tendo Achilles in the calcaneus. Using a tendon passer, bring the anterior tibial tendon through the interosseous membrane from anterior to posterior down to the level of this incision. Drill a large hole in the calcaneus, starting posteriorly and medially and exiting laterally and plantarward. After a Bunnell suture is passed through the tendon, use a Keith needle to draw the tendon through the hole. A button suture is not recommended because of pressure sores. Suture the tendon to the surrounding soft tissue structures at the level of its entrance into the calcaneus, as well as to the tendo Achilles. Close the wound, and apply a short-leg cast.

In severe calcaneus deformity in the older child with a major degree of structural deformity, simple tendon transfers or tenotomies seldom achieve correction and bony procedures are indicated, such as posterior wedge osteotomy of the calcaneus.

Hindfoot Valgus

Excessive hindfoot valgus often is associated with valgus deformity at the ankle joint, which exacerbates the hindfoot valgus. Initially, this deformity can be controlled with a well-fitted orthosis. Occasionally, to decrease the pressure over the head of the talus, the AFO should be made with the forefoot in slight supination. As the child becomes taller and heavier and control of the valgus deformity becomes more difficult, pressure sores over the medial malleolus and

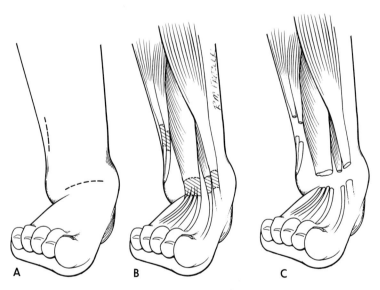

Fig. 12-7 Anterolateral release for calcaneus deformity (see text). **A,** Transverse and longitudinal incisions. **B** and **C,** Excision of portion of tendons and tendon sheaths.

head of the talus are common and surgical treatment is indicated. The Grice extraarticular arthrodesis (p. 100) is classic management of this problem, but frequent problems associated with the procedure include resorption of the graft, nonunion, varus overcorrection, and residual valgus. Recently Gallien et al reported their experience with subtalar arthrodesis in children with myelomeningocele. Of the 14 arthrodeses, 61% were successful. Unsatisfactory results were caused by overcorrection, residual valgus, and nonunion. Ross and Lyne, however, reported 80% unsatisfactory results in patients with myelomeningocele. Medial displacement osteotomy of the calcaneus has been reported by several authors as an effective means of correction of the hindfoot valgus, although few reports include patients with myelomeningocele. Clinical and roentgenographic measurements of hindfoot valgus (p. 695) should be obtained; more than 10 mm of "lateral shift" of the calcaneus is considered significant.

Medial displacement osteotomy of calcaneus

▶ *Technique.* With the patient supine on the operating table and the tourniquet inflated, make an incision beginning near the lateral Achilles tuberosity and extending distally parallel and plantar to the sural nerve. Split the soft tissue bluntly directly down to the bone. Reflect the peroneal tendons and sural nerve superiorly. Insert a Kirschner wire on the lateral surface of the calcaneus, parallel to the plantar surface of the foot. Obtain roentgenograms to determine the exact level of the osteotomy. Begin the osteotomy just behind the posterior subtalar articulation, and direct it plantarward toward the origin of the plantar aponeurosis (Fig. 12-8, *A*). Place retractors proximally to protect the insertion of the tendo Achilles in the calcaneus and distally proximal to the plantar fascia and short flexor musculature origin. A power saw can be used initially, but make the most medial cut with an osteotome. Because the medial extent of the osteotomy is not performed under direct vision, be careful not to penetrate the periosteum. After the osteotomy is completed, shift the loose proximal fragment medially to correct the lateral displacement of the calcaneus and use internal fixation to maintain correction. Insert a threaded Kirschner wire vertically through the distal fragment and across the proximal fragment, but do not enter the subtalar joint (Fig. 12-8, *B*). Because of the medial displacement of the calcaneus (Fig. 12-9), closure of the surgical wound will cause some tension at the suture line. To avoid wound healing problems, use nylon sutures. Leave a suction drain in place, and apply a short-leg cast.

▶ *Postoperative management.* If a Kirschner wire is used for internal fixation, the child is kept nonweight bearing for 2 weeks; then the cast and wire are removed, and a new short-leg walking cast is applied to be worn another 4 weeks.

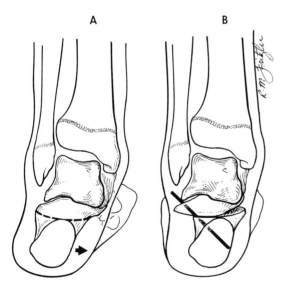

Fig. 12-8 Medial displacement of calcaneus for hindfoot valgus. **A,** Transverse osteotomy of calcaneus. **B,** Fixation with Kirschner wire after distal fragment is shifted medially to place calcaneus in weight-bearing line of tibia.

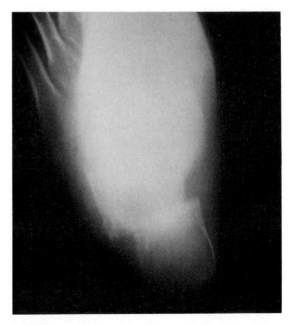

Fig. 12-9 Early follow-up with excellent medial displacement of calcaneus.

In patients with myelomeningocele it is important to recognize the combination of hindfoot and ankle valgus. If the valgus deformity at the ankle is more than 10 to 15 degrees, closing wedge osteotomy or hemiepiphysiodesis of the distal tibial physis is recommended in association with sliding osteotomy of the calcaneus.

Vertical Talus

Approximately 10% of children with myelomeningocele have a vertical talus deformity characterized by malalignment of the hindfoot and midfoot. The talus is in an almost vertical position, the calcaneus is in equinus and valgus, the navicular is dislocated dorsally on the talus, and at times the cuboid may be dorsally subluxated in relation to the calcaneus. The bone and joint abnormalities result from the soft tissue contractures and are caused by remodeling of bone and cartilage to adapt to abnormal forces. Two types of vertical talus deformities occur in children with myelomeningocele: developmental and congen-

ital. Neither type can be corrected by conservative means. In developmental vertical talus the foot is more supple and the talonavicular dislocation can be reduced by plantar flexion of the foot. In congenital vertical talus, manipulation and serial casting may partially correct the soft tissue contractures in preparation for complete posteromedial-lateral release (p. 84), which should be performed when the child is approximately 12 to 18 months old.

Pes Cavus Deformity

Cavus deformity, alone or in association with clawing of the toes or varus deformity of the hindfoot, occurs most often in children with sacral level lesions. The deformity may cause painful callosities under the metatarsal heads and rapid breakdown of shoes. As stressed by Paulos et al, failure to correct the plantar flexion of the first ray essentially eliminates any chance of success. Several procedures have been proposed for treatment of this deformity, but little has been written about its treatment in patients with myelomeningocele. For the cavus deformity alone, with no hindfoot varus, a radical plantar release is indicated. When varus deformity is present, medial subtalar release (p. 727) is indicated. After surgery a short-leg cast in applied, and 1 to 2 weeks after surgery, gradual correction of the deformity is obtained by means of weekly or every-other-week cast changes for approximately 6 weeks. In the older child with a rigid cavus deformity, anterior first metatarsal closing wedge osteotomy (p. 727) is indicated in addition to radical plantar release. For residual varus deformity, Dwyer closing-wedge osteotomy of the calcaneus (p. 90) is performed.

Toe Deformities

Claw toes or hammer toes occur most often in children with sacral-level lesions and may cause problems with shoe and orthotic fitting. For claw toe alone, simple tenotomy of the flexors at the level of the proximal phalanx usually is sufficient. The tendo suspension, as described by Jones (Fig. 12-10), is indicated when clawing of the toes is associated with cavus deformity. For clawing of the great toe, arthrodesis of the proximal interphalangeal joint (p. 676) or tenodesis of the distal stump of the extensor pollicis to the extensor pollicis brevis is recommended. An alternative method of correction of claw toes and cavus deformity is the Jones procedure (p. 728) for the great toe only and the Hibbs transfer (p. 728) for the remaining toes.

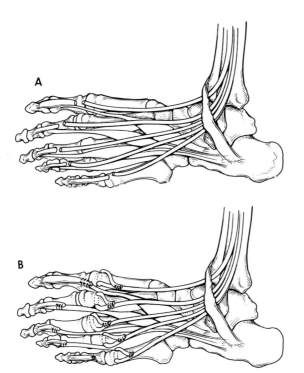

Fig. 12-10 Jones procedure for clawing of great toe. **A,** Extensor tendons are divided distally. **B,** Each tendon is passed through drill hole at neck of metatarsals and sutured to itself.

Ankle
Progressive Valgus Deformity

Progressive valgus deformity may occur at the ankle or in combination with hindfoot valgus. This deformity is most common in children with low lumbar–level lesions. Severe valgus deformity can cause significant problems with brace fitting. The medial malleolus is bulky, the head of the talus is shifted medially, and pressure ulceration of these areas is frequent. Clinically, a calcaneus foot is obvious, and often external tibial torsion also is present. The gastrocsoleus muscle strength is decreased or absent, and excessive laxity of the tendo Achilles is characterized by marked passive ankle dorsiflexion. The calcaneovalgus deformity appears quite early, but problems with orthotic fitting usually do not arise until after the child is 6 years of age. Fibular shortening is common in children with lesions of L4-5 or higher. In the paralytic limb, abnormal shortening of the fibula and lateral malleolus results in a valgus tilt of the talus with subsequent valgus deformity at the ankle (Fig. 12-11). Makin described a delay in the appearance of the fibular epiphysis in 10 children with myelomeningocele, all of whom had shortening of the fibula. With abnormal shortening of the fibula, normal distribution of forces on the distal tibial articular surface is altered, causing increased compression forces on the lateral portion of the tibial epiphysis and inhibiting growth. The decreased compression on the medial portion of the tibial epiphysis accelerated growth. Such imbalance causes the lateral wedging that leads to a valgus inclination of the talus. The degree of lateral wedging of the tibial epiphysis correlates well with the degree of fibular shortening (Fig. 12-12).

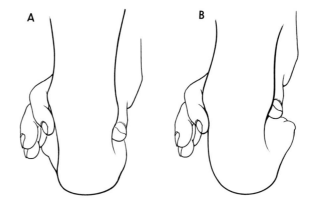

Fig. 12-11 **A,** Posterior view of right foot of normal child with correct alignment of malleoli and hindfoot. **B,** In child with myelomeningocele, medial malleolus is prominent and lateral malleolus is shortened, causing valgus deformity of ankle.

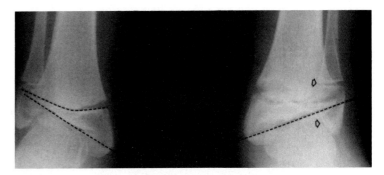

Fig. 12-12 Weight-bearing roentgenogram shows valgus deformity of ankle with severe shortening of fibula.

Accurate evaluation of valgus deformity in the child with myelomeningocele requires determination of three parameters: (1) the degree of fibular shortening, (2) the degree of valgus tilt of the talus in the ankle mortice, and (3) the amount of "lateral shift" of the calcaneus in relation to the weight-bearing line of the tibia. The amount of fibular shortening can be determined by measuring the distance between the distal fibular physis and the dome of the talus. In the normal ankle joint the distal fibular physis is 2 to 3 mm proximal to the dome of the talus in children up to 4 years of age (Fig. 12-13, *A*). Between the ages of 4 and 8 years the physis is at the same level as the talar dome (Fig. 12-13, *B*), and in children older than the age of 8 years, 2 to 3 mm distal to the talar dome (Fig. 12-13, *C*). A difference of less than 10 mm from normal is considered mild shortening, but differences greater than 10 mm are significant. The valgus tilt of the talus can be measured accurately on anteroposterior, weight-bearing roentgenograms.

Accurate measurement of the lateral shift of the calcaneus is more difficult. Stevens, as well as Busch et al., described roentgenographic techniques to evaluate valgus at the ankle joint and hindfoot alignment (Fig. 12-14, *A*). If talar tilt exceeds 10 degrees, Stevens recommends tilting the roentgen tube appropriately to obtain a true lateral weight-bearing view of the foot on which the weight-bearing line of the tibia is drawn, and the distance from this line to the center of the calcaneus is measured. Busch and Pozanski also use a weight-bearing anteroposterior roentgenogram, directing the beam horizontally and preserving the coronal relationship in both dimensions. They position the foot in slight dorsiflexion by placing a hard foam wedge under the plantar surface but not under the calcaneus and positioning the cassette behind the foot and ankle. The normal lateral shift of the calcaneus is from 5 to 10 mm (Fig. 12-14, *B*); if the center of the calcaneus is more than 10 mm lateral to the weight-bearing line, excessive valgus is present (Fig. 12-14, *C*). This technique is useful to determine preoperatively if the valgus deformity is at the ankle or subtalar level, and a nonweight-bearing roentgenogram can be used postoperatively to assess the correction obtained by sliding osteotomy of the calcaneus.

A   B   C

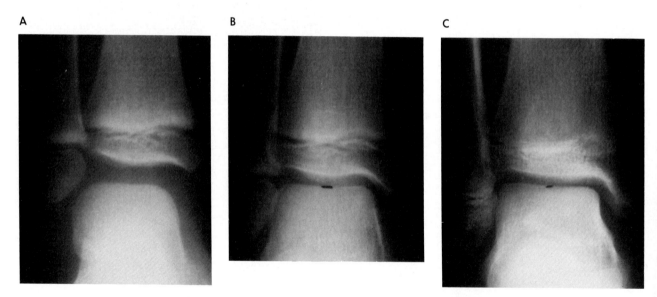

Fig. 12-13 Normal position of distal fibular physis. **A,** Proximal to dome of talus in children up to 4 years of age. **B,** Level with dome of talus in children between 4 and 8 years of age. **C,** Distal to dome of talus in children older than 8 years of age.

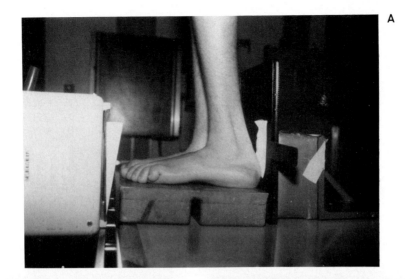

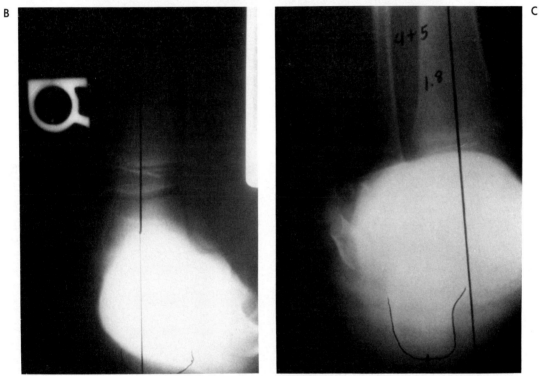

Fig. 12-14 Roentgenographic technique for evaluation of ankle valgus (see text). **A,** Normal ankle valgus on weight-bearing view. **B,** Normal shift of calcaneus is from 5 to 10 mm. **C,** Lateral shift of 15 to 18 mm indicates excessive valgus.

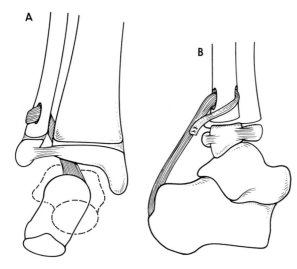

Fig. 12-15 **A,** Anterior and, **B,** lateral views of tenodesis of tendo Achilles to calcaneus.

Surgical treatment of ankle valgus deformity is indicated when the deformity causes problems with orthotic fitting and cannot be alleviated with orthoses. Tenodesis of the tendo Achilles to the fibula was first described by Westin and Defiore for patients with poliomyelitis. Dias, and more recently Stevens and Toomey, described this operation for patients with myelomeningocele (Fig. 12-15). Tendo Achilles tenodesis is indicated in patients between the ages of 6 and 10 years with valgus talar tilt between 10 and 25 degrees (Fig. 12-16). When significant bony deformities are present, other procedures may be indicated, such as hemiepiphysiodesis for mild deformity in a child with remaining growth potential or supramalleolar derotation osteotomy (p. 200) for severe bony angular deformity, which also may improve rotational alignment. If the valgus deformity is in the subtalar joint and calcaneus, a medial sliding osteotomy of the calcaneus (p. 693) may be indicated. Medial osteotomy is preferable to Grice subtalar arthrodesis, which results in a stiff subtalar joint. For valgus in both the ankle and subtalar joints, the calcaneal osteotomy can be done in conjunction with correction of the ankle.

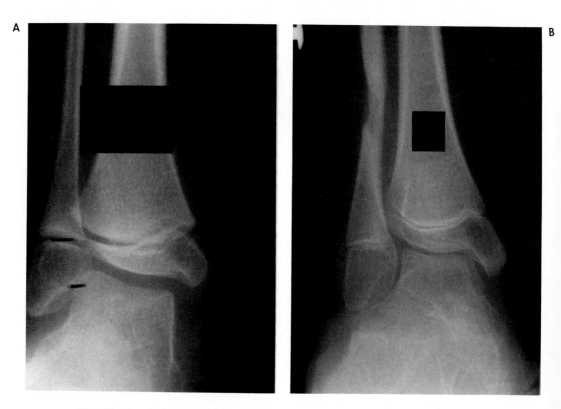

Fig. 12-16 **A,** Preoperative valgus deformity. **B,** Correction after tenodesis of tendo Achilles to fibula.

Tendo Achilles tenodesis

▲ *Technique.* Place the patient in the supine position, tilted toward the nonoperative side. Apply and inflate a pneumatic tourniquet. Make a posterolateral longitudinal skin incision just behind the posterior border of the fibula, beginning about 7 to 10 cm above the tip of the lateral malleolus and extending distally to the tendo Achilles insertion in the calcaneus. Expose the tendo Achilles, and section it transversely at the musculotendinous junction, usually 6 cm from its insertion. Stevens advised that the tendon be split eccentrically, leaving the lateral one fifth to prevent retraction. Transect the medial four fifths proximally. Expose the peroneus brevis and longus tendons, and if they are completely paralyzed or spastic, excise them. Expose the distal fibula, taking care not to damage the fibular physis. About 4 cm proximal to the distal physis, using a fine drill bit, make a longitudinal hole in the anteroposterior direction. The size of the hole should be such that the tendo Achilles can be passed easily through it (Fig. 12-17, *A*). If the tendon is too large, trim it longitudinally for about 2.5 cm. Bring the tendo Achilles through the hole, and suture it to itself under enough tension to limit ankle dorsiflexion to 0 degrees (Fig. 12-17, *B*). Do not suture the tendon in too much equinus because of the possibility of causing a fixed equinus deformity.

Westin and Defiore recommend a T-shaped incision in the periosteum instead of a drill hole with imbrication of the distal segment of the sectioned tendon below the periosteum with absorbable sutures. Stevens believes the hypoplastic fibula is too small to permit placing the tendon through a tunnel in the bone and that the periosteum is too flimsy to rely on periosteal sutures alone; he recommends that the tendon be sutured to the fibular shaft with absorbable sutures placed through two oblique drill holes.

In patients with active anterior tibial tendons, simultaneous transfer of this tendon through the interosseous membrane to the calcaneus is indicated to avoid stretching the tendo Achilles after surgery (Fig. 12-17, *C*).

▲ *Postoperative management.* Weight bearing is allowed in a short-leg cast with the ankle in 5 to 10 degrees of equinus. The cast is removed after 6 weeks, and an AFO with the ankle in neutral position is fitted.

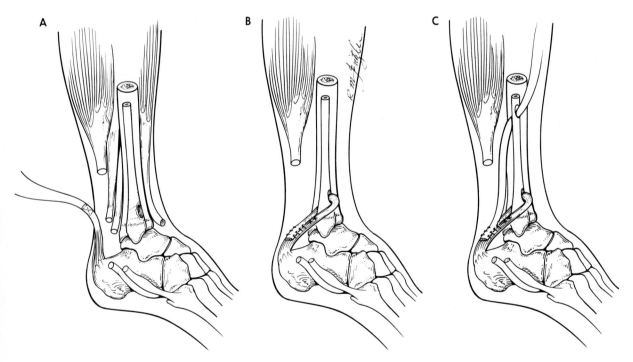

Fig. 12-17 Tenodesis of tendo Achilles. **A,** After division of tendo Achilles, tenotomy of peroneus brevis and longus, and detachment of anterior tibial tendon from its insertion, longitudinal hole is made in fibula 2 cm proximal to physis. **B,** Tendo Achilles is passed through hole in fibula and sutured to itself. **C,** If necessary, anterior tibial tendon may be passed through interosseous membrane and attached to calcaneus.

Hemiepiphysiodesis of distal tibial physis. Burkus et al in 1983 reported the use of hemiepiphysiodesis of the distal tibial physis for correction of the valgus deformity of the ankle in young children with myelomeningocele in whom lateral tibial epiphyseal growth remains and in whom the valgus deformity is less than 20 degrees and the fibular shortening is not severe. Through a medial incision at the ankle level, the medial aspect of the distal tibial physis is exposed and epiphysiodesis is performed either percutaneously or open as described by Blount and Phemister (Fig. 12-18). With the growth arrest on the medial aspect of the physis and continued growth on the lateral aspect, there is gradual correction of the lateral wedging of the tibial epiphysis, which corrects the valgus tilt. If overcorrection occurs, the epiphysiodesis should be completed laterally. This technique is simple and yields excellent results; however, it does not correct any rotational component of the deformity and derotation osteotomy of the distal tibia and fibula may be required.

Supramalleolar varus derotation osteotomy. In the older child (older than the age of 10 years) with a low lumbar level lesion who has severe fibular shortening (more than 10 to 20 mm), valgus tilt in the an-

kle mortice of more than 20 degrees, and external tibial torsion, the deformity can be corrected by supramalleolar varus derotation osteotomy.

▶ *Technique.* With the patient supine on the operating table, make an anterior longitudinal skin incision at the distal third of the leg. Expose the distal tibia and metaphyseal area, and identify the physis. Make a second incision over the distal third of the fibula, and perform an oblique osteotomy starting laterally and extending distally and medially, depending on the degree of valgus to be corrected (determined from preoperative weight-bearing, anteroposterior roentgenograms). Make the medial-based wedge osteotomy as distal on the tibia as possible (Fig. 12-19, *A*). At the time of correction of the valgus, rotate the distal fragment internally to correct external tibial torsion. Use two Kirschner wires to temporarily hold the osteotomy in place, and obtain roentgenograms to evaluate correction of the valgus deformity. The talus should be in a horizontal postion with the lateral malleolus lower than the medial malleolus. Powered staples or Kirschner wires (or in skeletally mature patients, a plate and screws) can be used for internal fixation (Fig. 12-19, *B*). Close the wound in the routine manner, and apply a long-leg cast with the ankle and foot in neutral position.

▶ *Postoperative management.* The child is allowed to partially bear weight with crutches immediately after surgery. Three weeks after surgery the cast is changed for a below-knee cast, and full weight bearing is allowed. Kirschner wire fixation may be removed 8 to 12 weeks after surgery.

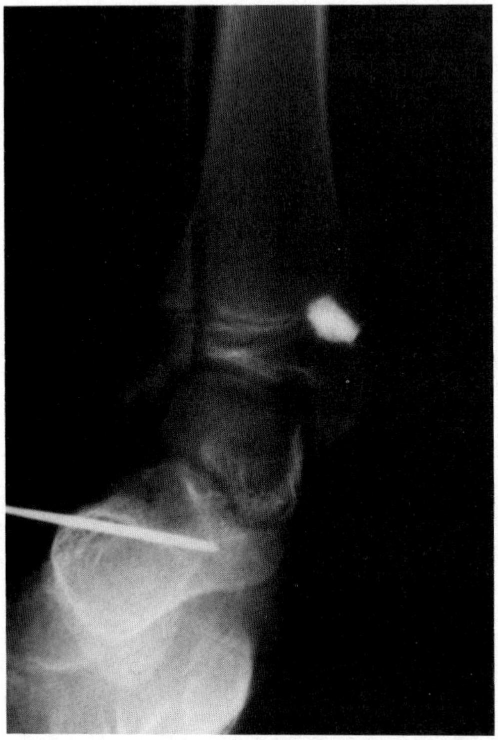

Fig. 12-18 Radiopaque dye shows extent of medial hemiepiphysiodesis of distal tibial physis.

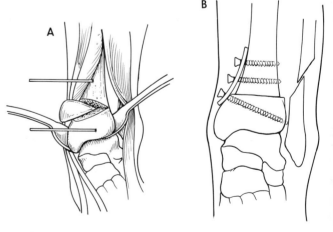

Fig. 12-19 Supramalleolar varus derotation osteotomy for severe ankle valgus deformity in adolescent (see text). **A,** Removal of medial bone wedge from distal tibial metaphysis. **B,** Fixation of osteotomy with plate and screws.

Knee

Four types of deformities involve the knee joint in patients with myelomeningocele: (1) flexion contracture, (2) extension contracture, (3) valgus deformity, and (4) varus deformity.

Muscle Contractures

Flexion contractures are the most common. Reports in the literature indicate that half the children with thoracolumbar level lesions have knee flexion contractures. A knee flexion contracture up to 20 degrees commonly is present at birth and generally corrects spontaneously. Factors that lead to a fixed knee flexion contracture in children with myelomeningocele are (1) the typical postion assumed in the supine position: hips in abduction, flexion, and external rotation, knees in flexion, and feet in equinus, (2) gradual contracture of the hamstring and biceps muscles with contracture of the posterior knee capsule from quadriceps weakness and prolonged sitting, (3) spasticity of the hamstrings, as in the tethered cord syndrome, and (4) paralysis of the gastrocsoleus and gluteus maximus muscles. Knee flexion contractures in children with high level lesions usually are caused by positioning and can be prevented by early splinting (total body splint) and a well-supervised home physical therapy program. In children with low lumbar level lesions, the flexion deformity usually occurs later, after the age of 10 years. With increasing height and weight, even the use of an orthosis to block ankle dorsiflexion does not prevent gradual development of knee flexion deformity. There is no obvious contracture of the hamstrings, but there is contracture of the posterior knee capsule. Radical flexor release generally is required for flexion contractures of 15 to 30 degrees, particularly in the child with a low lumbar level lesions who walks with a below-knee orthosis. Supracondylar extension osteotomy of the femur (p. 702) generally is required for contractures of more than 30 to 45 degrees. If hip flexion deformity is present, both hip and knee contractures should be corrected at the same time.

Radical flexor release

▶ *Technique.* Make a transverse incision just above the flexor crease. In the child with a high level lesion, identify and divide the medial hamstring tendons (semitendinosus, semimembranosus, gracilis, and sartorius). Resect part of each tendon (Fig. 12-20, *A*). Laterally, identify, divide, and resect the biceps tendon and iliotibial band. In the child with a low lumbar level lesion, intramuscularly lengthen the biceps and semimembranosus to preserve some flexor power. Next free the origin of the gastrocnemius from the medial and lateral femoral condyles, expos-

ing the posterior knee capsule, and perform extensive capsulectomy (Fig. 12-20, *B*). If full extension is not obtained, divide the medial and lateral collateral ligaments and the posterior cruciate ligament. Close the wound over a suction drain, and apply a long-leg cast with the knee in full extension. If the flexion contracture is greater than 45 degrees, because of the possibility of vascular problems, the first cast should be applied with the knee in some degree of flexion (20 to 30 degrees) and the knee gradually should be brought to full extension through serial cast changes.

▶ *Postoperative management.* The cast is removed after 14 days, and long-leg splints are used at night. In the child with a low lumbar–level lesion, intensive physical therapy for strengthening of the quadriceps mechanism is imperative after cast removal.

• • •

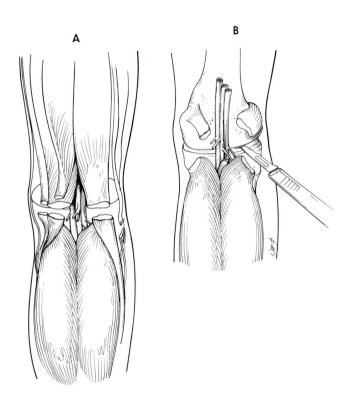

Fig. 12-20 Radical release of flexor tendons for flexion contracture of knee. **A,** All flexor tendons are divided, and about 3 cm of each is resected. **B,** Gastrocnemius origin from femoral condyle is divided and retracted; capsule is completely divided. If full extension is not obtained, posterior cruciate ligament is divided.

Supracondylar extension osteotomy of the femur is indicated in the older child who is a community ambulator and has a fixed knee flexion deformity of more than 15 to 20 degrees and in whom radical knee flexor release was unsuccessful (Fig. 12-21). In the older child who is not a community ambulator, no surgical treatment is indicated if the knee flexion contracture is not interfering with mobility.

Extension contracture of the knee is much less common than flexion contracture. The deformity usually is bilateral and frequently is associated with other congenital anomalies, such as dislocation of the ipsilateral hip, external rotation contracture of the hip, equinovarus deformity of the foot, and occasionally a valgus deformity of the knee. Knee extension contracture can seriously decrease ambulation, making wheelchair sitting and transfer in and out of a motor vehicle very difficult. Treatment with serial casting, attempting to flex the knee to at least 90 degrees, is successful in most patients. If conservative treatment does not correct the deformity, lengthening of the quadriceps mechanism (p. 736) is indicated. Several methods of lengthening have been reported, including "anterior circumcision" (Dupre and Walker), in which all the structures in front and at the side of the knee are divided by subcutaneous tenotomy, Z-plasty

of the extensor mechanism combined with anterior capsulotomy (Parsch and Manner), and V-Y quadriceps lengthening (Chapter 2) (Curtis and Fisher). Ninety degrees of knee flexion should be obtained before the quadriceps mechanism is sutured in its lengthened position. After surgery the knee is immobilized in a cast at 45 to 60 degrees of flexion for 2 weeks. After cast removal, active and passive range-of-motion exercises are begun.

Varus or Valgus Deformity

Varus or valgus deformity of the knee may be caused by malunion of a supracondylar fracture of the femur or proximal metaphyseal fracture of the tibia. Contracture of the iliotibial band also can cause a valgus deformity. For mild varus or valgus deformity, no treatment is indicated. If the iliotibial band is contracted, division of the distal portion is advised (Yount procedure, p. 704). More severe deformities that interfere with bracing and mobility require either supracondylar (p. 33) or tibial (p. 39) osteotomy with internal fixation.

Hip

Hip deformities and instability in the child with myelomeningocele can result from muscle imbalance or congenital dysplasia, or both. Nearly half the children with myelomeningocele have either hip subluxation or dislocation, and hip contractures can be more of a problem than the dislocation itself. Hip abduction or adduction contractures can cause infrapelvic obliquity, which may interfere with ambulation and bracing. The cause, prevention, and treatment of hip dislocations in these children are significantly different from those of congenital hip dislocation. Patients with myelomeningocele may have different levels of paralysis, and spasticity may be mixed with flaccid paralysis; thus treatment must be individualized.

Muscle Contracture

Flexion deformity of the hip is more frequent in children with high lumbar-thoracic level lesions and is caused by the unopposed action of the hip flexors (iliopsoas, sartorius, and rectus), by long periods of lying supine or sitting, or by spasticity of the hip flexors. Abduction-external rotation contractures also are frequently present. Hip flexion contractures must be distinguished from the physiologic flexion position. The amount of hip flexion contracture should be measured by the Thomas test. Shurtleff et al found

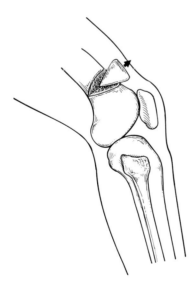

Fig. 12-21 Supracondylar extension osteotomy of femur for fixed knee flexion deformity in older child; removal of anterior wedge.

that in the first 27 months of life, the deformity decreased except in patients with lesions at T12 and above. Because of this tendency to decrease, hip flexion deformities rarely should be treated surgically in patients younger than 24 months of age. Surgical release is indicated to correct any hip flexion deformity that interferes with bracing and walking but rarely is required for contractures of less than 20 degrees. Associated knee flexion contractures are common in children with high level lesions and should be corrected at the same time as the hip contracture.

Correction of hip flexion contractures is performed through an anterior approach and involves the release of the sartorius, rectus femoris, iliopsoas, and tensor fasciae latae muscles and the anterior hip capsule, as well as the iliopsoas tendon. Anterior hip release should adequately correct flexion contractures up to 60 degrees. If hip deformity remains after release, subtrochanteric extension osteotomy is indicated (Fig. 12-22), but osteotomy should be postponed until near skeletal maturity to avoid recurrence of the deformity.

Anterior hip release

▶ *Technique.* Make a "bikini" skin incision slightly distal and parallel to the iliac crest, extending it obliquely along the inguinal crease. Identify and protect the neurovascular bundle medially. Identify the iliopsoas tendon as far distally as possible, and divide the tendon transversely. Divide the sartorius muscle from its origin in the superior iliac crest, and then identify the rectus insertion in the anteroinferior iliac crest and divide it. Identify laterally the tensor fasciae latae, and after carefully separating it from the fascia, divide the fascia transversely completely posteriorly to the anterior border of the glutei muscles to expose the anterior hip capsule. If any residual flexion contracture is present, open the joint capsule transversely about 2 cm from the acetabular labrum. Place a suction drain in the wound, suture the subcutaneous tissue with interrupted sutures, and approximate the skin edges with subcuticular nylon sutures. Apply a hip spica cast with the hip in full extension, 10 degrees of abduction, and neutral rotation.

In a child with a low lumbar level lesion the anterior hip release causes significant loss of hip flexor power and may impair mobility. A free tendon graft, using part of the tensor fascia, can be used to reattach the sartorius to the anterosuperior iliac crest and the rectus tendon can be sutured distal to the sartorius muscle in the hip capsule.

▶ *Postoperative management.* Early weight bearing, 2 to 3 hours a day, is encouraged. After removal of the hip spica cast at 4 to 6 weeks, a total body splint is fitted with the hip in the same position.

• • •

Flexion-abduction-external rotation contractures of the hip are common in children with thoracic-level lesions and complete paralysis of the muscles of the lower extremity. Continuous external rotation of the hip in the supine position causes contractures in the posterior hip capsule and in the short external rotator muscles. This deformity can be prevented by the use of night splints (total body splints) and range-of-motion exercises. Surgery is indicated only when the deformity interferes with bracing. This deformity frequently is bilateral, and both hips should be corrected at the same time.

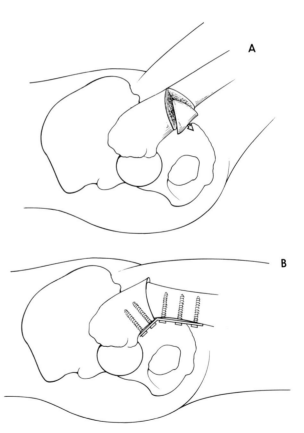

Fig. 12-22 Subtrochanteric extension osteotomy. **A,** Posterior closing wedge osteotomy. **B,** Application of plate.

Complete hip release for flexion-abduction-external rotation contracture

▶ *Technique* (Fig. 12-23). Place the patient in a lateral position. Make a transverse incision medial and distal to the anterosuperior iliac spine, extending it laterally above the greater trochanter. Divide the iliopsoas tendon distally, and excise 1 cm of it. Detach the sartorius from its origin in the anterosuperior iliac spine, detach the rectus from the anteroinferior iliac spine, and divide the tensor fasciae latae from its anterior border completely posteriorly. Detach the gluteus medius and minimus and the short external rotators from their insertions on the trochanter. Retract the sciatic nerve posteriorly. Then open the hip capsule from anterior to posterior, parallel with the acetabular labrum. Close the wound over suction drainage, and apply a hip spica cast with the hip in full extension, 10 degrees of abduction, and, if possible, internal rotation.

▶ *Postoperative management.* Two weeks after surgery the cast is removed, and a total body splint is fitted with the hip in the same position.

• • •

Isolated external rotation contracture of the hip occasionally occurs in children with low lumbar–level lesions. Initially, a twister cable attached to an AFO will help the child ambulate without major rotational malalignment. If, after the twister cable is removed (when the child is older than 5 or 6 years), the external rotation of the hip persists, subtrochanteric medial rotation osteotomy (p. 66) is indicated.

Isolated unilateral abduction contracture is a common cause of pelvic obliquity, causing scoliosis and difficulty in sitting and ambulation. This deformity generally is caused by contracture of the tensor fasciae latae, but it may occur after iliopsoas transfer. It occurs frequently in children with high level lesions and can be prevented by early splinting and physical therapy. Surgery is indicated when the abduction contracture causes pelvic obliquity and scoliosis and interferes with function.

Release of abduction contracture by fascial release

▶ *Technique.* Incise the skin along the anterior one half or two thirds of the iliac crest to the anterosuperior iliac spine. Divide all tight fascial and tendinous structures around the anterolateral aspect of the hip: fascia lata, fascia over the gluteus medius and minimus, and tensor fasciae latae. Do not divide muscle tissue, only the enveloping fascial structures. Fasciotomy of the fascia lata distally, as described by Yount, sometimes is required.

▶ *Technique (Yount).* Expose the fascia lata through a lateral longitudinal incision just proximal to the femoral condyle. Divide the iliotibial band and fascia lata posteriorly to the biceps tendon and anteriorly to the midline of the thigh at a level 2.5 cm proximal to the patella. At this level, incise a segment of the iliotibial band and lateral intermuscular septum 5 to 8 cm long. Before closing the wound, determine by palpation that all tight bands are divided. Close the wound over suction drainage. Apply a hip spica cast with the operated hip in neutral abduction and the opposite hip in 20 degrees of abduction, enough to permit perineal care.

▶ *Postoperative management.* Two weeks after surgery the cast is removed, and a total body splint is fitted.

• • •

Adduction contracture of the hip frequently occurs in association with hip subluxation and dislocation in children with high level lesions because of spasticity and contracture of the adductor muscles. Surgical treatment is indicated when the contracture causes pelvic obliquity and interferes with sitting or walking. Adductor release frequently is combined with the surgical treatment of subluxation and dislocation. If fixed deformities and hip dislocation are present, femoral osteotomy and pelvic osteotomy may be required.

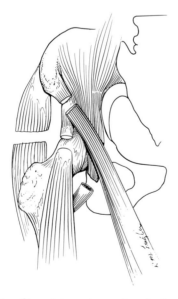

Fig. 12-23 Complete release for flexion-abduction-external rotation contracture of hip (see text).

Adductor release

▶ *Technique.* Make a transverse inguinal incision about 2 to 3 cm long, just distal to the inguinal crease over the adductor longus tendon. Open the superficial fascia, and expose the adductor longus tendon. Using electrocautery, divide the adductor longus tendon close to its insertion in the pubic ramus. Next, if needed, divide the muscle fibers of the gracilis proximally, and when necessary, after the anterior branch of the obturator nerve is protected, completely divide the adductor brevis muscle fibers. At least 45 degrees of abduction should be possible. Close the wound over suction drainage, and apply a spica cast with the hip in 25 to 30 degrees of abduction.

▶ *Postoperative management.* Two weeks after surgery the cast is removed, and a total body splint is fitted with the hip in 25 degrees of abduction.

Hip Subluxation and Dislocation

Hip subluxation and dislocation are common problems in children with myelomeningocele, occurring in more than half. At birth, congenital, teratologic, or paralytic dislocation may be present. Congenital hip dislocation occurs in children with sacral-level lesions without muscle imbalance. It should be treated conservatively by standard methods of treatment for congenital hip dislocation (Pavlik harness, traction plus closed reduction, and spica cast immobilization). Teratologic dislocations usually occur in children with high level lesions. Initial roentgenograms show a severely dysplastic acetabulum, with the head of the femur displaced proximally. Teratologic dislocations should not be treated initially.

The most common type of hip subluxation and dislocation is paralytic, which occurs in 50% to 70% of children with low level (L3 or L4) lesions because of imbalance between abduction and adduction forces. The dislocation occurs most frequently during the first 3 years of life; dislocations in older children usually are caused by contractures or spasticity of the unopposed adductors and hip flexors associated with tethered cord syndrome. Reduction of dislocated hips in children with myelomeningocele is controversial. In 1975 Barden et al noted no correlation between the status of the hip and the ability to walk in children followed up for 20 years. Feiwell et al reported that reducing the hip into the acetabulum did not improve hip range of motion, reduce pain, or reduce the amount of bracing needed, and that a few children had increased hip stiffness after surgery. They stressed that maintaining a level pelvis and flexible hips was more important than reduction of the hips. The goal of treatment should be maximum function, not roentgenographic reduction of the dislocated hip. Soft tissue release alone is indicated in patients without functional quadriceps muscles because only occasionally do they remain community ambulators as adults. Open reduction is appropriate only for those children with strong quadriceps muscles bilaterally, normal trunk balance, and normal upper extremity function. Bilateral or unilateral hip dislocation or subluxation in children with high level lesions does not require extensive surgical treatment, but soft tissue contractures should be corrected. Surgical treatment is indicated for unilateral or bilateral hip subluxation in children with low level lumbar lesions who are likely to maintain ambulatory potential.

Successful treatment of dislocated hips requires, in addition to open reduction of the femoral head into the acetabulum, correction of the muscle imbalance, release of contractures, correction of bony deformities such as acetabular dysplasia and coxa valga, and plication of capsular laxity (see Chapter 2). Lee and Carroll recommend iliopsoas transfer with adductor release, capsulorrhaphy, and acetabuloplasty in conjunction with open reduction. Of 53 hips they treated with this approach, 44 were considered normal at follow-up, 7 showed subluxation, and 2 were dislocated.

The Sharrad iliopsoas transfer through the posterolateral ilium is a modification of the Mustard procedure. Reported results of posterior iliopsoas transfer vary from a success rate of 95% to only 20%. In 1987 Roye et al advised against bilateral iliopsoas transfers because the resulting weakness of the hip flexors may impair ambulation. Although the transfer functions as a tenodesis, it does not allow continued active maintenance of hip abduction and extension. Posterior iliopsoas transfer should not be done prophylactically to prevent hip dislocation, but it may be combined with adductor release, capsulorrhaphy, and acetabuloplasty.

Iliopsoas muscle transfer

◣ *Technique (Sharrard).* Place the patient on the operating table, slightly tilted toward the nonoperative side. Through a transverse incision overlying the adductor longus, expose and divide the adductor muscles. Expose the lesser trochanter, and detach it from the femur (Fig. 12-24, *A*). Then clear the psoas muscle as far proximally as possible. Make a second incision just below and parallel to the iliac crest. Detach the iliac crest with the muscles of the abdominal wall, and open the psoas muscle sheath. Locate the insertion of the muscle with a finger tip. Through the first incision, grasp the lesser trochanter with a Kocher forceps and pull it upward, within the psoas sheath, and into the upper operative area (Fig. 12-24, *B*). Next expose the sartorius muscle, and divide its proximal half. Allow the sartorius muscle to remain in the cartilaginous portion of the anterosuperior iliac spine, which is retracted medially. Identify the direct head of the rectus femoris muscle, and divide it at its origin in the anteroinferior iliac spine. Identify the reflected head, dissect it free from the hip capsule, and elevate it posteriorly. Open the hip capsule anteriorly and laterally, parallel to the labrum, excise the ligamentum teres, and remove any hypertrophic pulvinar. Reduce the hip.

Now make a hole through the iliac wing just lateral to the sacroiliac joint. Make an oval, with its long axis longitudinal, its width slightly more than one third that of the iliac wing, and its length 1.5 times as long as its width. Then pass the iliopsoas tendon through the hole (Fig. 12-24, *C*). Pass a finger from the gluteal region distally and posteriorly into the bursa, deep to the gluteus maximus tendon, and identify by touch the posterolateral aspect of the greater trochanter. By referring to this point, expose the corresponding anterior aspect of the greater trochanter by dissecting through the fascia lata. Now, with awls and burrs, and from anteriorly and posteriorly, make a hole through the greater trochanter until it is big enough to receive the tendon. Then, while the hip is held in abduction, extension, and neutral rotation, pass the end of the tendon through the buttock and posteriorly to anteriorly through the tunnel in the greater trochanter (Fig. 12-24, *C*). Secure the psoas and lesser trochanter to the greater trochanter with sutures or a screw (Fig. 12-24, *D*).

For severe coxa valga or anteversion that requires more than 20 to 30 degrees of abduction for stability, varus derotation osteotomy with internal fixation can be performed before insertion and suturing of the iliopsoas tendon in the greater trochanter.

Wissinger et al described a modification of the Sharrard transfer in which a "gutter" or notch is cut into the posterolateral iliac crest rather than a window in the ilium. The musle and its tendon can be redirected laterally through the notch and inserted into the greater trochanter (Fig. 12-24, *E* and *F*). This is technically simpler because the iliac musle is not transferred to the outside of the pelvis.

◣ *Postoperative management.* The hip is immobilized for 6 weeks in an abduction spica cast.

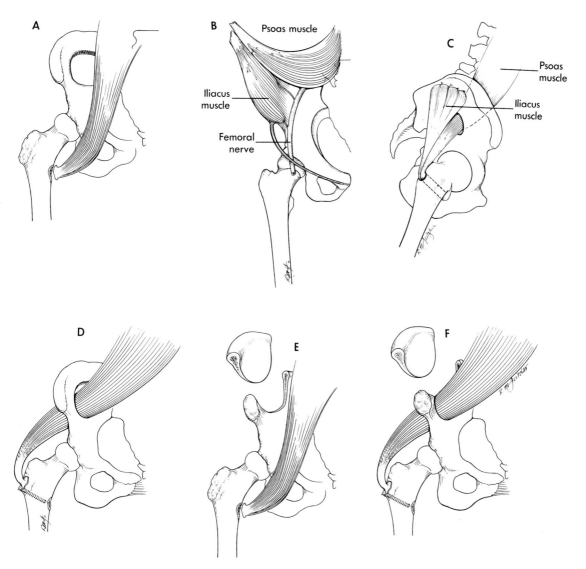

Fig. 12-24 Sharrard transfer of iliopsoas muscle. **A,** Iliopsoas tendon released from lesser trochanter. **B,** Iliopsoas tendon and lesser trochanter detached, iliacus and psoas muscles elevated, origin of iliacus freed, and hole made in ilium. **C,** Iliopsoas tendon passed from posterior to anterior through hole in greater trochanter. **D,** Iliopsoas muscle and lesser trochanter secured to greater trochanter with screw. **E** and **F,** Modification of technique in which muscle and tendon are redirected laterally through notch in ilium and inserted into greater trochanter, as described by Weisinger et al. (**B** and **C,** Redrawn from Sharrard WJW: J Bone Joint Surg 46B:426, 1964.)

External oblique transfer. Anatomically, the external oblique muscle is a good substitute for paralyzed abductors of the hip because its nerve supply is from a different spinal segment than that of the gluteus medius and minimus muscles and usually it is not paralyzed. Its aponeurosis is long and broad, its surfaces are well adapted for gliding movement, and after transfer its mechanical action on the greater trochanter is direct. Thomas et al in 1950 described a method of transferring the external oblique muscle to the greater trochanter. In 1977 McKay recommended transfer of the external oblique muscle in conjunction with femoral osteotomy for hip subluxation in patients with myelomeningocele. Lindseth recommends posterolateral transfer of the fascia in association with transfer of the adductor and external oblique muscles.

Transfer of the external oblique muscle has four advantages over transfer of the iliopsoas muscle: (1) the hip is not further weakened by eliminating the iliopsoas as a hip flexor, (2) muscle power is added to the hip by taking the muscle from the abdominal wall, where its absence is well tolerated, (3) external oblique transfer functions synergistically whereas iliopsoas transfer functions antagonistically, and (4) external oblique transfer does not violate the ilium, allowing pelvic osteotomy if necessary.

▶ *Technique.* With the patient lying supine and slightly tilted toward the nonoperative side, make a skin incision similar to that for the anterolateral approach to the hip (p. 140). Elevate the subcutaneous tissue from the external oblique aponeurosis all the way to the midline. Make an incision in the aponeurosis just at the level of the anterosuperior iliac spine, directed distally and medially parallel to the inguinal ligament. At this point, direct the aponeurosis incision medially and proximally parallel to the linea alba. Carefully detach the external oblique muscle fibers from their insertion in the ilium, freeing the muscle from the underlying tissues by blunt dissection (Fig. 12-25, *A*). Now fold under and suture together the cut edges of the muscle and its aponeurosis to form a cone-shaped structure. Beginning at the pubis, repair the remaining aponeurosis of the muscle as far laterally as possible. Suture the remaining free edge of the aponeurosis to the underlying internal oblique muscle.

Perform adductor myotomy or adductor transfer to the ischium through a transverse incision beginning just anterior to the tendon of the adductor longus and extending down to the ischium. If the adductor transfer is performed, detach the tendon of the adductor longus, brevis, and anterior third of the magnus from the pubis and transfer them to the ischium with nonabsorbable sutures.

Expose the greater trochanter through a separate lateral incision. The external oblique tendon aponeurosis can be inserted in the trochanter through either two holes, 1 cm in diameter and at right angles to each other, or through a posterolateral window

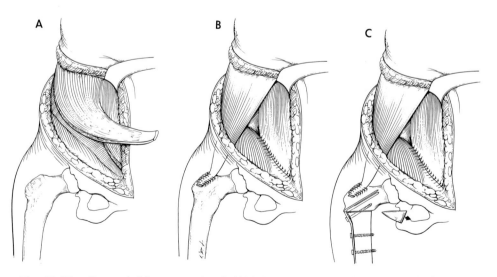

Fig. 12-25   External oblique transfer. **A,** With long oblique incision, muscle is freed distally. **B,** External oblique aponeurosis attached to greater trochanter. **C,** Varus femoral osteotomy may be performed if necessary (see text).

hinged posteriorly. Make a large subcutaneous tunnel extending proximally from the original incision as far posterior as possible. Now pass the cone-shaped strip of external oblique muscle distally through the tunnel, place the hip in 30 to 40 degrees of abduction, and pass the tendon aponeurosis through the holes or window in the trochanter and suture it firmly with nonabsorbable sutures and with wire sutures (Fig. 12-25, *B*). If necessary, reattach the rectus anterior to the anteroinferior iliac crest, and approximate and suture the iliac crest. Apply a hip spica cast with the hip in 25 to 30 degrees of abduction, extension, and internal rotation.

▶ *Postoperative management.* Six weeks after surgery, the spica cast is removed, the child is admitted to the hospital for intensive physical therapy, and a total body splint is made with the hip in 25 degrees of abduction and medial rotation.

• • •

If needed for acetabular dysplasia, a shelf procedure (p. 161) or Chiari pelvic osteotomy (p. 163) can be performed in conjunction with the transfer. If more than 20 to 30 degrees of abduction is necessary to maintain concentric reduction of the hip, a varus femoral osteotomy (Fig. 12-25, *C*) is advisable.

Proximal femoral resection and interposition arthroplasty. One of the most serious problems in hip surgery in patients with myelomeningocele is severe stiffness of the joint. This occurs for a variety of reasons and occasionally occurs after hip surgery. If the hip is stiff in extension, the child cannot sit; if it is stiff in flexion, the child cannot stand; if it is stiff "in between," the child can neither sit nor stand. Very little has been written about the management of this complication, but resection of the femoral head and neck is not effective. Proximal femoral resection and interposition arthroplasty, as reported by Castle and Schneider, have been used in severely retarded, multiply handicapped children with dislocated hips and severe adduction contractures of the lower extremity (Fig. 12-26). This procedure allows the child to sit comfortably and makes nursing care easier.

▶ *Technique (Baxter and D'Astous).* Position the patient with a sandbag beneath the affected hip. Make a straight lateral approach beginning 10 cm proximal to the greater trochanter and extending down the proximal femur. Split the fascia lata. Detach the vastus lateralis and gluteus maximus from their insertions. Detach the gluteus medius and minimus from the greater trochanter. Identify the psoas tendon, and detach its insertion on the lesser trochanter to expose

extraperiosteally the proximal femur. Incise the periosteum circumferentially just distal to the gluteus maximus insertion, and transect the bone at this level. Divide the short external rotators. Incise the capsule circumferentially at the level of the basal neck. Cut the ligamentum teres, remove the proximal femur, and test range of motion. If necessary, a proximal hamstring tenotomy may be performed through the same incision after identification of the sciatic nerve; adductor release also can be performed through a separate groin incision. Seal the acetabular cavity by oversewing the capsular edges. Cover the proximal end of the femur with the vastus lateralis and rectus femoris muscles. Interpose the gluteal muscles between the closed acetabulum and the covered end of the proximal femur to act as a further soft tissue cushion. Close the wound in layers over a suction drain.

▶ *Postoperative management.* The operated lower extremity is placed in Russell traction in abduction until the soft tissues are healed, and then gentle range-of-motion exercises are begun.

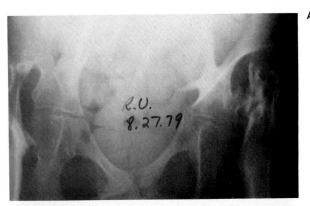

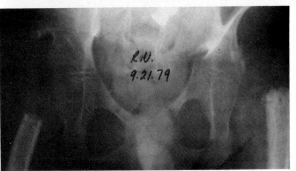

Fig. 12-26 **A,** Severe bilateral hip pain after Girdlestone procedure. **B,** After bilateral proximal femoral resection and interposition arthroplasty.

Pelvic Obliquity

Pelvic obliquity is frequent in patients with myelomeningocele. In addition to predisposing the hip to dislocation, pelvic obliquity interferes with sitting, standing, and walking, and it can lead to ulceration under the prominent ischial tuberosity. Mayer described three types of pelvic obliquity: (1) infrapelvic, caused by contracture of the abductor and tensor fasciae latae muscles of one hip and contracture of the adductors of the opposite hip, (2) suprapelvic, caused by uncompensated scoliosis resulting from bony deformity of the lumbosacral spine or severe paralytic scoliosis, and (3) pelvic, caused by bony deformity of the sacrum and sacroiliac joint, such as partial sacral agenesis. This bony abnormality leads to asymmetry of the pelvis itself. Infrapelvic obliquity can be prevented by splinting, range-of-motion exercises, and positioning, but when hip contractures are well established, soft tissue release is required to correct the contractures and level the pelvis. Occasionally, for more severe deformities, osteotomy of the proximal femur is required. Suprapelvic obliquity can be corrected by control of the scoliosis by orthoses or spinal fusion. If severe scoliosis cannot be completely corrected, bony pelvic obliquity is fixed and permanent.

Lindseth stated that obliquity of 20 degrees is sufficient to interfere with walking and to produce ischial decubitus ulcerations and recommended pelvic osteotomy for fixed pelvic obliquity of more than 20 degrees. He reported good results in nine patients after pelvic osteotomy. All had improved sitting balance, and standing balance also was improved in four ambulatory patients. No child had postoperative ischial ulceration or progressive dislocation of the hip. Before osteotomy, hip contractures should be released and maximal correction of the scoliosis should be obtained by spinal fusion. The degree of correction of pelvic obliquity is determined preoperatively from appropriate roentgenograms of the pelvis and spine (Fig. 12-27, A). The maximum correction obtainable with bilateral iliac osteotomies is 40 degrees.

Pelvic osteotomy

▶ *Technique (Lindseth).* The approach is similar to that described by O'Phelan for iliac osteotomy in correction of exstrophy of the bladder (p. 168). With the child prone on the operating table, make bilateral inverted L-shaped incisions starting above the iliac crest, proceeding medially to the posterosuperior iliac spine, then curving downward along each side of the sacrum to the sciatic notch. Detach the iliac apophysis by splitting it longitudinally, starting at the anterosuperior iliac spine and proceeding posteriorly (Fig. 12-27, B). Retract the paraspinal muscles, the quadratus lumborum muscle, and the iliac muscles medially along the inner half of the epiphysis and the inner periosteum of the ilium. After the sacral origin of the gluteus maximus has been detached from the sacrum, divide the outer periosteum of the ilium longitudinally just lateral to the posteromedial border of the ilium, extending from the posterosuperior iliac spine down to the sciatic notch. Strip the outer periosteum, along with the gluteus muscles and the outer half of the epiphysis, from the outer table of the ilium, taking care to avoid damaging the superior and inferior gluteal vessels and nerves. Retract the soft tissues down to the sciatic notch, and protect them by inserting malleable retractors. Next make bilateral osteotomies approximately 2 cm lateral to each sacroiliac joint. The size of this wedge is determined by the amount of correction desired and is limited to no more than one third of the iliac crest; the base of the wedge usually is about 2.5 cm long (Fig. 12-27, C).

After the wedge of bone is removed, correct the deformity by pulling on the limb on the short side and pushing up on the limb on the long side (Fig. 12-27, C). This usually closes the osteotomy site where the wedge of bone was removed on the long side. If upper migration of the ilium onto the sacrum is severe, trim the excess iliac crest. Close the wedge osteotomy with two threaded pins or sutures through drill holes. Then use a spreader to open the osteotomy on the opposite (short) side sufficiently to receive the graft. Use two Kirschner wires to hold the graft in place (Fig. 12-27, D). Close the wounds over suction-irrigation drains, and apply a double, full-hip spica cast.

▶ *Postoperative management.* The cast is worn for 8 weeks. The Kirschner wires are removed when roentgenograms show sufficient healing of the osteotomy.

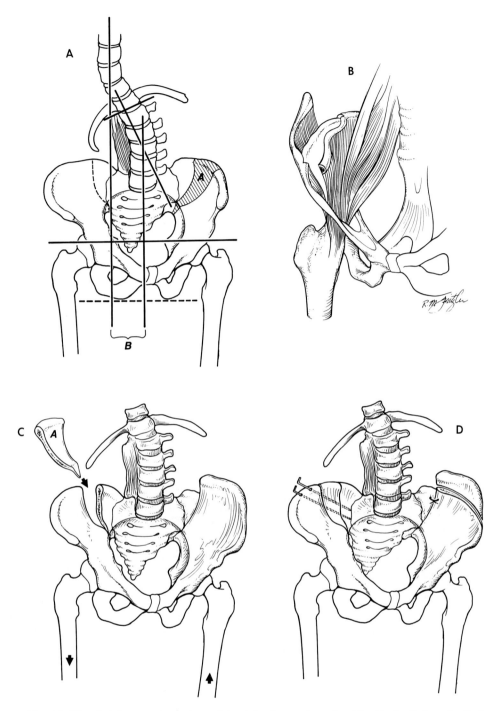

Fig. 12-27   Pelvic osteotomy for pelvic obliquity as described by Lindseth (see text). **A,** Preoperative determination of size of iliac wedge to be removed and transferred. **B,** Exposure of ilium. **C,** After bilateral osteotomies and removal of predetermined wedge from low side, deformity is corrected. **D,** Transferred iliac wedge fixed with two Kirschner wires. (Redrawn from Lindseth RE: J Bone Joint Surg 60A:17, 1978.)

Spine

Paralytic spinal deformities have been reported in up to 90% of patients with myelomeningocele. Scoliosis is the most common deformity and usually is relentlessly progressive. The incidence of scoliosis is related to the level of the bony defect. Moe et al noted a 100% incidence of scoliosis with T12 lesions, 90% with L1 lesions, 80% with L2 lesions, 70% with L3 lesions, 60% with L4 lesions, 25% with L5 lesions, and 5% with S1 lesions. The curves develop gradually before the child reaches the age of 10 years and increase rapidly with the adolescent growth spurt. Raycroft and Curtis divided scoliosis in patients with myelomeningocele into developmental or congenital curves. Congenital curves that involved structural disorganization of the vertebral bodies occurred in 48% of their patients, and 52% had developmental scoliosis without vertebral anomalies. The majority of developmental curves occurred between the ages of 5 and 10 years. Raycroft and Curtis suggested muscle imbalance and habitual posturing as causative factors in developmental scoliosis because 70% of patients also had dislocated hips and 83% had pelvic obliquity. Developmental curves occur later, are more flexible, and usually are in the lumbar area, with compensatory curves above and below.

A number of reports in the literature have suggested that some developmental scoliosis may be caused by hydromyelia or a tethered cord syndrome. In 1987 Riegel et al reviewed 104 patients with myelomeningocele who had undergone a tethered cord release. Curves greater than 30 degrees developed in only 20 (19.2%). The remaining 84 patients maintained normal spinal alignment after tethered cord release. Early onset of scoliosis (in the child younger than 6 years of age) frequently is related to some pathology at the spinal cord level (hydromyelia or tethered cord), and curves developing late in the child with a high-level lesion are most likely developmental paralytic curves.

Because of the frequency of scoliosis in patients with myelomeningocele, spinal roentgenograms should be obtained at least once a year, beginning when the child is 5 years of age. If any scoliosis is found, further evaluation is indicated. MRI of the spine is performed to determine if hydromyelia or a tethered spinal cord is present.

Orthotic treatment is advised when the curve is greater than 20 to 25 degrees. Although the majority of curves will progress despite bracing, bracing slows progression and delays surgical intervention. A molded, bivalved, polypropylene body jacket (a

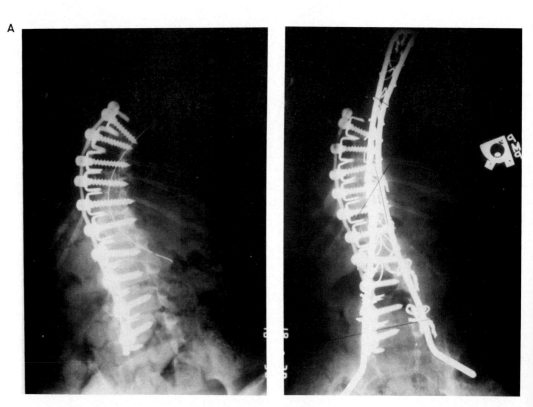

Fig. 12-28   Correction of severe scoliosis with anterior fusion with Dwyer instrumentation **(A),** followed by later posterior fusion with Luque rods **(B).**.

thoracic-lumbar-sacral orthosis) is worn during the daytime only. Indications for spinal fusion are a progressive increase in angular deformity that cannot be controlled by conservative means, the presence of unacceptable deformities, and progressive thoracic lordosis. For severe curves, anterior spinal fusion, followed by posterior spinal fusion, may be indicated (Fig. 12-28). Contraindications to surgery include short life expectancy, uncontrollable hydrocephalus, failure to thrive, and marked mental retardation with no hope of independent function.

• • •

Congenital kyphosis is the most severe spinal deformity in patients with myelomeningocele; it occurs in approximately 10% of patients. The kyphosis usually is present at birth and may make sac closure difficult. The curve generally extends from the lower thoracic level to the sacral spine, with the apex of the curve in the midlumbar region. The deformity is progressive throughout life and usually is greater than 90 degrees by the time the child is 2 years old.

Congenital kyphosis is completely unresponsive to bracing, and unless the deformity is mild, it must be corrected surgically. Lindseth and Seltzer advise early surgical treatment because a delay leads to increased deformity and disability during the formative years of the child's life. The goal of treatment of the kyphosis is not to obtain a normal spine but to provide sitting balance without the use of the arms or hands, to increase the lumbar height to allow room for abdominal contents and provide better mechanics for breathing, and to decrease the prominence of the kyphosis to prevent pressure sores. The degree of correction that can be obtained is limited.

Surgical techniques for spinal fusion in scoliosis and correction of kyphosis are described in Chapter 10. Complications of spinal surgery in patients with myelomeningocele are significantly greater than in patients with idiopathic scoliosis. The primary complication is failure of fusion, reported to occur in up to 40% of patients. The infection rate can be as high as 8%.

REFERENCES

General

Asher M and Olson J: Factors affecting the ambulatory status of patients with spina bifida cystica, J Bone Joint Surg 65A:350, 1983.

Barden GA, Meyer LC, and Stelling FH III: Myelodysplastics: fate of those followed for 20 years or more, J Bone Joint Surg 57A:643, 1975.

Bunch WH, Scarff TB, and Dvonch VM: Progressive loss in myelomeningocele patients, Orthop Trans 7:185, 1983.

Carroll NC: The orthotic management of the spina bifida child, Clin Orthop 102:108, 1974.

DeSouza LJ and Carroll N: Ambulation of the braced myelomeningocele patient, J Bone Joint Surg 58A:1112, 1976.

Dias LS, Jasty MJ, and Collins P: Rotational deformities of the lower limb in myelomeningocele: evaluation and treatment, J Bone Joint Surg 66A(2):215, 1984.

Douglas R et al: The LSU reciprocation—joint orthosis, Orthopedics 6:834, 1983.

Drennan JC et al: Symposium: current concepts in the management of myelomeningocele, Contemp Orthop 19:63, 1989.

Drummond DS Moreau M, and Cruess RL: Postoperative neuropathic fractures in patients with myelomeningocele, Dev Med Child Neurol 23:147, 1981.

Flandry F et al: Functional ambulation in myelodysplasia: the effect of orthotic selection on physical and physiologic performance, J Pediatr Orthop 6:661, 1986.

Hoffer M et al: Functional ambulation in patients with myelomeningocele, J Bone Joint Surg 55A:137, 1973.

Kumar SJ, Cowell HR, and Townsend P. Physeal, metaphyseal, and diaphyseal injuries of the lower extremities in children with myelomeningocele, J Pediatr Orthop 4(1):25, 1984.

Lock TR and Aronson DD: Fractures in patients who have myelomeningocele, J Bone Joint Surg 71A:1153, 1989.

Lorber J: Results of treatment of myelomeningocele: an analysis of 270 consecutive cases with criteria for selection for the future, Arch Dis Child 47:854, 1972.

Lorber J: Selective treatment of myelomeningocele: to treat or not to treat? Pediatrics 53:307, 1974.

Mazur JM, Stillwell A, and Menelaus M: The significance of spasticity in the upper and lower limbs in myelomeningocele, J Bone Joint Surg 68B(2):213, 1986.

Mazur JM et al: Hand function in patients with spina bifida cystica, J Pediatr Orthop 6(4):442, 1986.

Mazur JM et al: Orthopaedic management of high-level spina bifida: early walking compared with early use of a wheelchair, J Bone Joint Surg 71A:56, 1989.

McCall RE, Schmidt WT. Clinical experience with the reciprocal gait orthosis in myelodysplasia. J Pediatr Orthop 1986;6(2):157.

Menelaus MB: Orthopaedic management of children with myelomeningocele: a plea for realistic goals, Dev Med Child Neurol 18(suppl 37):3, 1976.

Menelaus MB: The orthopedic management of spina bifida cystica, ed 2, Edinburgh, 1980, Churchill-Livingstone.

Roberts JA, Bennet GC, and MacKenzie JR: Physeal widening in children with myelomeningocele, J Bone Joint Surg 71B:30, 1989.

Robinson JM, Hewson JE, and Parker PM: The walking ability of fourteen to seventeen year old teenagers with spina bifida: a physiotherapy study, Z Kinderchir 31:421, 1980.

Rose GK, Sankarankutt M, and Stallard J: A clinical review of the orthotic treatment of myelomeningocele patients, J Bone Joint Surg 65B:242, 1983.

Samuelsson L and Skoog M: Ambulation in patients with myelomeningocele: a multivariate statistical analysis, J Pediatr Orthop 8:569, 1988.

Schafer MF and Dias LS: Myelomeningocele: orthopaedic treatment, Baltimore, 1983, The Williams & Wilkins Co.

Stillwell A and Menelaus MB: Walking ability in mature patients with spina bifida, J Pediatr Orthop 3:184, 1983.

Swank SM et al: Spina bifida: a review of 10 years' experience with 198 children. Presented at the American Academy of Cerebral Palsy and Developmental Medicine, Toronto, Oct 26-29, 1987.

Yngve DA, Douglas R, and Roberts JM: The reciprocating gait orthosis in myelomeningocele, J Pediatr Orthop 4(3):304, 1984.

Foot

Banta JV, Sutherland DH, and Wyatt M: Anterior tibial transfer to the os calcis with Achilles tenodesis for calcaneal deformity in myelomeningocele, J Pediatr Orthop 2:125, 1982.

Crawford AH, Marxen JL, and Osterfield DL: The Cincinnati incision: a comprehensive approach for surgical procedures of the foot and ankle in childhood, J Bone Joint Surg 64A:1355, 1982.

Cyphers SM and Feiwell E: Review of the Gridlestone-Taylor procedure for clawtoes in myelodysplasia, Foot Ankle 8:229, 1988.

Dias LS: Valgus deformity of the ankle joint: pathogenesis of fibular shortening, J Pediatr Orthop 5:176, 1985.

Dias LS, Busch M, and Tachdjian MO: Surgical treatment of severe hindfoot valgus by medial displacement osteotomy of the os calcis
Orthop Trans 11(3):35, 1987.

Dias LS and Stern LS: Talectomy in the treatment of resistant talipes equinovarus deformity in myelomeningocele and arthrogryposis, J Pediatr Orthop 7:39, 1987.

Evans D: Calcanco-valgus deformity, J Bone Joint Surg 57B:270, 1975.

Gallien R, Morin F, and Marquis F: Subtalar arthrodesis in children, J Pediatr Orthop 9:59, 1989.

Gross PM, Lyne D. The Grice procedures: indications and evaluation of long-term results. Clin Orthop 1980;153:194.

Hayes JT and Gross HB: Surgery for paralytic defects secondary to myelomeningocele and myelodysplasia, J Bone Joint Surg 46A:1577, 1964.

Jones R: Certain operative procedures in the paralysis of children, with special reference to poliomyelitis, Br Med J 2:1520, 1911.

Levitt RL, Canale ST, and Gartland JJ: Surgical correction of foot deformity in the older patient with myelomeningocele, Orthop Clin North Am 5:19, 1974.

Lichtblau S: Medial and lateral release operation for clubfoot: preliminary report, J Bone Joint Surg 55A:1377, 1973.

Lindseth RE: Treatment of the lower extremity in children paralyzed by meningocele (birth to 18 months). In The American Academy of Orthopaedic Surgeons: instructional course lectures, vol 25, St Louis, 1976, The CV Mosby Co.

Menelaus MD: Talectomy for equinovarus deformity in arthrogryposis and spina bifida, J Bone Joint Surg 53B:468, 1971.

Olney BW and Menelaus MB: Triple arthrodesis of the foot in spina bifida patients, J Bone Joint Surg 70B:234, 1988.

Paulos L, Coleman SS, and Samuelson KM: Pes cavovarus, J Bone Joint Surg 62A:942, 1980.

Ross PM and Lyne D: The Grice procedure: indications and evaluation of long-term results, Clin Orthop 153:195, 1980.

Segal LS et al: Equinovarus deformity in arthrogryposis and myelomeningocele: evaluation of primary talectomy, Foot Ankle 10:12, 1989.

Sharrard WJW and Grosfield I: The management of deformity and paralysis of the foot in myelomeningocele, J Bone Joint Surg 50B:456, 1968.

Sherk HH and Amos MD: Talectomy in the treatment of the myelomeningocele patient, Clin Orthop 110:218, 1975.

Sherk HH et al: Ground reaction forces on the plantar surface of the foot after talectomy in the myelomeningocele, J Pediatr Orthop 9:269, 1989.

Stevens PM: Relative hypoplasia of fibula and associated ankle valgus, J Pediatr Orthop 7:605, 1987.

Stevens PM and Toomey E: Fibular-Achilles tenodesis for paralytic ankle valgus, J Pediatr Orthop 8:169, 1988.

Trieshmann H et al: Sliding calcaneal osteotomy for treatment of hindfoot deformity, Orthop Trans 4:305, 1980.

Trumble T et al: Talectomy for equinovarus deformity in myelodysplasia, J Bone Joint Surg 67A:21, 1985.

Westin GW and Defiore RJ: Tenodesis of the tendo-Achilles to the fibula for a paralytic calcaneus deformity, J Bone Joint Surg 56A:1541, 1975.

Ankle

Banta JV, Sutherland DH, and Wyatt M: Anterior tibial transfer to the os calcis with Achilles tenodesis for calcaneal deformity in myelomeningocele, J Pediatr Orthop 1:125, 1982.

Bliss HG and Menelaus MB: The results of transfer of the tibialis anterior to the heel in patients who have a myelomeningocele, J Bone Joint Surg 68A:1258, 1986.

Burkus JK, Moore DW, and Raycroft JF: Valgus deformity of the ankle in myelodysplastic patients: correction by stapling of the medial part of the distal tibial physis, J Bone Joint Surg 65A:1157, 1983.

Dias LS: Ankle valgus in children with myelomeningocele, Dev Med Child Neurol 20:627, 1981.

Makin M: Tibio-fibular relationship in paralysed limbs, J Bone Joint Surg 47B:500, 1965.

Malhotra D, Puri R, and Owen R: Valgus deformity of the ankle in children with spina bifida aperta, J Bone Joint Surg 66B:381, 1984.

Sanda JPS, Skinner SR, and Banto PS: Posterior transfer of tibialis anterior in low level myelodysplasia, Dev Med Child Neurol 26:100, 1984.

Sharrard WJW and Webb J: Supra-malleolar wedge osteotomy of the tibia in children with myelomeningocele, J Bone Joint Surg 56B:458, 1974.

Knee

Blount WP: Unequal leg length in children, Surg Clin North Am 38:1107, 1958.

Curtis PE and Fisher RL: Congenital hyperextension with anterior subluxation of the knee, J Bone Joint Surg 51A:255, 1969.

Dias L: Surgical management of knee contractures in myelomeningocele, J Pediatr Orthop 2:127, 1982.

Dupre P and Walker G: Knee problems associated with spina bifida, Dev Med Child Neurol Suppl 27:152, 1972.

Lloyd-Roberts CG, Williams DI, and Braddock GTF: Pelvic osteotomy in the treatment of ectopia vesicae, J Bone Joint Surg 41B:754, 1959.

Parsch K and Manner G: Prevention and treatment of knee problems in children with spina bifida, Dev Med Child Neurol Suppl 37:114, 1976.

Phemister DB: Operative arrestment of longitudinal growth of bones in the treatment of deformities, J Bone Joint Surg 15:1, 1933.

Hip

Baxter MP and D'Astous JL: Proximal femoral resection-interposition arthroplasty: salvage hip surgery for the severely disabled child with cerebral palsy, J Pediatr Orthop 6:681, 1986.

Bazih J and Gross RH: Hip surgery in the lumbar level myelomeningocele patient, J Pediatr Orthop 1:405, 1981.

Bunch WA and Hakala NM: Iliopsoas transfers in children with myelomeningocele, J Bone Joint Surg 66A:224, 1984.

Canale ST et al: Pelvic displacement osteotomy for chronic hip dislocation in myelodysplasia, J Bone Joint Surg 57A:177, 1975.

Carroll NC: Assessment and management of the lower extremity in myelodysplasia, Orthop Clin North Am 18:709, 1987.

Carroll NC and Sharrard WJ: Long-term follow-up of posterior iliopsoas transplantation for paralytic dislocation of the hip, J Bone Joint Surg 54A:551, 1972.

Castle ME and Schneider C: Proximal femoral resection interposition arthroplasty, J Bone Joint Surg 60A:1051, 1978.

Crandall RC, Birkebak RC, and Winter RB: The role of hip location and dislocation in the functional status of the myelodysplastic patient: a review of 100 patients, Orthopedics 12:675, 1988.

Dias LS and Hill JA: Evaluation of treatment of hip subluxation in myelomeningocele by intertrochanteric varus derotation femoral osteotomy, Orthop Clin North Am 11:31, 1980.

Drummond DS, Moreau M, and Cruess RL: The results and complications of surgery for the paralytic hip and spine in myelomeningocele, J Bone Joint Surg 62B:49, 1980.

Feiwell E: Surgery of the hip in myelomeningocele as related to adult goals, Clin Orthop 148:87, 1980.

Feiwell E, Sakai D, and Blatt T: The effect of hip reduction on function in patients with myelomeningocele: potential gains and hazards of surgical treatment, J Bone Joint Surg 60A:169, 1978.

Lee EH and Carroll NC: Hip stability and ambulatory status in myelomeningocele, J Pediatr Orthop 5:522, 1985.

Lindseth RE: Posterior iliac osteotomy for fixed pelvic obliquity, J Bone Joint Surg 60A:17, 1978.

McKay DW: McKay hip stabilization in myelomeningocele, Orthop Trans 1:87, 1977.

Menelaus MB: Progress in the management of the paralytic hip in myelomeningocele, Orthop Clin North Am 11:17, 1980.

Molloy MK: The unstable paralytic hip: treatment by combined pelvic and femoral osteotomy and transiliac psoas transfer, J Pediatr Orthop 6:533, 1986.

Mustard WT: Iliopsoas transfer for weakness of the hip abductors, J Bone Joint Surg 34A:647, 1952.

O'Phelan EH: Iliac osteotomy in exstrophy of the bladder, J Bone Joint Surg 45A:409, 1963.

Raycroft JF: Abduction splinting of the hip joints in myelodysplastic infants, J Pediatr Orthop 7:686, 1987.

Raycroft TF: Posterior iliopsoas transfer—long term results in patients treated at Newington Children's Hospital, Orthop Trans 11:454, 1987.

Roy DR and Crawford AH: Idiopathic chondrolysis of hip: management by subtotal capsulectomy and aggressive rehabilitation, J Pediatr Orthop 8:203, 1988.

Roye DP et al: Treatment of the hip in myelomeningocele: a review of 200 patients. Presented at the Annual Meeting of the Pediatric Orthopaedic Society of North America, Toronto, May 17-29, 1987.

Sharrard WJW: Paralytic deformity in the lower limb, J Bone Joint Surg 49B:731, 1967.

Sharrard WJW: Posterior iliopsoas transplantation in the treatment of paralytic dislocation of the hip, J Bone Joint Surg 52B:779, 1970.

Sherk HA, Melchionne J, and Smith R: The natural history of hip dislocation in ambulatory myelomeningoceles, Z Kinderchir 42(suppl 1):48, 1987.

Stillwell A and Menelaus MB: Walking ability after transplantation of the iliopsoas: a long-term follow-up, J Bone Joint Surg 66B(5):656, 1984.

Taylor LJ: Excision of the proximal end of the femur for hip stiffness in myelomeningocele, J Bone Joint Surg 68B:75, 1986.

Thomas LI, Thompson TC, and Straub LR: Transplantation of the external oblique muscle for abductor paralysis, J Bone Joint Surg 32A:207, 1950.

Weisl H, Fairclough JA, and Jones DG: Stabilisation of the hip in myelomeningocele: comparison of posterior iliopsoas transfer and varus-rotation osteotomy, J Bone Joint Surg 70B:29, 1988.

Wissinger HA, Tumer Y, and Donaldson WF: Posterior iliopsoas transfer: a treatment for some myelodysplastic hips, Orthopedics 3:865, 1980.

Yngve DA and Lindseth RE: Effectiveness of muscle transfers in myelomeningocele hips measured by radiographic indices, J Pediatr Orthop 2:121, 1982.

Yount CC: The role of the tensor fasciae femoris in certain deformities of the lower extremities, J Bone Joint Surg 8:171, 1926.

Spine

Allen BL and Fergusion RL: The operative treatment of myelomeningocele spinal deformity, Orthop Clin North Am 10:845, 1979.

Altman R and Altman DA: Imaging of spinal dysraphism, Am J Neurol Radiol 8:533, 1987.

Banta JV and Becker G: The natural history of scoliosis in myelomeningocele, Orthop Trans 10:18, 1986.

Banta JV and Park SM: Improvement in pulmonary function in patients having combined anterior and posterior spine fusion for myelomeningocele scoliosis, Spine 8:765, 1983.

Drennan JC: Orthotic management of the myelomeningocele spine, Dev Child Neurol 18 (suppl 37):97, 1976.

Hall PV et al: Myelodysplasia and developmental scoliosis: a manifestation of syringomyelia, Spine 1:48, 1976.

Hall JE and Poitras B: The management of kyphosis in patients with myelomeningocele, Clin Orthop 128:33, 1977.

Hedemann JS and Gillespie R: Management of myelomeningocele kyphosis in the older child by kyphectomy and segmental spinal instrumentation, Spine 12:37, 1987.

Hull WJ, Moe JN, and Winter RB: Spinal deformity in myelomeningocele: natural history, evaluation, and treatment, J Bone Joint Surg 56A:1767, 1974.

Letherman KD and Dickson RA: Congenital kyphosis in myelomeningocele: vertebral body resection and posterior spinal fusion, Spine 3:222, 1978.

Lindseth RE and Seltzer L: Vertebral excision for kyphosis in children with myelomeningocele, J Bone Joint Surg 61A:699, 1979.

Mayer L: Further studies of fixed pelvic obliquity, J Bone Joint Surg 18:27, 1936.

Mazur J et al: Efficacy of surgical management for scoliosis in myelomeningocele: correction of deformity and alteration of functional status, J Pediatr Orthop 6(5):568, 1986.

McLaughlin TP et al: Intraspinal rhizotomy and distal cordectomy in patients with myelomeningocele, J Bone Joint Surg 68(1):88, 1986.

McMaster MJ: Anterior and posterior instrumentation and fusion of thoracolumbar scoliosis due to myelomeningocele, J Bone Joint Surg 69B:20, 1987.

McMaster MJ: The long-term results of kyphectomy and spinal stabilization in children with myelomeningocele, Spine 13:417, 1988.

Moe JH et al: Scoliosis and other spinal deformities, ed 2, Philadelphia, 198, WB Saunders Co.

Osebold WR et al: Surgical treatment of paralytic scoliosis associated with myelomeningocele, J Bone Joint Surg 64A:841, 1982.

Piggott H: The natural history of scoliosis in myelodysplasia, J Bone Joint Surg 62B:54, 1980.

Raycroft JF and Curtis BH: Spinal curvature in myelomeningocele. In The American Academy of Orthopaedic Surgeons: Symposium on myelomeningocele, St Louis, 1972, The CV Mosby Co.

Samuelsson L and Eklof O: Scoliosis in myelomeningocele, Acta Orthop Scand 59:122, 1988.

Shurtleff DB et al: Myelodysplasia: the natural history of kyphosis and scoliosis. A preliminary report, Dev Med Child Neurol Suppl 18(suppl 37):126, 1976.

Winter RB and Carlson JM: Modern orthotics for spinal deformities, Clin Orthop 126:74, 1977.

13 Neuromuscular Disorders

James H. Beaty

Neuromuscular disease in children includes the generally hereditary conditions that affect the spinal cord, peripheral nerves, neuromuscular junctions, and muscles. Accurate diagnosis is essential because the procedures commonly used to treat deformities in patients with neuromuscular disease such as poliomyelitis or cerebral palsy may not be appropriate for hereditary neuromuscular conditions. The diagnosis is made on the basis of clinical history, detailed family history, physical examination, and laboratory testing (including serum enzyme studies, especially serum levels of creatinine phosphokinase and aldolase), electromyography, nerve conduction velocity studies, and nerve and muscle biopsies. Serum enzyme levels of creatinine phosphokinase are generally elevated, but the increase varies dramatically from levels of 50 to 100 times normal in patients with some dystrophic muscle conditions (such as Duchenne muscular dystrophy) to only slight increases (1 to 2 times normal) in some patients with congenital myopathy or spinal muscular atrophy.

Nerve or muscle biopsy, or both, is useful for precise diagnosis. The muscle to be biopsied must be involved but still functioning—usually the deltoid, quadriceps, or gastrocnemius muscles. The biopsy specimen should not be taken from the region of musculotendinous junctions because the normal fibrous tissue septa may be confused with the pathologic fibrosis. Specimens should be about 10 mm long and 3 mm deep and should be fixed in glutaraldehyde. For nerve biopsy, the sural nerve is usually chosen. This nerve can be accessed laterally between the tendo Achilles and the lateral malleolus just proximal to the level of the tibiotalar joint. The entire width of the nerve should be taken for a length of 3 to 4 cm. Atraumatic technique is essential in either type of biopsy for meaningful results.

Effective treatment for the primary process of childhood neuromuscular disease generally is not available, and orthopaedic treatment is aimed at supporting and aligning the musculoskeletal system. Orthopaedic treatment can improve the quality of life for most children, no matter how severely impaired. Louis et al reported 34 surgical procedures performed over a 12-year period to improve sitting posture, care, and comfort in a select population of individuals with severe multiple impairments. Significant improvement was found in most patients, and no patient was made worse. Bleck listed the priorities of patients with severe neuromuscular diseases: the ability to communicate with other people and the ability to perform many activities of daily living, mobility, and ambulation. The role of the orthopaedic surgeon in achieving these goals includes prescribing orthoses for lower extremity control to facilitate transfer to and from wheelchairs, preventing or correcting joint contractures, and maintaining appropriate standing and sitting postures. Treatment must be individualized for each patient. The choice and timing of the procedures depend on the particular disorder, the severity of involvement, the ambulatory status of the patient, and the experience of the physician. This chapter includes only the common neuromuscular disorders in children that frequently require surgical intervention.

GENERAL TREATMENT CONSIDERATIONS
Fractures

Fractures are common in children with neuromuscular disease because of disuse osteoporosis and frequent falls. Most fractures are nondisplaced metaphyseal fractures that heal rapidly. Minimally displaced metaphyseal fractures of the lower limbs should be splinted so that walking can be resumed quickly. If braces are in use, they may be enlarged to accommodate the fractured limb and allow progressive weight bearing. Displaced diaphyseal fractures may be treated with cast-braces or, rarely, open reduction and internal fixation to allow walking during fracture healing.

Orthoses

Spinal bracing is usually accomplished with a polypropylene plastic shell with a soft foam polyethylene lining, in the form of either an anterior and posterior (bivalved) total-contact orthosis or an anterior-opening Boston brace with lumbar lordotic contouring. Knee-ankle-foot orthoses provide stability for patients with proximal muscle weakness. A pelvic band with hip and knee locks can be added if necessary.

Seating Systems

For most children with severe neuromuscular disease, walking is difficult and frustrating and a wheelchair may be eventually needed. The chair—whether manual or electric—must be carefully contoured. A narrow chair with a firm seat increases pelvic support, and a firm back in slight extension supports the spine. Lateral spine supports built into the chair may help control scoliosis deformity. The sophisticated specialized seating clinics provide custom-fitted chairs with numerous options for daily use.

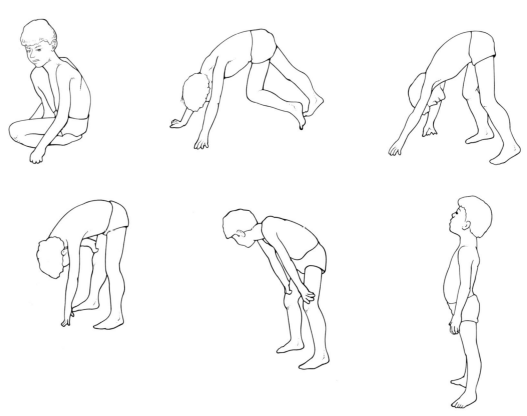

Fig. 13-1   Gower sign. Child must use hands to arise from sitting. (Redrawn from Siegel IM: Clinical management of muscle disease, London, 1977, William Heinemann Medical Books, Ltd.)

MUSCULAR DYSTROPHY

The muscular dystrophies are a group of hereditary disorders of skeletal muscle that produce progressive degeneration of skeletal muscle and associated weakness. The X-linked dystrophies are more common and include Duchenne muscular dystrophy and Becker muscular dystrophy, which differ primarily in severity—Duchenne muscular dystrophy being the more severe form of the disease. Limb-girdle muscular dystrophy and congenital muscular dystrophy are the two most common autosomal recessive muscular dystrophies. Facioscapulohumeral muscular dystrophy is inherited as an autosomal dominant trait.

Duchenne Muscular Dystrophy

Duchenne muscular dystrophy, a sex-linked recessive inherited trait, occurs in males and in females with Turner syndrome; carriers are female. It is reported to occur in one in 3000 live births. There is a family history in 70% of patients, and the condition occurs as a spontaneous mutation in about 30% of patients.

Children with Duchenne muscular dystrophy usually reach early motor milestones at appropriate times, but independent ambulation may be delayed and many are initially toe-walkers. Clinical features include large, firm calf muscles; the tendency to toe-walking; a widely-based, lordotic stance; a waddling Trendelenburg gait; and a positive Gower test indicative of proximal muscle weakness (Fig. 13-1). The diagnosis is usually obvious by the time the child is 5 or 6 years old. Diagnosis is confirmed by a dramatically elevated level of creatinine phosphokinase (50 to 100 times normal) and muscle biopsy characterized by variations in fiber size in internal nuclei, split fibers, degenerating or regenerating fibers, and fibro-fatty tissue deposition.

Physical Examination

The degree of muscular weakness depends on the age of the patient. Because the proximal musculature weakens before the distal muscles, examination of the lower extremities demonstrates an early weakness of gluteal muscle strength. The calf pseudohypertrophy is caused by infiltration of the muscle by fat and fibrosis, giving them the feel of hard rubber (Fig. 13-2). The extrinsic muscles of the foot and ankle retain their strength longer than the proximal muscles of the hip and knee. The posterior tibial muscle retains its strength for the longest time. This pattern of weakness causes an equinovarus deformity of the foot. Weakness of the shoulder girdle musculature can be demonstrated by the Meryon sign, which is elicited by lifting the child with one arm encircling the child's chest. Most children contract the muscles about the shoulder to increase shoulder stability and facilitate lifting. In the child with muscular dystrophy, however, the arms abduct because of the severe shoulder abductor muscle weakness until they eventually slide through the examiner's arms unless the chest is tightly encircled. Later in the disease process, the Thomas test demonstrates hip flexion contracture, and the Ober test demonstrates an abduction contracture of the hip.

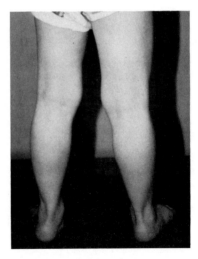

Fig. 13-2 Calf pseudohypertrophy in child with Duchenne muscular dystrophy.

Orthopaedic Treatment

The major goal of early treatment is to maintain functional ambulation as long as possible. This requires prevention or retardation of the development of contractures of the lower extremity, which would eventually prohibit ambulation. It is easier to keep patients walking than to induce them to resume walking once they have stopped. When children with Duchenne muscular dystrophy stop walking, they also become more susceptible to the development of scoliosis and severe contractures of the lower extremities. Cambridge and Drennan reported that scoliosis developed in 95% of their patients after loss of ambulation. Cessation of ambulation also results in rapid pulmonary deterioration. Generally, surgery is best performed when unassisted ambulation becomes difficult and the patient experiences frequent falls.

Equinus contractures of the feet should not be corrected early, since this equinus position helps force the knee into extension, which in turn helps prevent the knee buckling caused by severe weakness of the quadriceps. Stretching exercises and nightly bracing can be used to prevent the contractures from becoming severe. Flexion and abduction contractures of the hip, however, impede ambulation and should be minimized. Exercises to stretch the hip muscles and lower-extremity braces worn at night to prevent the child's sleeping in a frog position are helpful initially. When surgery is indicated, the foot and hip contractures should be released simultaneously, usually through percutaneous incisions. Ambulation should be resumed immediately after surgery if possible. Polypropylene braces are preferred to long-term casting. Prolonged immobilization must be avoided to prevent or limit the progressive muscle weakness caused by disuse.

Percutaneous release of hip flexion and abduction contractures and tendo Achilles contracture

▶ *Technique (Green).* With the child supine on the operating table, prepare and drape both lower extremities from the iliac crests to the toes. First flex and then extend the hip to be released, holding the hip in adduction to place tension on the muscles to be released; keep the opposite hip in maximum flexion to flatten the lumbar spine. Insert a No. 15 knife blade percutaneously just medial and just distal to the anterosuperior iliac spine (Fig. 13-3). Release the sartorius muscle first, then the tensor fasciae femoris muscle. Push the knife laterally and subcutaneously—without cutting the skin—to release the tensor fasciae latae completely. Bring the knife to the original insertion point and push it deeper to release the rectus femoris completely. Take care to avoid the neurovascular structures of the anterior thigh. Next, approximately 3 to 4 cm proximal to the upper pole of the patella, percutaneously release the fascia lata laterally through a stab wound in its midportion. Push the knife almost to the femur to release the lateral intermuscular septum completely. Now perform a percutaneous release of the tendo Achilles. Apply long-leg casts with the feet in neutral position and with the heels well-padded to prevent pressure ulcers.

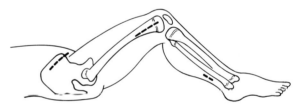

Fig. 13-3 Tenotomy sites for percutaneous release of hip flexion and abduction contractures and tendo Achilles contracture. (Redrawn from Siegel IM: Clin Pediatr 19:386, 1980.)

▶ *Postoperative management.* The child is transferred from the operating table to an electric bed that allows the patient to stand the same day as surgery. If tolerated, a few steps are allowed. Walker-assisted ambulation is begun as soon as possible, and once transfer is achieved, the patient is placed on a regular bed and physical therapy is continued. The casts are bivalved, and bilateral polypropylene long-leg orthoses are fitted as soon as possible. The patient is discharged from the hospital as soon as he can ambulate independently with a walker.

• • •

Although release of contractures usually allows another 2 to 3 years of ambulation, by the age of 12 to 13 years, most children with Duchenne muscular dystrophy can no longer walk, and spinal deformity becomes the primary problem. Scoliosis affects approximately 90% of children with Duchenne muscular dystrophy, and the curve is progressive in almost all of them (Fig. 13-4). Scoliosis produces pelvic obliquity, which makes sitting increasingly difficult and increases the deterioration of pulmonary function. Bracing and wheelchair spinal-support systems may slow progression of the curve somewhat, but spinal fusion is ultimately required for most patients. Fusion should not be delayed too long because decreasing pulmonary function might prohibit surgery. Most authors recommend that the forced vital capacity of the lungs should be 50% or more of normal to reduce pulmonary complications to an acceptable level. Cambridge and Drennan list forced vital capacity of less than 35% as a relative contraindication to surgery and as evidence of significant cardiomyopathy. Posterior spinal fusion should be performed when the scoliosis reaches 30 to 35 degrees if pulmonary function is adequate. The fusion of the entire thoracolumbar spine must extend to the proximal thoracic spine to prevent postoperative kyphosis above the fusion and usually should extend to the sacrum. Currently the use of Luque rods segmentally wired to the spine, and fixed to the pelvis by the Galveston technique if pelvic obliquity is severe, is the procedure of choice.

A
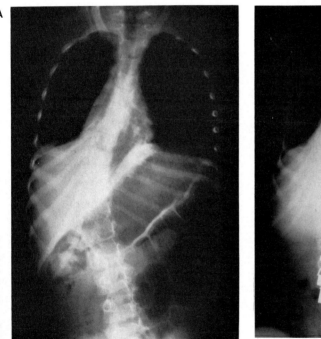

B
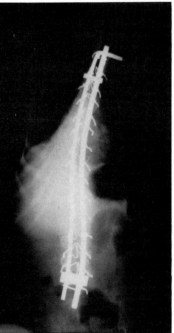

Fig. 13-4 **A,** Paralytic scoliosis in 12-year-old boy with Duchenne muscular dystrophy. **B,** After spinal fusion with Luque segmental instrumentation.

Other Variants of Muscular Dystrophy

Becker muscular dystrophy is a milder, slowly progressive form of sex-linked recessive muscular dystrophy occurring in about 10% to 20% of patients with sex-linked dystrophies. Serum creatine phosphokinase levels are highest before muscle weakness is clinically apparent and may be 10 to 20 times normal levels. Onset of symptoms usually occurs after the age of 7 years, and patients may live to their mid-40s or later. Cardiac involvement is much less frequent, and most patients do not require surgical intervention during childhood or adolescence.

Limb-girdle dystrophy is an autosomal recessive condition with a wide range of severity. The disease may occur in the first to fourth decades of life; the later the onset, the more rapid the progression. Weakness may be in the muscles of either the shoulders or the pelvis (Fig. 13-5). Lower extremity weakness may involve the gluteus maximus, the iliopsoas, and the quadriceps. Upper extremity weakness may involve the trapezius, the serratus anterior, the rhomboids, the latissimus dorsi, and the pectoralis major. Some weakness may develop in the prime movers of the fingers and wrists as well. Surgery is seldom required in patients with limb-girdle dystrophy. Sta-bilization of the scapula to the ribs may be required for winging of the scapula, and rarely muscle transfers about the wrist may be needed.

Facioscapulohumeral dystrophy is an autosomal dominant condition with characteristic weakness of the facial and shoulder-girdle muscles (Fig. 13-6). Onset of the disease may be in early childhood, in which case the disease runs a rapid, progressive course, confining most children to a wheelchair by the age of 8 to 9 years; or onset may occur in patients from 15 to 35 years of age, in which case the disease progresses more slowly. The most striking clinical manifestation is facial weakness with an inability to whistle, purse the lips, wrinkle the brow, or blow out the cheeks. The greatest functional impairment is the inability to to abduct and flex the arm at the glenohumeral joint. As the disease progresses, weakness of the lower extremities, especially the tibialis anterior, peroneal, and (sometimes) quadriceps muscles, requires the use of ankle-foot or knee-ankle-foot orthoses. Scapulothoracic fusion may be indicated for the high-riding, winged scapulae and an inability to abduct the arms fully. Rarely, spinal fusion may be required for progressive scoliosis.

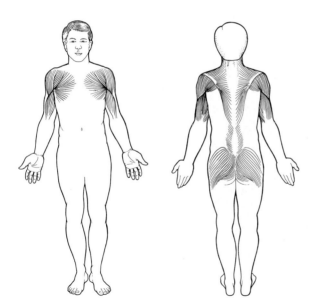

Fig. 13-5   Pattern of muscle weakness in limb-girdle dystrophy.

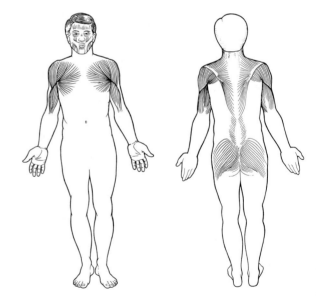

Fig. 13-6   Pattern of muscle weakness in facioscapulohumeral dystrophy.

Scapulothoracic fusion

▶ *Technique (Copeland and Howard).* The graft used for scapulothoracic fusion may be obtained from the tibia, or a full-thickness bicortical cancellous iliac crest graft may be used. Once the approximately 9-cm × 1-cm graft is obtained, prepare and drape the upper back, shoulder, and upper arm to allow movement of the arm and access to the thoracic spine; allow the arm to hang from the side of the table. Make an incision along the vertebral border of the scapula. Divide the underlying muscles, and denude a 2-cm width beneath the vertebral border of the scapula along most of its length.

Now denude by subperiosteal dissection the soft tissues of three ribs (usually the fourth, fifth, and sixth), including the periosteum, the intercostal muscle, and the parietal pleura. Expose enough of the ribs so that half the length of the cortical grafts (the original graft being divided into three 3-cm segments) will lie against the denuded ribs. Drill a hole in each end of the graft, and fix the grafts with screws to the three ribs and to the underside of the medial aspect of the scapula (Fig. 13-7). Protect the parietal pleura from penetration by a drill bit or screw. Fill any gap between the scapula and the chest wall with cancellous bone. Insert a drain, close the wound, and carefully turn the patient supine. Apply a shoulder spica cast with the arm in 30 degrees of forward flexion, 80 degrees of abduction, and the hand in front of the mouth.

▶ *Postoperative managment.* The patient is kept in a seated position. The arm section of the cast is removed at 3 months to allow abduction, and once abduction can be controlled the entire cast is removed. A triangular pillow is placed between the inner arm and the thorax, and its size is gradually decreased to allow gradual adduction of the arm to the side. As soon as the cast is removed, physical therapy is begun to help gain glenohumeral movement and deltoid strength.

• • •

Congenital dystrophies include relatively rare conditions such as nemaline dystrophy, central core myopathy, myotubular myopathy, congenital fiber disproportion, and multicore and minicore disease. Electron microscopy may be needed to differentiate some of the types; some show an inheritance pattern. Weakness and contractures at birth may cause hip dislocation, clubfeet, or other deformities. Respiratory weakness and difficulty with feeding and swallowing are common. The clinical appearance is one of dysmorphism, with kyphoscoliosis, chest deformities, a long face, and a high palate. Muscle tissue is gradually replaced with fibrous tissue, and contractures may become severe. Treatment is aimed at keeping the patient ambulatory and preventing contractures by exercises and orthotic splinting. Equinus and varus deformities of the feet may require releases if they interfere with ambulation. Congenital dislocation of the hip and clubfoot deformity are treated conventionally, but recurrence is frequent.

Myotonic dystrophy is characterized by an inability of the muscles to relax after contraction. It is progressive and usually is present at birth, although it may develop in childhood. Inheritance is most often autosomal dominant but may be autosomal recessive. In addition to the inability of the muscles to relax, muscle weakness causes the most functional impairment. Other defects may include hyperostosis of the skull, frontal and temporal baldness, gonadal atrophy, dysphasia, dysarthria, electrocardiographic abnormalities, and mental retardation. The characteristic clinical appearance is a tent-shaped mouth, facial diplegia, and dull expression. About half the children with myotonic dystrophy have clubfoot deformities, and hip dysplasia and scoliosis may exist. The hip dysplasia is treated conventionally, but because of capsular laxity may not respond as readily as in other children. Serial casting can correct equinovarus deformity early on, but recurrence is likely and extensile release is usually required; triple arthrodesis may be required at skeletal maturity if recurrence is frequent despite extensile releases. The high incidence of cardiac abnormalities and decreased pulmonary function in these patients may prohibit surgery.

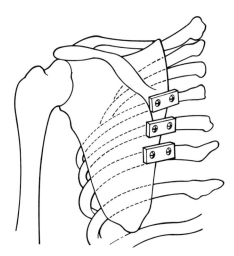

Fig. 13-7 Scapulothoracic fusion with strut grafts. (Redrawn from Copeland SA and Howard RC: J Bone Joint Surg 60B:549, 1978.)

CHARCOT-MARIE-TOOTH DISEASE (PERONEAL MUSCULAR ATROPHY)

Charcot-Marie-Tooth disease is an inherited degenerative disorder of the central and peripheral nervous systems that causes muscle atrophy and loss of proprioception. It is usually an autosomal dominant trait, but may be X-linked recessive or autosomal recessive. Muscle atrophy is steadily progressive in most patients with the autosomal dominant form; less often, the disease arrests completely or manifests intermittently. The recessive forms have an early onset (first or second decade) and are more rapidly progressive. Initial complaints are usually general weakness of the foot and an unsteady gait. Foot problems may include pain under the metatarsal heads, claw toes, foot fatigue, and difficulty in wearing regular shoes. Distal loss of proprioception and spinal ataxia are common. Charcot-Marie-Tooth disease should be suspected in patients with claw toes, high arches, thin legs, poor balance, and an unsteady gait. In addition to physical examination and family history, electromyograms and nerve-conduction studies should confirm the diagnosis.

Cavovarus Foot Deformity

Charcot-Marie-Tooth disease is the most common neuromuscular cause of cavovarus foot deformity in children. This is a complex deformity of the forefoot and hindfoot. Surgery is often required to stabilize the foot. Although there is little question that the cavovarus deformity is caused by muscle imbalance, theories explaining which muscles are involved and how the imbalances produce the rigid cavovarus deformity do not completely account for the clinical deformity. The neuropathic cavovarus deformity of Charcot-Marie-Tooth disease has been suggested to be caused by a combination of intrinsic and extrinsic weakness, beginning with weakness of the intrinsic foot muscles and the tibialis anterior, with normal strength of the tibialis posterior and peroneus longus. The triceps surae is also weak and may be contracted. The forefoot is pulled into equinus relative to the hindfoot, and the first ray becomes plantarflexed. The long toe extensors attempt to assist the weak tibialis anterior in dorsiflexion, but contribute to metatarsal plantarflexion, and the foot is pronated into a valgus position with mild adduction of the metatarsals. Initially the foot is supple and plantigrade with weight bearing, but as the forefoot becomes more rigidly pronated, the hindfoot assumes a varus position. Weight bearing becomes a "tripod" mechanism, with weight borne on the heel and the first and fifth metatarsal heads (Fig. 13-8).

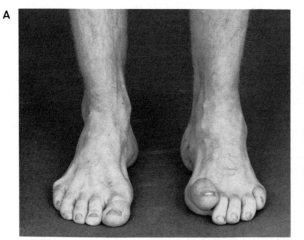
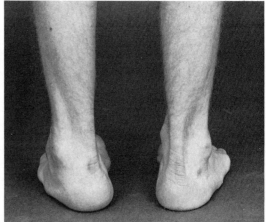
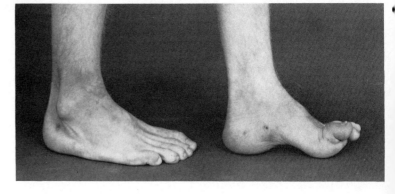

Fig. 13-8 Cavovarus foot deformity in Charcot-Marie-Tooth disease. **A,** Clawing of left great toe. **B,** Fixed varus deformity of left hindfoot. **C,** Supination and cavus deformity of forefoot. (Courtesy Dr Jay Cummings.)

Clinical and Roentgenographic Evaluation

Clinical evaluation of the cavovarus deformity includes determination of the rigidity of the hindfoot varus, usually with the block test of Coleman (Fig. 13-9), and assessment of individual muscle strength and overall balance. Careful examination of the peripheral and central nervous systems is required, including electromyography and nerve conduction velocity studies.

Standard anteroposterior, lateral, and oblique roentgenograms are the most useful methods of evaluating the child's foot; however, to determine any significant relationships between the bones, it is essential that the anteroposterior and lateral views be made with the foot in a weight-bearing or simulated weight-bearing position. Anteroposterior views document the degree of forefoot adduction. The degree of cavus can be estimated on the lateral view by determining Meary's angle, the angle between the long axis of the first metatarsal and long axis of the talus; the normal angle is 0 (Fig. 13-10). Roentgenograms using the Coleman block test demonstrate the correction of the varus deformity if the hindfoot is flexible.

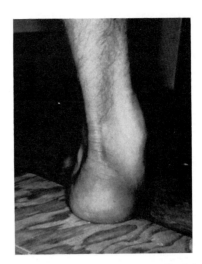

Fig. 13-9 Coleman block test shows flexible hindfoot. Heel placed on 1-inch block with plantar flexed forefoot on floor.

A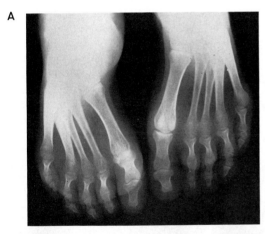

B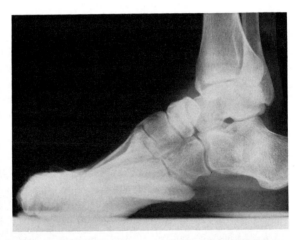

C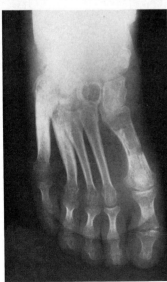

D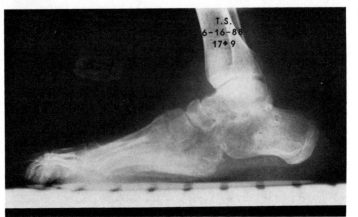

Fig. 13-10 Cavovarus deformity in Charcot-Marie-Tooth disease. **A** and **B,** Preoperative roentgenograms. **C** and **D,** After triple arthrodesis, tendo Achilles lengthening, posterior tibialis tendon transfer. (Courtesy Dr Jay Cummings.)

Orthopaedic Treatment

Treatment is determined by the age of the patient and the cause and severity of the deformity. Nonoperative treatment of the cavovarus foot has generally been unsuccessful. Surgical procedures are of three types: soft tissue (plantar fascia release, tendon release or transfer), osteotomy (metatarsal, midfoot, calcaneal), and joint stabilizing (triple arthrodesis). Children younger than 8 years with a supple hindfoot usually respond to plantar release and appropriate tendon transfers. Bradley and Coleman use a more extensive plantar-medial release for a rigid forefoot and osteotomy of the first metatarsal. In children younger than 12 years with a rigid hindfoot, radical plantar-medial release, first metatarsal osteotomy, and Dwyer calcaneal osteotomy may correct the deformity.

Triple arthrodesis is reserved for children older than 12 years with severe rigid deformity. Wukich and Bowen reported that only 14% of patients with Charcot-Marie-Tooth disease required triple arthrodesis and recommended soft tissue procedures and osteotomies in skeletally immature feet and those with less severe deformity. The Hoke arthrodesis or a modification of it is most often recommended. Appropriate wedge resections correct both the hindfoot varus and midfoot component of the cavus deformity; soft tissue release and muscle balancing are required for the forefoot deformity. Wukich and Bowen recommend restoring hindfoot stability with triple arthrodesis and transferring the posterior tibial tendon ante-

riorly to eliminate the need for a postoperative drop-foot brace. They reported good or excellent results in 88% of their patients treated with this method. McCluskey et al recommend tendo Achilles lengthening with triple arthrodesis after correction of the forefoot (Fig. 13-11).

Flexible clawtoe deformity is usually corrected without additional surgery when the midfoot deformity is corrected. For clawing in a young child without severe weakness of the anterior tibial muscle, the toe extensors can be transferred to the metatarsal necks with tenodesis of the interphalangeal joint of the great toe (Jones procedure). For adolescents or children with severe weakness of the anterior tibial muscle all the long toe extensors can be transferred to the middle cuneiform with fusion of the interphalangeal joint (Hibbs procedure). For severe deformity, the posterior tibial tendon may be transferred anteriorly to the middle cuneiform instead of the long toe extensors (p. 621).

Surgical procedures are usually staged. The initial procedure is a radical plantar or plantar-medial release, with dorsal closing wedge osteotomy of the first metatarsal base if necessary. Tendo Achilles lengthening should not be performed as part of the initial procedure because the force used to dorsiflex the forefoot would dorsiflex the calcaneus into an unacceptable position. If the hindfoot is flexible and a posterior release is not necessary, posterior tibial tendon transfer may be done as part of the initial procedure for severe anterior tibial weakness.

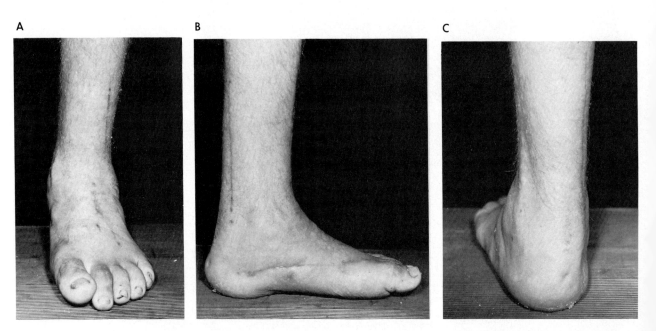

Fig. 13-11 Clinical appearance of foot after triple arthrodesis, tendo Achilles lengthening, and posterior tibialis tendon transfer. **A,** Anterior view. **B,** Medial correction of cavus. **C,** Posterior correction of hindfoot varus. (Courtesy Dr Jay Cummings.)

Radical plantar-medial release and dorsal closing wedge osteotomy

▶ *Technique (Coleman).* Make a curved incision over the medial aspect of the foot, extending anteriorly from the calcaneus to the base of the first metatarsal (Fig. 13-12, *A*). Identify the origin of the abductor hallucis and separate it from its bony and soft tissue attachments both proximally and distally, but leave it attached at its origin and insertion. Identify the posterior neurovascular bundle as it divides into medial and lateral branches and enters the intrinsic musculature of the foot. Identify the tendinous origin of the abductor at its attachment on the calcaneus between the medial and lateral plantar branches of the nerve and artery, and sever it to free the origin of the abductor hallucis. Identify the long toe flexors as they course along the plantar aspect of the foot, and section the retinaculum of the tendons. Sever the origins of the plantar aponeurosis, the abductor hallucis, and the short flexors from their attachments to the calcaneus (Fig. 13-12, *B*), and gently dissect this entire musculotendinous mass distally and extraperiosteally as far as the calcaneocuboid joint.

If the first metatarsal remains in plantarflexion after this release, make a dorsally based closing wedge osteotomy immediately distal to the physis, removing enough bone to correct the lateral talo–first metatarsal angle to 0. Fix the osteotomy with a smooth Steinmann pin or Kirschner wire. Close the wounds in routine fashion, and apply a short leg cast with the foot in the corrected position.

▶ *Postoperative management.* If there is excessive tension on the wound, the foot may be casted in slight plantarflexion. A new cast should be applied at 2 weeks with the foot in a fully corrected position. The pins and cast are removed at 6 to 8 weeks.

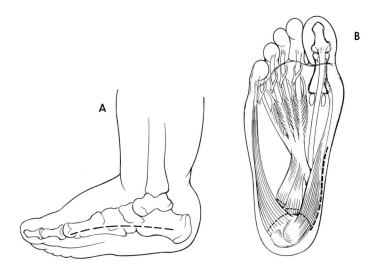

Fig. 13-12 Radical plantar-medial release and dorsal closing wedge osteotomy for cavovarus deformity. **A,** Incision. **B,** Release of musculotendinous mass. (Redrawn from Coleman SS: Complex foot deformities in children, Philadelphia, 1983, Lea & Febiger.)

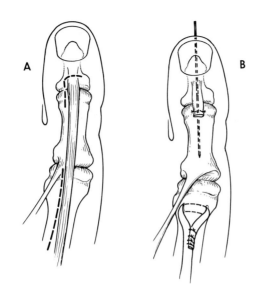

Fig. 13-13 Transfer of extensor hallucis longus tendon for clawtoe deformity (Jones procedure). **A,** Incisions. **B,** Completed procedure.

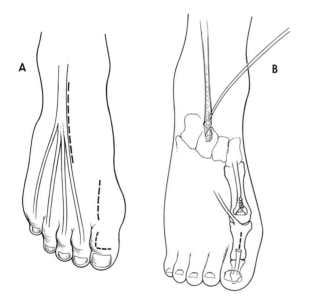

Fig. 13-14 Transfer of extensor tendons to middle cuneiform for clawtoe deformity (Hibbs procedure). **A,** Incisions. **B,** Completed procedure combined with Jones procedure.

Transfer of extensor hallucis longus tendon for clawtoe deformity

▶ *Technique (Jones).* Expose the interphalangeal joint of the great toe through an L-shaped incision (Fig. 13-13). Retract the flap of skin and subcutaneous tissue medially and proximally and expose the tendon of the extensor hallucis longus. Cut the tendon transversely 1 cm proximal to the joint and expose the joint. Excise the cartilage, approximate the joint surfaces, and insert a ⁵⁄₆₄-inch intramedullary Kirschner wire for fixation. Clip the wire off just outside the skin. Now expose the neck of the first metatarsal through a 2.5-cm dorsomedial incision extending distally to the proximal extensor skin crease. Dissect free the extensor hallucis longus tendon but protect the short extensor tendon. Cleanly and carefully excise the sheath of the long extensor tendon throughout the length of the proximal incision. Beginning on the inferomedial aspect of the first metatarsal neck, drill a hole transverse to the long axis of the bone to emerge on the dorsolateral aspect of the neck. Now pass the tendon through the hole and suture it to itself with interrupted sutures. The same procedure can be performed on adjacent toes with clawing. Close the wounds and apply a short-leg walking cast with the ankle in neutral position.

▶ *Postoperative management.* Walking with crutches is allowed in 2 to 3 days. At 3 weeks the cast and skin sutures are removed and a short-leg walking cast is applied. At 6 weeks the walking cast and Kirschner wire are removed, and active exercises are begun.

Transfer of extensor tendons to middle cuneiform

▶ *Technique (Hibbs).* Make a curved incision 7.5 to 10 cm long on the dorsum of the foot lateral to the midline and expose the common extensor tendons (Fig. 13-14). Divide the tendons as far distally as feasible, draw their proximal ends through a tunnel in the third cuneiform, and fix them with a nonabsorbable suture. As an alternative, use a plantar button and felt with a Bunnell pull-out stitch. Close the wounds and apply a plaster boot cast with the foot in the corrected position.

▶ *Postoperative management.* The cast and plantar button are removed at 6 weeks.

Spinal Deformities

Scoliosis is uncommon in association with Charcot-Marie-Tooth disease, occurring in only approximately 10% of patients. The curve is usually mild to moderate and often does not require any treatment. In patients with Charcot-Marie-Tooth disease, Hensinger and MacEwen reported associated kyphosis in half their patients with scoliosis. They reported that nonoperative treatment with a brace was well tolerated and successfully controlled the curve in many patients. Generally, spinal deformities in children with Charcot-Marie-Tooth disease can be managed by the same techniques used for idiopathic scoliosis.

Charcot-Marie-Tooth Variants

Roussy-Lévy syndrome (hereditary areflexic dystaxia) is an autosomal dominant disease with the clinical characteristics of classic Charcot-Marie-Tooth disease plus a static tremor in the hands. The disease is usually arrested at puberty.

Déjérine-Sottas syndrome (familial interstitial hypertrophic neuritis) is usually an autosomal recessive disease, but it may show an autosomal dominant inheritance with variable penetrance. The disease usually begins in infancy but may not appear until adolescence. Along with the classic pes cavus deformity, there is marked sensory loss in all four extremities, and patients may also have clubfoot or kyphoscoliosis.

Refsum disease is an autosomal recessive disorder beginning in childhood or puberty in which the spinal fluid protein is increased. It is accompanied by retinitis pigmentosa and is characterized by a hypertrophic neuropathy with ataxia and areflexia. There is distal sensory and motor loss in the hands and feet. The course is unpredictable, with repeated reactivations and remissions, but the prognosis is poor.

Neuronal type Charcot-Marie-Tooth disease is an autosomal dominant disease with a usually late onset (middle age or later). The small muscles of the hands are not as weak as in other forms of the disease, but the ankle muscles and plantar muscles of the feet are much weaker and more atrophic.

FRIEDREICH ATAXIA

Friedreich ataxia is an autosomal recessive condition characterized by spinocerebellar degeneration, which distinguishes it from Charcot-Marie-Tooth disease. Onset is generally between the ages of 6 and 20 years, and children with Friedreich ataxia are frequently wheelchair bound in the first and second decades of life. About two thirds have scoliosis, and many have a cardiomyopathy that often leads to death in the third or fourth decade of life. Primary symptoms are an ataxic gait and a cavovarus foot, which may be followed by clumsiness in the use of the hands, dysarthria, and nystagmus. Knee jerk and ankle jerk reflexes are lost quite early. As in Charcot-Marie-Tooth disease, the orthopaedist is concerned primarily with correction of the foot and spinal deformities, and treatment recommendations in patients with Friedreich ataxia are similar to those for patients with Charcot-Marie-Tooth disease. Sometimes in patients with Friedreich ataxia, the plantar reflex is so great that when standing is attempted, the feet and toes immediately plantarflex and the tibialis posterior tendon pulls the forefoot into equinovarus. If general anesthesia is contraindicated because of myocardial involvement or other medical conditions, tenotomies of the tendo Achilles, the tibialis posterior tendon at the ankle, and the toe flexors at the plantar side of the metatarsophalangeal joints can be performed with the patient under local anesthesia.

Labelle et al, in a study of 56 patients with Friedreich ataxia and scoliosis, found the curve patterns were similar to those of idiopathic scoliosis, many curves were not progressive, no relationship existed between muscle weakness and the curvature, and the onset of the scoliosis before puberty was the major factor in progression. They recommend that curves of less than 40 degrees should be observed and curves of more than 60 degrees should be treated surgically; treatment of curves between 40 and 60 degrees is based primarily on the patient's age at onset of the disease, age at which the scoliosis was first recognized, and evidence of the curve's progression.

SPINAL MUSCULAR ATROPHY

Spinal muscular atrophy is an inherited degenerative disease of the anterior horn cells of the spinal cord. It is generally transmitted by an autosomal recessive gene, but other hereditary patterns have been described. Hoffmann (1893) and Werdnig (1894) first described an infantile condition of generalized weakness that resulted in early death because of respiratory failure, and in 1956 Kugelberg and Welander described a similar condition of juvenile onset and less progressive nature. In the acute infantile type (type I) severe generalized weakness is manifest in patients younger than 6 months, and terminal respiratory failure occurs early. A chronic infantile type (type II) occurs during the middle of the first year and after initial progression of weakness may remain static for long periods. The juvenile type (type III) presents later with gradual onset of weakness and a slowly progressive course.

Clinical characteristics of spinal muscular atrophy include severe weakness and hypotonia, areflexia, fine tremor of the fingers, fasciculation of the tongue, and normal sensation. Proximal muscles are affected more than distal ones, and the lower extremities are usually weaker than the upper extremities. Evans et al proposed a functional classification to aid in planning long-term orthopaedic care: group I patients never develop the strength to sit independently and have poor head control; group II patients develop head control and can sit but are unable to walk; group III patients can pull themselves up and walk in a limited fashion, frequently with the use of orthoses; and group IV patients develop the ability to walk and run normally and to climb stairs before onset of the weakness.

Orthopaedic treatment is generally required for hip and spine problems. Many children with infantile spinal muscular atrophy (Werdnig-Hoffmann disease) are never able to walk even with braces, but most patients with the juvenile form (Kugelberg-Welander disease) are able to walk for many years. Gentle passive range-of-motion exercises and positioning instructions may be beneficial initially. Surgical release of contractures is rarely required. Because of the absence of movement and weight-bearing, coxa valga deformity of the hip is frequent and unilateral or bilateral hip subluxation may follow (Fig. 13-15). Since many of these children are sitters, a stable and comfortable sitting position is essential. In nonambulatory patients, proximal femoral varus derotational osteotomy (p. 17) produces a more stable sitting base; this procedure is not indicated if the child is ambulatory. Valgus subtrochanteric osteotomy or distal transfer of the greater trochanter may be indicated for severe coxa vara deformity in ambulatory patients.

Among children with spinal muscular atrophy who survive childhood, scoliosis becomes the greatest threat during adolescence. It is usually progressive and severe and may limit daily function and cause cardiopulmonary problems. Bracing may be indicated during the growing years to slow curve progression, but spinal stabilization is ultimately required in almost all adolescent patients. Several authors have emphasized the importance of early surgery before the curve becomes severe and rigid. Fusion should generally extend beyond that indicated for idiopathic scoliosis, since curve progression above the level of the fusion is likely, and fusion to the sacrum should be considered. Segmental spinal instrumentation (see p. 484) is most often advocated for paralytic scoliosis, but Piasecki et al list four problems associated with this technique in children with spinal muscular atrophy: (1) passage of multiple wires under the laminae increases the risk of neurologic complications, (2) classic posterior spinal fusion is technically impossible because of the spatial requirements of Luque instrumentation, (3) the lengthy procedure further complicates anesthesia and increases blood loss, and (4) long-term (at least 10 years) evaluation of the technique is not yet available. They recommend the use of a Harrington rod fixed with wires to the bases of adjacent spinous processes and laminae to prevent sublaminar passage of wires, reporting that this technique improves correction and stability and allows for use of adequate bone graft. Intraoperative and postoperative complications are frequent in these patients, and thorough preoperative evaluation is mandatory. Hensinger and MacEwen and Piasecki et al noted that the frequency of respiratory infections before surgery and the vital capacity of the lungs are good indicators of the patient's ability to tolerate surgery. Tracheostomy should be considered for any patient with frequent preoperative respiratory infections and a vital capacity of less than 35% of normal.

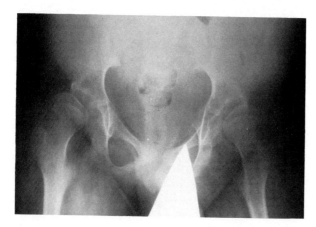

Fig. 13-15 Coxa valga deformity and subluxation in 12-year-old child with spinal muscular atrophy.

ARTHROGRYPOSIS MULTIPLEX CONGENITA

Arthrogryposis multiplex congenita, or multiple congenital contractures, is a nonprogressive syndrome characterized by deformed and rigid joints; atrophy or absence of muscles or muscle groups; cylindric, fusiform, or cone-shaped involved extremities with diminished skin creases and subcutaneous tissue; contracture of joint capsular and periarticular tissues; dislocation of joints, especially of the hip and knee; and intact sensation and intellect (Fig. 13-16).

More than 150 specific entities can be associated with what has been known as "arthrogryposis multiplex congenita"; because it is no longer considered a discrete clinical entity, the term *multiple congenital contractures* is preferred. Although the deformities may result from neurogenic, myogenic, skeletal, or environmental factors, most are neurogenic in origin and result from a congenital or acquired defect in the organization or number of anterior horn cells, roots, peripheral nerves, or motor end plates, producing muscular weakness and resultant joint immobility at critical stages of intrauterine development (Table 13-1). Myopathic multiple congenital contractures, accounting for 10% or less of patients, appear to be transmitted as an autosomal recessive disorder.

Neurologic assessment, electromyography and nerve-conduction studies, serum enzyme tests, and muscle biopsy may help determine the underlying diagnosis. Roentgenographic examination will assess the integrity of the skeletal system, especially the presence of dislocated hips or knees, scoliosis, and

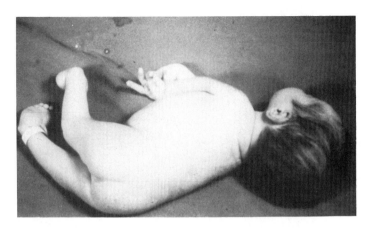

Fig. 13-16 Newborn with arthrogryposis multiplex congenita. Note orthopaedic conditions: congenital dislocation of knees, teratologic clubfeet, internal rotation contractures of shoulder, extension contractures of elbow, and flexion contractures of wrist.

other skeletal anomalies. The most common lower extremity deformities are rigid clubfeet and fixed extension or flexion contractures of the knees. Major problems in the upper extremity are usually immobile shoulders, elbow contractures, severe fixed palmarflexion deformities of the wrists, and contractures of the metacarpophalangeal and interphalangeal joints. Involvement is usually bilateral but not always symmetric. Scoliosis has been reported to occur in 10% to 30% of patients.

Table 13-1   Deformities found in patients with arthrogryposis multiplex congenita

Pattern of deformity	Level
Upper Limb	
Type I: adduction and/or medial rotation of shoulder, extension of elbow, pronation of forearm, flexion and ulnar deviation of wrist (in addition, two had weak intrinsic muscles of the hand, indicating T1 involvement)	C5, C6
Type II: adduction and/or medial rotation of shoulder, flexion deformity of elbow, flexion and ulnar deviation of wrist (in addition, two had weak intrinsic muscles indicating T1 involvement)	Partial C5, C6, partial C7
Lower Limb	
Type III: flexion and adduction of hip (with dislocation in five limbs), extension of knee, equinovarus of foot (in addition, two had weak intrinsic muscles indicating S3 involvement)	L4, L5, S1
Type IV: flexion of knee, equinovarus of foot	L3, L4, partial L5
Type V: flexion and abduction of hip, flexion of knee, equinovarus of foot	L3, L4, patchy S1-2
Type VI: flexion of hip, extension of knee with valgus, equinus of foot	L4, L5
Type VII: equinus of foot	L4
Type VIII: equinovarus of foot, weak intrinsic muscles of foot	L4, patchy L5, S3

From Brown LM, Robson MJ, and Sharrard WJW: J Bone Joint Surg 62B:4, 1980.

Treatment

Palmer et al devised a program of passive stretching exercises for each contracted joint to be followed by serial splinting with custom thermoplastic splints. Although they reported significant gains in extremity function and a reduction in the need for corrective surgery, most authors report that any improvement after physical therapy is transient at best and that recurrence of the deformity is likely. Drummond et al and Williams outlined the following principles for orthopaedic management of patients with multiple congenital contractures:

1. Muscle balance should be established, if functioning muscles are available for transfer.
2. Recurrence of the deformity is the rule because the dense, inelastic soft tissues about the joints do not properly elongate with growth.
3. Tenotomy should be accompanied by capsulotomy and capsulectomy on the concave side of the joint, followed by prolonged plaster support and then orthotic support to prevent, or at least delay, recurrence of deformity.
4. Maximal safely obtainable correction should be achieved at the time of surgery. The use of wedging or corrective casts after surgery is of little additional benefit.
5. Osteotomies to correct deformity or transfer the range of motion to a more useful arc are beneficial, but only in patients at or near skeletal maturity, or else the deformity promptly recurs with growth.

Lower Extremity

The rigid foot deformity in multiple congenital contractures is usually a clubfoot or congenital vertical talus. The goal of treatment is conversion of the rigid deformed foot into a rigid plantigrade foot; a normal foot is not a realistic goal of treatment. If the valgus foot is plantigrade, treatment is not usually required. The most common foot deformity is clubfoot. Serial casting is begun as soon after birth as possible, but surgery is eventually required in almost all patients, usually between the ages of 6 and 18 months. Extensive posteromedial and posterolateral release (p. 84) is recommended. If the deformity recurs in a young child or is so severe that it cannot be corrected by soft tissue release, talectomy is indicated. Gross described a technique of cancellectomy of the talus and cuboid in which a window is created in the dorsal cortex of the cuboid and lateral cortex of the neck and body of the talus (Fig. 13-17). All cancellous bone is carefully curetted, and the deformity is corrected by manual manipulation. He credits Verebelyi with the original description of the technique, and cites reports of Ogston and Kopits on its use in patients with myelomeningocele. Triple arthrodesis may be performed for rigid deformity in adolescents.

The most common knee deformity in multiple congenital contractures is a fixed flexion contracture. Initial treatment is serial splinting or casting in progres-

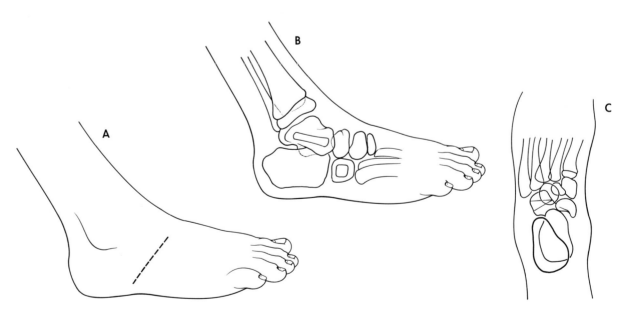

Fig. 13-17 Cancellectomy of talus and cuboid. **A,** Incision. **B,** Windows in talus and cuboid to expose cancellous bone. **C,** Closing wedge osteotomy in cuboid. (**A** redrawn from Gross RH: Clin Orthop 194:99, 1985. **B** and **C** redrawn from Spires TD et al: J Pediatr Orthop 4:706, 1984.)

sive degrees of extension. If complete correction has not been obtained by 6 to 12 months of age, posteromedia land lateral hamstring lengthening and knee capsulotomies are indicated. Supracondylar extension osteotomy of the distal femur may be required to correct a contracture of more than 25 degrees to allow the use of orthoses. Contracture of the quadriceps mechanism may cause hyperextension of the knee, which again is treated initially by serial casting. If the deformity does not respond to conservative treatment by 6 to 12 months of age, surgical correction by quadricepsplasty (p. 737) is recommended.

The hip is involved in approximately 80% of patients with multiple congenital contractures. In general, hip deformities should be treated by passive stretching exercises beginning in infancy. Intermittent skin traction may also be used. If conservative measures fail, as they do in approximately 25% of patients, surgical correction of the hip deformity should be delayed until deformities of the knees and then the feet are corrected. In general, most authors recommend that bilateral teratologic hip dislocations should not be reduced, since reduction may not improve function. If surgical intervention is chosen, the preferred combination is a one-stage open reduction, primary femoral shortening, and pelvic osteotomy between the ages of 12 and 36 months. Unilateral dislocation of the hip, whether flexible or rigid, should be reduced operatively and placed in a functional position to prevent potential pelvic obliquity and scoliosis.

Upper Extremity

Correction of upper extremity deformities should be delayed until ambulation has been achieved, usually until the age of 3 to 4 years. The goal of treatment of upper extremity deformities is to provide optimal function of the hand in the activities of daily living. Function may be adequate despite severe deformity, and operative intervention risks loss of function. Weakness and stiffness about the shoulder do not significantly impair function and usually require no treatment. Proximal humeral rotational osteotomy (p. 736) may be indicated for severe internal rotation deformity. Deformity of the elbow is usually severe limitation of either flexion or extension. The stiff flexed elbow is not a severe impairment, and surgery is not indicated (Fig. 13-18). Fixed-extension elbow deformity, especially if bilateral, is a severe functional impairment. Surgical options available for the fixed extended elbow are tricepsplasty, triceps transfer, Steindler flexorplasty, and pectoralis major transfer. Lengthening of the triceps mechanism and posterior capsulotomy are the most reliable and durable of

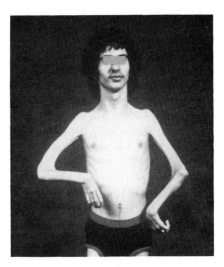

Fig. 13-18   Fixed elbow flexion contractures in adolescent with arthrogryposis multiplex congenita.

available surgical procedures. Triceps transfer is often unsatisfactory at long-term because of the gradual development of a flexion deformity. Tricepsplasty on one elbow and triceps transfer on the opposite side allows basic activities of feeding and toileting, as well as apposition of the hands for bimanual activities. Steindler flexorplasty is rarely indicated in children with multiple congenital contractures because the wrist flexors are usually both inactive and contracted.

Wrist stabilization at the optimal functional position is probably the single most beneficial procedure in patients with multiple congenital contractures, but determination of the best position for function must be made carefully. Mild ulnar deviation and dorsiflexion between 5 and 20 degrees will prove to be the most satisfactory position. After skeletal maturity, wrist fusion can be performed by traditional methods when required. In younger children, Williams recommended sacrificing the carpal bones and radius and inserting an intramedullary nail through the third metacarpal, the carpals, and the radius. If the wrist and hand need to be repositioned, a procedure analogous to centralization for radial clubhand (p. 268) can be performed.

Scoliosis

Scoliosis is reported to occur in 10% to 30% of patients with multiple congenital contractures, generally associated with neuromuscular weakness or pelvic obliquity. If the deformity is severe and progressive, early operative intervention is warranted. Indications and techniques for treatment of scoliosis in patients with multiple congenital contractures are the same as for patients with other neuromuscular disorders.

BRACHIAL PLEXUS PALSY

Brachial plexus palsy may be seen after injury of the brachial plexus during birth. Reported incidences range from 0.4 to 2.5 per 1000 live births. While the pathomechanics of these injuries are not fully understood, numerous risk factors have been identified, including large birth weight, breech presentation, and shoulder dystocia. The severity of the palsy depends on which roots of the brachial plexus have been injured and the extent of the injury.

Brachial plexus palsy is classified according to the location of injury of the brachial plexus. Seddon classified the injuries into three types and Sunderland into five. The most common types are: upper plexus palsy (Erb's palsy), in which the supraspinatus and infraspinatus muscles are the most frequently paralyzed, apparently because the suprascapular nerve is fixed at the suprascapular notch (Erb's point); whole plexus palsy ("mixed" palsy) in which complete sensory and motor paralysis of the entire extremity is caused by severe injury in all roots of the brachial plexus; and lower plexus palsy (Klumpke's palsy), in which the muscles of the forearm and hand together with parts served by the cervical sympathetic chain are paralyzed after injury of the eighth cervical and first thoracic nerve roots. Upper root-level injuries (C5-C6) occur most frequently (approximately 90% of patients) and have the best prognosis; lower plexus and whole plexus injuries have the worst prognosis, but are much less common. Narakas proposed a more detailed classification based on the clinical course of children with brachial plexus palsies during the first 8 weeks after birth. His classification includes a prognosis for each type of injury (Table 13-2).

Clinical Features

The diagnosis is usually evident at birth. In upper root involvement the arm is held in internal rotation and active abduction is limited. The elbow may be slightly flexed or in complete extension. The thumb is flexed, and occasionally the fingers will not extend. In complete paralysis, the entire arm is flail and the hand is clutched. Pinching produces no reaction. Vasomotor impairment may be indicated by the relative paleness of the involved extremity. Roentgenograms of the shoulder may reveal fracture of the proximal humeral physis or fracture of the clavicle.

Characteristic deformities usually develop promptly. The shoulder becomes flexed, internally rotated, and slightly abducted; active abduction of the joint decreases; and external rotation disappears. The shoulder may become posteriorly subluxed and eventually dislocated, or the humeral head becomes flattened against the glenoid. Evaluation of the brachial plexus injury may include clinical evaluation, electrical diagnostic studies, myelography, and computerized tomography.

Table 13-2 Classification and prognosis in obstetric palsy

	Clinical picture	Recovery
Type I	C5-C6	Complete or almost in 1-8 weeks
Type II	C5-C6	Elbow flexion: 1-4 wks
		Elbow extension: 1-8 wks
	C7	Limited shoulder: 6-30 wks
Type III	C5-C6	Poor shoulder: 10-40 wks
		Elbow flexion: 16-40 wks
	C7	Elbow extension: 16-20 wks
		Wrist: 40-60 wks
	C8-T1 (no Horner sign)	Hand complete: 1-3 wks
Type IV	C5-C7	Poor shoulder: 10-40 wks
		Elbow flexion: 16-40 wks
	C8	Elbow extension incomplete, poor: 20-60 wks or nil
	T1 (temporary Horner sign)	Wrist: 40-60 wks
		Hand complete: 20-60 wks
Type V	C5-C7	Shoulder and elbow as above
	C7	
	C8	Wrist poor or only extension; poor flexion or none
	T1	
	C8-T1 (Horner sign usually present)	Very poor hand with no or weak flexors and extensors; no intrinsics

Modified from Narakas AO: Injuries to the brachial plexus. In Bora FW Jr, editor: The pediatric upper extremity: diagnosis and management, Philadelphia, 1986, WB Saunders Co.

Treatment

Minimal injuries respond well to conservative treatment, and although recovery may require as long as 18 months, usually residual disability or deformity is slight. Most authors report significant recovery within the first 3 months, with slower recovery occurring within the next 6 to 12 months. Jackson et al reported that all of their patients who recovered fully did so within 1 year, and Greenwald et al reported complete recovery in 92% of patients within 3 months. Gilbert and Tassin, as well as Millesi, suggest that if no evidence of deltoid or biceps recovery is seen by the age of 3 months, surgical exploration should be considered.

The aim of treatment in the initial stages is prevention of contractures of muscles and joints. Gentle passive exercises are begun to maintain full range of passive motion in all joints of the upper extremity, especially full extension of the fingers, hand, and wrist, full pronation and supination of the forearm, full extension of the elbow, and full abduction, extension, and external rotation of the shoulder. Splinting is discouraged by most authors, but Perry et al recommend functional bracing to encourage early hand use. Early surgical intervention was long recommended, but results were disappointing. More recently, microsurgical nerve repair or grafting has been reported to give satisfactory results in carefully selected patients. Kawabata et al and others use CT scanning and myelography, followed by electromyographic and nerve conduction velocity studies. If these studies show root avulsion from the spinal cord, the authors recommend no surgery. If the CT scan and myelogram are normal, they recommend exploration of the brachial plexus and repair of any injuries. Many authors recommend electromyography and myelography and consider surgical exploration if significant recovery is not evident by the age of 3 months.

Surgery in unresolved brachial plexus palsy is usually directed toward improving shoulder function and joint contractures. Sever recommends anterior subscapularis release to correct mild to moderate internal rotation contracture. Wickstrom and others recommend external rotation osteotomy of the humerus for severe fixed rotation contracture. Any reconstructive surgery necessary to correct deformity and restore function of the shoulder should be delayed until the age of about 4 years unless the deformity is progressing rapidly despite physical therapy. Bayne and Costas recommend a subscapularis slide procedure for fixed contractures of 18 months' to 3 years' duration; however, they believe rotational osteotomy is preferable to and more predictable than soft tissue procedures for contractures of longer duration.

Anterior shoulder release

▶ *Technique (Fairbank, Sever).* Make an incision on the anterior aspect of the shoulder distally from the tip of the coracoid process to a point distal to the tendinous insertion of the pectoralis major muscle in the deltopectoral groove. Divide this tendon parallel to the humerus. Then retract the anterior margin of the deltoid laterally and the pectoralis major medially and expose the coracobrachialis muscle (Fig. 13-19). With the shoulder externally rotated and abducted, trace the coracobrachialis superiorly to the coracoid process. If the coracoid is elongated, resect 0.5 to 1 cm of its tip together with the insertions of the coracobrachialis, the short head of the biceps, and the pectoralis minor muscles; this resection increases the range of motion of the shoulder in external rotation and abduction. Now locate the inferior edge of the subscapularis tendon at its insertion on the lesser tuberosity of the humerus, elevate it with a grooved director, and divide it completely without incising the capsule. External rotation and abduction of the shoulder should then be almost normal. A curved prolongation of the acromion may interfere with abduction and with reduction of any mild posterior subluxation of the joint. If it does, either resect this obstructing part or divide the acromion and elevate this part.

▶ *Postoperative management.* An abduction splint that holds the shoulder in abduction and mild external rotation is applied and should be worn constantly for 2 weeks and intermittently for another 4 weeks. Active exercises are started early and are continued until the maximum of improvement occurs.

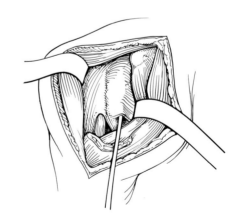

Fig. 13-19 Anterior shoulder release for internal rotation contracture in brachial plexus palsy.

Rotational osteotomy of humerus

▲ *Technique (Rogers).* Approach the humerus anteriorly between the deltoid and pectoralis major muscles. With the arm abducted, perform an osteotomy 5 cm distal to the joint. Under direct vision externally rotate the distal fragment of the humerus 90 degrees; be sure the fragments are then apposed. Kirschner wire fixation may be used if needed. Close the wound.

▲ *Postoperative management.* With the shoulder abducted 40 degrees, the elbow flexed 90 degrees, and the forearm supinated, a shoulder spica cast is applied and should be worn for 8 to 12 weeks. Kirschner wires, if used, are removed at the time of cast removal.

QUADRICEPS CONTRACTURE

In 1964 Lloyd-Roberts and Thomas and Gunn noted the relationship between the development of quadriceps contractures and intramuscular thigh injections in infancy or early childhood. The exact mechanism causing these contractures is still unclear, but suggested causes include compression of the muscle bundles and capillaries by the volume of medication injected and the local toxicity of the drug. Whatever the etiology, there is considerable delay between injection and contracture. Jackson and Hutton reported the average age of their patients at presentation to be 3 years. Quadriceps contracture may also occur in association with other conditions, including myelomeningocele, arthrogryposis, congenital dislocation of the knee, and fracture of the femoral shaft.

The most common symptom is a progressive, painless limitation of knee flexion. The child may have difficulty in squatting, kneeling, sitting cross-legged, running, or climbing stairs. A characteristic dimple usually exists on the thigh and becomes more pronounced when the knee is flexed. Williams reported that half his patients complained of habitual dislocation of the patella. Jackson and Hutton reported patella alta, fragmentation of the inferior pole of the patella, and hypoplastic patella.

If untreated, the muscle contractures may cause changes in the soft tissues and articular cartilage of the femur and tibia. In children in whom treatment was delayed for several years, Karlen found flattened femoral condyles, distortion of the knee joint, and chondromalacia patella. Although McCloskey and Chung emphasized the importance of early treatment and prevention through passive exercise while the child is receiving intramuscular injections, surgery is usually indicated once the contracture is well established. For the rare isolated contracture of the rectus femoris, proximal release, as described by Lenart and Kullmann, is preferred. Most patients, however, require distal quadricepsplasty. General principles of distal quadricepsplasty include placement of the skin incision to prevent problems in healing, excision of any scarred muscle or periosteum causing adhesions in the quadriceps muscle, realignment of the patella to allow normal tracking, and at least 90 degrees of passive motion intraoperatively. The patient should expect very slow return of active quadriceps extension. Most patients can expect improvement in range of motion of the knee after quadricepsplasty but should expect quadriceps weakness for 12 to 24 months. Some improvement in flexion may be lost in skeletally immature patients as growth occurs.

▲ *Technique (Thompson).* An electrocoagulation unit may be used throughout the operation. Make an anterior longitudinal incision through the skin and superficial fascia from the proximal third of the thigh to the distal pole of the patella (Fig. 13-20, *A*). The exact location of the incision depends on the position of any scars, but an anteromedial incision is preferred. Avoid placing the incision directly over the patella. Divide the deep fascia along each side of the rectus femoris muscle from the proximal end of the skin incision to the patella and separate this muscle from the vasti medialis and lateralis. Then divide the anterior part of the knee capsule, including the expansions of the vasti on both sides of the patella, far enough to overcome their contracture (Fig. 13-20, *B*). Excise any part of the quadriceps muscle complex that has scarred and prevents smooth motion of the remaining muscle. If the tendon of the rectus has been destroyed by injury, create a new one by making longitudinal incisions through the scar tissue at the distal third of the thigh.

Now slowly flex the knee to 110 degrees to release the remaining intraarticular adhesions. If the vasti medialis and lateralis are badly scarred, interpose subcutaneous tissue and fat between them and the rectus (Fig. 13-20, *C*). If these muscles are relatively normal, suture them to the rectus as far distally as the distal third of the thigh. If the rectus femoris is severely shortened, it may be lengthened by a Z-plasty; this should be avoided if possible to prevent long-term extension lag but may be required to obtain 90 to 110 degrees of flexion. If a tourniquet has been used, deflate it and obtain complete hemostasis before closing the wound.

▲ *Postoperative management.* The extremity is immobilized in a splint in 45 degrees of knee flexion. For the very young child a cast may be applied 2 weeks

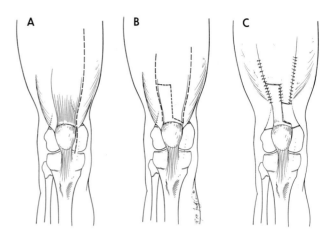

Fig. 13-20 Thompson quadricepsplasty. **A,** Incision. **B,** Division of vasti lateralis and medialis from rectus femoris. Note Z-plasty of rectus femoris. **C,** Vasti lateralis and medialis are sutured proximal to incision. Z-plasty of rectus femoris is repaired.

after surgery. This may done as an outpatient procedure with the child under general anesthesia to flex the knee to 90 degrees after the wound has healed and can tolerate more tension. For older, more cooperative adolescents, passive motion can start 3 days after surgery. The extremity is placed in a continuous passive motion machine, range of motion is begun, and the child remains hospitalized until 90 degrees of passive flexion is achieved. Passive and active exercises for the quadriceps and hamstrings continue and are of critical importance to the success of this procedure. The knee is splinted in flexion at night and is exercised during the day with active and active-assisted exercises. Casting and splinting are discontinued 3 months after surgery.

REFERENCES

General

Allen BL Jr and Ferguson RL: The Galveston technique of pelvic fixation with L-rod instrumentation of the spine, Spine 9:388, 1984.

Bleck EE: Orthopaedic management of cerebral palsy, Philadelphia, 1979, WB Saunders Co.

Drennan JC: Neuromuscular disorders. In Morrissy RT, editor: Lovell and Winter's pediatric orthopaedics, ed 3, vol 2, Philadelphia, 1990, JB Lippincott Co.

Drennan JC: Orthopaedic management of neuromuscular disorders, Philadelphia, 1983, JB Lippincott Co.

Ingram AJ: Paralytic disorders. In Crenshaw AH, editor: Campbell's operative orthopaedics, ed 7, St Louis, 1987, The CV Mosby Co.

Lonstein JE and Renshaw TS: Neuromuscular spine deformities. American Academy of Orthopaedic Surgeons: Instructional Course Lectures 36:285, 1987.

Louis DS et al: Surgical management of the severely multiply handicapped individual, J Pediatr Orthop 9:15, 1989.

O'Neill DL and Harris SR: Developing goals and objectives for handicapped children, Phys Ther 62:295, 1982.

Rinsky LA, Gamble JG, and Bleck EE: Segmental instrumentation without fusion in children with progressive scoliosis, J Pediatr Orthop 5:687, 1985.

Sage FP: Inheritable progressive neuromuscular diseases. In Crenshaw AH, editor: Campbell's operative orthopaedics, ed 7, St Louis, 1987, The CV Mosby Co.

Tachdjian MO: Pediatric orthopedics, ed 2, Philadelphia, 1990, WB Saunders Co.

Muscular dystrophy—general

Bailey RO, Marzulo DC, and Hans MB: Muscular dystrophy: infantile facioscapulohumeral muscular dystrophy—new observations, Acta Neurol Scand 74(1):51, 1986.

Becker PE: Two new families of benign sex-linked recessive muscular dystrophy, Rev Can Biol 21:551, 1962.

Berman AT et al: Muscle biopsy: proper surgical technique, Clin Orthop 198:240, 1985.

Bowker JH and Halpin PJ: Factors determining success in reambulation of the child with progressive muscular dystrophy, Orthop Clin North Am 9:431, 1978.

Copeland SA and Howard RC: Thoracoscapular fusion for facioscapulohumeral dystrophy, J Bone Joint Surg 60B:547, 1978.

Florence JM, Brocke MH, and Carroll JE: Evaluation of the child with muscular weakness, Orthop Clin North Am 9(2):49, 1978.

Gardner-Medwin D: Clinical features and classification of muscular dystrophies, Br Med Bull 36:109, 1980.

Green NE: The orthopaedic care of children with muscular dystrophy. In American Academy of Orthopaedic Surgeons: Instructional course lectures 36:267, 1987.

Lehman JB: Biomechanics of ankle-foot orthoses: prescription and design, Arch Phys Med Rehabil 60:200, 1979.

Shapiro F and Bresnan MJ: Current concepts review: orthopaedic management of childhood neuromuscular disease. Part II. Diseases of muscle, J Bone Joint Surg 64A:1102, 1982.

Siegel IM: The clinical management of muscle disease: a practical manual of diagnosis and treatment, London, 1977, William Heinemann Medical Books, Ltd.

Siegel IM: Diagnosis, management, and orthopaedic treatment of muscular dystrophy. In American Academy of Orthopaedic Surgeons: Instructional course lectures, vol 30, St Louis, 1981, The CV Mosby Co.

Duchenne muscular dystrophy

Bleck EE: Mobility of patients with Duchenne muscular dystrophy [letter], Dev Med Child Neurol 21:823, 1979.

Brown JC: Muscular dystrophy, Practitioner 226:1031, 1982.

Brownell AKW et al: Malignant hyperthermia in Duchenne muscular dystrophy, Anesthesiology 58:180, 1983.

Cambridge W and Drennan JC: Scoliosis associated with Duchenne muscular dystrophy, J Pediatr Orthop 7:436, 1987.

Cooper RR: Skeletal muscle and muscle disorders. In Cruess RL and Rennie WRJ: Adult orthopaedics, vol 1, New York, 1984, Churchill Livingstone.

Crisp DE, Ziter FA and Bray PF: Diagnostic delay in Duchenne's muscular dystrophy, JAMA 247:478, 1982.

Douglas R et al: The LSU reciprocation-gait orthosis, Orthopedics 6:834, 1983.

Drennan JC and Bondurant M: Paralytic disorders. In American Academy of Orthopaedic Surgeons: Atlas of orthotics, ed 2, St Louis, 1985, The CV Mosby Co.

Firth M et al: Interviews with parents of boys suffering from Duchenne muscular dystrophy, Dev Med Child Neurol 25:466, 1983.

Fletcher R et al: Malignant hyperthermia in a myopathic child: prolonged postoperative course requiring dantrolene, Acta Anaesth Scand 26:435, 1982.

Florence JM, Brooke MH, and Carroll JE: Evaluation of the child with muscular weakness, Orthop Clin North Am 9:409, 1978.

Fowler WM Jr: Rehabilitation management of muscular dystrophy and related disorders. Part 2. Comprehensive care, Arch Phys Med Rehabil 63:322, 1982.

Fowler WM Jr and Taylor M: Rehabilitation management of muscular dystrophy and related disorders. Part 1. The role of exercise, Arch Phys Med Rehabil 63:319, 1982.

Gardner-Medwin D and Johnston HM: Severe muscular dystrophy in girls J Neurol Sci 64:79, 1984.

Gibson DA et al: The management of spinal deformity in Duchenne's muscular dystrophy, Orthop Clin North Am 9:437, 1978.

Hsu JD: Management of foot deformity in Duchenne's pseudohypertrophic muscular dystrophy, Orthop Clin North Am 7:979, 1976.

Hsu JD: The natural history of spine curvature progression in the nonambulatory Duchenne muscular dystrophy patient, Spine 8:771, 1983.

Hsu JD and Hsu CL: Motor unit disease. In Jahss MH, editor: Disorders of the foot, Philadelphia, 1982, WB Saunders Co.

Hsu JD and Lewis JE: Challenges in the care of the retarded child with Duchenne muscular dystrophy, Orthop Clin North Am 12:73, 1981.

Hsu JD et al: Control of spine curvature in the Duchenne muscular dystrophy (DMD) patient. In Proceedings of the Scoliosis Research Society, Denver, Scoliosis Research Society, 1982.

Kelfer HM, Singer WD, and Reynolds RN: Malignant hyperthermia in a child with Duchenne muscular dystrophy, Pediatrics 71:118, 1983.

Kurz LT et al: Correlation of scoliosis and pulmonary function in Duchenne muscular dystrophy, J Pediatr Orthop 3:347, 1983.

Lane RJM, Robinow M, and Roses AD: The genetic status of mothers of isolated cases of Duchenne muscular dystrophy, J Med Genet 20:1, 1983.

Lutter LD et al: Spine curvatures in progressive muscular dystrophy. Presented at the Annual Meeting of the Pediatric Orthopaedic Society, Vancouver, BC, Canada, May 21-23, 1984.

Marchildon MB: Malignant hyperthermia: current concepts, Arch Surg 117:349, 1982.

Melkonian GJ et al: Dynamic gait electromyography study in Duchenne muscular dystrophy (DMD) patients, Foot Ankle 1:78, 1980.

Moser H: Duchenne muscular dystrophy: pathogenetic aspects and genetic prevention, Hum Genet 66:17, 1984.

Mubarak SJ et al: Correlating scoliosis and pulmonary function in Duchenne muscular dystrophy. Presented at the American Academy for Cerebral Palsy and Developmental Medicine Annual Meeting, Chicago, 1983.

Renshaw TS: Treatment of Duchenne's muscular dystrophy, JAMA 248:922, 1982.

Rochelle J, Bowen JR, and Ray S: Pediatric foot deformities in progressive neuromuscular disease, Contemp Orthop 8:41, 1984.

Seeger BR, Caudrey DJ, and Little JD: Progression of equinus deformity in Duchenne muscular dystrophy, Arch Phys Med Rehabil 66:286, 1985.

Seeger BR, Sutherland AD'A, and Clark MS: Orthotic management of scoliosis in Duchenne muscular dystrophy, Arch Phys Med Rehabil 65:83, 1984.

Siegel IM: Equinocavovarus in muscular dystrophy: treatment by percutaneous tarsal medullostomy and soft tissue release, Isr J Med Sci 13:198, 1977.

Siegel IM: Prolongation of ambulation through early percutaneous tenotomy and bracing with plastic orthoses, Isr J Med Sci 13:192, 1977.

Siegel IM: Maintenance of ambulation in Duchenne muscular dystrophy: the role of the orthopedic surgeon, Clin Pediatr 19:383, 1980.

Siegel IM, Miller JE, and Ray RD: Subcutaneous lower limb tenotomy in the treatment of pseudohypertrophic muscular dystrophy: description of technique and presentation of twenty-one cases, J Bone Joint Surg 50A:1437, 1968.

Smith AD, Koreska J, and Moseley CF: Progression of scoliosis in Duchenne muscular dystrophy, J Bone Joint Surg 71A:1066, 1989.

Sussman MD: Advantage of early spinal stabilization and fusion in patients with Duchenne muscular dystrophy, J Pediatr Orthop 4:531, 1984.

Sutherland DH, Olshen R, Cooper L, Wyatt M, Leach J, Mubarak S, Schultz P: The pathomechanics of gait in Duchenne muscular dystrophy, Dev Med Child Neurol 1981; 23:3.

Swank SM, Brown JC, and Perry RE: Spinal fusion in Duchenne's muscular dystrophy, Spine 7:484, 1982.

Vignos PJ et al: Predicting the success of reambulation in patients with Duchenne muscular dystrophy, J Bone Joint Surg 65A:719, 1983.

Weimann RL et al: Surgical stabilization of the spine in Duchenne muscular dystrophy, Spine 8:776, 1983.

Wilkins KE and Gibson DA: The patterns of spinal deformity in Duchenne muscular dystrophy, J Bone Joint Surg 58A:24, 1976.

Becker muscular dystrophy

Becker PE and Kiener F: Eine neue x-chromosomale Muskeldystrophie, Arch Psychiatr Nervenkr 193:427, 1955.

Emery AEH and Skinner R: Clinical studies in benign (Becker type) X-linked muscular dystrophy, Clin Genet 10:189, 1976.

Florence JM, Brooke MH, and Carroll JE: Evaluation of the child with muscular weakness, Orthop Clin North Am 9:409, 1978.

Fowler WM Jr: Rehabilitation management of muscular dystrophy and related disorders. II. Comprehensive care, Arch Phys Med Rehabil 63:322, 1982.

Grimm T: Genetic counseling in Becker type X-linked muscular dystrophy. I. Theoretical considerations, Am J Med Genet 18:713, 1984.

Grimm T: Genetic counseling in Becker type X-linked muscular dystrophy. II. Practical considerations, Am J Med Genet 18:719, 1984.

Herrmann FH and Spiegler AWJ: Carrier detection in X-linked Becker muscular dystrophy by muscle provocation test (MPT), J Neurol Sci 62:141, 1983.

Khan RH and MacNicol MF: Bilateral patellar subluxation secondary to Becker muscular dystrophy: a case report, J Bone Joint Surg 64A:777, 1982.

Kloster R: Benign X-linked muscular dystrophy (Becker type): a kindred with very slow rate of progression, Acta Neurol Scand 68:344, 1983.

Limb-girdle dystrophy

Fowler WM Jr: Rehabilitation management of muscular dystrophy and related disorders. II. Comprehensive care, Arch Phys Med Rehabil 63:322, 1982.

Fowler WM Jr and Nayak NN: Slowly progressive proximal weakness: limb-girdle syndromes, Arch Phys Med Rehabil 64:527, 1983.

Facioscapulohumeral dystrophy

Copeland SA and Howard RC: Thoracoscapular fusion for facioscapulohumeral dystrophy, J Bone Joint Surg 60B:547, 1978.

Fowler WM Jr: Rehabilitation management of muscular dystrophy, and related disorders. II. Comprehensive care, Arch Phys Med Rehabil 63:322, 1982.

McGarry J, Garg B, and Silbert S: Death in childhood due to facioscapulo-humeral dystrophy, Acta Neurol Scand 68:61, 1983.

Padberg G et al: Linkage studies in autosomal dominant facioscapulohumeral muscular dystrophy, J Neurol Sci 65:261, 1984.

Congenital dystrophy

Cornelio F and Di Donato S: Myopathies due to enzyme deficiencies, J Neurol 232:329, 1985.

Cunliffe M and Burrows FA: Anaesthetic implications of nemaline rod myopathy, Can Anaesth Soc J 32:543, 1985.

Eeg-Olofsson O et al: Early infant death in nemaline (rod) myopathy, Brain Dev 5:53, 1983.

Fowler WM Jr: Rehabilitation management of muscular dystrophy and related disorders. II. Comprehensive care, Arch Phys Med Rehabil 63:322, 1982.

Jones R et al: Congenital muscular dystrophy: the importance of early diagnosis and orthopaedic management in the long-term prognosis, J Bone Joint Surg 61B:13, 1979.

McComb RD, Markesbery WR, and O'Connor WN: Fatal neonatal nemaline myopathy with multiple congenital anomalies, J Pediatr 94:47, 1979.

McMenamin JB, Becker LE, and Murphy EG: Congenital muscular dystrophy: a clinicopathologic report of 24 cases, J Pediatr 100:692, 1982.

McMenamin JB, Becker LE, and Murphy EG: Fukuyama-type congenital muscular dystrophy, J Pediatr 100:580, 1982.

Ramsey PL and Hensinger RN: Congenital dislocation of the hip associated with central core disease, J Bone Joint Surg 57A:648, 1975.

Myotonic dystrophy

Begin R et al: Pathogenesis of respiratory insufficiency in myotonic dystrophy: the mechanical factors, Am Rev Respir Dis 125:312, 1982.

Bell DB and Smith DW: Myotonic dystrophy in the neonate, J Pediatr 81:83, 1972.

Carroll JE, Brooke MH, and Kaiser K: Diagnosis of infantile myotonic dystrophy, Lancet 2:608, 1975.

Harper PS: Myotonic dystrophy, ed 12, Philadelphia, 1979, WB Saunders Co.

Hawley RJ et al: Families with myotonic dystrophy with and without cardiac involvement, Arch Intern Med 143:2134, 1983.

O'Brien TA and Harper PS: Course, prognosis and complications of childhood-onset myotonic dystrophy, Dev Med Child Neurol 26:62, 1984.

Ray S, Bowen JR, and Marks HG: Foot deformity in myotonic dystrophy, Foot Ankle 5:125, 1984.

Winters JL and McLaughlin LA: Myotonia congenita, J Bone Joint Surg 52A:1345, 1970.

Zellweger H and Ionasescu V: Early onset of myotonic dystrophy in infants, Am J Dis Child 125:601, 1973.

Charcot-Marie-Tooth disease

Alexander IJ and Johnson KA: Assessment and management of pes cavus in Charcot-Marie-Tooth disease, Clin Orthop 246:273, 1989.

Bradley GW and Coleman SS: Treatment of the calcaneocavus foot deformity, J Bone Joint Surg 63A:1159, 1981.

Charcot JM and Marie P: Sur une forme particuliere d'atrophie musculaire souvent familiale debutant par les pied et les jambes et atteignant plus tard les mains, Rev Med p 96, 1886.

Coleman SS: Complex foot deformities in children, Philadelphia, 1983, Lea & Febiger.

Coleman SS and Chestnut WJ: A simple test for hind foot flexibility in the cavovarus foot, Clin Orthop 123:60, 1977.

Daher YH et al: Spinal deformities in patients with Charcot-Marie-Tooth disease: a review of 21 patients, Clin Orthop 202:219, 1986.

Dejerine J and Sottas J: Sur la neurite interstitielle hypertrophique et progressive de l'enfance, CR Soc Biol 45:63, 1893.

Dwyer FC: The treatment of relapsed club foot by the insertion of a wedge into the calcaneum, J Bone Joint Surg 45B:67, 1963.

Gartland JJ: Posterior tibial transplant in the surgical treatment of recurrent club foot, J Bone Joint Surg 46A:1217, 1964.

Gould N: Surgery in advanced Charcot-Marie-Tooth disease, Foot Ankle 4:267, 1984.

Hensinger RN and MacEwen GD: Spinal deformity associated with heritable neurologic conditions: spinal muscular atrophy, Friedreich's ataxia, familial dysautonomia, and Charcot-Marie-Tooth disease, J Bone Joint Surg 58A:13, 1978.

Hibbs RA: An operation for "claw-foot," JAMA 73:1583, 1919.

Jones R: The soldier's foot and the treatment of common deformities of the foot. Part II. Claw-foot, Br Med J 1:749, 1916.

Kumar SJ et al: Hip dysplasia associated with Charcot-Marie-Tooth disease in the older child and adolescent, J Pediatr Orthop 5(5):511, 1985.

Levitt RL and Gartland JJ: The role of foot surgery in progressive neuromuscular disorders in children, J Bone Joint Surg 55A:1396, 1973.

McCluskey WP, Lovell WW, and Cummings RJ: The cavovarus foot deformity: etiology and management, Clin Orthop 247:27, 1989.

Medhat MA and Krantz H: Neuropathic ankle joint in Charcot-Marie-Tooth disease after triple arthrodesis of the foot, Orthop Rev 17:873, 1988.

Miller GM et al: Posterior tibial tendon transfer: a review of the literature and analysis of 74 procedures, J Pediatr Orthop 2:363, 1982.

Paulos L, Coleman SS, and Samuelson KM: Pes cavovarus: review of a surgical approach using selective soft-tissue procedures, J Bone Joint Surg 62A:942, 1980.

Refsum S: Heredopathia atactica polyneuritiformis: a familial syndrome not hitherto described, Acta Psych Neurol Suppl 38:1, 1946.

Rochelle J, Bowen JR, and Ray S: Pediatric foot deformities in progressive neuromuscular disease, Contemp Orthop 8:41, 1984.

Roussy G and Levy G: Sept case d'une maladie familiale particuliere: troubles de la marche, pieds, bots et areflexie tendineuse generalisee, avec accesoirement, Rev Neurol 54:427, 1926.

Sabir M and Lyttle D: Pathogenesis of Charcot-Marie-Tooth disease: gait analysis and electrophysiologic, genetic, histopathologic, and enzyme studies in a kinship, Clin Orthop 184:223, 1984.

Samilson RL and Dillin W: Cavus, cavovarus, and calcaneocavus: an update, Clin Orthop 177:125, 1983.

Sherman FC and Westin GW: Plantar release in the correction of deformities of the foot in childhood, J Bone Joint Surg 63A:1382, 1981.

Siffert RS and del Torto U: "Beak" triple arthrodesis for severe cavus deformity, Clin Orthop 181:64, 1983.

Steindler A: Stripping of the os calcis, J Orthop Surg 2:8, 1920.

Tooth HH: The peroneal type of progressive muscular atrophy, London, 1886, HK Lewis.

Wukich DK and Bowen JR: A long-term study of triple arthrodesis for correction of pes cavovarus in Charcot-Marie-Tooth disease, J Pediatr Orthop 9:433, 1989.

Friedreich ataxia

Cady RB and Bobechko WP: Incidence, natural history, and treatment of scoliosis in Friedreich's ataxia, J Pediatr Orthop 4:673, 1984.

Hensinger RN and MacEwen GD: Spinal deformity associated with heritable neurologic conditions: spinal muscular atrophy, Friedreich's ataxia, familial dysautonomia, and Charcot-Marie-Tooth disease, J Bone Joint Surg 58A:13, 1978.

Labelle H et al: Natural history of scoliosis in Friedreich's ataxia, J Bone Joint Surg 68A:564, 1986.

Levitt RL et al: The role of foot surgery in progressive neuromuscular disorders in children, J Bone Joint Surg 55A:1396, 1973.

Paulos L, Coleman SS, and Samuelson KM: Pes cavovarus: review of a surgical approach using selective soft-tissue procedures, J Bone Joint Surg 62A:942, 1980.

Rochelle J, Bowen JR, and Ray S: Pediatric foot deformities in progressive neuromuscular disease, Contemp Orthop 8:41, 1984.

Rothschild H, Shoji H, and McCormick D: Heel deformity in hereditary spastic paraplegia, Clin Orthop 160:48, 1981.

Shapiro F and Bresnan MJ: Current concepts review: orthopaedic management of childhood neuromuscular disease. Part II. Peripheral neuropathies, Friedreich's ataxis, and arthrogryposis multiplex congenita, J Bone Joint Surg 64A:949, 1982.

Spinal muscular atrophy

Aprin H et al: Spine fusion in patients with spinal muscular atrophy, J Bone Joint Surg 64A:1179, 1982.

Daher YH et al: Spinal surgery in spinal muscular atrophy, J Pediatr Orthop 5:391, 1985.

Drennan JC: Skeletal deformities in spinal muscular atrophy. In Abstracts of Association of Bone and Joint Surgeons, Clin Orthop 133:266, 1978.

Evans GA, Drennan JC, and Russman BS: Functional classification and orthopaedic management of spinal muscular atrophy, J Bone Joint Surg 63B:516, 1981.

Ferguson RL and Allen BL: Segmental spinal instrumentation for routine scoliotic curve, Contemp Orthop 2:450, 1980.

Hensinger RN and MacEwen GD: Spinal deformity associated with heritable neurological conditions: spinal muscular atrophy, Friedreich's ataxia, familial dysautonomia, and Charcot-Marie-Tooth disease, J Bone Joint Surg 58A:13, 1976.

Hoffmann J: Ueber chronische spinale Muskelatrophie im Kindersalter, auf familiarer Basis, Dtsch Z Nervenheulkd 3:427, 1893.

Hsu JD et al: The orthopaedic management of spinal muscular atrophy, J Bone Joint Surg 55B:663, 1973.

Kugelberg E and Welander L: Heredofamilial juvenile muscular atrophy simulating muscular dystrophy, Arch Neurol Psychiatry 75:500, 1956.

Piasecki JO, Mahinpour S, and Levine DB: Long-term follow-up of spinal fusion in spinal muscular atrophy, Clin Orthop 207:44, 1986.

Shapiro F, and Bresnan MJ: Current concepts review: orthopaedic management of childhood neuromuscular disease. Part I. Spinal muscular atrophy, J Bone Joint Surg 64A:785, 1982.

Werdnig G: Die fruhinfantile progressive spinale Amyotrophie, Arch Psychiatr Nervenkr 26:706, 1894.

Arthrogryposis multiplex congenita

Atkins RM, Bell MJ, and Sharrard WJ: Arthrogryposis: pectoralis major transfer for paralysis of elbow flexion in children, J Bone Joint Surg 67B:640, 1985.

Banker BQ: Neuropathologic aspects of arthrogryposis multiplex congenita, Clin Orthop 194:30, 1985.

Bayne LG: Hand assessment and management in arthrogryposis multiplex congenita Clin Orthop 194:68, 1985.

Brown LM, Robson MJ, and Sharrard WJW: The pathophysiology of arthrogryposis multiplex congenita neurologica, J Bone Joint Surg 62B:291, 1980.

Carlson WO et al: Arthrogryposis multiplex congenita: a long-term follow-up study, Clin Orthop 194:115, 1985.

Diamond LS and Alegado R: Perinatal fractures in arthrogryposis multiplex congenita, J Pediatr Orthop 1:189, 1981.

Drummond DS and Cruess RL: The management of the foot and ankle in arthrogryposis multiplex congenita, J Bone Joint Surg 60B:96, 1978.

Drummond DS, Siller TN, and Cruess RL: The management of arthrogryposis multiplex congenita. In American Academy of Orthopaedic Surgeons: Instructional course lectures, vol 23, St Louis, 1974, The CV Mosby Co.

Friedlander HL, Westin GW, and Wood WL Jr: Arthrogryposis multiplex congenita, J Bone Joint Surg 50A:89, 1968.

Green ADL, Fixsen JA, and Lloyd-Roberts GC: Talectomy for arthrogryposis multiplex congenita, J Bone Joint Surg 66B:697, 1984.

Gross RH: The role of the Verebelyi-Ogston procedure in the management of the arthrogrytotic foot, Clin Orthop 194:99, 1985.

Guidera KJ and Drennan JC: Foot and ankle deformities in arthrogryposis multiplex congenita, Clin Orthop 194:93, 1985.

Hahn G: Arthrogryposis: pediatric review and habilitative aspects, Clin Orthop 194:104, 1985.

Hall JG: Genetic aspects of arthrogryposis multiplex congenita, Clin Orthop 194:44, 1985.

Herron LD, Westin GW, and Dawson EG: Scoliosis in arthrogryposis multiplex congenita, J Bone Joint Surg 60A:293, 1978.

Hoffer MM et al: Ambulation in severe arthrogryposis, J Pediatr Orthop 3:293, 1983.

Hsu LCS, Jaffray D, and Leong JCY: Talectomy for clubfoot in arthrogryposis, J Bone Joint Surg 66B:694, 1984.

Huurman WW, and Jacobsen ST: The hip in arthrogryposis multiplex congenita, Clin Orthop 194:81, 1985.

Palmer PM et al: Passive motion for infants with arthrogryposis, Clin Orthop 194:54, 1985.

St Clair HS and Zimbler S: A plan of management and treatment results in the arthrogrytotic hip, Clin Orthop 194:74, 1985.

Staheli LT et al: Management of hip dislocations in children with arthrogryposis, J Pediatr Orthop 7:681, 1987.

Swinyard CA and Bleck EE: The etiology of arthrogryposis (multiple congenital contracture), Clin Orthop 194:15, 1985.

Thomas B et al: The knee in arthrogryposis, Clin Orthop 194:87, 1985.

Thompson GH and Bilenker RM: Comprehensive management of arthrogryposis multiplex congenita, Clin Orthop 194:6, 1985.

Wenner SM and Saperia BS: Proximal row carpectomy in arthrogrytotic wrist deformity, J Hand Surg 12A:523, 1987.

Williams PF: The management of arthrogryposis, Orthop Clin North Am 6:967, 1978.

Williams PF: Management of upper limb problems in arthrogryposis, Clin Orthop 194:60, 1985.

Wynne-Davis R, Williams PF, and O'Connor JC: The 1960s epidemic of arthrogryposis multiplex congenita: a survey from the United Kingdom, Australia and the United States of America, J Bone Joint Surg 63B:76, 1981.

Brachial plexus palsy

Brown KLB: Review of obstetrical palsies: nonoperative treatment, Clin Plast Surg 11:181, 1984.

Buschmann WR and Sager G: Orthopaedic considerations in obstetric brachial plexus palsy, Orthop Rev 16:290, 1987.

Chung SMK and Nissenbaum MM: Obstetrical paralysis, Orthop Clin North Am 6:393, 1975.

Déjerine-Klumpke A: Des polynévrites en général et des paralysies et atrophies saturnines en particulier: etude clinique et anatomo-pathologique, Paris, 1889, Ancienne Librairie Germer Bailliére et Cie.

Erb W: Ueber eine eigenthiumliche Localization von Lachmungen in Plexus Brachialis, Verhandl Naturhist Med Verin 1:130, 1874.

Fairbank HAT: Birth palsy: subluxation of the shoulder-joint in infants and young children, Lancet 1:1217, 1913.

Gilbert A, Razabone R, and Amar-Khodja S: Indications and results of brachial plexus surgery in obstetrical palsy, Orthop Clin North Am 19:91, 1988.

Gilbert A and Tassin JL: Surgical repair of the brachial plexus in obstetric paralysis, Chirurgie 110(1):70, 1984.

Green WT and Tachdjian MO: Correction of residual deformity of the shoulder from obstetrical palsy, J Bone Joint Surg 45A:1544, 1963.

Greenwald AG, Schute PC, and Shiveley JL: Brachial plexus birth palsy: a 10-year report on the incidence and prognosis, J Pediatr Orthop 4:689, 1984.

Hardy AE: Birth injuries of the brachial plexus: incidence and prognosis, J Bone Joint Surg 63B:98, 1981.

Hoffer MM, Wickenden R, and Roper R: Brachial plexus birth palsies: results of tendon transfers to the rotator cuff, J Bone Joint Surg 60A:691, 1978.

Jackson ST, Hoffer MM, and Parrish N: Brachial-plexus palsy in the newborn, J Bone Joint Surg 70A:1217, 1988.

Jones SJ: Diagnostic value of peripheral and spinal somatosensory evoked potential in traction lesions of the brachial plexus, Clin Plast Surg 2:167, 1984.

Kawabata H et al: Early microsurgical reconstruction in birth palsy, Clin Orthop 215:233, 1987.

Klumpke A: Paralysies radiculaires du plexus brachial; paralysies radiculaires totales; paralysies radiculaires inferieures; de la partipation des filets sympathiques oculopupillaires dan ces paralysies, Rev Med 5:739, 1885.

Meyer RD: Treatment of adult and obstetrical brachial plexus injuries, Orthopedics 9:899, 1986.

Millesi H: Surgical management of brachial plexus injuries, J Hand Surg 2:367, 1977.

Narakas A: Brachial plexus surgery, Orthop Clin North Am 12:303, 1981.

Narakas AO: Injuries to the brachial plexus. In Bora FW Jr, editor: The pediatric upper extremity: diagnosis and managment, Philadelphia, 1986, WB Saunders Co.

Perry J et al: Orthoses in patients with brachial plexus injuries, Arch Phys Med Rehabil 55:132, 1974.

Rogers MH: An operation for the correction of the deformity due to "obstetrical paralysis," Boston Med Surg J 174:163, 1916.

Seddon HJ: Brachial plexus injuries, J Bone Joint Surg 31B:3, 1949.

Sever JW: The results of a new operation for obstetrical paralysis, Am J Orthop Surg 16:248, 1918.

Sever JW: Obstetric paralysis, JAMA 85:1862, 1925.

Sever JW: Obstetrical paralysis, Surg Gynecol Obstet 44:547, 1927.

Solonen KA, Telaranta T, and Ryoppy S: Early reconstruction of birth injuries of the brachial plexus, J Pediatr Orthop 1:367, 1981.

Sugioka H: Evoked potentials in the investigation of traumatic lesions of the peripheral nerve and the brachial plexus, Clin Orthop 184:85, 1984.

Tada K, Tsuyuguchi Y, and Kawai H: Birth palsy: natural recovery course and combined root avulsion, J Pediatr Orthop 4:279, 1984.

Zancolli EA: Classification and management of the shoulder in birth palsy, Orthop Clin North Am 12:433, 1980.

Quadriceps contracture

Alvarez EV et al: Quadriceps myofibrosis: a complication of intramuscular injections, J Bone Joint Surg 62A:58, 1980.

Bose K and Chong KC: The clinical manifestations and pathomechanics of contracture of the extensor mechanism of the knee, J Bone Joint Surg 58B:478, 1976.

Chiu SS et al: Contracture of the quadriceps caused by injections, Acta Orthop Belg 41:306, 1975.

Engel WK: Focal myopathic changes produced by electromyographic and hypodermic needles: "needle myopathy," Arch Neurol 16:509, 1967.

Euliano JJ: Fibrosis of the quadriceps mechanism in children, Clin Orthop 70:181, 1970.

Fairbank TJ and Barrett AM: Vastus intermedius contracture in early childhood: case report in identical twins, J Bone Joint Surg 43B:326, 1961.

Hnevkovsky O: Progressive fibrosis of the vastus intermedius in children: a cause of limited knee flexion and elevation of the patella, J Bone Joint Surg 43B:318, 1961.

Jackson AM and Hutton PAN: Injection-induced contractures of the quadriceps in childhood: a comparison of proximal release and distal quadricepsplasty, J Bone Joint Surg 67B:97, 1985.

Karlen A: Congenital fibrosis of the vastus intermedius muscle, J Bone Joint Surg 46B:488, 1964.

Lenart G and Kullmann L: Isolated contracture of the rectus femoris muscle, Clin Orthop 99:125, 1974.

Lloyd-Roberts GC and Thomas TG: The etiology of quadriceps contractures in children, J Bone Joint Surg 46B:498, 1964.

McCloskey J and Chung S: Quadriceps contracture as a result of multiple intramuscular injection, Am J Dis Child 131:416, 1977.

Thompson TC: Quadricepsplasty to improve knee function, J Bone Joint Surg 26:366, 1944.

Williams PF: Quadriceps contractures, J Bone Joint Surg 50B:278, 1968.

14 Osteochondroses

S. TERRY CANALE

Osteochondrosis includes a number of clinical entities characterized by pain and roentgenographically indicated abnormality in the growing child. It is not a part of the normal pattern of growth and development but is considered a developmental abnormality that usually resolves with conservative treatment. In the consideration of all forms of osteochondrosis, approximately two thirds to three quarters of patients have satisfactory results. However, treatment of Legg-Calvé-Perthes disease of the hip, osteochondrosis of the elbow, Osgood-Schlatter disease of the tibial tubercle, Kohler's disease of the tarsal navicular, and Freiberg's disease of the metatarsal head may result in less than satisfactory results in approximately 25% of patients. Surgical intervention therefore is directed toward improvement of the poor results in these children.

LEGG-CALVE-PERTHES DISEASE

Legg-Calvé-Perthes disease (LCPD) was described in the literature in 1910 by Legg, Calvé, and Perthes individually. Each recognized this deformity of the hip in children as a separate entity from the more common tuberculosis of the hip, partly because of the absence of other local and systemic signs of tuberculosis but primarily because of the characteristic roentgenographic appearance of the proximal femoral epiphysis. LCPD is not a static condition but rather a chronic sequence of changes initiated by an avascularity of the femoral head. The disease, which occurs in approximately 1 in 1500 children, is about six times more frequent in boys than in girls. With few exceptions LCPD is limited to children between the ages of 3 and 13 years; more than half those affected are between the ages of 5 and 7 years. Approximately 15% of affected children have bilateral disease.

The specific cause of the avascular necrosis of the femoral head is still unproved, although both genetic and environmental factors have been implicated. Metabolic bone disease, thrombotic vascular insults, trauma, infection, and transient synovitis all have been suggested as possible causes. There is no clear genetic pattern in LCPD, although several investigators have found significant numbers of patients with retarded growth and delayed skeletal maturation. LCPD is familial in approximately 20% to 24% of patients.

The natural history of LCPD is sequential progression through four stages: condensation, fragmentation (lytic), reossification, and remodeling. Once the vascular compromise has occurred, from whatever cause, the involved bone of the femoral epiphysis and sometimes the metaphysis becomes necrotic. Growth ceases in the involved bone, and in severe cases a metaphyseal cyst forms. The necrosis may involve only a small part of the femoral head or all of the femoral head, the epiphyseal line, and metaphysis. As the dead bone is resorbed and fragments, revascularization is initiated. During this stage the femoral head may become deformed and the acetabulum flattened. Gradually, the deformed head reossifies from the periphery to the center. Finally, there is some remodeling of the femoral head and acetabulum, and slight improvement in the congruity of the hip joint may gradually occur. The femoral head always revascularizes, but it is almost always deformed to some extent.

Almost 90% of patients with LCPD have retardation of skeletal age. A high incidence of genitourinary anomaly and inguinal hernia has been reported in patients with LCPD, and there have been a few re-

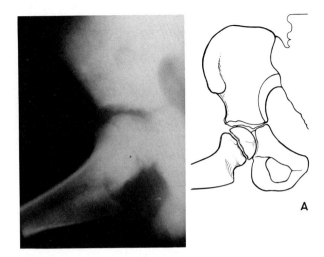

A, *Type I,* less than 25% involvement of femoral head.

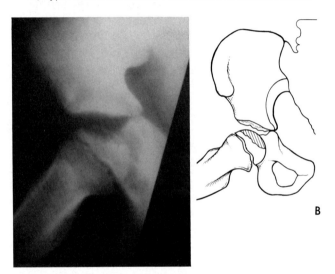

B, *Type II,* 50% involvement of femoral head, with sparing of lateral border.

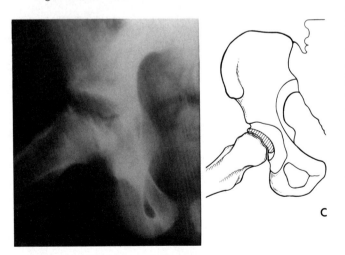

C, *Type III,* 75% involvement with lateral head significantly involved and collapsed.

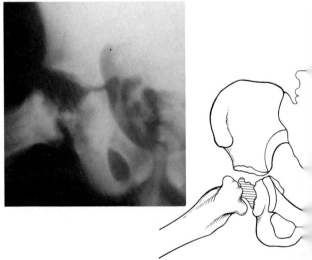

D, *Type IV,* total femoral head involvement.

Fig. 14-1 Catterall classification of LCPD.

ports of renal rickets and chronic glomerulonephritis associated with LCPD.

Clinical and Roentgenographic Findings

The clinical findings in LCPD are variable and often correlate poorly with roentgenographic changes. Early in the disease process, limping and hip pain are the most common symptoms. Adductor and iliopsoas muscle spasm may be present, and passive motion may be limited and painful. There often is tenderness to palpation over the hip joint. Later, hip flexion contractures may develop, medial rotation and abduction are restricted, and the pain may be referred to the thigh and knee. A positive Trendelenburg sign is common. With long-standing disease and significant femoral head involvement, passive abduction and rotation may become markedly restricted and leg length discrepancy may become apparent.

Because the same clinical symptoms may be present in other disorders of the hip in children, such as transient synovitis and infection, it is the roentgenographic appearance of the hip joint that is diagnostic. Catterall lists four roentgenographic signs as valuable markers in the early diagnosis of LCPD: lateral displacement of the femoral head, a subchondral fracture line, increased epiphyseal density, and a smaller epiphyseal nucleus in the involved hip than in the normal hip. Initially described by Waldenström in 1920, lateral displacement of the femoral head appears on roentgenogram as a widening between the medial margin of the metaphysis and the tear drop of the acetabulum. The subchondral fracture line is present in 25% to 33% of patients and is best seen on the Lauenstein lateral view; it begins at the anterior margin of the epiphysis and passes posteriorly in the subchondral zone. A small epiphyseal nucleus is seen in approximately half the patients with LCPD. Roentgenographic changes later in the disease process become more obvious: fragmented appearance of the ossification center, the radiolucent metaphyseal "cyst," flattening of the acetabulum, and deformation of the femoral head. In severe involvement the femoral head may become irregular and mushroom-shaped, with large extraarticular prominences that restrict motion (hinged abduction). Growth of the proximal femur may be affected, with shortening and varus deformity of the femoral neck. Trochanteric overgrowth may be pronounced.

Technetium bone scanning is useful in the diagnosis of LCPD when initial roentgenograms are normal. Paterson and Savage reported a sensitivity rate of 98% in examinations of 131 children. This is, however, a relatively invasive procedure, and some false-negative results may be obtained in children with synovitis in addition to the necrosis of the femoral head. If used, specific techniques should include pinhole collimation of both hips 1.5 to 3 hours after injection. Magnetic resonance imaging (MRI) also provides early diagnosis of LCPD when roentgenograms are normal, but false-negative results have been reported. MRI is, however, expensive and it is often difficult for the younger child to remain still in an enclosed unit for

periods of 30 to 45 minutes. Like arthrography, MRI may be useful in the diagnosis of hinge abduction. Computerized tomographic scanning is of limited value for either diagnosis or prognosis but is useful in evaluating the rare sequela of osteochondritis dissecans of the femoral head in LCPD. The roles of bone scanning and MRI in assessment of femoral head revascularization are still unclear.

Classification

Catterall classified LCPD into four types according to the amount of capital femoral epiphysis involved in the disease process: type I, less than 50% of the femoral head is involved (Fig. 14-1, *A*); type II, 50% of the femoral head is involved (Fig. 14-1, *B*); type III, 75% of the femoral head is involved (Fig. 14-1, *C*); and type IV, the entire epiphysis is involved (Fig. 14-1, *D*). Catterall also found that the presence of two or more roentgenographic signs of LCPD correlated with poor results, and he called these *head-at-risk* signs: lateral subluxation of the femoral head from the acetabulum, calcification lateral to the capital epiphysis, metaphyseal cyst, a more horizontal growth plate than the contralateral hip, and Gage's sign, a radiolucent V-shaped defect in the lateral epiphysis and adjacent metaphysis (see Fig. 14-7). Green and Griffin noted that lateral subluxation may be determined by measuring the distance between the medial inferior border of the femoral head and the inferior acetabular wall and that the greater this distance, the poorer the prognosis (Fig. 14-2).

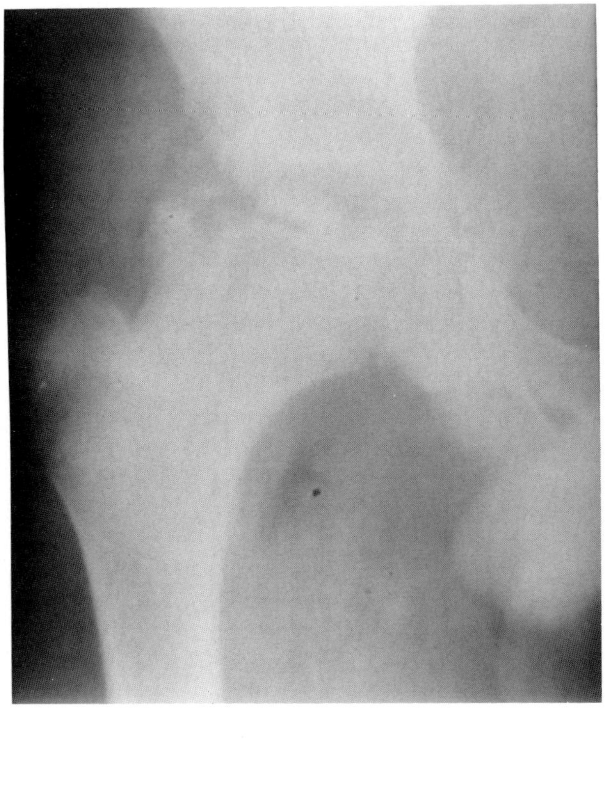

Fig. 14-2 Lateral subluxation of femoral head from acetabulum. This is considered "head-at-risk" sign, which portends worst prognosis.

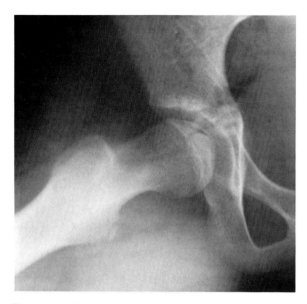

Fig. 14-3 Subchondral fracture of femoral head. Extent of early fracture determines amount of femoral head involved in LCPD.

Salter and Thompson described a subchondral fracture in the superolateral portion of the femoral head (Fig. 14-3) that can be detected earlier than the amount of femoral head involvement and the head-at-risk signs described by Catterall and thus allows earlier treatment decisions. They classified LCPD into two groups, depending on the extent of this subchondral fracture: type A, less than 50% of the superior dome of the femoral head, and type B, more than 50%. They report good results in type A involvement and poor results in type B. Although this classification is reliable, subchondral fracture occurs in only one third of children with LCPD, and the Catterall classification must be used for the other two thirds.

Because approximately 8.1 months are required to make an accurate Catterall classification on the basis of routine roentgenograms, bone scanning can be used to help determine femoral head involvement, comparing the uptake to the contralateral hip, as described by several authors, but not attempting to quantitate this definitively. Generally, if the uptake in the affected hip is decreased less than 50% as compared with the contralateral hip, it is considered Catterall type I or II and if the uptake is decreased more than 50%, Catterall type III or IV (Fig. 14-4).

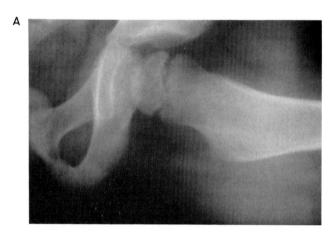
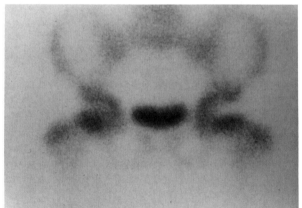

Fig. 14-4 **A,** Subchondral lucency in superolateral aspect of femoral head on lateral roentgenogram. **B,** Technetium bone scan shows significantly decreased uptake in anterolateral portion of right femoral head indicative of more than 50% involvement.

TREATMENT

Between 60% and 75% of children with LCPD will have satisfactory results if the only treatment is careful observation; however, in those children with poor results LCPD is a debilitating disease and the reconstruction of the damaged hip joint requires an extensive procedure such as hip fusion or total hip replacement; both are undesirable in a young, active person. Determining early which children will benefit from treatment is difficult and imprecise. The various classification systems offer some assistance. Catterall recommends containment for children with types II, III, or IV involvement of the femoral head with two or more head-at-risk signs. Salter and Thompson recommend innominate osteotomy for children with type B subchondral fractures. The age of the child at onset of the disease also has been used as a treatment criterion, with most authors recommending conservative treatment for children younger than 6 years. Snyder, however, has reported poor results in children as young as 4 years with untreated LCPD. Because the consequences of a poor result are so disastrous and because the prognosis is so difficult to determine accurately, all children aged 4 years or older with LCPD should be treated with containment or noncontainment methods. Children aged 2 to 3 years may be observed, with aggressive treatment instituted if sudden, significant loss of motion or lateral subluxation occurs.

According to Moseley the goals of treatment of LCPD are good containment and congruence and reduction of weight on the affected area of the femoral head. Coleman, Gross, and others also have suggested that range of motion should be maintained during the active phase of the disease, not only to preserve adequate function but also to serve as an indicator of the severity of the disease process. They note that a sudden, significant loss of motion indicates impending problems: lack of congruity and containment and lateral subluxation. They recommend a supervised range of motion program, surgical adductor tenotomy if necessary, and, with the patient under general anesthesia, even manipulation to regain motion.

Treatment for LCPD has ranged from bed rest to noncontainment or "weight-relieving" bracing to containment obtained by bracing or surgery. The concept of containment is that the femoral head lies more concentrically in the acetabulum in the abducted and internally rotated position and that the femoral head can reform spherically because of what Salter calls "biological plasticity." Roberts, as well as Bellyei and Milke, recently reported that, in addition to femoral head reformation, congruity may be achieved in younger children by conformation of the superior dome of the acetabulum to any flatness or irregularity of the femoral head. After the child is 6 or 7 years old, the acetabulum appears to lose this biologic plasticity and retains its fixed contour, sometimes forming a trough in the laterally subluxed femoral head. As flexion and abduction take place, the femoral head hinges on the trough, resulting in "hinged abduction" as described by Yngve and Roberts (Fig. 14-5).

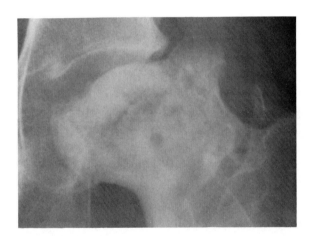

Fig. 14-5 "Hinged abduction" resulting from trough formed in laterally subluxed femoral head.

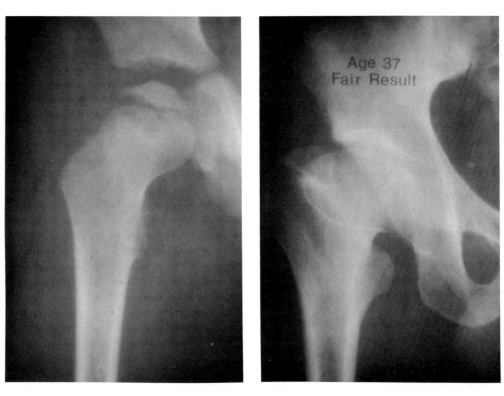

Fig. 14-6 "Congruous incongruity" described by Ratliff. **A,** At age 6 years, patient had lateral calcification, metaphyseal cyst, and lateral subluxation. **B,** At age 37 years, patient had excellent function but unsatisfactory roentgenographic result, with coxa plana and a large mushroom-shaped femoral head.

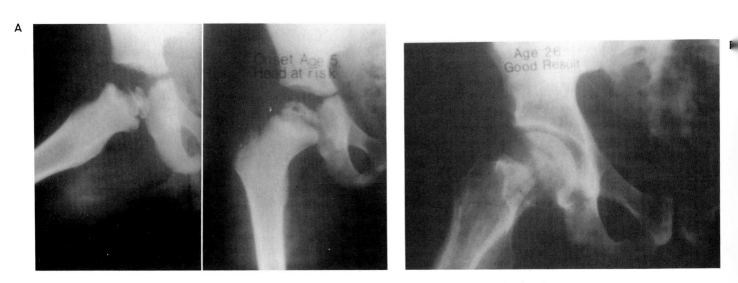

Fig. 14-7 **A,** At age 5 years, patient had head-at-risk signs, including metaphyseal cyst, more horizontal epiphysis, Gage's sign (translucent V at lateral epiphyseal margin), and lateral subluxation. **B,** At age 26 years, patient had a good result both clinically and roentgenographically.

Because containment often requires prolonged brace wear—with all its psychosocial implications—or surgery (varus or innominate osteotomy), noncontainment treatment was reviewed by Kelly et al. In 80 children, 80% had good results, 12% fair results, and 8% poor results. The patients with fair results had satisfactory motion at an average of 33 years despite an unsatisfactory roentgenographic appearance of their hips (Fig. 14-6), because of the "congruous incongruity" described by Ratliff. Over half the patients with two or more head-at-risk signs (see p. 745) had good results (Fig. 14-7). Although 80% had good results with this method, it must be remembered that 60% to 75% of children have good results with no treatment, and the slightly higher percentage of good results do not outweigh the disadvantages of prolonged crutch ambulation required with noncontainment methods.

Containment of the femoral head within the acetabulum requires abduction of the hip, with or without internal rotation. Several orthoses are available that achieve this result, many of which are cumbersome, heavy, and interfere with the child's daily activities and often social development. The least restrictive brace in current use is the Scottish Rite brace popularized by Purvis and Lovell (Fig. 14-8). This orthosis does not internally rotate the hip but holds it in abduction and slight flexion. If the hip does not sublux, the femoral head is congruously reformed and hinged abduction is avoided. Other braces currently used include ambulatory abduction frames such as the Newington brace and the Petrie cast (Fig. 14-9). An experimental brace, worn on the uninvolved extremity to fix the knee and ankle in extension and elevate the foot 4.5 to 6 cm, has been used in the treatment of 12 children, most with Catterall grade III or IV LCPD. Time of brace-wear ranged from 3 to 19 months, with an average of 11 months. The brace tilts the pelvis into relative abduction to contain the involved femoral head within the acetabulum. The advantages of this polypropylene, unilateral, "relative abduction" brace are that it causes less restriction of daily activities and is more cosmetically and socially acceptable (Fig. 14-10). At an average follow-up time of almost 8 years, all 12 patients were active with little pain or limitation of motion. Only two reported being limited in sports activities. Although these early results are promising, long-term follow-up is necessary to establish the efficacy of this containment method.

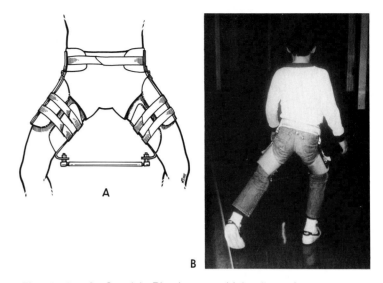

Fig. 14-8 **A,** Scottish Rite brace, which allows free knee and ankle motion and flexion of hip with telescoping abduction bar. **B,** Ambulation in brace.

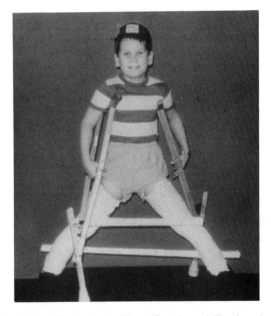

Fig. 14-9 Petrie cast without foot immobilization does not allow internal rotation of hip.

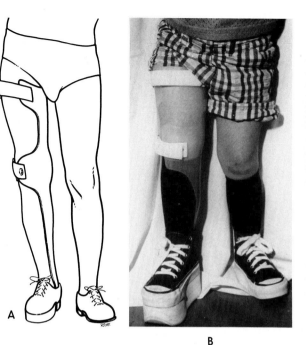

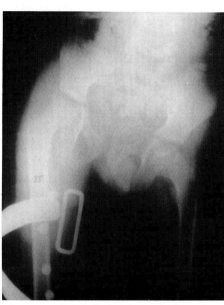

Fig. 14-10 A, Dynamic abduction brace. **B,** Brace is worn on uninvolved extremity to tilt pelvis into relative abduction. **C,** Roentgenogram of patient in brace shows pelvis tilted over femoral head.

One of the disadvantages to any containment orthosis is the length of time the brace must be worn before the femoral head is reformed. The natural course of LCPD has been documented to require from 24 to 36 months, which has been the usual length of brace wear, but Thompson and Westin have reported equally satisfactory results in patients wearing containment orthoses for only 12 to 18 months. Bracing is recommended for 12 to 15 months in children with Catterall type I or II involvement and for 15 to 18 months in those with Catterall type III or IV. Another hindrance to successful containment treatment is that it requires compliance and cooperation from the patient and the parents, which often are difficult to monitor and enforce.

Surgical containment is indicated when bracing is contraindicated because of a noncompliant patient or parents, because of bilateral involvement at different stages that would require an unreasonably long stint of brace wear, or because coverage of the femoral head in abduction cannot be obtained. Surgery has the advantage of directly covering the femoral head and often is attractive to the patient and parents when the 3-month postoperative immobilization in a spica cast is compared with the 12 to 18 months of brace wear; however, all the complications of major hip surgery should be explained thoroughly (Fig. 14-11), including the need for a second surgical procedure to remove any internal fixation devices and the risks associated with anesthesia and possible blood transfusion.

Surgical containment of the femoral head may be obtained by altering either the acetabular or femoral configuration, and there are advocates for each. Salter, Moseley, Coleman, and Maxted and Jackson have had good results with pelvic osteotomy, whereas Axer, Craig et al, Green and Griffin, Somerville, Lloyd-Roberts et al, Catterall, and Serlo et al reported good results with varus derotational femoral osteotomy. The choice of a particular technique depends on the individual patient and the experience of the surgeon. Regardless of which technique is chosen, preoperative arthrography generally is advisable to rule out any flattening of the femoral head that would contraindicate osteotomy and to determine how much subluxation is present and how much containment is necessary.

Using osteovenography, Serlo et al, as well as Green and Griffin, noted increased intraosseous pressures in affected hips. Green and Griffin believe that intertrochanteric varus osteotomy may decrease this pressure and lead to more rapid and complete reformation of the femoral head. Serlo et al found that intraosseous pressures decreased significantly after 14 to 17 days of Russell traction and recommended its use preoperatively to ensure a better surgical result.

Although both pelvic and femoral osteotomies should be aimed at containing the femoral head before permanent malformation occurs, there are several procedures for reconstruction of the severely damaged hip: valgus (abduction) osteotomy as described by Quain and Catterall for hinge abduction, Garceau cheilectomy, Chiari pelvic osteotomy, and trochanteric transfer.

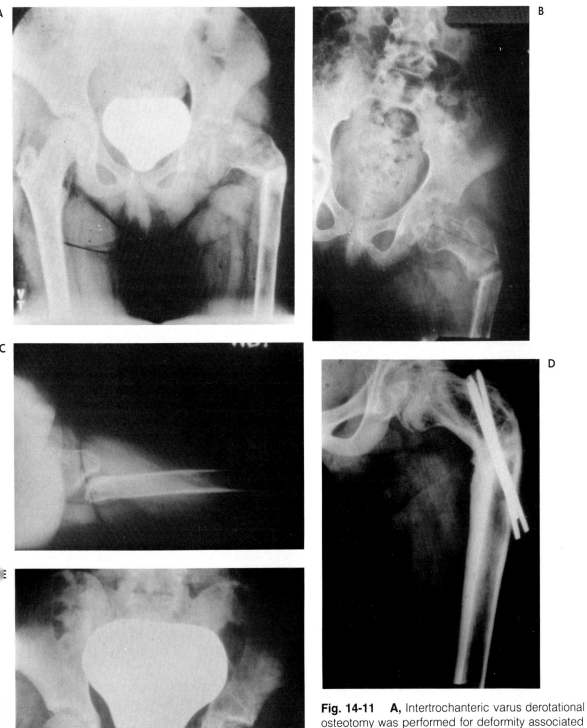

Fig. 14-11 **A,** Intertrochanteric varus derotational osteotomy was performed for deformity associated with LCPD. **B** and **C,** Six months after osteotomy, nonunion was obvious. **D,** Bone grafting and internal fixation in a varus position achieved union. **E,** After pin removal the involved extremity was 3.4 cm shorter than the opposite leg; epiphysiodesis of the uninvolved extremity was performed.

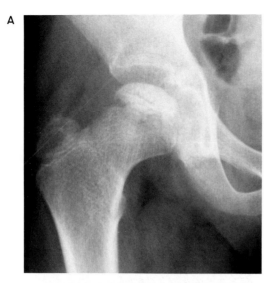

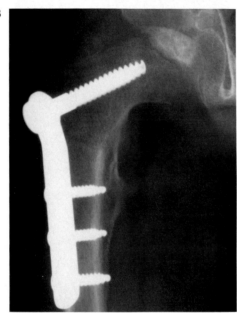

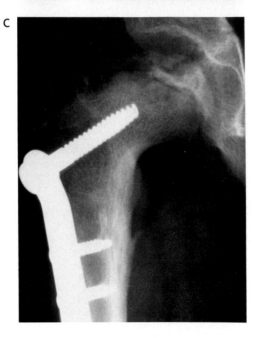

Varus Derotational Osteotomy

The advantages of varus derotational osteotomy include maximum coverage of the femoral head, especially in the older child, and correction of excessive femoral anteversion with the same osteotomy (Fig. 14-12). Disadvantages include excessive varus angulation that may not correct with growth (especially in the older child), further shortening of an already shortened extremity, the possibility of a gluteal lurch produced by increasing the length of the lever arm of the gluteal musculature, the possibility of nonunion of the osteotomy, and the need for a second operation to remove the internal fixation. Indications for varus derotational osteotomy include inability to obtain containment by bracing for psychosocial or other reasons, the age factor in children from 8 to 10 years old, the absence of leg length inequality, arthrographic evidence that most of the femoral head is uncovered, a decrease in the angle of Wiberg, and significant femoral anteversion. Axer performs a subtrochanteric osteotomy early in the course of LCPD and uses the following plan.

An anteroposterior roentgenogram of the pelvis is taken with the lower extremities in internal rotation and parallel to each other (no abduction). If satisfactory containment of the femoral head is noted, derotational osteotomy alone is carried out. The degree of derotation is roughly estimated from the amount of internal rotation of the extremity, but further adjustments are made during the operation. Significant anteversion and internal rotation of the extremity should be confirmed and measured by computed tomography or other means; otherwise, derotation will cause excessive external rotation of the leg.

When internal rotation is seriously limited and remains so preoperatively after a 4-week period of bed rest with traction, varus osteotomy is carried out with the addition of extension that is produced by a slight backward tilt of the proximal fragment.

When femoral anteversion is not present, abduction of the extremity will bring about the desired containment of the femoral head. The degree of abduction is expressed by the angle formed by the shaft of the femur and a vertical line parallel to the midline of the pelvis. This angle represents the desired angle

---

Fig. 14-12 A, Legg-Calvé-Perthes disease with total femoral head involvement 6 months after onset of disease. **B,** After subtrochanteric varus derotational osteotomy. **C,** In view 18 months after osteotomy, early healing is evident with good hip joint congruity and some mild remodeling into more nearly normal, valgus neck-shaft angle.

of the osteotomy (see technique described below). Because derotational osteotomy alone may result in lengthening of the extremity from stimulation of growth, a varus angle of 5 degrees to 10 degrees may be added.

Reliable information on acetabular containment of the femoral head, the size of the head, the flattening of the epiphysis, and the width of the medial joint space can be obtained from preoperative arthrography. The osteocartilaginous head of the femur should be covered adequately by the acetabular roof as the femur is abducted and the flattened segment of the femoral head is rotated into the depths of the acetabular fossa.

Axer performs a lateral opening wedge osteotomy on children 5 years of age and younger. A prebent plate is used to hold the cortices apart laterally the measured amount. The defect laterally fills in rapidly in young children, but the open wedge may result in delayed union or nonunion in children older than 5 years of age. Because few children with LCPD younger than 5 years are treated surgically in this country, indications for this procedure are rare. Axer's reversed wedge modification uses the removal of a wedge one half the calculated height based medially and its reversal for insertion laterally before fixation with the prebent plate. This method produces approximately the same amount of shortening as the opening wedge but not as much as complete removal and closure of the full height of the wedge medially.

▶ *Technique (Axer).* With the patient supine on the operating table, drape the lower limb free for manipulation. Make a straight lateral incision beginning at the level of the middle of the greater trochanter, and continue it distally 10 to 13 cm. Expose subperiosteally the proximal part of the femur up to the origin of the vastus lateralis muscle. Apply a self-retaining bone clamp vertically on the femoral shaft

as distally as possible while the lower extremity is held in full internal rotation. This clamp serves as an efficient retractor and enables the surgeon to control the distal fragment after osteotomy. Choose two Sherman bone plates of identical size so that one half the length of the plate reaches from the base of the trochanter to the osteotomy site. Prebend one of them in the middle to the desired osteotomy angle, and hold the other against the lateral aspect of the femur so that its proximal end reaches to the base of the greater trochanter. Make a transverse mark on the femoral shaft at the level of future osteotomy, corresponding with the midpart of the plate. Insert two long ⁷⁄₆₄ -inch (2.8 mm) drill points through the two proximal plate holes and through both femoral cortices and leave them there. Remove the plate and measure with calipers the width of the femoral shaft at the level of the subtrochanteric osteotomy. Read the length of the base of the wedge to be opened from the table credited by Axer to Orkan and Roth (Table 14-1). Then select either an opening wedge or reversed wedge technique for the osteotomy as indicated.

Opening wedge technique. While the extremity is held in internal rotation, divide the bone with an oscillating saw at the previously marked level. Hold the proximal fragment in slightly less than full internal rotation and in abduction with the help of the protruding long drill points. Bring the medial cortices of the distal and proximal fragments together after rotating the distal fragment externally until the patella points straight forward. Slip the prebent bone plate over the drill points, and fix it to the proximal and distal fragments of the femoral shaft with two self-retaining bone clamps. Pay attention to the contact of the medial cortices and to an accurate fit of the plate to the outer surface of the bone so that the required varus angle is established. Carefully attempt to inter-

Table 14-1   Table for calculating the height of the base of the wedge to be removed for varus osteotomy*

Desired angulatory change (degrees)	Femoral shaft width at osteotomy site (mm)												
	10	12.5	15	17.5	20	22.5	25	27.5	30	32.5	35	37.5	40
10	1.5	2.0	2.5	3.0	3.5	4.0	4.5	5.0	5.5	6.0	6.5	7.0	7.5
15	2.0	3.0	4.0	4.5	5.0	6.0	6.5	7.5	8.0	9.0	10.0	10.5	11.5
20	3.0	4.0	5.0	6.0	7.0	8.0	9.0	10.0	11.0	12.0	13.0	14.0	15.0
25	4.5	5.0	6.5	7.5	9.0	10.0	11.5	12.5	14.0	15.0	16.0	17.5	18.5
30	5.5	6.5	8.0	10.0	11.5	12.5	14.0	15.5	17.0	18.5	20.0	22.0	23.0
35	6.5	8.0	10.0	12.0	13.5	14.0	17.0	18.3	21.0	22.0	24.0	26.0	27.5
40	8.0	10.0	12.5	14.5	16.5	18.5	20.0	23.0	25.0	27.0	29.0	31.5	33.5

The height of the base of the wedge in millimeters is read at the junction of the horizontal axis (desired degrees of angulatory change) and the vertical axis (width of the femoral shaft at the osteotomy site).
*Credited to Orkan and Roth. Data from Axer, A.: Personal communication, 1978.

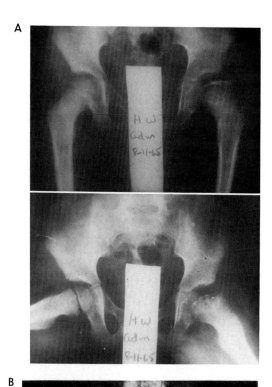

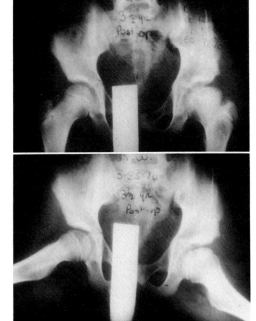

Fig. 14-13 **A,** Despite total femoral head involvement and lateral subluxation, this child had good motion. **B,** Three and one-half years after innominate osteotomy, there is excellent coverage of the femoral head.

nally rotate the extremity. It should be possible for a few degrees. Check the position of the patella to be sure that there is not too much external rotation of the foot at the midposition of the joint. Insert screws of proper length into the distal fragment and then into the proximal one, replacing the long drill points.

Reversed wedge technique. After calculating from the table the height of the base of the wedge to be removed, hold the extremity in internal rotation at the hip and mark a wedge one half of this height over the anterior surface of the femur with the base medially. Remove this wedge with an oscillating saw, rotate the distal fragment externally to the desired degree, turn the bone wedge 180 degrees, and insert it in the osteotomy with its base lateral or reversed. Since its base now is lateral, the varus angle obtained equals the angle that would be obtained with complete removal of a full-height bone wedge medially. Fix the bone fragments with the prebent plate as previously described with all cortices in contact. When the reversed bone wedge is not stable enough, fix it to the distal or proximal fragment with small Kirschner wires.

▶*Postoperative management.* A double spica plaster cast is applied and removed after 6 to 8 weeks or when union is confirmed by roentgenography. The child is encouraged to walk, in water initially if increased joint stiffness is noted. No restrictions are imposed on the child except for follow-up every 3 months in the first year.

Innominate Osteotomy

The advantages of innominate osteotomy by either Salter's method or the Elizabethtown method (Fig. 14-13) include anterolateral coverage of the femoral head, lengthening of the extremity (possibly shortened by the avascular process), and avoidance of a second operation for plate removal. The disadvantages of innominate osteotomy include the inability sometimes to obtain proper containment of the femoral head, especially in older children, an increase in acetabular and hip joint pressure that may cause further avascular changes in the femoral head, and an increase in leg length on the operated side as compared with the normal side that may cause a relative adduction of the hip and uncover the femoral head.

In surgically treated patients older than 6 years of age with total head involvement and subluxation Cotler and Wolfgang reported no further embarrassment of vascularity of the femoral head as indicated by avascular necrosis or chondrolysis. A faster healing rate (progression from one stage to the next in a shorter period of time) was not found after osteotomy; rather a change from one stage of the disease to the next was determined earlier, probably by the more frequent roentgenograms of hips that had been operated on. Clancy and Steel performed incomplete intertrochanteric osteotomies on 53 patients with Perthes' disease and compared the "healing" time roentgenographically with that of 36 patients who had nonoperative treatment. They concluded that intertrochanteric osteotomy also did not alter the rate of healing of the disease.

Innominate osteotomy as described by Salter is included in the discussion of congenital deformities (Chapter 2). It should be remembered that Salter's procedure includes iliopsoas release.

▲ *Technique (Canale et al)*. Through a Smith-Petersen approach to the hip, release the sartorius, tensor fasciae latae, and rectus femoris muscles, and expose the anterosuperior iliac spine. Release the psoas tendon from its insertion and dissect subperiosteally on the inner and outer walls of the ilium down to the sciatic notch. Using retractors in the sciatic notch, with a right-angle clamp pass a Gigli saw through the sciatic notch. With the saw carefully cut horizontally and anteriorly through the ilium as close as possible to the capsular attachment of the acetabulum. Maximally flex the knee and then flex and abduct the hip to open the osteotomy. Use a towel clip to pull the distal fragment of the osteotomy anteriorly and laterally. Take a full-thickness quadrilateral graft approximately 2 × 3 cm from the wing of the ilium according to the size of the space produced by opening the osteotomy (Fig. 14-14). Predrill or precut the outline of the graft on the surfaces of the ilium to prevent fracture of the inner and outer cortices. Shape the quadrilateral graft carefully to fit the space produced, and impact it into the osteotomy site. Use one or more threaded pins for fixation, and leave the ends subcutaneous so that they can be removed later with the patient under local anesthesia.

Use the center edge angle of Wiberg in the weight-bearing position at this time to assess by roentgenography the coverage and containment of the femoral head.

▲ *Postoperative management*. The patient is immobilized for 10 to 12 weeks in a spica cast before the pins are removed. Range-of-motion exercises and full weight-bearing ambulation are then started and roentgenographic assessment is repeated.

Reconstructive Surgery
Valgus Osteotomy for Hinge Abduction

Quain and Catterall and Roberts described hinge abduction of the hip as an abnormal movement of the hip that occurs when the femoral head, deformed from LCPD, fails to slide within the acetabulum. A trench is formed laterally, adjacent to a large uncovered portion of the deformed femoral head anterolat-

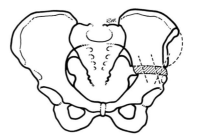

Fig. 14-14 Innominate osteotomy using quadrangular graft (see text). (Redrawn from Canale ST et al: J Bone Joint Surg 54A:25, 1972.)

erally. Clinically, flexion and abduction are limited, the extremity is shortened, and often there is a painful, clunking sensation. Pelvic osteotomy (Chiari or shelf procedure) has been recommended, but although these operations improve lateral coverage they do not reduce lateral impingement during abduction. Quain and Catterall reported satisfactory results in 26 of 27 patients after abduction (valgus) extension osteotomy (Fig. 14-15). They recommend arthrography of the hip with the patient under general anesthesia. Moving the hip through a range of motion will determine both the limitations of motion and where hinge abduction occurs—usually between 15 and 30 degrees of abduction and 10 to 30 degrees of flexion. Abduction extension osteotomy is then performed to align the leg to this position of congruity, and a pediatric lag screw is used for fixation (see subtrochanteric valgus and varus osteotomy using the Campbell screw, p. 146).

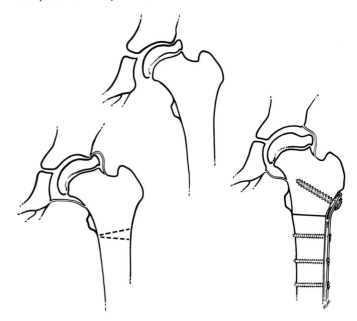

Fig. 14-15 Valgus femoral osteotomy to reduce hinged abduction and increase flexion of hip. Osteotomy is fixed with Campbell cannulated pediatric lag screw.

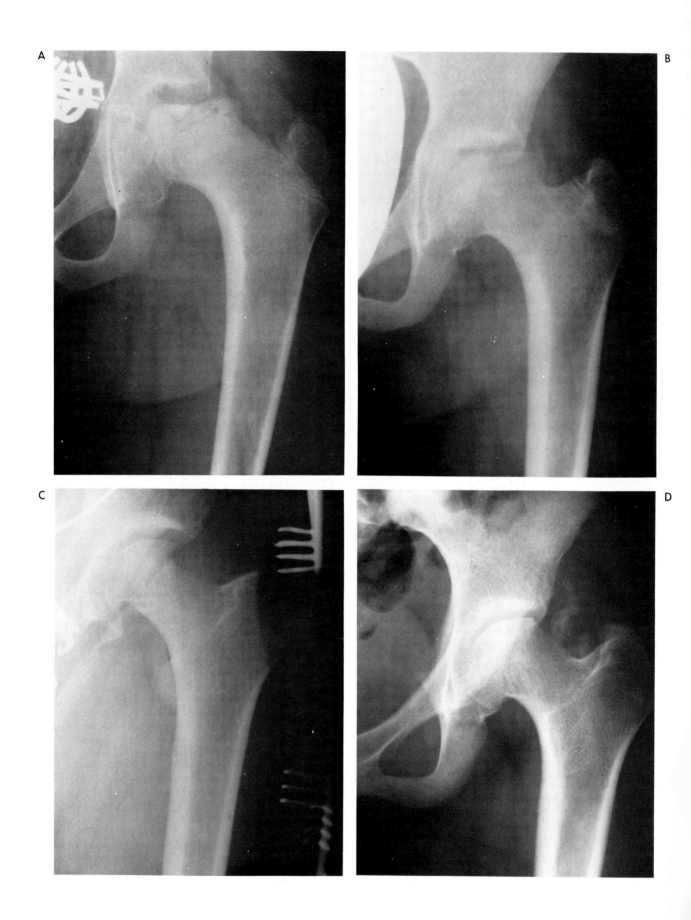

Cheilectomy

Occasionally, as a late residual effect of LCPD, a child will be left with a malformed femoral head, usually either a large mushroom-shaped (coxa plana) head or a lateral protuberance of the head outside the acetabulum. For this lateral protuberance on the head, when the hip is painful and has a lack of abduction or a clicking sensation on abduction, Garceau recommended a cheilectomy for its removal (Fig. 14-16). When the head is mushroom-shaped as in coxa plana and subluxating from the acetabulum and when the hip is painful, coverage can be achieved by a Chiari osteotomy.

Preoperative evaluation for cheilectomy includes determination as to whether the protuberance is anterior or posterior; it usually is anterior and lateral, and for this reason a lateral approach generally is used.

▶ *Technique (Sage and Clark).* With the patient supine and the involved hip on a sandbag, begin an incision laterally approximately 5 cm proximal to the greater trochanter and carry it distally for 7.5 to 10 cm. Locate the interval between the gluteus medius and tensor fasciae latae muscles, and carry the dissection proximally to expose the inferior branch of the superior gluteal nerve. Retract this nerve carefully because it innervates the tensor fasciae latae muscle. Complete the separation of the interval and expose the hip capsule. Open the capsule longitudinally along the anterosuperior surface of the femoral neck. Because the protuberance almost always lies laterally, it then can be seen either anteriorly or posteriorly. When it is more posterior, detach a small portion of the fibers of the gluteus medius tendon from the trochanter for exposure. Excise the entire protuberance with a sharp osteotome. Direct the osteotome away from the lateral edge of the proximal femoral physis to avoid its excision. Slipping of the capital femoral epiphysis has followed cheilectomy and may be related to excision of the lateral portion of the physis and the adjacent cortex of the neck. Check the range of motion, especially abduction, to be sure that a sufficient cheilectomy has been performed.

▶ *Postoperative management.* The extremity is placed in balanced suspension, and over the next 2 to 3 weeks range-of-motion exercises, especially hip abduction, are carried out.

Chiari Osteotomy

The pelvic osteotomy described by Chiari (Fig. 14-17) has been used as a salvage procedure to accomplish coverage of a large flattened femoral head in the older child when the femoral head is subluxating and painful. The addition of a supplemental bone graft was suggested by Graham et al for severely dysplastic hips. The technique of Chiari osteotomy is described in detail in Chapter 2.

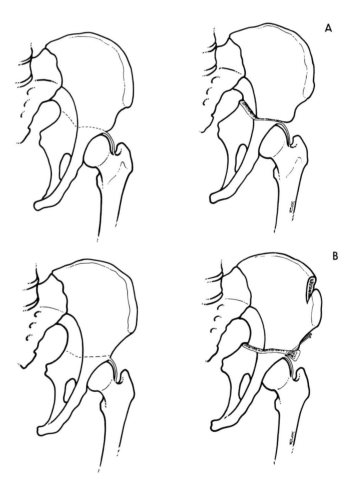

Fig. 14-17 **A,** Ideal Chiari osteotomy with 15-degree upslope cut and coverage obtained in mild dysplasia. **B,** Chiari osteotomy with supplemental bone graft for severely dysplastic, subluxed hip. (Redrawn from Graham S et al: Clin Orthop 208:149, 1986.)

Fig. 14-16 Cheilectomy for LCPD. **A,** Roentgenogram of left hip of 7-year-old boy with LCPD who had been treated without containment and developed lateral subluxation of femoral head (late group III). **B,** Same patient in residual stage with coxa plana and lateral protuberance of femoral head outside acetabulum. Patient had pain and limited abduction of hip. **C,** Roentgenogram made during surgery for cheilectomy. Large protruding area of bone has been excised. **D,** At follow-up several years later there is no pain. Motion, including abduction, is increased. There is area of myositis ossificans or calcification in superior capsule of hip joint.

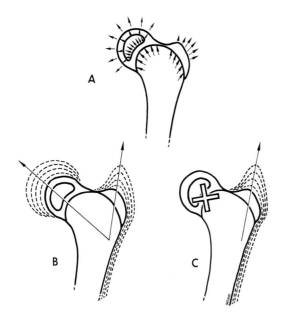

Fig. 14-18 Growth of proximal femur. **A** and **B,** Arrows indicate site and direction of growth. **C,** If growth potential is impaired, longitudinal growth is arrested but greater trochanter continues to grow. (Redrawn from Wagner H and Holder J. In Schatzker J, editor: The intertrochanteric osteotomy, Berlin, 1984, Springer-Verlag.)

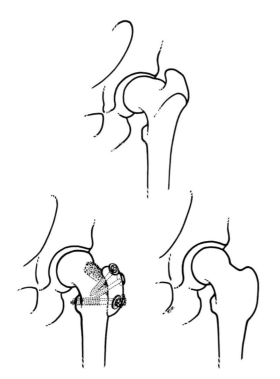

Fig. 14-19 Transfer of greater trochanter improves mechanical function after trochanteric overgrowth. (Redrawn from Wagner H and Holder J. In Schatzker J, editor: The intertrochanteric osteotomy, Berlin, 1984, Springer-Verlag.)

Trochanteric Transfer (Advancement)

Although trochanteric overgrowth may be caused by a number of conditions, including osteomyelitis, fracture, or congenital dysplasia, it occurs in LCPD when the disease causes premature closure of the capital femoral epiphysis. Whatever the mechanism the result is the same: arrest of longitudinal growth of the femoral neck with continuation of growth of the greater trochanter (Fig. 14-18). According to Wagner the functional consequences are always the same: elevation (overgrowth) of the trochanter decreases tension and mechanical efficiency of the pelvic and trochanteric muscles; shortening of the femoral neck moves the greater trochanter closer to the center of rotation of the hip, decreasing the lever arm and mechanical advantage of the muscles and impairing muscular stabilization of the hip; the line of pull of the muscles becomes more vertical, increasing the pressure forces concentrated over a diminished area of hip joint surface; and impingement of the trochanter on the rim of the acetabular roof during abduction limits range of motion. Transfer of the greater trochanter distally restores normal tension to the trochanteric muscles and improves mechanical efficiency, puts a more horizontal pull on the pelvic-trochanteric muscle action to more uniformly distribute forces over the hip joint, and increases the length of the femoral neck to increase abduction and decrease acetabular impingement (Fig. 14-19).

▶ *Technique (Wagner).* With the patient supine, approach the hip through a lateral incision. Excise the fascia lata longitudinally, and release the vastus lateralis muscle from the greater trochanter. Retract the gluteus medius muscle posteriorly, and insert a Kirschner wire superiorly parallel to the femoral neck and greater trochanteric apophyseal line pointing toward the trochanteric fossa (Fig. 14-20, *A*). Confirm the placement of the guide pin by image intensification. Internally rotating the hip slightly will facilitate placement of the pin and allow better imaging. Make the osteotomy parallel to the Kirschner wire with a low-speed oscillating saw, completing it proximally with a flat osteotome (Fig. 14-20, *B*); pry open the osteotomy until the medial cortex fractures (Fig. 14-20, *C* and *D*). Mobilize the greater trochanter first cephalad, and with dissecting scissors remove any adhesions, joint capsule, and soft tissue flush with the medial surface of the trochanter, taking care to spare the blood vessels in the trochanteric fossa (Fig. 14-20, *E*). Once the greater trochanter is freed, transfer it distally and laterally. If excessive anteversion is present, it also may be transferred anteriorly. Using an osteotome, freshen the lateral femoral cortex to which the trochanter is to be attached. Place the trochanter against the lateral femoral cortex, and check the posi-

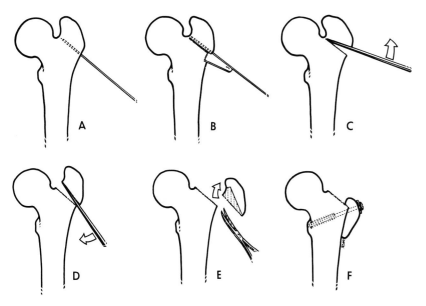

Fig. 14-20   Trochanteric transfer (advancement) for trochanteric overgrowth (see text). (Redrawn from Wagner H and Holder J. In Schatzker J, editor: The intertrochanteric osteotomy, Berlin, 1984, Springer-Verlag.)

tion with image intensification. According to Wagner the tip of the greater trochanter should be level with the center of the femoral head, and the distance between them should be 2 to 2.5 times the radius of the femoral head. When proper position is confirmed, fix the greater trochanter with two screws inserted in a cephalolateral to caudad direction (Fig. 14-20, *F*). These screws, with washers, should compress an area of bony contact between the trochanter and femur. Bury the screw heads by retracting all soft tissue so that soft tissue necrosis and local mechanical irritation will not occur postoperatively. Wagner uses a supplemental strong tension band suture that he believes helps absorb tensile forces from the pelvic and trochanteric muscles and prevents trochanteric avulsion. No postoperative immobilization is required if the patient is compliant and the fixation is secure.

▲ *Postoperative management.* Ambulation on crutches is begun 7 days after surgery, but active exercises of the pelvic and trochanteric muscles are not permited until 3 weeks after surgery. Sitting upright and flexing the hip also should be avoided because overpull of the gluteus medius muscle may cause loss of fixation.

▲ *Technique (Lloyd-Roberts et al).* Approach the trochanter through a "goblet incision" or a long lateral incision. Place a Gigli saw deep to the gluteus medius and minimus muscles, and divide the trochanter at its base. Then mobilize the gluteus muscles anteriorly and posteriorly as they are dissected off the joint capsule, and strip them for a short distance from the ilium above. Displace the detached trochanter with its attached muscles distally to the lateral cortex of the

femur while the hip is abducted (Fig. 14-21). Bevel the femoral cortex to help reduce tension and improve placement of the trochanter. Secure the trochanter by screw or wire to the femur, and suture the femoral periosteum and vastus lateralis.

▲ *Postoperative management.* The hip is protected by a plaster spica cast in abduction for 8 weeks. In the neutral position, the fixation is under unacceptable tension until bony union is secure (Fig. 14-21).

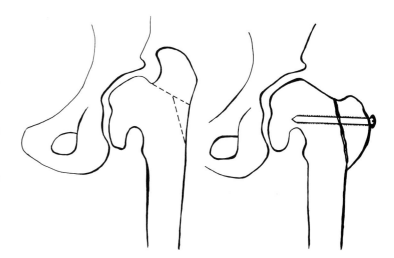

Fig. 14-21   Operative technique for advancement of trochanter. Trochanter is divided at its base and displaced distally onto beveled lateral cortex of femur. Note that relationships within joint are unaffected. (From Lloyd-Roberts GC, Wetherill MH, and Fraser M: J Bone Joint Surg 67B:20, 1985.)

OSTEOCHONDRITIS DISSECANS OF THE HIP

The term *osteochondritis dissecans* indicates the presence of an osteocartilaginous fragment in the joint, an occurrence more frequent in the knee and ankle joints than in the hip joint. Several etiologic factors have been implicated, including trauma, endocrine abnormalities, ossification anomalies, and familial predilection, but most authors agree that the cause is probably multifactorial. Osteochondritis dissecans of the hip may be associated with avascular necrosis, sickle cell disease, multiple epiphyseal dysplasia, and in adults, Gaucher disease and occult trauma. It occurs in approximately 3% of patients treated for LCPD. Ratliff described the osteochondritic fragment as an unhealed necrotic bony fragment that persists from the time of active disease until adulthood. Hallel and Salvati distinguished osteochondritis dissecans after LCPD from idiopathic osteochondritis dissecans of adulthood.

Clinical and Roentgenographic Findings

Osteochondritis dissecans of the hip after LCPD has variable symptoms. Patients may have no symptoms, minimal symptoms, or severely disabling symptoms. The most common are arthralgia, limping and snapping, catching, locking, or a sensation of giving way of the hip joint, which may be caused by loose body formation or secondary degenerative joint changes.

Diagnosis of osteochondritis dissecans of the hip usually can be made from plain roentgenogram (Fig. 14-22), with the osteochondritis fragment appearing in the superior portion of the femoral head (on the weight-bearing surface area). Tomography, arthrography, and CT scanning may be useful to confirm the diagnosis or better outline the lesion.

Treatment

Treatment of osteochondritis dissecans of the hip has been varied and confusing, ranging from observation to symptomatic treatment to removal of the loose fragment and drilling of the bed to internal fixation of the fragment with bone pegs. Kahmi and MacEwen, as well as other authors, described satisfactory results in children who had no treatment; they noted that operative treatment required dislocation of the hip joint with the attendant risk of further vascular damage to the head of the femur. In the symptom-free child with osteochondritis dissecans of the hip, restriction of activity and prolonged observation are indicated to allow healing and revascularization.

Surgical treatment is indicated for severe lesions with disabling symptoms. The choice of operative procedure depends on the extent of the lesion, its lo-cation, the age and activity expectations of the patient, and the presence of degenerative joint changes. Flashman and Ghormley reported that, in their small series of adults, excision of the fragment was as successful as arthroplasty. They drilled the lesion to promote revascularization and recommended packing large craters with cancellous bone to retain the articular surface contour. Removal of the loose fragment with curettage of the bed to bleeding bone obtained good results in two patients reported by Hallel and Salvati. Lindholm and Osterman reported good results with internal fixation of the fragment with cortical bone pegs. More recently, Bowen et al reported arthroscopic removal of the loose osteocartilaginous fragment in four patients, all of whom were symptom free or had improvement approximately 1 year after the procedure. None of the preceding procedures are recommended if severe osteoarthritic changes are present, and a procedure to redirect the femoral head (such as valgus extension osteotomy) is preferred.

Arthroscopy of the hip. Arthroscopy of the hip joint is not a simple procedure and should not be undertaken lightly. In addition to removal of an osteochondritic lesion, arthroscopy of the hip may be indicated for synovial biopsy, removal of loose bodies, removal of debris and inspection of the labrum after fracture-dislocation, and partial or total synovectomy. If the lesion is not anterior or anterolateral, it is very difficult to see, and longitudinal traction should be used to increase the visibility of posterior or posterolateral lesions. A fracture table and image intensification are helpful in judging the correct amount of distraction and joint penetration. The anterior portals are most often used for arthroscopy of the hip joint, as described by Bowen et al, but the lateral portals, as described by Glick et al, may be necessary for lesions that are more posteriorly located.

Anterior approach

◣ *Technique (Bowen et al).* Place the patient, who is under general endotracheal anesthesia, on the fracture table. Using image intensification, apply traction in the neutral position on the involved extremity until the hip joint is distracted approximately 1 cm. Introduce a 21-gauge spinal needle into the hip and confirm its intraarticular location by injecting 1 ml of contrast (Renografin-60, E.R. Squibb & Sons, Inc.). Distend the joint with approximately 15 ml lactated Ringer's solution and 1% lidocaine (Xylocaine) with 1:100,000 epinephrine at a 1:1 dilution. Under image intensification introduce a 5-mm arthroscope with a 30-degree angular lens through an anterolateral portal just lateral to the sartorius muscle. Pay special attention to the introduction of the arthro-

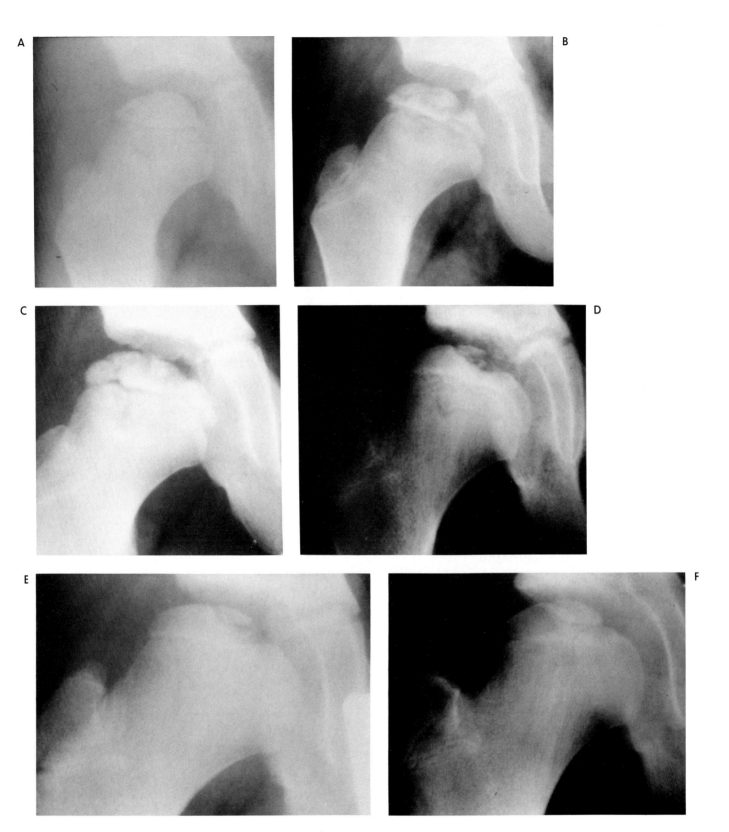

Fig. 14-22 **A,** Early total head involvement in LCPD. **B,** Six months later, Catterall type III or IV involvement. **C,** LCPD healing at 18 months. **D,** Three years after onset of LCPD, there is persistent central defect. **E,** Five years after LCPD, osteochondritis dissecans is obvious. **F,** Seven years after LCPD, osteochondritis dissecans persists with what appears to be a loose body within a crater in superior middle portion of femoral head.

scopic trocar, directing the tip beneath the lateral acetabular labrum, through the capsule, and into the distracted space in the hip joint. The hip capsule should be penetrated only once because multiple punctures will allow the irrigation solution to escape from the joint space. Withdraw the trocar and insert the arthroscope. During the entire procedure, irrigate the joint with lactated Ringer's solution; if bleeding occurs, add 2 ml of 1% Xylocaine with 1:100,000 epinephrine to the irrigant. Examine the hip joint and locate the osteochondritic fragment; an arthroscope with multiple-angled lenses is necessary to evaluate the joint.

When indicated, remove the osteochondritic fragment through a second portal just anterior and distal to the first. Introduce the trocar through the second portal as previously described and place the intraarticular cutter. Under image intensification, debride and extract the loose body. Debride the bed of the osteochondritis dissecans fragment to bleeding bone. At the end of the procedure, inject contrast medium with the irrigant to detect any residual fragments. Remove the arthroscope and cutter, and close the wounds with simple sutures.

Lateral approach

▶ *Technique (Glick et al).* Place the patient, who is under general anesthesia, on the fracture (traction) table in the lateral decubitus position. Carefully pad the perineal post of the traction table to prevent pressure areas. Extend the affected hip but do not flex it. Apply sufficient traction to create a space that will accommodate a 5-mm arthroscope and arthroscopic instruments. Image intensification is helpful to verify the amount of hip distraction. Because of stretch neurapraxias to the nerves of the extremity, Glick et al use

a spring-loaded scale to measure the amount of traction placed on the hip. They recommend 25 to 30 pounds of traction to distract a loose, abnormal hip and 50 to 65 pounds to distract a tight, normal adult hip. Releasing the traction at intervals during the surgery also will help avoid a neurapraxia. Once correct traction has been verified, prepare and drape the lateral aspect of the leg about the greater trochanter and hip.

Make two portals directly over the greater trochanter and a third portal anteriorly (Fig. 14-23). This anterolateral portal is necessary to inspect the anterior corners of the hip joint. Insert a long, 18-gauge, spinal needle at the anterior point over the superior edge of the greater trochanter, and maneuver it into the hip joint, using image intensification if necessary. Distend the joint with 30 to 50 ml of irrigating solution. Reverse flow of the fluid verifies entrance into the joint. Next, through this same area, make a stab incision and place the arthroscopic sheath in the same direction as the needle. Use a sharp trocar to pass smoothly through the abundant tissue and strong capsular structure; then use a blunt trocar.

Now introduce an inflow-outflow cannula by first inserting a spinal needle anteriorly. Angle the needle about 45 degrees cephalad and 20 degrees medial, or triangulate the needle toward the arthroscope. Make a small stab incision at the needle site, and insert a 5.25-inch inflow-outflow cannula. Avoid the lateral femoral cutaneous nerve in this area by making a shallow incision and passing the trocar and sheath only once through the underlying tissues. Locate by palpation and carefully avoid the femoral artery and nerve, which also lie medially in this area (Fig. 14-23).

The inflow-outflow cannula and the surgical instruments can be changed from portal to portal as necessary, and extra portals can be made in the manner described; however, instrument crowding may become a problem. A complete inspection of the hip joint can be made by rotating the leg to expose the femoral head and moving the arthroscope to each portal. Biopsy or removal of loose bodies can be performed from these portals. Complications reported by Glick et al are nerve traction palsies and scuffing of the joint surfaces.

▶ *Postoperative management.* After routine diagnostic arthroscopy of the hip the patient is allowed to bear weight to tolerance on crutches for 1 week. Strengthening exercises for the hip and quadriceps musculature are begun immediately after surgery. After operative arthroscopy for either excision of the osteochondritic lesion or partial synovectomy, nonweight bearing on crutches is recommended for 4 to 6 weeks, supplemented by a strengthening exercise program for the hip and quadriceps muscles.

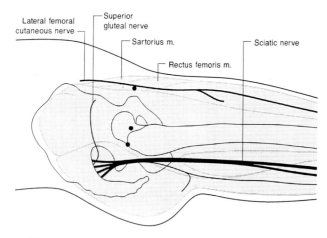

Fig. 14-23 Arthroscopic incisions around hip joint and their relationship to nerves in vicinity. Femoral nerve is too medial to depict in this diagram. (From Glick JM et al: J Arthroscopy 3:4, 1987.)

OSGOOD-SCHLATTER DISEASE

Osgood-Schlatter is a disease of adolescence, generally affecting children between the ages of 11 and 15 years; however, it may persist into adulthood. It occurs most frequently in boys who participate in sports, and there may be a history of a rapid growth spurt before the onset of symptoms. Most authors believe this osteochondrosis or "epiphysitis" is caused by prolonged overuse and chronic avulsion of the patellar tendon at its insertion into the tibial tubercle.

Clinical and Roentgenographic Findings

The clinical picture is that of a low-grade inflammatory process. Patients usually describe discomfort that is aggravated by running, jumping, going up and down stairs, or direct pressure such as falling on or being kicked in the area. Point tenderness and swelling over the insertion of the patellar tendon and excessive enlargement of the proximal tibial tubercle are dependable diagnostic signs of this disease. Roentgenograms may show chronic hypertrophy in the area, with excessive bone formation and multiple ossicles, which suggests the chronic, repetitive nature of the process. If the area of chronic avulsion is significant and displaced proximally, the patella may be slightly higher and more proximal than the contralateral patella. Woolfrey and Chandler described three distinct roentgenographic types of Osgood-Schlatter disease. In type I the tibial tuberosity is prominent and irregular, in type II it is prominent and irregular with a small free particle of bone anteriorly, and in type III there is a free particle of bone anterior and superior but the tuberosity is otherwise apparently normal.

Treatment

Rest, decreased activity, and immobilization will resolve the acute symptoms, but symptoms often recur when sports activities are resumed. Surgery rarely is indicated for Osgood-Schlatter disease. When symptoms recur despite conservative treatment and interfere significantly with daily and sports activities, surgery may be considered. Thompson and Dickinson and Ferciot recommend excision of the bony prominence through a longitudinal incision of the patellar tendon. Longitudinal growth of the tibia was not disturbed by this procedure in 41 patients in Thompson and Dickinson's series and in 11 in Ferciot's series. Bosworth recommends insertion of bone pegs into the tibial tuberosity, a simple procedure that he reports almost always relieves symptoms. It does not, however, remove the unsightly prominence, which still may be painful when fallen on or bumped. Any surgery should be done only in the older child at about 15 years of age when the tibial tubercle normally ossifies to the proximal tibia.

Ogden and Roberts both have reported complications of Osgood-Schlatter disease, treated conservatively and surgically, including subluxation of the patella, patella alta, nonunion of the bony fragment of the tibia, and premature fusion of the anterior part of the epiphysis with resulting genu recurvatum.

Insertion of Bone Pegs

▲ *Technique (Bosworth).* Make a longitudinal midline incision 7.5 cm long beginning at the distal part of the patellar tendon and continuing distally over the tibial tuberosity and tibial shaft (Fig. 14-24). Incise the periosteum longitudinally distal to the tuberosity. With an electric saw cut two matchstick pegs 4 cm long from the tibia; make the base of each peg larger than its tip. Then drill two holes through the tibial tuberosity: one near but not in contact with the proximal tibial physis and slanting proximally and laterally and the other distal to the physis and slanting proximally and medially. Insert the pegs into these holes and resect their projecting ends.

▲ *Postoperative management.* A cast is applied from groin to toes and is worn for 2 weeks. A cylinder walking cast then is worn for 4 more weeks.

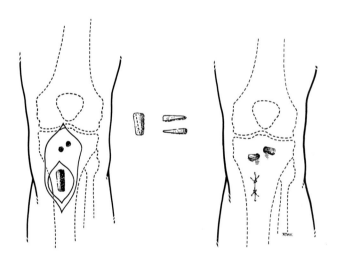

Fig. 14-24   Insertion of bone pegs into tibial tuberosity for Osgood-Schlatter disease (see text). (Redrawn from Bosworth DM: J Bone Joint Surg 16:829, 1934.)

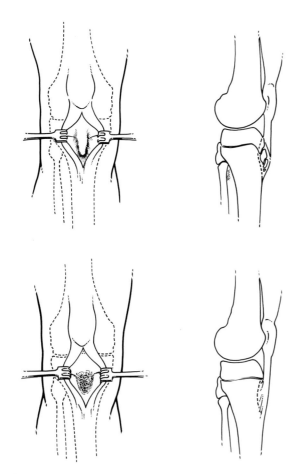

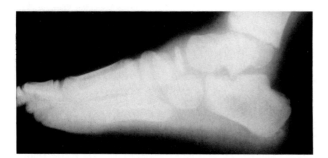

Fig. 14-25 Excision of ununited tibial tuberosity for Osgood-Schlatter disease (see text). (Redrawn from Ferciot CF: Clin Orthop 5:204, 1955.)

Fig. 14-26 Köhler's disease of tarsal navicular bone. The small sclerotic navicular characteristic of this disease has been described as an "Alka-Seltzer on end."

Excision of Ununited Tibial Tuberosity

▶ *Technique (Ferciot, Thompson, and Dickinson).* Make a longitudinal incision over the tibial tuberosity. Expose the patellar tendon, and incise it longitudinally (Fig. 14-25). Elevate the tendon laterally and medially, and excise any loose fragments of bone and enough tibial cortex, cartilage, and cancellous bone to remove completely any bony prominence. Do not disturb the peripheral and distal margins of the insertion of the patellar tendon. Close the wound.

▶ *Postoperative management.* A cylinder walking cast is applied and worn for 2 to 3 weeks. Exercises then are begun.

KÖHLER'S DISEASE

Köhler's disease is an uncommon and self-limiting disease of the tarsal navicular bone. It occurs more often in boys than in girls, and the average age of onset is 4 to 5 years. One third of patients are affected bilaterally.

Clinical and Roentgenographic Findings

Clinical signs include an antalgic limp, with the child walking on the lateral side of the foot to relieve the pain. The dorsum and the arch of the foot usually are extremely painful, and pain may be elicted by exertion of the posterior tibialis tendon. The subtalar joint range of motion is normal, which helps differentiate Köhler's disease from other inflammatory processes in the subtalar joint. Roentgenograms show a characteristic sclerotic, smaller-than-normal navicular bone, especially on the lateral view (Fig. 14-26). There are multiple centers of ossification in the navicular bone, which ossifies later than most bones in the foot, and delayed ossification is not uncommon; this should not be mistaken for Köhler's disease.

Treatment

Conservative treatment, such as decreased activity and immobilization, usually is sufficient for Köhler's disease. Karp reported 45 children with osteochondrosis of the tarsal navicular bone treated with arch supports in whom the bone regenerated to nearly normal 2 to 3 years after the onset of symptoms.

Surgery is rarely indicated, only for disabling symptoms that persist after the osteochondrosis has resolved, usually caused by a distorted, sclerotic navicular bone. The head of the talus may become flattened on its articular surface, and the two bones become fibrillated with osteophytes forming on the margin of the articular surface. Arthrodesis is the only procedure of value for this condition. Calcaneocuboid fusion should be performed in addition to the talonavicular arthrodesis because most of its function is lost when the talonavicular joint is fused. Excellent results usually can be obtained with the use of arthrodesis techniques similar to those for deformities in poliomyelitis. Most patients become free of symptoms, although they may lose some lateral motion of the foot. When symptoms arise from the naviculocuneiform joint, this joint should be included in the fusion. Arthrodesis is difficult here, and metallic internal fixation and inlay grafts of autogenous cancellous bone may be helpful. Triple arthrodesis should be reserved for the older child, aged 11 years or older, because extensive cartilage in the growing bone makes fusion difficult and because of the possibility of growth arrest with ultimate shortening of the foot.

FREIBERG'S INFRACTION

Freiberg's infraction most commonly involves the second metatarsal head, although involvement of other metatarsal joints has been reported. The acute form of the disease occurs in adolescence, more often in girls than in boys, and sequelae of a malformed metacarpal joint may be present into adulthood. The exact cause is unknown, but a lack of blood supply to the area, often associated with trauma, appears to be the main factor.

Clinical and Roentgenographic Findings

The primary symptom is pain, and roentgenograms show the flattened, deformed metacarpal joint.

Treatment

Conservative measures, such as metatarsal relief pads, may relieve the pain. Occasionally, a loose body is present (Fig. 14-27), and simple removal of the loose body will relieve the symptoms. More extensive surgery is not recommended during the acute phase, which may persist for 2 years, but surgery may be indicated later because of pain, deformity, and disability. Procedures recommended for treatment of Freiberg's infraction include resection of the metatarsal head (Giannestras), elevation of the depressed fragments of the metatarsal head and bone grafting of the defect (Smillie), resection of the base of the proximal phalanx with creation of a syndactyly of the second and third toes (Trott), dorsal closing wedge osteotomy of the metatarsal head (Gauthier and Elbaz), and joint debridement and metatarsal head remodeling (Freiberg and Mann). Because proximal resection shortens the toe significantly, it should be avoided in young patients. Resection of the head of the second metatarsal also should be avoided because hallux valgus may develop after the shifting of the first toe into the vacancy created by resection of the second metatarsal head, along with loss of plantar support across the base of the foot and metatarsalgia of the third, fourth, and fifth metacarpal bones.

Joint debridement and metatarsal head remodeling

▸ *Technique.* Make an angled incision at the apex of lateral margin of the metatarsophalangeal joint, and expose the extensor hood by sharp dissection. Make a longitudinal incision through the extensor hood a few millimeters plantar and parallel to the extensor digitorum longus muscle as it crosses the metatarsophalangeal joint. Elevate the extensor hood, and retract it medially to expose the underlying capsule. Through a transverse incision, open the capsule from one collateral ligament to the other. Note the degree of degeneration of the metatarsal head, which may be striking compared with the roentgenographic appearance. Remove all osteochondral fragments. Manually distract the toe, and flex it acutely to expose the entire metatarsal head. Remodel the metatarsal head with a rongeur, and remove any osteophytes on its plantar surface. The surface of the metatarsal head usually is depressed dorsally and centrally; round the remainder of the head to this depth, which may require removal of 3 to 4 mm of bone circumferentially. Irrigate the joint copiously to remove any loose fragments or bone or cartilage. Secure hemostasis, close the appropriate layers, and apply a sterile compression dressing.

▸ *Postoperative management.* The foot should be elevated continuously for 48 hours after surgery, followed by walking in a wooden-soled shoe. Two weeks after surgery the skin sutures are removed and the foot is redressed, with the toe held in the desired position. Toe motion is begun. Four weeks after surgery the patient may wear a wide toe–box shoe with a metatarsal bar, and toe exercises are continued three or four times a day for another 8 to 12 weeks.

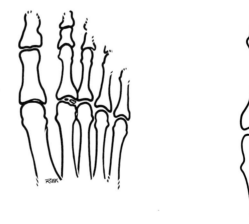

Fig. 14-27 Excision of loose body in Freiberg's infraction of bone.

OSTEOCHONDROSIS AND OSTEOCHONDRITIS DISSECANS OF THE CAPITELLUM

The term *Little League elbow* often is used to describe symptoms in the area of the capitellum that occur as a result of overuse. Adams coined the name when he noted that the symptoms occurred after strenuous pitching by youngsters in Little League baseball competition. Others have pointed out that this is a misnomer because the condition occurs more commonly in children older than Little League players.

Osteochondrosis of the capitellum usually is a diffuse reaction in the entire capitellum that occurs in a younger age-group. It is relieved by decreasing the activity that causes it, such as pitching, and will resolve over a period of 1 to 2 years. Conversely, osteochondritis dissecans usually is a discrete area in the capitellum that may be an impending loose body and crater. It occurs in the older child and does not resolve so dramatically. Further loose body formation may result in changes in the radial head.

Clinical and Roentgenographic Findings

The common symptoms of both osteochondrosis and osteochondritis dissecans of the capitellum are an inability to extend the elbow and the presence of pain over the radial head. Roentgenographic findings include "diffuse reaction" and "discrete areas."

Treatment

If there is relationship between osteochondrosis and osteochondritis dissecans of the capitellum, it is not known. Osteochondrosis appears to be a diffuse condition that may lead to the more discrete osteochondritis dissecans and possibly a loose body. Regardless of the sequence of events, Woodward and Bianco and Tullos and King recommend excising loose fragments only in osteochondritis dissecans and allowing the osteochondrosis to resolve spontaneously. Woodward and Bianco reported no better results with drilling, curettage, or trimming of the crater than with simple removal of the loose body in 38 patients with osteochondritis dissecans of the capitellum. They reported that range of motion of the elbow increased for several years after loose body removal until elbow function was essentially normal.

Micheli reported that nonsurgical treatment usually is satisfactory when no loose body is present. Arthroscopy and arthrogram may be indicated when a loose body is suspected but not seen on plain roentgenograms. Surgical and arthroscopic techniques for osteochondritis dissecans of the elbow are described in Chapter 15.

BLOUNT'S DISEASE (OSTEOCHONDROSIS DEFORMANS TIBIAE, TIBIA VARA)

Blount's disease is included in this chapter because it has long been believed to be an osteochondrosis, although it now is most commonly considered a developmental condition that affects the medial side of the proximal tibial epiphysis and causes a varus deformity of the tibia. The exact cause is unknown, but there appears to be an alteration of endochondral ossification. Suggested causative factors include infection, trauma, avascular necrosis, or a latent form of rickets, although none of these have been proved. A combination of hereditary and developmental factors is the most likely cause. Boys and girls are affected equally, and black children are affected more frequently than those of other races. The relationship of early walking and obesity to Blount's disease has been clearly documented.

Two distinct forms of the disease are manifested at different ages. Infantile Blount's disease affects children between the ages of 1 and 3 years, and the adolescent form affects children older than 8 years. The infantile form is difficult to differentiate from physiologic bowing common in this age-group, especially before the age of 2 years. Infantile Blount's disease is bilateral and symmetric in approximately 60% of children; physiologic bowing almost always is bilateral. In Blount's disease the varus deformity becomes progressively severe, whereas physiologic bowing tends to resolve with growth. The tibia alone is angulated in Blount's disease; both the femur and tibia are angulated in physiologic bowing. Adolescent Blount's disease has been attributed to occult trauma, formation of a bony bar, and even very slowly progressive infantile disease that does not become apparent until adolescence.

Roentgenographic and Pathologic Findings

The roentgenographic changes associated with Blount's disease were classified by Langenskiöld in 1952 into six stages (Fig. 14-28) and included the characteristic medial metaphyseal fragmentation, depression, and beaking that progress with age. Because of the difficulty of distinguishing roentgenographically between Blount's disease and physiologic bowing, other diagnostic and prognostic measures have been sought. Vankka and Salenius described the normal progression of the tibiofemoral angle from pronounced varus before the child is 1 year old to valgus between the ages of 18 months and 3 years. Several reports have suggested that deviation from normal tibiofemoral angle development is indicative of Blount's disease. Levine and Drennan reported that the metaphyseal-diaphyseal angle is an earlier indicator of Blount's disease. In their study Blount's disease developed in most children with metaphyseal-diaphyseal angles of 11 degrees or more, whereas children with angles of less than 11 degrees had physiologic bowing that resolved with growth. This measurement is not totally reliable or an absolute prognosticator of Blount's disease, but a metaphyseal-diaphyseal angle of more than 11 degrees warrants close observation. O'Neill and MacEwen examined roentgenographically 39 knees in bowlegged children younger than 30 months and found a poorer prognosis associated with a longer fibula than tibia and more acute proximal tibial angulation than distal femoral angulation. They emphasized the importance of comparing the degree of bowing with the normal developmental pattern and noted that a significant deviation suggests a poor prognosis for spontaneous resolution.

In adolescent Blount's disease the roentgenographic signs are more obvious. The epiphysis appears slightly wedged, sloped, and even cupped, although there generally is no severe (90-degree) sloping deformity. This form is unilateral more often than the infantile form.

Arthrography has the advantage of outlining the tibial plateau and may indicate the hypertrophied,

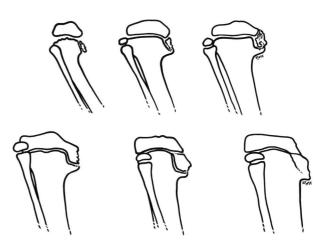

Fig. 14-28 Langenskiöld classification of roentgenographic changes in Blount's disease. Stages show progressively increasing deformity of proximal tibia. In stage 5, physis is angulated 90 degrees, and in stage 6, physis is fused. (Redrawn from Langenskiöld A: Acta Chir Scand 103:1, 1952.)

nonossified cartilage not visible on plain roentgenograms. The use CT scanning and magnetic resonance imaging in Blount's disease has been reported, but their efficacy has not been established.

Siffert and Katz, in a study of the pathologic changes in the medial aspect of the proximal tibial epiphysis, noted a posteromedial depression on the articular surface and a hypermobile meniscus. Because of the delayed ossification of the medial aspect of the epiphysis, early walking and increased weight produce abnormal stress on the medial plateau, which, according to Heuter, inhibits growth on the medial side of the bone. Cook et al analyzed the static forces that produce the varus deformity in Blount's disease and reported that as the varus deformity increases, the stress on the medial plateau increases, in turn causing an increase in varus. This interdependent cause-and-effect relationship between varus deformity and abnormal stress is responsible for the increasing severity of the deformity.

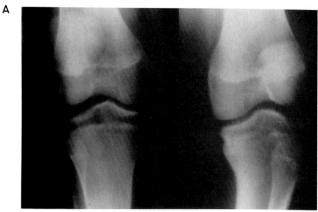

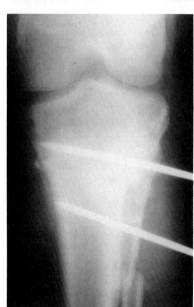

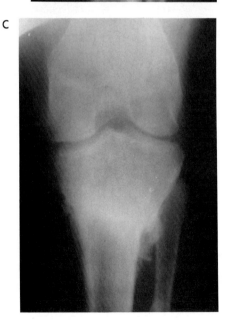

Treatment

The treatment of Blount's disease depends on the age of the child and the severity of the varus deformity. Some very young children with Langenskiöld grade I or II involvement have spontaneous resolution of the deformity without any treatment, whereas in others the deformity progresses to Langenskiöld grade V or VI even with brace treatment. Generally, for children between the ages of 2 and 5 years, observation or a trial of bracing is indicated, but progressive deformity usually requires osteotomy. Beaty et al reported that early osteotomy (children aged 2 to 4 years) gave the best results, with only 1 of 10 patients having recurrence of the deformity. Conversely, of 12 patients in whom osteotomy was performed after the age of 5 years, 10 (83%) had recurrence of the deformity that required repeat osteotomy. Valgus osteotomies of both the proximal tibia and fibula are recommended, with mild overcorrection in young children (Fig. 14-29).

In children older than 9 years of age with Langenskiöld grade V or VI involvement, osteotomy alone, with bony bar resection, or with epiphysiodesis of

Fig. 14-29   A, Older child with Blount's disease. **B,** Closing wedge high tibial osteotomy. **C,** At follow-up, with no signs of recurrence of deformity.

the lateral tibial and fibular epiphyses may be indicated. Physeal bar resection alone has been reported effective when premature closure of the epiphysis was evident, but significant angular deformity will not be corrected by resection alone. Epiphysiodesis should be performed when the child is older than 9 years but before skeletal maturity. In unilateral involvement, epiphysiodesis of the uninvolved leg may be indicated to correct leg length discrepancy.

Ingram, Siffert, and others described epiphyseal-metaphyseal osteotomy for significant sloping deformity (Fig. 14-31, *A*). The aims of this combined procedure are restoration of knee articular anatomy to nearly normal and prevention of posterior subluxation with knee flexion. Again, this is indicated only in the child older than 9 years with Langenskiöld grade V or VI involvement, a severe sloping deformity, or premature closure of the medial epiphysis (Fig. 14-30).

The techniques for high tibial and fibular osteotomies and for bony bar resection are described on pp. 44 and 51, respectively.

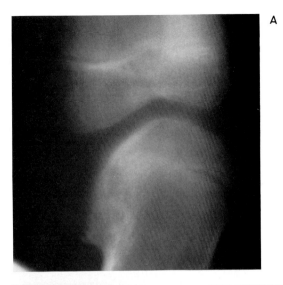

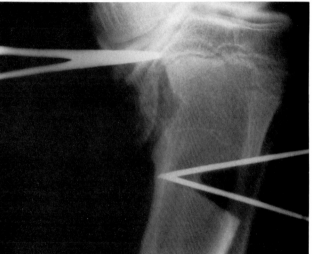

Fig. 14-30   A, Tomogram of severe Blount's disease with closure of physis. **B,** Closing wedge metaphyseal osteotomy. **C,** Epiphyseal elevation.

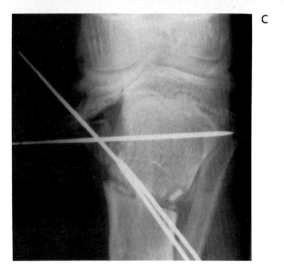

◤ *Epiphyseal-metaphyseal osteotomy technique (Ingram, Canale and Beaty).* Determine preoperatively the amount of wedge to be removed from the epiphyseal and metaphyseal areas (Fig. 14-31, *A*) and whether a graft will be taken from the fibula or tibia. Prepare and drape the patient in the usual manner, and apply and inflate a tourniquet. Expose the proximal tibia through a vertical incision approximately 10 cm long at the lateral border of the proximal tibia in the area of the epiphyseal plate. Carry the dissection down through the soft tissue to expose the physis (Fig. 14-31, *B*). Continue subperiosteal exposure distally, and place reverse retractors in the metaphyseal area of the bone into the area of the medial collateral ligament attachment on the tibia. Make a short incision in the proximal third of the lateral compartment, and carry soft tissue dissection down to the fibula, taking care to avoid the peroneal nerve. Remove a segment of the fibula approximately 1.5 cm long. If a graft is to be used beneath the tibial plateau, a longer segment of fibula may be required. Fasciotomy may be performed through this incision or through the tibial incision. With an osteotome and mallet, make

an osteotomy through the physis, resecting any bony bar (Fig. 14-31, *C*). Complete the osteotomy from the periphery to the center of the knee anteriorly to posteriorly, taking care to avoid vessels and nerves posteriorly. Place an elevator in the osteotomy site, and gently pry open and elevate the medial tibial plateau until it is as nearly parallel as possible to the lateral tibial plateau (Fig. 14-31, *D*). If there is any offset of the osteotomy in the middle of the joint, arthrotomy may be performed to inspect the joint; the abundant soft tissue and cartilage in the area of the tibial eminence usually acts as a hinge, preventing any offset. Now cut the appropriate closing lateral wedge in the metaphysis and insert two parallel Steinmann pins. Place this wedge (or bone graft from the fibula) beneath the elevated tibial plateau (Fig. 14-31, *E*). The graft helps elevate the tibial plateau and may be placed under compression (Fig. 14-31, *F*). Insert crossed Steinmann pins through the epiphysis and proximal tibial graft. Close the wound and apply a long-leg, bent-knee cast incorporating the pins in the plaster (Fig. 14-31, *G*).

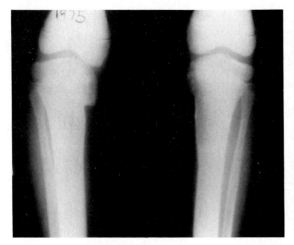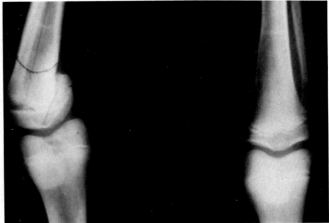

Fig. 14-31 Epiphyseal-metaphyseal osteotomy. (See text.)

A, Before osteotomy (*left*) and recurrence of deformity 4 years after osteotomy (*right*).

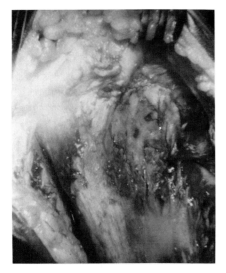

B, Exposure of physis.

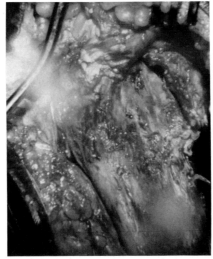

C, Osteotomy through physis.

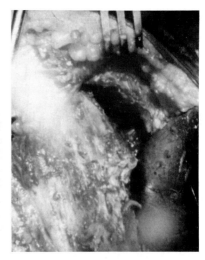

D, Elevation of tibial plateau.

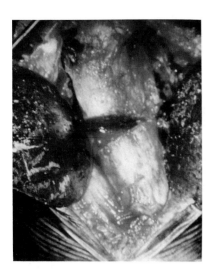

E, Lateral closing metaphyseal osteotomy.

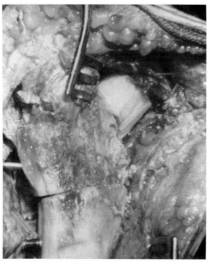

F, Graft placed beneath tibial plateau.

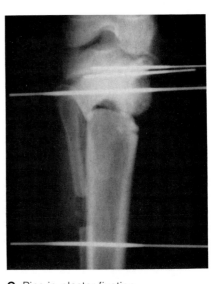

G, Pins in plaster fixation.

Continued.

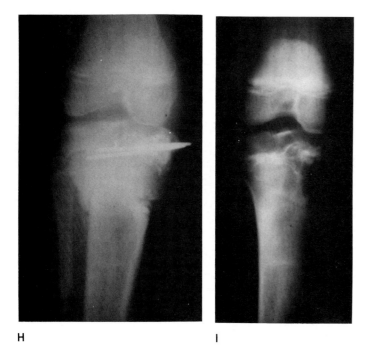

H   I

Fig. 14-31, cont'd.   H, Metaphyseal osteotomy healed; epiphyseal osteotomy still held with pins. **I,** Results at 1 year after surgery.

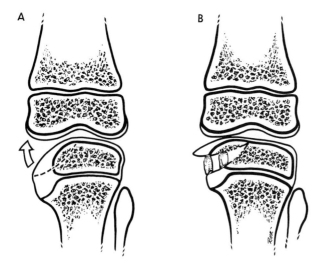

A   B

Fig. 14-32 Epiphyseal-metaphyseal osteotomy. **A,** Curved osteotomy of epiphysis. **B,** Elevation of tibial condyle. (See text.) (From Siffert RS: J Pediatr Orthop 2:81, 1982.)

▶ *Postoperative management.* The pins in the osteotomy site are removed 6 weeks after surgery; the pins in the medial plateau are removed 12 weeks after surgery. Cast immobilization is discontinued at 12 weeks and range of motion exercises are begun (Fig. 14-31, *H* and *I*).

▶ *Technique (Siffert, Støren).* With the knee in extension, begin a medial longitudinal incision at the medial femoral condyle, extending distally and anteriorly and ending 2 cm medial and distal to the tibial tuberosity. (Siffert prefers a transverse incision along the medial joint line, curved distally to the tibial tuberosity.) Take care to preserve the infrapatellar branch of the saphenous nerve at the inferior aspect of the incision. Expose the knee joint through a capsular incision anterior to the tibial collateral ligament to allow inspection of the articular surface of the tibia. Try to preserve the medial meniscus, even if it is hypertrophied. With a scalpel, make a circumferential incision through the physis down to the primary ossification center of the proximal tibial epiphysis, extending from the posteromedial corner of the tibia to the anteromedial corner, midway between the articular surface and the prominent vascular ring that penetrates the epiphysis just proximal to the physis. Then, with an 18-mm (¾-inch) curved osteotome, make an osteotomy through the medial aspect of the primary ossification center of the epiphysis. Because of the abnormal slope of the medial tibial plateau, the osteotomy parallels the articular surface medially and should reach subchondral bone in the intercondylar area adjacent to the anterior cruciate ligament (Fig. 14-32). Gently elevate the segment to bring the medial tibial plateau congruent with the medial femoral condyle and level with the lateral tibial plateau. Insert small cortical grafts from the medial proximal tibia (or from the bone bank) into the osteotomy. Because the articular depression usually is more anterior than posterior, grafts of different sizes and shapes are needed to maintain articular congruity and contact through a normal range of motion. Place the grafts only in the opened wedge of the epiphysis, not in the cartilage medially. A medial opening wedge may be required to correct varus deformity of the tibia.

Now through a lateral incision, perform osteotomy of the proximal fibula and subcutaneous fasciotomy, taking care to protect the superficial peroneal nerve. Smooth Steinmann pins may be used proximally and distally to the osteotomy and in the epiphyseal osteotomy to hold the grafts in place; these are incorporated in a long-leg plaster cast.

▶ *Postoperative management.* Cast immobilization is continued for 12 weeks. Pins are removed at 6 weeks.

REFERENCES

General

Green WT and Banks HH: Osteochondritis dissecans in children, J Bone Joint Surg 35A:26, 1953.

Roberts JM: Fractures and dislocations of the knee. In Rockwood CA Jr, Wilkins KE, and King RE, editors: Fractures in children, Philadelphia, 1984, JB Lippincott, Co.

Legg-Calvé-Perthes disease

Axer A: Subtrochanteric osteotomy in the treatment of Perthes' disease, J Bone Joint Surg 47B:489, 1965.

Bellyei A and Milke G: Acetabular development in Legg-Calvé-Perthes disease, Orthopedics 11:407, 1988.

Bowen JR, Foster BK, and Hartzell CR: Legg-Calvé-Perthes disease, Clin Orthop 185:97, 1984.

Bowen JR et al: Premature femoral neck physeal closure in Perthes' disease, Clin Orthop 171:24, 1982.

Calvé J: Sur une forme particulare de pseud-coxalgia greffée sur des deformations caracteristiques de l'extremité superieur du fémur, Rev Chir [Orthop] 30:54, 1910.

Canale ST et al: Use of innominate osteotomy in Legg-Calvé-Perthes disease, J Bone Joint Surg 54A:25, 1972.

Catterall A: The natural history of Perthes' disease, J Bone Joint Surg 53B:37, 1971.

Catterall A: Legg-Calvé-Perthes' disease, Edinburgh, 1982, Churchill Livingstone.

Catterall A: Adolescent hip pain after Perthes' disease, Clin Orthop 209:65, 1986.

Chairi K: Medial displacement osteotomy of the pelvis, Clin Orthop 98:55, 1974.

Clancy M and Steel HH: The effect of an incomplete intertrochanteric osteotomy on Legg-Calvé-Perthes disease, J Bone Joint Surg 67A:213, 1985.

Clarke NMP and Harrison MHM: Painful sequelae of coxa plana, J Bone Joint Surg 65A:13, 1983.

Coleman SS: Legg-Calvé-Perthes disease: Observations on proximal femoral osteotomy and pelvic osteotomy, Orthop Rev 8:139, 1979.

Cotler JM: Surgery in Legg-Calvé-Perthes syndrome. In The American Academy of Orthopaedic Surgeons: Instructional course lectures, vol 25, St Louis, 1976, The CV Mosby Co.

Cotler JM and Wolfgang G: Femoral head containment following innominate osteotomy for coxa plana: a radiologic evaluation, Orthop Rev 5:27, March 1976.

Craig WA, Pinder RC, and Kramer WG: A review of one hundred hips operated on for Legg-Calvé-Perthes syndrome, J Bone Joint Surg 51A:814, 1969 (abstract).

Crider RJ and Schlesinger I: Gage's sign revisited, J Pediatr Orthop 8:210, 1988.

Garceau GJ: Surgical treatment of coxa plana, J Bone Joint Surg 46B:779, 1964.

Graham S et al: The Chiari osteotomy: a review of 58 cases, Clin Orthop 208:149, 1986.

Green NE and Griffin PP: Intraosseous venous pressure in Legg-Perthes disease, J Bone Joint Surg 64A:666, 1982.

Gross RH: Arthroscopy and hip disorders in children, Orthop Rev 6:43, 1977.

Gross RH and Gruel CR: Legg-Calvé-Perthes disease: ambulatory treatment without bracing, Orthop Trans 7:143, 1983.

Gross RH and Harry JD: New method for evaluating Legg-Calvé-Perthes syndrome, Orthop Trans 9:497, 1985.

Hall DJ: Genetic aspects of Perthes' disease: a critical review, Clin Orthop 208:100, 1986.

Harrison MHM: A preliminary account of the management of the painful hip originating from Perthes' disease, Clin Orthop 209:57, 1986.

Hogersson S et al.: Arthroscopy of the hip in juvenile chronic arthritis, J Pediatr Orthop 1:273, 1981.

Ikeda T et al: Torn acetabular labrum in young patients. Arthroscopic diagnosis and management, J Bone Joint Surg 70B:13, 1988.

Ippolito E, Tudisco C, and Farsetti P: Long-term prognosis of Legg-Calvé-Perthes disease developing during adolescence, J Pediatr Orthop 5:652, 1985.

Karpinski MRK, Newton MB, and Henry APJ: The results and morbidity of varus osteotomy for Perthes' disease, Clin Orthop 209:30, 1986.

Kelly FB, Canale ST, and Jones RR: Long-term evaluation of non-containment treatment of Legg-Calvé-Perthes disease, J Bone Joint Surg 62A:400, 1980.

Kendig RJ and Evans GA: Biologic osteotomy in Perthes' disease, J Pediatr Orthop 6:278, 1986.

Legg AT: An obscure affection of the hip joint, Boston Med Surg J 162:202, 1910.

Lloyd-Roberts GC, Catterall A, and Salamon PB: A controlled study of the indications for and the results of femoral osteotomy in Perthes disease, J Bone Joint Surg 58B:31, 1976.

Lloyd-Roberts GC, Wetherhill MH, and Fraser M: Trochanteric advancement for premature arrest of the capital femoral epiphysis, J Bone Joint Surg 67B:20, 1985.

Lovell WW et al: Legg-Perthes disease in girls, J Bone Joint Surg 64B:637, 1982.

Maxted MJ and Jackson RK: Innominate osteotomy in Perthes disease. A radiological survey of results, J Bone Joint Surg 67B:399, 1985.

McAndrew MP and Weinstein SL: A long-term follow-up of Legg-Calvé-Perthes disease, J Bone Joint Surg 66A:860, 1984.

Menelaus MD: Lessons learned in the management of Legg-Calvé-Perthes disease, Clin Orthop 209:41, 1986.

Mirovsky Y, Axer A, and Hendel D: Residual shortening after osteotomy for Perthes' disease. A comparative study, J Bone Joint Surg 66B:184, 1984.

Moseley CF: The biomechanics of the pediatric hip, Orthop Clin North Am 11:3, 1980.

Perthes GC: Juvenile osteoarthritis, Dtsch Z Chir 107:111, 1910.

Purvis JM et al: Preliminary experience with the Scottish Rite Hospital abduction orthosis for Legg-Perthes disease, Clin Orthop 150:49, 1980.

Quain S and Catterall A: Hinge abduction of the hip, J Bone Joint Surg 68B:61, 1986.

Ratliff AHC: Perthes' disease—a study of sixteen patients followed up for forty years (abstract). In Proceedings and Reports of Universities, Colleges, Councils, and Associations, J Bone Joint Surg 59B:248, 1977.

Roy D and Crawford AH: Idiopathic chondrolysis of the hip: management by subtotal capsulectomy and agressive rehabilitation, J Pediatr Orthop 8:203, 1988.

Sage FP and Clark MS: Personal communication.

Salter RB: Current concepts review. The present status of surgical treatment for Legg-Perthes disease, J Bone Joint Surg 66A:961, 1984.

Salter RB and Thompson GH: Legg-Calvé-Perthes disease. The prognostic significance of the subchondral fracture and a two-group classification of the femoral head involvement, J Bone Joint Surg 66A:479, 1984.

Schatzker J, editor: The intertrochanteric osteotomy, Berlin, 1984, Springer-Verlag.

Schlesinger I and Crider RJ: Gage's sign—revisited, J Pediatr Orthop 8:201, 1988.

Scoles PV et al: Nuclear magnetic resonance imaging in Legg-Calvé-Perthes disease, J Bone Joint Surg 66A:1357, 1984.

Serlo W, Heikkinen E, and Puranen J: Progressive Russell traction in Legg-Calvé-Perthes disease, J Pediatr Orthop 7:288, 1987.

Snyder CR: Legg-Perthes disease in the young hip: does it necessarily do well? J Bone Joint Surg 57A:751, 1975.

Somerville EW: Perthes disease of the hip, J Bone Joint Surg 53B:639, 1971.

Thompson GH and Salter RB: Legg-Calvé-Perthes disease: current concepts and controversies, Orthop Clin North Am 18:617, 1987.

Thompson GH and Westin GW: Legg-Calvé-Perthes disease: results of discontinuing treatment in the early reossification phase, Clin Orthop 139:70, 1979.

Wagner H: Trochanteric advancement in the intertrochanteric osteotomy. In Schatzker J editor: The intertrochanteric osteotomy, Berlin, 1984, Springer-Verlag.

Wagner H and Holder J: Treatment of osteoarthritis of the hip by corrective osteotomy of the greater trochanter. In Schatzker J, editor: The intertrochanteric osteotomy, Berlin, 1984, Springer-Verlag.

Waldenström H: Coxa plana, osteochondritis deformans coxae, Calvé-Perthessche Krankhert, Legg disease, Zentr Chir 47:539, 1920.

Yngve DA and Roberts JM: Acetabular hypertrophy in Perthes disease, J Pediatr Orthop 5:416, 1985.

Osteochondritis dissecans of the hip

Bowen JR et al: Osteochondritis dissecans following Perthes disease. Arthroscopic-operative treatment, Clin Orthop 209:49, 1986.

Flashman FL and Ghormley RK: Osteochondritis dissecans of the head of the femur, West J Surg 57:221, 1949.

Glick JM et al.: Hip arthroscopy by the lateral approach, Arthroscopy 3:4, 1987.

Hallel T and Salvati E: Osteochondritis dissecans following Legg-Calvé-Perthes disease, J Bone Joint Surg 58A:708, 1976.

Kahmi E and MacEwen GD: Osteochondritis dissecans in Legg-Calvé-Perthes disease, J Bone Joint Surg 57A:506, 1975.

Lindholm TS and Osterman K: Internal fixation of the fragments of osteochondritis dissecans in the hip using bone transplants, J Bone Joint Surg 62B:43, 1980.

Ratliff AHC: Perthes' disease—a study of sixteen patients followed up for forty years (abstract). In Proceeding and Reports of Universities, Colleges, Councils, and Associations, J Bone Joint Surg 59B:248, 1977.

Osgood-Schlatter disease

Batten J and Menelaus MB: Fragmentation of the proximal pole of the patella: another manifestation of juvenile traction osteochondritis? J Bone Joint Surg 67B:249, 1985.

Bosworth DM: Autogenous bone pegging for epiphysitis of the tibial tubercle, J Bone Joint Surg 16:829, 1934.

Ferciot CF: Surgical management of anterior tibial epiphysis, Clin Orthop 5:204, 1955.

Ogden JA: Skeletal injury in the child, Philadelphia, 1982, Lea & Febiger.

Thompson MS and Dickinson PH: Osgood-Schlatter's disease in the army, Int Surg 23:170, 1955.

Woolfrey BF and Chandler EF: Manifestations of Osgood-Schlatter's disease in late teenage and early adulthood, J Bone Joint Surg 42A:327, 1960.

Zimbler S and Merrow S: Genu recurvatum: a possible complication after Osgood-Schlatter disease, J Bone Joint Surg 66A:1129, 1984.

Köhler's disease

Karp MG: Kohler's diease of the tarsal scaphoid: an end-result study, J Bone Joint Surg 19:84, 1937.

Freiberg's infarction of bone

Freiberg AH: The so-called infarction of the second metatarsal bone, J Bone Joint Surg 8:257, 1926.

Gauthier G and Elbaz R: Freiberg's infarction: a subchondral bone fatigue fracture: a new surgical treatment, Clin Orthop 142:93, 1979.

Giannestras NJ: Foot disorders: medical and surgical management, ed. 2, Philadelphia, 1973, Lea & Febiger.

Helal B and Gibb P: Freiberg's disease: a suggested pattern of management, Foot Ankle 8:94, 1987.

Mann RA, editor: DuVries surgery of the foot, ed. 4, St Louis, 1978, The CV Mosby Co.

Richardson EG: The foot in adolescents and adults. In Crenshaw AH, editor: Campbell's operative orthopaedics, ed 7, St Louis, 1987, The CV Mosby Co.

Smillie IS: Freiberg's infarction (Kohler's second disease), J Bone Joint Surg 39B:580, 1957.

Trott AW: Developmental disorders. In Jahss MH, editor: Disorders of the foot, Philadelphia, 1982, WB Saunders Co.

Osteochondrosis and osteochondritis dissecans of the capitellum

Adams JE: Injury to the throwing arm: a study of traumatic changes in the elbow joints of boy baseball players, Calif Med 102:127, 1965.

Adams JE: Bone injuries in very young athletes, Clin Orthop 58:129, 1968.

Micheli LJ: Overuse injuries in children's sports: the growth factor, Orthop Clin North Am 14:337, 1983.

Tullos JS and King JW: Lesions of the pitching arm in adolescents, JAMA 220:264, 1972.

Woodward AH and Bianco AJ Jr: Osteochondritis dissecans of the elbow, Clin Orthop 110:35, 1975.

Blount's disease (tibia vara)

Bateson EM: Non-rachitic bow leg and knock-knee deformities in young Jamaican children, Br J Radiol 39:92, 1966.

Bathfield CA and Beighton PH. Blount disease: a review of etiological factors in 110 patients, Clin Orthop 135:29, 1978.

Beaty JH, Coscia MF, and Holt M: Blount's disease. Paper presented at the Southern Orthopaedic Association, Edinburgh, Scotland, Sept 1988.

Beck CL et al: Physeal bridge resection in infantile Blount's disease, J Pediatr Orthop 7:161, 1987.

Beskin JL et al: Clinical basis for a mechanical etiology in adolescent Blount's disease. Orthopedics 9:365, 1986.

Blount WP: Tibia vara: osteochondrosis deformans tibiae, J Bone Joint Surg 19:1, 1937.

Blount WP: Tibia vara, osteochondrosis deformans tibiae. Curr Pract Orthop Surg 3:141, 1966.

Bradway JK, Klassen RA, and Peterson HA: Blount disease: a review of the English literature, J Pediatr Orthop 7:472, 1987.

Bright RW: Operative correction of partial epiphyseal plate closure by osseous-bridge resection and silicone-rubber implant, J Bone Joint Surg 56A:655, 1974.

Bunch WH: Decision analysis of treatment choices in the osteochondroses, Clin Orthop 158:91, 1981.

Canale ST and Harper MC: Biotrigonometric analysis and practical applications of osteotomies of tibia in children. In The American Academy of Orthopaedic Surgeons: Instructional course lectures, vol 30, St Louis, 1981, The CV Mosby Co.

Catonne Y et al: Blount's disease in the Antilles: review of 26 cases, Rev Chir Orthop 69:131, 1983.

Cook SD et al: A biomechanical analysis of the etiology of tibia vara, J Pediatr Orthop 3:449, 1983.

Dalinka MK et al: Arthrography in Blount's disease, Radiology 113:161, 1974.

Dietz WH Jr, Gross WL, and Kirkpatrick JA Jr: Blount disease (tibia vara): another skeletal disorder associated with childhood obesity, J Pediatr 101:735, 1982.

Foreman KA and Robertson WW Jr. Radiographic measurement of infantile tibia vara, J Pediatr Orthop 5:452, 1985.

Gregosiewicz A et al: Double-elevating osteotomy of tibiae in the treatment of severe cases of Blount's disease, J Pediatr Orthop 9:178, 1989.

Herring JA and Ehrlich MG: Instructional case: valgus knee deformity—etiology and treatment, J Pediatr Orthop 3:527, 1983.

Heuter C: Anatomische Studien an den Extremitätengelanken Neugeborener und Erwachsener, Virchows Arch 25:572, 1862.

Hofmann A, Jones RE, and Herring JA: Blount's disease after skeletal maturity, J Bone Joint Surg 64A:1004, 1982.

Hutter CG Jr, Scott W: Tibial torsion, J Bone Joint Surg 31A:511, 1949.

Ingram AJ: Personal communication.

Johnston CE II: Late onset tibia vara (adolescent Blount's disease), Orthopedics 7:734, 1984.

Kling TF Jr, Hensinger RN: Angular and torsional deformities of the lower limbs in children, Clin Orthop 176:136, 1983.

Knight RA: Developmental deformities of the lower extremities, J Bone Joint Surg 36A:521, 1954.

Langenskiöld A: Tibia vara (osteochondrosis deformans tibiae): a survey of 23 cases, Acta Chir Scand 103:1, 1952.

Langenskiöld A: An operation for partial closure of an epiphysial plate in children, and its experimental basis, J Bone Joint Surg 57B:325, 1975.

Langenskiöld A: Tibia vara: osteochondrosis deformans tibiae: Blount's disease, Clin Orthop 158:77, 1981.

Langenskiöld A and Riska EB: Tibia vara (osteochondrosis deformans tibiae): a survey of seventy-one cases, J Bone Joint Surg 46A:1405, 1964.

Levine AM and Drennan JC: Physiological bowing and tibia vara: the metaphyseal-diaphyseal angle in the measurement of bowleg deformities, J Bone Joint Surg 64A:1158, 1982.

Lichtblau PO and Waxman BA: Blount's disease: review of the literature and description of a new surgical procedure, Contemp Orthop 3:526, 1981.

Mitchell EI et al: A new radiographic grading system for Blount's disease evaluating the epiphyseal metaphyseal angle, Orthop Rev 9(Sept):27, 1980.

Mycoskie P: Complications of osteotomies about the knee in children, Orthopedics 4:1005, 1981.

O'Neill DA and MacEwen GD: Early roentgenographic evaluation of bowlegged children, J Pediatr Orthop 2:547, 1982.

Sasaki T et al: Transepiphyseal plate osteotomy for severe tibia vara in children: follow-up study of four cases, J Pediatr Orthop 6:61, 1986.

Schoenecker PI et al: Blount's disease: a retrospective review and recommendations for treatment, J Pediatr Orthop 5:181, 1985.

Shelton WR and Canale ST: Fractures of the tibia through the proximal tibial epiphyseal cartilage, J Bone Joint Surg 61A:167, 1979.

Siffert RS: Intraepiphyseal osteotomy for progressive tibia vara: case report and rationale of management, J Pediatr Orthop 2:81, 1982.

Siffert RS and Katz JF: The intra-articular deformity in osteochondrosis deformans tibiae, J Bone Joint Surg 52A:800, 1970.

Smith CF: Current concepts review: tibia vara (Blount's disease), J Bone Joint Surg 14A:630, 1982.

Steel HH, Sandrow RE, and Sullivan PD: Complications of tibial osteotomy in children for genu varum or valgum, J Bone Joint Surg 53A:1629, 1971.

Støren H: Operative elevation of the medial tibial joint surface in Blount's disease, Acta Orthop Scand 40:788, 1969.

Tachdjian MO: Pediatric orthopedics, Philadelphia, 1972, WB Saunders Co.

Thompson GH, Carter JR, and Smith CW: Late-onset tibia vara: a comparative analysis, J Pediatr Orthop 4:185, 1984.

Vankka E and Salenius P: Spontaneous correction of severe tibiofemoral deformity in growing children, Acta Orthop Scand 53:567, 1982.

Volkmann R: Chirurgische erfahrungen uber knocheneur brigungen und Knochenwachsthum, Arch Pathol Anat 24:512, 1862.

Wenger DR, Mickelson M, and Maynard JA: The evolution and histopathology of adolescent tibia vara, J Pediatr Orthop 4:78, 1984.

15 Sports Medicine

S. Terry Canale

The field of pediatric sports medicine is relatively new. Until the last two decades most children did not take part in organized sporting events. Recent studies, however, estimate that approximately 50% of boys and 25% of girls between the ages of 8 and 16 years now participate in some type of competitive, organized sport. The incidence of sports-related injuries in children and adolescents has increased in proportion to this increase in participation. Zaricznyj et al reported a sports injury rate of 3 per 100 children in primary school and 7 and 11 per 100 in junior high and high school, respectively. In a review of Massachusetts emergency room visits over 1 year, Gallager et al found that 1 of every 14 adolescents seen for an acute injury sustained that injury in sports. The benefits of participation—physical conditioning, accomplishment, and pleasure—relative to the risk of injury are controversial. The vast majority of sports-related injuries in children are minor and cause no lasting sequelae. Apple and McDonald reported that chronic, repetitive, cyclic loading in the lower extremity produced no harmful effect on the epiphyses and that no more injuries occurred in young runners than in adult runners. Micheli also found no deleterious effects from weight training in immature athletes. Tursz and Crost, however, reported that 12% of the children in their study who required hospitalization for a sports injury experienced angulation or shortening of a limb or limited joint motion.

Although acute trauma (such as sprain, ligament injury, epiphyseal injury, and fracture) produces the most debilitating injuries, the majority of sports injuries in children are overuse syndromes caused by repetitive frictional, tractional, or cyclic loading forces. Some recent investigators have suggested that the articular surface in the growing child is less able to withstand repetitive microtrauma than that of the adult. Frictional microtrauma may produce chondromalacia, whereas repetitive traction on a ligament or tendon may be responsible for Osgood-Schlatter disease, epiphysitis of the base of the fifth metatarsal (Iselin's disease) (Fig. 15-1), plantar fasciitis, or other avulsion injuries. Cyclic loading forces produce shin splints, stress fractures, or stress reactions. Bone scanning may reveal multiple stress fractures in the lower extremities of even very young athletes (Fig. 15-2).

Besides the risk of physical injury associated with sports participation, the psychologic impact of excessive competition and emphasis on winning is of concern. Many children suffer "burn-out" early and never return to sports activities as adolescents or adults. The "Little Leaguer's" or "John Deere hat" syndrome results from stress caused by excessive parental en-

777

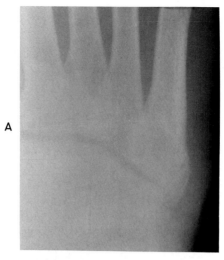

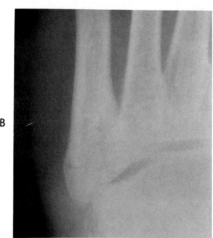

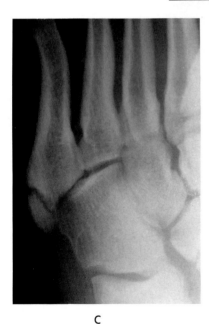

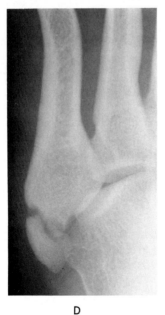

couragement of the child's participation in a sport as a form of delayed parental gratification. This parental pressure to return to competition often exacerbates or prevents healing of a minor injury and should be considered in recommending treatment. Although the child complains of pain in the elbows and shoulders, no musculoskeletal cause can be determined. The symptoms usually occur during the hottest part of the summer, when the child is physically and psychologically "burned out." The parents of these children, especially the father, usually are extremely aggressive and competitive. The father, in his John Deere baseball cap, demands to know exactly what is wrong and how soon his son will be able to pitch seven innings. In this situation it usually is best to protect the child by prescribing rest for 2 to 3 weeks, then allowing him to play a less stressful position, if he wants to play at all, until the parental pressure resolves or counseling can be arranged.

Fortunately, the vast majority of sports-related injuries in children require neither hospitalization nor surgery; the percentage of patients who require operative treatment ranges from 4.7% to 6.9% in most studies. The immature athlete cannot, however, be treated as a small adult athlete. The unique skeletal characteristics of the child—hyperelastic joints, malleable bones, physes, and apophyseal traction epiphyses—must be considered in the diagnosis and treatment of sports injuries in children, as well as the psychologic implications of participation in the sport. Children rarely exhibit symptoms of injury, such as a limp or pain, for secondary gain, as sometimes occurs with mature athletes, and any complaints should be thoroughly investigated before return to sport is allowed.

Fig. 15-1 **A** and **B,** Evidence of delayed union and epiphysitis (Iselin's disease) at bases of both left and right fifth metatarsals in a 14-year-old male after injury during basketball game. **C** and **D,** Roentgenograms made 5 years later still show evidence of nonunion; right foot is symptom free, but left foot is occasionally painful.

GENERAL MUSCULOSKELETAL INJURIES
Stress Fractures

Stress fractures result from abnormal stress or torque on a bone with normal elastic resistance. They often are caused by muscular action on a bone, rather than by direct impact. Chronic repetitive microtrauma results in cortical bone fatigue and small cortical cracks that progress as the microtrauma increases or continues. The most common sites of stress fractures in children are the tibia and the fibula, but stress fractures may occur in the metatarsals, the ribs, the pelvis, the femur, and the humerus. Any persistent, activity-related pain of the foot, leg, hip, knee, or ankle should suggest the possibility of a stress fracture. Differential diagnoses include benign or malignant bone tumors and osteomyelitis. Stress fractures often are not visible on plain roentgenograms for 6 to 8 weeks after the onset of pain. Bone scanning usually will identify the lesion much earlier. Most stress fractures can be treated by activity modification. Metaphyseal stress fractures, such as in the proximal tibia, generally heal rapidly, but stress fractures through the diaphyseal area, as in the anterior bow of the tibia, may be more difficult to treat (Fig. 15-3).

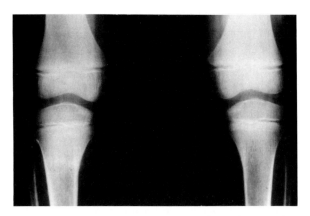

Fig. 15-2 Bone scan shows metaphyseal stress fracture of proximal tibia in 9-year-old child as result of overuse syndrome.

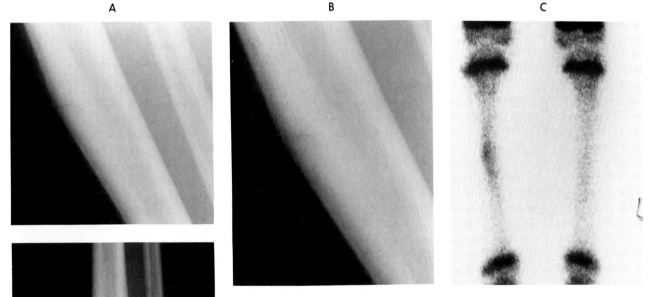

Fig. 15-3 **A,** Diaphyseal stress fracture at acute angle of tibia in 9-year-old child. **B,** Tomogram shows fracture of anterior cortex. **C,** Bone scan may be used as screening technique to aid in diagnosis of stress fracture. Note increased uptake at all physes. **D,** At follow-up there is evidence of callus and healing of fracture.

Myositis Ossificans

Traumatic myositis ossificans is the formation of heterotopic bone in injured muscle or around a joint. This occurs most commonly in adolescents but has been reported in children as young as 3 years. Myositis ossificans in children is most frequent around the elbow, after dislocation or fracture, and in the thigh in adolescent athletes, but it also occurs around the hip, knee, and ankle joints after trauma. The heterotopic bone usually is visible on roentgenogram 3 to 4 weeks after the initial injury (Fig. 15-4). Periarticular ossification gradually may be resorbed when motion of the joint is resumed, but resorption is less likely if the ossification is adjacent or attached to the diaphysis. Excision of the heterotopic bone rarely is indicated and only if it causes pain or disability, and excision should be delayed until the process has completely matured, usually 9 to 12 months after injury.

Compartment Syndromes

Compartment syndromes occur when increased tissue pressure in a closed fascial space compromises circulation to nerves and muscles within the compartment. In young athletes the increase in pressure may be caused by fracture, severe contusion, or even vigorous exercise. Pain with muscle stretching, swelling, and palpable tension over a muscle compartment should suggest compartment syndrome. Measurement of compartment pressures and treatment of compartment syndromes are discussed in Chapter 16.

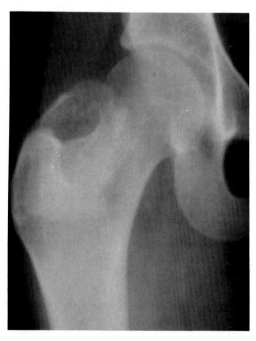

Fig. 15-4 Myositis ossificans of hip in 13-year-old with vague history of trauma.

ANKLE JOINT INJURIES
Acute Ligamentous Injuries

Ankle "sprains" are less frequent in children than in adults because of the ligamentous laxity and the pliability of cartilage in the child's foot and ankle. In adolescents, however, ankle sprains are relatively frequent. Smith and Reischl, in a study of 84 varsity basketball players, found that 70% had suffered an ankle sprain and 80% of those had multiple sprains. Almost half the athletes had residual symptoms. Ankle sprain in the child usually is a significant injury and actually may be an epiphyseal injury. Congenital or developmental conditions (such as tarsal coalition), osteochondritis dissecans, or osteochondral fracture also may be present. Because the physis is weaker than the ankle ligaments, Salter-Harris type I epiphyseal injuries are common in the ankle; if the fracture is nondisplaced, diagnosis may be difficult. Spinella and Turco described a juvenile Tillaux (Salter-Harris type III) fracture occurring in adolescent athletes when the medial part of the distal tibial epiphysis is fused while the lateral part is still open. Ossification of coalitions of the subtalar joint usually occurs in the second decade, according to Snyder, and may cause limitation of subtalar and foot motion, making the child more prone to ankle sprain. Just as in the adult, treatment depends on the magnitude of the injury; the number of ligaments, especially laterally, that are partially or completely ruptured must be determined. Inversion and eversion stress testing, as well as anterior and posterior drawer tests, usually are helpful in determining if the sprain is grade II or III. Because of the ligamentous laxity in the child, there is more tilting of the talus on stress testing than in the adult. Results should be compared with the appearance of the contralateral ankle; an increase of 8 to 10 degrees of talar tilt over the noninjured ankle indicates a significant lateral ligament injury. Anterior and posterior drawer tests will determine rupture of the anterior talofibular ligament, as well as capsular tears and the rare rupture of the calcaneofibular ligament. Momentary anterior subluxation of the talus within the ankle joint is indicative of talofibular ligament disruption. Arthrographic examination has been recommended to demonstrate capsular and ligamentous tears, especially anteriorly and posteriorly, and to determine the necessity of surgical treatment. Surgery rarely is needed for ankle sprain in the child, however, and arthrography is not routinely indicated.

Deltoid Ligament Ruptures

In the older adolescent, gross medial instability, abnormal tilt or shift of the talus in the ankle mortise, and occasionally a palpable defect indicate acute rupture of the deltoid ligament. Isolated tear of the deltoid is rare and usually is associated with a lateral malleolar fracture. The malleolar fracture should be reduced by open or closed methods; if closed reduction is accomplished, the deltoid rupture can be treated closed also. Even if open reduction of the fracture is necessary, the deltoid ligament generally does not require repair. Baird and Jackson and Harper reported satisfactory results with open reduc-

tion and internal fixation of the fibular fracture and closed reduction of the ankle joint without deltoid ligament repair (Fig. 15-5). If satisfactory closed reduction of the ankle joint cannot be obtained, soft tissue interposition is likely and open reduction and repair of the ligament are indicated. Care should be taken not to place drill holes for internal fixation through the tibial physis.

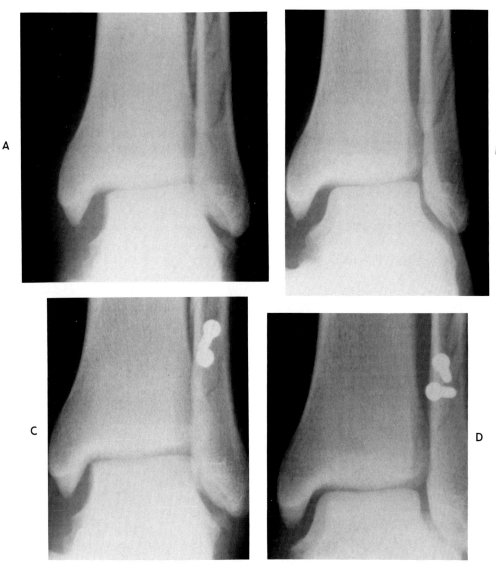

Fig. 15-5   Tear of deltoid ligament associated with fibular fracture. **A,** Anteroposterior view shows small fragment off medial malleolus and shift of talus within ankle mortise. **B,** Oblique view shows widening of joint space on medial side of ankle. **C** and **D,** Open reduction and internal fixation of fracture of lateral malleolus, with reduction of talus into ankle mortise; deltoid ligament tear was not repaired.

Repair of deltoid ligament

▶ *Technique.* Make an anteromedial incision over the ankle joint, running slightly more distally than for internal fixation of the medial malleolus. Identify the two parts of the deltoid ligament: the fan-shaped, superficial portion and the short, heavy, deep portion. The superficial portion almost always is torn across the middle or avulsed from the medial malleolus; the fanned-out inferior attachment makes inferior tear less likely. Open the sheath of the tibialis posterior tendon, and displace this tendon to allow examination and repair of the deep portion of the deltoid ligament. This deep portion may be torn from the tip of the malleolus, avulsed from the side of the talus, or torn in the middle; most often it is avulsed from the medial aspect of the talus. If so, place two nonabsorbable sutures through the ligament and pass them through holes drilled diagonally across the body and neck of the talus, exiting at the sinus tarsi. If the lateral malleolus is fractured, leave these sutures untied until the fracture has been reduced and fixed, then tie them snugly. Replace the tibialis posterior tendon in its sheath and close the sheath. Repair the superficial portion of the deltoid ligament with multiple interrupted, nonabsorbable sutures.

If the entire ligament is avulsed from the medial malleolus, drill two or three small holes in the malleolus, place sutures through them and the avulsed end of the ligament, and tie the sutures. Be sure the drill holes in the malleolus do not involve the physis. Apply a long-leg, bent-knee cast (30 to 45 degrees) with the ankle in neutral position.

▶ *Postoperative management.* The nonwalking cast is worn for 4 weeks, and a short-leg walking cast is worn an additional 4 weeks.

Acute Rupture of Lateral Ligaments

Surgical repair of acute lateral ligamentous injuries generally is advocated for mature athletes but rarely is required in the child or adolescent. The ankle must be immobilized adequately to allow healing of the ligaments in the correct position, usually for a period of 3 to 6 weeks. If surgical repair is performed, care must be taken to avoid damage to the distal fibular physis. Cedell and Anderson et al, among others, believe the anterior talofibular ligament is the most important stabilizing force in the ankle joint and that isolated ruptures of this ligament can be treated by immobilization. Immobilization also is recommended by Freeman, who noted that the cause of functional instability of the ankle after ligament injury is unknown. Some of his patients had lateral pain and swelling after healing of a ruptured anterior talofibular ligament, even though they returned to full activity. He postulated that these sequelae may have been caused by localized synovitis, scarring of the ligament, weakening of the peroneal musculature, or proprioceptive defect of the nerves of the ankle joint. Vahvanen et al, on the other hand, recommend repair of isolated talofibular ligament tears in children as young as 5 years of age.

Surgical repair may be appropriate when both the talofibular and the calcaneofibular ligaments are torn. Staples reported only 58% satisfactory results with immobilization in a group of young athletes with this injury; in a later report 88.9% of a group of similar patients had good results after surgical repair of the talofibular and calcaneofibular ligaments. Eyring and Guthrie also believe that acute complete disruption of both ligaments warrants surgery in most patients who participate in athletics, but they treat the injury conservatively in very young patients, reserving surgery for chronic, painful instability. They augment ligament repair with a peroneus brevis graft, similar to procedures described by Evans and Watson-Jones. Evans et al, however, compared their results with surgical and nonsurgical treatment in 100 randomly selected adults (not necessarily athletes) with acute isolated talofibular rupture and with associated rupture of the calcaneofibular ligament and found that operative repair resulted in a higher incidence of early complications and produced no better functional result than nonoperative treatment at 2-year follow-up. Surgical repair is not indicated in the child except for gross lateral instability or in unusual circumstances.

▶ *Technique (Staples and Bröstrom).* Begin a curved incision 5 cm proximal to the distal tip of the fibula and 1.5 cm anterior to its margin, and curve it distally and then posterior and distal to the fibula, half the distance from the tip of the fibula to the tip of the heel. Identify and resect the branches of the superficial peroneal nerve anteriorly and the sural nerve distally, preserving as many superficial veins as possible. Section the aponeurotic tissue overlying the tibiofibular and ankle joint capsule, and expose the tears in these areas by blunt dissection. Excise the peroneal sheath, and retract the peroneal tendons to expose the calcaneofibular ligament and the anterior portion of the posterior talofibular ligament. Test the stability of the lateral ligaments at the ankle and subtalar joints by forcibly inverting the foot while observing the ligaments. With nonabsorbable sutures approximate the torn ends of the ligaments, or if the ligaments are avulsed from the bone, suture the ends of the ligaments to the adjacent aponeurotic tissue or through small drill holes in the bone, taking care to avoid the physis. If the subtalar joint is unstable, suture the calcaneofibular ligament only and, if necessary, reinforce it with a flap of adjacent aponeurotic tissue. Repair the joint capsule and peroneal sheath, close the wounds, and apply a short-leg cast closed to the tibial tuberosity with the ankle in neutral position.

▶ *Postoperative management.* Sitting, with the leg dependent, is allowed for 30 to 60 seconds each half hour. When dependency can be tolerated, crutch walking is begun. Sutures are removed, and the initial cast is changed 2 weeks after surgery. After 2 more weeks, weight bearing with crutches is begun. Six weeks after surgery the cast is removed, and range-of-motion (dorsiflexion and plantar flexion) and manual stretching exercises are begun.

Acute Rupture of Interosseous (Syndesmosis) Ligaments

▶ *Technique.* With the ankle in 30 degrees of dorsiflexion, insert a screw transversely through the fibula and into the tibia approximately 1 to 1.5 cm proximal to the ankle joint through the lateral incision. Use roentgenographic or image intensification control to make sure the transverse screw does not penetrate the ankle joint or physis. Place the screw with the ankle held just above the position of dorsiflexion. If the foot is held in equinus during screw fixation, the narrowest part of the talus is engaged in the ankle mortise, and when the ankle is in dorsiflexion, the widest part of the talus is forced into the narrow space between the malleoli. Confirm the position of the screw and reduction of the talus by roentgenograms in the operating room; if the talus is not placed precisely next to the medial malleolus, it is likely that some soft tissue structure, such as a tendon or the deltoid ligament, is caught between these bones. Close the wound, and apply a cast from the base of the toes to the tibial tuberosity.

▶ *Postoperative management.* Three weeks after surgery the cast is removed, and a walking cast is applied to be worn for 4 weeks. The screw across the syndesmosis is removed no later than 8 weeks after surgery to prevent breakage of the screw between the syndesmosis of the tibiofibular joint during ankle motion.

Chronic Instability

Chronic instability of the ankle is rare in children but may occur after improper immobilization of ligamentous injuries. Reconstruction of the medial deltoid ligament rarely is necessary for chronic instability in children, but surgical intervention may be indicated for lateral instability. Pain and recurrent instability should be evaluated using inversion and eversion stress testing and special roentgenographic views similar to those used for acute injuries (p. 780). Reconstructive procedures, such as those described by Watson-Jones, Elmslie, Evans, and Chrisman and

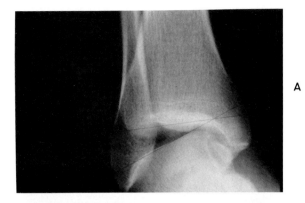

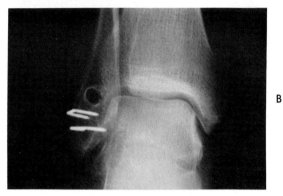

Fig. 15-6   A, Stress roentgenogram showing lateral tilt of talus caused by chronic lateral instability of ankle joint. **B,** Two years after Chrisman-Snook procedure.

Snook, should be delayed until the child has reached skeletal maturity because each requires a number of drill holes in the area of the physis of the fibula and through the growing cartilage of the talus and calcaneus (Fig. 15-6). The procedure described by Chrisman and Snook provides stability for the subtalar joint as well as the ankle and, if there is any question of subtalar stability, is preferable to the Watson-Jones procedure, which stabilizes only the anterolateral ankle joint. In young children, drill holes should avoid the fibular physis.

Eyring and Guthrie described augmentation of the collateral ligament system by passing the anterior portion of the peroneus brevis tendon forward to the fibula and securing it to the talocalcaneal interosseous ligament (Fig. 15-7). Of 107 ankles treated with this procedure, 97 (91%) obtained clinical stability. The authors recommend the procedure for patients of all ages and cite advantages of technical simplicity, preservation of potentially useful tendons, and avoidance of postoperative stiffness. Of the eight patients who required repeated surgery, however, seven were adolescent girls with chronic instability.

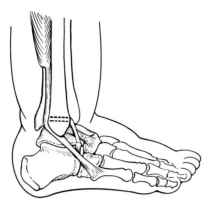

Fig. 15-7 Augmentation of collateral ligaments with peroneus brevis. (Redrawn from Eyring EJ and Guthrie WD: Clin Orthop 206:185, 1986.)

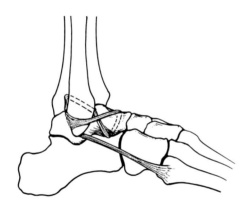

Fig. 15-8 Modified Watson-Jones technique for reconstruction of lateral ligaments of the ankle (see text).

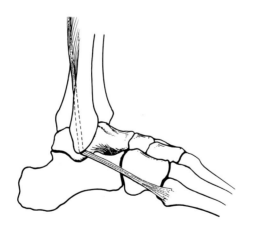

Fig. 15-9 Evans technique for reconstruction of lateral ligaments of the ankle (see text).

▲ *Technique (Watson-Jones, modified).* Make a lateral incision over the ankle beginning proximally at the junction of the middle and distal thirds of the fibular shaft; continue it distally along the anterior border of the shaft; curve it gently anteriorly; and end it 5 cm anterior to the tip of the lateral malleolus. Open the peroneal sheath as far proximally as possible, sharply separate the peroneus brevis tendon from the muscle, and dissect proximally an extension of the muscle fascia with the tendon to make the transfer long enough. Then suture the severed end of the muscle to the adjacent peroneus longus tendon. Free the peroneus brevis tendon as far distally as the lateral malleolus, but do not disturb the peroneal retinaculum. Now drill two tunnels through the bone as follows, making them large enough to receive the tendon. Drill the first tunnel in an oblique anteroposterior direction through the lateral malleolus about 2.5 cm proximal to its tip (Fig. 15-8). Drill the second in the longitudinal axis of the leg through the lateral part of the neck of the talus just anterior to the talofibular joint; here it is easier to drill a hole in the superolateral margin of the neck and another in the inferolateral margin so that they join to form the tunnel. Next guide the peroneus brevis tendon through the first tunnel from posterior to anterior and then through the second from inferior to superior; finally unroll the remainder of the tendon to make it flat and carry it posteroinferiorly across the lateral surface of the malleolus after making an oblique incision through the periosteum at this level. Suture the tendon to itself and to the periosteum on the posterior aspect of the malleolus. Then suture the periosteum to the tendon on the lateral side of the malleolus.

▲ *Postoperative management.* A cast is applied from the base of the toes to the tibial tuberosity and is worn for 8 weeks. After the second or third week the cast is altered to permit walking, and weight bearing is begun.

▲ *Technique (Evans).* Approach, divide, and mobilize the peroneus brevis tendon as described in the Watson-Jones technique. Suture the free end of the peroneus brevis muscle to the peroneus longus tendon. Then drill a tunnel through the fibula large enough to receive the tendon, beginning at the tip of the fibula and emerging posteriorly 3.2 cm proximal to the tip. Then guide the tendon through the tunnel from inferior to superior (Fig. 15-9), and suture it under tension to the adjacent soft tissue at both ends of the tunnel.

▲ *Postoperative management.* See discussion of postoperative management for the modified Watson-Jones technique.

▲ *Technique (Chrisman-Snook).* Make a long, curved incision over the course of the peroneal tendons from their musculotendinous junctions to the base of the fifth metatarsal. Divide the ligament holding the tendons in their groove behind the fibula. Identify the sural nerve and dissect it from above downward, leaving some fatty subcutaneous tissue about it. Free the nerve sufficiently to allow gentle retraction. Retract the peroneus longus tendon, which overlies the peroneus brevis tendon in the groove, and expose the peroneus brevis. Split the peroneus brevis in half longitudinally from its insertion upward to its musculotendinous junction. Leave the anterior and posterior halves of the tendon attached to the base of the fifth metatarsal. Then divide the half with the longest tendon component at the musculotendinous junction. Clean most of the muscle tissue away from the cut end proximally. Drill a hole 0.6 to 0.9 cm in diameter through the fibula in an anteroposterior direction at or just proximal to the level of the tibiotalar joint (Fig. 15-10, *A*). Thread the graft through this hole from anterior to posterior. Make the hole slightly larger than the diameter of the graft. Pass a suture through the end of the graft, and use a suture passer to thread it through the hole. After the tendon graft has been pulled through the hole, place the ankle in neutral position and the foot in mild eversion, obtained by gentle manual positioning. Pull the graft taut and, using chromic catgut or Dexon sutures, suture the graft to the periosteal ligamentous tissues adjacent to the anterior end of the drill hole (Fig. 15-10, *B*). This portion of the tendon graft replaces the anterior talofibular ligament. If a stump of the original ligament on the talus remains, suture it firmly to the contiguous tendon graft. Return the peroneus longus tendon and the remaining half of the peroneus brevis tendon to the fibular groove, allowing the graft to pass superficial to them to prevent dislocation of the tendons. Expose by dissecting distally and somewhat posteriorly the lateral border of the calcaneus. Periosteal elevation will reveal a constant vertical ridge. Drill two holes, 1.5 cm apart and of the same size as the hole in the fibula, anterior and posterior to the ridge, and then join them using curved curets. Pass the tendon through this tunnel from posterior to anterior, and place sutures at both ends of the tunnel through the graft and adjacent soft tissues. The posterior and inferior direction of the graft from the fibula to the calcaneus duplicates that of the original fibulocalcaneal ligament. If the graft is short, drill a single hole completely through the calcaneus from the lateral to the medial side; then make a stab wound on the medial side of the heel, and use the suture to pull the graft tautly into the hole. Tie the suture to a padded button on the medial side of the heel. If, however, the remaining graft is long enough, suture it at the insertion of the peroneus brevis on the fifth meta-

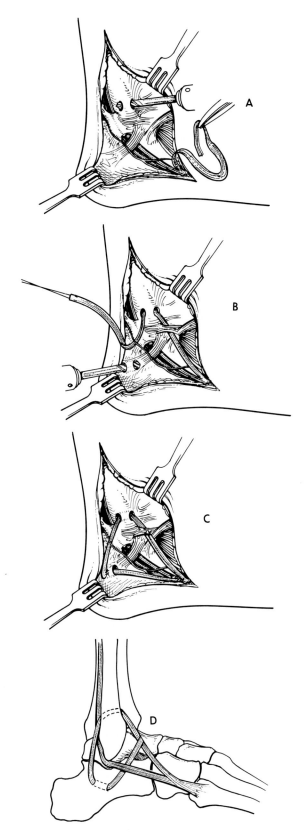

Fig. 15-10   *Chrisman-Snook technique for reconstruction of lateral ligaments of the ankle (see text). (Redrawn from Yocum LA. In Shields CL Jr editor: Manual of sports surgery, New York, 1987, Springer-Verlag.)*

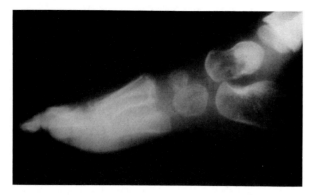

Fig. 15-11 Eosinophilic granuloma in body of talus, which produced symptoms of sprained ankle.

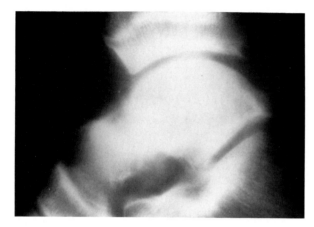

Fig. 15-12 Pigmented villonodular synovitis in anterior neck of talus; ankle joint was swollen and "boggy," and patient reported multiple ankle sprains.

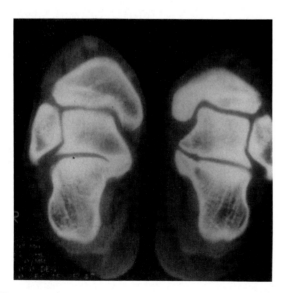

Fig. 15-13 CT scan shows medial facet tarsal coalition of calcaneus and talus in young patient with frequent ankle sprains.

tarsal (Fig. 15-10, *C*), as Chrisman and Snook originally described, or suture it onto itself at the anterior end of the fibula tunnel, as is now recommended to gain additional support (Fig. 15-10, *D*). After the graft is sutured in place, close the fascia and ligament over the fibular groove and close the skin in a routine fashion.

▶ *Postoperative management.* A walking cast is applied and worn for 8 weeks, followed by an elastic support for at least 4 months. Lateral heel wedges or suitable shoes are recommended for 6 more months.

▶ *Technique (Eyering and Guthrie).* Make a curved posterolateral incision approximately 5 inches long centered just behind the lateral malleolus. Reflect the skin and subcutaneous fat to expose the anterolateral aspect of the ankle; then open the sinus tarsi to expose the interosseous talocalcaneal ligament. Place a suture in this ligament. Next expose the peroneus brevis tendon, and isolate its anterior two thirds approximately 3 inches proximal to the lateral malleolus. Open the tendon sheath distal to the retinaculum. Place a hemostat behind the malleolus, and pull the free portion of the tendon down to the level of the fifth metatarsal to create a separate ligament. Then pass the tendon behind the lateral retinaculum, and place a retention suture in its free end. Drill a hole through the distal fibula, taking care to avoid the physis. Remove the periosteum and soft tissue from the posterior opening of the drill hole in the fibula, and then pass the detached portion of the peroneus brevis tendon from behind and forward through the drill hole. A bent Keith needle is helpful to retrieve the retention suture in the tendon and pull it through the fibula. Secure the new "ligament" to the anterior periosteum with one or two sutures. Fix the remaining portion of the reconstruction to the suture in the sinus tarsi (Fig. 15-7). While an assistant holds the foot in neutral flexion, close the peroneal tendon sheath, subcutaneous tissues, and skin. Infiltrate the entire wound and ankle with approximately 10 ml of a mixture of four parts 0.5% bupivacaine (Marcaine) and one part 4 mg/ml dexamethasone (Decadron) to reduce postoperative pain. Apply a light compression dressing and a well-molded short-leg cast with the foot in neutral position.

▶ *Postoperative management.* Ambulation with partial weight bearing is begun as soon as tolerated, usually within 2 days. Full weight bearing is encouraged during the last 10 to 14 days of cast immobilization. The cast is removed 4 weeks after surgery, and an active exercise program is begun. A stiff canvas ankle support is worn for 3 weeks, and additional brace support is used during vigorous activities for 3 to 4 months.

Osteochondritis Dissecans of the Talus

Many lesions of the ankle joint mimic ankle sprain, including neoplasms such as osteoid osteoma, eosinophilic granuloma (Fig. 15-11), and pigmented villonodular synovitis (Fig. 15-12). Snyder et al also reported a high incidence of tarsal coalition associated with ankle sprains in children and adolescents, including fibrous coalitions, cartilaginous coalitions, and bony coalitions (Fig. 15-13). Osteochondral fracture also may mimic ankle sprain. Ankle symptoms that do not resolve after 4 to 5 weeks of conservative treatment should initiate appropriate roentgenograms and further evaluation to rule out tarsal coalition or osteochondral fracture.

Impingement syndromes do occur in adolescent athletes. The anterior impingement syndrome occurs frequently in runners and jumpers, most commonly in the distal tibia, where it is always anterior and usually lateral. Restriction of activities usually is sufficient treatment in younger patients, although older children may benefit from antiinflammatory medication or cortisone injection. Only rarely is arthroscopy or arthrotomy required for excision of a bony spur or osteophyte in the talar neck or distal tibia. A similar posterior syndrome (talar compression syndrome or os trigonum syndrome) occurs quite often in ballet dancers and runners. It is always posterolateral and also can be effectively treated by activity restrictions and antiinflammatory medication.

Occult avulsions or stress fractures also occur in this area. The os trigonum is believed by many to be an old fracture rather than a separate ossicle of bone, and fractures of the adjacent posterior process of the lateral tubercle may be difficult to recognize. Another difficult fracture to ascertain on plain roentgenograms is that of the lateral process of the inferior body of the talus (Fig. 15-14). Bone scanning is helpful to identify these fractures, and a positive bone scan should be followed by computed tomography (CT) scanning or possibly tomographic examination to determine the extent of the fracture (Fig. 15-15). If possible, these occult fractures in the talus and ankle should be treated nonsurgically.

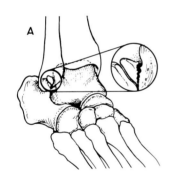

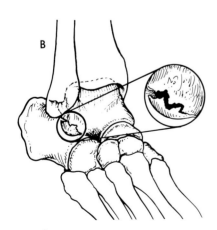

Fig. 15-14   A, Fracture of posterior process of talus. **B,** Displaced fracture of lateral process of talus. (Redrawn from Amis JA and Gangl PM: J Musculoskel Med, Sept 1987, p. 68.)

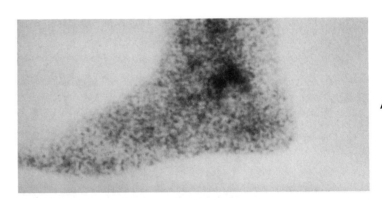

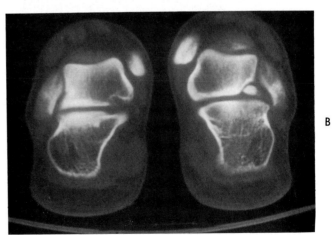

Fig. 15-15   A, As a screening method, lateral bone scanning produces "hot spot" in talus. **B,** Follow-up CT scan shows fracture of inferolateral process of talus on the right.

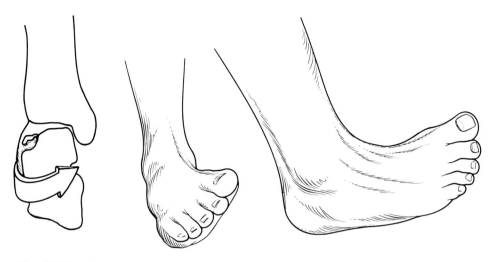

Fig. 15-16 Inversion injury resulted in lateral osteochondral fracture of talus; trauma caused osteochondritis dissecans of talus. (From Nash WC and Baker CL: South Med J 77:560, 1984.)

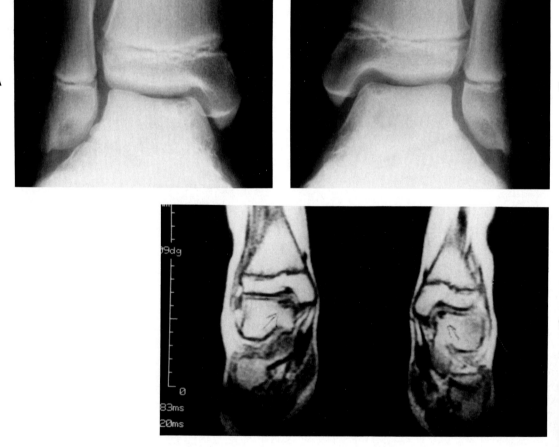

Fig. 15-17 Bilateral osteochondritis dissecans of talus in child with open physes. **A** and **B,** Roentgenograms. **C,** Magnetic resonance image.

In any ankle sprain that does not resolve, osteochondral fracture (osteochondritis dissecans) should be considered. Baker et al reported that 80% of patients with traumatic osteochondritis dissecans have a history of seemingly benign ankle sprain (Fig. 15-16). Of 31 lesions treated at the Campbell Clinic, 25 were caused by trauma, most commonly the lateral lesions. Nontraumatic lesions were more common on the medial side, especially in bilateral lesions (Fig. 15-17) and in adult female patients.

Berndt and Harty defined the mechanism of injury in osteochondral fractures and described four stages (Fig. 15-18): stage 1, a "blister" with no detachment; stage II, an elevated, but attached, fragment; stage III, a totally detached fragment in the crater; and stage IV, a displaced fragment loose in the joint. The lesions also differ in morphology depending on their location in the talus. Medial lesions are more cup-shaped, deeper, and resemble osteochondritis dissecans; lateral lesions are more wafer-shaped, shallow, and resemble an osteochondral fracture (Fig. 15-19). Medial lesions tend to stay within the crater and produce fewer symptoms than do lateral lesions, which tend to become detached.

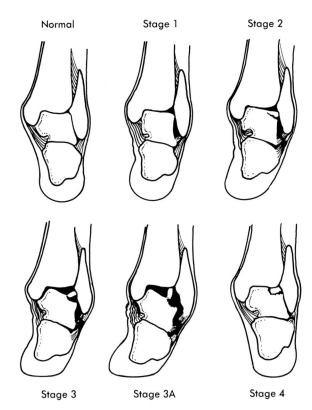

Fig. 15-18 Four stages of osteochondritis dissecans as described by Berndt and Harty. (Redrawn from Berndt AL and Harty M: J Bone Joint Surg 41A:988, 1959.)

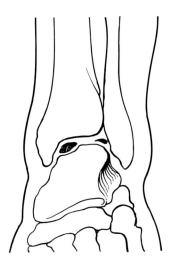

Fig. 15-19 Medial lesion of osteochondritis dissecans is cup-shaped and deep, compared with lateral lesion, which is more shallow and wafer-shaped.

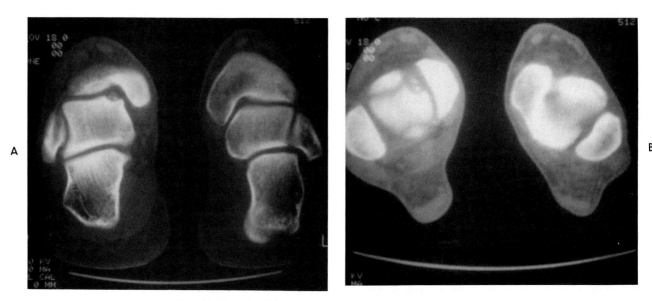

Fig. 15-20 **A,** CT scan shows medial lesion in sagittal plane. **B,** CT scan in coronal plane helps determine if lesion is anterior, medial, or posterior.

Fig. 15-21 "Floating fragment" in osteochondritis dissecans; fragment actually is inverted within crater. **A,** Roentgenographic appearance. **B,** Graphic illustration. **C,** At surgery.

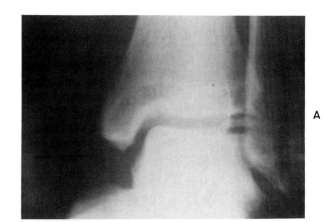

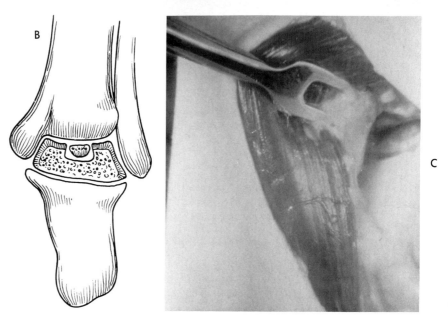

Diagnosis

If there is persistent effusion, delayed synovitis, or locking or giving way of the joint, roentgenographic examination should be performed 4 to 5 weeks after injury. Oblique and plantarflexion views that avoid tibial overlap generally show the lesion more clearly than plain films. If osteochondral fracture is suspected, bone scanning with the use of a pinhole collimator should be done. Once the lesion is localized, tomograms can determine its depth and size. If surgery is considered, preoperative planning can be aided by CT scanning; axial cuts (Fig. 15-20, *A*) determine the location of the lesion (anterior, medial, or posterior) and the necessity of osteotomy of the medial malleolus (Fig. 15-20, *B*). If the fragment appears to be floating in the crater (Fig. 15-21, *A*), it usually is inverted (Fig. 15-21, *B*) so that cartilage apposes the crater and cancellous bone apposes the ankle joint (Fig. 15-21, *C*). Tomograms and MRI are helpful to localize the floating lesion (Fig. 15-22).

Treatment

Stages I and II lesions, either medial or lateral, usually heal spontaneously and can be treated conservatively. Stage III medial lesions have fewer symptoms and result in traumatic arthritis less frequently than do stage III lateral lesions. Stage III medial lesions generally can be treated conservatively, but stage III lateral lesions often require excision in adults because they are less likely to heal, cause more symptoms, and more often result in traumatic arthritis. In children with open physes, however, a trial period of conservative treatment is warranted to avoid producing a crater in the talus (Fig. 15-23).

If necessary, the fragment can be excised either by arthrotomy or by arthroscopy. Parisien, Drez et al, Guhl, and Baker et al all have described arthroscopic techniques for treating osteochondritis dissecans of the ankle joint, but this is difficult and requires considerable expertise with arthroscopic instrumentation. A well-performed arthrotomy is preferable to a poorly done arthroscopic procedure. If excision of the entire fragment is not certain after arthroscopy, arthrotomy should be performed immediately. A small, 2-inch arthrotomy of the ankle results in less morbidity than does arthrotomy of the knee joint and often can be performed as an outpatient procedure in older children.

Arthroscopic principles for the ankle are the same as those for the knee, but a small-joint system is used that includes a 4-mm arthroscope with 30- and 70-degree angles. Shaving the synovium anteriorly and using some form of ankle distraction provide better visibility. Ankle distraction can be obtained with an external fixator by securing a skeletal traction pin

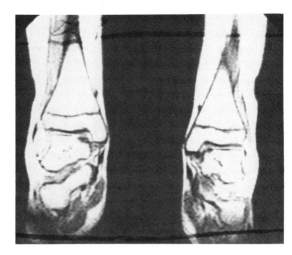

Fig. 15-22 MRI shows bilateral osteochondritis dissecans of medial talus.

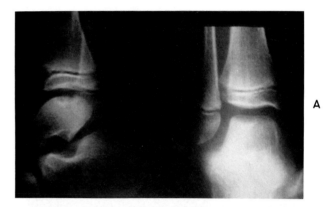
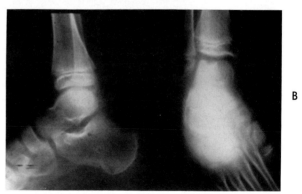

Fig. 15-23 **A,** Early evidence of osteochondritis dissecans of talus in child with open physes. **B,** After 6 months of conservative treatment, area of osteochondritis is smaller and appears to be consolidating.

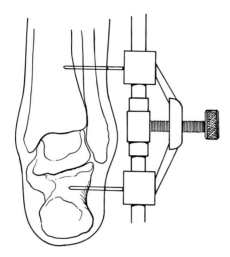

Fig. 15-24 Uniplaner distractor used for distraction of ankle joint during arthroscopy.

through the distal tibia and a parallel skeletal traction pin through the calcaneus. Applying longitudinal traction through the external fixator will open the joint sufficiently to expose all but the most posterior lesions. A "uniplaner" distractor on the appropriate side usually is sufficient for medial or lateral lesions (Fig. 15-24), and two distractors can be used for central or multiple lesions. If skeletal traction is used for ankle distraction, pins must avoid the tibial and fibular physes. In adolescent athletes, drill holes in the distal tibia, calcaneus, or talus may serve as stress risers, and return to strenuous activity should be delayed to avoid pathologic fracture. Neurologic complications also have been reported after overzealous distraction.

Arthroscopy of the ankle

▶ *Technique.* Place the patient in the lateral decubitus position on the operating table with a sandbag under the hip to internally rotate the foot slightly (Fig. 15-25, *A*). After sterile preparation, place a large, 14-gauge needle into the medial ankle joint between the

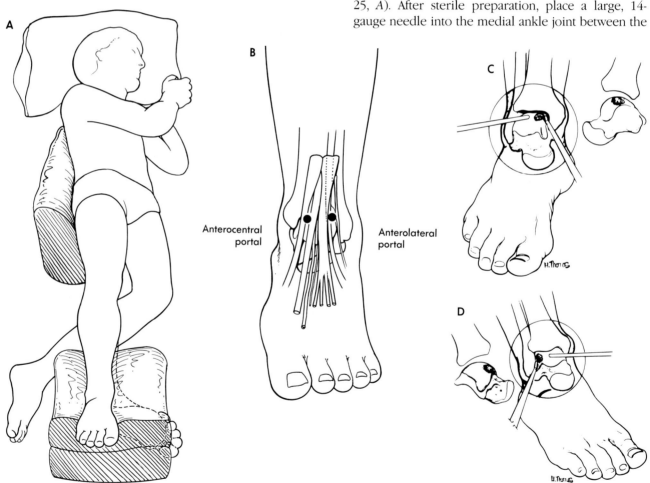

Fig. 15-25 Arthroscopy of ankle joint. **A,** Positioning of patient. **B,** Central and anterolateral portals. **C,** Lateral portal for viewing medial lesions. **D,** Medial portal for viewing and removing lateral lesions. (**A** and **B** redrawn, **C** and **D** from Parisien JS: Bull Hosp Jt Dis 45:38, 1985.)

medial malleolus and medial aspect of the talus (Fig. 15-25, *B*). Distend the ankle with fluid through this needle. Make a small puncture wound over the lateral aspect of the ankle, between the lateral malleolus and the lateral dome of the talus, and insert a 4-mm, 30-degree arthroscope. Examine the anterior synovium, the talus, the posterior aspect of the lateral border of the talus, and the lateral recess (Fig. 15-25, *C*). The anterior and medial aspects of the talus can be examined superficially through this portal. Place the foot in plantar flexion to increase visibility. Place the light source of the scope against the skin to outline the saphenous vein and nerve to avoid these structures when making the medial portal. Reverse the inflow by attaching the inflow tube to the scope, and introduce the scope through the medial portal, avoiding the saphenous area. Shave any anterior synovium that impedes vision. Locate the osteochondral defect with a probe, and attempt to completely outline the area of the defect. With graspers, remove the loose fragment or fragments (Fig. 15-25, *D*). Shave

any cartilaginous flaps around the edges of the crater. Then, using the arthroscope for guidance, introduce a small-caliber drill through the skin or through the malleoli into the crater and drill three holes about 1.5 cm in depth in three different directions to allow later ingrowth of vessels. If there is any doubt that all fragments have been removed, arthrotomy should be performed.

Arthrotomy of the ankle. Arthrotomy can be performed initially or in conjunction with arthroscopy. Lateral lesions are more easily exposed than medial lesions because the lateral malleolus is more posterior than the medial malleolus. CT scanning is helpful in locating medial lesions; in posterior lesions, medial malleolar osteotomy may be necessary, but this should be avoided if possible when the distal tibial physis is open. Osteotomy of the medial malleolus is fraught with complications such as malunion, nonunion, and necessity of later screw removal (Fig. 15-26). Extensive plantar flexion of the toes should be avoided, and the incision should be extended care-

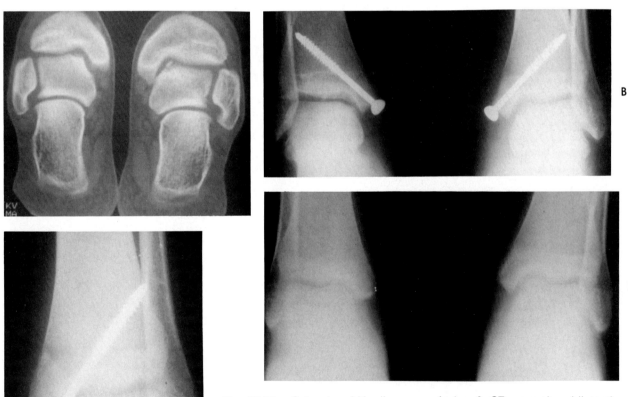

Fig. 15-26 Osteochondritis dissecans of talus. **A,** CT scans show bilateral medial lesions. **B,** After osteotomies of both medial malleoli and excision of osteochondritic fragments. **C,** Cancellous screw protruding into joint. **D,** six months after surgery, cancellous screws are removed and lesions appear to be healing.

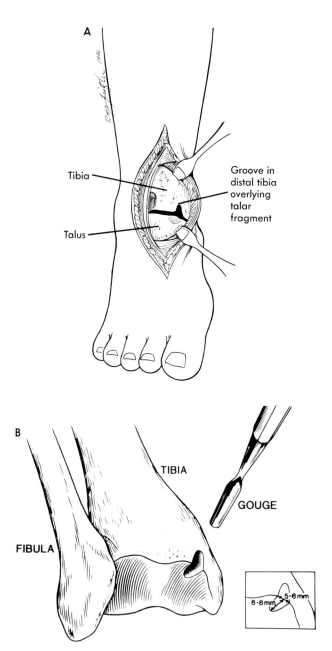

A

Tibia

Talus

Groove in
distal tibia
overlying
talar
fragment

B

FIBULA

TIBIA

GOUGE

5-6 mm
6-8 mm

fully to prevent rupture or cutting of the extensor tendons. Arthrotomy most commonly is performed through an anteromedial approach, but Thompson described a posteromedial approach to be used if the osteochondral fragment cannot be exposed through an anteromedial incision. In his technique a flap is reflected anteriorly through the anteromedial incision, avoiding the neurovascular bundle and tendinous structures behind the posterior medial malleolus, and a capsular incision is made to expose the posterior aspect of the talus. Flick and Gould described tibial "grooving" in which a small area is grooved out of the distal tibia with a gouge to expose the posteromedial lesion (Fig. 15-27). Regardless of the type of procedure, a patellar tendon weight-bearing cast is used postoperatively for several weeks, and then a patellar tendon weight-bearing brace is worn for 8 to 12 weeks to unload the ankle joint.

Fig. 15-27 Tibial grooving, as advocated by Flick and Gould, to better expose osteochondral lesion of talus. **A,** Groove on lateral aspect to expose posterolateral lesion. **B,** Groove on medial apsect to expose posteromedial lesion. (From Flick AB and Gould N: Foot Ankle 5:165, 1985.)

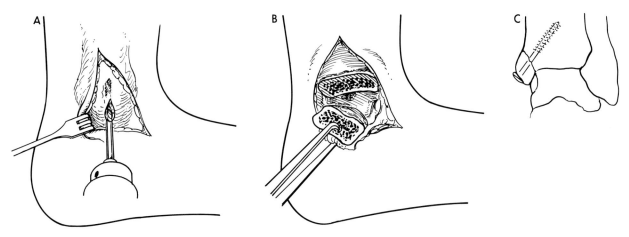

Fig. 15-28   Technique of arthrotomy for osteochondritis dissecans of talus. **A,** Predrilling of talus. **B,** Osteotomy of medial malleolus. **C,** Fixation of osteotomy with cancellous screw. (Redrawn from Yocum LA. In Shield CL Jr: Manual of sports surgery, New York, 1988, Springer-Verlag.)

▶ *Technique.* If arthrotomy is performed after arthroscopy, apply a second sterile drape, change gloves and gowns, and proceed with the arthrotomy through either the anterolateral or the anteromedial arthroscopy portal. Otherwise, make a vertical incision approximately 1.5 inches long either anterolaterally or anteromedially, taking care to avoid the extensor tendons and neurovascular bundle. Place the foot in plantar flexion to expose the lesion, and excise it with a grasper or curet. Curet the area down to bleeding bone, and drill three or four holes with a small drill bit. This can be accomplished through a transmalleolar approach under direct vision if necessary. If the lesion is difficult to locate, use a 4-mm gouge in the distal tibia directly superior to the lesion to resect the bone for better exposure. Medial malleolar osteotomy rarely is necessary and is required primarily for medial lesions. If needed, predrill the medial malleolus with a cancellous screw (Fig. 15-28, *A*); then perform an osteotomy on the medial malleolus obliquely through metaphyseal bone and retract it to expose the lesion (Fig. 15-28, *B*). After the lesion is resected and the crater drilled, secure the osteotomy site with the cancellous bone screw (Fig. 15-28, *C*). Close the wounds, and apply a sterile dresing and a short-leg, patellar tendon weight-bearing cast.

▶ *Postoperative management.* After 2 weeks of non-weight bearing in the cast, the cast and sutures are removed and a patellar tendon weight-bearing brace is fitted and is worn for 10 weeks (Fig. 15-29).

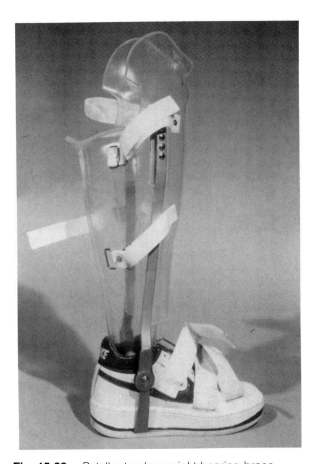

Fig. 15-29   Patellar tendon weight-bearing brace.

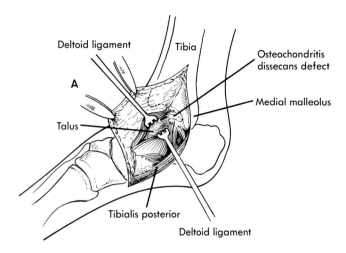

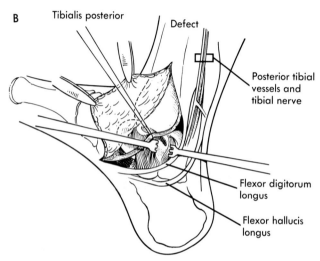

Fig. 15-30 Technique of excision of osteochondral lesions of talus. **A,** Anteromedial exposure with foot in maximum plantar flexion. **B,** Posteromedial exposure through same skin incision with foot in maximum dorsiflexion. (Redrawn from Thompson JP and Loomer RL: Am J Sports Med 12:460, 1984.)

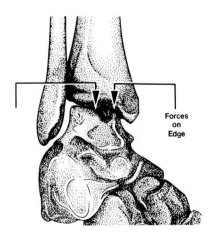

Fig. 15-31 Tibia may articulate with edge of talar crater without significantly damaging joint cartilage.

▶ *Technique (Thompson and Loomer).* Make a 10-cm curved incision, convex posteriorly, centered posterior to the medial malleolus, and expose the medial capsule. Make a 2-cm longitudinal incision in the anteromedial capsule, extending from the tibia to the talus (Fig. 15-30, *A*). Place the foot in maximum plantar flexion, and inspect the anterior half to two thirds of the superomedial rim of the talus. If the defect cannot be completely inspected, curetted, and drilled from this approach, make a curved incision directly over the tibialis posterior tendon. Retract it anteriorly and make an incision in the deep surface of the flexor retinaculum (Fig. 15-30, *B*). Do not expose or examine, but retract gently posteriorly, the remainder of the contents of the tarsal tunnel. By maximum dorsiflexion of the foot, observe the posterior one half of the superomedial border of the talus, inspect the lesion, and treat it appropriately by excision and curettage.

▶ *Postoperative management.* A soft dressing is used. Immediate range-of-motion exercises are begun, and weight bearing and return to function are allowed as soon as tolerated.

• • •

Whether open or arthroscopic techniques are used, the best results are obtained with excision and drilling of the crater. In the Campbell Clinic series 87% of patients had satisfactory results with this procedure (Fig. 15-31), and recurrences were rare. Transmalleolar retrograde drilling (proximal to distal) can be performed arthroscopically or percutaneously with the aid of image intensification (Fig. 15-

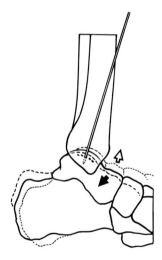

Fig. 15-32 Percutaneous transmalleolar drilling of medial osteochondral defect with use of multiple Kirschner wires. Single wire and drill hole through tibia can produce multiple holes in talus when talus is flexed. (Redrawn from Gepstein R et al: Clin Orthop 213:197, 1986.)

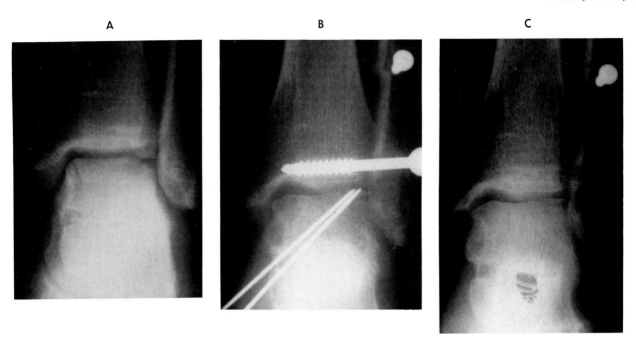

Fig. 15-33 **A,** Large lateral osteochondral lesion in talus. **B,** After fibular osteotomy and fixation of fragment with two small Kirschner wires. **C,** One year after removal of wires and syndesmosis screw, lesion appears to have healed.

32). Multiple drill holes should be avoided if the distal tibial physis is open.

Large lesions can be replaced and fixed with pinning and grafting similar to the techniques used for osteochondral lesions in the knee (p. 801), but the fragment must have viable subchondral cancellous bone (Fig. 15-33). Pinning and grafting are technically difficult, and nonunion may necessitate later removal of the pins and the fragment. Harper and other authors have described a fibrous cement that is not available commercially but has been used in Europe to "spot weld" a small portion of the fragment into the crater, leaving the periphery of cancellous bone to ossify in the crater (Fig. 15-34).

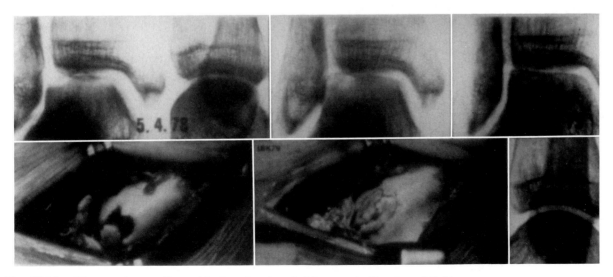

Fig. 15-34 Fibrogen "cement" used to fix osteochondral fragment. (Courtesy J Bohler, M.D.)

KNEE INJURIES

Although knee injuries in children are similar to those in adults, treatment may be radically different. In children the better choice is to attempt healing of abnormal tissue rather than to create a surgical defect that may cause later degenerative changes. This is particularly important in the treatment of meniscal injuries and osteochondritis dissecans. Although it is important to the young athlete to return to competitive activity as soon as possible, the treating physician must remember that the present sports endeavor is not as important as the lifelong ability of the patient to participate in competitive and recreational sports. All applicable methods should be used to determine the diagnosis, and treatment should be conservative whenever possible, even if surgical treatment might yield a quicker "cure." The diagnosis may be made more difficult because children are poor historians. Complaints of vague, generalized symptoms around the knee may indicate a pathologic condition in the hip joint, with pain referred to the knee. Transient synovitis or infection of the hip should be considered in children younger than age 4 years, Legg-Calvé-Perthes disease in children from 3 to 10 years of age, and slipped capital femoral epiphysis in children aged 11 to 14 years.

Sudeck's atrophy (reflex sympathetic dystrophy)

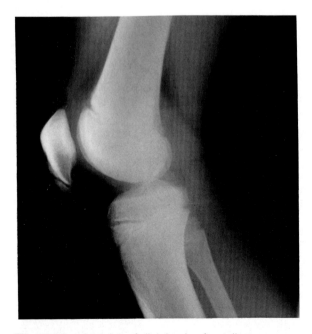

Fig. 15-35 Avulsion of distal pole of patella may cause chronic patellar tendonitis (Sinding-Larsen-Johansson disease) in immature athlete.

has been reported to occur more frequently in adults than previously appreciated, generally after significant trauma, immobilization, or knee surgery. Reflex sympathetic dystrophy also occurs in children and is compounded by the fear factor. Most children overcome this syndrome with compassion and understanding and an appropriate physical therapy program. Sympathetic blocks and other methods are seldom necessary. Psychologic burn-out also may initiate complaints of knee pain, either acute or chronic, and should be considered when no physical cause can be determined. The child should be taken out of the sport and the parents and child counseled to pursue other less stressful activities (see "John Deere hat" syndrome, p. 777).

The most common injuries of the knee in children and adolescents are overuse or quadriceps malalignment syndromes (Fig. 15-35), including chondromalacia, recurrent patellar dislocation, symptoms of bipartite patella, Baker's cyst, osteochondritis dissecans, and Osgood-Schlatter disease (p. 763). Acute injuries include sprains of the medial and lateral collateral ligaments, disruptions of the anterior cruciate ligaments (tibial spine fractures), and meniscal lesions, including discoid menisci.

Osteochondritis Dissecans of the Knee

The term *osteochondritis dissecans of the knee* is used loosely to describe any condition in which there is separation of bone or articular cartilage from the underlying femoral condyle. Attempts to clarify the definition have included Smillie's description of four patterns of osteochondritis dissecans, including an adult form that occurs after physeal closure. Green and Banks reported their results with the condition in children. Bradley and Dandy reviewed 5000 lesions of the femoral condyles and classified them as developing and late osteochondritis dissecans, acute and old osteochondral fractures, chondral separations, chondral flaps, and idiopathic osteonecrosis (Fig. 15-36). They limited the term *osteochondritis dissecans* to expanding concentric lesions on the medial femoral condyle that appeared during the second decade of life and progressed to a concave steep-sided defect. *Developing osteochondritis dissecans* was defined as an expanding concentric lesion at the margin of an otherwise normal epiphysis. Patients with loose bodies were diagnosed as having *late osteochondritis dissecans.* Bradley and Dandy found developing osteochondritis dissecans only in patients from 10 to 19 years of age and late osteochondritis dissecans only in patients older than 18 years.

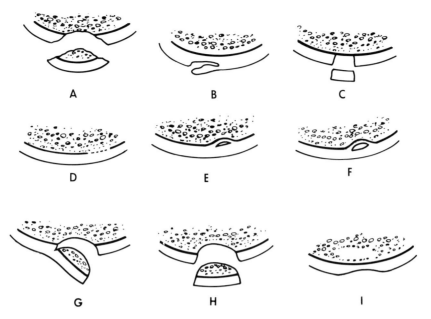

Fig. 15-36   Classification of osteochondral lesions of knee proposed by Bradley and Dandy. **A,** Osteochondral fracture; **B,** chondral flap; **C,** chondral separation; **D, E,** and **F,** developing osteochondritis dissecans; **G,** separating osteochondritis dissecans; **H,** loose body from osteochondritis dissecans; **I,** spontaneous osteonecrosis. (Redrawn from Bradley J and Dandy DJ: J Bone Joint Surg 71B:518, 1989.)

Etiology

The etiology of osteochondritis dissecans is not clearly defined. Although most agree that ischemia and avascular necrosis are major factors, there is no consensus concerning the initiating process. Suggested causes include traumatic osteochondral fracture, repetitive microtrauma that interrupts the intraosseous blood supply to the subchondral area of the epiphysis, anatomic variations in the knee, and congenitally abnormal subchondral bone. In the Campbell Clinic series of 256 patients treated for osteochondritis dissecans of the knee, 95 of which were observed for an average of 10.5 years, 45% reported a history of trauma, 37% denied any prior trauma, and 18% were uncertain. The two most common locations for osteochondritis dissecans of the knee are the medial femoral condyle (69% of Campbell Clinic series) and the lateral femoral condyle (19%) (Fig. 15-37); osteochondritis dissecans of the patella is uncommon (6%). Osteochondritis dissecans of the knee should not be confused with anomalous ossification centers, as described by Smillie, which may cause transient symptoms but which usually coalesce within 6 to 12 months. These anomalous ossification centers are frequently bilateral; thus comparison roentgenograms are helpful to differentiate these from osteochondritis dissecans.

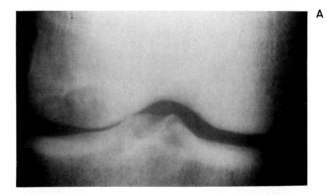

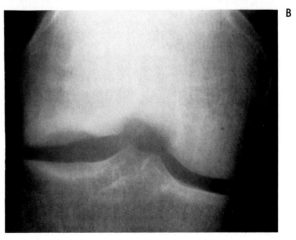

Fig. 15-37   **A,** Osteochondritis dissecans of lateral femoral condyle. **B,** Five years after excision of defect.

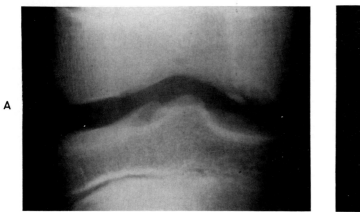
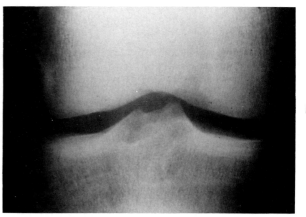

Fig. 15-38   A, Osteochondritis dissecans of medial femoral condyle in child with open physis. **B,** Four years later, physis is closed and lesion has healed.

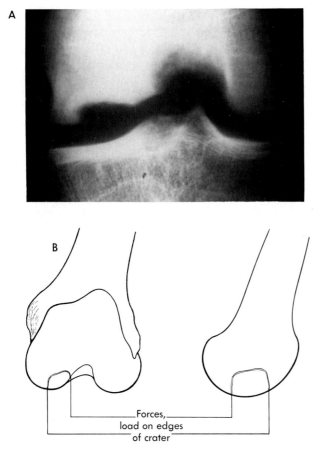

Fig. 15-39   A, Large crater in femoral condyle after removal of osteochondral lesion. **B,** Articular surface of tibia articulates with edge of crater, distributing weight-bearing forces around sides of crater rather than in defect.

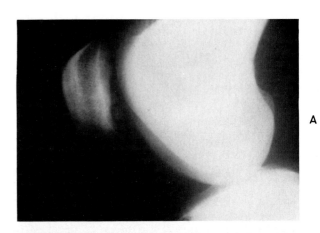
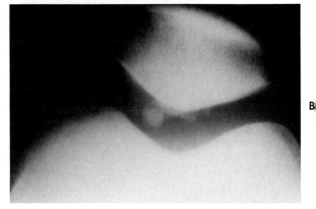

Fig. 15-40   A, Anteroposterior view. **B,** Skyline view of patella shows multiple ossific irregularities consistent with osteochondritis dissecans of patella.

Treatment

Treatment of osteochondritis dissecans is almost as controversial as its cause. In younger children with open physes, nonsurgical treatment generally is successful (Fig. 15-38). After physeal closure, best results are obtained from surgical treatment, usually excision, curettage, and drilling of the crater (Fig. 15-39). Lesions of the medial femoral condyle had more good results in the Campbell Clinic series than did

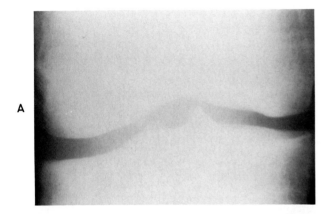

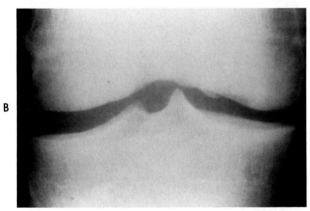

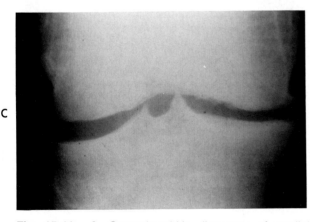

Fig. 15-41 **A,** Osteochondritis dissecans of medial femoral condyle after long period of conservative treatment. **B,** Fragment was excised 2 years later. **C,** Five years after excision, joint is narrowed and flattened with early arthritic changes.

lesions in the lateral femoral condyle or patella (Fig. 15-40). The worst results occurred in patients initially treated nonsurgically and later surgically, especially when nonoperative treatment was begun after physeal closure, which indicates that prolonged nonoperative treatment after physeal closure actually may promote degenerative joint disease (Fig. 15-41). Gepstein et al reported better results in patients with closed physes when surgery was performed early than when surgery was delayed; they obtained 83% satisfactory results with early shaving and drilling of the lesion. Outerbridge recommends drilling and bone grafting of femoral condylar lesions in all patients older than 15 years. Hughston et al recommend arthrotomy to determine if the osteochondral fragment can be pinned or excised. If the articular surface is intact, they advise drilling of the crater to promote revascularization. Guhl recommends arthroscopic drilling of the lesion if the fragment is larger than 1 cm and is located in a weight-bearing region in a child older than 12 years. The treatment of lesions larger than 2.5 cm is more difficult. Excision and drilling give good results initially, but the long-term results of removing large weight-bearing areas is not established; the development of traumatic arthritis seems likely. The lesions can be replaced and pinned with small wooden (Fig. 15-42) or metal pins, as described by Collie and Smillie (Fig. 15-43), or

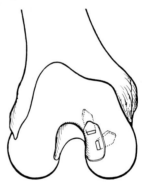

Fig. 15-42 Bone pegs used as cortical struts for internal fixation of osteochondral fragment.

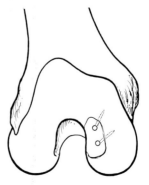

Fig. 15-43 Pinning of fragment with Smillie pins.

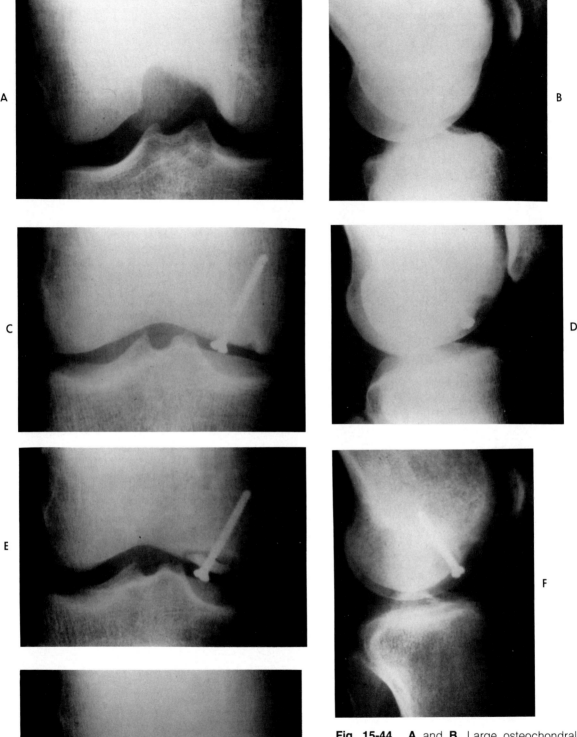

Fig. 15-44 **A** and **B,** Large osteochondral lesion in weight-bearing portion of knee joint. **C** and **D,** After internal fixation of fragment with cortical screw. **E** and **F,** One year after surgery, fragment is smaller and sclerotic and screw is loose. **G,** Two years after removal of screw and fragment and curettage and drilling of the crater.

with cortical screws (Fig. 15-44). Wombell and Nunley recently reported the use of a Herbert screw for pinning of the osteochondritic fragment in one patient. The advantage of this type of screw is its small size and ability to compress tightly. Viable subchondral bone must be present on the fragment for healing to occur. Retrograde drilling, pinning, or bone grafting should not cross the physis (Fig. 15-45). The advantage of pegging and grafting of these larger lesions is the preservation of more normal anatomy. Disadvantages include the possibility of resorption of the fragment, failure of the fragment to heal, and the possibility that a second procedure may be required for removal of the fragment and internal fixation. Removal of loose bodies without curettage and drilling of the crater produced better results in the Campbell Clinic series than did screw fixation of large fragments; however, because internal fixation was used for the most difficult cases, the results in this group of patients would be expected to be less satisfactory. Postoperative complications included peroneal nerve palsy, superficial infection, subcutaneous hematoma, synovial fistula, keloid formation, and backing out of the screw.

In general, nonsurgical treatment is indicated in children with open physes, and surgical treatment is indicated after physeal closure. Specific indications for surgical treatment of osteochondritis dissecans in children are prolonged pain without evidence of healing during a 6-month period, an unhealed lesion in which symptoms persist after physeal closure, a sclerotic lesion in the crater, and a troublesome loose body. Guhl outlined treatment recommendations based on the arthroscopic appearance of the lesion: (1) intact lesions can be treated with multiple drilling of the lesion and crater; (2) lesions with early separation and some movement of the fragment can be pinned with multiple pins (Fig. 15-46); (3) partially detached fragments with a hinge can be curetted at the base and pinned with multiple pins or screws and bone grafted; and (4) loose bodies should be removed and the crater drilled. Guhl recommends pinning a loose fragment only when there is viable metaphyseal bone at its base. Whether the lesion is drilled, excised, curetted, replaced and pinned, or bone grafted depends on the size and weight-bearing nature of the lesion, factors that can be confirmed only at surgery. Either arthroscopy or arthrotomy may be chosen, but arthroscopy may be difficult if the lesion is posterior or on the patella. A well-performed arthrotomy is preferable to a poorly done arthroscopic procedure.

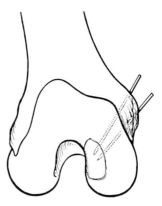

Fig. 15-45 Fragment fixed with retrograde pins; in young children pins should not cross physis.

The general technique of knee arthroscopy is described on p. 819, but some specific details concerning arthroscopic treatment of osteochondritis dissecans are important. In drilling an intact lesion the full extent of the lesion should be determined and a 0.062-cm Kirschner wire should be used to drill the area through both the medial and lateral portals if possible. The drill holes should be 1 to 1.5 cm deep to promote vascular ingrowth; the drill holes should not violate the physis (Fig. 15-47).

For lesions with early separation the edge of the lesion should be debrided and two or three 0.062-mm Kirschner wires should be inserted in a retrograde manner flush with the joint (Fig. 15-48); motion is restricted and weight bearing prohibited until the pins are removed 4 to 8 weeks after surgery. The flap of a partially detached lesion should be lifted on its hinge to allow the base of the crater to be curetted and then replaced; if there is a step-off, bone graft should be packed in the area or placed retrograde and pinned with two or three threaded pins (Fig. 15-49). The partially detached lesion also may be bone grafted in a retrograde manner, avoiding the physis in the child. A cannulated reamer is used to perforate the sclerotic base, with the use of image intensification to determine the depth of the lesion; cancellous bone then is packed into the channel (Fig. 15-50). For excision of a loose body the portal must be large enough to allow removal of the fragment with a gentle turning motion. The crater then is contoured to make both sides stable and remove any tags. Weight bearing is begun immediately after surgery.

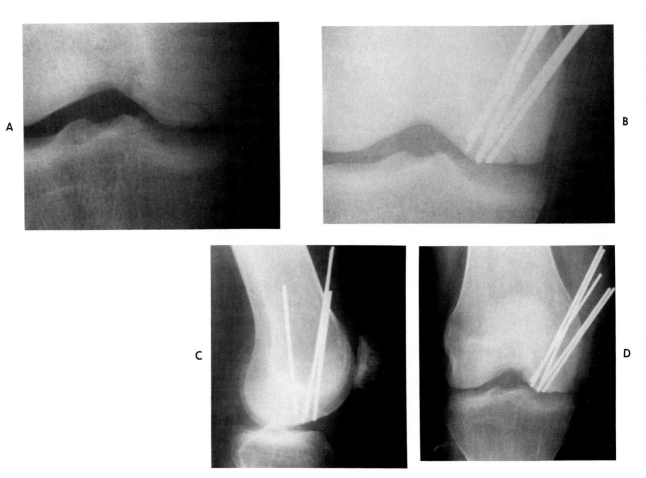

Fig. 15-46 Osteochondritis dissecans of medial femoral condyle. **A,** After 10 months of conservative treatment, there is no evidence of healing. **B** and **C,** After arthroscopic pinning of lesion. **D,** At time of pin removal the lesion has healed.

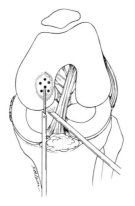

Fig. 15-47 Arthroscopic inspection and drilling of osteochondral lesion.

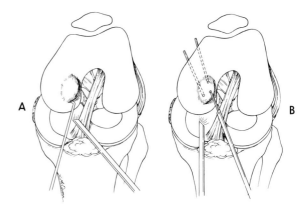

Fig. 15-48 Arthroscopic retrograde pinning of fragment. **A,** Probing lesion of medial femoral condyle showing early detachment. **B,** Insertion of multiple Kirschner wires for fixation of early separated lesion of medial femoral condyle.

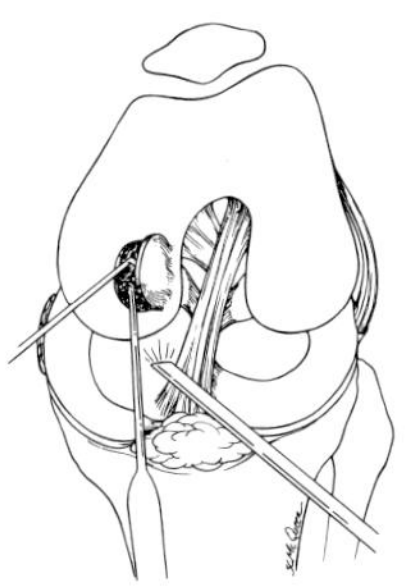

Fig. 15-49 Arthroscopic curettage and debridement of crater and pinning of fragment.

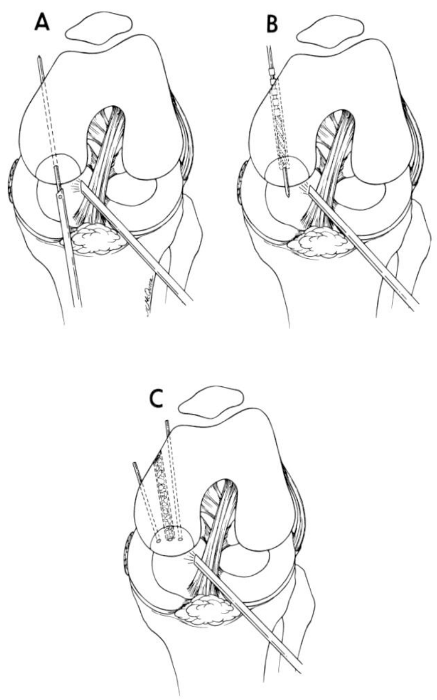

Fig. 15-50 Arthroscopic bone grafting of lesion with use of cannulated reamer. **A,** Placement of Kirschner wire through center of lesion to be internally fixed and bone grafted. **B,** Cannulated reamer over wire creates tunnel through femoral condyle to point immediately behind osteochondritis dissecans fragment. **C,** Bone grafts packed down tunnel to defect. Fixation of fragment with multiple Kirschner wires.

Arthrotomy and excision of osteochondritis dissecans fragment

▲ *Technique.* Prepare and drape the knee in the usual fashion, and exsanguinate the knee with a compression bandage or use a tourniquet for hemostasis. Make a medial joint-line arthrotomy incision about 2.5 inches vertically. Carry the dissection down to the joint capsule and incise it sharply. Beginning proximally, open the joint near the patella to avoid damage to the medial meniscus located distally. With the anterior edge of the cartilage in view, incise the capsule and synovium down to the edge of the meniscus. Insert right-angle retractors into the joint, and flex the knee to approximately 80 degrees to expose the most posterior portion of the osteochondral defect in the medial femoral condyle. With a hemostat or Kirschner wire, delineate the margins of the lesion. Often the nonviable cartilage is yellowish-brown over the defect and may be softer and more pliable than adjacent normal cartilage. If the lesion is not detached, make three or four drill holes 1 cm to 1.5 cm in depth. If it is partially detached, curet and drill the base of the crater; if the fragment is large (greater than 2.5 cm) and has viable subchondral bone, replace the fragment and reattach it with two or three 0.62-mm Kirschner wires exiting medially and avoiding the physis. Cut the wires so that they do not protrude through the skin but will allow easy removal. If the lesion is loose, excise the entire lesion down to bleeding bone and curet the crater, and with a small hand or power drill, make four or five holes of no more than 2.5 cm in depth at different angles into the crater. Irrigate the joint thoroughly, and close both the synovial and capsular layer and then the skin. Apply a sterile dressing and release the tourniquet.

▲ *Postoperative management.* After simple exision of the lesion, weight bearing and range-of-motion exercises are begun 1 week after surgery. After reattachment, drilling, and pinning or grafting of the lesion, the knee is immobilized in the flexed position in a cast or knee brace for 6 to 12 weeks, after which pins are removed if healing is evident.

Chondromalacia

Although many theories have been proposed, the exact etiology of chondromalacia still is unknown. It occurs more often in adolescent girls than in adolescent boys and produces significant pain. Symptoms are aggravated by going up and down stairs or hills, flexing the knee more than 90 degrees, and chronic, repetitive overuse. Malalignment of the quadriceps mechanism has been implicated in chondromalacia, as have genu valgum, patella alta, abnormalities of the patellar tracking mechanism in the intercondylar groove, rudimentary small patella, and bipartite patella. Chondromalacia also has been reported to occur after patellar dislocation or habitual subluxation, which causes secondary changes on the undersurface of the patella. Insall described four stages of chondromalacia: stage I, swelling and softening of the cartilage; stage II, fissuring within the softened areas; stage III, breakdown of the surface (fasciculation); and stage IV, osteoarthritis with erosive changes and exposure of the subchondral bone. Stage IV often involves the femoral intercondylar groove. Chondromalacia in most children involves the medial facet and does not cause joint effusion. As the patient ages, however, symptoms, including effusion, often are in the lateral facet, and the condition is better termed osteoarthritis of the patella than chondromalacia.

Accurate diagnosis and identification of any contributing conditions are mandatory. In addition to malalignment syndromes (including patellar subluxation and dislocation), external rotation of the leg, genu valgum, and patella alta, Hungerford and Barry described excessive lateral pressure syndromes caused by shortening of the lateral retinaculum that required lateral retinacular release. Direct trauma may cause a small osteochondral fracture, which can produce acute chondromalacia.

The major clinical signs of patellar disorders are fairly characteristic, and most diagnostic errors are caused by overlooking the patella as a possible cause of symptoms. Pain usually is anteromedial and aggravated by activities that require knee flexion. Locking, clicking, catching, and giving way of the knee joint also are common symptoms and may simulate tear of the medial meniscus. The most reliable sign of chondromalacia is retropatellar pain that can be elicited by direct compression against the femur or by displacing the patella medially and laterally and applying direct pressure beneath the medial and lateral facets. According to Insall, quadriceps atrophy, a consistent finding in meniscal tears, is unusual in patellar disorders. Roentgenograms should reveal any loose bodies, osteochondritis dissecans of the patella, osteochondral fractures, patella alta, squinting of the patella (on Hughston views), or patellofemoral incongruence.

Conservative treatment is successful in most children with chondromalacia. Modification of sports activity and counseling concerning the specific activity that causes symptoms constitute initial treatment. Nonsteroidal antiinflammatory medication may help relieve acute symptoms, and a Neoprene elastic brace with a cut-out for the patella may be beneficial physically and psychologically. A short-arc, isometric exercise program will benefit the tracking mechanism of the patella, and improvements can be measured objectively by Cybex or KinCom testing. Diagnostic arthroscopy usually is not required for chondromalacia, and shaving or chondroplasty of the undersurface of the patella is contraindicated in children. Lateral release, which may be indicated for subluxation of the patella or malalignment tracking syndrome, rarely is indicated for chondromalacia alone.

Patellar Subluxation

Subluxation of the patella is difficult to diagnose and may be confused with meniscal injury, chondromalacia, or patellar tendinitis. Because subluxation occurs after an initial dislocation has been undetected or untreated, there frequently is no history of acute dislocation before episodes of subluxation. Pain is localized to the medial aspect of the patella and the patellar retinaculum or beneath the patella as a result of chondromalacia and patellofemoral changes. The patella may be lateral riding and "squinting," and the patient may exhibit apprehension when subluxation of the patella from the intercondylar groove is attempted. Patella alta (high-riding patella), genu valgum, femoral anteversion, or external tibial torsion also may be present.

Several roentgenographic and clinical signs help identify a high-riding, maltracking patella. A useful clinical sign is the Q angle, which is formed by the line of pull of the quadriceps mechanism and that of the patellar tendon. Lines drawn from the anterosuperior iliac spine and from the center of the tibial tuberosity to the center of the patella intersect to form the Q angle, normally at the center of the patella (Fig. 15-51). Q angles of 10 degrees in boys and approximately 15 degrees (plus or minus 5 degrees) in girls are considered normal; Q angles greater than these are abnormal. Abnormal Q angles may be caused by femoral anteversion, abnormal quadriceps muscle alignment or function, external tibial torsion, lateral position of the tibial tuberosity, or genu valgum. Roentgenographic examination consists of skyline (Hughston) views of the patella made with the knee flexed 50 to 60 degrees and the roentgen beam angled 45 degrees from vertical, pointed down toward the infrapatellar region (Fig. 15-52). On lateral views, patella alta has been diagnosed if the patella is proximal to Blumensatt's line, but this method is inexact, and the ratio of the length of the patella to the length of the patellar tendon is a more exact measurement. Normally this ratio is one to one, and variation of more than 20% indicates an abnormal, high-riding position of the patella (Fig. 15-53).

Distal transposition of a high-riding patella is fraught with problems. Even in adults, distal transposition of the patella has been reported to increase pathologic pressure (torsion) on the articular surface at the intercondylar groove and patella and cause patellofemoral joint pain. Heywood warned against transferring the patella distally in children because continued growth increases tension in the patellar tendon, causing severe chondromalacia.

According to Insall, chronic patellar subluxation is best treated conservatively. He reported that children with no surgical treatment of subluxation had less pain and osteoarthritis and fewer recurrences than did those who had proximal or distal realignment procedures. In patients treated conservatively, the number of subluxations decreased dramatically as they approached the age of 30 years. Early degenerative patellofemoral joint changes developed in those with distal realignment. Those with proximal realignment had fewer patellofemoral changes, but the recurrence rate was 25%. In distal realignment procedures in the child the transfer of the patellar tendon away from the tibial apophysis prevents normal growth at the proximal tibial apophysis but allows

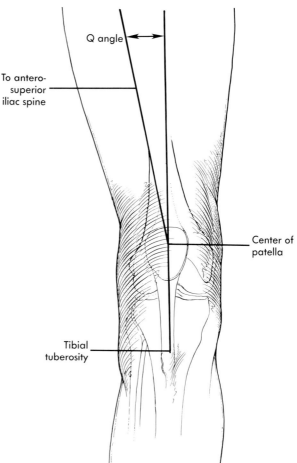

Fig. 15-51   The Q angle (see text). (Redrawn from Insall JA et al: J Bone Joint Surg 58A:1, 1976.)

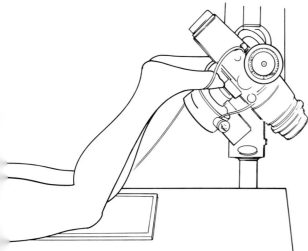

Fig. 15-52   Technique for infrapatellar view of knee. Cassette is placed beneath knees and distal thighs, feet rest on roentgen tube, legs are in neutral rotation, and knees are flexed 50 to 60 degrees. (Redrawn from Hughston JC: J Bone Joint Surg 50A:1003, 1968.)

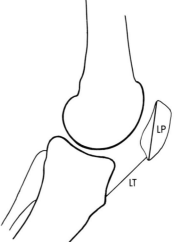

Fig. 15-53   Insall method of determining patella alta. Length of patella (LP) and length of patellar tendon (LT) have normal ratio of 1:0. Variation of more than 20% indicates abnormal position. (Redrawn from Insall J and Salvati E: Radiology 101:101, 1971. Reproduced in Clin Orthop 88:67, 1972.)

continued growth at the proximal tibial epiphysis, resulting in a distal insertion of the patellar tendon (patella baja) and causing shortening of the patellar mechanism and extreme pressure over the intercondylar groove. Premature closure of the tibial physis, anteriorly, also can result in a hyperextension deformity of the tibia and knee. Most children and adolescents with chronic patellar subluxation can be treated with a short-arc exercise program, monitored by Cybex testing, and a Neoprene brace reinforced over the lateral side of the patella. Surgery should be delayed until all conservative methods have been exhausted.

Persistent and frequent subluxation or dislocation causes traumatic chondromalacia and may be an indication for a realignment procedure. Frequently used techniques include lateral release, open or arthroscopic; proximal realignment, as described by Insall; and tenodesis of the semitendinosus tendon to the patella. Patellar shaving and debridement, distal realignment procedures, patellar replacement, and excision of the patella generally are contraindicated in children (Fig. 15-54). Supracondylar or tibial osteotomy for femoral anteversion, genu valgum, or external tibial torsion generally have not been successful in preventing subluxation of the patella; Haywood et al reported failure in five of seven patients.

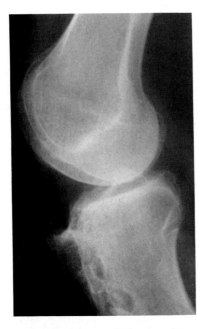

Fig. 15-54 Patellectomy and distal realignment of the tibial tuberosity were performed in this young girl for recurrent patellar dislocations and severe degenerative joint changes. At 5-year follow-up, patient had severe anterior knee pain.

Lateral release. Because lateral release, either open or arthroscopic, is considered a "minor" procedure, it probably is overused, especially in patients with mild symptoms who generally respond well to conservative treatment. Numerous complications may be associated with lateral release, including the formation of large hematomas from bleeding of the lateral geniculate vascular system. If the procedure is done arthroscopically, the geniculate vessels cannot be identified and an adequate compression dressing over the femoral condyle is mandatory to minimize bleeding. Some authors have argued that scar formation on the lateral patellar retinaculum causes fibrotic shortening that actually shifts the patella more laterally. Release of not only the lateral retinaculum and capsule but also the synovium distally to the edge of the meniscus should be performed to obtain maximum medial shift and to prevent the development of scar tissue. Results are better when lateral release is performed for patellar subluxation than for chondromalacia.

▲ *Technique.* Prepare and drape the patient in the usual manner, and apply and elevate a tourniquet. Place sandbags under the hip for internal rotation and better exposure of the lateral side of the femur. Make a vertical incision approximately 3 to 4 cm proximal to the lateral border of the patella, just lateral to the tendinous portion of the vastus lateralis muscle. Carefully retract down to the fascial retinaculum and capsule, and release this sharply for 1 inch. Then with a long pair of heavy scissors, release the retinaculum, capsule, and synovium all the way distally to and adjacent with the lateral meniscus; be sure that one blade of the scissors is in the joint. Perform an identical release proximally for several more centimeters. Insert a gloved finger into the joint, and palpate the undersurface of the patella for any softening or defect, checking for soft tissue bands that restrict medial movement of the patella. Close the soft tissue and skin, but leave the synovium and capsule open laterally. Apply a soft dressing and large spongelike bandage to the lateral aspect of the femur for compression. Release the tourniquet, and apply a knee immobilizer.

▲ *Postoperative management.* The knee immobilizer is worn for 1 week, and the knee is inspected frequently for increased hemarthrosis. Aspiration of the hematoma, which is not indicated unless pain is severe, should be avoided if possible. After 1 week range-of-motion and short-arc exercises are begun, and weight bearing is allowed when the patient can control the knee. Physical therapy is continued for 3 months.

Lateral release with proximal soft tissue realignment. Insall reported long-term follow-up of 81 knees treated surgically and 26 treated conservatively for recurrent dislocation of the patella. Satisfactory results were obtained in 65% of patients treated without surgery, in 59% treated with distal realignment, and in 75% treated with proximal realignment. Moderate or severe osteoarthritis was more common in those treated with distal realignment than in those with proximal aligment and did not occur in those treated nonsurgically. Complications of distal realignment included genu recurvatum caused by the formation of a bony bar anteriorly in 5 of 27 children younger than 14 years of age. Insall recommends conservative management in all children if possible and proximal realignment and lateral release when surgery is required.

▶ *Technique (Insall).* Make a straight line incision just medial to the patellar tendon and quadriceps mechanism, beginning proximal to the vastus medialis muscle and ending distal to the tibial tubercle (Fig. 15-55, *A*). Free the soft tissue over the patella, patellar tendon, and quadriceps mechanism. Carry soft tissue dissection superficially and laterally to expose the lateral retinaculum. Beginning proximally, release for 8 to 10 cm the vastus lateralis and lateral retinaculum capsule and synovium distally down to, but not including, the lateral meniscus (Fig. 15-55, *B*). Avoid the lateral geniculate vessels if possible. Now make a straight-line incision over the medial third of the patella, patellar tendon, and quadriceps mechanism, and "shell out" the retinaculum on the superior surface of the patella (Fig. 15-55, *C*). Continue distally to include the patellar tendon, capsule, and synovium. Inspect the joint for intraarticular disease, and palpate the undersurface of the patella for chondromalacia or soft spots. Then imbricate in a pants-over-vest manner the medial 1 to 1.5 cm of the quadriceps mechanism (vastus medialis muscle, patellar retinaculum, and patellar tendon), making the medial flap lie superior and overlap the lateral flap by 1 cm (Fig. 15-55, *D*). Move the knee through a range of motion to check for proper tracking, close the soft tissue wounds, and apply a soft, sterile dressing.

▶ *Postoperative management.* The knee is immobilized in extension for 2 weeks, during which straight-leg raises are performed. After 2 weeks a range-of-motion exercise program is begun.

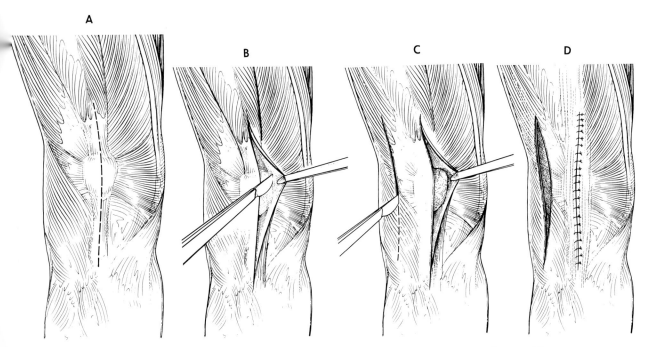

Fig. 15-55 Insall technique for lateral release and proximal soft tissue realignment (see text). (Redrawn from Insall JN: AAOS Instructional Course Lectures 30:342, 1981.)

Tenodesis of the semitendinosus tendon to the patella. Baker, Carroll, Dewer, and Hall have popularized a procedure described by Galeazzi in which tenodesis of the semitendinosus tendon to the patella is performed. They reported good results in young patients with open physes and recommend that the procedure be combined with lateral release of the patella.

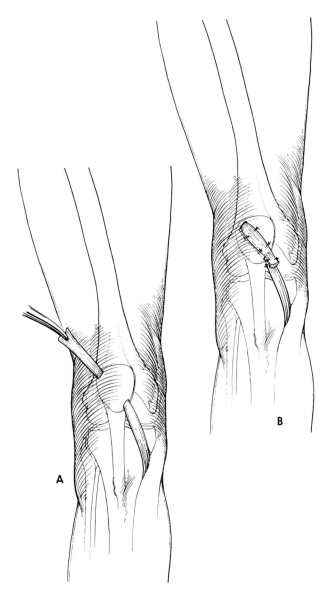

Fig. 15-56   Modified Galeazzi technique for semitendinosus tenodesis (see text). (Redrawn from Baker RH et al: J Bone Joint Surg 54B:103, 1972.)

▶ *Technique.* Use two separate skin incisions. Make the first on the posteromedial aspect of the distal thigh over the pes anserinus tendons (gracilis, semimembranosus, and semitendinosus). Deepen the incision down to these tendons, and identify the semitendinosus tendon. It is most distal and most posterior of the three and usually is large and at least 13 cm long. Divide the semitendinosus tendon at its musculotendinous junction, leaving as much tendon distally as possible. Suture its muscle belly to the semimembranosus tendon, make a medial parapatellar incision, identify the semitendinosus tendon in its distal end, and pull the cut tendon into the wound. Expose the anterior surface of the patella and the quadriceps mechanism by mobilizing the lateral skin flap with subcutaneous dissection. Open the joint through a medial parapatellar capsular incision, and inspect it for intraarticular changes, especially on the patellar, femoral, and tibial surfaces. Repair the capsular incision by plication. Mobilize the patella by complete release of the lateral capsule, fascial bands, and vastus lateralis insertion. Drill a tunnel obliquely, inferomedial to superolateral, through the patella, using successively larger drill bits. Take care to avoid disrupting the anterior and posterior articular surfaces of the patella. Pass the tendon through the tunnel, using sutures in the tendon to facilitate passage (Fig. 15-56, *A*). Using the transferred tendon, pull the patella distally and medially and with the patella held in this position, suture the tendon back onto itself (Fig. 15-56, *B*). Apply sufficient tension to the semitendinosus tendon to leave the patellar tendon slack. Do not repair the lateral capsular incision. Close the wound in layers over drains, or release the tourniquet and obtain hemostasis before closure. Apply a plaster cylinder cast, extending from groin to ankle.

▶ *Postoperative management.* If any neurovascular complications arise, the cast is bivalved and the posterior half used as a splint. Weight-bearing ambulation with crutches is permitted during the first week after surgery. The cast is changed or windowed for suture removal at 2 weeks, but casting is maintained for a total of 6 weeks. Exercises are begun in the hospital and are continued throughout rehabilitation of the knee.

Acute dislocations of the patella, even with tears of the retinaculum, should be treated with immobilization to allow healing of the medial soft tissues. Surgical repair of soft tissues usually is not indicated for acute patellar dislocations in children. If osteochondral fracture of the patella or lateral femoral condyle is suspected, arthroscopic excision of the loose body (p. 803) should be considered.

Acute Ligamentous Injuries

Because of the pliable cartilage and hyperelasticity in children, ligamentous injuries are less frequent than in adults. It generally is accepted that severe twisting injuries in children with open physes will first produce fractures of the physes, but ligament injuries do occur with these fractures or even as isolated injuries. Because the medial collateral ligament attaches proximal to the distal femoral physis, the physis separates more readily than the ligament (Fig. 15-57). The anterior cruciate ligament attaches at the intercondylar eminence or adjacent to it, and fracture through the intercondylar eminence is more common than midsubstance disruption of the anterior cruciate ligament. Bradley et al, however, reported medial collateral ligament injuries in children as young as 4 years, and midsubstance tears of the anterior cruciate ligament have been reported in children as young as 9 years, although these are more frequent in adolescents.

An accurate history is mandatory. Acute hemarthrosis suggests intraarticular injury, such as a torn anterior cruciate ligament, whereas a slowly developing hematoma suggests an extraarticular injury. Localizing the area of point tenderness may be difficult in the frightened child, but gentle palpation and noting the location of ecchymosis are helpful. If possible, clinical stress testing for medial, lateral, posterior, and anterior laxity should be performed. Because children often have more ligamentous laxity than do adults, the contralateral extremity should be tested for comparison. Stress roentgenograms should be obtained to differentiate epiphyseal separation from purely ligamentous injury.

Medial Collateral Ligament Injuries

Medial collateral ligament disruptions may be mild (grade 1), moderate (grade 2), or severe (grade 3). Grades 1 and 2 sprains of the medial collateral ligament can be treated conservatively by short periods of immobilization, followed, if necessary, by the use of a dial-locked hinged knee brace that allows flexion but blocks extension. Grade 3 injuries involve complete disruption of the ligament and are more difficult to treat. It is important to localize the area of the medial collateral ligament disruption and determine the severity of the injury. Point tenderness and swelling over the adductor tubercle are frequent in proximal avulsions, which may be difficult to differentiate from a distal femoral epiphyseal fracture. Valgus stress roentgenograms are helpful to delineate any joint line or physeal opening in cases of medial instability. In general, avulsions from the adductor tubercle, which results in one-plane instability, can be treated conservatively if there is no evidence of dis-

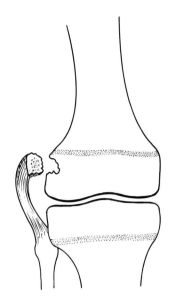

Fig. 15-57 Avulsion of attachment of fibular collateral ligament at physis, which can cause peripheral growth arrest and severe angular deformity. (Redrawn from Weber BG, Brunner G, and Freuler F: Treatment of fractures in children and adolescents, New York, 1980, Springer-Verlag.)

ruption of other structures. A long-leg, bent-knee cast, which is applied with the knee in 60 degrees of flexion and the leg in 15 to 20 degrees of internal rotation, is worn for 4 to 6 weeks.

Grade 3 midsubstance or distal tears are more complex. Occasionally, the ligament becomes incarcerated in the joint and requires surgical release. Midsubstance, and especially distal, tears have a tendency to retract and seldom heal without some residual instability. In the child, however, one-plane instability should be treated conservatively. Conversely, multiplane instability that indicates disruption of the anterior cruciate ligament and posterior capsule may require surgical treatment, especially in adolescents with high athletic expectations. A common combination of injuries includes fracture of the intercondylar eminence and tears of the anterior cruciate ligament, medial collateral ligament, and posteromedial capsule, resulting in multiplane anteromedial instability. In adolescents, repair of the medial structures, as well as the anterior structures, should be considered. In younger children complete repair or reconstruction generally should be avoided if possible because of the possibility of damage to the physis. The medial collateral ligament tear, especially if avulsed from the adductor tubercle, can be treated conservatively, and, after arthroscopic examination for meniscal injury, reconstruction of the anterior cruciate ligament tear can be delayed until the child is older; reconstruction then can be performed if instability persists. Clanton et al reported surgical treatment of nine children younger than 14 years of age (average age, 10.4 years) with knee ligament injuries. Five also had fractures of the tibial eminence. These authors emphasized that, despite thorough physical and roentgenographic evaluation, the extent of the injury was determined only at surgery in seven of the nine patients. In spite of surgical repair, all nine patients had some degree of ligamentous instability after surgery; the instability was greatest in patients in whom meniscectomy had been performed at the time of ligament repair.

Bradley et al recommend examination with the child under anesthesia and surgical repair of confirmed medial collateral ligament tears; they list gross instability to valgus stress as the indication for surgery. Clanton et al recommend repair if the joint line opening is 8 mm or more on stress roentgenograms compared with the opposite extremity. Recent reports of successful nonsurgical treatment of medial collateral ligament injuries in adults give promise that such results also can be obtained in young patients. Magnetic resonance imaging currently is being evaluated to determine if imaging can pinpoint the ligament tear and allow limited repair through a small medial incision.

If the medial collateral ligament is repaired, sutures at the adductor tubercle should be placed in the soft tissues, avoiding the physis, because premature closure of the periphery of the physis will cause marked angular deformity. Staples should be placed distal to the physis rather than proximal. Proximal stapling may place the physis under tension and cause a tethering effect that may slow or prohibit growth. A staple in the area of insertion of the collateral ligament into the tibia (distal to the physis) returns the ligament to its anatomically correct location and is less likely to cause tethering of the tibial physis. Midsubstance tears can be repaired with sutures in the deep and superficial portions of the medial collateral ligaments.

▶ *Technique.* Make a long, median, parapatellar incision, curving the proximal and distal ends posteriorly. Completely dissect a large posterior flap. Dissect the soft tissue anteriorly to expose the vastus medialis muscle and the medial border of the patella and the patellar tendon, and dissect posteriorly to expose the posteromedial corner of the knee. Identify and protect the large sartorial branch of the saphenous nerve as it exits from the sartorius and gracilis muscles. If the injury is acute, a hematoma may identify the area of disruption. Inspect the entire medial side of the knee by excising the medial retinaculum along the anterior edge of the sartorius from its tibial insertion

posteriorly to the posteromedial corner. Make longitudinal and transverse incisions so that a triangle of retinaculum can be elevated to expose the superficial portion of the medial collateral ligament. Acutely flex the knee, place retractors beneath the pes anserinus, and examine the insertion of the medial collateral ligament onto the tibia. Now deepen the anterior longitudinal incision, and carry it into the joint. Inspect both menisci and the anterior cruciate ligament. Examine the medial collateral ligament at its origin at the adductor tubercle, including the semitendinosus complex and the posterior oblique ligament.

Stress testing the knee in flexion will help in identifying the ligament injury. Midsubstance tears of the superficial portion of the medial collateral ligament usually are readily identified; tears of the deep portion may be more difficult to ascertain. Placing a retractor deep to the medial collateral ligament may expose an area of bone avulsed from the femoral condyle, as well as avulsion of the capsular ligament and synovium.

If the disruption cannot be identified in the superficial portion of the ligament, make a vertical incision through the superficial portion to expose a tear in the deep (meniscotibial and meniscofemoral) portions of the ligament. If a meniscotibial tear is peripheral enough, suture the ligament to the medial meniscus, leaving the meniscus undisturbed. If necessary, expose the posterior capsule by locating the interval between the medial head of the gastrocnemius and semimembranosus muscles, incise the sheath of the semimembranosus, and dissect the posterior capsule off the medial head of the gastrocnemius. With the patient's knee flexed, expose the posterior capsule to the midline. Posteromedial capsular tears may extend well around the posteromedial corner to involve the posterior capsule at its tibial insertion.

After examination of the cruciate ligaments, the tibial insertion of the superficial and deep layers of the medial collateral ligament, the posterior capsule, and the proximal origin of the medial collateral ligament, repair or reconstruct the cruciate ligament by passing sutures through drill holes in the epiphysis (but not across the physis), but do not tie the sutures. Repair the posterior capsular structures with heavy, nonabsorbable sutures, augmented if necessary by passing heavy sutures posterior to anterior through drill holes and tying them over bone. Now repair the deep portion of the medial collateral ligament and its meniscotibial attachment at the periphery, maintaining the knee in 60 degrees of flexion and the limb in internal rotation. If the cruciate ligament has been repaired through drill holes in the epiphysis, tie the sutures. To avoid difficulty in closing the anteromedial arthrotomy incision, close this before completing the collateral ligament repairs. Repair midsubstance tears of the superficial collateral ligament with heavy, non-absorbable sutures. Reattach with a staple tears at the insertion of the medial collateral ligament onto the tibia, and proximally reattach with sutures the origin of the medial collateral ligament, avoiding the physis. Replace the triangular position of the medial patellar retinaculum, and close it with absorbable sutures. Close the soft tissues over drains, close the skin with skin staples, and apply a long-leg, bent-knee cast with the knee in 60 degrees of flexion and the leg in internal rotation or apply a commercial dial-lock knee brace.

▲ *Postoperative management.* The knee is kept flexed and internally rotated for 6 weeks. If necessary, depending on the age and compliance of the child, a dial-lock brace may be fitted with the knee in this position but allowing 30 degrees more flexion. Active progressive resistance exercises are begun immediately after surgery, and physical therapy is continued for 6 months, with progress documented by Cybex testing if possible.

Lateral Collateral Ligament Injuries

Tears of the lateral collateral ligaments are rare in children. Because the child's ligaments often are more lax than the adult's, both knees should be examined to evaluate lateral ligamentous instability. Stress testing will confirm that the injury is ligamentous rather than physeal separation (Fig. 15-58). The integrity of the lateral collateral ligament can be assessed by flexing the knee into a figure-4 position and palpating the entire length of the ligament. Occasionally, a lateral capsular sign may be seen on roentgenogram, which suggests that the capsule, along with a small piece of bone, has been torn off the lateral side of the knee, usually from the tibial insertion. Rupture of the lateral collateral ligament seems to be associated more frequently with an avulsed fragment of bone from the fibula than from the femur; midsubstance tears also are less common.

Anterolateral instability, which suggests lateral instability and a deficient anterior cruciate ligament, is more common in adolescents than in children. Arthroscopy generally is indicated for significant injuries to determine if the anterior cruciate ligament has been disrupted. In adolescents with serious athletic ambitions, exploration of the lateral side of the knee and repair or reconstruction of the cruciate ligament and lateral structures should be considered.

▲ *Technique.* Place a sandbag under the ipsilateral hip to tilt the patient medially and to facilitate lateral exposure. Made a long parapatellar incision over Gerdy's tubercle proximal to the patella, curving the ends posteriorly. Dissect the subcutaneous tissue and superficial fascia down to deep fascia. Hematoma formation may identify areas of significant injury. Identify, expose, and protect the common peroneal nerve, noting any damage to the nerve; usually primary repair is not performed, but microsurgical repair may be indicated later. Stress the knee to further delineate the area of ligament injury. Then incise deep through the vertical limb of the parapatellar incision into the joint, and carefully and systematically inspect both

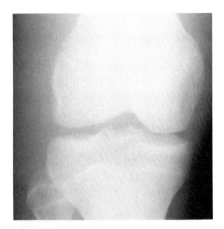

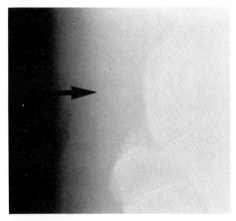

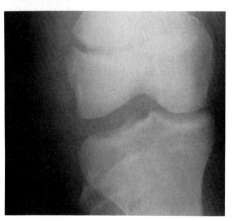

Fig. 15-58   Stress view of knee.

menisci and cruciate ligaments. If necessary, repair or reconstruct the anterior cruciate ligament with sutures passed through drill holes in the epiphysis, but do not tie the sutures. For midsubstance or complex anterior cruciate ligament tears, make a midline parapatellar incision to facilitate repair or reconstruction. Make any necessary repairs of the posterior cruciate ligament in the same manner. Now locate the separation between the posterior portion of the iliotibial band and the anterior portion of the biceps muscle. Retract the iliotibial band anteriorly and the biceps muscles with the common peroneal nerve posteriorly. Incise the iliotibial band if it cannot be retracted. Make a vertical incision in the capsule between the fibular collateral ligament and the popliteal tendon to examine the posterior capsule and popliteal tendon for tears; do not confuse the capsular hiatus of the popliteus tendon with disruption of the posterior capsule. Examine the posterior horn of the meniscus and the posterior cruciate ligament that inserts onto the tibia.

If necessary, repair the posterolateral capsule with sutures passed posterior to anterior through drill holes in the tibia. Roughen the back of the tibia with an osteotome before securing the sutures. Examine the fibulocollateral ligament, popliteus and biceps tendons, arcuate ligament, and lateral capsular and collateral ligaments. Close the anterolateral capsular incision at this point because closure may be impossible after repair. Repair any proximal tears of the popliteus tendon; more distal tears in its muscle or musculotendinous junction may be difficult to repair.

If the popliteus tendon is torn from the femur along with the fibulocollateral ligament, reattach these structures to the femur, distal to the physis, with sutures passed through drill holes in the femur and tied over bone on the medial side, taking care to avoid the physis. Repair the fibulocollateral ligament by reattaching it to the fibula or femur with Bunnell-type nonabsorbable sutures or, if avulsed with a bony fragment, with a screw or staple, avoiding the physes of the fibula and proximal tibia. Repair tears of the midlateral capsular ligament (lying just anterior to the fibulocollateral ligament) with nonabsorbable sutures, passed through drill holes in the tibial plateau if necessary for stability. Repair the arcuate ligament complex next; tension may be increased by advancing its lateral edge anteriorly around the posterolateral corner and suturing it to the posterior edge of the lateral capsule and posterior edge of the fibulocollateral ligament. If the iliotibial band was incised, repair it. Close the soft tissue over drains, and test the knee for anterior and anterolateral stability. Close the skin incisions, and apply a long-leg, bent-knee cast with the the knee in external rotation and 60 degrees of flexion.

▶ *Postoperative management.* Two weeks after surgery, compliant patients may be fitted with a dial-lock brace that allows flexion, but blocks extension beyond 50 degrees. A vigorous physical therapy program is begun 6 to 8 weeks after surgery and continued for at least 6 months, with progress documented by Cybex testing if possible.

Anterior Cruciate Ligament Injuries

The anterior cruciate ligament is the main intraarticular stabilizer of the knee and, combined with the posterior cruciate ligament, prevents anterior and posterior instability and contributes to rotary stability. Anterior cruciate ligament injuries in preadolescent children are most commonly avulsion fractures of the tibial insertion of the ligament and usually are associated with medial collateral ligament injuries. The avulsion of the tibial eminence or spine should be treated as described in Chapter 16. Midsubstance ruptures of the anterior cruciate ligament are most common in adolescents involved in contact sports. Lipscomb and Anderson reported reconstruction of 24 anterior cruciate ligament injuries in patients between the ages of 12 and 15 years. Most authors agree that repeated trauma to an anterior cruciate–deficient knee in this age-group eventually will cause further meniscal damage and later degenerative changes in the knee and may result in chronic instability and recurrent injury. If participation in athletics is to be continued, reconstruction is necessary. Reconstruction of the anterior cruciate ligament in children and adolescents has not been widely recommended because of the possibility of physeal injury from drilling across open tibial and femoral epiphyses. Lipscomb and Anderson, however, reported significant growth disturbance in only one of their 24 patients whose anterior cruciate ligament was reconstructed with the use of the semitendinosus and gracilis tendons along with an extraarticular reconstruction (Losee or Ellison procedure). The drill holes were placed in the center of the knee so that any growth disturbance would produce uniform shortening rather than angular deformity.

McCarroll et al compared their results in 16 adolescents with open physes and anterior cruciate ligament injuries treated conservatively with rehabilitation, bracing, and counseling on activity modification with a similar group of 24 patients who had arthroscopic examination and extraarticular or intraarticular reconstructions. Younger patients had extraarticular procedures, and older patients with physes near closure had intraarticular procedures, including drill holes across the physes. Of the 16 patients treated nonsurgically, 6 later had arthroscopic surgery for meniscal tears and only 7 returned to sports; all experienced recurrent episodes of giving way, effusion, and pain. Of the 24 patients treated surgically, torn menisci were found in 18 at arthroscopy and 22 had satisfactory results. For young patients with anterior cruciate ligament tears McCarroll et al recommend arthroscopic examination of the anesthetized patient. Reconstruction should be considered on the basis of the amount of instability, the presence of meniscal tears, and the expectations of the patient concerning participation in athletics. Lynch et al reported only one growth disturbance in 33 children with anterior cruciate ligament reconstructions. They recommend an over-the-top procedure with special precautions when performing a notchplasty or drilling across the tibial epiphysis. Although Clanton et al found results of anterior cruciate ligament reconstruction to be no better in children than in adults, they recommend surgical treatment of knee ligament injuries because of the possibility of repairable meniscal injuries.

Significant ligamentous disruption that involves two or more ligaments in two planes requires surgical repair. If possible, it is preferable to convert multiplane instability to one-plane instability, such as repair of the cruciate ligament with augmentation or reconstruction and conservative treatment of the medial collateral ligament, especially if it is avulsed at the medial femoral condyle. Conversely, if the medial collateral ligament is injured at the medial femoral condyle and the anterior cruciate ligament also is injured, closed treatment of the medial femoral condyle can be carried out to convert the two-plane instability to anterior stability only; at a later date reconstruction of the anterior cruciate ligament can be considered if necessary. Use of the central third of the patellar tendon is preferred for reconstruction in adolescents. Also, arthroscopically assisted reconstruction is preferred to facilitate postoperative rehabilitation.

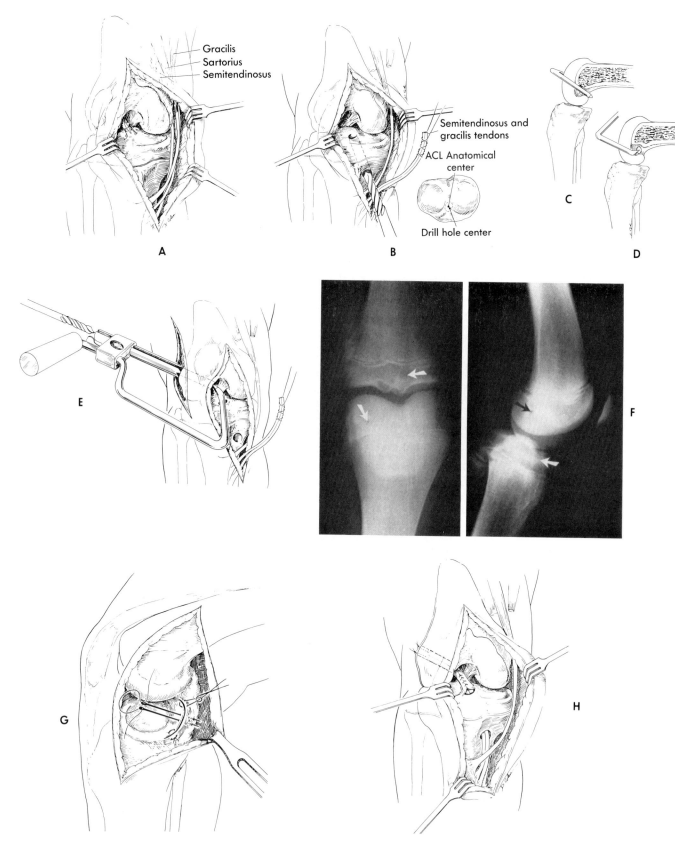

Fig. 15-59 Technique for reconstruction of anterior cruciate ligament with use of semi-tendinosus and gracilis tendons (see text). (Redrawn from Lipscomb AB and Anderson AF: J Bone Joint Surg 68A:19, 1986.)

◣ *Technique (Lipscomb and Anderson).* With the patient's knee flexed to 90 degrees, make a long medial parapatellar incision, perform a medial arthrotomy, and dislocate the patella laterally. Incise the synovial sleeve of the torn anterior cruciate ligament along its entire length for suture around the new ligament (Fig. 15-59, *A*). Dissect free the semitendinosus and gracilis tendons in the distal thigh, divide them at the musculotendinous junction, suture them together, and place a Bunnell suture in the tendon ends. Allow the muscle bellies to retract. Make a 0.64-cm drill hole through the anteromedial aspect of the tibia, beginning 3.8 cm distal to the joint, crossing the tibial physis, and penetrating the knee joint medial and anterior to the anatomic insertion of the anterior cruciate ligament (Fig. 15-59, *B*). This allows the new ligament to lie in its correct anatomic position and prevents impingement on the lateral femoral condyle.

Now make a long, curved, lateral incision ending over Gerdy's tubercle for both the drill hole in the lateral femoral condyle and the Losee procedure. Identify the distal femoral physis with a Keith needle. Insert the point of a drill guide through the slit in the synovial sleeve into the posterior compartment of the knee (Fig. 15-59, *C*). Draw the point back into the notch over the posterior ridge of the lateral femoral condyle by about 1.3 cm. Then secure the point in bone just posterior and superior to the anatomic origin of the anterior cruciate ligament (Fig. 15-59, *D*), holding the point of the drill guide securely in bone to prevent slipping. Push the points of the barrel into the surface of the lateral femoral condyle for fixation. Begin a 0.8-cm (⁵⁄₁₆-inch) drill hole in the lateral femoral condyle at a point just proximal to the insertion of the fibular collateral ligament (Fig. 15-59, *E*), directing it at a 70- to 90-degree angle to the long axis of the femur to avoid drilling across the femoral physis and entering the joint just posterior and superior to the anatomic insertion of the anterior cruciate ligament (Fig. 15-59, *F*). Make any necessary meniscal repairs (Fig. 15-59, *G*).

Next, pass the semitendinosus and gracilis tendons through the tibial and femoral drill holes. Suture them to the periosteum of the lateral femoral condyle under moderate tension, with the patient's knee flexed 45 degrees and the tibia posterior to the femur. If a substantial portion of the torn anterior cruciate ligament is present, place a gathering suture in its end, draw this through the femoral drill hole, and suture it to the periosteum. Make no attempt to primarily repair tears that disrupt the substance of the ligament; instead, suture the fibers around the newly reconstructed anterior cruciate ligament along with the synovial sleeve (Fig. 15-59, *H*). Use the same technique for acute and chronic tears. For chronic tears,

if the synovial sleeve has been attenuated or scarred, draw a pedicle of the infrapatellar fat pad through the femoral drill hole and suture it around the new anterior cruciate ligament intraarticularly.

To prevent anterolateral rotatory instability, perform a Losee reconstruction of the lateral compartment. Take a strip of iliotibial tract, 3.8 cm wide and 23 cm long from proximal to distal, leaving it attached to Gerdy's tubercle. Route it front to back through the femoral condyle and posterior part of the joint capsule, running just superior to the drill hole for the anterior cruciate. Then bring it around the arcuate complex, pass it under the fibular collateral ligament, and secure it to Gerdy's tubercle superiosteally with nonabsorbable sutures.

◣ *Postoperative management.* The knee is immobilized for 6 weeks in 15 degrees of flexion, and touch-down weight bearing with crutches is permitted. Full weight bearing in the immobilizer is begun at 6 weeks, as are range-of-motion exercises.

Meniscal Injuries

Although rarer than in adults, tears of both the medial and lateral menisci have been reported in children. Making the correct diagnosis often is the most difficult aspect of treatment. Medial or lateral joint line pain and effusion do not necessarily indicate meniscal tear. Bergstrom et al and Juhl and Boe reported diagnostic accuracy in approximately 20% of children believed to have meniscal injury; abnormality of the patellofemoral articulation was the most common pathologic finding. They emphasized that whereas hemarthrosis indicates significant injury to the knee, meniscal lesions in children are relatively rare. King also noted differences in presentation of mensical injuries in children and adults. History, physical examination, prolonged observation, and even direct inspection by arthrotomy may not be reliable in determining the exact pathologic condition. King, as well as Juhl and Boe, recommend arthroscopy if necessary for definitive diagnosis.

Although previous studies reported lateral lesions more common in children, King found more medial lesions in his patients, most commonly peripheral detachment of the posterior portion. He also noted that the younger the patient, the more peripheral the tear. Conversely, bucket handle tears occurred most often in older children and adolescents.

Meniscectomy once was believed to be a benign procedure in children. Recent reports, however, have proved this false. King, Juhl and Boe, Zaman and Leonard, and Manzione et al are among those reporting poor long-term results in children with total meniscectomy. Baratz et al showed in cadaver studies that the meniscus carries a weight-bearing load and that contact stresses are increased proportional to the amount of the meniscus removed and the degree of disruption of the meniscal structure. They also found no difference in the weight-bearing characteristics of the meniscus whether repair was performed by open or arthroscopic technique.

As King pointed out, removal of a damaged meniscus to minimize irreversible damage to the joint is advisable, but every effort should be made to spare the meniscus in children. A longer period of observation is indicated for children and adolescents than for adults. Arthroscopic determination of the exact meniscal pathology and the potential for repair is helpful to formulate treatment plans. Zaman and Leonard recommend observation of small peripheral tears, repair of larger peripheral tears, and partial meniscectomy leaving as much of the meniscus as possible; they believe that total meniscectomy is contraindicated in young patients. Manzione et al reported 60% poor results in their 20 children and adolescents with meniscectomy and found no correlation with the site of meniscectomy, type of meniscal tear, severity of roentgenographic changes, or type of meniscectomy (partial or total).

The appropriate treatment of meniscal injuries in children and adolescents begins with an accurate diagnosis, with arthroscopic examination if necessary. Small peripheral tears should be given a chance to heal without surgical treatment, and large peripheral tears should be repaired. Partial meniscectomy, removing as little of the meniscus as possible, is preferable to total meniscectomy, which should be avoided if at all possible.

Discoid Lateral Meniscus

Discoid meniscus is a relatively common cause for meniscal surgery in children. Symptoms may be similar to those of a tear of the lateral meniscus, except for a prominent "snap" felt in the lateral compartment as the knee is extended. Roentgenograms may show widening of the lateral compartment, squaring of the femoral condyle, hypoplasia of the lateral tibial spine, tilting of the tibial articular surface, and apparent elevation of the fibular head. Arthrographic examination may be helpful in establishing the diagnosis.

DeLee and Dickhaut reported two types of discoid lateral meniscus found at surgery: (1) stable with intact peripheral attachments and (2) Wrisberg-type with no peripheral attachments and only the hypertrophic ligament of Wrisberg attaching posteriorly. The Wrisberg-type discoid lateral meniscus is believed to be a congenital abnormality. Of DeLee and Dickhaut's 18 patients 12 had complete or stable discoid lateral menisci with intact ligamentous attachments; the lesion was an incidental finding at arthroscopic examination in all 12; and 10 of the 12 had no symptoms, meniscal tears, or ligamentous laxity. Six patients had Wrisberg-type discoid lateral menisci in which the meniscus was abnormally mobile; all 6 patients had symptoms and reported "snapping" of their knees.

Differentiation between the two types of discoid lateral meniscus at surgery is mandatory. Good results have been reported with saucerization and partial meniscectomy of asymptomatic, stable lesions, but partial meniscectomy in the hypermobile, Wrisberg type results in an unstable meniscal rim. DeLee and Dickhaut recommend total meniscectomy of symptomatic Wrisberg-type lesions, despite the fact that later degenerative changes are likely, because the "snapping" and occasional blocking of knee extension are disabling to the young athlete.

Arthroscopic Techniques for Diagnosis, Meniscectomy, and Meniscal Repair

General anesthesia is preferred because total muscle relaxation allows the best exposure. A tourniquet and leg-holding device also are helpful. A surgical assistant is indispensable to apply varus and valgus stress at different degrees of flexion and extension, to apply digital pressure to the joint line to expose the meniscus, and to hold the arthroscope while other instruments are used for surgery. The use of the "flat table" technique, without bending the patient's knee 90 degrees, allows the surgeon to control varus and valgus stress by placing the leg across his or her body and using a footstool for support. The tourniquet is inflated before the leg is prepared to avoid iodine or povidone-iodine (Betadine) leakage, which may cause "tourniquet burn."

Anterolateral, anteromedial, and posteromedial portals are used most commonly, although suprapatellar and transpatellar portals may be necessary. The transpatellar portal allows access through the middle of the knee into the intercondylar notch. The posteromedial portal is useful for examining the posterior cruciate ligament, posterior meniscus, and posterior portion of the intercondylar notch. Portal placement is critical. Portal sites are located with the patient's knee flexed to 45 degrees after the joint has been distended with saline solution through a large inflow cannula placed on the medial side of the joint into the suprapatellar space. The patella, patellar tendon, and medial joint line are outlined on the skin with a marking pen. The anterolateral portal is made 1 cm above the lateral joint line adjacent to the patellar tendon. The anteromedial portal is made 1 cm above the medial joint line adjacent to the patellar tendon.

Most children's knee joints easily accommodate a 4.5-mm arthroscope, as used in adult patients, and it is familiar to most practitioners. A 30-degree angle scope is most commonly used, but scopes of 0 degrees and 70 degrees can be used as needed. The scope is introduced into the joint through one of the portals and a sterile hand-held or nonsterile draped camera is attached.

Diagnostic arthroscopy

▸ *Technique.* First introduce the scope into the anterolateral portal to examine the suprapatellar area, the area beneath the patella, and the intercondylar notch, before moving into the medial compartment to locate the meniscus. With the use of arthroscopic observation, introduce a spinal needle through the area of the anteromedial portal into the medial joint. When the spinal needle is in the proper position, make the anteromedial incision and introduce a probe through this portal. Use the probe to examine the medial meniscus, noting any inferior or superior tears and testing meniscal stability by grasping and pulling forward the posterior rim. Observe the medial femoral condyle for any areas of osteochondritis dissecans (p. 798). Flexing the patient's knee to approximately 70 degrees will help identify any areas of osteochondritis. Then move the scope into the intrapatellar notch to examine the anterior cruciate ligament, examining it with the probe for tears. Perform a manual drawer test while observing with the arthroscope. Now examine the medial meniscus by flexing the patient's knee and externally rotating the foot. Examine the posterior horn of the mensicus through the intercondylar notch. Examine the anteromedial gutter and the suprapatellar area for any loose bodies. Examine the tracking mechanism by flexing the knee from 0 to approximately 70 degrees. Note any defect or fibrillation from chondromalacia on the inferior surface of the patella, as well as any plica formation crossing the medial femoral condyle.

Move the scope to the anteromedial portal and place the leg in the figure-4 position to expose the lateral meniscus for examination with the probe inserted in the anterolateral portal. Lifting the patient's heel in this position further distends the joint. The lateral meniscus generally is more mobile than the medial meniscus, with a more anterior border. Identify the popliteal hiatus, making sure not to confuse this with a tear of the lateral meniscus. After thorough inspection of the joint, perform any arthroscopic repair or excision that is required. If the procedure is to be terminated without further procedures, remove the scope and the inflow cannula and express the saline through the outflow cannula. With a separate needle, inject a long-acting local anesthetic such as bupivacaine (Marcaine) into the joint, close each portal with one suture, and apply a sterile dressing and elastic bandage.

▸ *Postoperative management.* Full weight bearing is allowed immediately after surgery, and patients usu-

ally are dismissed within 3 or 4 hours of the procedure. The patient is instructed to change the bandage twice a day and to begin straight-leg raising exercises The sutures are removed 1 week after surgery, and a short-arc exercise program is begun.

Arthroscopic meniscectomy. Partial meniscectomy is indicated only for unrepairable, unstable meniscal tears. Rosenberg et al stress that arthroscopic meniscectomy should excise only the damaged, unstable portion of the meniscus, leaving the maximum amount of the stable portion intact (Fig. 15-60). The transition from the area of excision to the remaining meniscus must be tapered or contoured to avoid leaving an edge or lip that will propogate the tear.

Availability of the proper instruments is mandatory, including arthroscopic punch forceps, right-angle rotary cutters, scissors, and knives. The safest and most commonly used cutting instrument is the punch forceps. Smaller sizes (2.7 mm) are available for use in children, as are small scissors. Back-cutting, banana, and Smillie knives are useful but must be handled carefully to avoid damaging the articular cartilage. Motorized cartilage cutters, shavers, and synovial cutters are hand- or foot-controlled and range from slow, side-cutting blades to high-speed (3000 rpm) auger-style blades. Rosenberg et al reported the full-radius cutter useful for shaving synovium, cartilage, and meniscus, but any motorized instrument must be used carefully and requires experience to be used safely. Inflow must be increased to the maximum because motorized instruments require outflow suction.

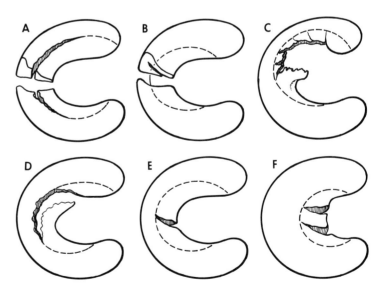

Fig. 15-60 Types of meniscal tears with proposed partial meniscectomy shown in dotted lines. **A,** Bucket handle. **B,** Horizontal. **C,** Degenerative flap. **D,** Flap. **E,** Radial. **F,** Radial tear in discoid meniscus. (Redrawn from Rosenberg TD et al. In The American Academy of Orthopaedic Surgeons: Instructional course lectures, vol 38, St Louis, 1988, The CV Mosby Co.)

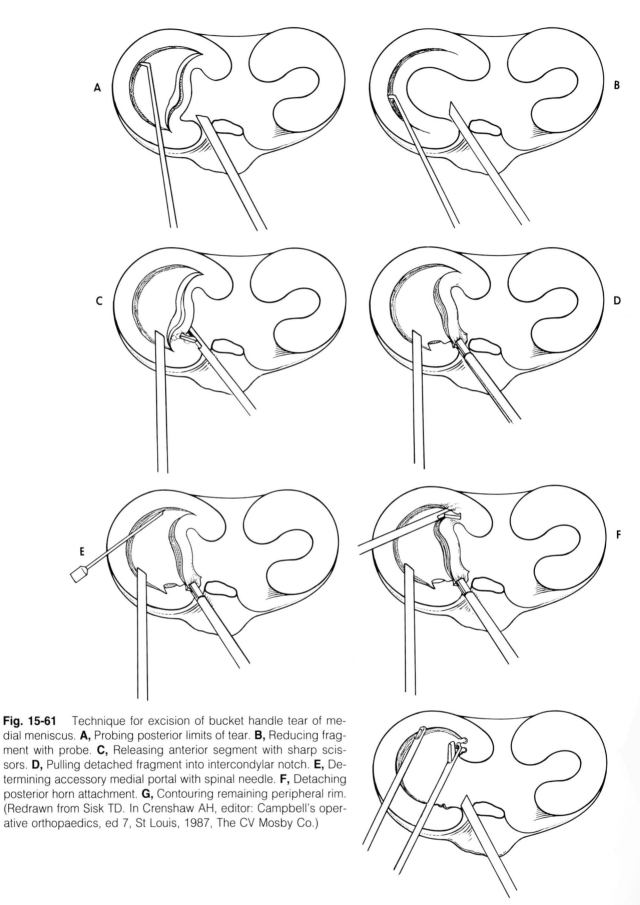

Fig. 15-61 Technique for excision of bucket handle tear of medial meniscus. **A,** Probing posterior limits of tear. **B,** Reducing fragment with probe. **C,** Releasing anterior segment with sharp scissors. **D,** Pulling detached fragment into intercondylar notch. **E,** Determining accessory medial portal with spinal needle. **F,** Detaching posterior horn attachment. **G,** Contouring remaining peripheral rim. (Redrawn from Sisk TD. In Crenshaw AH, editor: Campbell's operative orthopaedics, ed 7, St Louis, 1987, The CV Mosby Co.)

Excision of bucket handle tears of the medial meniscus

▶ *Technique.* With the scope in the anterolateral portal, examine the entire meniscus. Use a probe through the anteromedial portal to determine the limits of the tear (Fig. 15-61, *A*). If the bucket handle portion of the tear is displaced into the intercondylar notch, reduce it with the probe (Fig. 15-61, *B*). First release the anterior segment of the tear with sharp scissors inserted through the anteromedial portal (Fig. 15-61, *C*). This sometimes is difficult and requires a good deal of expertise. If the segment cannot be released in this manner, move the scope to the anteromedial portal or to a suprapatellar portal and insert the scissors through the anterolateral portal. After the anterior segment is detached, with the scope in the anteromedial portal and the grasper in the anterolateral portal, grasp the segment with a clamp and pull it into the intercondylar notch (Fig. 15-61, *D*). If a more medial accessory portal is needed, again determine its location with a spinal needle (Fig. 15-61, *E*). Introduce the scissors through this accessory portal to detach the posterior horn (Fig. 15-61, *F*); then round it off with basket forceps or a motorized trimmer. Probe the meniscus for any other tears, especially cleavage tears, complete contouring (Fig. 15-61, *G*), and check for stability. Close each portal with one absorbable suture, and apply a sterile dressing and elastic bandage.

Partial excision of discoid lateral meniscus

▶ *Technique.* Observe the meniscus through the anteromedial portal. With a probe through the anterolateral portal determine the stability of the meniscus (type I or II tear) and the extent of the tear, and, depending on the nature of the tear, use scissors, basket forceps, or graspers to remove portions of the meniscus (Fig. 15-62, *A* and *B*). It may be necessary to alternate the scope and instruments in the anterolateral and anteromedial portals for better vision and excision. Trim the discoid meniscus so that its contour is similar to the normal lateral meniscus, taking special care to balance the rim with the thickness of the inner edge (Fig. 15-62, *C*). Close each portal with one absorbable suture and apply a sterile dressing and elastic bandage.

▶ *Postoperative management.* Quadriceps-strengthening exercises (straight-leg raising) are begun immediately after surgery. Sutures are removed 1 week after surgery, and a progressive-resistance, short-arc exercise program is begun.

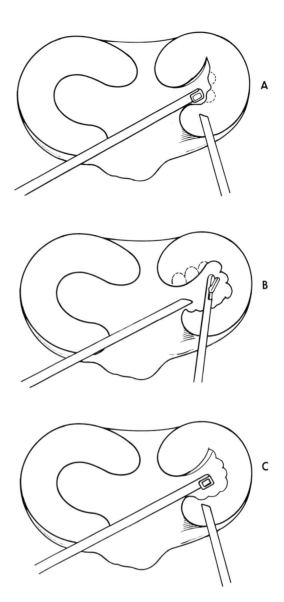

Fig. 15-62 Technique for excision of discoid lateral meniscus. **A** and **B,** Removing portions of meniscus with basket forceps. **C,** Contouring rim. (Redrawn from Sisk TD. In Crenshaw AH, editor: Campbell's operative orthopaedics, ed 7, St Louis, 1987, The CV Mosby Co.)

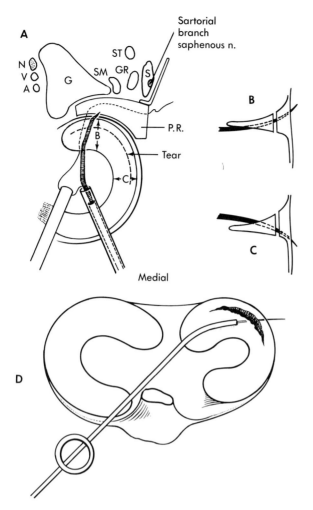

Sartorial
branch
saphenous n.

P.R.

Tear

Medial

Fig. 15-63 Medial meniscus repair. **A,** Repair of medial meniscus with arthroscope in anterolateral portal, intraarticular needle-holder in anteromedial portal, and popliteal retractor in posteromedial incision. Note that needle is bent to be directed away from midline neurovascular structures; needle-holder is directed toward intercondylar notch, with slight bend in needle at junction with needle-holder, thus directing tip of needle into space of popliteal retractor. *N,* Tibial nerve; *V,* popliteal vein; *A,* popliteal artery; *G,* gastrocnemius, *SM,* semimembranosus; *GR,* gracilis, *ST,* semitendinosus, *S,* sartorius; *PR,* popliteal retractor. **B,** Cross section. First arm of mattress suture is in place on inferior surface of meniscus, directed inferiorly. Second needle is engaged in inferior surface of meniscus, directed superiorly. **C,** Cross section. When tear extends anterior into middle and anterior one third of meniscus, mattress suture is placed on superior surface of meniscus, with arms of suture diverging superiorly and inferiorly. **D,** Suture of peripheral tear of medial meniscus, using single curved cannula technique. Anteromedial and midmedial sutures are inserted with cannula through contralateral portal. Cannula passed posterior to medial tibial emmence from contralateral portal. (**A to C** redrawn from Scott GA et al: J Bone Joint Surg 68A:847, 1986. **D** from Rosenberg TD et al: Arthroscopy 2:14, 1986.)

Repair of torn meniscus. In the child, preservation of meniscal tissue is extremely important to prevent unicompartmental arthritis. Repair of the meniscus generally is successful, especially if the tear is within the outer one third of the meniscus. A significant percentage of acute meniscal tears in this peripheral area have been reported to heal after suturing and immobilization. According to Sisk, meniscoplasty should be limited to the most peripheral 10% to 25% of the meniscus. Several recent reports indicate that repair also can be successful in chronic and less peripheral tears. Some authors prefer open repair to arthroscopic techniques, citing advantages of better preparation of the repair site and more precise placement of vertical sutures. Those advocating arthroscopic repair cite advantages of results equal to open technique with less morbidity and easier repair of certain tears (posterolateral tears and tears central to the meniscosynovial junction). Because of the danger of damage to the neurovascular structures on the medial and lateral sides of the knee during blind placement of sutures with large needles, arthroscopic techniques commonly are combined with a posterior incision. Rosenberg et al and Henning et al described an "inside-to-outside" technique using a posterior incision.

According to Sisk, arthroscopic meniscal repair consists of three steps: (1) documentation of a single, vertical, longitudinal tear in the outer one third of the meniscus that is capable of healing, (2) debridement of the tear and abrasion of the meniscus, synovium, and capsule to stimulate a proliferative fibroblastic healing response, and (3) appropriate suture placement to reduce and stabilize the meniscus.

Medial meniscus repair

▶ *Technique (Rosenberg et al and Scott et al).* Either a single or double cannula system can be used; varying the suture angle is easier with a single cannula system and it can be used with a posterior incision. Introduce the arthroscope in the anterolateral or suprapatellar portal. Acute peripheral tears require little preparation before suturing; however, if the tear is chronic, excoriate and abrade the torn surfaces with basket forceps, motorized shaver, scissors, or angled rasp before suturing. A small skeletal distractor device, as described by Wagner, may be useful for posterior lesions. Once debridement and freshening of the tear have been accomplished, reduce the meniscus and prepare for suturing. Place the arthroscope in the anteromedial portal and the single cannula for suturing in the anterolateral portal crossing under the arthroscope (Fig. 15-63). If necessary for tears in the posterior third of the meniscus, reverse the positions of the scope and the cannula. Make a posteromedial 4-cm incision, and retract posteriorly the sartorius muscle, the sartorial branch of the saphenous nerve, the medial hamstring muscles, and the medial half of the medial head of the gastrocnemius muscle. Because of the very tight insertion of the semimembranosus tendon into the posterior capsule and the slip to the oblique popliteal ligament, medial dissection may be difficult. Place a popliteal retractor in the posterior incision to protect the vessels as needles and suture materials are passed from within the joint, through the meniscus and capsule, and out in the popliteal space. During suturing, keep the patient's knee at 10 to 20 degrees of flexion as the sutures are passed through the posterior capsule; greater degrees of flexion cause laxity in the posterior capsule, and when the knee is extended, the capsule will become taut and place too much tension on the suture line. Place the cannula and the suturing material in the desired position against the meniscus after reduction into an anatomically correct position. Load the cradle with the first needle, and pass the needle through the cannula and the tear and out through the capsule. Remove the needle cradle after loosening the suture from the handle, and load the second needle with the other end of the suture while the cannula remains in the joint. Move the cannula 2 to 3 mm, and pass the second needle in a similar fashion through the meniscal tear and out through the capsule. Place three or four sutures in the posterior third of the medial meniscus. Depending on the type of tear, place sutures on the inferior surface at 4-mm intervals. In these intervals, place sutures on the superior surface of the meniscus so that top and bottom sutures are alternated. Scott et al described schematically the repair of single longitudinal, double longitudinal, radial, flap, and horizontal split tears (Fig. 15-64). The number of sutures needed depends on the length of the tear. Once all sutures are passed into the medial incision posteriorly, tie them over the posterior capsule, closing the meniscal tear as the sutures are tied. Close the posterior skin incision and the arthroscopic portals, and apply a sterile dressing and a long-leg cylinder cast with the knee in 10 degrees of flexion.

▲ *Postoperative management.* Straight leg–raising exercises are begun immediately and continued for 6 weeks. A progressive resistance range-of-motion exercise program is then begun and continued for 6 months. The cast is removed at 6 weeks, and weight bearing is allowed. Cutting, contact, or collision sports are prohibited for 6 more months.

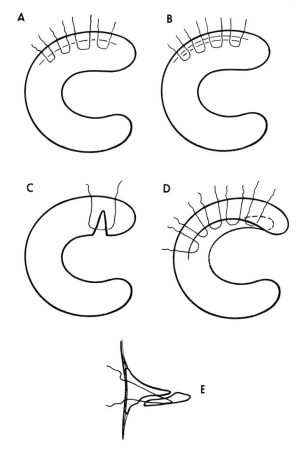

Fig. 15-64 Repair techniques for different types of meniscal tears. **A,** Single longitudinal tear. **B,** Double longitudinal tear. **C,** Radial tear. **D,** Flap tear. **E,** Horizontal split. (Redrawn from Scott GA et al: J Bone Joint Surg 68A:847, 1986.)

Bipartite Patella

Bipartite patella usually causes no symptoms and often is a coincidental finding on roentgenograms obtained for some other reason. It may be confused with acute fracture of the superolateral portion of the patella, and patellar fractures may simulate bipartite patella. Bipartite patella has been reported to be bilateral in approximately 40% of patients, and anteroposterior and skyline views of the contralateral patella are helpful in distinguishing it from an acute fracture. Complaints of pain in the superolateral pole of the patella usually indicate an overuse syndrome such as chondromalacia rather than bipartite patella. Restriction of competitive activity, use of nonsteroidal antiinflammatories, and short-arc exercises generally allow resolution of symptoms. Excision of the lateral portion of the patella rarely is indicated for persistent pain in older adolescents and young adults who wish to continue competitive sports.

The diagnosis can be confirmed and the joint examined arthroscopically before open excision is performed. Arthroscopic examination of the bipartite patella reveals a smooth cleft at the area of the separation with a slight (10- to 15-degree) sloping angle, often resembling grade 1 to grade 3 chondromalacia.

▰ *Technique.* Through an anteromedial or suprapatellar portal, examine the lateral portion of the bipartite patella for roughening or chondromalacia on the undersurface of the patella at the cleft and medial and lateral to this. If excision is deemed necessary, apply new sterile drapes and instruct operating room personnel to reglove. Make a small 3-cm lateral incision adjacent to the bipartite portion of the patella. Make the arthrotomy incision in the lateral portion of the suprapatellar pouch. At this point the cleft should be visible or palpable. Carry subperiosteal dissection superiorly to an area adjacent to the cleft, and with sharp dissection excise the bipartite portion from superior to inferior. Smoothe the remaining superior portion with a rasp. Remove any ragged edges on the inferior intraarticular surface and any other roughened areas on the remaining adjacent articular surface. Lateral retinacular release may be performed, but usually it is not necessary. Irrigate the wound copiously with antibiotic solution, and close in the standard manner. Apply a sterile dressing and a knee immobilizer.

▰ *Postoperative management.* Quadriceps exercises are begun 1 week after surgery, and full weight bearing without crutches is allowed. Range-of-motion and short-arc exercise programs are added at 3 weeks.

Popliteal Cyst (Baker's Cyst)

Popliteal cysts, or Baker's cysts, occur under or adjacent to the medial head of the gastrocnemius muscle in the posteromedial aspect of the knee. The lesion is prominent when the knee is hyperextended and usually is distal to the popliteal crease. The usual distention by fluid of the cyst implies knee joint irritation and fluid accumulation at the weakest point of the posterior capsule of the knee. Although this is true in adults and in some children, the majority of these cysts in children are isolated bursal sac formations and are not related to pathologic findings in the knee joint. A detailed history should be obtained, however, to ascertain that there has been no internal derangement of the knee joint. Rarely, discoid meniscus, torn medial meniscus, or patellar pathology can cause a popliteal cyst in the child. The posteromedial mass, which usually causes no symptoms, is noticed by the parents. Symptoms of knee derangement usually are absent, although occasionally there may be a sense of fullness or stiffness in the posterior aspect of the knee.

Treatment is conservative and surgery is not indicated for popliteal cysts in children. If present, any underlying pathology such as discoid meniscus or meniscal tear should be treated appropriately. Aspiration of the cyst and injection of cortisone are not indicated because recurrences are frequent after these procedures. Dinham reported that children with popliteal cysts who were treated nonsurgically remained symptom free and the cyst ultimately resolved, in contrast to children treated with surgical resection in whom the cyst recurred in over half. Excision is indicated only if the cyst is painful or irritating to the child and no knee joint pathology is found. Excision can be performed in conjunction with diagnostic arthroscopy with the patient in the supine position, although this is difficult; if excision is performed primarily, the prone position facilitates the procedure.

Excision of popliteal cyst without arthroscopy

▶ *Technique.* Place the patient prone on the operating table, and prepare and drape the posterior aspect of the knee in the usual manner. Apply a tourniquet to the proximal thigh. Make a zig-zag incision on the posterior aspect of the knee, with the 7 cm horizontal limb in the popliteal crease and the 6 cm vertical limbs medial and lateral (Fig. 15-65, *A*). Carry soft tissue dissection down toward the popliteal space. Divide the subcutaneous fascia, and locate the protruding cyst (Fig. 15-65, *B*). Identify and protect the deeper neurovascular bundle; do not expose these structures. Try not to rupture the cyst, but outline its borders, including the pedicle extending toward the joint. Continue dissection, taking care not to incise the sac of the cyst, which usually is located between the semimembranosus muscle and the medial side of the gastrocnemius. Retract both these muscles medially and laterally to expose the pedicle of the cyst where it enters the posterior aspect of the capsule (Fig. 15-65, *C*). With a sharp knife divide the pedicle at its communication with the posterior capsule, and then excise the entire cyst (Fig. 15-65, *D*). If possible, close any defects in the capsule with nonabsorbable suture (Fig. 15-65, *E*). Close the soft tissue and skin in the usual manner, and apply a sterile dressing.

▶ *Postoperative management.* Full weight bearing is allowed immediately after surgery. Sutures are removed at 2 weeks, and a range-of-motion exercise program is begun.

SHOULDER AND HUMERUS INJURIES

Most throwing-type injuries in the shoulder area of children and adolescents do not require surgical intervention. They are primarily sprains of the anterior and posterior capsular structures of the shoulder and can be treated with rest and restriction of activity to eliminate the chronic repetitive stresses. Areas of point tenderness do not require steroid injection. Steroid injections into the biceps tendon and groove proximally have been reported to cause iatrogenic rupture of the biceps tendon in young adults.

Proximal humeral epiphyseal injuries have been reported in adolescent pitchers, as have fractures of the humerus in shot-putters. Rettig and Beltz reported delayed union of a stress fracture of the humerus in an adolescent tournament tennis player. These uncommon injuries rarely require any surgical treatment.

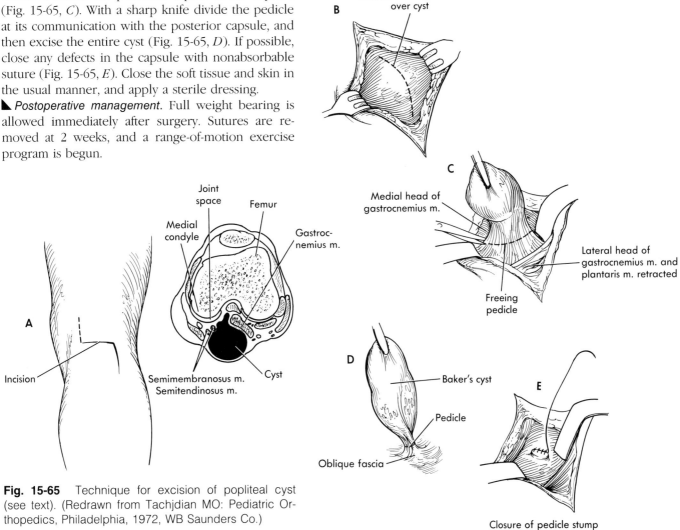

Fig. 15-65 Technique for excision of popliteal cyst (see text). (Redrawn from Tachjdian MO: Pediatric Orthopedics, Philadelphia, 1972, WB Saunders Co.)

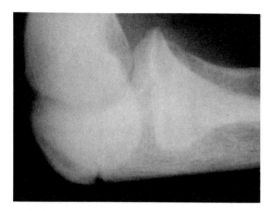

Fig. 15-66   Lucency in posterior aspect of olecranon may be confused with fracture but is normal ossification.

ELBOW INJURIES

Injuries to the elbow usually are traumatic (fractures and dislocations) in the young child, but they are predominantly overuse injuries in the adolescent, particularly those involved in repetitive, throwing-type activities. These injuries are not identical to those in adults because of the differences in anatomy. First, there appears to be a differential rate of growth of muscle and bone in the child, causing traction apophysitis. Second, cartilaginous traction apophyses that occur in children weaken these areas of the bone. Third, the open physis in children is vulnerable to injury. Generally, the majority of growth centers in the elbow close at age 17 years in boys and 14 years in girls. The physis of the radial head and olecranon close at about age 15 years in boys and 14 years in girls; the medial epicondylar physis closes later, at around 18 years in boys and 15 years in girls. Silberstein et al have noted several "vagaries" of the physes of the elbow. At the olecranon the proximal physis closes later in adolescence and may simulate a fracture line (Fig. 15-66). Furthermore, it closes later posteriorly than anteriorly, and this irregular ossification also may be mistaken for a fracture. The radial head often has the appearance of a "compressed" fracture because of a notch on the lateral aspect of the radial metaphysis, which is a normal variant rather than a fracture (Fig. 15-67). During late adolescence a spike of bone from the lateral epicondyle that is progress-

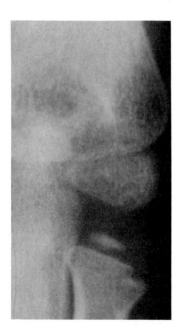

Fig. 15-67   Notched aspect of radial neck and metaphysis simulates fracture but is a normal growth variant. (From Silberstein MJ et al: J Bone Joint Surg 64A:1153, 1982.)

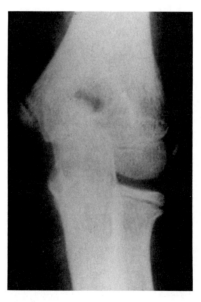 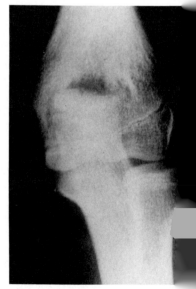

Fig. 15-68   Fleck of bone that appears to be a fracture of the lateral epicondyle is actually normal variation in ossification. (From Silberstein MJ et al: J Bone Joint Surg 64A:444, 1982.)

ing to fusion with the capitellum may appear similar to an avulsion fracture (Fig. 15-68). Multiple ossification centers in the medial epicondyle also may be confused with a fracture (Fig. 15-69). Roentgenograms of the contralateral elbow should be taken for comparison to distinguish these normal variants from a fracture.

Four types of injuries that result from throwing are common in adolescents: (1) traction apophysitis of the medial epicondyle, (2) avulsion of the medial epicondyle, (3) osteochondrosis of the capitellum, and (4) osteochondritis dissecans of the capitellum. These injuries occur through a valgus stress mechanism in which the medial collateral ligament may be stretched, causing apophysitis or avulsion of the medial epicondyle (Fig. 15-70). On the lateral side the valgus stress produces compression, which may cause osteochondrosis or osteochondritis dissecans of the capitellum or even secondary changes in the radial head (Fig. 15-71). Adams originally described these injuries as *Little League elbow,* and this term has become common, although many argue that most children in whom these overuse problems develop are older than Little League age; whether the problems actually begin in Little League and cause symptoms later is unknown. Regardless of the exact age at which the injury occurs, chronic repetitive valgus stress from throwing-type activities does produce orthopaedic problems in adolescent athletes.

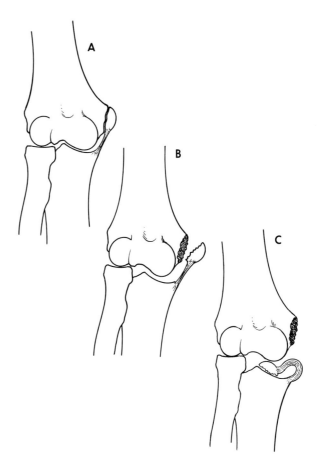

Fig. 15-70   Valgus stress may cause traction on medial side of elbow resulting in apophysitis **(A),** displacement of medial epicondyle **(B),** fracture or dislocation of elbow joint **(C)** with entrapment of medial epicondyle. (Redrawn from Schwab HG et al: Clin Orthop 146:42, 1980.)

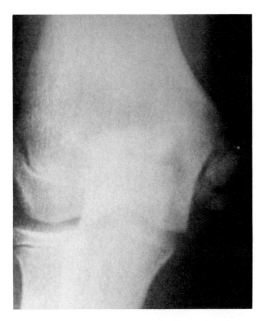

Fig. 15-69   Multiple ossification centers in the medial epicondyle may be mistaken for a fracture but are normal variations in ossification. (From Silberstein MJ et al: J Bone Joint Surg 63A:524, 1981.)

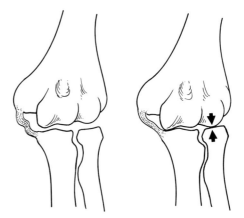

Fig. 15-71   Changes in capitellum and radial head caused by compression forces. (Redrawn from Bennett JB and Tulbs HS: In Morrey BF, editor: The elbow and its disorders, Philadelphia, 1985, WB Saunders Co.)

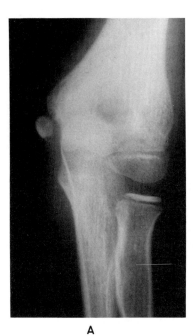
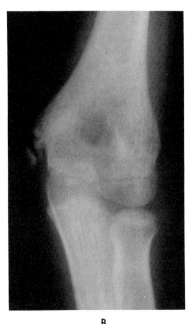

A   B

Fig. 15-72 **A,** Medial epicondylitis began as mild separation with chronic inflammation. **B,** Eight weeks later, callus formation is present, as after fracture; there is minimal widening of joint, and multiple ossification centers are visible.

Fig. 15-73 **A,** Severely displaced fracture of medial epicondyle. **B** and **C,** After open reduction and internal fixation with cancellous bone screws.

Medial Epicondylitis and Avulsion of the Medial Epicondyle

Medial epicondylitis produces slowly increasing point tenderness over the medial epicondyle and pain on throwing, with decreased effectiveness and distance. Mild flexion contracture of about 15 degrees is common, and roentgenograms usually show minimal widening of the medial epicondylar apophysis (Fig. 15-72). Treatment consists of restriction of activity until acute symptoms resolve, then resumption of limited activity (such as moving a pitcher to the outfield), with physical therapy to stretch and strengthen the elbow.

Avulsion of the medial epicondyle produces acute symptoms of pain, effusion, and flexion contracture. Roentgenograms show displacement of the apophysis. If the fragment is minimally displaced, immobilization generally is sufficient treatment; however, if the fragment is rotated or displaced more than 1 cm,

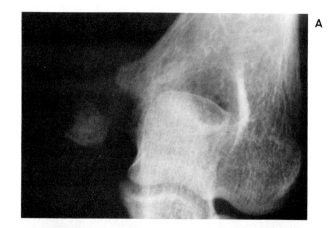

A

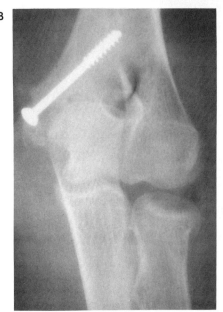

B

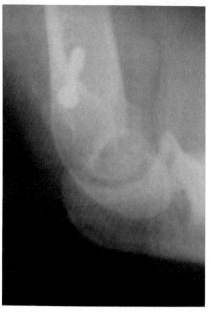

C

or if it is unstable, open reduction and internal fixation are recommended (Fig. 15-73). Valgus stress testing, as described by Woods and Tullos, is helpful to determine stability. If further distal displacement of the fragment occurs when gravity or weights are used to produce a valgus mechanism, the fracture is considered unstable (Fig. 15-74).

Woods and Tullos classified unstable fractures of medial epicondyle into two types, based primarily on the age of the patient. Type I occurs in children younger than 15 years of age, and the large fragment is made up of the entire epiphysis, which is displaced and/or rotated more than 1 cm (Fig. 15-75, *A*). Type II occurs in adolescents 15 years of age or older in whom the physis is closed; it also consists of a large fragment; and it may be associated with avulsion of the anterior oblique ligament (Fig. 15-75, *B*). In either type the large epicondylar fragment should be surgically reattached or, if extremely small, excised. The anterior oblique ligament and flexor muscles should be reattached if avulsed. Smooth or threaded pins may used for fixation because (1) the medial epicondyle is an apophyseal center rather than a primary growth center and (2) this injury usually occurs in older children and the apophysis contributes nothing to longitudinal growth. This relatively common fracture of the medial epicondyle should not be confused with the rare fracture of the medial condyle; fixation should not cross the medial condyle in young children for fear of growth arrest.

Occasionally, the medial epicondylar fragment becomes entrapped in the elbow joint and causes persistent elbow dislocation. Often closed reduction with a valgus stress will dislodge the fragment from the joint; if this is not successful, open reduction, removal of the fragment from the joint, and excision or pinning of the fragment should be performed (see Chapter 16).

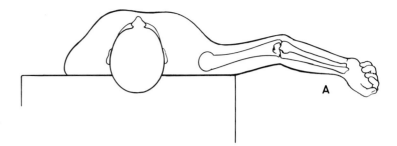

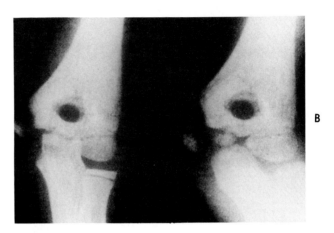

Fig. 15-74 **A,** Gravity test uses weight of forearm to determine displacement of fracture fragment with valgus stress. **B,** Positive result of gravity test. Note displacement of fracture with valgus stress *(right)* compared with view taken without stress *(left).* (**A** redrawn from Schwab GH et al: Clin Orthop 146:42, 1980.)

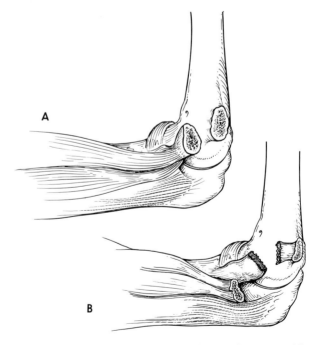

Fig. 15-75 Rupture of anterior oblique ligament with displaced avulsion fracture of medial epicondyle (see text). (Redrawn from Woods GS and Tullos HS: Am J Sports Med 5:23, 1977.)

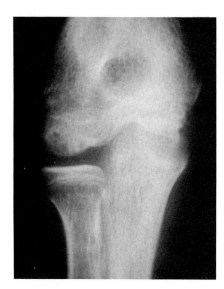

Fig. 15-76 Osteochondrosis involving entire capitellum.

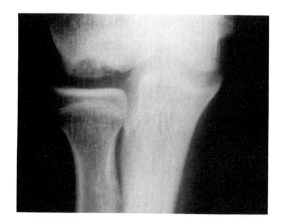

Fig. 15-77 Early osteochondritis dissecans involves only small area of capitellum.

Osteochondrosis and Osteochondritis Dissecans of the Capitellum

There is much discussion and confusion surrounding the entities of osteochondrosis and osteochondritis dissecans of the capitellum. Are they really different entities, and does it really matter? Osteochondrosis generally is believed to occur because of avascularity of the capitellum, usually when the child is about 10 years old; there is fragmentation of the entire capitellum (Fig. 15-76) and a mild, 10- to 15-degree flexion contracture. It sometimes is bilateral and often causes secondary changes in the radial head. Osteochondrosis of the capitellum generally can be treated with rest, stretching exercises, and moderation of sports activities to exclude throwing. Osteochondritis dissecans of the capitellum, on the other hand, is believed to be caused by trauma, avascularity, or a recalcitrant form of osteochondrosis. It usually occurs in adolescents, involves a discrete focal area of the capitellum (Fig. 15-77), and causes a lack of elbow extension. Because it sometimes involves multiple joints, some authors have suggested that osteochondritis dissecans is a variant of multiple epiphyseal dysplasia. The treatment of osteochondritis dissecans of the capitellum generally consists of observation. Surgical treatment, arthroscopic or open, should be reserved for fragments that are loose in the joint or that produce symptoms such as locking of the elbow joint. By either method the fragment should be excised and the crater drilled. Arthroscopy of the elbow requires expertise and should be attempted only by surgeons experienced in the techniques of arthroscopy. The lesion in the capitellum usually can be seen, and posterior loose bodies are easily excised arthroscopically; anterior or lateral loose bodies may be more difficult to locate and excise. Although several authors have reported success with pinning or bone grafting of the lesion, McManama et al reported that the majority of patients do well after simple excision of the fragment.

Arthroscopy of the elbow

▶ *Technique.* Elbow arthroscopy is performed on a routine operating table, with the patient under general anesthesia and in the supine position. Place a tourniquet around the proximal humerus, being sure to leave sufficient room in the elbow area to ensure sterility. Suspend the arm so that the shoulder is abducted 90 degrees and the elbow is flexed 90 degrees. Use sterile procedure to drape the entire arm and hand after routine preparation.

Sit with the patient's elbow in front of you at chest level; the viewing monitor is on the opposite side of the patient. Use a standard 4.0- to 4.5-mm arthroscope with a 25- to 30-degree lens angle. Interchangeable cannulas are recommended to allow easy movement of the arthroscope, inflow tube, and instruments around the different elbow compartments. A one-piece immersible camera-scope unit is preferred to avoid water fogging the system.

Identify with a pen all portal sites and bony landmarks before beginning the procedure because any fluid extravasation may alter the topical anatomy. Mark the medial epicondyle, lateral epicondyle, and olecranon, and outline the radial head. Locate three portals—anteromedial, anterolateral, and posterolateral—by measuring a specified distance from the adjacent bony landmarks. The distances for each patient will vary, depending on the child's size. The values given in this section are for average adults and should be scaled down according to the size of the patient. The other common portals are direct lateral and straight posterior. The anteromedial portal in the adult is located 2 cm distal and 2 cm anterior to the medial epicondyle. The anterolateral portal in the adult in located 3 cm distal and 1 cm anterior to the lateral epicondyle. The direct lateral portal lies within the lateral soft spot between the lateral epicondyle, radial head, and olecranon tip. An effusion is most easily palpated here and the joint aspirated. Establishment of the posterolateral portal and straight posterior portal requires prior extension of the elbow to approximately 30 degrees of flexion. This maneuver relaxes the triceps muscle, which will allow distention of the posterior capsule. The adult posterolateral portal is located 3 cm proximal to the olecranon tip and immediately lateral to the triceps tendon. The straight posterior portal is located 2 cm medial to the posterolateral portal in a triceps-splitting fashion.

Distend the elbow joint with saline by inserting an 18-gauge spinal needle into the direct lateral portal. With the joint maintained maximally distended, introduce a second 18-gauge spinal needle through the anterolateral portal. Once satisfactory position is confirmed by the free return of saline, make an incision through the skin only. Then insert a sharp trocar, aiming back toward the center of the joint. At the level of the joint capsule, exchange the sharp trocar for the blunt one and then enter the joint. Connect the arthroscope to the cannula with inflow through the scope. From this portal the medial side of the joint, the trochlear ridges, the coronoid process, and a small part of the radial head are visible (Fig. 15-78, A).

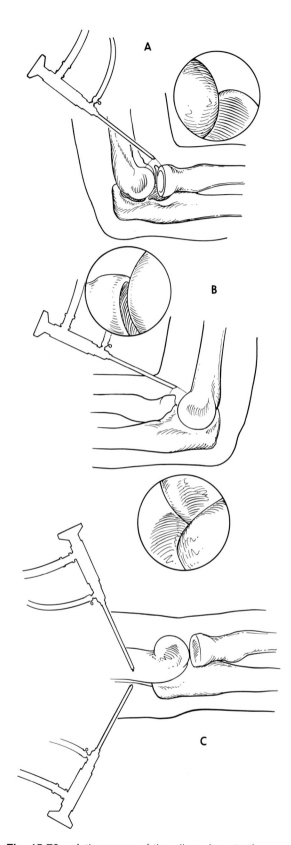

Fig. 15-78   Arthroscopy of the elbow (see text).

Establish the anteromedial portal under arthroscopic observation from the anterolateral side. First insert an 18-gauge spinal needle and confirm satisfactory position to protect the nearby median nerve and brachial artery. Then follow the same procedure of skin incision, using sharp and dull trocars. The arthroscope may be placed anteromedially and the inflow cannula anterolaterally. From this vantage point the lateral structures (radial head and capitellum) are best seen (Fig. 15-78, *B*). With pronation and supination of the patient's forearm, more of the radial head is visible. If posterior portals are to be established, the anteromedial cannula usually is used for inflow. Leave all cannulas in place to prevent extravasation of fluid and to allow easy return anteriorly if the need arises.

The direct lateral portal is at the soft spot where the 18-gauge spinal needle was first introduced. Use the same sequence of trocars through the skin incision. This is a tight space, and inadvertent withdrawal from the joint can occur. From this site the posterior aspects of the radial head and capitellum are visible. The arthroscope may be moved from anterior to posterior to inspect the articular surface of the olecranon and trochlea. At the tip of the olecranon the surgeon's view is in the direction of the posterolateral portal. After extending the elbow, introduce an 18-gauge spinal needle through the posterolateral portal while viewing from the direct lateral portal. After ensuring satisfactory position, make an incision through the skin and capsule similar to those in the knee. With the arthroscope in this site the olecranon fossa, olecranon tip, and posterior trochlea can be examined (Fig. 15-78, *C*). If an additional portal is needed for removal of a loose body, establish a straight posterior portal. Use an 18-gauge spinal needle first to confirm that the loose body can be reached from the chosen site. Make an incision through skin, tendon, and capsule in line with the tendon fibers, and insert the operating instrument. Be aware that the ulnar nerve is just medial to the straight posterior portal.

▶ *Postoperative management.* Range-of-motion exercises are begun on the first postoperative day, and biceps and triceps setting exercises, as well as strength gripping of the wrist and hand, are added on the second postoperative day. On the third day, curls of the wrist are added to increase flexor and extensor strength. Progressive resistance exercises with weights up to 5 pounds are begun at 1 week. For persistent stiffness a Dynasplint (Fig. 15-79) may be helpful; this device allows active range of motion and constant pressure to achieve an increased passive range of motion.

Removal of loose bodies by arthrotomy

▶ *Technique (Tibone and Collins).* With the patient supine, apply and inflate a tourniquet on the upper portion of the arm and drape the arm free. Begin the incision approximately 3 cm proximal to the lateral epicondyle of the humerus in line with the lateral border of the humerus and the triceps. Extend the incision distally over the lateral epicondyle, curving it between the radial head and the ulna. Develop the interval between the anconeus muscle and the extensor carpi ulnaris muscle, and expose the underlying elbow capsule. Then open the capsule of the radioulnar joint with a longitudinal incision. Loose bodies usually can be removed through the small incision, but if wider exposure is necessary, carry the incision up proximally along the epicondylar ridge until the triceps is identified. Then with sharp dissection, displace the triceps posteriorly to expose the tip of the olecranon and the olecranon fossa. For wider exposure place a varus stress on the elbow joint. After thorough irrigation close the capsule and the interval between the epicondylar ridge and the triceps. Then close the anconeus, extensor carpi ulnaris fascia, subcutaneous tissues, and skin. Release the tourniquet, obtain hemostasis, and apply a compression dressing and a posterior molded plaster splint with the arm in approximately 90 degrees of flexion.

▶ *Postoperative management.* The splint is removed at 1 week, and range-of-motion exercises are begun. At 3 weeks a strengthening program is begun, and return to sports usually can be accomplished within 3 months.

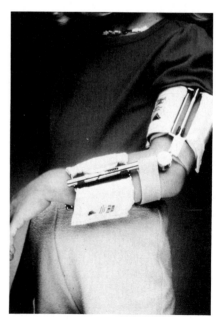

Fig. 15-79 Dynasplint.

REFERENCES

General

Apple DF Jr and McDonald A: Long-distance running and the immature skeleton, Orthopedics 3:929, 1981.

Baxter MP and Dulberg C: "Growing pains" in childhood: a proposal for treatment, J Pediatr Orthop 8:402, 1988.

Gallagher SS et al: The incidence of injuries among 87,000 Massachusetts children and adolescents: results of the 1980-81 statewide childhood injury prevention program surveillance system, Am J Public Health 74:1340, 1984.

Goldberg B, Rosenthal P, and Robertson LS: Injuries in youth football, Pediatrics 81:255, 1988.

Gugenheim JJ et al: Little League survey: the Houston study, Am J Sports Med 4:189, 1976.

Harvey JS Jr: Overuse syndromes in young athletes, Pediatr Clin North Am 29:1369, 1982.

Kannus P, Nittymaki S, and Jarvinen M: Athletic overuse injuries in children: a 30-month prospective follow-up study in an outpatient sports clinic, Clin Pediatr 27:333, 1988.

Lehman RC, Gregg JR, and Torg E: Iselin's disease, Am J Sports Med 14:494, 1986.

Micheli LJ: Overuse injuries in children's sports: the growth factor, Orthop Clin North Am 14:337, 1983.

Ogden JA: Skeletal injury in the child, ed 2, Philadelphia, 1990, WB Saunders Co.

O'Neill DB and Micheli LJ: Overuse injuries in the young athlete, Clin Sports Med 7:591, 1988.

Pillemer FG and Micheli LJ: Psychological considerations in youth sports, Clin Sports Med 7:679, 1988.

Sewall L and Micheli LJ: Strength training for children, J Pediatr Orthop 6:143, 1986.

Shields CL Jr, editor: Manual of sports surgery, New York, 1987, Springer-Verlag.

Stanitski CL: Management of sports injuries in children and adolescents, Orthop Clin North Am 19:689, 1988.

Tursz A and Crost M: Sports-related injuries in children: a study of their characteristics, frequency, and severity, with comparison to other types of accidental injuries, Am J Sports Med 14:294, 1986.

Watson AWS: Sports injuries during one academic year in 6799 Irish school children, Am J Sports Med 12:65, 1984.

Wenger HA and Collis ML: The effects of resistance training on aerobic and anaerobic power of young boys, Med Sci Sports Exerc 19:389, 1982.

Zaricznyj B et al: Sports-related injuries in school-aged children, Am J Sports Med 8:318, 1980.

Ankle

Amis JA and Gangl PM: When inversion injury is more than a "sprained ankle," J Musculoskel Med, Sept 1987, p. 68.

Anderson KJ, LeCocq JF, and Clayton ML: Athletic injury to the fibular collateral ligament of the ankle, Clin Orthop 23:146, 1962.

Baird RA and Jackson ST: Fractures of the distal part of the fibula with associated disruption of the deltoid ligament: treatment without repair of the deltoid ligament, J Bone Joint Surg 69A:1346, 1987.

Baker CL, Andrews JR, and Ryan JB: Arthroscopic treatment of transchondral talar dome fractures, Arthroscopy 2:82, 1986.

Berndt AL and Harty M: Transchondral fracture of the talus, J Bone Joint Surg 41A:988, 1959.

Boccanera L, Laus M, and Lelli A: Chronic lateral instability of the ankle, Ital J Orthop Traumatol 8:315, 1982.

Bröstrom L: Sprained ankles. VI. Surgical treatment of chronic ligament ruptures. Acta Chir Scand 132:551, 1966.

Canale ST and Beaty JH: Osteochondral lesions of the talus. In Hamilton WC, editor: Traumatic disorders of the ankle, New York, 1984, Springer-Verlag.

Cedell CA: Supination-outward rotation injuries of the ankle, Acta Orthop Scand Suppl 110, 1967.

Chrisman OD and Snook GA: Reconstruction of lateral ligament tears of the ankle, J Bone Joint Surg 51A:904, 1969.

Davidson AM et al: A review of twenty-one cases of transchondral fractures of the talus, J Trauma 7:378, 1967.

Drez D, Guhl JF, and Gollehan DL: Ankle arthroscopy—technique and indications, Foot Ankle 2:138, 1981.

Elmslie RC: Recurrent subluxation of the ankle-joint, Ann Surg 100:364, 1934.

Evans DL: Recurrent instability of the ankle—a method of surgical treatment, Proc R Soc Med 46:343, 1953.

Evans GA, Hardcastle P, and Frenyo AD: Acute rupture of the lateral ligaments of the ankle: to suture or not to suture, J Bone Joint Surg 66B:209, 1984.

Eyring EJ and Guthrie WD: A surgical approach to the problem of severe lateral instability at the ankle, Clin Orthop 206:185, 1986.

Flick AB and Gould N: Osteochondritis dissecans of the talus (transchondral fractures of the talus): review of the literature and new surgical approach for medial dome lesions, Foot Ankle 5:165, 1985.

Freeman MA: Instability of the foot after injuries to the lateral ligament of the ankle, J Bone Joint Surg 47B:669, 1965.

Freeman MA: Treatment of ruptures of the lateral ligament of the ankle, J Bone Joint Surg 47B:661, 1965.

Gepstein R et al: Closed percutaneous drilling for osteochondral dissecans of the talus, Clin Orthop 213:197, 1986.

Guhl JF: New techniques for arthroscopic surgery of the ankle: preliminary report, Orthopedics 9:261, 1986.

Harper MC: The deltoid ligament: an evaluation of need for surgical repair, Clin Orthop 226:156, 1988.

Jackson DW, Ashley RL, and Powell JW: Ankle sprains in young athletes: relation of severity and disability, Clin Orthop 101:201, 1974.

Lehman RC and Gregg JR: Osteochondritis dissecans of the midfoot, Foot Ankle 7:177, 1986.

McManama GB: Ankle injuries in the young athlete, Clin Sports Med 7:547, 1988.

Nash WC and Baker CL Jr: Transchondral talar dome fractures: not just a sprained ankle, South Med J 77:560, 1984.

O'Neill DB and Micheli LJ: Tarsal coalition: a follow-up of adolescent athletes, Am J Sports Med 17:544, 1989.

Parisien JS: Diagnostic and surgical arthroscopy of the ankle: technique and indications, Bull Hosp J Dis 45:38, 1985.

Parisien JS: Arthroscopic treatment of osteochondral lesions of the talus, Am J Sports Med 14:211, 1986.

Pritsch M, Horoshovski H, and Farine I: Arthroscopic treatment of osteochondral lesions of the talus, J Bone Joint Surg 68A:862, 1986.

Ramsey PL and Hamilton W: Changes in tibiotalar areas of contact caused by lateral talar shift, J Bone Joint Surg 58A:356, 1976.

Rubin G and Witten M: The talar-tilt angle and the fibular collateral ligaments: a method for the determination of talar tilt, J Bone Joint Surg 42A:311, 1960.

Smith RW and Reischl SF: Treatment of ankle sprains in young athletes, Am J Sports Med 14:465, 1986.

Snook GA, Chrisman OD, and Wilson TC: Long-term results of Chrisman-Snook operation for reconstruction of the lateral ligaments of the ankle, J Bone Joint Surg 67A:1, 1985.

Snyder RB, Lipscomb AB, and Johnston RK: The relationship of tarsal coalitions to ankle sprains in athletes, Am J Sports Med 9:313, 1981.

Spinella AJ and Turco VJ: Avulsion fracture of the distal tibial epiphysis in skeletally immature athletes (juvenile Tillaux fracture), Orthop Rev 17:1245, 1988.

Staples OS: Injuries to the medial ligaments of the ankle: result study, J Bone Joint Surg 42A:1287, 1960.

Staples OS: Ruptures of the fibular collateral ligaments of the ankle: result study of immediate surgical treatment, J Bone Joint Surg 57A:101, 1975.

Thompson JP and Loomer RL: Osteochondral lesions of the talus in a sports medicine clinic—a new radiographic technique and surgical approach, Am J Sports Med 12:460, 1984.

Vahvanen V, Westerlund M, and Kajarti M: Sprained ankle in children—a clinical follow-up study of 90 children treated conservatively and by surgery, Am Chir Gynaecol 72:71, 1983.

Watson-Jones R: Fractures and joint injuries, ed 3, Baltimore, 1946, Williams & Wilkins Co.

Yocum LA: Treatment of osteochondritis dissecans of the talus. In Shields CL Jr: Manual of sports surgery, New York, 1987, Springer-Verlag.

Knee

Andrews JR and Axe MJ: The classification of knee ligament instability, Orthop Clin North Am 16:69, 1985.

Andrish JT: Ligamentous injuries of the knee, Orthop Clin North Am 16:273, 1985.

Baratz ME, Fu HF, and Mengate R: Meniscal tears: the effect of meniscectomy and repair of intraarticular contact areas and stress in the human knee, Am J Sports Med 14:270, 1986.

Bergström R et al: Arthroscopy of the knee in children, J Pediatr Orthop 4:542, 1984.

Bradley GW, Shives TC, and Samuelson KM: Ligament injuries in the knees of children, J Bone Joint Surg 61A:588, 1979.

Bradley J and Dandy DJ: Osteochondritis dissecans and other lesions of the femoral condyles, J Bone Joint Surg 71B:518, 1989.

Bright R and Green W: Freeze-dried fascia lata allografts: a review of 47 cases, J Pediatr Orthop 1:13, 1981.

Cahill BR and Berg BC: 99m-Technetium phosphate compound joint scintigraphy in the management of juvenile osteochondritis dissecans of the femoral condyles, Am J Sports Med 11:329, 1983.

Cerullo G et al: Evaluation of the results of extensor mechanism reconstruction, Am J Sports Med 16:93, 1988.

Clanton TO and DeLee JC: Osteochondritis dissecans: history, pathophysiology, and current treatment concepts, Clin Orthop 167:50, 1982.

Clanton TO et al: Knee ligament injuries in children, J Bone Joint Surg 61A:1195, 1979.

Collie L: Personal communication, 1978.

Cox JS: Chondromalacia of the patella: a review and update. I. Contemp Orthop 6:17, 1983.

Cox JS: Chondromalacia of the patella: a review and update. II. Contemp Orthop 7:35, 1983.

Crosby EB and Insall J: Recurrent dislocation of the patella: relation of treatment to osteoarthritis, J Bone Joint Surg 58A:9, 1976.

DeLee J and Curtis R: Anterior cruciate ligament insufficiency in children, Clin Orthop 172:112, 1983.

DeLee JC and Dickhaut SC: The discoid lateral meniscus syndrome, J Bone Joint Surg 64A:1068, 1982.

Desai SS et al: Osteochondritis dissecans of the patella, J Bone Joint Surg 69B:320, 1987.

Dinham JM: Popliteal cysts in children: the case against surgery, J Bone Joint Surg 57B:69, 1975.

Ehrlich MG and Zaleske DJ: Pediatric orthopedic pain of unknown origin, J Pediatr Orthop 6:460, 1986.

Eiskjar S and Larsen ST: Arthroscopy of the knee in children, Acta Orthop Scand 58:273, 1987.

Ellison AE: Distal iliotibial-band transfer for anterolateral rotatory instability of the knee, J Bone Joint Surg 61A:330, 1979.

Falstie-Jensen S and Sondergard-Peterson PE: Incarceration of the meniscus in fracture of the intercondylar eminence of the tibia in children, Injury 15:236, 1984.

Ficat RP, Phillipe J, and Hungerford DS: Chondromalacia patellae: a system of classification, Clin Orthop 144:55, 1979.

Green WT and Banks HH: Osteochondritis dissecans in children, J Bone Joint Surg 35A:26, 1953.

Guhl JF: Arthroscopic treatment of osteochondritis dissecans, Clin Orthop 167:65, 1982.

Hamberg P, Gillquist J, and Lysholm J: Suture of new and old peripheral meniscus tears, J Bone Joint Surg 65A:193, 1983.

Hawkins RJ, Bell RH, and Anisette G: Acute patellar dislocations, Am J Sports Med 14:117, 1986.

Henning CE et al: Arthroscopic meniscus repair with a posterior incision. In The American Academy of Orthopaedic Surgeons: Instructional Course lectures, vol 37, St Louis, 1988, The CV Mosby Co.

Heywood AWB: Recurrent dislocation of the patella: a study of its pathology and treatment in 106 knees, J Bone Joint Surg 43B:508, 1961.

Huberti HA and Hayes WC: Patellofemoral contact pressures: the influence of Q-angle and tendofemoral contact, J Bone Joint Surg 66A:715, 1984.

Hughston JC et al: Classification of knee ligament instabilities. I. The medial compartment and cruciate ligaments, J Bone Joint Surg 58A:159, 1976.

Hughston JC et al: Classification of knee ligament instabilities. II. The lateral compartment, J Bone Joint Surg 58A:173, 1976.

Hungerford DS and Barry M: Biomechanics of the patellofemoral joint, Clin Orthop 144:9, 1979.

Indelicato PA: Non-operative treatment of complete tears of the medial collateral ligament of the knee, J Bone Joint Surg 65A:323, 1983.

Insall, JN: Current concepts review: patellar pain, J Bone Joint Surg 64A:147, 1982.

Insall JN: Patella pain syndromes and chondromalacia patellae, In The American Academy of Orthopaedic Surgeons: Instructional course lectures, 30:342, 1981.

Insall, JN, Falvo KA, and Wise DW: Chondromalacia patellae: a prospective study, J Bone Joint Surg 58A:1, 1976.

Jakob RP et al: Arthroscopic meniscal repair, Am J Sports Med 16:137, 1988.

Jones RE, Henley B, and Francis P: Nonoperative management of isolated grade III collateral ligament injury in high school football players, Clin Orthop 213:137, 1986.

Juhl M and Boe S: Arthroscopy in children, with special emphasis on meniscal lesions, Injury 17:171, 1986.

King AG: Meniscal lesions in children and adolescents: a review of the pathology and clinical presentation, Injury 15:105, 1983.

Lindholm S, Pylkkanen P, and Osterman K: Fixation of osteochondral fragments in the knee joint, Clin Orthop 126:256, 1977.

Lipscomb AB and Anderson AF: Tears of the anterior cruciate ligament in adolescents, J Bone Joint Surg 68A:19, 1986.

Losee RE, Johnson TR, Southwick WO: Anterior subluxation of the lateral tibial plateau: a diagnostic test and operative repair, J Bone Joint Surg 60A:1015, 1978.

Lynch MA, Henning CE, and Glick KR Jr: Knee joint surface changes: long-term follow-up meniscus care, treatment, and stable anterior cruciate ligament reconstructions, Clin Orthop

Manzione M et al: Meniscectomy in children: a long-term follow-up study, Am J Sports Med 11:111, 1983.

McCarroll JR, Rettig AC, and Shelbourne DK: Anterior cruciate ligament injuries in the young athlete with open physes, Am J Sports Med 15:44, 1988.

McDaniel WJ and Dameron TB: Untreated ruptures of the anterior cruciate ligament, J Bone Joint Surg 62A:696, 1980.

Medlar RC, Mandibery JJ, and Lyne ED: Meniscectomies in children, Am J Sports Med 8:87, 1980.

Metcalf RW: An arthroscopic method for lateral release of the subluxating or dislocating patella, Clin Orthop 167:9, 1982.

Metcalf RW: Operative arthroscopy of the knee. In The American Academy of Orthopaedic Surgeons: Instructional course lectures, vol 30, St Louis, 1982, The CV Mosby Co.

Micheli IJ and Stanikski CL: Lateral patellar retinacular release, Am J Sports Med 9:330, 1981.

Morrissy RT et al: Arthroscopy of the knee in children, Clin Orthop 162:103, 1982.

Mubarak SJ and Carroll NC: Juvenile osteochondritis dissecans of the knee: etiology, Clin Orthop 157:200, 1981.

Nichols JA: Bracing the anterior cruciate ligament deficient knee using the Lenox Hill derotation brace, Clin Orthop 172:137, 1983.

Noyes FR et al: The symptomatic anterior cruciate deficient knee. II. The results of rehabilitation, activity modification, and counseling on functional disability, J Bone Joint Surg 65A:163, 1983.

Ogilivie-Harris DJ and Jackson RW: The arthroscopic treatment of chondromalacia patellae, J Bone Joint Surg 66B:660, 1984.

Outerbridge RE: The etiology of chondromalacia patellae, J Bone Joint Surg 43B:752, 1961.

Outerbridge RE: Osteochondritis dissecans of the posterior femoral condyle, Clin Orthop 175:121, 1983.

Paulos L, Noyes FR, and Malek M: A practical guide to the initial evaluation and treatment of knee ligament injuries, J Trauma 20:498, 1980.

Price CT and Allen WC: Ligament repair in the knee with preservation of the meniscus, J Bone Joint Surg 60A:61, 1978.

Rosenberg TD, Metcalf RW, and Gurley WD: Arthroscopic meniscectomy. In The American Academy of Orthopaedics Surgeons: Instructional course lectures, vol 37, St Louis, 1988, The CV Mosby Co.

Sandow MJ and Goodfellow JW: The natural history of anterior knee pain in adolescents, J Bone Joint Surg 67B:36, 1985.

Scott GA, Jolly BL, and Henning CE: Combined posterior incision and arthroscopic intra-articular repair of the meniscus, J Bone Joint Surg 68A:847, 1986.

Sisk TD: Arthroscopy of knee and ankle. In Crenshaw AH, editor: Campbell's operative orthopaedics, ed 7, St Louis, 1987, The CV Mosby Co.

Smillie IS: Treatment of osteochondritis dissecans, J Bone Joint Surg 39B:248, 1957.

Smillie IS: Injuries of the knee joint, ed 4, Baltimore, 1970, Williams & Wilkins Co.

Steiner ME and Grana WA: The young athlete's knee: recent advances, Clin Sports Med 7:527, 1988.

Stewart MJ: Athletic injuries, particularly to the ligaments of the knee: diagnosis, repair, and physical rehabilitation, Am J Orthop 3:52, 1961.

Thompson NL: Osteochondritis dissecans and osteochondral fragments managed by Herbert compression screw fixation, Clin Orthop 224:71, 1987.

Torg JS, Conrad W, and Kalen V: Clinical diagnosis of anterior cruciate ligament instability in the athlete, Am J Sports Med 4:84, 1976.

Vahvanen V and Aalto K: Meniscectomy in children, Acta Orthop Scand 50:791, 1979.

Wombell JH and Nunley JA: Compressive fixation of osteochondritis dissecans fragments with Herbert screws, J Orthop Traum 1:74, 1987.

Woods GW, Stanley RF, and Tullos HS: Lateral capsular sign: x-ray clue to a significant knee instability, Am J Sports Med 7:27, 1979.

Zaman M and Leonard MA: Meniscectomy in children: a study of fifty-nine knees, J Bone Joint Surg 60B:436, 1978 (abstract).

Zarins B: Combined intra-articular and extra-articular reconstructions for anterior tibial subluxation, Orthop Clin North Am 16:223, 1985.

Ziv I and Carroll NC: The role of arthroscopy in children, J Pediatr Orthop 2:243, 1982.

Shoulder

Bennett GE: Elbow and shoulder lesions of baseball players, Am J Surg 98:484, 1959.

Rettig AC and Beltz HF: Stress fracture in the humerus in an adolescent tennis tournament player, Am J Sports Med 13:55, 1985.

Elbow

Adams JE: Injury of the throwing arm: a study of traumatic changes in the elbow joints of boy baseball players, Calif Med 102:127, 1965.

Andrews JR: Bony injuries about the elbow in the throwing athlete. In The American Academy of Orthopaedic Surgeons: Instructional course lectures, vol 34, St. Louis, 1985, The CV Mosby Co.

Andrews JR and Carson WG: Arthroscopy of the elbow, Arthroscopy 1:97, 1985.

Barnes DA and Tullos HS: An analysis of 100 symptomatic baseball players, Am J Sports Med 6:62, 1978.

Bennett JB and Tullos HS: In Morrey BF: The elbow and its disorders, Philadelphia, 1985, WB Saunders Co.

DeHaven KE and Evarts CM: Throwing injuries of the elbow in athletes, Orthop Clin North Am 4:301, 1973.

Guhl J: Arthroscopy and arthroscopic surgery of the elbow, Orthopaedics 8:1290, 1985.

Johnson LL: Elbow joint. In Johnson LL, editor: Diagnostic and surgical arthroscopy: the knee and other joints, ed 2, St Louis, 1981, The CV Mosby Co.

McManama GB et al: The surgical treatment of osteochondritis of the capitellum, Am J Sports Med 13:11, 1985.

Morrey BF: Arthroscopy of the elbow. In Marreg BF, editor: The elbow and its disorders, Philadelphia, 1985, WB Saunders Co.

Schwab GH et al: Biomechanics of elbow instability: the role of the medial collateral ligament, Clin Orthop 146:42, 1980.

Silberstein MJ, Brodeur AE, and Graviss ER: Some vagaries of the medial epicondyle, J Bone Joint Surg 63A:524, 1981.

Silberstein MJ, Brodeur Ae, and Graviss ER: Some vagaries of the olecranon, J Bone Joint Surg 63A:722, 1981.

Silberstein MJ, Brodeur AE, and Graviss ER: Some vagaries of the radial head and neck, J Bone Joint Surg 64A:1153, 1982.

Slocum DB: Classification of the elbow injuries from baseball pitching, Am J Sports Med 6:62, 1978.

Tibone JE and Collins HR: Elbow debridement. In Shields CL, Jr: Manual of sports surgery, New York, 1987, Springer-Verlag.

Tivnon MC, Anzel SH, and Waugh TR: Surgical management of osteochondritis dissecans of the capitellum, Am J Sports Med 4:121, 1976.

Torg JS: Little League: "the theft of a carefree youth," Phys Sports Med 1:72, 1978.

Wilson FD et al: Valgus extension overload in the pitching elbow, Am J Sports Med 11:83, 1983.

Woods GW and Tullos HS: Elbow instability and medial epicondyle fractures, Am J Sports Med 5:23, 1977.

Woodward AH and Bianco AJ: Osteochondritis dissecans of the elbow, Clin Orthop 110:35, 1975.

Yocum LA: Elbow arthroscopy. In Shields CL Jr: Manual of sports surgery, New York, 1987, Springer-Verlag.

16 Fractures and Dislocations

S. TERRY CANALE

Surgical treatment rarely is indicated for fractures or dislocations in children. Thompson et al, in a study of 4411 consecutive fractures in children and adolescents, found that only 3.6% required any form of internal fixation. Indications for internal fixation, with open or closed techniques, have been described by several authors. The most common indications include (1) displaced physeal fractures, (2) displaced intraarticular fractures, (3) unstable fractures, (4) fractures in children with multiple injuries, especially concomitant neurologic injuries, and (5) open fractures with extensive soft tissue damage.

Fractures in children differ from those in adults in several ways. In addition to their greater potential for remodeling, children's bones are more malleable, allowing a plastic type of "bowing" injury and absorption of more energy before breaking. The periosteum is thicker than in adults, usually remaining intact on one side of the fracture and helping to stabilize reduction and decrease displacement. Nonunion is rarely a problem in fractures in children, but angular or rotational deformities are frequent. In a young child, growth of the bone will compensate for imperfections in apposition and, to some extent, alignment and length. The older the child the less that spontaneous correction can be expected. Blount (1955) established general rules concerning the prognosis of fractures of the shafts of long bones in children, basing his principles on the age of the child, the location of the fracture, and the degree of angulation. Greater angulation is acceptable in a young child with a deformity near the end of the bone. If the child is near maturity or if the fracture is near the middle of the bone, reduction must be almost perfect. Spontaneous correction of angular deformity is greatest when the angulation is in the plane of motion of a nearby hinged joint. Angulation in any other direction usually persists to some extent. Rotational deformities are permanent. Some varus or valgus angulation may correct spontaneously after fractures of long bones, but excessive angulation will not correct spontaneously and may cause significant cosmetic and functional problems. Valgus angulation of the long bones is more readily tolerated than varus angulation, especially in the lower extremities.

PHYSEAL INJURIES

The most significant difference in pediatric and adult fractures is the presence of the epiphyses and physes in the long bones of children, the latter probably the weakest point in the child's skeleton. Approximately 15% of all injuries to the long bones during childhood involve the physis. Injuries to the physis may occur at any age but are more common during rapid skeletal growth, such as in the first year of life and during the prepubertal growth spurt. The physes that provide the most longitudinal growth are the most commonly injured. Separation of the distal radial physis is by far the most common, followed by the distal ulnar, distal humeral, proximal radial, distal tibial, distal femoral, proximal humeral, proximal femoral, proximal tibial, and phalangeal physes. The normal anatomy of the physes must be preserved to ensure normal growth of the bones, and this consideration, coupled with the fact that many fractures occur through the physes in children, makes treatment difficult.

Injuries that involve the physes and epiphyses have long been recognized to cause cessation of growth and resultant angular deformities, and several investigators have devised classification systems by which prognosis of different fractures can be made. Epiphyseal injuries have been classified by Weber, Poland, Ogden, and others, but the most commonly used classification is that of Salter and Harris, which is based on the roentgenographic appearance of the fracture (Fig. 16-1). The Salter-Harris classification reflects the amount of involvement of the physis, the epiphysis, and the joint. The higher the classification the more likely physeal arrest or joint incongruity. Type I fractures are epiphyseal separations through the physis only, with or without displacement. Type II fractures have a metaphyseal spike attached to the separated epiphysis (Thurston Holland sign), with the separation also through the physis. Type III is a physeal separation with a fracture through the epiphysis into the joint, with joint incongruity when the fracture is displaced. Type IV is a fracture through the metaphysis, through the physis, through the epiphysis, and into the joint, also with possible joint incongruity. Type V fracture, which can be diagnosed only in retrospect, is a compression fracture of the physis that produces permanent damage. Peterson and Burkhart have questioned the validity of the Salter-Harris type V compression fracture of the physis be-

cause they found no evidence of physeal injury resulting from pure compression unassociated with some other fracture pattern in the physis. Rang added to the classification system a "bruise" or contusion to the periphery of the physis, causing scarring, tethering, and arrest of the periphery, which may be the most critical area in angular deformities. Ogden's classification is more complicated but fits almost every fracture pattern in every physis. The first five classes are basically the same as those of Salter and Harris, but subclasses are added for peculiar fracture patterns in special joints such as the hip and for certain traction epiphyses. Type VI fractures in the Ogden system are similar to the bruise injury described by Rang. Type VII fracture is an intraarticular osteochondral fracture, and types VIII and IX are not epiphyseal or physeal fractures but appear to stimulate the physes and contribute to horizontal bone growth. Chadwick and Bentley added four subclasses (Fig. 16-2) to Salter-Harris type IV fractures of the distal tibial physis, which reflects the mechanism of injury and which they believe is a more precise predictor of growth disturbance.

Physeal injury results in growth disturbance, most commonly after Salter-Harris types III, IV, and V fractures. Most types I and II fractures can be treated by closed reduction. Types III and IV fractures often require open reduction and internal fixation to reposition the fragments anatomically and fix them securely to allow continued growth in the physis and joint congruity. In type V fractures the cartilage cells of the physis are crushed and growth disturbance may occur regardless of the type of treatment; in fact type V fractures usually are diagnosed only in retrospect when growth disturbance occurs. These guidelines are not absolute, and some fractures do not behave as predicted by their classification. For example, significantly displaced type II fracture of the the distal femoral epiphysis quite often results in growth arrest and angular deformity because of premature physeal closure. Some authors advocate closed reduction of nondisplaced types III and IV fractures, but Bright (1974) reported displacement in the cast of nondisplaced distal tibial fractures, which resulted in bony bar formation, and he recommends open reduction and internal fixation regardless of the amount of displacement. Indications for open reduction of specific physeal injuries are given in the appropriate sections of this chapter.

Type	Poland	Salter-Harris	Ogden

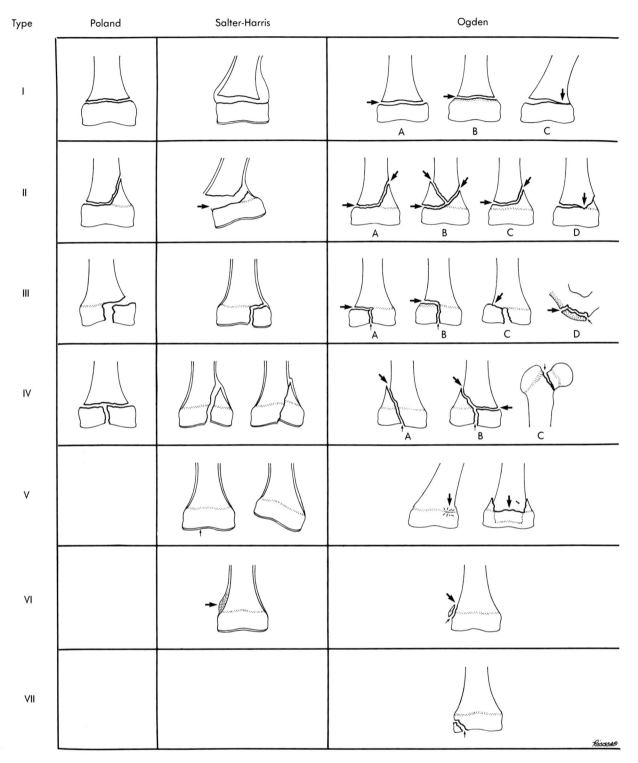

Fig. 16-1 Classification of physeal injuries by Poland, Salter and Harris, Weber, and Ogden. All four systems are similar, but from *left* to *right* are increasingly complex. Salter-Harris classification is a refinement of Poland's system; Weber classification adds extraarticular and intraarticular designations to Salter-Harris system; and Ogden's classification, which is all-inclusive, adds more subclasses to simpler systems.

Because of the rapidity of repair in this area, physeal separations should be reduced as soon as possible after injury. All reductions of physeal fractures should be performed gently to prevent further damage to the germinal cells in the physis. Crossing the physis with any form of fixation should be avoided if at all possible. In types III and IV fractures the pins should cross the epiphysis in the fractured areas, and in types II and IV pins should cross the metaphyseal spike rather than the physis if at all possible.

Complete or partial premature closure of the physis and formation of bony bars result in growth arrest and angular deformity. In the older child resection of the bony bar, with or without corrective osteotomy, is indicated; in younger children, bony bar resection, with various interposition materials, is appropriate (see Chapter 1). In general, more angular deformity can be tolerated in the upper extremity than in the lower, more valgus deformity can be tolerated than varus deformity, and more flexion deformity can be tolerated than extension deformity. In the lower extremity more deformity can be tolerated proximally than distally (the same varus angle in the hip can be better compensated than in the knee and least well compensated in the ankle). Symmetric growth arrest across the physis can cause significant limb shortening in the younger child; epiphysiodesis of the opposite limb can be performed by several techniques (see Chapter 3). In the older child, femoral and tibial shortening or lengthening may be used for leg length inequality (see Chapter 3).

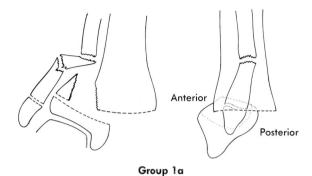

Group 1a
Abduction injury

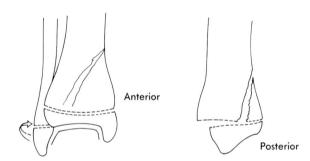

Group 1b
Supination/hyper plantarflexion injury

Group 1c
Supination/external rotation injury

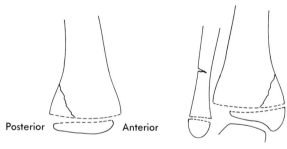

Group 1d
Rare adduction injury

Fig. 16-2 Chadwick and Bentley's classification of distal tibial physeal injuries. (Redrawn from Chadwick JD and Bentley G: Injury 18:157, 1987.)

OPEN FRACTURES

Treatment and classification of open fractures in children are essentially the same as those for open fractures in adults. Young children, however, may not give as accurate or reliable a history concerning the mechanism of injury and the environment in which it occurred. When the history is questionable, the open fracture should be treated as if contaminated. Seemingly innocuous Gustilo type I puncture wounds in both-bone forearm fractures may become sealed over with a seroma, producing a perfect medium for *Bacillus clostridium* and gas gangrene. Fee et al reported five cases of gas gangrene after both-bone fractures in which the proximal fragment protruded and became contaminated by the soil. As a general rule all compound wounds should be irrigated and debrided thoroughly in the operating room with the patient under general or regional block anesthesia, and the child should be hospitalized for observation and intravenous antibiotic treatment. Treatment of the fracture depends on the age of the child, the severity of the soft tissue injuries, and other associated injuries. Often standard traction and casting techniques are most appropriate, especially in younger children with minimal soft tissue injury. In older children with clean wounds, intramedullary nailing has been reported to be successful, but it should not be used in children with open physes. External fixation may be appropriate, especially for lower extremity open fractures, if there is extensive soft tissue damage or associated head injury. Several recent reports have indicated good results with external fixation of children's fractures, but all stress the necessity of avoiding the physis with the transfixing pins and the use of adequate incisions for pin insertion to prevent skin necrosis and infection. Tolo reported external fixation of 14 acute fractures in children, 11 of which were open fractures. All fractures healed, but three children had refractures after apparent union. Three patients had leg length discrepancies of 2 cm or more. Reff reported treatment of 10 open fractures in children, all of which healed without infection, malunion, or pseudarthrosis.

OTHER SPECIAL FRACTURES

Pathologic fractures that result from neoplasms or dysplasia or from metabolic, genetic, or systemic conditions usually benefit from open reduction and internal fixation because these procedures prevent long periods of immobilization that make the bones more osteoporotic. Intramedullary fixation of pathologic fractures adds strength to the weakened bone and helps prevent rotational or angular malunion. Techniques for treating pathologic fractures of different bones are discussed in the appropriate chapters in this text.

Fractures of the clavicle, humerus, hip, and femur are sometimes present at birth. These fractures rarely require surgery but should be recognized because they frequently are misdiagnosed as pseudopalsy, infection, or dislocation.

Fractures caused by child abuse usually occur between birth and 2 years of age. Most do not require surgical treatment, but any child suspected of being a victim of abuse should be protected, if necessary by hospitalization. Child abuse should be suspected in any child younger than 2 years with a significant fracture and a questionable history of its occurrence. Bone scan or skeletal survery usually is indicated to rule out this possibility. Multiple fractures in different stages of healing are almost always indicative of child abuse, as are multiple areas of large ecchymoses in different stages of resolution.

GENERAL PRINCIPLES OF SURGICAL TREATMENT OF FRACTURES IN CHILDREN

Although few children's fractures require open reduction and internal fixation, when surgical treatment is indicated, it is imperative to adhere to some basic principles of treatment:

1. Do not fail to obtain adequate reduction in the belief that all children's fractures will remodel completely.
2. Consider the unique anatomy of the physis; each physis has its own particular contour and configuration.
3. Reposition the fracture fragments as anatomically as possible, especially at the physis.
4. Use adequate, but not excessive, fixation.
5. Use fixation that can be easily removed.
6. Use smooth rather than threaded pins (Fig. 16-3).

7. Do not cross the physis with fixation, but rather parallel it or place pins in the metaphyseal spike (Fig. 16-4).
8. Avoid unnecessary drill holes that cause pathologic fracture.
9. Do not penetrate the joint with pins.
10. Use plastic type closure with absorbable suture.
11. Use adequate immobilization after the reduction in the noncompliant patient, especially the young child.
12. Watch for neurovascular insufficiency in the convalescent period.
13. Warn parents before surgery of the possibility of early and late complications such as bony bar formation, angular deformity, and avascular necrosis.

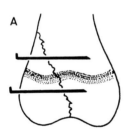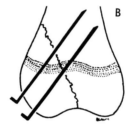

Type 4 fixation methods

Fig. 16-3 Fixation of epiphyseal fracture. **A,** Correct placement of parallel smooth pins across epiphysis and metaphysis. **B,** Smooth pins should cross physis only if necessary to hold reduction. (From Ogden JA: Skeletal injury in the child, Philadelphia, 1982, Lea & Febiger.)

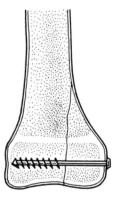

Fig. 16-4 Fixation of epiphyseal fracture. If threaded pins or cancellous screws are used, they should cross epiphysis or metaphysis and not physis. (From Weber BG: Treatment of fractures in children and adolescents, New York, 1980, Springer-Verlag.)

FOOT FRACTURES
Metatarsal and Phalangeal Fractures

Metatarsal and phalangeal fractures are fairly common in children, but they usually heal uneventfully and rarely require surgical treatment. Because of the strong interosseous ligaments, fractures of the proximal metatarsals usually are not significantly displaced unless produced by severe trauma. Swelling generally is extensive because of considerable damage to the soft tissues. Elevation and observation are appropriate initial treatment; a circumferential cast should not be applied. Once swelling has resolved, longitudinal traction may be used for reduction of a displaced fracture, or open reduction and smooth pin fixation may be performed if necessary for multiple fractures with significant displacement. This procedure occasionally is needed in fractures of the first metatarsal in older children in which little remodeling can be expected (Fig. 16-5). Most displaced fractures of the metatarsal neck heal and remodel quite well in young children, but significant displacement and deformity, especially in the anteroposterior plane, and multiple fractures may require open reduction and internal fixation with longitudinal wires.

Stress fractures of the metatarsal shaft or neck may occur in children, particularly those involved in sports that demand chronic, repetitive, stressful activity. Bone scanning may be helpful in the diagnosis of these fractures, and treatment should be limitation of activity, with a period of nonweight bearing until pain subsides; a short-leg cast may be applied for 1 to 2 weeks if pain is severe. Jones fractures, fractures of the base of the fifth metatarsal, were originally described in 1902 by Robert Jones as a diaphyseal avulsion fracture caused by overpull of the peroneus brevis muscle. Kavanaugh et al, however, reported that of 16 Jones fractures in older adolescents, most were stress fractures and were not caused by inversion or overpull of the peroneus brevis. Because of the uncertainty of healing of this diaphyseal fracture, they suggested open reduction and internal fixation with a medullary screw for high-performance athletes, recreational athletes, and patients with delayed union. Avulsions of the most proximal base of the fifth metatarsal also occur in children and heal uneventfully, except for some bony hypertrophy at the fracture site.

Fractures of the phalanges are caused primarily by hitting a hard object with the toe or dropping a heavy object on the toe. Dislocations usually are dorsal and can be reduced easily. Fractures must be distinguished from developmental disorders of the phalanges. Lyritis noted frequent fragmentation of the proximal epiphysis of the hallux (Fig. 16-6), in which the epiphysis may be fissured, compressed, or fragmented without fracture of the physis. Fractures and dislocations of the phalanges should be reduced by longitudinal traction and held by "buddy" taping to the next toe. Open reduction and internal fixation rarely are indicated. *Pseudomonas* infection should be suspected if the phalangeal fracture is caused by a penetrating wound, such as a nail puncture wound, and the infection should be treated by irrigation, debridement, and appropriate intravenous antibiotic therapy. Severe open fractures in the forefoot and phalanges from bicycle spoke or lawn mower injuries are treated by debridement and delayed closure.

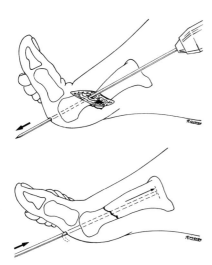

Fig. 16-5 Method of open pinning of metatarsal shaft or neck fractures in retrograde fashion through first metatarsal head. (Redrawn from Cehner J: Fractures of the tarsal bones, metatarsals, and toes. In Weber BG, Brunner C, and Freuler F, editors: Treatment of fractures in children and adolescents, New York, 1980, Springer-Verlag.)

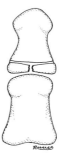

Fig. 16-6 Fissuring of epiphysis of proximal phalanx of great toe, which is not a fracture. (Redrawn from Lyritis G: Skeletal Radiol 10:250, 1983.)

Tarsal Fractures

Because of the flexibility of the child's foot, fractures of the tarsal bones are uncommon in children and are usually part of a severe injury to the entire foot, such as a wringer, severe compression, or lawn mower injury. Wiley (1981) described 19 tarsometatarsal joint injuries in adults and children, pointing out that the second metatarsal is the cornerstone of the foot and that strong ligamentous attachments are present between the metatarsals themselves and between the cuneiforms. He emphasized that fracture of the base of the second metatarsal, with or without a "buckle" fracture of the cuboid, indicates significant tarsometatarsal joint injury, and he noted that even fractures with intraarticular components will heal if joint incongruity is not severe, but subluxation or dislocation does not remodel. Persistent dorsal dislocation, even in children, will produce a painful hypertrophic osseous area on the dorsum of the foot, often with associated varus angulation. Therefore, with the patient under general anesthesia, any dislocated tarsometatarsal joints should be reduced. If this cannot be accomplished closed, then open reduction and internal fixation are indicated, with care taken to avoid injury to the proximal physis of the first metatarsal.

Johnson described a pediatric Lisfranc fracture that he called a "bunk bed" fracture and noted that this fracture of the tarsometatarsal area produces a subtle deformity that may be overlooked. Fracture-dislocation or fracture-subluxation of the first tarsometatarsal often is associated with the fracture, and the first and second metatarsals may be involved. According to Johnson, this injury occurs from a twisting force when the foot is extended, producing soft tissue injury that is more severe than indicated by the bony injury evident on roentgenograms.

Calcaneal Fractures

Although not infrequent in adults, calcaneal fractures are rare in children. These fractures in children tend to have less intraarticular involvement than the adult counterpart, are less severe because of the elasticity of the involved structures in the child, and will remodel. Schmidt and Weiner classified 62 calcaneal fractures in children, using a system similar to that of Essex-Lopresti. They included epiphyseal fractures at the tuberosity and a fracture almost unique to children that involves significant loss of bone at the posterior aspect of the calcaneus and occurs in lawn mower injuries. Of the 62 fractures 63% were extraarticular and 37% intraarticular, the reverse of the ratio in adult calcaneal fractures. Displacement of intraarticular fractures was minimal compared with adult fractures, and only two required open reduction and internal fixation. In several older children, however, the subtalar joint was involved, with a decreased "crucial" angle and a joint compression fracture (similar to Essex-Lopresti type II fracture). Schmidt and Weiner reported that most calcaneal fractures in children can be expected to heal without functional loss because of the rarity of displacement in both intraarticular and extraarticular fractures, the exception being fractures associated with severe loss of bone and soft tissue from the heel resulting from lawn mower injuries.

Harris views (ski-jump views) of the heel should be obtained, and CT scanning may be helpful to delineate the minimal disturbance in the bony architecture, which often is difficult to determine because of the high percentage of cartilage in the calcaneus in children. Stress fractures of the calcaneus in children have been reported, and bone scanning may be helpful in diagnosing these. Trott noted that cysts in the triangular space of the calcaneus can become large enough to result in pathologic fracture of the calcaneus. Surgical treatment of calcaneal fractures in children almost never is indicated.

Talar Fractures

There are three basic types of fractures of the talus: (1) fractures of the neck, (2) fractures of the body and dome, and (3) transchondral (osteochondral) fractures. Vertical fracture through the neck of the talus is the most common injury in children. In general, talar fractures in children heal with fewer complications than in adults.

Talar Neck Fractures

The most important factor in the prognosis of talar neck fractures is the retrograde blood supply to the talus, which is present in a sling fashion around the talar head and neck. This blood supply enters the bone in three principal ways: through the neck, through the foramina in the sinus tarsi and tarsal canal, and deep into the foramina in the medial surface of the body. The most commonly used fracture classification is that proposed by Hawkins, which is based on the amount of disruption of the blood supply to the talus. A type I lesion is a fracture through the neck of the talus with minimal displacement and minimal damage to the blood supply of the talus, theoretically damaging only one vessel, the one entering through the neck (Fig. 16-7). In type II lesions the subtalar joint is subluxated or dislocated and at least two of the three sources of blood supply may be lost, that through the neck and that entering the tarsal canal and sinus tarsi (Fig. 16-8).

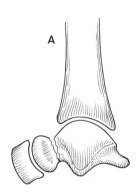

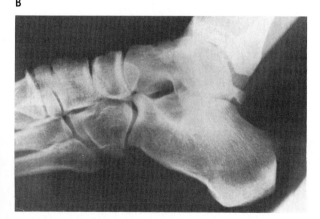

Fig. 16-7 Type I talar neck fracture. **A,** Drawing and, **B,** roentgenogram of fracture with minimal displacement.

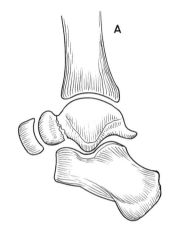

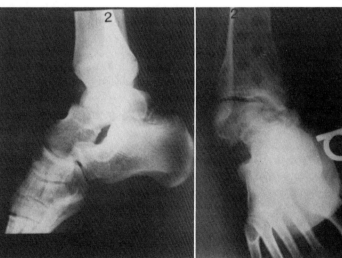

Fig. 16-8 Type II talar neck fracture. **A,** Drawing and, **B,** roentgenogram of fracture of neck and dislocation of subtalar joint.

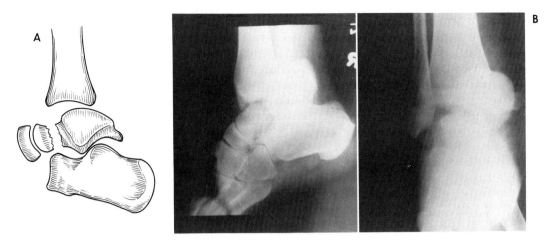

Fig. 16-9   Type III talar neck fracture. **A,** Drawing and, **B,** roentgenogram of neck fracture and dislocation of talus from tibia and calcaneus.

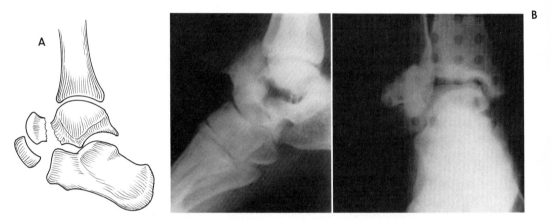

Fig. 16-10   Type IV talar neck fracture. **A,** Drawing and, **B,** roentgenogram of neck fracture with dislocation of talus from tibia and calcaneus and dislocation of talar head from navicular.

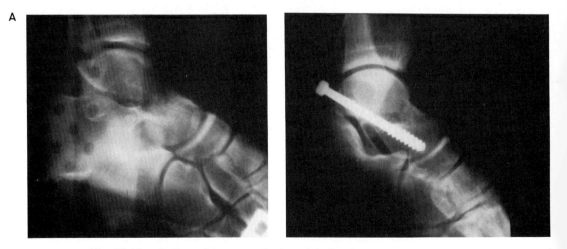

Fig. 16-11   **A,** Type II fracture of talar neck. **B,** After open reduction and posterior percutaneous pin fixation.

In type III lesions the body of the talus is dislocated from the tibia and the calcaneus, and all three sources of blood supply may be disrupted (Fig. 16-9). The incidence of avascular necrosis is high in type III fractures. A type IV fracture, unrelated to the blood supply, also has been described. In this injury the body of the talus is dislocated or subluxated at the subtalar joint, the body of the talus is dislocated at the ankle joint, the talar neck is fractured, and the head of the talus is dislocated at the talonavicular joint (Fig. 16-10).

Closed reduction followed by nonweight bearing is the preferred treatment for type I mildly or moderately displaced fractures. If adequate reduction cannot be obtained or maintained, open reduction and internal fixation are indicated. A reduction of less than 5 mm of displacement and less than 5 degrees of malalignment is considered adequate. Types II, III, and IV fractures often require open reduction, with or without internal fixation, because of the difficulty of maintaining adequate reduction by closed means in fractures with significant displacement. Open fractures are treated by irrigation, debridement, and delayed closure, and internal fixation is used if required for stability of reduction. Open reduction is performed through an anteromedial approach with lateral retraction of the neurovascular bundle. A cancellous screw inserted from medial to lateral usually is used for fixation. As an alternative a cancellous lag screw can be inserted percutaneously from posterior to anterior (Fig. 16-11).

The frequent problem of varus malalignment can be alleviated by the use of a special roentgenographic technique to determine the amount of varus angulation in the anteroposterior plane. A cassette is placed directly under the foot, and the ankle is placed in maximum equinus position, the usual position after reduction of the fracture of the talar neck. This position can be maintained more easily with maximum flexion of the hip and knee. The foot then is pronated 15 degrees, and the roentgen tube is directed cephalad at a 75-degree angle from the horizontal table top. This view will help detect any offset or varus deformity of the head and neck of the talus.

Complications after talar neck fracture include avascular necrosis of the talar body, malunion, traumatic arthritis of the ankle and subtalar joint, and infection. The presence of a subchondral lucency in the talar dome (Hawkins' line) 12 weeks after injury is an indication that avascular necrosis will not occur (Fig. 16-12), but this is not an absolute prognosticator.

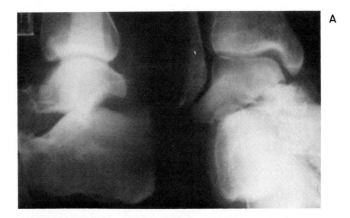

A

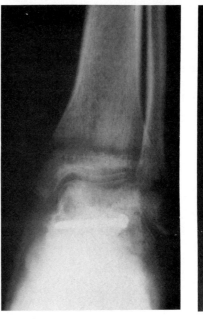

B

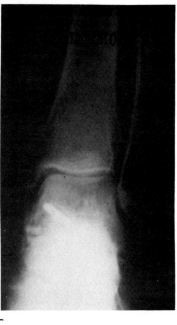

C

Fig. 16-12   A, Type II fracture of talar neck. **B,** Three months after open reduction and internal fixation, Hawkins' line is evident in subchondral dome of talus. **C,** Eighteen years after fracture, there is no evidence of avascular necrosis.

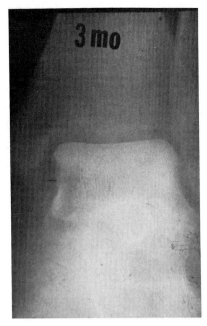

Fig. 16-13 Absence of subchondral lucency (Hawkins' line) 3 months after injury. Patient later developed avascular necrosis.

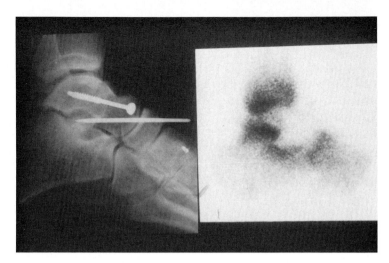

Fig. 16-14 Bone scan obtained 8 days after open reduction of type IV talar neck fracture with talonavicular dislocation showing decreased uptake.

Fig. 16-15 **A,** Type III fracture of talar neck with posteromedial displacement in 9-year-old child. **B,** After closed reduction and casting. Note also fracture of medial malleolus. **C,** Nine months after fracture, there is evidence of healing, but also avascular necrosis of talus with sclerotic and cystic changes. **D,** Six years after fracture, physis is still open and there is some healing of the avascular necrosis of talus; patient is asymptomatic.

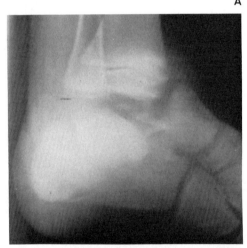

A

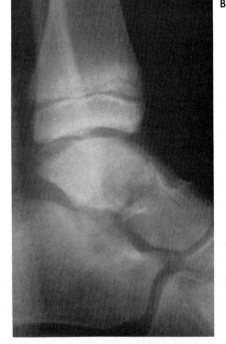

B

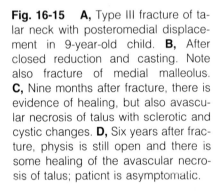

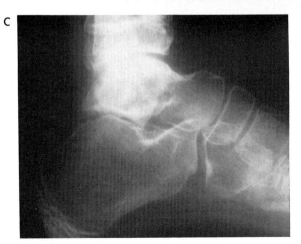

C

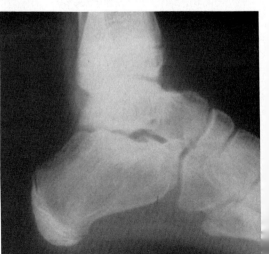

Conversely, lack of this subchondral lucency at 3 months (Fig. 16-13) indicates that avascular necrosis has occurred, and bone scanning may show decreased uptake (Fig. 16-14). The avascular process in children is different from that in adults in that it generally progresses from a sclerotic lesion in the dome and body of the talus to a cystic lesion on roentgenogram to spontaneous resolution 2 to 3 years after injury (Fig. 16-15). Most children with avascular necrosis after talar neck fracture do not require surgery, and either nonweight bearing or a patellar tendon–bearing brace should be tried before surgery is considered. Malunion of talar neck fractures, although frequent in adults, is uncommon in children. Malunion usually occurs with the distal fragment in dorsiflexion or in a varus position and with the fibula rotated more anteriorly than normal. Traumatic arthritis in the ankle and subtalar joint after talar neck fracture develops in only a few children. Persistent drainage from infection in the talus can be a difficult problem, and established osteomyelitis may be resistant to treatment because of the cancellous nature of the bone and the disruption of the blood supply to the talus.

Operations, when necessary for avascular necrosis, malunion, or infection, include triple arthrodesis (p. 106), Blair fusion, and talocalcaneal fusion, all of which produce better results than talectomy alone.

Talar Dome and Body Fractures

Fractures of the dome and body of the talus rarely occur in children, and most are shearing injuries caused by lawn mowers, bicycle spokes, or other degloving injuries. Excision of part of the talus often is required in severe, compound shearing injuries from lawn mowers and other power equipment. The wound should be irrigated, debrided, and left open; delayed closure and skin grafting, if necessary, are performed later. The primary goal of treatment is to salvage as much length and function of the foot and ankle as possible. Large, nondisplaced, closed talar dome or body fractures can be treated satisfactorily by closed methods. If the fracture is significantly displaced, is intraarticular, and has cancellous bone attached to the fragment, open reduction and internal fixation through an anteromedial approach usually are necessary (Fig. 16-16). Osteotomy of the medial malleolus rarely is necessary for exposure of the fracture site. Care should be taken to avoid the physis in this area. Oblique or transverse cancellous screws are inserted across the body of the talus, usually without medial malleolar osteotomy. Small, displaced fragments often can be removed.

A
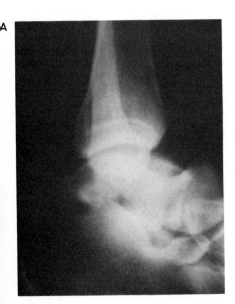

B
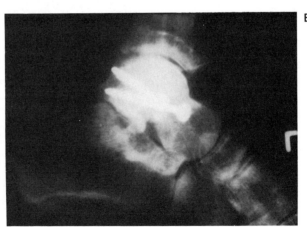

Fig. 16-16   A, Severely comminuted fracture of talar body. **B,** Eight years after open reduction and internal fixation.

Talar Osteochondral Fractures

Osteochondral lesions of the talus are primarily lesions of adolescence, often noted after a "sprained" ankle does not heal. The system of Berndt and Harty is the most commonly used classification of these fractures: stage I, a small area of subchondral compression; stage II, a partially detached fragment; stage III, a completely detached fragment remaining in the crater; and stage IV, a fragment that is detached and loose in the joint (Fig. 16-17). Lesions also are classified by location as medial, lateral, or central. Lateral lesions, which usually are related to trauma, are thin and wafer-shaped and resemble osteochondral fractures. Medial lesions generally are deep and cup-shaped and do not resemble a traumatic fracture (Fig. 16-18). Lateral lesions seem to produce more persistent symptoms and degenerative changes than medial lesions and require surgery more often.

Initial treatment should be cast immobilization (approximately 12 weeks): double, upright, patellar tendon weight-bearing brace; arch supports; or leather, lace-up ankle corsets. Surgery is performed for persistent symptoms or a loose body in the ankle joint.

Most stages I and II lesions, regardless of location, can be treated successfully without operation. Stage III medial lesions generally can be treated nonsurgically, but stage III lateral lesions have better results after surgical excision. Stage IV lesions, with the fragment loose in the joint, almost always require surgical treatment.

Three technical points are important in surgical treatment of osteochondral fractures of the talus. (1) When the osteochondral fragment appears on roentgenogram to be floating in its crater, with a proximal flake of bone that appears to be in the joint, the fragment probably is inverted in the crater, with the subchondral bone proximal in the ankle joint and the cartilaginous portion in the crater (Fig. 16-19). The cartilaginous fragment will not heal to the bone in the crater in this position, and excision is indicated. (2) The location of medial and lateral lesions, and the determination of whether they are anterior, in the middle, or posterior, are difficult to assess on lateral roentgenograms. CT scanning in the coronal (axial) plane with coronal sections through the dome and body of the talus will reveal the exact location of the

Fig. 16-17 Four types or stages of osteochondral fractures (osteochondritis dissecans of talus). Stage I, "blister"; stage II, elevated fragment but attached; stage III, fragment detached but still in crater; stage IV, displaced fragment.

Stage I

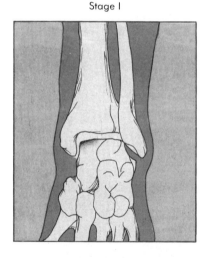

Stage II

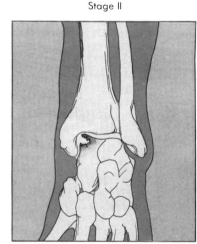

Stage III

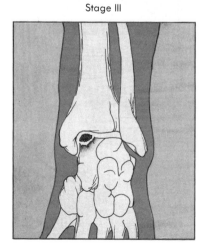

Stage IV

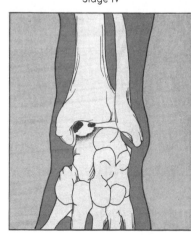

lesion and help in planning the surgical approach (Fig. 16-20). (3) Malleolar osteotomy rarely is needed to reach lateral lesions because the fibula is more posterior than the medial malleolus, but it often is necessary for medial lesions located in the middle or posterior part of the talus. The osteotomy should be made horizontally or obliquely at the plafond, and the malleolus should be predrilled to accept a cancellous screw. The malleolar fragment can be displaced with a towel clip to expose the medial osteochondral lesion.

Large fragments may be replaced and held with subchondral pins, similar to the technique used for osteochondritis of the knee (p. 801); there are, however, no long-term results of this technique and short-term results have been variable. Harper and Ralston reported experimental work with "fibrinogen" cement, in which a small amount of cement is placed in a small subchondral bony area of a large fragment and the fragment is replaced in the crater. The concept is that the uncemented peripheral edges of the fragment will unite with the underlying talus.

Types I, II, and III lesions often are difficult to see at surgery, and palpation or ballottement may be required to determine the exact location. A Keith needle or hemostat used for ballottement helps outline the extent of the lesion. Arthroscopy has been used, but it is difficult to find and define the margins of occult lesions and an arthroscope with more than 30 degrees of angulation is recommended (see discussion of arthroscopy of the ankle joint in Chapters 14 and 15). Parisien described a technique for arthroscopic excision of osteochondral lesions of the talus and reported 88% good or excellent results in 18 patients. Arthroscopic and open surgical techniques for treatment of osteochondral fractures of the talus are described in detail in Chapters 14 and 15.

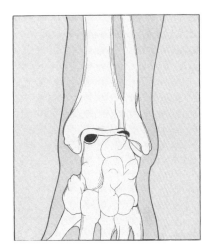

Fig. 16-18   Morphology of medial and lateral lesions (see text).

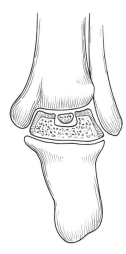

Fig. 16-19   "Floating" fragment in reality is loose fragment turned upside down in crater.

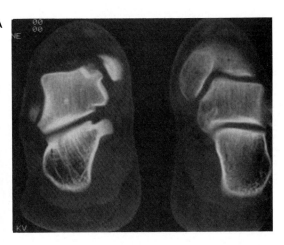

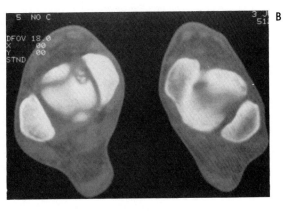

Fig. 16-20   Osteochondral lesion in anteromedial dome of talus. Crater seen in, **A**, CT scan in axial plane shows crater and fragments. **B**, Coronal CT scan will locate lesion whether anterior, middle, or posterior, which is often difficult to do on roentgenogram.

TIBIAL AND FIBULAR FRACTURES

Most fractures of the tibia and fibula can be treated with closed methods. Surgical treatment is required only when the fracture cannot be reduced, when it is open, or occasionally when it occurs in the proximal or distal tibial epiphysis. Special attention should be paid to distal tibial and fibular epiphyseal fractures because if not treated properly these fractures may result in varus and valgus angulation in older children or formation of a bony bar, causing angular deformity in younger children. In addition, incomplete metaphyseal fracture of the proximal tibia is of special concern, and fractures of the proximal tibial epiphysis also deserve special attention because of the proximity of the popliteal artery, which may be injured when the tibial shaft is posteriorly displaced.

Distal Tibial and Fibular Epiphyseal Fractures

Carothers and Crenshaw related the mechanisms of injury of distal tibial epiphyseal fractures to the Salter-Harris classification system. They found that abduction, external rotation, and plantar flexion frequently produce Salter-Harris types I and II epiphyseal fractures (Fig. 16-21), adduction produces type III or IV fractures (Fig. 16-22), and axial compression produces type V fractures. In a review of 100 ankle fractures in children, the most common fracture was the Salter-Harris type II fracture (26), followed by type III fractures (19); type I (9) and type IV (6) were relatively rare. Triplane and Tillaux fractures accounted for 12 fractures. The remaining 28 fractures were distal fibular fractures, and all were Salter-Harris type I or II, except for one type IV fracture. Most fractures of the fibular epiphysis occur in conjunction with distal tibial fractures; type III fractures usually are isolated injuries.

Fractures of the fibular epiphysis are treated for 3 to 6 weeks in a short-leg cast. Salter-Harris types I and II fractures of the distal tibial epiphysis usually are treated by closed reduction and the application of a bent-knee, long-leg cast. In young children moderate displacement after closed reduction, especially in the anteroposterior plane, is acceptable, but varus or valgus angulation in older children with type I or II fractures will not correct spontaneously (Fig. 16-23).

Most types III and IV fractures, as well as triplane and Tillaux fractures, require open reduction and internal fixation. Acceptable displacement after closed reduction of these fractures has not been established, although surgery has been recommended for displacement of 2 to 3 mm or more. Open reduction and internal fixation are justified if they can improve a less than satisfactory closed reduction (Fig. 16-24). The use of tomograms and CT scanning can help determine acceptable displacement.

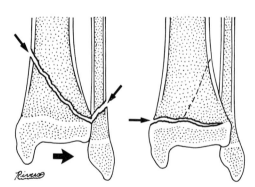

Fig. 16-21 Salter-Harris type II epiphyseal fractures are produced by external rotation, abduction, and plantar flexion forces. (Redrawn from Ogden JA: Skeletal injury in the child, Philadelphia, 1982, Lea & Febiger.)

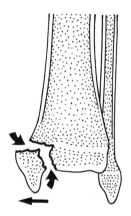
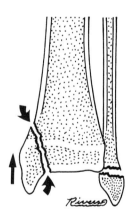

Fig. 16-22 Salter-Harris types III and IV fractures are produced by adduction forces (supination inversion). (Redrawn from Ogden JA: Skeletal injury in the child, Philadelphia, 1982, Lea & Febiger.)

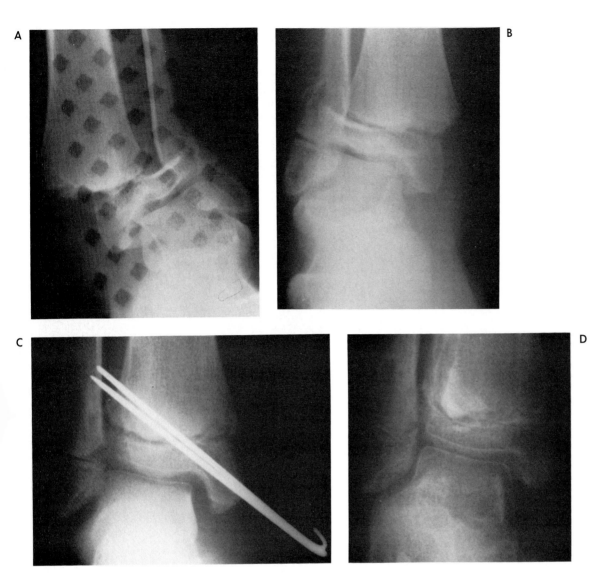

Fig. 16-23 Open reduction of Salter-Harris type I fracture. **A,** Before treatment. **B,** After closed reduction residual angulation is 17 degrees in this older child, **C,** After open reduction and internal fixation with smooth pins; flap of periosteum was found caught in fracture. **D,** At early follow-up no evidence of bony bridge is seen.

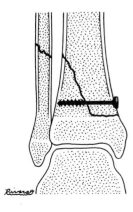

Fig. 16-24 Cancellous screw fixing large metaphyseal spike of Salter-Harris type II fracture, treated by open reduction and internal fixation because closed reduction was unacceptable. (Redrawn from Weber, BG, and Sussenbach, F: Malleolar fractures. In Weber BG, Brunner C, and Freuler F, editors: Treatment of fractures in children and adolescents, New York, 1980, Springer-Verlag.)

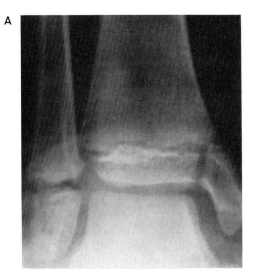
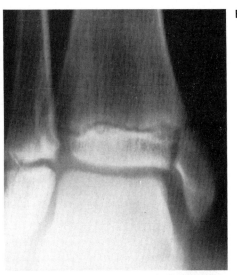
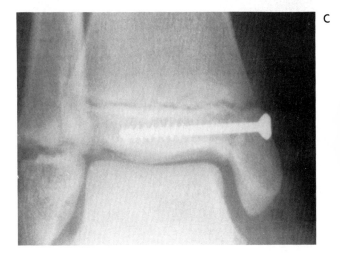

Fig. 16-25 **A** and **B,** Roentgenogram and tomogram of displaced type III fracture of the medial malleolus and type I fracture of lateral malleolus. **C,** After open reduction of medial malleolar fracture fixed with threaded screw through only the physis.

Fig. 16-26 Pins inserted across physis. **A,** Smooth pins cross physis in Salter-Harris type III fracture. **B,** At time of union and pin removal. **C,** At 2 years, symmetric growth (note parallel "injury line" proximally) and no bony bridge formation. However, parallel transverse pins are preferred when possible.

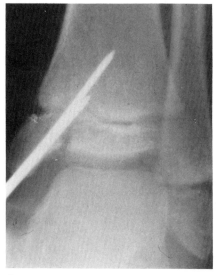
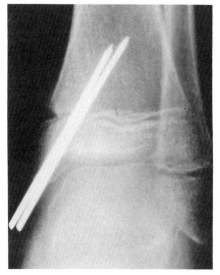
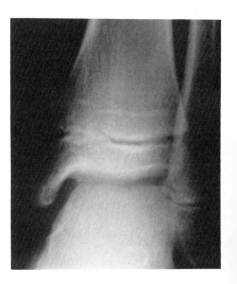

A

B

C

A

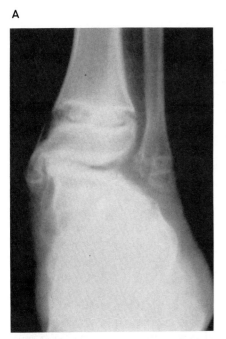

B

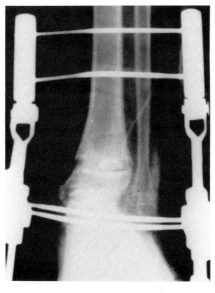

C

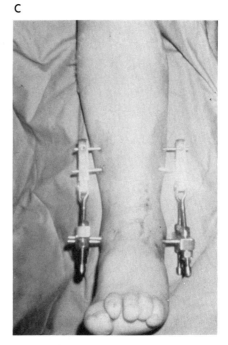

D

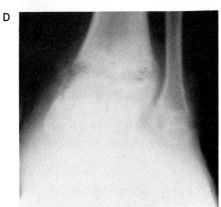

Fig. 16-27   Severe epiphyseal injury caused by lawn mower. **A,** Severe injury with loss of talar dome and part of distal tibia and separation of distal tibial physis. **B** and **C,** Roentgenogram and photograph at time of compression arthrodesis with use of Calandruccio triangular compression clamp. **D,** Solid fusion with physis still open.

Types III and IV fractures are almost always medial at the plafond. Often a tiny triangular piece of bone is present on the metaphyseal side in type IV fractures. This piece of bone should be removed at open reduction to aid exposure of the physis and perhaps prevent the formation of a bony bar in this area. Pins should not cross the physis unless absolutely necessary for fixation (Fig. 16-25). According to Rang and to Weber and Sussenbach, the perichondral ring may be avulsed by a minor fracture or ligamentous injury and may cause peripheral growth arrest and angular deformity.

Hynes and O'Brien, in a study of 26 Salter-Harris types II and III distal tibial epiphyseal fractures, noted the development of a sclerotic line of growth disturbance that appeared 6 to 12 weeks after fracture, and they suggest that the likelihood of growth arrest can be determined from the presence and displacement of these lines. In their series, if the line extended across the whole width of the metaphysis in both planes, and if the line continued to grow away from the physis remaining parallel to it, growth disturbance did not occur (Fig. 16-26). Patients without this formation and displacement of the line had abnormal growth resulting in varus angulation. They point out that previous reports have indicated that growth arrest cannot be determined before 18 months after injury, and they believe their method can predict the growth pattern of the physis as early as 3 months after injury.

Severe open ankle fractures often are produced by high-velocity motor vehicular accidents or lawn mower injuries and may involve the distal tibial epiphysis and the body of the talus. The result is epiphyseal arrest and joint roughening. Infection may develop after open fractures, and external fixators can be used initially until the wound is clean. Bony bar resection (p. 67) or osteotomy (p. 55) may be required for angular deformity, and ankle fusion may be required for severe joint involvement or infection (Fig. 16-27). If fusion is required, the physis should be preserved by using compression clamps proximal to the physis (p. 73). Interposition of iliac bone graft, as described by Chuinard and Peterson (p. 74), may be added to the fusion technique.

Open reduction and internal fixation

▶ *Technique.* Place the patient supine on the operating table; prepare and drape in the usual fashion and use a tourniquet. Make a straight longitudinal incision over the medial malleolus, anteriorly and slightly laterally, for approximately 4 cm. Carry the soft tissue dissection down to the fracture. Clear all soft tissue from the area, but preserve the periosteum if possible. Gently expose the fracture. Remove any interposed soft tissue from within the fracture, especially periosteum and small bony fragments. Expose the ankle joint anteriorly, and with the aid of a bone holder, reduce the fracture anatomically. If the fracture is a Salter-Harris type IV with a small metaphyseal spike, remove the spike to better see the reduction and prevent a later bony bridge at the periphery. Insert small, parallel, smooth Steinmann pins horizontally across the fracture. Do not cross the physis unless necessary. Use a cancellous screw if desired, making sure, however, that the threads do not damage the physis and the screw is horizontal across the fracture (Fig. 16-28). Check the reduction and pin or screw placement with roentgenograms. Reduce manually any fibular fracture, close the wound, and apply a long-leg, bent-knee cast with the ankle in neutral position.

▶ *Postoperative management.* Weight bearing is not permitted for 4 to 6 weeks, depending on the age of the patient. Then a short-leg, weight-bearing cast is worn for 3 weeks. The pins or screw can be removed at 6 to 8 weeks.

Triplane Fractures

Triplane fractures are caused by an external rotational force and are considered a combination of Salter-Harris types II and III fractures (Fig. 16-29). Marmor first coined the term *triplane fracture of the distal part of the tibia* in 1970 in his description of lesions consisting of three fragments: (1) the anterolateral portion of the distal tibial epiphysis, (2) the remainder of the epiphysis (anteromedial and posterior portions) with an attached posterolateral spike of the distal tibial metaphysis, and (3) the remainder of the distal tibial metaphysis and tibial shaft. The fracture lines run in three planes: coronal, transverse, and sagittal. Cooperman et al in 1978 called attention to two-part fractures with fracture lines in three planes. Dias and Giegerich related both these lesions to pure external rotation of the foot without pronation or supination and classified them as grade I (triplane fracture) and grade II (triplane fracture with fibular fracture). They found that three-part fractures occurred in younger patients and required surgical treatment more often than did two-part fractures.

Closed reduction usually can be achieved by internal rotation of the foot and immobilization in a long-leg cast. If closed reduction cannot be achieved, open reduction and internal fixation are indicated. Because of the complex fracture pattern and large fragments, reduction often is difficult and extensive dissection is necessary. For three-part fractures, open reduction of both the Salter-Harris type II and type III components is necessary. Physeal arrest and angular deformity are uncommon after triplane fractures because they generally occur in older children, but these complications may occur.

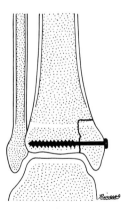

Fig. 16-28 Salter-Harris type III or IV fracture should be fixed by horizontal pins or cancellous bone screws not involving physis. (Redrawn from Weber BG and Sussenbach F: Malleolar fractures. In Weber BG, Brunner C, and Freuler F, editors: Treatment of fractures in children and adolescents, New York, 1980, Springer-Verlag.)

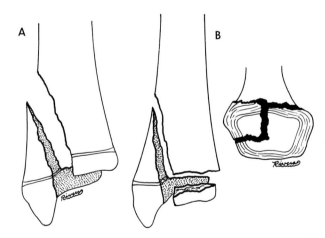

Fig. 16-29 **A,** Example of two-fragment triplane fracture, which is Salter-Harris type IV fracture. **B,** Example of three-fragment triplane fracture, consisting of Salter-Harris type II and III fractures. (Redrawn from Rockwood CA, Jr, Wilkins KE, and King RE: Fractures in children, Philadelphia, 1984, JB Lippincott Co.)

Open reduction and internal fixation

▲ *Technique (Dias and Giegerich).* Make a medial longitudinal incision over the distal metaphyseal area of the tibia down to the ankle joint. Expose the fracture fragments, but do not resect any periosteum. Examine the fracture gap, and make sure that no periosteum is inverted into it. Reduce the metaphyseal fragment. If the reduction is not anatomic, do not use internal fixation at this time, but proceed to the lateral fragment. If, however, the reduction is satisfactory, insert two cancellous screws parallel and transverse across the metaphyseal fragment. The triplane fracture now has been converted to a Tillaux fracture, or a Salter-Harris type III fracture laterally. Make an an-

terolateral longitudinal incision, expose the lateral fragment, and reduce it anatomically, making sure no periosteum is caught within the fracture. Insert smooth pins transversely across the fracture, or use a cancellous bone screw making sure the threads do not damage the physis (Fig. 16-30). Confirm the reduction by inspecting the joint. Also confirm the reduction and the placement of the pins by roentgenograms. Close the wounds, and apply a long-leg cast.

▲ *Postoperative management.* Weight bearing is not permitted for 8 weeks. At 6 weeks the long-leg cast is removed and a short-leg, nonweight-bearing cast is applied. The pins are removed at 8 weeks if necessary.

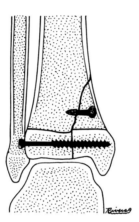

Fig. 16-30 Example of triplane fracture with medial metaphyseal spike and lateral Tillaux fracture both fixed with transverse screws.

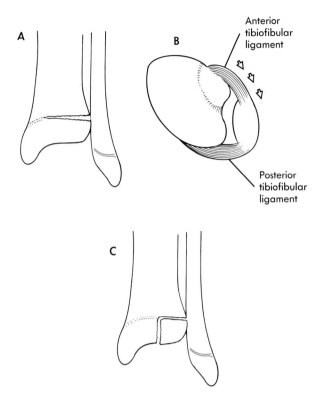

Fig. 16-31 Mechanism of injury in Tillaux fracture. **A,** Physis in older child closing medially but still open laterally. **B,** External rotational force causes anterior tibiofibular ligament to avulse epiphysis anterolaterally. **C,** Avulsion produces Salter-Harris type III fracture because medial part of physis is closed. (From Rang M: Children's fractures, ed 2, Philadelphia, 1983, JB Lippincott Co.)

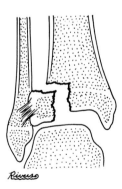

Fig. 16-32 Tillaux fracture. See Fig. 16-31 for mechanism of injury. (Redrawn from Weber BG and Sussenbach F: Malleolar fractures. In Weber BG, Brunner C, and Freuler F: Treatment of fractures in children and adolescents, New York, 1980, Springer-Verlag.)

Tillaux Fracture

A fracture that occurs primarily in older adolescents was originally described by Tillaux and is caused by the same external rotational mechanism as the triplane fracture. The external rotation places stress on the anterior tibiofibular ligament, causing avulsion of the distal tibial physis anterolaterally (Fig. 16-31). This fracture occurs after the medial part of the physis has closed (Fig. 16-32) but before the lateral part closes. The fracture line runs through the physis, across the epiphysis, and distally into the joint, creating a Salter-Harris type III or IV fracture. Most juvenile Tillaux fractures can be reduced with gentle internal rotation, but displaced fractures (Fig. 16-33) usually require open reduction and internal fixation. The fracture fragment pulled off by the anterior tibiofibular ligament is almost always anterior, and osteotomy of the fibula is not necessary for exposure.

Open reduction and internal fixation

▶ *Technique.* Expose the type III or IV fracture anterolaterally through a 6-cm anterolateral incision. Gently clean and observe the fracture fragments. Take care not to disrupt the periosteum, but remove it from within the fracture site. Then with a bone holder, gently reduce the fracture. Check the reduction by examining the fragment in the ankle joint. Insert two smooth pins parallel or a small cancellous screw transversely across the fracture but not penetrating the physis. Check the reduction with roentgenograms, close the wound, and apply a long-leg cast with the knee bent.

▶ *Postoperative management.* Weight bearing is prohibited for 6 to 10 weeks, and any subcutaneous smooth pins should be removed at 4 to 6 weeks, depending on the age of the child.

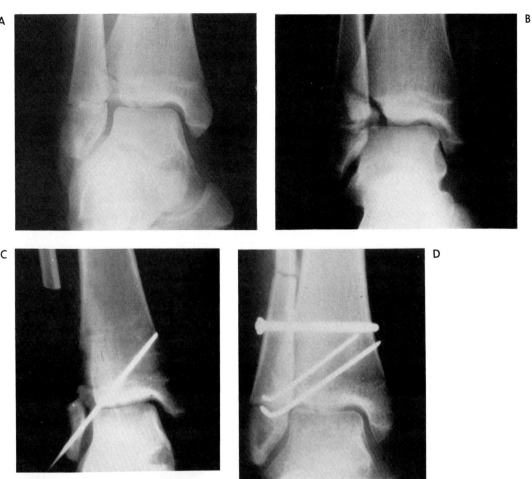

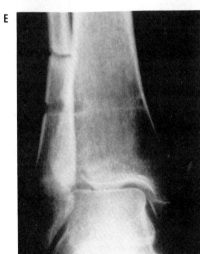

Fig. 16-33 Tillaux fracture. **A,** Fracture at time of injury. **B,** At 6 weeks there is no evidence of union and joint is incongruous. **C,** Open reduction was carried out through posterolateral approach of Gatellier and Chastang. Fibular fragment was removed unintentionally because iatrogenic fracture occurred through physis distally. This approach, for this reason, and because this fracture is almost always anterior, should not be used in children. **D,** Fixation of fracture with two smooth pins and fibular fragment with diastases screw. **E,** At 1 year, fracture has healed with good alignment.

Middle and Distal Tibial Shaft Fractures

Fractures of the shaft of the tibia, with or without associated fibular fractures, usually can be treated by closed reduction and casting, as can distal tibial metaphyseal fractures. Because of the possibility of compartment syndromes, tibial and fibular fractures should not be treated casually. If vascular injury is suspected, a soft tissue dressing should be applied instead of a circular cast and the extremity should be monitored with a wick catheter or some other compartment-pressure measuring device. If swelling is extreme and compartment syndrome seems imminent, an external fixator may be used to stabilize the fracture. Surgical treatment of tibial and fibular fractures in the child is indicated for fractures that cannot be managed by closed means, open tibial fractures, or nonunion of tibial fractures (Fig. 16-34). Shannak, in a study of 117 tibial shaft fractures treated by above-knee casts (with or without traction), found that initial shortening of up to 10 mm was compensated wholly or partially by growth acceleration, varus deformities up to 15 degrees underwent spon-

taneous correction, valgus deformity and posterior angulation persisted to some degree, and rotational deformities, particularly internal rotation, persisted.

Rarely, intramedullary nailing may be indicated because of inability to obtain or maintain reduction in the older child or for multiple pathologic fractures in the younger child, such as occur in osteogenesis imperfecta or congenital pseudarthrosis of the tibia. The proximal and distal physes, if open, must be avoided. Intramedullary nailing has been reported to be successful in stabilizing severely comminuted tibial fractures so that union is obtained without angular deformity. If possible, closed techniques of nail insertion should be used, with a small incision over the fracture site if necessary for adequate reduction of the fracture. Bailey-Dubow rods (p. 379) or larger intramedullary nails (p. 28) may be used, but the intramedullary canal of the tibia must be carefully measured because the smallest commercially available intramedullary rod at present is 9 mm in diameter (Russell-Taylor Delta tibial nail).

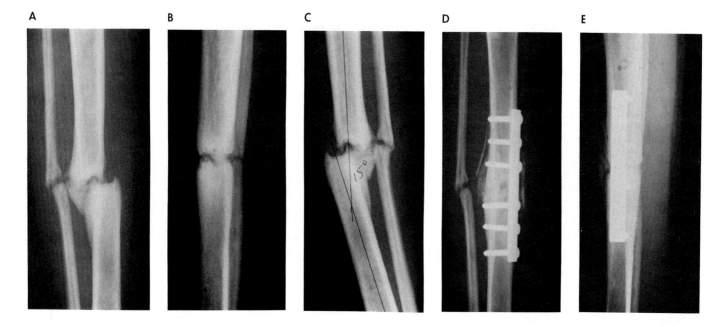

Fig. 16-34   Nonunion of tibia and fibula in child. **A** and **B,** Nonunion before treatment. **C,** Stress roentgenogram showing motion at fracture. **D** and **E,** Early union after bone grafting and compression plate fixation.

Proximal Tibial Metaphyseal Fractures

The initial concern in displaced fractures of the proximal tibial metaphysis is the proximity of the posterior tibial artery and the possibility of damage to the vasculature of the leg (see p. 864). The most serious concern after reduction is the development of a valgus angular deformity, which may occur after nondisplaced fractures of the proximal tibial metaphysis, with or without an associated proximal fibular fracture. Roentgenograms show a benign greenstick nondisplaced fracture in a child between the ages of 3 and 8 years that heals uneventfully with apparently satisfactory alignment after cast immobilization. Later, significant valgus angulation of the tibia is noted in comparison with the opposite extremity.

Numerous theories have been advanced to explain the development of this valgus angulation:

1. Inadequate reduction of fractures initially angulated by trauma. Rang believes that the valgus angulation occurs at the time of fracture and that roentgenograms taken in the cast do not reveal the valgus angulation, especially when comparison with the contralateral extremity is not made. Bahnson and Lovell stressed the importance of accurate initial assessment and reduction.

2. Deforming forces produced by early weight bearing. Pollen postulated that weight bearing before solid union of the fracture produced the valgus angulation, and this was supported by Salter and Best.

3. Soft tissue imbalance or interposition. Tibial fractures angulate toward the side with the intact soft tissues. Houghton and Rooker showed that in rabbits division of the periosteum at certain levels can lead to valgus deformity. Weber and others believe soft tissue such as the pes anserinus interposed between the fracture fragments prevents adequate reduction and complete healing of the fracture, which causes an exaggerated stimulation of the physis on the medial side of the tibia and results in overgrowth and valgus deformity (Fig. 16-35).

4. Tethering by an intact fibula or by overgrowth of the tibia. Taylor suggested that valgus angulation does not develop when the fibula is fractured, because in his series of patients genu valgum did not develop when the fibula was involved. Other authors, including Jackson and Cozen, believe that the tibial physis is stimulated more or longer than the fibular physis, which may or may not have been fractured, causing a tethering effect as the tibia overgrows more medially than the fibula laterally.

5. Asymmetric growth of the proximal tibial physis caused by premature arrest of the lateral portion. Ogden suggested that during injury compressive forces laterally cause a Salter-Harris type V injury to the lat-

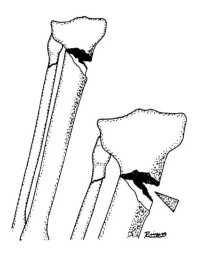

Fig. 16-35 Opening of fracture gap medially showing that periosteum or pes anserinus could be interposed. (Redrawn from Weber BG, Brunner C, and Freuler F, editors: Fractures in children and adolescents, New York, 1980, Springer-Verlag.)

eral physis, resulting in asymmetric growth between the medial and lateral aspects of the lateral tibia.

6. Asymmetric growth stimulation of the medial proximal tibia caused by asymmetric vascular response. Several authors, including Green, Herring, and Moseley, Ogden, and Jordan et al, have postulated that an unbalanced vascular healing response occurs after injury to the metaphysis, causing the medial side of the tibia to outgrow the lateral side. Zionts et al reported that technetium bone scanning in one patient 5 months after injury demonstrated increased uptake at the proximal tibial physis with proportionally greater uptake on the medial side, which suggests a relative increase in vascularity and consequent overgrowth of the medial portion of the proximal tibial metaphysis.

Although no one of these proposed etiologic factors can be implicated definitively, all may be contributing factors to the development of valgus deformity after proximal tibial metaphyseal fractures. This controversy about the cause of the deformity has led to conflicting treatment recommendations. For most nondisplaced fractures a straight-leg cast should be applied and frequent roentgenograms of the fractured tibia should be compared with the contralateral tibia to detect any valgus angulation. The cast should be wedged into a corrected position if valgus angulation occurs. Robert et al recommend reduction with the patient under general anesthesia for any fracture with a break in the medial cortex and even minimal valgus deformity. If the medial gap and valgus angulation persist, they recommend open reduction through a medial approach. Skak et al also suggest that the only indication for surgical treatment is a wide medial gap that persists after closed reduction. Because these fractures usually occur in children between the ages of 3 and 8 years, when physiologic valgus is at a maximum, the placement of the fractured tibia in slightly less valgus than the opposite tibia sometimes is appropriate. If interposition of soft tissues is strongly suspected or is confirmed by appropriate valgus stress roentgenograms that show gapping of the fracture site, removal of the soft tissues, including the periosteum and pes anserinus, as advocated by Weber et al (p. 861), is indicated.

Regardless of the method of treatment, valgus angulation may increase after union of the fracture, even as late as 12 months after treatment. Some spontaneous correction can be expected in most young children for as long as 3 years after injury, most probably because of the normal correction of physiologic valgus in children between the ages of 3 and 8 years. Bracing may augment this natural correction of physiologic genu valgum, and Skak reported bracing to be of some benefit in several of his patients. Robert et al found that the valgus tended to stabilize within a year after its appearance and recommended observation as initial treatment. Osteotomy of the proximal tibia (p. 50) should be performed only for significant deformity (more than 15 degrees of valgus angulation on standing roentgenogram compared with opposite tibia) and should be correlated to the age of the child, the normal physiologic valgus, and the severity of the deformity. Osteotomy will correct the angular deformity but also may stimulate the medial side of the tibia and cause the deformity to recur. Of 15 tibial valgus deformities treated by osteotomy reported in the literature (Aadalen, Parsch et al, Jackson and Cozen, Balthazar and Pappas, and Robert et al), 14 (93%) recurred (Fig. 16-36). Because of this high incidence of recurrence and the risks associated with osteotomy, Roberts et al do not recommend osteotomy but prefer correction of persistent deformity by medial tibial epiphysiodesis (p. 219) at puberty. Bo-

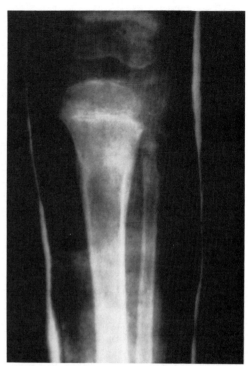

A

Fig. 16-36 **A,** Undisplaced proximal tibial fracture in 4-year-old immediately after casting. **B,** At 16 months, standing roentgenogram shows significant valgus deformity compared with opposite limb. **C,** After varus osteotomy. **D,** At time of healing of osteotomy. **E,** At 4 years, standing roentgenogram reveals acceptable result, but valgus deformity has recurred mildly.

wen et al reported good results with 16 unilateral partial epiphysiodeses for genu varum and genu valgum. They used both open and percutaneous techniques to ablate a peripheral 1 cm margin of the physis, allowing normal growth of the remainder of the physis to correct the angular deformity. Their best results were obtained when a predictive growth chart was used to determine appropriate bone age for the procedure.

B

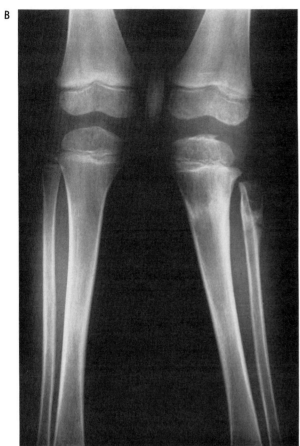

C

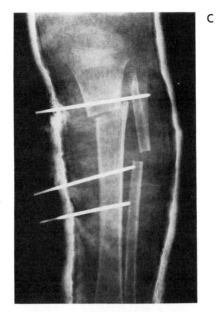

E

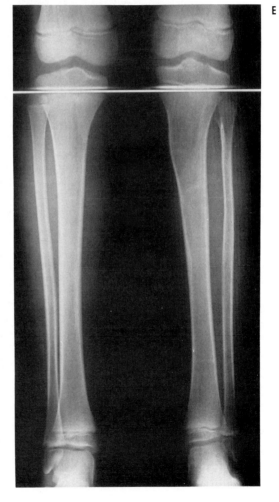

D

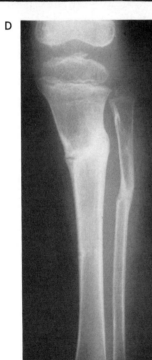

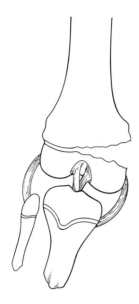

Fig. 16-37   Major ligamentous attachments of distal femoral and proximal tibial epiphyses.

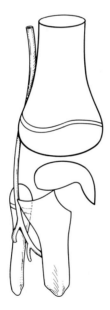

Fig. 16-38   Salter-Harris types I and II fractures with posterior displacement of tibial shaft may injure popliteal artery.

Proximal Tibial Epiphyseal Fractures

Separations of the proximal tibial epiphysis (Fig. 16-37) are much less common than those of the distal femoral epiphysis because there are fewer ligamentous attachments to the proximal tibial epiphysis than to the distal femoral epiphysis. They occur most often in adolescents, particularly those engaged in athletics. The primary concern in these fractures is the status of the popliteal artery, which may be injured in Salter-Harris types I and II fractures because of the close proximity of the posteriorly displaced tibial shaft (Fig. 16-38). Roentgenograms may not accurately reveal the extent of injury, but CT scanning and tomographic examination will help determine the amount of displacement. Stress roentgenograms also may help in the diagnosis of nondisplaced type I fractures (Fig. 16-39). Types I and II fractures generally can be treated with closed reduction and cast immobilization in a bent-knee cast. Type III fractures are of two types: one basically a tibial plateau fracture (Fig. 16-40, *A*) and the other a type III fracture beginning at the epiphysis of the tibial tuberosity and extending up into the joint and across the proximal tibial epiphysis (Fig. 16-40, *B*). The latter are large tongue-type fractures extending from the medial to lateral side of the knee, lifting the tibial tuberosity and proximal tibial epiphysis anteriorly. A rare Salter IV fracture is a more extensive type of plateau fracture or tongue type with a metaphyseal extension (spike) (Fig. 16-41). These fractures almost always require open reduction and internal fixation. For both type III fractures the exposure required is extensive and should be undertaken only after complete understanding of the anatomy. Fixation with cancellous or cannulated screws is used for most fractures (Fig. 16-42).

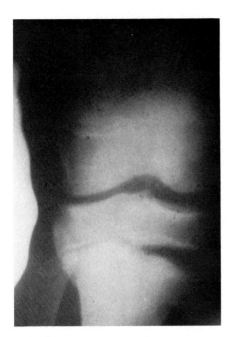

Fig. 16-39   Stress anteroposterior roentgenogram revealing Salter-Harris type I fracture that was undisplaced and unrecognizable otherwise.

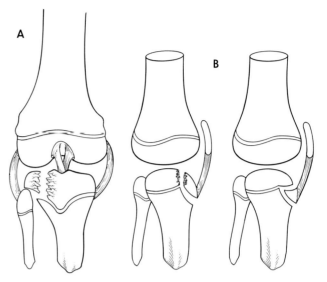

Fig. 16-40   Salter-Harris type III fracture of proximal tibial epiphysis. **A,** Fracture analogous to tibial plateau fracture. **B,** *left,* Fracture through tibial tuberosity and across epiphysis into knee joint somewhat similar to, but with different prognosis from, *right,* avulsion of epiphysis of tibial tuberosity.

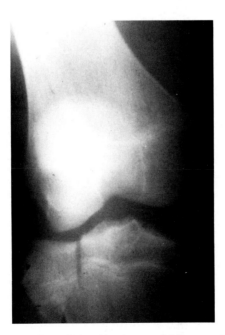

Fig. 16-41   Rare Salter-Harris type IV fracture is more extensive type of plateau fracture or tongue type with a metaphyseal extension (spike).

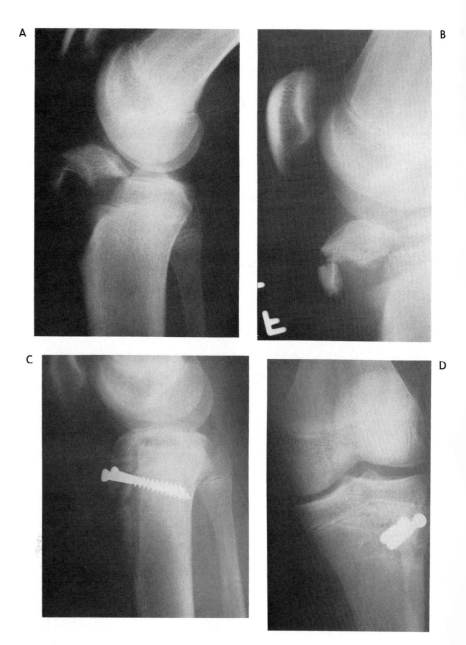

Fig. 16-42   Salter-Harris type III fracture of proximal tibial epiphysis. **A** and **B,** Oblique and lateral roentgenograms before treatment show severe displacement. **C** and **D,** After open reduction and internal fixation with cancellous screws.

Open reduction and internal fixation

▲ *Technique.* Prepare and drape the knee in the usual fashion. Inflate the tourniquet. Make a long medial or lateral parapatellar incision, depending on the location of the fracture. Carry the soft tissue dissection down to the fracture site and expose the fracture widely. The Salter-Harris type III or IV injury frequently is a tongue type of fracture anteriorly with the entire tibial tuberosity elevated and hinged posteriorly. Dissect both medially and laterally into the joint until the epiphyseal fracture is seen. It may be located in the midportion of the joint or even posteriorly. Elevate the entire epiphyseal fragment. Wash out any debris, and remove all soft tissues such as periosteum from the fracture site so they do not impede the reduction. Now reduce the fracture anatomically. This should be similar to closing a hinge, and if any soft tissue is entrapped, the hinge will not close completely when the knee is extended. After the reduction, observe for joint congruity and reduction of the fracture at its peripheral margins.

In a vertical fracture, insert transverse pins for fixation. Because the patient usually is an older child, threaded pins, cannulated screws, or cancellous bone screws can be used. In younger children use smooth pins transversely or horizontally. Irrigate the wound copiously with saline. Close the wound in the usual manner, and apply a bent-knee cast.

▲ *Postoperative management.* The cast remains in place for 4 to 6 weeks. At 2 weeks a window should be made in it for removal of sutures and change of dressing. Gentle mobilization of the knee should be started between 4 and 6 weeks, depending on the age of the child.

• • •

Complications of proximal tibial epiphyseal fractures include anterior compartment syndrome, transient and permanent peroneal nerve palsy, arterial thrombosis, angular deformity, and leg length inequality. Any suggestion of ischemic changes, compartment syndrome, or peroneal palsy requires immediate action, including bivalving of the cast and appropriate testing or consultations. Anterior compartment syndrome usually is indicated by pain out of proportion to the severity of the injury, especially when, after the cast is bivalved, the most tender area is over the muscles rather than over the fracture site. The anterior compartment muscles may be very hard on palpation; other signs may include sensory deficit in the dorsum of the foot and weakness or paralysis of the extensor hallucis longus, extensor digitorum longus, and anterior tibial muscles. Passive plantar flexion of these muscles elicits extreme pain. Measurement of compartment pressures should be instituted, and if there is a pressure rise to 30 mm Hg, fasciotomy is indicated. Posterior compartment syndrome is characterized by pain, plantar hyperesthesia, weakness of toe flexion, pain on passive toe extension, and tension of the fascia between the tibia and the triceps surae muscles in the distal medial part of the leg.

Double-incision fasciotomy. Mubarak and Hargens believe that a double-incision fasciotomy is preferable to fibular ostectomy-fasciotomy because it is simpler (requiring minimal dissection), faster, and relatively safer and it leaves the fibula intact. They believe the use of two incisions also has several advantages over fasciotomy performed through a single, long skin incision: better cosmesis, accessibility to any specific combination of fewer than four compartments through any portion of the double-incision technique, possibility of double-compressive dermotomy if required, and ease of debridement of necrotic muscle if needed. A fasciotome designed to incise the fascia without a long skin incision is commercially available. Mubarak and Hargens recommend intraoperative measurement of compartment pressure to verify complete decompression. Limited skin incisions (approximately 15 cm in length) may be used if compartment pressure is monitored during surgery; if not, longer skin incisions (20 to 25 cm in length) should be used.

▶ *Technique (Mubarak and Hargens).* To approach the anterior and/or lateral compartments, place the anterolateral incision halfway between the fibular shaft and tibial crest, approximately over the anterior intermuscular septum dividing the anterior and lateral compartments (Fig. 16-43). Undermine the skin edges proximally and distally to allow wide exposure of the fascia. Make a transverse incision just through the fascia to identify the anterior intermuscular septum separating the anterior compartment from the lateral compartment. Locate and protect the superficial peroneal nerve lying in the lateral compartment next to the septum. Using 12-inch Metzenbaum scissors, open the anterior compartment fascia. With the tips opened slightly, push the scissors in the direction of the great toe distally and proximally toward the patella. If there is any question that the tip of the scissors has strayed from the fascia, leave the instrument in place and make a small incision over the tip of the scissors; if the fasciotomy is incomplete, further re-

lease can be performed through this incision. Make the lateral compartment fasciotomy in line with the fibular shaft, directing the scissors proximally toward the fibular head and distally toward the lateral malleolus (posterior to the superficial peroneal nerve). Both compartments should now be widely decompressed, and the superficial peroneal nerve should be intact.

Approach the superficial and deep posterior compartments through a posteromedial incision slightly distal to the first incision and 2 cm posterior to the posterior tibial margin; this location will avoid injury to the saphenous nerve and vein. Undermine the skin edges, and retract the saphenous nerve and vein anteriorly. Make a transverse incision in the fascia, and identify the septum between the deep and superficial posterior compartments. Identify the tendon of the flexor digitorum longus in the deep compartment and the tendo Achilles in the superficial posterior compartment. Decompress the superficial posterior compartment first by extending the fasciotomy proximally as far as possible and distally behind the medial malleolus. Release the deep posterior compartment distally, then proximally under the soleus bridge.

If intraoperative pressure monitoring is used, make a final pressure check of each compartment. Then pack the wounds open and apply a dressing. Immobilize the leg in a posterior splint.

▶ *Postoperative management.* Five to 7 days after fasciotomy, irrigation and debridement are performed, and generally secondary closure can be obtained. Vertical mattress sutures are best for skin closure after fasciotomy. Split-thickness skin grafting may be necessary if there is considerable swelling or further delay in closing the wound. Development of contractures is treated by posterior splinting of the ankle in neutral position.

Angular deformity can be treated by epiphysiodesis, osteotomy, or bony bar resection (see Chapter 1). Treatment of leg length inequality is discussed in Chapter 3.

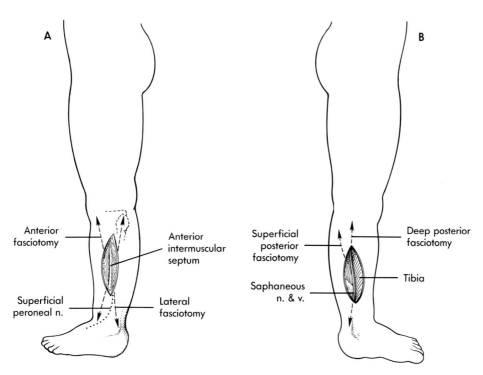

Fig. 16-43   **A,** Anterolateral incision for decompression of anterior and lateral compartments. **B,** Posteromedial incision for decompression of superficial and deep posterior compartments. (Redrawn from Mubarak SJ and Hargens AR: Diagnosis and management of compartment syndromes. In Moore IM, editor: AAOS symposium on trauma to the leg and its sequelae, St Louis, 1981, The CV Mosby Co.)

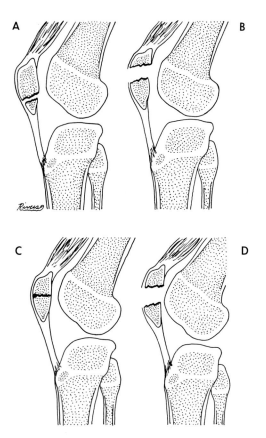

Fig. 16-44 Types of patellar fracture. **A,** Inferior pole. **B,** Superior pole. **C,** Transverse undisplaced midsubstance. **D,** Transverse displaced midsubstance. (Redrawn from Ogden JA: Skeletal injury in the child, Philadelphia, 1982, Lea & Febiger.)

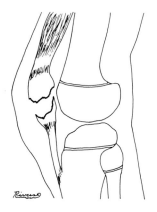

Fig. 16-45 Substantial sleeve of avulsed cartilage when seen on roentgenogram appears as only a "fleck" of bone and produces a benign appearance. (Redrawn after Houghton GR and Ackroyd CE: J Bone Joint Surg 61B:165, 1979.)

KNEE FRACTURES AND DISLOCATIONS
Patellar Fractures

Fractures of the patella are rare in children and usually occur in adolescents and older children. Osteochondral fractures, small peripheral fractures, and "sleeve"-type fractures can occur in association with acute dislocation of the patella. In adolescents, jumper's knee and Sinding-Larsen-Johansson syndrome may cause the same fractures. These are avulsion injuries of the proximal and distal poles of the patella and should be differentiated from chronic ligamentous injuries. Bipartite patella also must be distinguished from a patellar fracture. In bipartite patella the edges of the defect usually are rounded, the condition is bilateral in approximately half of children, and it is always in the superolateral quadrant of the bone. Congenital absence or hypoplasia of the patella, as seen in onychodysplasia, osteodysplasia, or nail-patella syndrome, also may be confused with patellar fracture.

Patellar fractures are classified according to location, type, and amount of displacement (Fig. 16-44). Houghton and Ackroyd described a sleeve-type fracture of the distal pole of the patella in which only a fleck of bone appears on roentgenograms, giving a falsely benign appearance. A large cartilaginous "sleeve" actually is attached to the patellar tendon and if not replaced properly, when healed and ossified, will be malaligned and will produce an abnormally elongated patella and patellar mechanism (Fig. 16-45). Transverse fractures are best seen on lateral roentgenograms with the knee flexed 30 degrees; longitudinally oriented marginal fractures are best seen on axial or skyline views.

Closed treatment is recommended for nondisplaced fractures, particularly if active extension is possible before treatment. Rang states that most patellar fractures in children can be treated with aspiration of effusion and application of a compression dressing with medial and lateral slab splints. Open reduction and internal fixation are indicated for displaced fractures with loss of active knee extension. The internal fixation may consist of a circumferential wire loop, nonabsorbable sutures through longitudinally drilled holes, screws, threaded pins, or AO tension band. Each method of fixation has its advocates, but all agree that meticulous repair of the adjacent retinacular tear is as important as accurate reduction and stable fixation of the bone fragments. In sleeve fractures the distal pole with its attached sleeve of cartilage should be carefully reduced to the main body of the patella. Houghton and Ackroyd recommend internal fixation with a modified tension-band technique.

Open reduction and internal fixation of sleeve fracture

▶ *Technique (Houghton and Ackroyd).* Place the patient supine on the operating table, and prepare the leg in the usual fashion; use a tourniquet. Approach the inferior pole of the patella through a 7-cm medial parapatellar incision, using only the distal portion. Expose the distal pole patellar fracture. Irrigate the fracture copiously with saline, and with a small curet remove any clots and loose cancellous bone. Reduce the fragment with a small bone holder. Observe the fracture fragments anteriorly, and try to observe the reduction posteriorly on the articular surface. If this is not possible, use a gloved finger to feel for any angulation or offset on the articular surface. Then perform a tension band wiring with two Kirschner wires. After reduction of the fracture, place two parallel longitudinal Steinmann pins across the fracture site. Leave them protruding approximately ¼ inch (0.5 cm) distally for easy removal. Then place a tension band wire from the superior to the inferior pole of the patella, crossing itself and incorporating the parallel pins. Tighten the wire sufficiently but not enough to overly compress and angulate the fracture fragments. Close the wound in layers and apply an appropriate cast with the knee in mild flexion.

▶ *Postoperative management.* At 3 to 4 weeks the cast is removed and range-of-motion exercises are started. The AO group recommends early motion in flexion after tension band wiring, which according to the tension band principle holds the reduction. However, this is unnecessary in a young child.

Tibial Intercondylar Eminence Fractures

The intercondylar eminence is the nonarticular bony prominence between the articular surfaces of the medial and lateral plateaus of the knee to which the anterior cruciate ligaments are attached. Meyers and McKeever classified fractures of the tibial intercondylar eminence into three types: type I, little or no displacement; type II, partially displaced with cartilaginous hinge; and type III, complete displacement (Fig. 16-46). Placement of the knee joint in full extension usually will reduce the fragment in types I and II fractures. Aspiration of the hemarthrosis from a tense knee joint also may be beneficial. A cylinder or long-leg cast is applied with the knee in full extension. Interposition of a meniscus, usually the lateral, may prevent reduction and necessitate open reduction in some type II fractures. Type III fractures also are treated initially by aspiration and extension. If reduction is achieved, a long-leg cast is applied; if not, open reduction and internal fixation are performed. A medial parapatellar incision will allow exposure of the tibial spine, anterior cruciate ligament, and anterior horns of both menisci to make sure they are not trapped beneath the fragment. Arthroscopic techniques (Chapter 15) can be used. Drill holes for the sutures should not cross the physis.

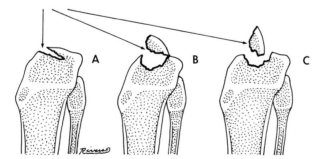

Fig. 16-46 Fractures of intercondylar eminence of tibia. **A,** Type I, avulsion fracture, nondisplaced. **B,** Type II, hinged fracture, displaced but posterior rim remains intact. **C,** Type III, completely displaced fracture. (Redrawn from Roberts JM: Fractures and dislocations of the knee. In Rockwood CA, Jr, Wilkins KE, and King RE, editors: Fractures in children, Philadelphia, 1984, JB Lippincott Co.)

Open reduction and internal fixation

▲ *Technique.* Expose the knee through the distal portion of an anteromedial parapatellar incision. Open the capsule medially to expose the fracture fragments and the defect in the proximal tibia. Examine the medial meniscus, and then with retraction examine the anterior horn of the lateral meniscus to make sure the menisci are not impeding the reduction. Place the knee in extension, and reduce the fragment after any clots and cancellous bone have been removed from the defect. Drill two holes from distal to proximal through the tibial epiphysis. Take care to drill the holes proximal to the physis. The holes should enter the joint (1) just medial and lateral to the fracture fragments or (2) into the defect and into the fragment itself if it is large enough. Pass either a 19-gauge or an 18-gauge wire, or a 1-0 nonabsorbable suture, through the distalmost portion of the anterior cruciate ligament just proximal to the fracture fragment. Now with suture carriers pass the ends of the suture through the drill holes, and tie them on themselves after the reduction is satisfactory. Flex and extend the knee to make sure the reduction is stable. Irrigate and close the wound.

▲ *Postoperative management.* A cast is applied with the knee in full extension. At 4 to 6 weeks, the cast is removed and range-of-motion exercises are started.

• • •

The most serious consequence of fractures of the intercondylar eminence of the tibia is disruption of the integrity of the cruciate ligaments. An increasing number of reports have associated ligament injuries in children with fractures of the tibial intercondylar eminence. Several authors have reported variable amounts of ligamentous laxity after these fractures, regardless of treatment methods. Baxter and Wiley, in a study of 45 fractures, reported that 51% of patients showed positive results of an anterior drawer test at follow-up and that all patients had a measurable loss of extension, ranging from 4 to 15 degrees; 64% were aware of the difference between their knees. Baxter and Wiley found that open reduction did not eliminate the cruciate laxity or persistent loss of extension.

Tibial Tuberosity Fractures

Fractures of the tibial tuberosity usually occur in older children, most often during sports or play activities and usually from sudden acceleration or deceleration of the knee extensor mechanism. By far the greatest number of these injuries occur in boys between the ages of 14 and 16 years. Watson-Jones classified these fractures as type I, a small fragment that is displaced superiorly; type II, a larger fragment involving the secondary center of ossification and the proximal tibial epiphysis, which is hinged upward; and type III, a fracture that passes proximally and posteriorly across the physis and proximal articular surface of the tibia (a Salter-Harris type III epiphyseal fracture) (Fig. 16-47). Ogden et al refined the classification, describing three types, depending on the distance of the separation from the distal tip, and two subtypes in each category, depending on the severity of displacement.

Roberts (1979) pointed out the difficulty of distinguishing this injury from Osgood-Schlatter disease and outlined differences between Osgood-Schlatter disease and traumatic avulsion of the tibial tuberosity. In Osgood-Schlatter disease the onset often is insidious, the symptoms are mild and intermittent and cause only partial disability, symptomatic and supportive treatment is all that is required, and the prognosis usually is good. In contrast, traumatic avulsions of the tibial tuberosity usually are acute injuries with immediate marked pain and swelling that make walking and standing impossible; open reduction and internal fixation often are required, with rapid healing and return to full activities.

Many of these fractures, especially types I and II fractures with minimal displacement, can be treated closed. Reduction should be performed with the knee in extension, followed by casting; if displacement of more than 0.5 cm persists, then open anatomic reduction is indicated. If closed reduction is used, serial roentgenograms, especially in the lateral plane, must be made frequently to ensure that proximal displacement does not occur because of quadriceps pull. Roberts recommends open reduction and internal fixation of all but the smallest, most minimally displaced fragment. Hand et al recommend open reduction and internal fixation in types II and III fractures and note that a large periosteal flap can prevent adequate closed reduction. Ogden et al recommend surgery for significant displacement of one or more fragments of the tuberosity anteriorly and superiorly and for extension of the fracture through the proximal tibial epiphysis into the knee joint, with disruption of the joint surface (Salter-Harris type III fracture). Displaced Salter-Harris type III fractures should be treated by open reduction and internal fixation as described for proximal tibial epiphyseal fractures (p. 867). Screw fixation can be used in large fragments in Watson-Jones types I and II avulsions of the tibial tuberosity in older children, but smooth wires or pins should be used in smaller or comminuted fragments in younger children (Fig. 16-48). A large periosteal flap may be avulsed from the adjacent metaphysis medially, laterally, or distally and should be sutured in its original position at the time of reduction. According to Ogden et al, this adds intrinsic stability to the reduction.

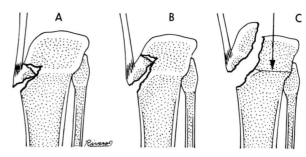

Fig. 16-47　Types of avulsion fracture of tibial tuberosity. **A,** Type I, through secondary ossification center. **B,** Type II, at junction of primary and secondary ossification centers. **C,** Type III, across primary ossification center (Salter-Harris type III) with physis near closing posteriorly. (Redrawn from Roberts JM: Fractures and dislocations of the knee. In Rockwood CA, Jr, Wilkins KE, and King RE, editors: Fractures in children, Philadelphia, 1984, JB Lippincott Co.)

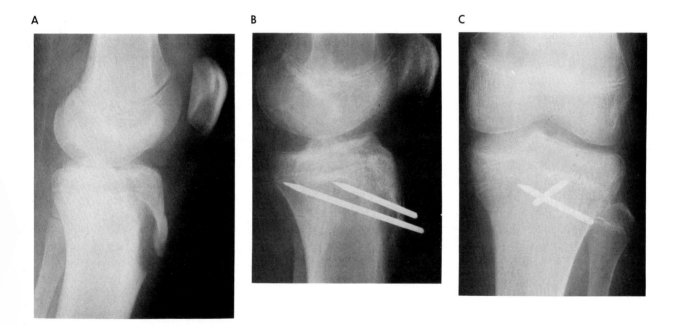

Fig. 16-48　Tibial tuberosity fracture. **A,** Watson-Jones type III fracture (Salter-Harris type III) extending into knee joint. **B** and **C,** After open reduction and internal fixation with smooth pins, avoiding physis.

Open reduction and internal fixation

▶ *Technique.* Make an anteromedial incision 5 cm long adjacent to the tibial tuberosity and parallel to the patellar tendon. Carry the dissection laterally over the tibial tuberosity and the insertion of the patellar tendon. Expose the fracture and clean its base with a curet. Do not dissect completely free the attachments of the tibial tuberosity. Identify any large periosteal flap, which may be avulsed medially, laterally, or distally. If it is frayed, resect some of it. If not, retain it for stability. Reduce the fracture with the knee in full extension. Insert two small pins across the fracture. If the fragment is large, a cancellous bone screw can be used quite satisfactorily; make sure the head of the screw is buried deeply enough not to cause chronic discomfort from contusions in the area. Check the reduction with roentgenograms. Suture any periosteal flap and close the wound in layers.

▶ *Postoperative management.* A cylinder cast is applied with the knee in full extension. At 4 to 6 weeks the cast is removed, and if smooth pins have been used, they also are removed at that time.

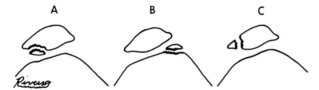

Fig. 16-49   Three locations of osteochondral fractures caused by dislocation of patella. **A,** Inferior surface of patella. **B,** Femoral condyle. **C,** Medial surface of patella. (Redrawn from Rang M: Children's fractures, Philadelphia, 1981, JB Lippincott Co.)

Osteochondral Fractures

Osteochondral fractures of the knee occur primarily on the cartilaginous surfaces of the medial or lateral femoral condyle or the patella. They may be caused by a direct blow to the front of the knee, such as a fall or kick, by tibiofemoral compression or rotation, or by acute patellar dislocation (Fig. 16-49). Most patients report hearing and feeling a distinct snap in the knee, followed by severe pain and extensive swelling. Usually a significant hemarthrosis occurs after the traumatic episode. If ligamentous instability is not present and the aspirate of the knee is sanguineous, then osteochondral fracture should be suspected, even though quite often the fragment is not bony and cannot be seen on roentgenograms. Occasionally, only a faint density or fleck of subchondral bone can be identified. This small osseous fragment usually is part of an osteocartilaginous loose body that is much larger than it appears on roentgenogram. Arthroscopic examination (p. 819) is indicated to locate, identify, and remove the loose body and to identify the defect in the patella or femur. All but exceptionally large fragments should be excised. Fragments recently displaced from the osseous crater can be replaced and fixed internally as for osteochondritis dissecans (p. 801).

"Floating Knee" Injuries

Although not actually an injury of the knee joint, floating knee describes the flail knee joint segment that results from a fracture of the shaft or adjacent metaphysis of the ipsilateral femur and tibia (Fig. 16-50). This uncommon injury in children, which results mostly from motor vehicle accidents, usually is associated with major soft tissue damage, open fractures, and head injuries. Letts et al proposed a five-part classification of these injuries (Fig. 16-51): type A, both femoral and tibial fractures are closed diaphyseal fractures; type B, one fracture is diaphyseal, one is metaphyseal, and both are closed; type C, one fracture is diaphyseal, the other is an epiphyseal displacement; type D, one fracture is open with major soft tissue injury; and type E, both fractures are open with major soft tissue injury. Their basic recommendation for treatment of these injuries is that at least one fracture (usually the tibia) must be rigidly fixed by open reduction and internal fixation. If mobilization of the child is essential, internal fixation of both fractures may be indicated. In older children intramedullary nailing may be more appropriate than plate fixation. Open fractures with major soft tissue injury should be left open and stabilized with external fixation.

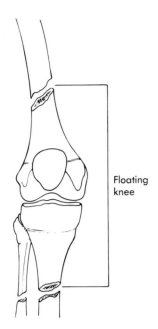

Fig. 16-50 Floating knee injury. (Redrawn from Letts M, Vincent N, and Gouw G: J Bone Joint Surg 68B:442, 1986.)

Acute Knee Dislocations

Acute dislocations of the knee and proximal tibiofibular joint are rare in children because the force necessary to produce dislocation is more likely to cause fracture of the distal femoral or proximal tibial epiphysis. In the young child dislocations of the knee seldom require surgical treatment, and closed reduction followed by cast immobilization usually yields good results. Acute knee dislocations in adolescents should be treated as those in adults; surgery is determined by the stability of the reduction. Most tibiofibular dislocations also can be treated closed. Ogden (1974) reported 43 subluxations and dislocations of the proximal tibiofibular joint, most of which were treated successfully with closed reduction. Eight patients with anterolateral dislocations, however, required arthrodesis or resection of the fibular head for persistent pain and instability. Five of six children with subluxation were successfully treated with cylinder cast immobilization for 2 to 3 weeks; the only child with recurrent symptoms had muscular dystrophy.

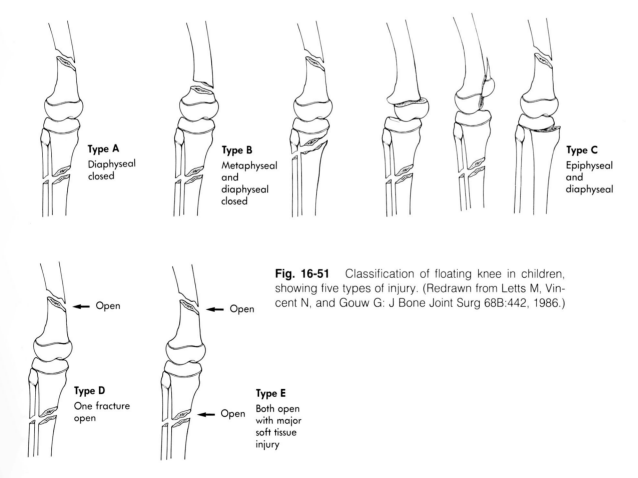

Fig. 16-51 Classification of floating knee in children, showing five types of injury. (Redrawn from Letts M, Vincent N, and Gouw G: J Bone Joint Surg 68B:442, 1986.)

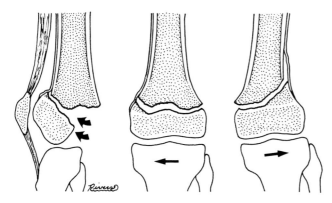

Fig. 16-52 Various angulations of distal femoral epiphyseal fractures, including posterior angulation, varus angulation, and valgus angulation. (Redrawn from Ogden JA: Skeletal injury in the child, Philadelphia, 1982, Lea & Febiger.)

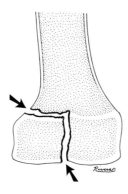

Fig. 16-53 Salter-Harris type III distal femoral epiphyseal fracture that requires anatomic reduction. (Redrawn from Ogden JA: Skeletal injury in the child, Philadelphia, 1982, Lea & Febiger.)

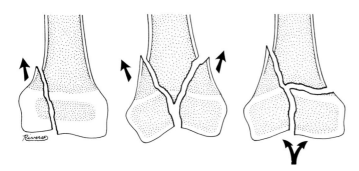

Fig. 16-54 Various types of Salter-Harris III and IV fracture-separations, including unicondylar, bicondylar, and combination of types III and IV, which is triplane fracture. (Redrawn from Ogden JA: Skeletal injury in the child, Philadelphia, 1982, Lea & Febiger.)

FEMORAL FRACTURES
Distal Femoral Epiphyseal Fractures

Fractures of the distal femoral epiphysis are less common than other epiphyseal injuries, but Salter-Harris type II fractures of the distal femoral epiphysis cause more severe epiphyseal arrests than in other parts of the skeleton. Occult Salter-Harris type V compression fractures with premature closure of the physis also are more frequent in this location, usually as the result of a "dashboard" injury.

Salter-Harris type I fractures of the distal femoral epiphysis rarely require surgical treatment. In the past many of these fractures were wagon "spoke wheel" injuries and were displaced anteriorly. Today most are nondisplaced and result from varus or valgus forces encountered in athletic activities (Fig. 16-52). Stress roentgenograms may be helpful in differentiating a collateral ligament tear from a type I epiphyseal separation.

Salter-Harris type II fractures are the most common in this location, occurring primarily in older children. Displacement is frequent, usually in the coronal plane, and physeal arrest is more frequent than in type II fractures in other locations. Makela et al, in an experimental study in rabbits, found that destruction of as little as 7% of the cross-sectional area of the distal femoral physis caused permanent growth disturbance and shortening of the femur. Roberts reported that the portion of the physis beneath the metaphyseal fracture spike (Thurston Holland sign) usually is spared. If the metaphyseal spike is medial, lateral closure of the physis may cause valgus deformity; if the spike is lateral, varus deformity may occur. Czitrom et al, in their review of distal femoral epiphyseal fractures, concluded that the Salter-Harris classification is a good indicator of the mechanism of injury and of the prognosis. Most types I and II fractures in their series did well, with an average loss of length of only 1 cm, and they attributed poor results in type II fractures to inadequate reduction or associated injuries.

Salter-Harris types III and IV fractures of the distal femoral epiphysis are rare, but exact anatomic reduction is critical in these fractures to prevent joint incongruity and bony bar development (Fig. 16-53). The metaphyseal spike of bone that occurs in Salter-Harris type IV fractures may be of various configurations (Fig. 16-54). Salter-Harris type V compression fractures usually are either unrecognized or misdiagnosed as type I fractures, and the correct diagnosis is made only after premature physeal closure.

Roberts and Rang, as well as others, have reported an avulsion injury at the edge of the physis, especially on the medial side. A small fragment, including a portion of the perichondrium and underlying bone, may be torn off the femur when the proximal attachment of the collateral ligament is avulsed. Although seemingly innocuous, this injury can result in severe angular deformity if a bony bar is formed at the most peripheral edge of the physis (Fig. 16-55).

Types I and II fractures of the distal femoral epiphysis, even if displaced, usually can be reduced closed without excessive trauma to the physis, but forceful or repeated manipulation should be avoided. Stephens et al believe that repeated manipulations, especially of type II fractures, grind the distal portion of the proximal fragment of the metaphysis into the cartilage of the physis on the distal fragment, causing premature physeal closure. After reduction with the patient under general anesthesia, a spica cast is applied. These fractures frequently redisplace, especially if initially displaced anteriorly, and varus and valgus types should be watched closely while in the cast. Closed reduction can be facilitated by the use of a traction bow on a Kirschner wire in the proximal tibia; the wire can be incorporated into the cast to maintain the reduction. Reduction should be 90% by traction or distraction and only 10% by leverage or manipulation. Perfect anatomic reduction is not required in types I and II fractures because they occur through the zone of provisional calcification of the physis, sparing the cells responsible for growth with the ossified epiphysis. If acceptable general alignment and position are obtained, then union and satisfactory growth and remodeling usually follow. Salter et al believe it better to accept less than anatomic reduction than to use forceful manipulation. Often in older children, closed reduction can be obtained but, because of inherent instability, cannot be maintained, and percutaneous cross-wire fixation inserted with the aid of image intensification may be necessary (Fig. 16-56). Occasionally, interposition of soft tissue may prevent closed reduction and necessitate open reduction and internal fixation. Several authors, however, have reported unsatisfactory results of closed reduction of displaced types I and II fractures and recommend anatomic reduction and more frequent use of internal fixation (Fig. 16-57). Lombardo and Harvey reported unsatisfactory results in type II fractures. Cassebaum and Patterson reported significant and measurable growth disturbance in 40% of distal femoral epiphyseal injuries, especially in types I and II fractures. Riseborough et al also concluded that results can be improved with more frequent use of internal fixation in these fractures.

Salter-Harris types III and IV fractures require anatomic reduction. If this cannot be achieved by closed methods, open reduction and internal fixation are in-

dicated. The amount of displacement acceptable has not been definitively determined, but most authors consider 2 mm or less acceptable for closed reduction. If displacement can be reduced by open reduction, this should be done. CT scanning and tomographic examination are helpful for determining the amount of displacement.

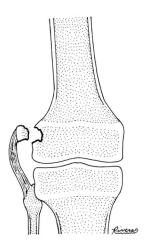

Fig. 16-55 Avulsion of attachment of fibular collateral ligament at physis, which can cause peripheral growth arrest and severe angular deformity. (Redrawn from Weber BG, Brunner C, and Freuler F: Treatment of fractures in children and adolescents, New York, 1980, Springer-Verlag.)

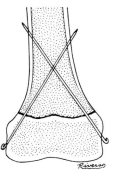

Fig. 16-56 Cross wire fixation with aid of image intensifier. Smooth pins should be used, and should penetrate opposite cortex. (Redrawn from Weber BG, Brunner C, and Freuler F: Treatment of fractures in children and adolescents, New York, 1980, Springer-Verlag.)

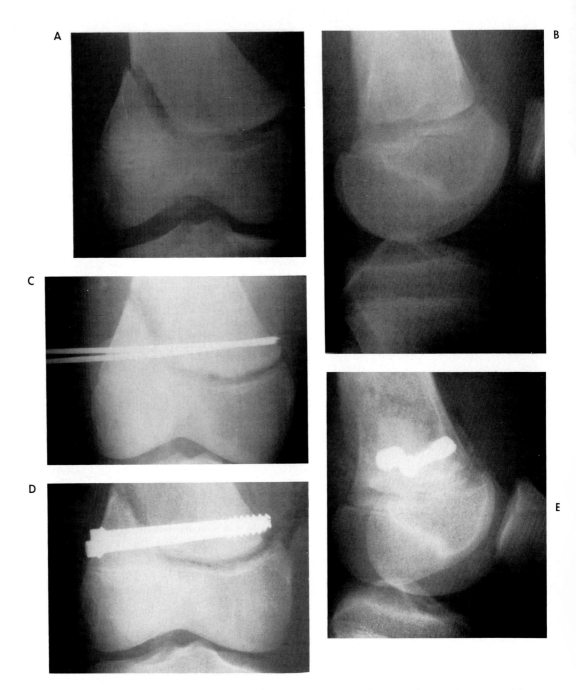

Fig. 16-57 **A** and **B**, Displaced Salter-Harris type II fracture of distal femoral epiphysis could be reduced by closed means, but reduction could not be maintained. **C**, Guide wires hold fracture reduction before placement of cannulated screw. **D** and **E**, Fixation with cannulated screw.

Closed or open reduction

▶ *Technique.* Carry out closed reduction for Salter-Harris types I and II fractures. If the reduction is satisfactory, apply a spica or long-leg cast, depending on the direction of the original displacement. If reduction cannot be maintained, insert crossed smooth 2.4-mm (3/32-inch) unthreaded Steinmann pins through the medial and lateral condyles and into the metaphysis (see Fig. 16-56).

If the Salter-Harris I or II fracture cannot be reduced closed, then expose the epiphysis through a lateral longitudinal incision. Reduce the separation as gently and completely as possible by manual traction and a minimal amount of leverage. If the use of instruments is necessary, avoid injury to the physis. Remove any interposed soft tissue, and gently maneuver the epiphysis into position. Once reduction is achieved, drill 2.4-mm (3/32-inch) unthreaded pins through the medial and lateral condyles so that they cross near the center of the physis and enter the metaphysis. Cut the pins off beneath the skin. If the pins are inserted as described and removed at 4 to 6 weeks, they are unlikely to cause any growth disturbance. If a type II or IV fracture has a large metaphyseal spike, then rather than using smooth crossed pins, drill two 2.4-mm (3/32-inch) threaded pins or a cancellous screw (Fig. 16-58) through the metaphysis of the spike into the proximal metaphyseal portion of the fracture. This should provide good stability and avoids crossing the physis (Fig. 16-59). If the fragment is too small, then cross the physis with smooth crossed pins.

If the injury is a displaced Salter-Harris type III fracture, expose the displaced condyle through either an anteromedial or anterolateral incision, depending on which condyle is involved. An arthrotomy is necessary to ensure an anatomic reduction of the articular surface. Drill a large smooth pin, a Knowles pin, or a cancellous screw into the displaced condyle to manipulate it. Gently and carefully reduce the displaced condyle into position with the pin or screw. Then insert the pin or screw transversely into the intact opposite condyle without crossing the physis. Confirm the reduction by roentgenograms. Threaded or cancellous screws can be used across the epiphysis, as long as they do not involve, penetrate, or cross the physis; however, smooth pins are preferable. These pins should be cut off beneath the skin for easy removal later.

Growth disturbance occurs frequently in type IV

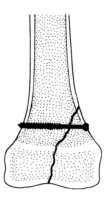

Fig. 16-58 Salter-Harris type IV fracture metaphyseal spike is secured transversely with cancellous screw. (Redrawn from Weber BG, Brunner C, and Freuler F: Treatment of fractures in children and adolescents, New York, 1980, Springer-Verlag.)

fractures if an anatomic reduction is not achieved and fixation is not secure. Arthrotomy usually is required to ensure anatomic reduction at the articular surface. Approach the fracture either anteromedially or anterolaterally, depending on which condyle is involved or on which side the metaphyseal spike is present. Reduce the articular surface and the physis precisely with smooth pins or cancellous or cannulated screws. Secure the fragment to the intact condyle, again with transverse fixation, without crossing the physis if possible. If, as in type II fractures, a large displaced metaphyseal spike is present, reduce the fracture anatomically with traction and secure the metaphyseal spike to the proximal metaphyseal fragment with threaded pins, screws, or cancellous bone screws. If the metaphyseal spike is not large enough to ensure rigid fixation or if transverse fixation of the epiphysis cannot be secured, then smooth pins can be inserted across the physis.

▶ *Postoperative management.* When the initial displacement was anterior, a single spica cast is applied with the knee in 45 degrees of flexion. These fractures are comparable to supracondylar fractures of the humerus in that the quadriceps and flexed knee are comparable to the triceps and flexed elbow in the maintenance of reduction. If the initial displacement was posterior, then the knee should be immobilized in extension. Union usually occurs at 4 to 6 weeks. The cast and Steinmann pins may then be removed and an exercise program is begun. Weight bearing can be permitted at 8 to 10 weeks.

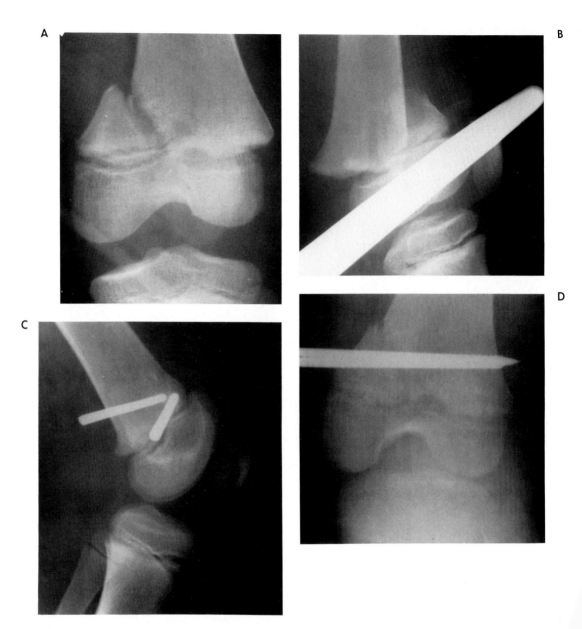

Fig. 16-59 Salter-Harris type II displaced distal femoral epiphyseal fracture. **A** and **B,** Before treatment. **C** and **D,** Closed reduction and transverse pin fixation through metaphyseal spike.

Femoral Shaft Fractures

Fractures of the femur in children generally result from high-energy trauma, such as motor vehicle accidents, and often are associated with other significant injuries. Femoral fractures can occur at birth, can be caused by child abuse, or can be pathologic. These fractures generally are classified according to location: subtrochanteric, proximal, middle, and distal thirds of the shaft, supracondylar, and distal femoral epiphyseal. The most common location is the middle third of the shaft. In proximal third and subtrochanteric fractures the proximal fragment usually is in a position of flexion, abduction, and external rotation because of the unopposed pull of the iliopsoas, abductor, and short external rotator muscles (Fig. 16-60). The adductors and extensors are intact in midshaft fractures, and the distal fragment usually is in satisfactory alignment except for some external rotation. In supracondylar fractures the distal fragment is in a position of hyperextension because of the overpull of the gastrocnemius (Fig. 16-61). These muscle imbalances are important in the alignment of the distal fragment to the proximal fragment in traction or spica cast.

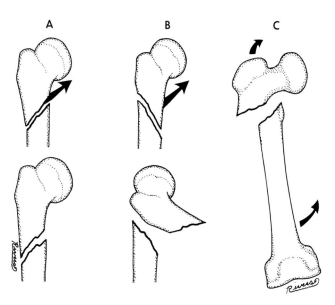

Fig. 16-60 Subtrochanteric fracture may be stable or unstable. **A,** If proximal spike of bone is posterior, often fracture is stable. **B,** Conversely, if proximal spike is anterior, often the fracture is unstable and 90-90 traction is necessary. **C,** Proximal third fracture with shaft in adducted position. (Redrawn from Rang M: Children's fractures, Philadelphia, 1981, JB Lippincott Co.)

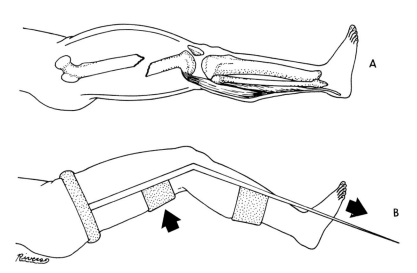

Fig. 16-61 Hyperextension of distal fragment. **A,** In supracondylar or distal third fracture, overpull of gastrocnemius hyperextends distal fragment. **B,** Thomas splint aids in reduction. (Redrawn from Rang M: Children's fractures, Philadelphia, 1981, JB Lippincott Co.)

Most femoral fractures in children are closed injuries and can and should be treated closed. A multitude of reports in the literature attest to the success of closed treatment of femoral fractures in children. Satisfactory results have been reported with cast bracing, immediate spica cast application, longitudinal skin traction, ordinary Russell traction, split Russell traction, and 90-90 skeletal traction. Staheli defines the ideal treatment of femoral fractures in children as one that controls alignment and length, does not compress or elevate the extremity excessively, is comfortable for the child and convenient for the family, and causes the least negative psychologic impact possible. Determining the ideal treatment for each child depends on the age of the child, location and type of fracture, family environment, and knowledge and ability of the surgeon, but some general guidelines can be formulated.

In children younger than 2 years of age, skeletal or skin traction is applied, depending on the size of the child and the level of the fracture. When stability, length, and alignment are achieved, a spica cast is applied. In children between the ages of 2 and 10 years, the age at which most femoral fractures occur, skeletal traction usually is appropriate, with application of a spica cast after approximately 3 weeks of traction. Aronson et al reported excellent results in 54 children with femoral fractures treated with 90-90 skeletal traction and spica casting. Their study showed that pins for skeletal traction should be placed parallel to the axis of the knee joint (Fig. 16-62) and that fractures in children older than 11 years should be reduced without overriding. The average time in traction of their patients was 24 days and the hip-spica cast was worn an average of 58 days. Guttmann and Simon described a modified pantaloon walking cast that they applied to 28 children with middle and proximal femoral shaft fractures. Their patients were treated for a mean of 20.5 days with skin or skeletal traction; all proximal fractures were treated with 90-90 traction. The walking spica cast was worn a mean of 48 days. They reported union in all fractures, minimal shortening (mean, 0.62 cm) and no lengthening, and resumption of a normal gait pattern in all children.

Immediate spica casting of femoral fractures in children has been recommended by several authors, including Clement and Colton, Griffin et al, Irani et

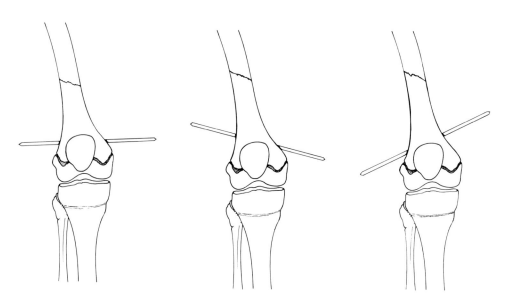

Fig. 16-62   Position of pin in traction is classified as either horizontal (optimal) or oblique. Oblique pins were further classified as *to varus* or *to valgus,* reflecting resultant pull of traction bow. (Redrawn from Aronson DD et al: J Bone Joint Surg 69A:1435, 1987.)

al, Neer and Cadman, and Staheli and Sheridan; best results with this method seem to be obtained in infants and very young children. Criticisms of its use in older children note its failure to control angulation and shortening. Cast bracing of femoral shaft fractures has been reported to give good results in children, but several studies indicate that its use should be restricted to fractures of the distal third of the shaft because of the difficulty in controlling varus and anterior angulation in proximal shaft fractures.

The treatment of femoral shaft fractures in adolescents is somewhat controversial. Historically, these fractures have been treated by nonsurgical methods, but adolescents tolerate prolonged immobilization less well than younger children, and Humberger and Eyring reported a high incidence of knee pain, angulation at the fracture site, and difficulty in maintaining length when 90-90 traction treatment was used in children older than 10 years. Recent reports indicate that intramedullary fixation of femoral shaft fractures in adolescents results in high rates of union with short hospital stays and brief periods of immobilization (Fig. 16-63). Kirby et al reported excellent results with Küntscher nailing of 13 fractures in patients with

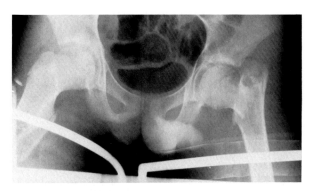

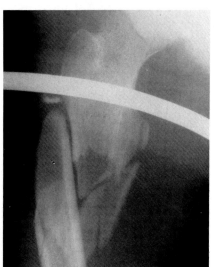

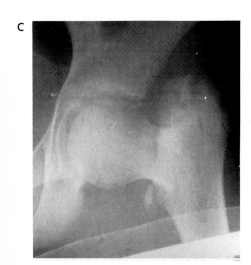

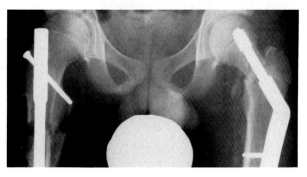

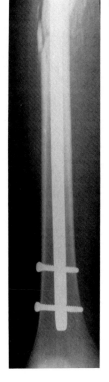

Fig. 16-63 **A,** Comminuted fracture of proximal third of left femur and cervicotrochanteric (type III) fracture of right hip in 14-year-old male involved in motor vehicle accident. **B** and **C,** Roentgenograms show comminution of femoral fracture and displacement of hip fracture. **D** and **E,** After closed reduction and intramedullary fixation of femoral fracture and internal fixation of hip fracture.

an average age of 12 years 7 months, and Mann et al successfully used Ender nailing in 16 patients of the same average age (Fig. 16-64). Ligier et al reported the use of elastic stable intramedullary nails in 123 fractures of the femoral shaft in patients ranging from 5 to 16 years of age; all fractures united and no patient complained of disability or had gait abnormalities at follow-up. Herndon et al compared nonsurgical treatment with intramedullary nailing in 45 femoral fractures and found that the incidence of malunion was significantly decreased in the fractures treated surgically. They used Küntscher nails, Ender nails, Rush rods, and interlocking nails, and although they do not recommend one device over another, they prefer interlocking nails for comminuted fractures and Ender nails in younger patients. They now prefer closed intramedullary nailing for virtually all femoral shaft fractures in patients older than 10 years. The primary difficulty with interlocking intramedullary nails is that the diameter of the nail precludes its use in small medullary canals; however, this problem is being overcome by the development of smaller-diameter interlocking nails. If intramedullary nailing is performed, the proximal and distal physes should be avoided, especially in children younger than age 10 years. As in the adult the fracture should be pulled out to length before closed nailing. If the fracture is anatomically reduced, some overgrowth of the femur can be expected in the younger child. The technique of intramedullary nailing of the femur is described on p. 29.

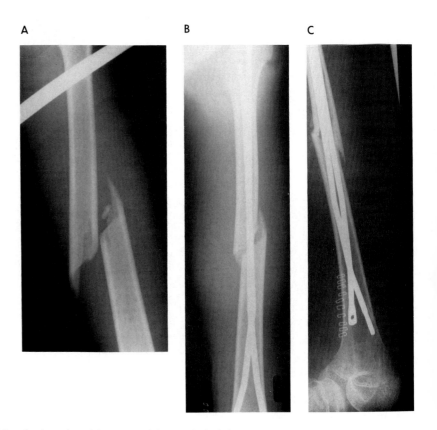

A   **B**   **C**

Fig. 16-64   **A,** Angulated fracture of femoral shaft in severely spastic 9-year-old child with extreme flexion contractures. **B** and **C,** After fixation with percutaneous intramedullary Enders pins avoiding the proximal and distal physes.

HIP FRACTURES AND DISLOCATIONS

Hip fractures include fractures of the head, neck, and intertrochanteric region of the femur and account for fewer than 1% of all children's fractures. Hip fractures in children differ from those in adults because of the presence of the physis, the vulnerability of the blood vessels to the femoral head, and the high incidence of avascular necrosis and angular deformity after fracture. Treatment of children's hip fractures also differs from that in adults because of the child's ability to better tolerate immobilization, making the options of traction, spica casting, and bed rest available. More aggressive, surgical treatment may be indicated in some types of children's hip fractures to prevent late complications of coxa vara, nonunion, and premature physeal closure.

The most commonly used classification of children's hip fractures is that proposed by Delbet and popularized by Colonna: type I, transepiphyseal separations with or without dislocation of the femoral head from the acetabulum; type II, transcervical fractures, displaced and nondisplaced; type III, cervicotrochanteric fractures, displaced and nondisplaced; and type IV, intertrochanteric fractures (Fig. 16-65).

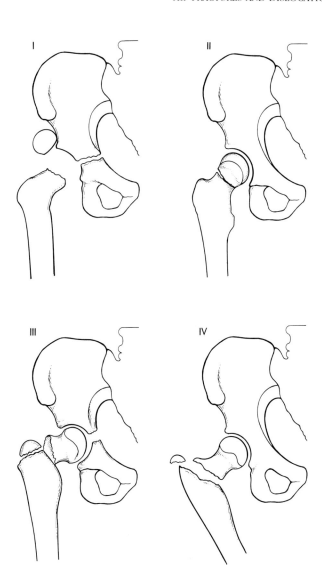

Fig. 16-65 Classification of hip fractures in children: *I,* transepiphyseal, with or without dislocation from the acetabulum; *II,* transcervical; *III,* cervicotrochanteric; *IV,* trochanteric.

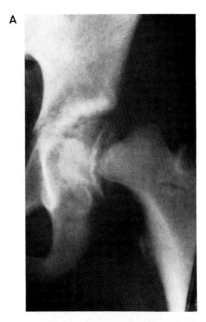

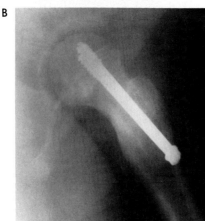

Fig. 16-66 Type I, transepiphyseal separation. **A,** Before treatment. **B,** After closed reduction and fixation with cannulated hip screws.

Type I: Transepiphyseal Separations

Transepiphyseal separations are the most prone to complications, with avascular necrosis and premature physeal closure rates ranging from 80% to 100% reported in the literature. Many of these fractures are associated with dislocation of the femoral head from the acetabulum. Closed reduction and fixation with pins inserted through a short lateral incision should be performed in the older child if possible; however, many fractures will require open reduction. The physis should be crossed only by smooth pins in the young child; threaded pins can be used in the older child because the capital femoral physis contributes only 15% of the total growth of the extremity and premature physeal closure in the child older than 9 years has little consequence. If the femoral head is not dislocated from the acetabulum, closed reduction can be obtained by longitudinal traction in abduction and internal rotation, and internal fixation through a small lateral incision with cannulated hip screws or smooth pins can be performed (Fig. 16-66). The number of pins needed varies with the size of the child and the size of the pin, but generally two or three pins are adequate. Swiontkowski and Winquist recommend gentle closed reduction of type I fractures if the physis is not completely displaced. If this fails or if displacement is complete, they recommend immediate open reduction and pin or screw fixation. CT scanning is helpful to verify dislocation and determine direction of the dislocation. For anterior dislocations an anterior Watson-Jones approach allows reduction and insertion of internal fixation under direct vision; for posterior dislocations a modified Gibson approach should be used.

Proximal femoral epiphysiolysis is an epiphyseal separation that occasionally occurs in newborns. It may be confused with congenital hip dislocation or infection of the hip, and an arthrogram usually is required for definitive diagnosis. Callus may be seen along the medial border of the femoral neck (Fig. 16-67) approximately 2 weeks after the separation. Surgical treatment is not required for this condition.

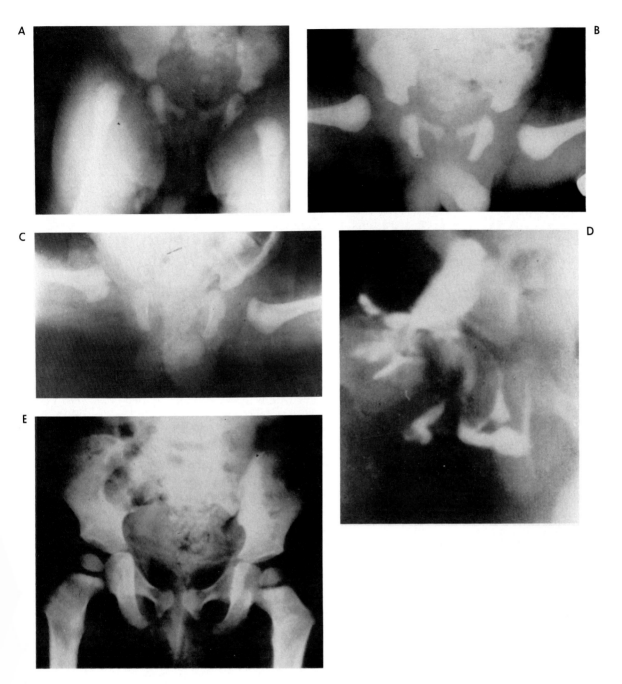

Fig. 16-67   Proximal femoral epiphysiolysis. **A** and **B,** Anteroposterior and frog-leg roentgenograms of new-born showing right hip standing wide and asymmetric in abducted position, simulating congenital hip dislocation. **C,** Roentgenogram made 3 weeks later showing early callus formation. **D,** Arthrogram outlining femoral head within acetabulum and showing obvious separation of capital femoral epiphysis. **E,** Roentgenogram made at 2 years showing good results after little treatment. (Courtesy Dr. RE Lindseth.)

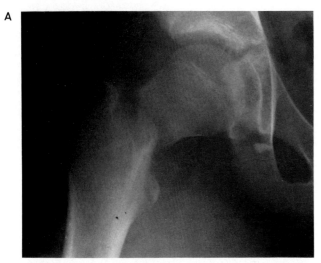

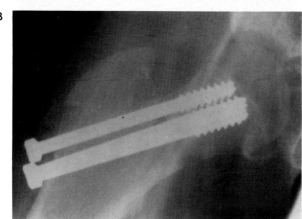

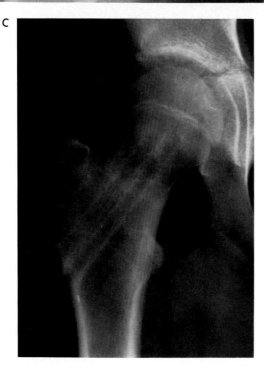

Fig. 16-68 **A,** Type II, transcervical fracture. **B,** After closed reduction and internal fixation with Asnis connulated screw system. **C,** One year later after removal of screws: no evidence of avascular necrosis.

Type II: Transcervical Fractures

Transcervical fractures are the most common type of hip fractures in children (Fig. 16-68). Most of these fractures are displaced, and the amount of displacement appears to be directly related to the development of avascular necrosis. Reports in the literature indicate a 50% incidence of avascular necrosis after type II fractures in most series. Boitzy, however, reported no avascular necrosis in 11 patients with type II fractures treated with early evacuation of the hematoma by either aspiration or capsular release (Fig. 16-69). Swiontkowski and Winquist also reported excellent functional and roentgenographic results in six displaced types II and III fractures treated with emergency open reduction, internal fixation with threaded pins or screws, and anterior capsulotomy for evacuation of intracapsular hematoma. Gerber et al, however, reported a 30% incidence of avascular necrosis in 28 femoral neck fractures despite early open reduction and internal fixation; avascular necrosis occurred after half the type II fractures. Internal fixation is recommended for all type II fractures because of the frequent instability. Almost invariably, both displaced and nondisplaced transcervical fractures "drift" into coxa vara if treated only by external fixation or by closed reduction and external fixation (spica cast). Nonunion also is frequent without internal fixation. Gentle closed reduction should be attempted with longitudinal traction, abduction, and internal rotation, followed by internal fixation with Knowles pins. Swiontkowski and Winquist recommend 4.5-mm AO cortical screws inserted short of the physis overdrilled in the distal fragment for a lag effect.

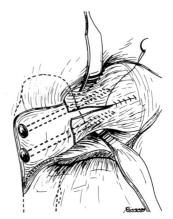

Fig. 16-69 Capsular release: evacuation of hematoma, open reduction and internal fixation with pins, and repair of capsule done as emergency. (Redrawn from Boitzy A. In Weber BG, Brunner CH, and Freuler F: Treatment of fractures in children and adolescents, New York, 1980, Springer-Verlag.)

Type III: Cervicotrochanteric Fractures

Cervicotrochanteric fractures in children are similar to those that occur at the base of the femoral neck in adults, but avascular necrosis after this fracture is more common in children than in adults. Nondisplaced type III fractures can be treated in an abduction spica cast after a period of traction; displaced fractures require closed reduction, or occasionally open reduction, and internal fixation. If there is any question about displacement, the fracture should be treated as if displaced. In both types II and III fractures the fracture is distal and pin fixation without crossing the physis is recommended (Fig. 16-70).

Type IV: Intertrochanteric Fractures

Type IV fractures generally result in fewer complications than do other types. Union is rapid, usually within 6 to 8 weeks, because of the child's osteogenic potential in the trochanteric area. Skeletal traction should be used initially to obtain an acceptable reduction, approximately 2 to 3 weeks, depending on the age of the child. Then an abduction spica cast is applied and worn for 6 to 12 weeks. If reduction cannot be achieved with traction, closed manipulation can be used; internal fixation may be necessary. In the older child and adolescent, intertrochanteric femoral fractures should be treated as in adults with open reduction and internal fixation, avoiding the proximal femoral physis if possible.

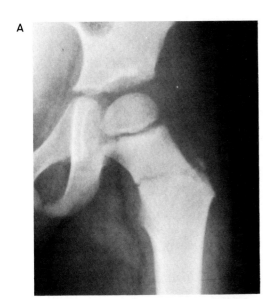
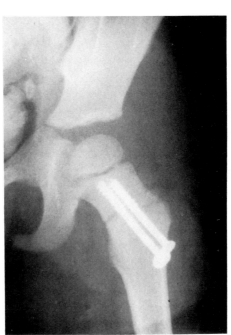
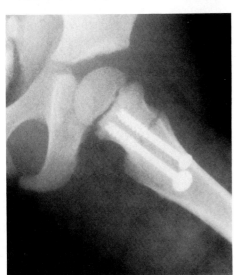

Fig. 16-70 A, Distal type II transcervical or proximal type III cervicotrochanteric fracture in very young patient. **B** and **C,** Fixation with cannulated, threaded, pediatric hip screws avoiding physis.

Complications

The most common and most serious complication of hip fractures in children is avascular necrosis. That this occurs primarily after displaced fractures seems to indicate that avascular necrosis is directly related to initial displacement of the fracture and to compromise of the blood supply at the time of fracture. The first physical symptoms of avascular necrosis may be pain and limitation of motion as a result of synovitis. Roentgenographic signs may be seen as early as 1.5 months after fracture, and radioisotopic scan with the use of a pin-hole collimator will show decreased uptake in the involved femoral head compared with the contralateral hip long before roentgenographic signs are evident. Roentgenographic changes include sclerosis of the femoral head with widening of the joint space, followed by fragmentation, and gross deformity of the femoral head.

Ratliff (1970) described three types of avascular necrosis: type I, whole head involvement; type II, partial head involvement; and type III, an area of avascular necrosis from the fracture line to the physis (Fig. 16-71). The prognosis of avascular necrosis is directly related to the severity of involvement: in type I avascular necrosis results are generally poor, whereas types II and III have better results. If remodeling occurs, it usually is prolonged, continuing for as long as 5 years after fracture. Younger children have a higher percentage of good results because of their potential for repair and remodeling. Treatment of avascular necrosis has ranged from bed rest to nonweight bearing to surgery, including osteotomy, arthrodesis, and arthroplasty. In children younger than 10 years, removal of the internal fixation and application of an "abduction containment" orthosis may be beneficial. When the first signs of avascular necrosis are noted, nonweight bearing on the involved hip is instituted; after fracture healing the internal fixation is removed and the child is fitted for an ambulatory containment orthosis, which is worn for approximately 1 year (Fig. 16-72).

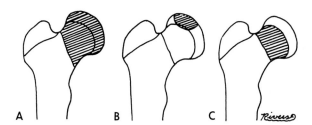

Fig. 16-71 Three types of avascular necrosis. **A,** Type I, total head involvement. **B,** Type II, segmental involvement. **C,** Type III involvement from fracture line to physis. (Redrawn from Ratliff AHC: J Bone Joint Surg 44B:528, 1962.)

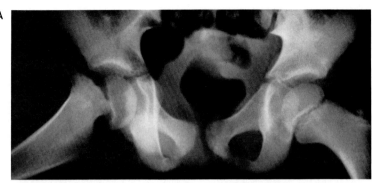

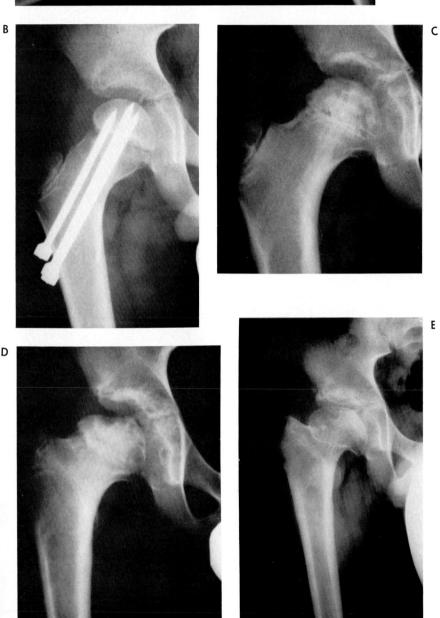

Fig. 16-72 Containment for avascular necrosis of femoral head. **A,** Type I, transepiphyseal fracture in child 6 years old. **B,** After closed reduction and smooth pin fixation. **C,** At 1 year after fracture, pins have been removed and avascular necrosis has developed. **D,** During course of abduction treatment. **E,** At 4 years after treatment for avascular necrosis, femoral neck is short because of premature physeal closure. However, head is reasonably shaped and result is acceptable.

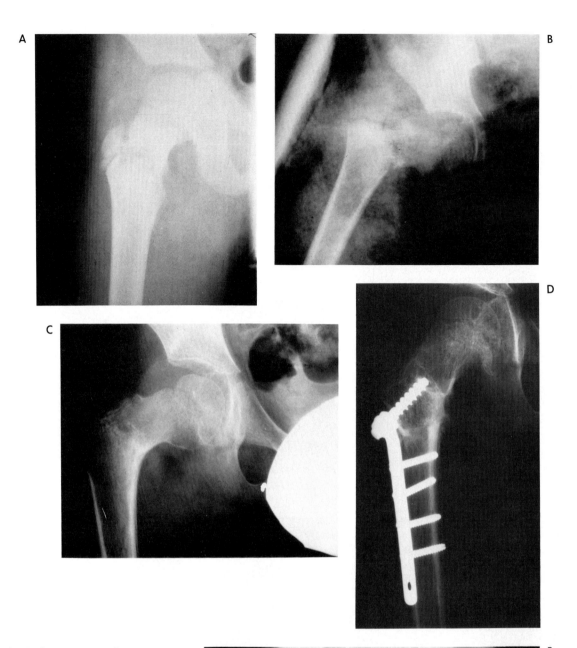

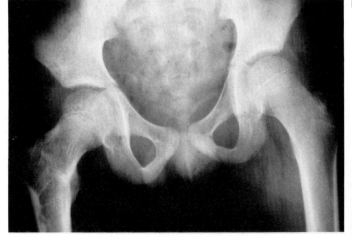

Fig. 16-73 Subtrochanteric osteotomy for coxa vara deformity. **A,** Type III, cervicotrochanteric fracture apparently nondisplaced. **B,** Fracture displaced into unaccepted varus in spica cast. **C,** Fracture united in unacceptable varus position. **D,** Following valgus subtrochanteric osteotomy. **E,** After removal of plate and screws position is acceptable.

The use of internal fixation has reduced the incidence of coxa vara after hip fractures in children, but premature physeal closure with overgrowth of the greater trochanter also can result in a varus deformity. Partial premature physeal closure may result in either a varus or a valgus deformity. Significant coxa vara shortens the affected extremity, causes an abductor or gluteal lurch, and results in later degenerative changes about the hip. If the neck-shaft angle is more than 120 degrees in a young child, some remodeling can be expected and disability will be minimal; however, if the neck-shaft angle is between 100 and 110 degrees, the deformity will persist. Subtrochanteric valgus osteotomy is recommended for persistent coxa vara deformity (Fig. 16-73), with the closing wedge removed just distal to the greater trochanter and the osteotomy fixed with a pediatric lag screw (p. 16).

Reported incidences of nonunion of hip fractures in children are approximately 6% to 10%, and lower incidences seem to follow the use of internal fixation. Unlike avascular necrosis and coxa vara, observation is not appropriate for nonunion; surgical treatment should be undertaken as soon as possible. Subtro-chanteric valgus osteotomy (p. 166) may be used, as recommended by Ratliff (1970), to make the nonunion more horizontal and to allow compressive vertical forces to aid in union (Fig. 16-74). Bone grafts can be used if necessary to augment the osteotomy, and internal fixation should be used across the nonunion site; a spica cast is worn for 12 weeks after osteotomy.

The exact reason for premature physeal closure after fracture is unknown, but it may be caused by avascular necrosis or by pins penetrating or completely crossing the physis. Because the capital femoral physis contributes only 15% of the growth of the entire extremity and normally closes earlier than most other lower extremity physes, shortening usually is less than 2 cm, depending on the age of the child; more significant shortening generally is associated with avascular necrosis, especially in younger children. Regardless of the amount of shortening, children with premature physeal closure should be observed closely, with frequent leg length scanograms and wrist roentgenograms to determine bone age. Epiphysiodesis of the opposite extremity can be performed if necessary.

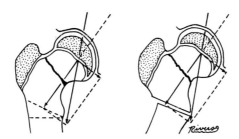

Fig. 16-74 Valgus subtrochanteric osteotomy places line of fracture or nonunion in more horizontal position so that compressive forces will aid in healing. (Redrawn from Ogden JA: Skeletal injury in the child, Philadelphia, 1982, Lea & Febiger.)

Stress Fractures

Stress fractures of the femoral neck can occur in children, especially in adolescents, as noted by Wolfgang. Devas described two types: transverse, in the superior portion of the femoral neck, which may become displaced and cause severe morbidity, and compression, in the inferior portion of the femoral, which rarely becomes displaced, although mild varus deformity may occur in young patients (Fig. 16-75). Knowles pin fixation is recommended for transverse stress fractures; compression stress fractures may be treated by nonweight bearing and limitation of activities.

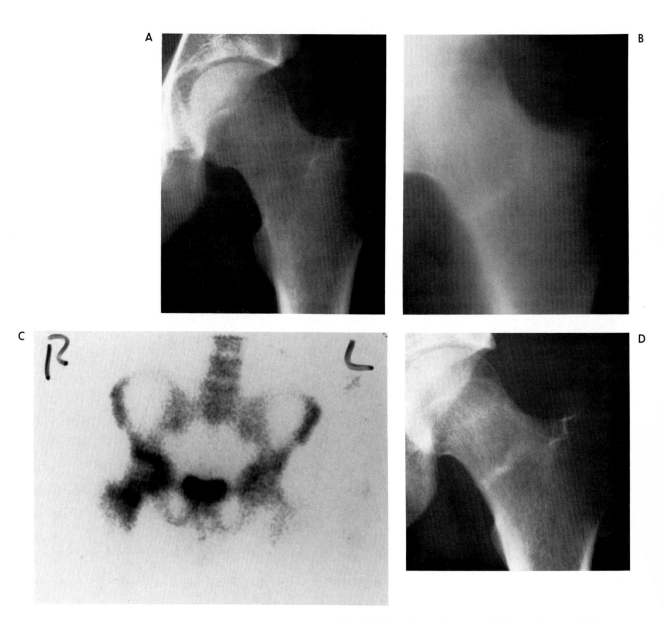

Fig. 16-75 Stress fracture of femoral neck. **A,** Roentgenogram showing possible faint inferior femoral neck fracture. **B,** Tomograms showing definite evidence of compression type of stress fracture in inferior femoral neck. **C,** Bone scan showing increased uptake in this area. **D,** Roentgenogram made 3 weeks later revealing callus formation in inferior neck at stress fracture.

Treatment
Closed reduction and internal fixation

▶ *Technique.* Place the child supine on a fracture table, and attach the feet to the traction stirrups. Carry out a gentle closed reduction by applying longitudinal traction, abduction, and internal rotation. Check the reduction with anteroposterior and lateral roentgenograms or with an image intensifier. If reduction is satisfactory, prepare and drape the involved hip. Make a 7-cm incision just distal to the greater trochanter, and dissect through the fascia lata. Reflect the vastus lateralis muscle anteriorly, exposing the proximal femoral shaft. Elevate the periosteum and place reverse retractors around the proximal femur to aid in exposure. With an image intensifier, determine the correct placement for a drill hole in the lateral shaft of the femur. With a power drill and a ⁹⁄₆₄ -inch drill bit, drill a hole in the lateral cortex. Through the hole drill a guide pin across the fracture site and proximally into the femoral neck. In the young child it is important to avoid penetrating the physis, if possible. Verify the correct position of the guide pin with the image intensifier. Measure the exact length of the portion of the guide pin in the bone. Then drill a Knowles pin or cannulated cancellous pediatric hip screw the same length as the measured length of the guide pin parallel to or over it across the fracture site. Remove the guide pin, and place a second pin or screw parallel to the first through the guide pin hole. Use a minimum of two Knowles pins; three or even four Knowles pins may be used, depending on the size of the child and the femoral neck. Place the Knowles pins parallel and in a "cluster" formation. Close the incision and apply a 1½ spica cast with the hip in the abducted position.

▶ *Postoperative management.* The spica cast is worn for 6 weeks, and then the patient progresses to weight bearing on crutches during the next 6 weeks. The Knowles pins or hip screws should be removed at 1 year when the fracture has united or when there is evidence of avascular necrosis.

Open reduction and internal fixation

▶ *Technique (Weber et al and Boitzy).* Place the patient supine, and drape the limb so that it may be moved freely during the operation. Use a Watson-Jones approach to the hip joint. Incise the hip joint capsule longitudinally, and evacuate and flush out the hematoma, which is usually under pressure. Reduce the fracture with a periosteal elevator. This may be made easier by appropriate traction and internal rotation of the extremity. Temporarily stabilize the fracture with Kirschner wires, and check the reduction in the region of the calcar. Then fix the fracture permanently with cancellous screws fitted with washers. The screw threads should be only in the proximal fragment and not across the physis of the femoral head. Confirm the reduction roentgenographically, and close the hip capsule.

An anterior approach, such as the Watson-Jones, can be used for displaced types II and type III fractures and for type I transepiphyseal separations when the femoral head is dislocated from the acetabulum anteriorly. When the femoral head is dislocated posteriorly, a modified Gibson approach is used. The femoral head may be devoid of all blood supply. However, it should be replaced in the acetabulum, making sure there are no cartilaginous or osseous fragments in the joint, and then fixed to the femoral neck with Knowles pins or cancellous screws.

▶ *Postoperative management.* A below-knee cast with a transverse bar is applied with the leg in 10 to 15 degrees of internal rotation. At 2 weeks the cast is removed and the patient begins active mobilization without weight bearing. A Thomas weight-relieving caliper is worn for 8 to 10 months, and the pins are removed at 12 months.

Traumatic Hip Dislocations

Traumatic hip dislocations in children are more common than hip fractures, but they are still relatively rare injuries, accounting for less than 10% of all hip dislocations. MacFarlane noted that half the hip dislocations in children occurred between the ages of 12 and 15 years, but Gartland and Brenner found an equal age distribution in 248 patients. Libri et al reported that their 22 patients fell into two distinct groups: those between 2 and 5 years of age (8 patients) and those between 11 and 15 years of age (14 patients). Because the young child's acetabulum is primarily soft, pliable cartilage and generalized joint laxity is common, minor trauma can cause hip dislocation in these children. As the child ages, more severe trauma, such as athletic activities or motor vehicle accidents, is required to dislocate the hip joint and associated injuries are more common. As in adults, posterior dislocations are 7 to 10 times more common than anterior dislocations.

With posterior hip dislocation the child holds the leg in flexion, adduction, and internal rotation; with anterior dislocation the leg is held extended, abducted, and externally rotated. The sciatic nerve may be involved, and thorough neurologic evaluation should be performed before and after treatment. Roentgenograms should be made before and after reduction.

Several factors contribute to the final result after hip dislocation: (1) severity of the injury, (2) interval between injury and reduction, (3) type of treatment, (4) period of nonweight bearing, (5) development of recurrent dislocation, (6) development of avascular necrosis, and (7) incomplete reduction because of capsular soft tissue or osseous cartilaginous interposition. As would be expected, the severity of the injury is the most crucial factor in prognosis: the more severe the injury the worse the results. The interval between injury and reduction, a critical factor in adult dislocations, seems less important in children's hip dislocations. Gartland and Brenner, Petrini and Grassi, and Libri et al found little correlation between the time to reduction and final result. Successful closed reduction produces better results than open reduction, but open reduction may be necessary for more severe injuries. Although most recent articles indicate no correlation between final result and the period of nonweight bearing, Libri et al reported better results in patients who were not allowed full weight bearing until full painless motion of the hip was achieved.

Recurrent dislocation is more common in children than in adults because of cartilaginous pliability and ligamentous laxity (Fig. 16-76). Rang and Bennet et al noted a higher incidence of recurrent dislocation in children with hyperlaxity syndromes, especially Down syndrome, and recommended posterior plication of the capsule combined with a bony procedure, such as innominate or varus osteotomy (Fig. 16-77). Recurrent dislocations of the hip also may be caused by a tear in the capsule or by attenuation of the capsule; arthrographic examination may be helpful in differentiating a capsular tear. Open reduction and surgical repair of the capsular defect, followed by 6 weeks of spica cast immobilization, may be indicated for persistent recurrent dislocations.

Fig. 16-76 A, Recurrent traumatic dislocation of hip with obvious avascular necrosis of femoral head. **B,** Stable and painless hip after hip arthrodesis.

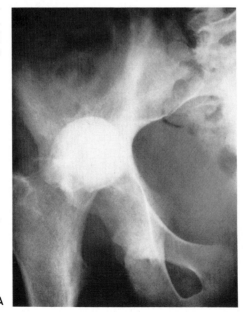
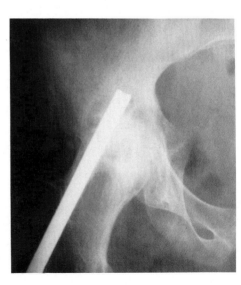

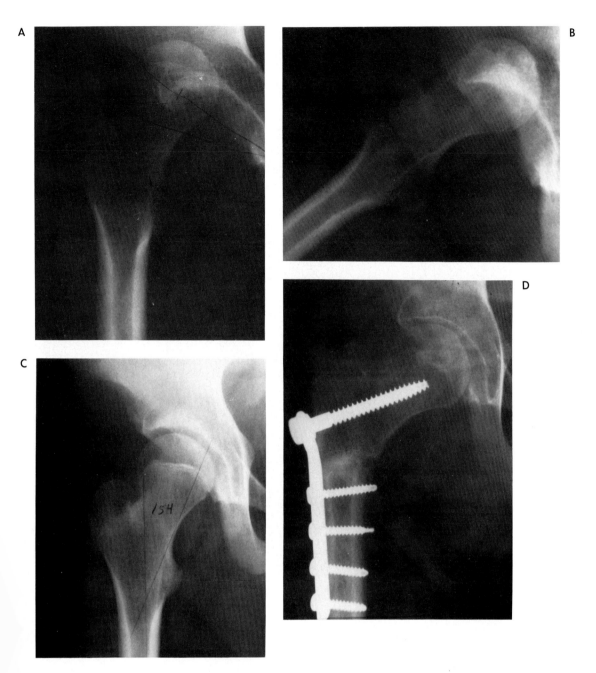

Fig. 16-77 Chronic recurrent dislocation of hip in child with Down syndrome. **A** and **B,** At age 8 years, posterior plication of capsule was performed but recurrent dislocation persisted at age 15 years. **C,** Valgus deformity of 154 degrees after reduction; CT scan shows little femoral anteversion. **D,** One year after second posterior plication of capsule and varus femoral osteotomy; no further dislocations have occurred.

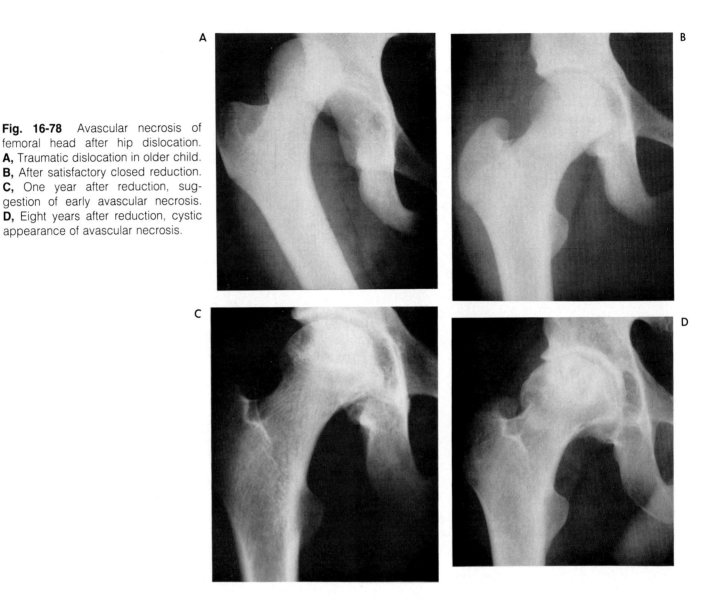

Fig. 16-78 Avascular necrosis of femoral head after hip dislocation. **A,** Traumatic dislocation in older child. **B,** After satisfactory closed reduction. **C,** One year after reduction, suggestion of early avascular necrosis. **D,** Eight years after reduction, cystic appearance of avascular necrosis.

Fig. 16-79 Incongruous reduction of hip. Roentgenogram of both hips after what was thought to be successful closed reduction of traumatic dislocation of right hip in adolescent. However, reduction is incongruous as shown by break in Shenton's line and increase in width of joint space.

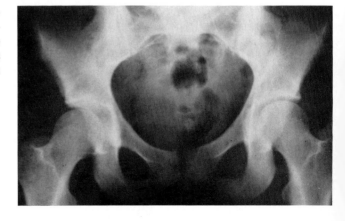

Avascular necrosis occurs after approximately 8% to 10% of simple hip dislocations in children (Fig. 16-78), compared with 10% to 25% in adults. The severity of the injury and the age of the child seem to be the most important contributing factors to the development of avascular necrosis, with severe trauma in older children more likely to result in this complication. The interval between injury and reduction and the type of treatment also are contributory.

Complete reduction of the dislocation may be prevented by interposition of the capsule, labrum, other soft tissue, or an osteocartilaginous fragment (Fig. 16-79). Roentgenograms of both hips should be made and compared after closed reduction. If the involved joint space is wider and Shenton's line is broken, an incongruous reduction should be suspected (Fig. 16-80, *A* and *B*). The interposed object may be disengaged by moving the hip through a full range of motion, with care taken not to completely dislocate the femoral head. If this is not successful, CT scanning may reveal the entrapped structure (Fig. 16-80, *C*). Open reduction and removal of the loose bony fragment, inverted limbus, or other soft tissue should be performed if necessary to achieve congruous reduction and to prevent degenerative changes in the hip joint. After reduction, roentgenograms should be taken in the operating room to confirm restoration of normal joint space.

When the hip dislocation occurs in association with an ipsilateral femoral shaft fracture, the hip should be reduced closed if possible. Watson-Jones suggested that, if necessary, a Steinmann pin can be driven into the trochanteric area of the femur and used to manipulate the dislocation. If this procedure fails, the hip joint itself must be exposed and reduced, but this should be avoided if at all possible because of the risk of avascular necrosis.

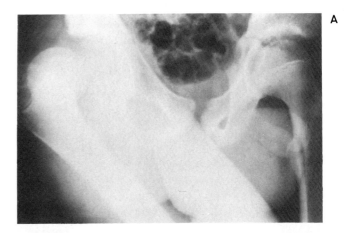
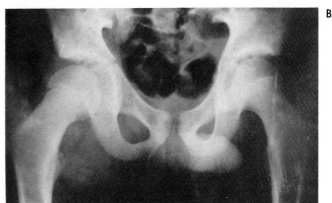
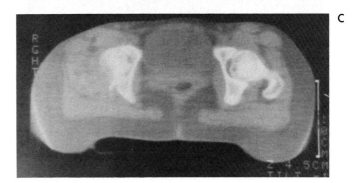

Fig. 16-80   Incongruous reduction of hip. **A,** Traumatic hip dislocation in adolescent. **B,** After two attempts at closed reduction joint space is still too wide and Shenton's line is broken. **C,** CT scan shows osteocartilaginous fragment in acetabulum impeding reduction; open reduction was necessary.

Open reduction and removal of interposed structures

▶ *Technique.* If an obstruction can be identified anteriorly, use the anterior iliofemoral approach, but usually a posterior or lateral approach is indicated because most of the injury is located posterior to the hip. Expose the acetabulum through a T-shaped incision in the capsule, and clear it of blood and debris. Move the femur and locate its head proximal and posterior to the acetabulum. The head will have penetrated the capsule, and usually a mass of capsule will be found around the femoral neck. The head also may have penetrated the abductor or short external rotator muscles. Occasionally the sciatic nerve will have become looped across the anterior surface of the head and neck. Carefully protect this nerve, and remove the muscles and other structures from the head and neck area. The edges of the torn capsule may have caught the femoral neck in such a way that reduction, even under direct vision, is impossible without enlarging the tear. After all obstructions have been removed from the acetabulum, replace the head within the capsule and reduce the dislocation, pulling on the thigh in its long axis with the hip flexed 90 degrees and adducted.

▶ *Postoperative management.* A Thomas splint or Buck's traction is usually enough to immobilize the hip when the reduction is stable. Active and passive exercises and physical therapy are begun at 2 weeks. Weight bearing gradually is resumed at 3 to 4 weeks.

SLIPPED CAPITAL FEMORAL EPIPHYSIS

Although slipped capital femoral epiphysis (SCFE) technically is not a fracture, it produces the same lesion as a type I transepiphyseal fracture-separation; however, the pathogenesis and natural histories of the two entities make them very different. Type I transepiphyseal separations usually are traumatic injuries in younger children; SCFE is a lesion of uncertain etiology that occurs in adolescence. It is the most common disorder of the hip in adolescents, with an incidence of approximately two cases per 100,000 persons. Skeletally mature, obese adolescents appear to be at greatest risk. The "slipping" is caused by dehiscence through the physis; the weakening of the perichondral ring allows the epiphysis and metaphysis gradually to slip away from each other. This process frequently is chronic and insidious, but minor trauma can cause acute slipping of the epiphysis. The left hip is more frequently involved, especially in boys, and bilateral SCFE occurs in approximately one third of patients. Posterior displacement is usual, although anterior displacement has been reported.

The etiology of SCFE is unknown. Suggested causes include trauma, mechanical factors, inflammation, endocrine disorders, nutritional deficiencies, and renal and irradiation therapy. Several conditions have been reported to be associated with SCFE, including Down syndrome, sarcoidosis, multiple sclerosis, Gilbert disease, cretinism, Legg-Calvé-Perthes disease, hypothyroidism, hypopituitarism, and chronic renal disease. The disorder is autosomal dominant with variable penetrance, and it carries a 7.1% risk to a second family member. Fewer than 3% of children with SCFE have parents who had the disorder.

Classification

SCFE generally is classified by severity as acute (sudden onset with symptoms for 2 weeks or less), chronic (symptoms existing more than 2 weeks and roentgenograms that show a combination of callus formation and attempted remodeling or bending of the femoral neck), acute-on-chronic (symptoms for longer than 1 month and a recent sudden exacerbation of pain after a relatively trivial injury), or preslip (essentially a roentgenographic finding manifested by irregularity, widening, and indistinctness of the physis). In addition to the type of slip, SCFE is classified by the amount of displacement of the femoral neck. The normal femoral head-shaft angle is 145 degrees on the anteroposterior roentgenographic projection; on the lateral projection it is 170 degrees or more. Mild slipping is defined as displacement of less than one third of the diameter of the femoral head or deviation of the head-shaft angle from normal by 30 degrees or less on either projection (Fig. 16-81). In moderate slipping the neck is displaced between one third and one half the diameter of the femoral head, or the head-shaft angle deviates between 30 and 60 degrees from normal on either projection. Severe slipping is characterized by neck displacement of more than one half the diameter of the head, or deviation of the head-shaft angle of more than 60 degrees from normal. This classification on the basis of degrees of slipping eliminates the problem of "bending" of the femoral neck in chronic slips.

Signs and Symptoms

The clinical symptoms and roentgenographic signs of SCFE vary according to the type of slip but usually include pain in the groin, medial thigh, or knee and limitation of hip motion, especially internal rotation. Patients with chronic slips may have mild or moderate shortening of the affected extremity. Roentgenograms of the patient with preslip show the widening of the physis, and bone scanning shows increased uptake in this area, but actual slipping cannot be appreciated. In acute slips, roentegenograms show displacement of the epiphysis from the metaphysis through the physis. Subtle slipping is best appreciated on "frog-leg" lateral comparison roentgenograms. In acute-on-chronic slips, roentgenograms show the acute physeal separation superimposed on osseous remodeling in the metaphysis. In chronic slips the patient complains of intermittent pain in the groin and thigh, which has been present for weeks to years. The leg may be in fixed external rotation and mildly or moderately shortened.

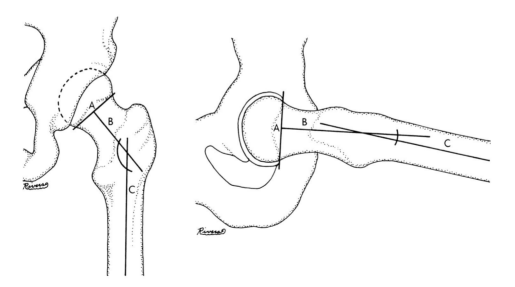

Fig. 16-81   Measurement of head-shaft angle on anteroposterior and lateral roentgenogram. Line *A* connects peripheral portions of physis. Line *B* is perpendicular to line *A*, and line *C* is in long axis of femoral shaft. Intersection of lines *B* and *C* forms head-shaft angle in both views. (Redrawn from Rao JP, Francis AM, and Siwek CW: J Bone Joint Surg 66A:1169, 1984.)

Treatment

The goals of treatment of SCFE are stabilization and prevention of additional slipping, stimulation of early closure of the physis, and prevention of avascular necrosis, chondrolysis, and osteoarthritis. The first two goals are easily obtainable by a variety of methods; the prevention of complications, however, has proved extremely difficult. Nonsurgical treatment of SCFE has not been particularly successful. Ordenberg et al confirmed the inadequacy of closed reduction and casting in their study of 72 patients 25 to 72 years after treatment. Most patients had pain and limited hip function, and 35% had required surgery for osteoarthritis as adults, compared with an untreated group in which only 2 of 49 (4%) required subsequent operation. Methods of surgical treatment of SCFE have included percutaneous and open in situ pinning, open reduction and internal fixation, epiphysiodesis, osteotomy, and reconstruction by arthroplasty, arthrodesis, or cheilectomy. Each technique has its proponents and opponents, and the choice of treatment must be individualized for each child, depending on age, type of slip, and severity of displacement (Table 16-1).

In Situ Pinning

Most authors agree that mild, moderate, and some severe acute or chronic slipping should be treated with closed in situ pinning. Open in situ pinning may be indicated for more severe acute or acute-on-chronic slipping. Several techniques of pinning have been described with the use of Knowles pins, triflanged nails, hip compression screws, and the newer cannulated hip screw systems. Knowles pins cause less trauma to the physis than triflanged nails or large hip compression screws, and generally they prevent further slipping and induce early closure of the physis. The development of pediatric cannulated screws for insertion over guide pins has improved fixation of SCFE by this method (Fig. 16-82).

In addition to the type of fixation the number of pins needed has been of some debate. Most earlier reports indicated that two or three pins were necessary for stability and the results of multiple pinning generally have been satisfactory, but more recent reports recommend the use of a single larger-diameter central pin or screw, a technically simpler procedure than insertion of multiple pins. O'Beirne et al reported single-pin fixation of 18 slipped epiphyses (8 acute and 10 chronic; 15 mild, 2 moderate, and 1 severe) and prophylactic pinning of 15 contralateral hips. All patients had satisfactory clinical results, with no slip progression, no pin breakage, and no late reslips. Morrissy described a technique for percutaneous in situ fixation of chronic SCFE with a single cannulated screw (Asnis), giving as criteria for successful pinning location of the pin in the central axis of the femoral head and avoidance of pin penetration into the joint.

Pin penetration has been the most serious disadvantage of in situ pinning. Adverse effects attributed to unrecognized pin penetration include joint sepsis, localized acetabular erosion, synovitis, postoperative hip pain, chondrolysis, and late degenerative osteoarthritis. The incidence of pin penetration has been reported to range from 14% to 60%. Various techniques have been recommended to lower this incidence. Volz and Martin, Walters and Simon, Rooks and Schmitt, and Cowell, among others, have described complex mathematical formulas for determining accurate pin placement, as well as roentgenographic techniques and templates (Fig. 16-83). Others, including Menche and Lehman, have emphasized the use of a rotating fluoroscopic beam to detect penetration. Lehman et al (1984) and Shaw recommend the use of a cannulated hip screw with injection of radiopaque dye to detect pin penetration. More recently, based on roentgenographic measurements and a mathematical formula, Rooks et al, as a practical clinical guide, recommended that the pin tip be ad-

Table 16-1 Treatment choices for severity of slip as compared with the temporal relationship

Time	Severity (degrees)		
	Mild <30	Moderate 30-60	Severe >60
Preslip	Pin in situ	—	—
Acute <2 wk	Pin in situ	Reduce/pin or pin in situ	Reduce/pin
Acute-on-chronic <2 wk	Pin in situ	Reduce/pin or pin in situ	Reduce/pin
>2 wk	Reduce/pin		Osteotomy
Chronic >2 wk	Pin in situ	Osteotomy or pin in situ	Osteotomy

Reduce/pin, Indicates SCFE can be reduced or just pinned in situ, depending on surgeon's preference.

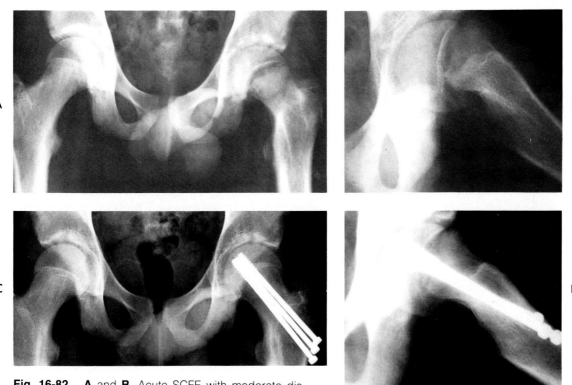

Fig. 16-82 **A** and **B,** Acute SCFE with moderate displacement. **C** and **D,** After in situ pinning with cannulated cancellous hip screws.

vanced to 8 mm or one third of the femoral head radius from subchondral bone, whichever projection is the closest. This places the actual tip 7 to 18 mm from the subchondral bone, leaving a safe margin.

As Morrissy emphasizes, in situ pinning is a roentgenographic technique, and good quality roentgenograms or image intensification must be available for successful pinning. He notes two common errors made in in situ pinning: passing the pin obliquely toward the anterior surface rather than the center of the femoral head and passing the pin out the posterior neck and into the head. His solution is to select the starting point of the fixation device on the basis of the position of the femoral head, starting the device on the femoral neck so that when it leaves the neck, it enters the femoral head perpendicular to the physeal surface and in its center. He contends that this starting point is on the anterior rather than lateral aspect of the femoral neck and the further the femoral head has slipped posteriorly, the more anterior this starting position must be.

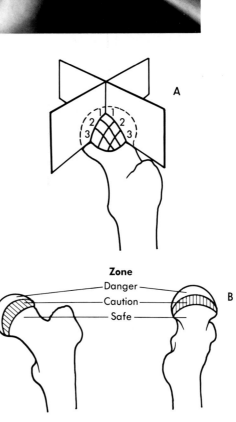

Fig. 16-83 **A,** Illustration of femoral head being an ellipse in three dimensions with three different quadrants outlined *(1-2-3).* **B,** Safe, caution, and danger zones as pins are inserted away from center of femoral head. (**A** redrawn from Walters R and Simon SR: The hip, St Louis, 1980, The CV Mosby Co.)

Knowles pinning

▲ *Technique.* Make a short, longitudinal incision over the lateral aspect of the thigh beginning just distal to the tip of the greater trochanter. In the proximal part of the incision, divide the fascia lata posterior to the tensor fasciae latae muscle to avoid splitting the muscle. This brings the vastus lateralis muscle into view. Beginning at the proximal part of its origin, divide the vastus lateralis longitudinally for about 4 cm along the lateral surface of the femoral shaft, and reflect the muscle to expose the bone. Now insert three Knowles pins through the femoral neck and into the epiphysis, as follows. Insert a guide wire through the lateral femoral cortex and the femoral neck and into the epiphysis, as for nailing of a fractured femoral neck. Check the position of the wire with roentgenograms or an image intensifier. When the wire is in satisfactory position, estimate the correct lengths for three Knowles pins. Using the wire as a guide, insert the Knowles pins through the lateral aspect of the femur into the epiphysis: one through the anterosuperior aspect of the femoral neck, a second through the posterosuperior aspect, and a third through the inferior aspect. The pins need not be parallel, but they should penetrate the physis and the area of the subchondral bone without piercing the articular surface of the epiphysis.

▲ *Postoperative management.* A cast is not necessary. The patient is kept in bed for 2 to 3 weeks, but quadriceps setting exercises are begun 2 to 3 days after surgery. Active flexion and extension of the hip and knee are started during the second week. At 4 weeks, walking with crutches is permitted with touchdown weight bearing on the affected limb. Partial weight bearing is permitted 2 to 4 weeks later and is continued until the physis begins to fuse, usually at 4 to 6 months.

Cannulated hip screw

▲ *Technique (Asnis).* Place the patient supine on a fracture table. Reduce the fracture or SCFE if necessary, and confirm the reduction by two-plane roentgenograms or image intensification. Make an 8-cm lateral incision, starting at the prominence of the greater trochanter and extending distally. Split the fasciae latae and vastus lateralis muscles in line with the incision, and retract their edges. Select a point 3 to 4 cm below the greater trochanter, midway between the anterior and posterior femoral cortices. Then at this point drive a two-part guide pin assembly into the lateral femoral neck, and direct it across the fracture site, or the physis in an SCFE, and into the femoral head. Confirm the position of the pin assembly with roentgenograms or an image intensifier. If the position is not acceptable, estimate the angle between this pin and another necessary for correction (Fig. 16-84, *A*), and insert another guide pin assembly. Place an adjustable pin guide system (Fig. 16-84, *B*) over the malaligned guide pin assembly, and using the estimated angle, insert another guide pin assembly in the proper location. Release both friction locks, and remove the malaligned guide pin assembly.

Next, use the fixed pin guide, which contains a grid of different-sized triangles. Select the desired triangle depending on the size of the femoral neck (Fig. 16-84, *C* and *D*). Drive two more guide pin assemblies into the femoral head with the aid of the fixed pin guide. Check the length and position of the guide pin assemblies with roentgenograms or the image intensifier. Place the tips of the guide pin assemblies 7 to 10 mm from the subchondral bone. Then tap the inner pin of each guide pin assembly gently with a mallet until its lateral end is flush with the lateral end of the outer component (Fig. 16-84, *E*). Remove each outer component with the power driver, leaving the inner guide pin in place (Fig. 16-84, *F*). For each guide pin determine the screw length by holding the depth gauge against the femoral cortex along the pin and reading off the depth of penetration of the pin (Fig. 16-84, *G*). Tap the outer femoral cortex at each guide pin with a cannulated tap placed over the pin. Now insert a cannulated screw over each guide pin, and tighten each with the cannulated screwdriver (Fig. 16-84, *H*). Check the placement of the screws by image intensification, and if a screw is not of ideal length remove it over the guide pin and replace it with one of appropriate length. Now remove the guide pins and close the wound.

▲ *Postoperative management.* A spica cast is generally unnecessary unless any large drill holes are not filled with screws, thereby acting as "stress risers." The patient should be nonweight bearing on crutches for 4 to 6 weeks.

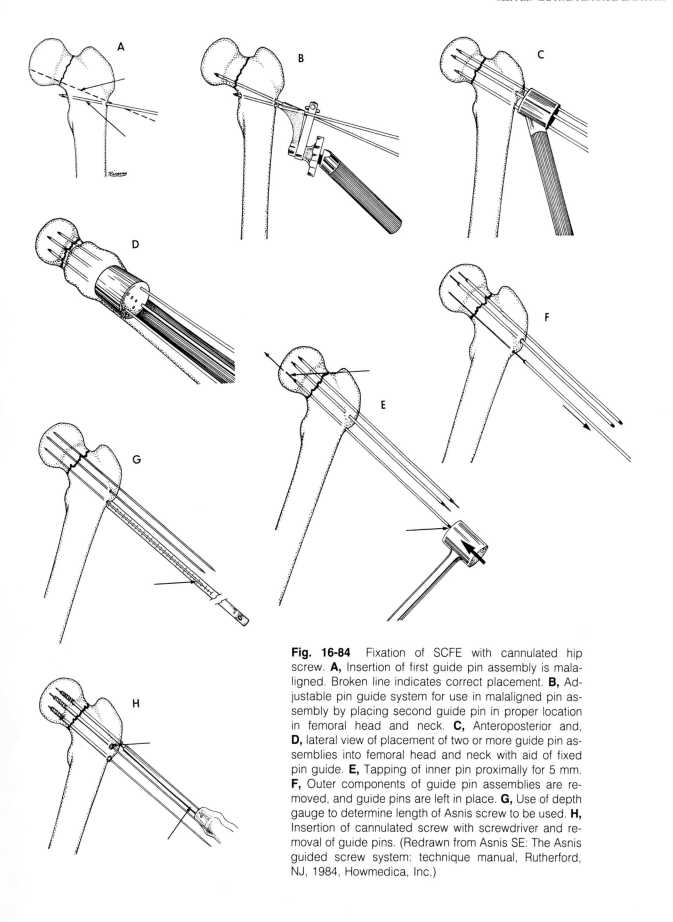

Fig. 16-84 Fixation of SCFE with cannulated hip screw. **A,** Insertion of first guide pin assembly is malaligned. Broken line indicates correct placement. **B,** Adjustable pin guide system for use in malaligned pin assembly by placing second guide pin in proper location in femoral head and neck. **C,** Anteroposterior and, **D,** lateral view of placement of two or more guide pin assemblies into femoral head and neck with aid of fixed pin guide. **E,** Tapping of inner pin proximally for 5 mm. **F,** Outer components of guide pin assemblies are removed, and guide pins are left in place. **G,** Use of depth gauge to determine length of Asnis screw to be used. **H,** Insertion of cannulated screw with screwdriver and removal of guide pins. (Redrawn from Asnis SE: The Asnis guided screw system: technique manual, Rutherford, NJ, 1984, Howmedica, Inc.)

▶ *Technique (Lyden; Lehman et al).* Place the patient supine, and drape the affected hip in the usual manner. Reduce the fracture or the SCFE if required, and verify the position roentgenographically. Then with a standard lateral approach, open the skin, fascia, and muscle down to the lateral femur. Make a hole in the lateral cortex of the femur with a 4.8-mm (3/16-inch) diameter "trocar pointed" Steinmann pin. This cortical aperture should be 40 to 50 mm below the crest of the greater trochanter (or opposite the middle of the lesser trochanter) to allow pin placement at 135 degrees (Fig. 16-85, *A*). Next introduce a 2.4-mm (3/32-inch) smooth guide pin across the fracture or across the slipped epiphysis in an acceptable position and depth in the femoral head. The tip should engage subchondral bone (Fig. 16-85, *B*). If the pin is poorly positioned, withdraw and reinsert it parallel to the axis of the femoral neck and central in the head. If more than one screw is used, the second and third pins should parallel the first, with their threads not touching. A triangular configuration is preferred. Use a measuring gauge to determine the length of the cannulated screw required (Fig. 16-85, *C*), or merely hold a second guide wire along the initial one to measure the length. Then connect the winch to the cannulated screw of appropriate length by means of a threaded winch stabilizer (Fig. 16-85, *D*). Place the

screw over the guide pin and insert it into the femur (Fig. 16-85, *E*). The flutes of the cannulated screw will cut through the cancellous bone until the beveled shoulders are seated on the lateral cortex. If self-tapping of the bone is difficult, especially in the femoral head, an appropriate reamer and tap should be used first. After the first screw is satisfactorily positioned, insert additional screws with or without the use of an alignment guide (Fig. 16-86). The number of screws chosen depends on the stability of the fracture or "slip," the quality of bone, and the adequacy of pin placement. Subsequent screws can be inserted with the initial guide wire protruding distally to act as an insertion guide and using the alignment guide and then the cannulated screw. Alternatively, if the correct length of the subsequent screw is ensured, follow the initial screw with a 4.8-mm (3/16-inch) parallel Steinmann pin to create a femoral hole, and then insert the subsequent cannulated screws directly without the intermediate guide alignment.

Lehman has modified this technique somewhat for SCFE. If self-tapping of the cannulated bone is difficult, use a reamer over the guide wire first; then use a tap before inserting the screws of appropriate size. Because the reamer or tap may advance the guide wire across the femoral head into the hip joint, remove the guide wire as the reamer or tap reaches the

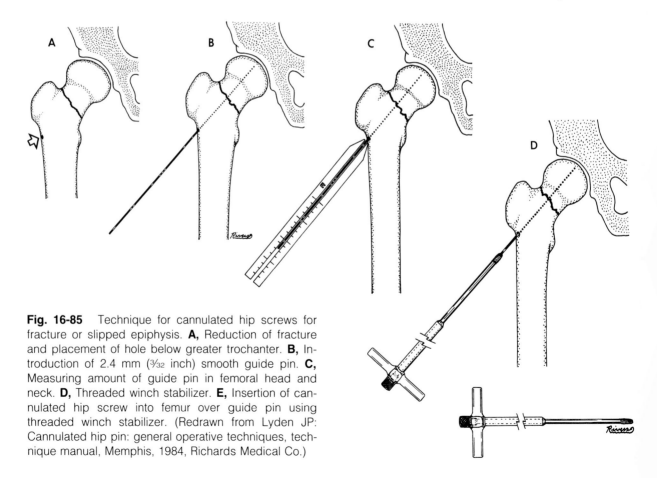

Fig. 16-85 Technique for cannulated hip screws for fracture or slipped epiphysis. **A,** Reduction of fracture and placement of hole below greater trochanter. **B,** Introduction of 2.4 mm (3/32 inch) smooth guide pin. **C,** Measuring amount of guide pin in femoral head and neck. **D,** Threaded winch stabilizer. **E,** Insertion of cannulated hip screw into femur over guide pin using threaded winch stabilizer. (Redrawn from Lyden JP: Cannulated hip pin: general operative techniques, technique manual, Memphis, 1984, Richards Medical Co.)

epiphysis. If the guide wire is not removed at this point, roentgenographic control is absolutely necessary during the advancement of the reamer or tap to be certain that the guide wire does not advance through the femoral head.

To make sure the screws have not penetrated the hip joint, screw the adapter into the cannulated hip screw (Fig. 16-87). Place about 30 mm of radiographic water-soluble dye, using one part 60% Hypaque to one part sterile saline, in a sterile beaker. Fill a 12-mm syringe with the dye, and remove all air from the syringe. Snap the syringe-tubing assembly to the adapter by pushing a coupler onto the adapter. Next inject the dye into the pin under pressure and view the hip with an image intensifier (Fig. 16-88). As soon as the dye is seen entering the femoral head or hip joint, stop further injection. Disassemble the dye injector, and unscrew the adapter from the hip screw. If the arthrogram shows dye in the hip joint, the femoral head has been penetrated (Fig. 16-89). In this event, remove the screw entirely and select a more desirable site to insert the screw. If an arthrogram shows negative findings (dye only in the femoral head), take final roentgenograms and close the wound in the usual manner.

▶ *Postoperative management.* Postoperative management is similar to that described for the Asnis technique.

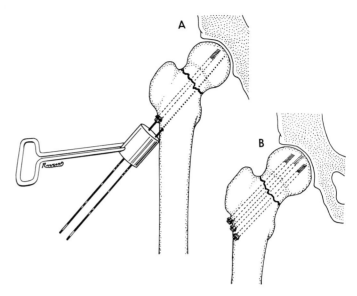

Fig. 16-86 **A,** Insertion of guide pins through alignment guide. **B,** Three cannulated screws have been inserted. (Redrawn from Lyden JP: Cannulated hip pin: general operative techniques, technique manual, Memphis, 1984, Richards Medical Co.)

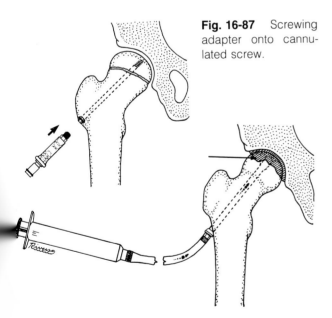

Fig. 16-87 Screwing adapter onto cannulated screw.

Fig. 16-88 Injection of appropriate dye under pressure into femoral head and hip joint viewed by image intensification, signifying pin penetration. (Redrawn from Lehman WB, Frant AD, and Rose D: Cannulated hip pin: modified technique for slipped capital femoral epiphysis, technique manual, Memphis, 1984, Richards Medical Co.)

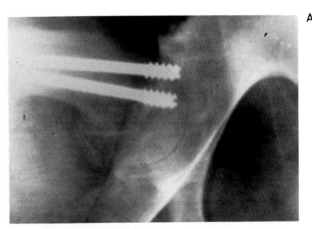

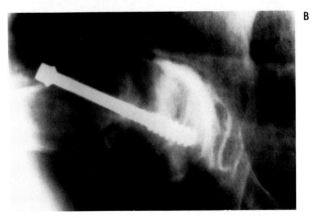

Fig. 16-89 Use of dye in pin penetration. **A,** Penetration with cannulated pediatric hip screw shown on lateral roentgenogram. **B,** Presence of roentgenographic dye in joint confirms penetration.

Percutaneous single screw fixation

In situ fixation of chronic slips with a single cannulated screw placed into the center of the proximal epiphysis has the advantage of requiring only a small, stab-wound incision for insertion of the screw—but if this starting point is not precisely determined, multiple stab wounds or a large incision may increase operative time and fluoroscopy exposure, may cause difficulty in screw placement, and may compromise cosmetic results. A fluoroscopic technique based on geometric axioms has been used in more than 30 children to determine preoperatively the appropriate site to allow the guide wire for the cannulated screw system to be placed through a minimal incision or a simple stab (puncture) wound. The geometric principles concern the intersection of skin planes with the line of correct insertion of the screw (Fig. 16-90, *A* and *B*).

▲ *Technique of determining insertion sites.* Position the patient supine so the anteroposterior and lateral fluoroscopic views can be obtained without repositioning the patient or the extremity; a fracture table can be used. The entire proximal femoral epiphysis and hip joint space should be clearly visible on both views. Prepare and drape the extremity to allow free access to the entire anterior surface of the thigh as far medial as the pubis in the inguinal area. Use a fluoroscopic C-arm for anteroposterior and exact lateral images. On the lateral view the femoral neck should be parallel to the femoral shaft.

Place a guide wire on the anterior aspect of the thigh (Fig. 16-90, *C*) so that the anteroposterior image shows in the desired varus-valgus position (Fig. 16-90, *D*); this indicates plane A. Mark the position of the guide wire on the anterior surface of the thigh with a marking pen to represent the intersection of plane A with the skin. Then place the guide wire along the lateral aspect of the thigh (Fig. 16-90, *E*) so that it is in the correct anteroposterior position on lateral fluoroscopic image (Fig. 16-90, *F*); this indicates plane B. Mark the position of the wire on the skin to represent the intersection of plane B with the skin. In SCFE the proximal femoral epiphysis is displaced posteriorly relative to the femoral neck, and this lateral guide wire angles from anterior to posterior and appears on fluoroscopic image to enter at the anterior femoral neck. The two skin lines should intersect on the anterolateral aspect of the thigh (Fig. 16-90, *G*). The greater the degree of the slip (the more posterior the epiphysis), the more anterior is the intersection (Fig. 16-90, *H*).

Place a guide wire, drill, or pin through either a small incision or a simple stab (puncture) wound (Fig. 16-90, *I*) at the intersection of the two skin lines. Monitor proper alignment, position, and depth of insertion in the proximal femoral epiphysis on anteroposterior and lateral fluoroscopic images. Insert internal fixation in the routine manner.

There are some limitations in exactness of this technique, because the skin lines and their intersection are made on mobile soft tissue and the guide wires are flexible. Also, the guide wire or pin may "walk" along the cortical bone to an unacceptable position. Thus the starting point and alignment must be confirmed fluoroscopically before advancing the wire. This technique simply aids in localizing and minimizing the skin incision and helps determine the approximate angle of the guide wire and pin, but does not prevent technical errors of pin placement.

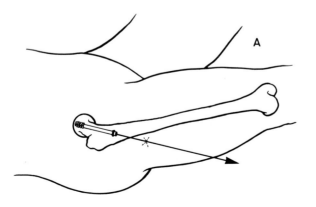

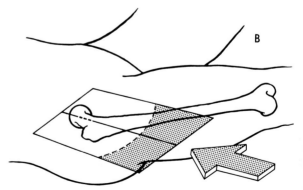

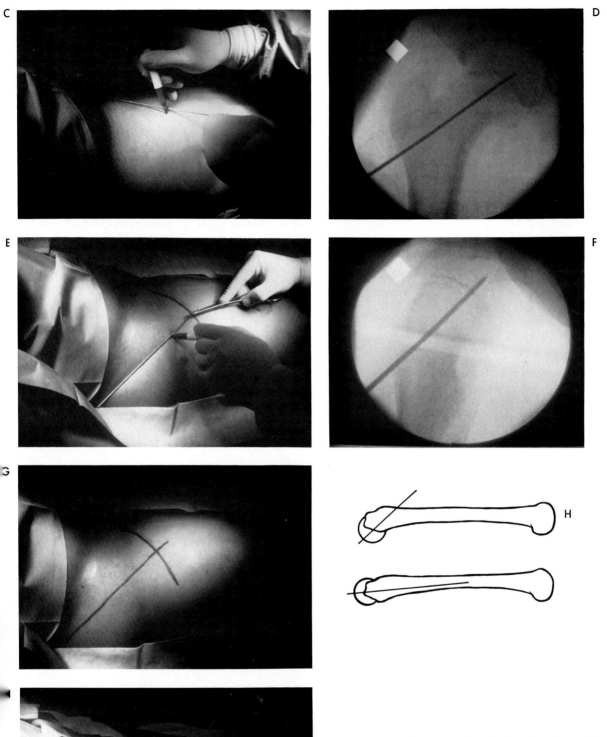

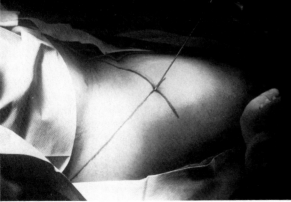

Fig. 16-90   Fluoroscopic technique for determining insertion site for cannulated screw (see text). **A,** Single line perpendicular to center of physis. **B,** Intersection of screw or guide wire with skin planes. **C,** Placement of guide wire on anterior thigh. **D,** Anteroposterior fluoroscopic image. **E,** Placement of guide wire on lateral thigh. **F,** Lateral fluoroscopic image. **G,** Intersection of planes *A* and *B*. **H,** Line of fixation in minimally displaced (*left*) and more severely displaced (*right*) slip. **I,** Insertion of guide wire at intersection of *A* and *B*.

▲ *Technique (Morrissy).* Place the patient on the fracture table with the affected leg abducted 10 to 15 degrees and internally rotated as far as it will go without force. This brings the femoral neck as close as possible to parallel to the floor to assist in obtaining true anterior and lateral views. Position the image intensifier between the legs so that anteroposterior and lateral views can be obtained by moving the tube around the arc of the machine (Fig. 16-91, *A*). After standard preparation and draping and with the use of image control, insert a Kirschner wire percutaneously through the anterolateral area of the thigh down to the femoral neck (Fig. 16-91, *B*), adjusting the guide wire on the anteroposterior projection to ascertain the axis of the femoral neck. Obtain a lateral view to determine the amount of posterior inclination necessary. When the starting point on the femoral neck and amount of posterior inclination have been estimated, insert the guide assembly through a small puncture wound. Advance the guide assembly to the physis, and confirm placement in the central axis of the femoral head by image intensification. If the position is correct, advance the guide assembly across the physis. (If positioning is incorrect, insert a second guide assembly using the first to determine what correction in the starting point or angulation is necessary.) When the proper depth is reached (at least 0.5 cm from subchondral bone), remove the cannula, leaving the guide wire in the bone. Determine the correct screw length by passing a guide wire of identical length along the one in the bone and measuring the difference. Advance the correct length screw over the guide pin, and then remove the guide pin. Remove the leg from the traction device and move it in multiple directions, using both anteroposterior and lateral views to confirm that the screw does not penetrate the joint. Close the stab wound with a single subcuticular suture.

If two screws are deemed necessary for an acute slip, the first screw should lie in the central axis of the femoral head and the second below it, avoiding the superolateral quadrant. The second screw should remain at least 8 mm from subchondral bone.

▲ *Postoperative management.* Range of motion exercises are begun the day after surgery. Most patients begin ambulation with a three-point partial weight-bearing crutch gait on the first postoperative day and are discharged the same day. Crutches are used until all signs of synovitis are gone and motion is free and painless (usually 1 week). All rigorous sports and activities are forbidden until the physes have closed. The screws are removed when there is roentgenographic evidence of physeal closure. The easiest method of removal is to pass a guide wire into the cannula of the screw with the use of image control to allow the screwdriver to be guided into the head of the screw over the guide wire.

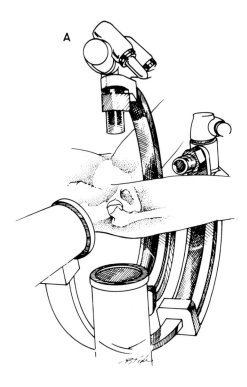
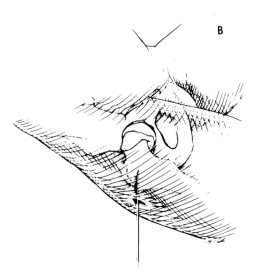

Fig. 16-91 Percutaneous in situ fixation of slipped capital femoral epiphysis. **A,** Positioning of image intensifier to allow rotation necessary to obtain lateral and anteroposterior views. **B,** Kirschner wire passed percutaneously to estimated starting point on femur. (From Morrissy RT: J Pediatr Orthop 10:347, 1990.)

Bone Peg Epiphysiodesis

Proponents of bone peg epiphysiodesis, initially reported by Ferguson and Howorth in 1931, recommend it as a safe, reliable method of treating mild, moderate, or even severe SCFE, with early physeal closure and low incidences of chondrolysis and avascular necrosis. Other advantages are the direct approach to the pathology of SCFE and the avoidance of a second operation to remove a fixation device. Weiner et al (1984) reported 185 bone peg epiphysiodeses performed over a 30-year period, noting avascular necrosis in only 2 of 26 children with acute slips and chondrolysis in one. In 159 chronic slips, four had further slipping caused by acute trauma in two, graft absorption occurred in one, and malplacement of the graft occurred in one. Avascular necrosis developed in only one child, and none had chondrolysis. Roberts and Bloom and Crawford believe long-term results are better after bone peg epiphysiodesis,

especially in moderate and severe slips, but recommend in situ pinning for mild acute or chronic slips. Zahrawi et al, however, after reviewing 105 patients, concluded that pinning in situ was more predictable, had fewer complications, and produced better long-term results than bone peg epiphysiodesis. The disadvantages of open bone peg epiphysiodesis are the longer operating time and the instability of the epiphysis until the graft heals, making postoperative spica casting necessary for acute slips. A major drawback has been a lack of familiarity with the anterior (iliofemoral) approach to the hip joint usually recommended for this procedure; however, Weiner et al recently described an anterolateral approach that simplifies the technique. In a report of 32 epiphysiodeses performed with the anterolateral approach, they cited advantages of reduced operating time, less blood loss, avoidance of damage to the lateral femoral cutaneous nerve, and improved wound healing.

Iliofemoral approach

▶ *Technique.* Make the skin incision along the anterior third of the iliac crest and then along the anterior border of the tensor fasciae latae muscle (Fig. 16-92, *A*); curve it posteriorly across the insertion of this muscle into the iliotibial band in the subtrochanteric region (usually at a point 8 to 10 cm below the base of the greater trochanter). Incise the fascia along the anterior border of the tensor fasciae latae muscle. Identify and protect the lateral femoral cutaneous nerve, which usually is medial to the medial border of the tensor fasciae latae and close to the lateral border of the sartorius muscle. Now cleanly incise the muscle attachments to the lateral aspect of the ilium along the iliac crest to make reflection of the periosteum easier. Reflect it as a continuous structure, without fraying, distally to the superior margin of the acetabulum. Now divide the muscle attachments between the anterosuperior iliac spine and the acetabular labrum. The flap thus reflected consists of the tensor fasciae latae, the gluteus minimus, and the anterior part of the gluteus medius muscles. Inferiorly carry the fascial incision across the insertion of the tensor fasciae latae into the iliotibial band, and expose the lateral part of the rectus femoris and the anterior part of the vastus lateralis muscles. Open the capsule in an H-shaped fashion. Use two large cobra retractors around the femoral neck to expose the femoral head and neck (Fig. 16-92, *B*) and the area of slipping. Fashion a square or rectangular window in the anterior surface of the femoral neck. Then insert a large, hollow "mill" through the window, and drill it across the physis into the epiphysis under image intensifier control (Fig. 16-92, *C*). Remove a cylindric core, consisting of metaphyseal bone, physis, and a portion of the epiphyseal bone, thereby guaranteeing passage of the mill across the physis and into the epiphysis. Enlarge the cylindric tunnel with a curet, and remove more of the physis. Remove sections of corticocancellous bone from the outer layer of the ilium. Sandwich them together and drive this composite bone peg across the physis into the epiphysis (Fig. 16-92, *D*).

▶ *Postoperative management.* In acute slips when there is considerable femoral head mobility, a spica cast should be applied with the femoral head in the reduced position with the graft in place. The cast is worn for 6 weeks and then touchdown weight bearing is allowed. In chronic slips, after bed rest for 48 to 96 hours, the patient ambulates on crutches. Weight bearing can be started at approximately 10 weeks.

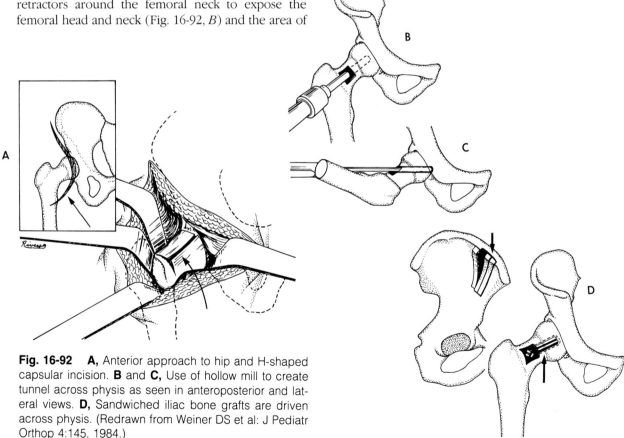

Fig. 16-92 **A,** Anterior approach to hip and H-shaped capsular incision. **B** and **C,** Use of hollow mill to create tunnel across physis as seen in anteroposterior and lateral views. **D,** Sandwiched iliac bone grafts are driven across physis. (Redrawn from Weiner DS et al: J Pediatr Orthop 4:145, 1984.)

Anterolateral approach

▲ *Technique (Weiner et al).* Make a midlateral incision beginning 4 to 5 inches (10 to 12 cm) below the level of the greater trochanter in the lateral midline of the upper portion of the thigh, proceeding proximally to the greater trochanter, and then angling obliquely to the anterosuperior iliac spine (Fig. 16-93, *A*). Split the tensor fasciae femoris proximally to the level of the anterosuperior iliac spine. Retract the tensor anteriorly and posteriorly to expose the underlying anterior portion of the gluteal musculature. Retract poste-

riorly the most anterior fibers of the gluteus medius to expose the joint capsule. Make an H-shaped incision in the capsule, and place large cobra retractors around the femoral neck (Fig. 16-93, *B*). If a bony prominence ("hump") on the anterolateral metaphyseal region resulting from the slipping is severe enough to act as an impediment to motion, remove it with an osteotome. Continue with grafting as already described (see Fig. 16-92, *D*).

▲ *Postoperative management.* Postoperative management is the same as after epiphysiodesis through an iliofemoral approach.

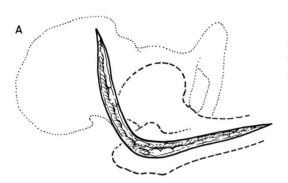

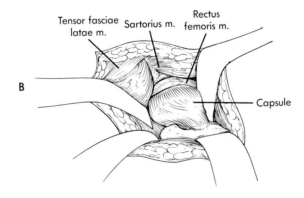

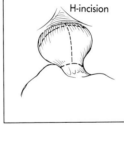

Fig. 16-93 Bone peg epiphysiodesis through anterolateral approach (see text for details). (Redrawn from Weiner DS, Weiner SD, and Melby A: J Pediatr Orthop 8:349, 1988.)

Closed or Open Reduction and Internal Fixation

Manipulative reduction has been reported for acute and acute-on-chronic slips with moderate and severe displacement by Fairbanks, Aadalen et al, and Griffith, among others. Although an association of avascular necrosis with manipulative reduction has been suggested, the development of avascular necrosis may be related to the severity of the slip rather than to the manipulative reduction, provided that only a very gentle reduction is performed. It probably is best, however, to manipulate only severe, acute slips that may be technically difficult to pin in situ.

Closed reduction

▶ *Technique (Boyd et al).* With the patient on the fracture table, apply internal rotation, abduction, and traction simultaneously by a continuous, smooth motion with the child's foot tied to the foot plate. If reduction is not accomplished by this maneuver, flex the hip to 10 to 20 degrees above a right angle with the thigh adducted and apply pressure downward on the flexed knee, forcing the anteriorly and slightly proximally displaced femoral neck back into the concavity of the distal surface of the epiphysis. Then internally rotate, extend, and abduct the thigh with one continuous, smooth motion. Extend the knee with the same movement, and secure the foot to the foot plate with the extremity in abduction, internal rotation, and moderate traction. Following either technique, check the reduction with roentgenograms or the image intensifier and fix the epiphysis with Knowles pins or a cannulated pediatric hip screw (p. 16). If the slip is acute-on-chronic, manipulate it into the position it occupied before the recent injury.

▶ *Postoperative management.* Postoperative management is the same as for pinning of an acute slip (p. 904). If closed reduction of a severe acute or acute-on-chronic slip cannot be obtained, open reduction and internal fixation rarely may be indicated, despite the high incidence of associated avascular necrosis.

Osteotomy

Chronic slips with moderate or severe displacement produce permanent irregularities in the femoral head and acetabulum, and some form of reconstructive procedure often is indicated. The goals of osteotomy are restoration of the normal relationship of the femoral head and neck and delay of the onset of degenerative joint disease. Carney et al, however, reported that at long-term follow-up patients with osteotomy fared worse on the Iowa hip rating with each passing decade compared with patients whose hips were not realigned; they recommended in situ fixation regardless of the severity of slip. Crawford recommends delaying realignment for 1 year after stabilization because of the capacity of the SCFE to remodel. His indications for osteotomy are problems with gait, sitting, or cosmetic appearance after 1 year. Osteotomy also may be indicated for malunion of a chronic slip in poor position; malunited slipped epiphysis differs from a chronic slip only in that in the former the physis has fused and further slipping will not occur.

There are two basic types of osteotomy: closing wedge osteotomy through the femoral neck, usually near the physis to correct the deformity, and compensatory osteotomy through the trochanteric region to produce a deformity in the opposite direction (Fig. 16-94). The advantage of osteotomy through the femoral neck is correction of the deformity itself, but incidences of avascular necrosis ranging from 2% to 100% have been associated with this procedure. Dunn emphasized the need to shorten the femoral neck to prevent tension on the posterior vessels when the epiphysis is reduced to prevent avascular necrosis. Szypryt et al compared the results of Dunn's open reduction with the more conservative Heyman-Herndon epiphysiodesis and concluded that whereas the Heyman-Herndon procedure gave consistently good results for moderate slips, Dunn's technique gave better results for severe slips. They recommend a realignment procedure for slips of more than 50%. Fish, however, reported cuneiform osteotomy just distal to the physis in 42 patients with severe displacement; avascular necrosis developed in only one and osteoarthritis in one, whereas the other 40 hips were reported as having excellent results.

Cuneiform osteotomy of femoral neck

▶ *Technique.* Expose the hip joint through an anterior iliofemoral approach. Incise the anterior capsule longitudinally, parallel to the axis of the femoral neck, and then detach the capsule from the rim of the acetabulum, for about 1 cm on each side of the incision. Place small retractors around the femoral neck to expose its proximal end. The epiphysis will be found medially, posteriorly, and distally, with the proximal neck positioned laterally, anteriorly, and proximally. Externally rotate the thigh, and bring the anterior margin of the epiphysis into view. Insert a Knowles pin through the anterior edge of the epiphysis and into its center; then use the pin as a lever to manipulate the epiphysis as the thigh is internally rotated. If the slip has been gradual before an acute separation, remove some of the new bone at the anterosuperior margin of the neck to obtain an accurate reduction. After completing the reduction, make a short longitudinal skin incision laterally over the base

of the greater trochanter, and insert three Knowles pins across the physis by the technique described for acute mild slips. Check the position of the epiphysis and the pins with roentgenograms in two planes or with an image intensifier.

▶ *Postoperative management.* In a reliable mature child, if internal fixation is secure, putting the extremity in balanced suspension for early motion is preferred. Otherwise, with the hip in 20 degrees of flexion but otherwise in a neutral position, a cast is applied from the nipple line to the toes on the affected side and to just above the knee on the opposite side. The cast is removed at 2 to 4 weeks. Active and passive motion of the hip is then started and is gradually increased. Walking with crutches is started gradually. The patient is allowed at first to place the weight of the extremity on the floor but should not bear full weight on the hip for 4 to 6 months. Then weight bearing is gradually resumed without crutches.

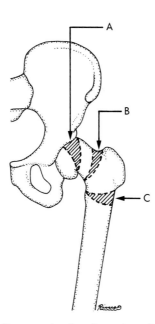

Fig. 16-94 Osteotomies for slipped capital femoral epiphysis. *A,* Through neck near epiphysis. *B,* Through base of neck. *C,* Through trochanteric region. (Redrawn from Crawford AH: In The American Academy of Orthopaedic Surgeons: Instructional course lectures, vol 33, St. Louis, 1984, The CV Mosby Co.)

▲ *Technique (Fish).* Place the patient supine on a standard operating table with a radiolucent roll beneath the involved side of the pelvis to elevate it. Drape the limb free to allow manipulation of the hip during the osteotomy and to facilitate roentgenographic determination of the position of the head of the femur and the pins used for internal rotation (gentle manipulation under anesthesia is done only for patients with an acute slip). Make an anterolateral approach to the hip (p. 913), and carry the dissection between the tensor fasciae latae and gluteus medius muscles to the anterior aspect of the capsule of the hip joint. Generously expose the capsule proximal to the rim of the acetabulum. Open the capsule longitudinally, and then make transverse incisions at each end of the longitudinal incision to expose the neck of the femur (Fig. 16-95, *A*). Carefully retract the capsule with either appropriate clamps or Meyerding retractors. Identify the capital femoral epiphysis, which usually is barely visible at the rim of the acetabulum. The projecting portion of the neck should be obvious. Locate the physis with the aid of a Keith needle or small, sharp, curved osteotome. Determine the size of the wedge to be removed by noting the degree of slip and the position of the epiphysis. Remove enough bone to allow effortless anatomic reduction of the head and neck. Make the base of the wedge anteriorly and superiorly for correct positioning of the epiphysis. Generally, a wider wedge superiorly is necessary in a more severe slip. Shape the wedge of the bone to be removed so that the curved contour of the epiphysis will match the corresponding curved cancellous surface of the femoral neck. After determining the size of the wedge, remove the bone gently in small pieces with an osteotome and mallet (Fig. 16-95, *B* and *C*). Approach the posterior aspect of the neck with caution to avoid vascular damage. This area can be cleared by using a small curet or a hand-held curved osteotome (Fig. 16-95, *D* and *E*). After removing sufficient bone, reduce the epiphysis by flexion, abduction, and internal rotation of the limb. If insufficient bone has been removed and the reduction is forceful, too much tension may be placed on the posterior periosteum, capsule, and vessels. After reduction, fix the epiphysis to the neck with three or four pins. Use pins that are 6 inches (15.2 cm) long, and threaded on one half of their lengths, with a knurled nut on the threads. Do not allow the pins to penetrate the articular cartilage of the epiphysis, but do penetrate the epiphysis deeply enough to obtain firm fixation. Determine, by anteroposterior and frog-leg lateral roentgenograms, the position of the pins. Screw down the knurled nuts to the femoral cortex, and cut the pins next to the nuts (Fig. 16-95, *F*).

▲ *Postoperative management.* The patient should be able to move freely in bed, with the involved limb supported on pillows, and when comfortable, allowed out of bed using crutches with only touch-down weight bearing on the involved limb. Full weight bearing is permitted after roentgenograms show the osteotomy to be completely healed, at approximately 5 months. Then the pins are removed, and full activity is allowed 2 months later.

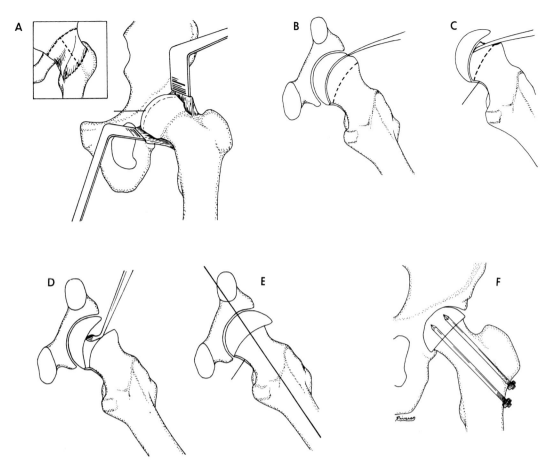

Fig. 16-95   **A,** Fish technique for cuneiform osteotomy of femoral neck. Femoral head and neck are exposed. **A** and *inset,* Joint capsule is incised longitudinally, and then transverse incision is made at each end of longitudinal incision, so that physis can be identified. **B,** Osteotomy is made distal to physis. **C,** Wedge of bone is removed in small pieces with osteotome and mallet. **D,** More bone is removed with small curet or curved osteotome. **E,** Anatomic alignment is obtained. After wedge is removed, diameter of femoral head is often greater than that of femoral neck. **F,** Epiphysis is fixed to femoral neck with three or four pins. (Redrawn from Fish JB: J Bone Joint Surg 66A:1153, 1984.)

Basilar neck osteotomy. Kramer et al described a compensatory osteotomy of the base of the femoral neck that corrects the varus and retroversion components of moderate or severe chronic SCFE, which they believe is safer than osteotomy near or at the physis because it is distal to the major blood supply in the posterior retinaculum. Threaded pins are used for fixation of the osteotomy and the epiphysis, thus preventing further slipping, as well as restoring the anatomic relationship of the proximal femur. The disadvantage of base-of-the-neck osteotomies is that the maximum correction can be obtained only in slips of 35 to 55 degrees. In patients with marked varus deformity the size of the wedge required for correction may cause shortening for which trochanteric osteotomy or epiphysiodesis of the opposite leg may be indicated. Sugioka described a transtrochanteric rotational osteotomy that theoretically corrects deformities of more than 60 degrees, but this has been associated with unacceptably high rates of avascular necrosis (up to 40%).

▶ ***Technique (Kramer et al).*** Determine preoperatively the size of wedge to be removed by measuring the degree of the slip. Determine on anteroposterior roentgenograms the head and neck angle (measure-

ment of this is identical to that described on p. 920). Use paper tracings of the anteroposterior and lateral roentgenograms, and cut with scissors the wedge on the tracing paper to determine the amount of bone to be removed and the results to be obtained.

Approach the hip laterally. Begin the skin incision 2 cm distal and lateral to the anterosuperior iliac spine, and curve it distally and posteriorly over the greater trochanter and then distally along the lateral surface of the femoral shaft to a point 10 cm distal to the base of the trochanter. Incise longitudinally the fascia lata. Develop the interval between the gluteus medius and tensor fasciae latae muscle. Carry the dissection proximally to the inferior branch of the superior gluteal nerve, which innervates the latter muscle. Incise the capsule of the hip joint longitudinally along the anterosuperior surface of the femoral neck. Release widely the capsular attachment along the anterior intertrochanteric line. Reflect distally the vastus lateralis muscle to expose the base of the greater trochanter and the proximal part of the femoral shaft. With the capsule of the hip joint open, identify the junction between the articular cartilage of the femoral head and the callus and the junction of the callus with the normal cortex of the femoral neck. Compare the distance between these two junctions with the calculations made from the paper cutouts of the roentgenograms. The widest part of the wedge will be in line with the widest part of the slip, in the anterior and superior aspects of the neck (Fig. 16-96, *A* and *B*). Make the more distal osteotomy cut first, per-

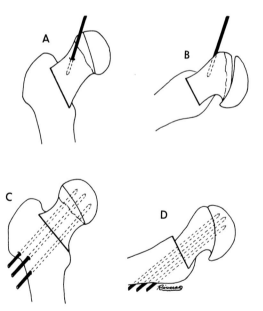

Fig. 16-96 **A** and **B,** Widest part of wedge (at base of neck) is in line with widest part of slip, correcting both varus retroversion components, and Steinmann pin is inserted into femoral neck to control proximal fragment. If wedge is too wide anteriorly, retroversion will be overly corrected. Most common mistake is to make wedge too narrow superiorly so that the varus is incompletely corrected. **C** and **D,** Osteotomy is closed and 5 mm threaded Steinmann pins are inserted from outer cortex of femoral shaft through femoral neck, across osteotomy site, and into head. Pins fix osteotomy, and because they cross physis they prevent any further slip. (Redrawn from Kramer WG, Craig WA, and Noel S: J Bone Joint Surg 58A:796, 1976.)

pendicular to the femoral neck and following the anterior intertrochanteric line from proximal to distal. Extend this osteotomy cut to the posterior cortex, but leave this cortex intact. Make the second osteotomy cut with the blade of the osteotome directed obliquely so that its cutting edge stays distal to the posterior retinacular blood supply. The capsule with the blood supply reaches to the intertrochanteric line anteriorly, but posteriorly the lateral third of the neck is extracapsular. Therefore according to Kramer et al an osteotomy made through the region of the anterior intertrochanteric line lies distal to the posterior retinacular vessels. Drill one or two 5-mm threaded Steinmann pins into the femoral neck proximally to ensure that the proximal portion of the femur is kept under control before completing the osteotomy (Fig. 16-96, *A* and *B*). Complete the osteotomy, taking care that the osteotome does not fully penetrate the posterior cortex. Insert several 5-mm threaded Steinmann pins from the outer cortex of the femoral shaft through the femoral neck. Complete the osteotomy by greensticking the posterior cortex and removing the wedge of bone. Advance the threaded Steinmann pins across the osteotomy site and the physis to prevent further slipping (Fig. 16-96, *C* and *D*). Close the capsule of the hip with interrupted sutures. Clip off the pins close to the femoral shaft. Close the wound in layers. If epiphysiodesis of the greater trochanter is necessary, do it at this time.

▲ *Postoperative management.* Bed rest is prescribed, followed by nonweight bearing for 2 to 3 weeks. Partial weight bearing is allowed according to the stability of the osteotomy and the weight of the patient. The threaded Steinmann pins should be removed only after the epiphyseal plate has fused.

Ball-and-socket and biplane wedge osteotomy. Correction of a deformity that consists of coxa vara, hyperextension, and moderate or severe internal rotation is more difficult. Ball-and-socket osteotomy or biplane wedge osteotomy (as described by Southwick) at the level of the lesser trochanter may correct this triple deformity. Both procedures are technically difficult and require careful planning. The modification of the Southwick procedure by Clark et al decreases the geometric requirements and makes the procedure somewhat simpler. A compression hip screw with side plate or a blade plate bent to the proper angle before surgery may be used for fixation.

This device must be inserted at exactly the same angles as the osteotomy; if inserted at only slightly different angles, alignment of the apposed surfaces of the osteotomy will be incorrect.

Ball-and-socket trochanteric osteotomy

▲ *Technique.* Plan carefully before surgery. Make tracings of anteroposterior and lateral roentgenograms, and measure them accurately to determine exactly the severity of the deformity. With paper cutouts determine the position in which the fragments should be fixed.

Through a lateral approach expose the trochanteric region and the proximal 7.5 to 10 cm of the femoral shaft. Insert a guide pin transversely through the femur at the level of the lesser trochanter, and verify its position by roentgenograms. Now with an osteotome make reference marks on the trochanter and the proximal shaft to be used in determining how much to rotate, flex, and abduct the distal fragment at the time of internal fixation. At the level of the lesser trochanter outline on the bone an osteotomy convex proximally. Along this outline make multiple holes in the cortices with a drill and complete the osteotomy with an osteotome directed proximally. Now the distal fragment is convex and the proximal fragment is concave. Next abduct, flex, and internally rotate the distal fragment appropriately as determined before surgery, and fix the fragments with a blade plate or compression hip screw as in a trochanteric fracture.

▲ *Postoperative management.* Whether a spica cast is applied depends on the firmness of fixation. Usually a cast is unnecessary. The care after surgery is usually about the same as that outlined for other trochanteric osteotomies.

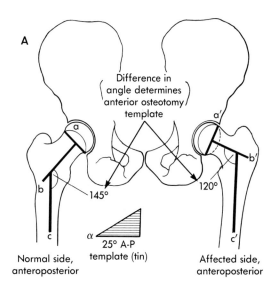

Fig. 16-97 Southwick technique for trochanteric osteotomy in slipped capital femoral epiphysis. Determination of measurements from roentgenograms for correction of slipped epiphysis. **A,** On anteroposterior roentgenogram of hips, angle of femoral neck with femoral shaft is measured on each side. Difference between these two angles determines angle of anterior osteotomy template. **B,** On frog-leg lateral roentgenogram, posterior angulation of neck on shaft is measured on each side. Posterior angulation on affected side minus normal angulation on unaffected side determines angle of lateral osteotomy template. **C,** Wedges of bone to be removed are marked on anteroposterior and lateral roentgenograms of affected hip. **D,** Appearance after wedges have been removed and surfaces of osteotomy have been approximated. (Modified from Southwick WO: J Bone Joint Surg 49A:807, 1967.)

Wedges marked on preoperative roentgenograms

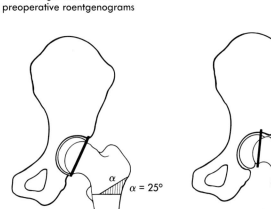

Anteroposterior wedge of 25 cuts through about two thirds of shaft

Lateral wedge of 50 cuts through about one half of shaft

Roentgenographic appearance after proper correction

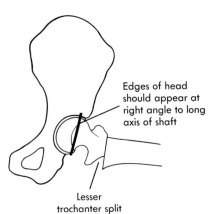

Anteroposterior correction

Lateral correction (frog leg)

Biplane wedge osteotomy

▶ *Technique (Southwick, revised).* Careful planning is necessary before surgery. Make an anteroposterior roentgenogram of the pelvis showing the hips in a position as nearly neutral as possible (the patellas facing upward) and another showing the hips in the frog-leg lateral position (maximum abduction and external rotation). Measurements made on the first roentgenogram determine the amount of varus deformity, and those made on the second determine the amount of posterior tilting (Fig. 16-97, *A* and *B*). Mark the wedges of bone to be removed on both roentgenograms of the affected hip (Fig. 16-97, *C* and *D*). Then using the angle of the wedges as determined on the roentgenograms, cut out of tin a template to be used during the operation in outlining the size and shape of a single wedge (the two wedges combined) to be removed (Fig. 16-98). Southwick noted that the necessary angles are usually 20 to 30 degrees anteriorly and 45 degrees laterally, and sterile commercial templates are available with these angles.

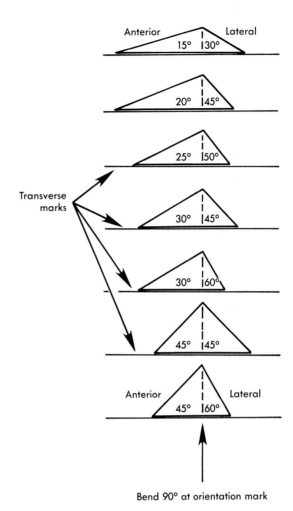

Fig. 16-98   Same as Fig 16-97. Template models (actual size) recommended for patient about 5½ feet tall. (Redrawn from Southwick WO: J Bone Joint Surg 49A:807, 1967.)

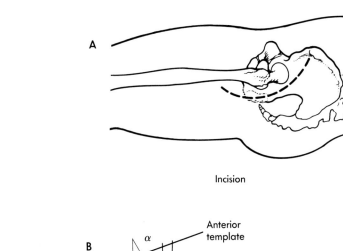

Incision

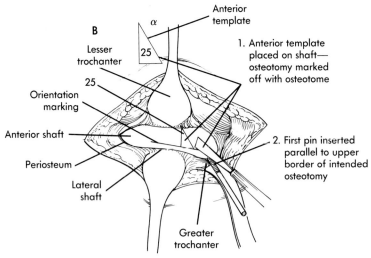

B

α

25

Lesser
trochanter

25

Orientation
marking

Anterior shaft

Periosteum

Lateral
shaft

Anterior
template

Greater
trochanter

1. Anterior template
placed on shaft—
osteotomy marked
off with osteotome

2. First pin inserted
parallel to upper
border of intended
osteotomy

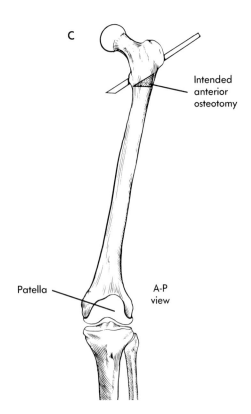

C

Intended
anterior
osteotomy

Patella

A-P
view

Place the patient on the operating table, and drape the affected limb free. Make a slightly curved lateral incision 15 to 20 cm in length along the posterior border of the greater trochanter (Fig. 16-99, *A*). Then incise the tensor fasciae latae and vastus lateralis along the line of the skin incision down to the lateral surface of the femoral shaft. Expose subperiosteally the femoral shaft, and identify the lesser trochanter. Next insert a Bennett or other retractor medially and detach the insertion of the psoas muscle with a sharp periosteal elevator, keeping close to the bone; take care not to injure the nearby vessels or the sciatic nerve. Identify the junction of the flat anterior surface of the femur and the slightly curved lateral surface, and along this junction make a longitudinal orientation mark with a sharp osteotome (Figs. 16-99, *B* and *C,* and 16-100, *A*). This mark identifies the anterolateral edge of the femur; it corresponds to the lateral edge of the bone as seen in the anteroposterior roentgenogram and the anterior edge of the bone as seen in the frog-leg lateral roentgenogram. After making the orientation mark, make a transverse mark with an osteotome at the level of the lesser trochanter.

The template consists of two right triangles (see Fig. 16-98). Bend it 90 degrees and superimpose the appropriate legs of each triangle on the orientation and transverse marks. The hypoteneuses of the triangles are proximal, and they intersect at the orientation mark. Then wrap the template around the anterior and lateral surfaces of the femur. With a sharp osteotome mark the outlines of the template on the bone (Fig. 16-100, *A*). Next drill a 7/32-inch (5.6-mm) Haynes pin into the greater trochanter parallel to the hypoteneuse of the anterior triangle. Place the pin about 6 mm proximal to the hypoteneuse, and drill it toward the lesser trochanter. Use this pin and the T-handle chuck with which it is inserted to control the proximal fragment.

Fig. 16-99 Same as Fig. 16-97. **A,** Skin incision. **B,** Anterior and lateral surfaces of proximal femur have been exposed. Longitudinal *orientation mark* at junction of anterior and lateral surfaces of femur and *transverse mark* at level of lesser trochanter have been made. Anterior part of template has been outlined and first pin has been inserted. **C,** Intended anterior osteotomy. (Redrawn from Southwick WO: J Bone Joint Surg 49A:807, 1967.)

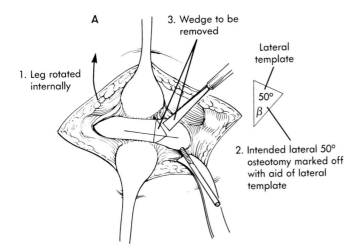

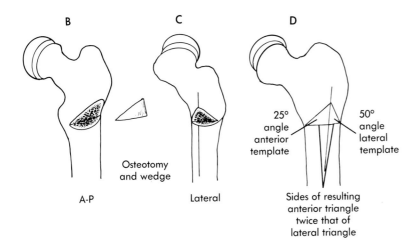

Fig. 16-100   Same as Fig. 16-97. **A,** Both anterior and lateral parts of template have been outlined, indicating wedge of bone to be removed. **B,** Wedge has been removed. **C,** Wedge removed should be large enough so that surface contact between two fragments is sufficient when osteotomy is closed. **D,** Anterior and lateral parts of template meet at orientation mark. (Redrawn from Southwick WO: J Bone Joint Surg 49A:807, 1967.)

Now with a sharp osteotome, following the outlines of the template, remove the wedge of bone consisting of the anterior and lateral cortices of the femur. The proximal oblique surface thus created is flat and is angled by the calculated amounts in both the sagittal and frontal planes (Fig. 16-100, *B*). Continue the transverse cut of the osteotomy through the posterior and medial cortices at the level of the lesser trochanter. Now stabilize the proximal fragment with the Haynes pin, and abduct and flex the distal fragment to place the oblique proximal surfaces of the osteotomy against the transverse end of the distal fragment; the orientation marks on both fragments should meet. As the osteotomy is closed anterolaterally, the transected halves of the lesser trochanter separate, thus adding length to the limb (Fig. 16-101). Posterior tilting and external rotation are related, and internal rotation of the shaft in relation to the proximal fragment rarely is necessary or desirable except in severe deformity.

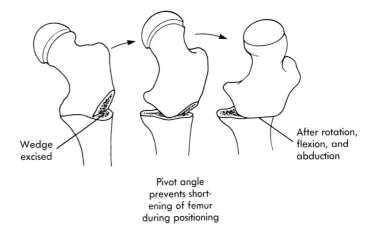

Fig. 16-101   Osteotomy closes anterolateral wedge and opens posteromedial wedge at lesser trochanter. (Redrawn from Southwick WO: J Bone Joint Surg 49A:807, 1967.)

To apply a temporary compression jig to the pin, bend a special side plate to fit, and apply it to the posterolateral surface of the greater trochanter and across the osteotomy while the compression device holds the fragments firmly in contact (Fig. 16-102, *A*). Insert two cancellous bone screws 5 cm in length into the proximal fragment through large holes in the plate. Engage the calcar with at least one of the cancellous screws, and insert one up to the neck of the femur. Secure the distal portion of the plate to the shaft with screws, and remove the Haynes pins and the compression device (Fig. 16-102, *B*). It is not necessary to transfix the capital femoral epiphysis with a screw unless the physis is still open. Make an anteroposterior roentgenogram to check the position of the osteotomy and the plate and screws.

◤ *Postoperative management.* The extremity is placed in balanced suspension for 2 to 4 weeks with the hip at 30 degrees of flexion to relax the capsule. Following this, sitting and standing at the bedside with weight bearing on the uninvolved side are encouraged, and slight active flexion of the hip and knee is encouraged to regain muscle control. After the patient has regained sufficient muscle control, crutch walking with toe touching is begun. No weight is borne on the operated hip until the physis has fused and the osteotomy is solid.

Complications

The two most serious complications of SCFE are chondrolysis and avascular necrosis. Various treatment factors have been implicated as causes, including manipulative or open reduction, spica cast immobilization, penetration of pins into the joint, and osteotomy; however, these complications also have been reported in patients who had no surgical treatment.

Chondrolysis is a rapid progressive narrowing of the hip joint as a result of the loss of articular cartilage, with a reported incidence ranging from 1% to 40% (average 7%). Ingram et al found that chondrolysis occurred more often in black persons and women than in white persons and men and more often in chronic or acute-on-chronic slips than in acute slips. Chondrolysis occurred after trochanteric osteotomy (59%) (Fig. 16-103), open reduction (55%), and femoral neck osteotomy (37%) but also after closed reduction and in situ fixation (13%). Pin penetration into the joint was associated with a 51% incidence of chondrolysis. Chondrolysis was present in 12% of patients before any treatment.

Recovery of the width of the joint space has been reported to occur 1 to 2 years after the onset of chondrolysis, and Southwick recommends that surgical treatment not be considered until at least a year elapses. Bed rest, traction, salicylates, antiinflammatories, steroids, and physical therapy all have been recommended for treatment of chondrolysis, but they do not appear to alter its course. Crawford recommends subtotal circumferential capsulectomy, intraoperative manipulation, and postoperative continued passive motion with bupivacaine analgesia for problems unresponsive to traction and physical therapy. If severe joint space narrowing persists with limitation of joint motion, arthrodesis or arthroplasty should be considered.

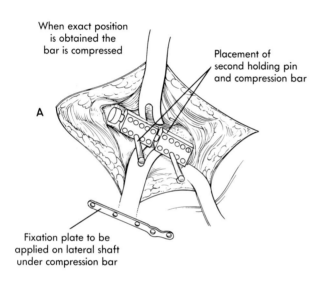

When exact position is obtained the bar is compressed

Placement of second holding pin and compression bar

A

Fixation plate to be applied on lateral shaft under compression bar

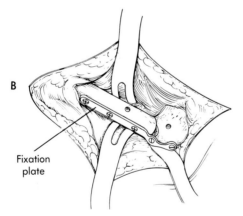

B

Fixation plate

Fig. 16-102 Southwick technique of compression fixation through biplane osteotomy of proximal femur for slipped capital femoral epiphysis. **A,** Compression device is shown in place over two holding pins in femur. **B,** Shaped side plate has been attached with screws and holding pins and compression device removed. (Redrawn from Southwick WO: J Bone Joint Surg 55A:1218, 1973.)

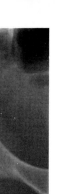
A

Fig. 16-103 Moderate slip of capital femoral epiphysis. **A,** Pinning in situ. **B,** Subtrochanteric osteotomy was followed by development of chondrolysis. Motion was limited and joint space of involved hip measured 1.5 mm compared with 4 mm in the uninvolved hip. **C,** One year following onset of chondrolysis. Internal fixation has been removed. Joint space and motion are unchanged.
Continued.

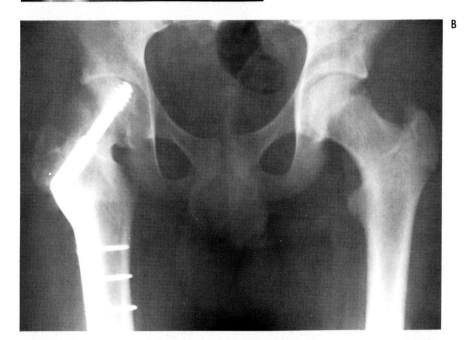
B

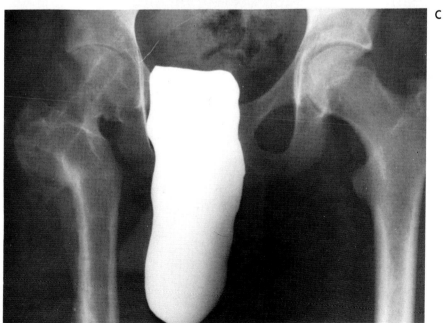
C

Avascular necrosis is rare in untreated patients and probably results from interruption of the retrograde blood supply by the original injury (if any), by forceful repetitive manipulations, by open reduction, or by osteotomy of the femoral neck. Ingram et al found avascular necrosis more common with moderate and severe displacement and after femoral neck osteotomy (33%), open reduction and pinning (27%), and closed reduction with Knowles pinning (27%). It was less common with mild displacement and after in situ fixation (1.5%) and trochanteric osteotomy (10%). Although tamponade of the blood supply to the proximal femoral epiphysis as a result of acute hemorrhage within the capsule of the hip has been sug-

gested as a cause of avascular necrosis, there seems to be no evidence that immediate aspiration of the hip joint is effective in preventing avascular necrosis. Superolateral placement of pins also has been associated with the development of avascular necrosis or at least with exacerbation of the process. Treatment guidelines are essentially the same as for treatment of avascular necrosis after hip fracture (p. 890).

Other complications that may occur include continued slipping in the absence of internal fixation or with incorrect pin placement or pin length or too early removal of pins (Fig. 16-104) and fracture distal to the internal fixation.

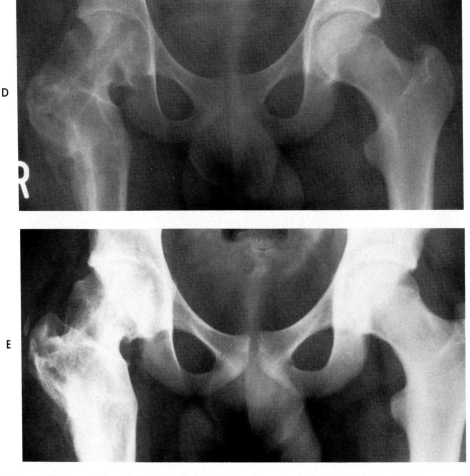

Fig. 16-103, cont'd **D,** Twenty-four months after onset of chondrolysis. Joint space is now 2.5 mm wide, but hip motion is only slightly improved. **E,** Thirty-six months after onset. Joint space on involved side measures 3.5 mm and is almost equal to opposite hip. Motion in hip is still decreased.

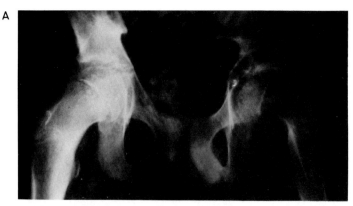

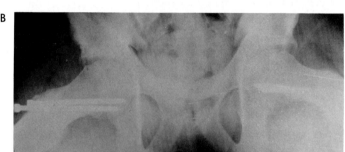

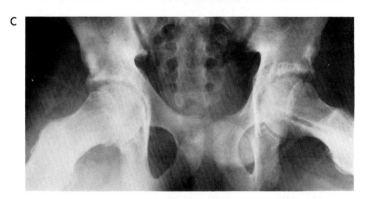

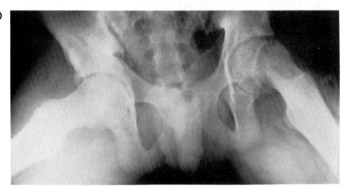

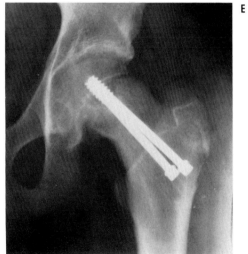

Fig. 16-104 **A,** Bilateral slipped femoral epiphysis. **B,** After internal fixation. **C,** One year after fixation, pins have been removed. **D,** Progression of slipping 18 months after fixation. **E,** Percutaneous pinning with cannulated pediatric hip screw to prevent further slipping.

PELVIC FRACTURES

Pelvic fractures are rare in children and rarely require surgical treatment. Because of the remodeling potential of the pelvis in children, conservative treatment generally yields satisfactory results. The child's pelvis is more malleable than an adult's, the joints are more elastic, and the cartilaginous structures are able to absorb more energy. The elasticity of the joints around the pelvis in children allows significant displacement, and a single break in the pelvic ring is frequent in children, rather than the double break most often seen in adults. The cartilage at the physes, however, is inherently weaker than bone, and avulsion fractures occur more frequently in children than in adults. Fractures into the triradiate cartilage may cause growth arrest, leg length inequality, and abnormal development of the acetabulum.

Because pelvic fractures in children generally are associated with high-energy trauma, such as motor vehicle accidents, the associated injuries often are severe and life-threatening; the mortality rate in children with pelvic fractures ranges from 9% to 18%. Bryan and Tullos reported that more than half of 52 children with pelvic fractures had prolonged hospitalization because of associated trauma. Torode and Zieg reported 11 deaths in 141 patients with pelvic fractures, and 40% of patients with type IV injuries (bilateral pubic rami fractures, fracture of the pubic rami or pubic symphysis, fractures through the posterior elements or disruption of the sacroiliac joint on the contralateral side, or fracture involving the anterior structures and acetabular portion of the pelvic ring) required laparotomy for associated injuries. Commonly associated injuries include fractures of the skull, cervical spine, facial bones, and long bones of the extremities; subdural hematomas, cerebral contu-

sions and concussions; lung contusions; hemothorax; hemopneumothorax; ruptured diaphragm; and lacerations of the spleen, liver, and kidney. Injuries adjacent to the pelvic fracture may include damage to major blood vessels, retroperitoneal bleeding, rectal tears, and rupture or laceration of the urethra or bladder. These injuries require immediate, definitive treatment.

Classification

The classification of pelvic fractures introduced by Key and Conwell is the most commonly used:

I. Fractures without a break in the continuity of the pelvic ring
  A. Avulsion fractures (Fig. 16-105)
    1. Anterior superior iliac spine
    2. Anterior inferior iliac spine
    3. Ischial tuberosity
  B. Fractures of the pubis or ischium
  C. Fractures of the wing of the ilium (Duverney) (Fig. 16-106)
  D. Fractures of the sacrum or coccyx
II. Single break in the pelvic ring
  A. Fracture of two ipsilateral rami (Fig. 16-107)
  B. Fracture near or subluxation of the symphysis pubis
  C. Fracture near or subluxation of the sacroiliac joint
III. Double break in the pelvic ring
  A. Double vertical fractures or dislocation of the pubis (straddle fractures)
  B. Double vertical fractures or dislocation (Malgaigne)
  C. Severe multiple fractures
IV. Fractures of the acetabulum
  A. Small fragment associated with dislocation of the hip (Fig. 16-108)

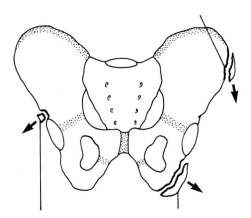

Fig. 16-105 Various avulsion fractures of pelvis. (Redrawn from Ogden JA: Skeletal injury in the child, Philadelphia, 1982, Lea & Febiger.)

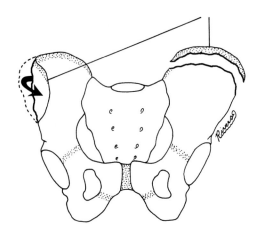

Fig. 16-106 Types of fractures of iliac wing. (Redrawn from Ogden JA: Skeletal injury in the child, Philadelphia, 1982, Lea & Febiger.)

B. Linear fracture associated with nondisplaced pelvic fracture
C. Linear fracture associated with hip joint instability
D. Fracture resulting from central dislocation of the acetabulum.

Torode and Zieg proposed a four-part classification (Fig. 16-109): type I, avulsion of bony elements of the pelvis; type II, iliac wing fractures; type III, simple ring fracture, including fractures involving the pubic rami or disruptions of the pubic symphysis; and type IV, ring disruption fractures that create an unstable segment of the pelvic ring, including bilateral pubic rami fracture (straddle), fractures involving either the right or left pubic rami or the pubic symphysis and fractures through the posterior elements or disruption of the sacroiliac joint, and fractures including the anterior structures and acetabular portion of the pelvic ring.

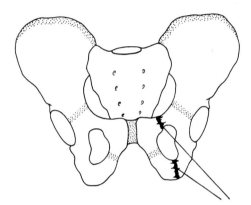

Fig. 16-107 Single break in pelvic ring, with two ipsilateral rami fractures. (Redrawn from Ogden JA: Skeletal injury in the child, Philadelphia, 1982, Lea & Febiger.)

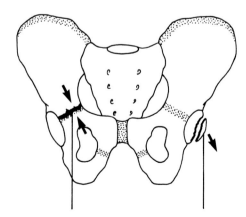

Fig. 16-108 Small acetabular rim fracture *(right)* and triradiate cartilage compression fracture *(left)*. (Redrawn from Ogden JA: Skeletal injury in the child, Philadelphia, 1982, Lea & Febiger.)

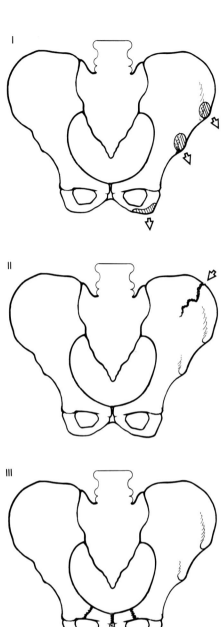
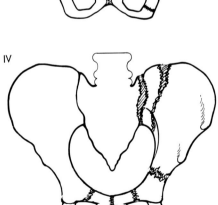

Fig. 16-109 Classification of pelvic fractures (see text for details). (Redrawn from Torode I and Zieg D: J Pediatr Orthop 5:76, 1985.)

Fractures of individual bones without a break in the continuity of the pelvic ring are most common in children (Table 16-2), accounting for approximately 67% of pelvic fractures. Of the individual bones the pubis and ischium are the most frequently fractured. Avulsion fractures occur most often in the anterosuperior and anteroinferior iliac spines and the ischial tuberosity and are caused by overpull of the sartorius muscle, rectus femoris muscle, and hamstring muscles, respectively. These avulsion fractures are most common in adolescent athletes. Fernbach and Wilkinson reported 20 avulsion fractures of the apophyses of the pelvis and proximal femur, most of which occurred in male adolescents engaged in competitive sports. Six of these fractures involved the ischial tuberosity, five the lesser femoral trochanter, four the anteroinferior iliac spine, four the anterosuperior iliac spine, and one the anterior iliac apophyses. Single and double breaks in the pelvic ring each account for approximately 12% of fractures, and fractures of the acetabulum are the least common. Few pelvic fractures in children are seriously displaced, and most are stable because of the relatively thick periosteum in children.

Signs and Symptoms

Three physical signs commonly associated with pelvic fractures were described by Milch: (1) Destot's sign, a large hematoma formation superficially beneath the inguinal ligament or in the scrotum; (2) Roux's sign, a decrease in the distance from the greater trochanter to the pubic spine on the affected side in lateral compression fractures; and (3) Earle's sign, a bony prominence or large hematoma and tenderness on rectal examination, indicating a significant pelvic fracture. Posterior pressure on the iliac crest will cause pain at the fracture site as the pelvic ring is opened, and compression of the pelvic ring at the iliac crest from lateral to medial will cause pain and possibly crepitation. Downward pressure on the symphysis pubis and posteriorly on the sacroiliac joints will cause pain and motion if there is a break in the pelvic ring. Pain in the inguinal area may be noted with flexion and extension of the hips.

Anteroposterior roentgenograms may be sufficient for diagnosis of a pelvic fracture, but the inlet and tilt views recommended by Judet et al give a more accurate picture of the amount of internal or external rotational deformity and the amount of displacement (Fig. 16-110), especially in fractures of the acetabulum and pelvic outlet. Comparison views of the contralateral apophysis are helpful in the diagnosis of avulsion fractures. Tomograms may be necessary to determine a nondisplaced pelvic fracture, especially in the pubic rami, and a CT scan may be beneficial in also determining disruption or incongruity of the sacroiliac joint, sacrum, or acetabulum. Radioisotopic bone scanning, several days after injury, may identify nondisplaced fractures, stress fractures, and fractures of the sacrum and coccyx.

Table 16-2 Distribution of pelvic fractures in children, Campbell Clinic series (134 patients)*

I—Individual bones 66.5%				II—Single break 11.9%			III—Double break 11.9%			IV—Acetabulum 9.7%			
A	B	C	D	A	B	C	A	B	C	A	B	C	D
13.4%	33.6%	18%	1.5%	8.2%	3%	0.7%	3%	8.2%	0.7%	0.7%	6%	0	3%

Comparison With Other Series

	Dunn† (115 patients)	Peltier† (186 patients)	Reed† (84 patients)	Hall, Klassen, Ilstrup‡ (204 patients)	Campbell Clinic‡ (134 patients)
I—Individual bones		10%	60.5%	24.5%	66.5%
II—Single break	70% (stable)	39%	2.5%	18.6%	11.9%
III—Double break	30% (unstable)	27%	32%	31.9%	11.9%
IV—Acetabulum	Not included	24%	5%	7.8% (17.2% acetabulum and pelvis)	9.7%

From Rockwood CA Jr, Wilkins KD, and King RE, editors: Fractures in children, vol 3, Philadelphia, 1984, JB Lippincott Co.
*Classification of Key and Conwell.
†Adult series.
‡Children's series.

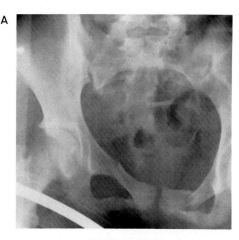

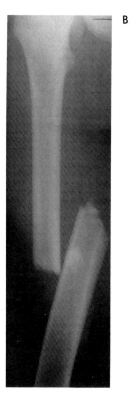

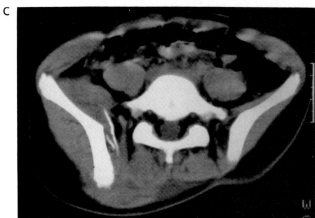

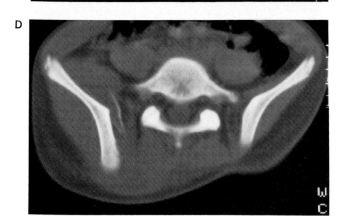

Fig. 16-110   **A,** Fracture of symphysis pubis, disruption of sacroiliac joint *(left),* and, **B,** fracture of femoral shaft in 12-year-old child. **C** and **D,** CT scanning shows fracture of ilium and gross disruption of the sacroiliac joint. **E** and **F,** At follow-up, good alignment of pelvis and fusion of sacroiliac joint with intramedullary rod fixation of femoral shaft fracture.

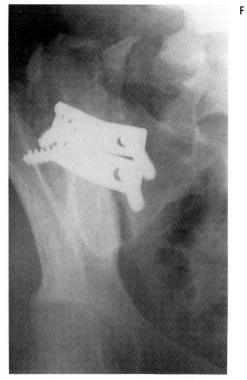

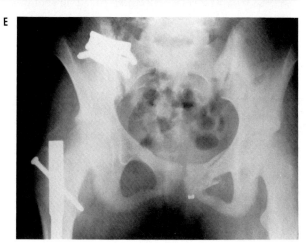

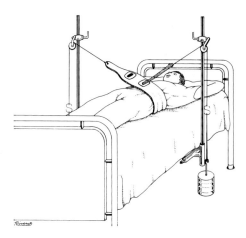

Fig. 16-111 Pelvic sling with crossed straps for treatment of diastasis of symphysis pubis. (Redrawn from Weber BG, Brunner CH, and Freuler F, editors: Treatment of fractures in children and adolescents, New York, 1980, Springer-Verlag.)

Fig. 16-112 Treatment of diastasis of symphysis pubis by external fixator. **A,** Wide diastasis of symphysis pubis seen on inlet view. **B,** Intraoperative roentgenogram shows closed reduction of diastasis and external fixator in place. **C,** At 8 months slight diastasis persists.

A
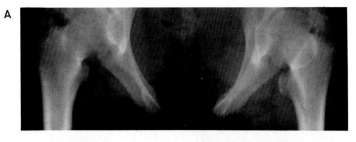

B
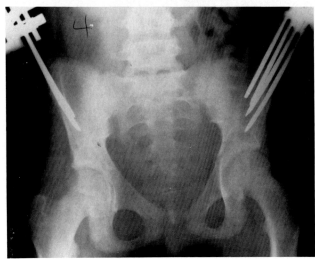

C
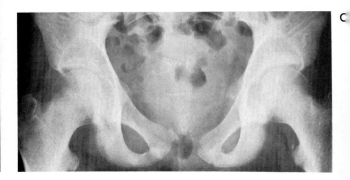

Treatment

Nearly all fractures of individual bones of the pelvis or single breaks in the pelvis in children can be treated with bed rest and protected ambulation. Fernbach and Wilkinson recommend conservative treatment of all avulsion fractures and, despite reports to the contrary, found no decrease in athletic ability in their patients. A pelvic sling occasionally may be required for significant diastasis of the symphysis (Fig. 16-111), followed by a spica cast in the reduced position. External fixation may be used to close the diastasis (Fig. 16-112). Mears and Fu recommend aggressive treatment of subluxations of the symphysis pubis and sacroiliac joint because little or no remodeling occurs to compensate for joint subluxations or dislocations. Malgaigne fractures (double vertical fractures or fractures with dislocation) generally can be treated with skeletal traction and a pelvic sling; to adequately reduce the fracture the pelvic sling should have enough traction weight applied to lift the buttocks slightly off the bed. The straps of the sling can be crossed to further close the pelvic ring, and occasionally the incorporation of the pelvic sling in a spica cast with the pelvic traction still in place is useful. If this does not adequately reduce the fracture, external fixation may be indicated. Bryan and Tullos emphasize the importance of maintaining a symmetric pelvis to prevent cephalad translation or anteroposterior hemipelvis rotation to avoid late complications. They recommend a combination of skeletal traction or pelvic sling, followed by spica casting or the use of an external fixation device for unstable fractures. Alonzo and Horowitz reported the use of AO-AISF external fixation in three children and recommend it for unstable pelvic fractures to align the fracture components, decrease blood loss, and permit early mobilization. Open reduction and internal fixation rarely are needed to stabilize a posterior column fracture because of persistent bleeding or significant malalignment.

Acetabular Fractures

Acetabular fractures occur in 0.8% to 15% of pelvic fractures in children. In contrast to pelvic fractures they may be caused by trivial trauma, and damage to the triradiate cartilage may cause growth arrest and a shallow, dysplastic acetabulum (Fig. 16-113). The classification of acetabular fractures is based on the extent of acetabular involvement and femoral head stability: (1) small fragments most often associated with dislocation of the hip, (2) linear fractures associated with pelvic fractures without displacement, (3) large linear fractures with hip joint instability, and (4) central fracture-dislocations. CT scanning may be helpful in determining the extent of acetabular involvement and stability of the femoral head.

A small, chip fracture from the posterior margin of the acetabulum may be found during reduction of a hip dislocation, but the hip usually is stable. Prereduction roentgenograms often better reveal the occult fragment than films made after reduction. Stable linear fractures of the acetabulum require only a period of nonweight bearing on crutches. Linear fractures that produce hip joint instability require skeletal traction and an accurate reduction. Skeletal traction has been recommended for 6 to 12 weeks in adults, but, depending on the skeletal age of the child, this lengthy period of traction usually is not necessary. Heeg et al (1989) reported good results in minimally displaced fractures with an average of 4.2 weeks of traction.

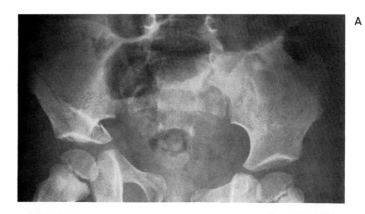

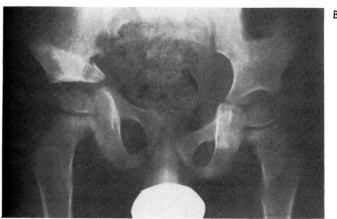

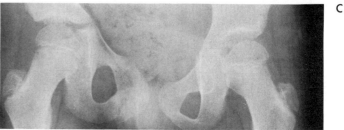

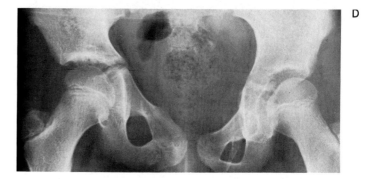

Fig. 16-113   Premature closure of triradiate cartilage. **A,** Fracture of right ilium is obvious. Fracture on left was not identified. **B,** At 4 months fracture on right again seen. In left acetabulum increased sclerosis caused by ischial fracture into acetabulum is noted. **C,** At 5 years premature closure of left triradiate cartilage. **D,** At 6 years premature closure of left triradiate cartilage and subluxation of femoral head caused by shallow acetabulum.

Central fracture-dislocations should be reduced promptly because the triradiate cartilage may be involved, and premature fusion of the triradiate cartilage can have devastating consequences. Gepstein et al found that after surgically induced premature fusion in young rabbits, acetabular dysplasia occurred 5 weeks after operation in all animals and hip dislocation occurred in 9 weeks in half. Heeg et al (1988) reported that of four patients with injuries of the triradiate cartilage, three had premature fusion of the cartilage, and acetabular deformity and hip subluxation developed in two of these. Because injury to the triradiate cartilage is easily missed on initial roentgenograms, they recommend that all patients with pelvic trauma be observed clinically and roentgenographically for at least 1 year. Bucholz et al noted two main patterns of physeal disruption in nine patients with triradiate cartilage injury: a Salter-Harris type I or II injury that had a favorable prognosis for continued normal acetabular growth and a Salter-Harris type V crushing injury that had a poor prognosis because of premature closure of the triradiate physes as a result of formation of a medial osseous bridge. In both patterns the prognosis was dependent on the age of the patient at the time of injury. In younger children, especially those younger than 10 years of age, abnormal acetabular growth was frequent and resulted in a shallow acetabulum. By skeletal maturity disparate growth increased the incongruity of the hip joint and led to progressive subluxation. The authors recommend acetabular reconstruction for correction of the gradual subluxation of the femoral head. Heeg et al found that surgical reduction, although required for unstable posterior fracture-dislocations and irreducible central fracture-dislocations, did not improve results in their patients, particularly those with type V fractures.

SPINE FRACTURES AND DISLOCATIONS
Cervical Spine Fractures

Cervical spine fractures are uncommon in children, but they do occur in infants from child abuse, in young children in association with congenital anomalies such as Down syndrome, and in older children from trauma such as diving accidents. Because the cervical spine is more flexible in children than in adults, it often is difficult to differentiate the normal from the abnormal on flexion and extension roentgenograms of the child's cervical spine. Fielding determined that anterior displacement of the atlas of up to 3 mm is normal in adults. A distance of 3 to 5 mm between the odontoid process and the arch of C1 indicates rupture of the transverse ligaments, and a distance greater than 10 to 12 mm indicates failure of all ligaments. Cattell and Filtzer, in a study of 14 symptom-free children aged 1 to 7 years, determined that a minimum of 3 mm and even more of anterior displacement of the atlas in flexion was a normal variation (Fig. 16-114), probably because of the increased mobility and ligamentous laxity in children as compared with adults. They also noted that pseudosubluxation was a common variant and that significant anterior displacement of C2 on C3 in flexion occurred in young children without symptoms. Fielding outlined the normal roentgenographic variations that may be misinterpreted as acute injuries: (1) the apical ossification center of the odontoid, which may be confused with an acute fracture; (2) secondary ossification centers at the tips of the transverse and spinous processes, which may be confused with avulsion fractures; (3) incomplete ossification, especially of the odontoid process, with apparent superior sub-

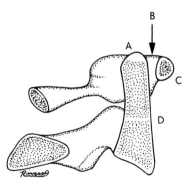

Fig. 16-114 Relationships of atlas and axis. *A,* Apical epiphysis. *B,* Space between odontoid and atlas anteriorly, which may be more than 3 mm in children. *C,* Anterior arch of atlas. *D,* Basilar odontoid synchondrosis or cartilaginous plate, which may fuse between 7 and 10 years of age. (Redrawn from Cattell HS and Filtzer DL: J Bone Joint Surg 47A:1295, 1965.)

luxation of the anterior arch of C1; (4) persistence of the synchondrosis (physis) at the base of the odontoid; (5) anterior wedging in a vertebral body, which may be misinterpreted as a compression fracture or a subluxation; (6) hypermobility "pseudosubluxation," especially of C2 anterior to C3; (7) increase in the atlanto-dens interval of up to 4 mm; (8) absence of the ossification of the anterior arch of C1 in the first year of life, which suggests posterior displacement of C1 on the odontoid; (9) physiologic variations in the width of the soft tissue swelling anterior to the cervical spine; (10) overlying anatomy, such as the ears, braided hair, teeth, or the hyoid bone; (11) horizontally placed facets in the normal child, which create the illusion of a pillar fracture; (12) congenital anomalies such as os odontoideum, spina bifida, and lack of segmentation; and (13) less-than-normal lateral lordotic posture of the neck. Bone scans, tomograms, CT scans, and MRI of the neck now make the various diagnoses much easier and may be helpful in distinguishing normal growth variants from traumatic injuries in the cervical spine.

Herzenberg et al recently described modifications necessary to the standard backboard for safer alignment of the spine during transport of young children with cervical spine injuries. In their study of 10 children younger than 7 years, they found that unstable injuries of the cervical spine had anterior angulation or translation, or both, and that extension was the proper position for reduction in all 10 children. Because young children have a large head in comparison with the rest of the body, positioning on a standard backboard may force the neck into relative kyphosis. They recommend the use of a recess for the occiput to lower the head or a double mattress pad to raise the chest and prevent undesirable cervical flexion.

Atlantoaxial Fracture-Dislocations

Lesions in the area from the occiput to the atlas or C1 are extremely rare and usually lethal. More injuries occur in children from C1 to C4, in contrast to adults in whom most cervical spine injuries occur from C3 to C7. Fielding described four lesions that occur at the C1-C2 interval in children: (1) ligamentous laxity related to inflammation or other local affliction, (2) rotary deformity, (3) traumatic ligamentous disruption, and (4) odontoid fracture.

Ligamentous laxity. Atlantoaxial displacement caused by inflammation may follow an upper respiratory viral infection, tuberculosis, syphilis, poliomyelitis, juvenile rheumatoid arthritis, or ankylosing spondylitis, or it may occur in association with Down syndrome or eosinophilic granuloma. This type of displacement should not be confused with traumatic ligamentous disruption. A thorough history and physical and roentgenographic examinations, including CT scanning, should determine if the displacement is traumatic. Appropriate treatment of the inflammation and cervical traction in extension to stabilize the vertebrae are successful in treating most atlantoaxial displacement. Marar and Balachandran, however, reported that 3 of 12 children with nontraumatic atlantoaxial dislocations required posterior cervical spine fusion because of persistent pain and neurologic signs.

Rotary deformity. Lateral rotary displacement of the odontoid-axial area is relatively common and is one of the most common causes of traumatic torticollis. Often the stiff neck and slightly twisted head resolve spontaneously, and most rotary deformities require little more than head-halter traction, muscle relaxants, and bed rest. Occasionally the rotary displacement, especially if significant, becomes fixed, and Fielding lists four indications for C1 to C2 fusion: (1) persistent neurologic involvement, (2) significant anterior rotary displacement, (3) failure to achieve or maintain correction of a deformity present for more than 3 months, and (4) recurrence of the deformity after an adequate trial of conservative management (at least 6 weeks of immobilization).

Traumatic ligamentous disruption. Traumatic ligamentous disruption is difficult to diagnose in children because in flexion there may be 3 mm or more of anterior displacement of the atlas on the axis without significant trauma. According to Fielding, evidence of significant trauma and more than 5 mm of displacement are indicative of ligamentous rupture. Acute ruptures should be treated by reduction in extension by traction; a Minerva jacket or halo cast is used to hold the reduction for 8 to 12 weeks, when flexion and extension roentgenograms should be obtained. If displacement and symptoms persist, fusion of C1 to C2 should be performed.

Odontoid fracture. The synchondrosis (physis) of the base of the odontoid usually is fused by the time the child is 7 years of age, but it can persist roentgenographically for 2 to 4 years longer. As a result most fractures of the odontoid process in children occur around the age of 7 years or earlier and almost invariably occur between the odontoid process and the body of the second cervical vertebra, at or near the synchondrosis (Fig. 16-115). Failure of ossification of the apical odontoid process or lack of synchondrotic fusion at the base of the odontoid should not be confused with a fracture (see Fig. 16-114). Sherk et al reported that prompt treatment of odontoid fractures in children younger than 7 years usually results in healing without sequelae. Reduction usually can be obtained by passive manipulation or recumbency and head-halter traction in extension, and it should be maintained for 2 to 3 months in a Minerva jacket or halo cast; a halo cast should not be applied until the fracture is reduced. If the fracture cannot be reduced, skeletal traction with tongs or even closed manipulative reduction with the patient under general anesthesia may be necessary.

Congenital anomalies such as an os odontoideum or rudimentary odontoid may contribute to C1-C2 instability in adolescent athletes; treatment of these conditions is discussed in Chapter 9.

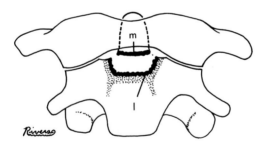

Fig. 16-115 Pattern of odontoid fractures. *M* marks level of usual adult fractures. *I* marks area of childhood fractures at synchondrosis. (Redrawn from Ogden JA: Skeletal injury in the child, Philadelphia, 1982, Lea & Febiger.)

Open reduction and C1-C2 fusion

▶ ***Technique (Rogers).*** Make an incision in the midline from the prominent spinous process of the seventh cervical vertebra to the easily palpable spinous process of the second (Fig. 16-116, *A*). When the first, second, or third vertebra is involved, extend the incision toward the occiput. Identify the spinous processes in preparation for subperiosteal exposure of the posterior aspect of one vertebra above and one below the involved vertebra. Insert a needle or pin into this spinous process, and check its location by a lateral roentgenogram. Expose by sharp subperiosteal dissection the spinous processes, laminae, and posterior articulations; if the neural arch has been fractured, be careful during the exposure to prevent cord damage. Steady the spinous process of the unstable vertebra with forceps during this dissection. Then accomplish the reduction by gentle traction with forceps. If the articular facets are dislocated, manipulate them into position using the procedure just described for dislocation.

Fix the fracture internally as follows. Usually two and sometimes three vertebrae are included in the internal fixation and fusion. If it is a dislocated vertebra only, fix the involved vertebra to the one below. Sometimes, however, the spinous processes (especially of the third, fourth, and fifth vertebrae) are small and fixation is insecure. In these instances, fix three or four vertebrae. When a fusion is being done for a fracture-dislocation, extend the fusion area from the first intact vertebra above to the first intact vertebra below the level of injury. Make a hole in the base of the spinous process of each vertebra to be included in the fusion. Use a towel clip to start the hole, and complete it with a Lewin clamp. This is safer than using a drill that can slip and damage the cord. By sharp dissection, remove all soft tissue from the spinous process and lamina of each vertebra to be fused; a small rongeur or pituitary forceps is helpful. Loop a wire through these holes as illustrated in Fig. 16-116, *B*. Place the wire around the superior border of the superior process, and insert the ends in opposite directions through the hole in this process. Then pass the ends of the wires distally and parallel along the spinous processes to the last process to be fused, and then through the hole in this spinous process in opposite directions, and loop them around the distal border of this process. Now lay transversely two iliac grafts bridging each interspace and tighten the wire. Force the edges of the graft beneath the wire to ensure maintenance of position (Fig. 16-116, *C*). Pack multiple chips of cancellous bone wherever possible to reinforce the larger grafts. When the spine is unstable, subperiosteal exposure is dangerous, and decortication of the laminae is even more so. The latter is unnecessary because the cancellous grafts will fuse satisfactorily to the laminae and spinous processes without this additional step.

▶*Postoperative management.* Postoperative management is the same as described for open reduction of dislocations.

Fig. 16-116 Rogers technique for open reduction of fracture-dislocation of cervical spine. **A,** *1,* Incision; *2,* subperiosteal approach to posterior aspect of vertebrae. **B,** *1,* Hole is drilled in bone on each side of base of spinous process; *2* and *3,* hole through base is completed with vulsellum forceps and small hook; *4,* vertebrae are fixed with wire loop as described in text. **C,** Iliac grafts are applied (see text). (Redrawn from Rogers WA: J Bone Joint Surg 24:245, 1942.)

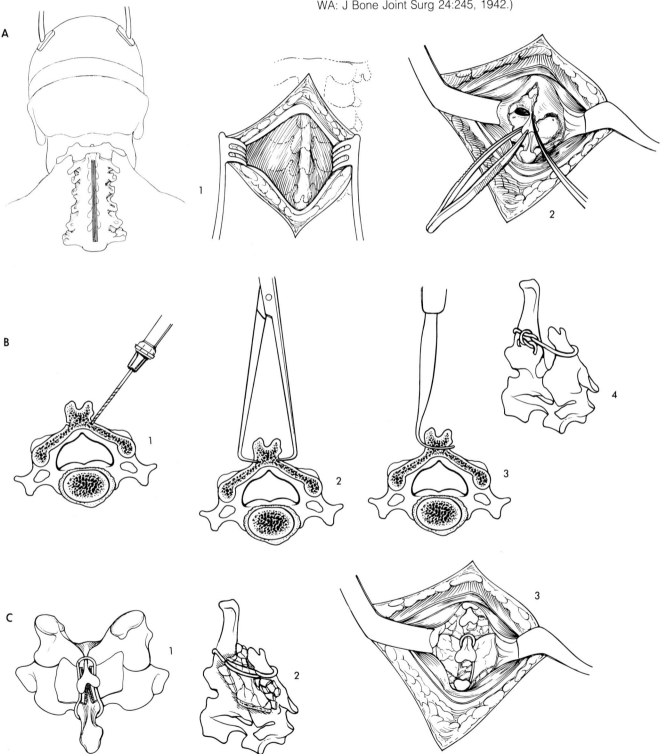

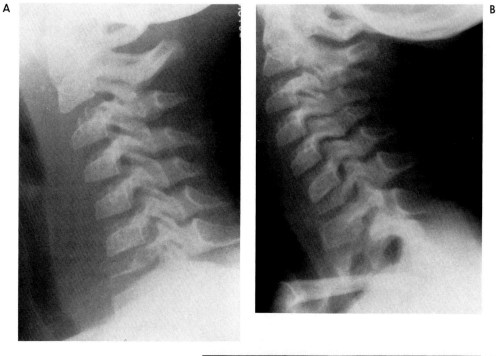

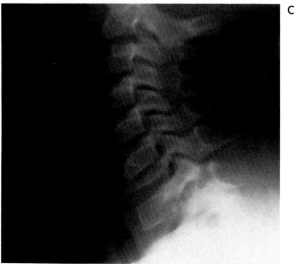

Fig. 16-117 **A,** Compression of C7 thought to be fracture or tumor. **B,** Evidence of vertebra plana, classic sign of eosinophilic granuloma of spine; biopsy of C7 was performed and diagnosis of eosinophilic granuloma confirmed. **C,** Six months later, patient is asymptomatic.

Fractures and Dislocation from C3 to C7

Fractures below C2 are extremely rare in young children and often are difficult to diagnose because anterior wedging of an end plate may simulate anterior compression fracture of a vertebral body. The more horizontal facets, ligamentous laxity, and increased anterior displacement of the superior vertebra in the child may simulate dislocation (pseudodislocation). Eosinophilic granuloma and vertebra plana are pathologic collapses and should not be mistaken for traumatic fractures; the collapses will heal uneventfully without treatment (Fig. 16-117). Significant fracture or fracture-dislocation of the cervical spine in this area may require stabilization as in adults, with reduction, wire fixation, and limited cervical fusion.

Several authors have reported that fusion of the cervical spine occurs more rapidly and profusely in children than in adults, making it prudent to explore only the area in which fusion is indicated to prevent fusion from occurring above or below the area of fracture or dislocation. This is especially true in C1 to C2 arthrodesis, in which a generous superior and inferior exposure will result in an occiput to C3 fusion, which is unnecessary.

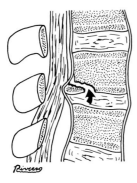

Fig. 16-118 Posterior epiphyseal injury that may mimic ruptured disk. Avulsion of ring epiphysis has produced displaced fragment that presses on nerve root. (Redrawn from Ogden JA: Skeletal injury in the child, Philadelphia, 1982, Lea & Febiger.)

Thoracic and Lumbar Spine Fractures

Fractures in the thoracic and lumbar spines are even rarer in children than fractures in the cervical spine. In infants they may be due to child abuse, in older children to motor vehicle accidents, and in adolescents and young adults to sports and recreational activities. Several entities may mimic traumatic compression fractures in the child, including eosinophilic granuloma, Gaucher disease, metastatic disease, osteogenesis imperfecta, idiopathic juvenile osteoporosis, and Scheuermann disease. Hensinger also described an anterior wedge compression fracture that simulates Scheuermann disease; he believes these are actually microfractures that may occur in adolescent weight lifters and female gymnasts. Lowery noted that a displaced fragment of a lumbar vertebral ring epiphysis may simulate disk rupture (Fig. 16-118) and reported three adolescents who, when operated on for suspected lumbar intervertebral ruptures, were found to have displaced bony fragments from the epiphyseal ring.

In a review of 97 children with spinal cord trauma (most of whom had complete spinal cord lesions), Kewalramani and Tori found that 35 (37.6%) had injuries in the thoracic and lumbar spine. Most of the fractures complicated by cord injuries occurred from T1 to T12. Because of the elasticity of the child's spine and the cartilaginous nature of the vertebrae, forces are transmitted over many segments and multiple fractures may occur. Most thoracolumbar fractures with neurologic loss are associated with vertebral body fractures; some have neural arch fractures and subluxation rather than dislocation. Hypervascularity of the reparative response and stimulation of the physis partly account for the restoration of height of a compressed vertebra in children and probably account for the rarity of kyphosis in children with multiple compression fractures. Several days to several weeks of bed rest usually is all that is necessary for symptoms to disappear completely. According to Hensinger, surgical treatment in the young child is indicated only for significant neurologic involvement, persistent frank dislocation, or block of dye on the myelogram.

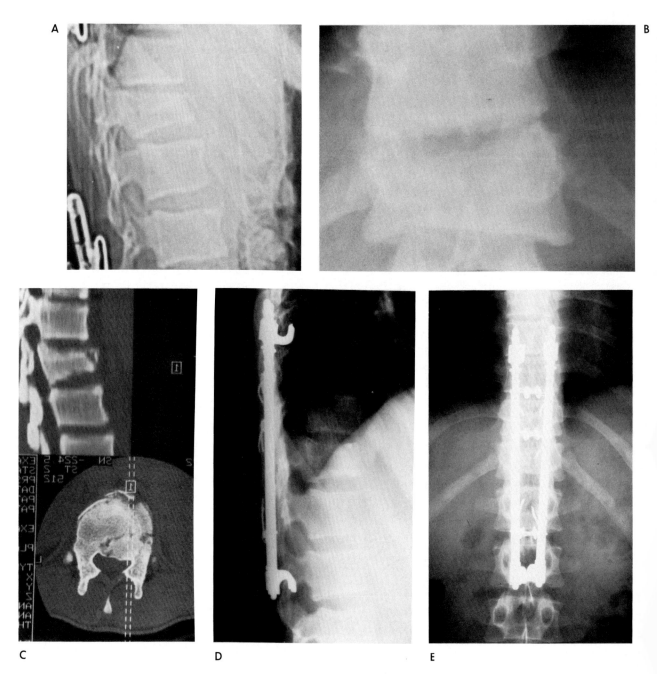

Fig. 16-119   **A** and **B,** Burst compression fracture of T12 in 14-year-old child. **C,** CT scan shows over 50% compromise of spinal canal. **D** and **E,** After open reduction and fixation with Harrington rods, vertebral height is restored.

More complex fractures, such as burst fractures with fragments that protrude into the spinal canal, the rare Chance fracture, and fracture-dislocations should be managed similarly to those in adults. If neurologic deficits follow a burst fracture-dislocation or Chance fracture, open reduction and internal fixation with Harrington or Luque rods should be performed (Chapter 10). Open reduction must be accompanied by posterior spine fusion at least one level above and below the fracture site (Fig. 16-119). Indications for immediate surgical decompression are an open wound, progressive neurologic deficit in an incomplete injury, and reduction of an unstable fracture-dislocation. Laminectomy rarely is indicated.

The major complication of thoracic spine fracture in children is paraplegia. Hensinger, as well as others, have described the sequelae of paraplegia: (1) increase in the number of long bone fractures, (2) paralytic hip dislocation, (3) decubitus ulcers, (4) flexion contractures, (5) genitourinary complications, and (6) progressive spinal deformity, including scoliosis, kyphosis, and lordosis. The most important factors in the development of significant spinal deformity are age, type of injury, and amount of spasticity. The management of paralytic kyphoscoliosis is described in Chapter 10.

FRACTURES AND DISLOCATIONS OF THE SHAFT AND EPIPHYSIS OF THE CLAVICLE

Fractures of the clavicle are classified by location: outer (distal), middle, and proximal (medial) (Fig. 16-120). The middle area is by far the most frequently fractured. Fractures of the distal or outer third of the clavicle generally heal satisfactorily without surgical treatment because the periosteal tube and the ligamentous attachments remain intact. Remodeling of the fracture occurs along the intact periosteal tube (Fig. 16-121). Surgery rarely is indicated. Havranek reported 10 distal epiphyseal clavicular injuries, 9 of

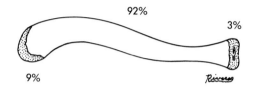

Fig. 16-120 Location of clavicular fractures in children: middle area is much more commonly fractured than distal and proximal areas. (Redrawn from Ogden JA: Skeletal injury in the child, Philadelphia, 1982, Lea & Febiger.)

Fig. 16-121 Distal clavicle fracture with coracoclavicular and coracoacromial ligaments still intact or at least attached to periosteal tube. Fracture in child will remodel satisfactorily without surgery. (Redrawn from Rockwood CA, Jr. In Rockwood CA, Jr, Wilkins KE, and King RE, editors: Fractures in children, Philadelphia, 1984, JB Lippincott Co.)

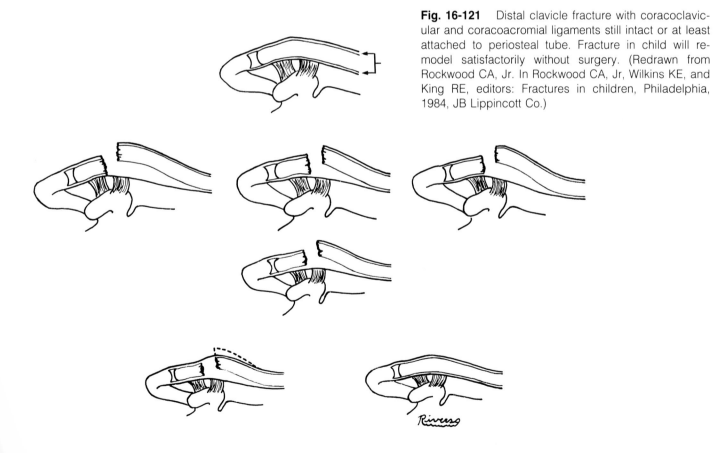

which were treated conservatively by closed reduction, by figure-8 bandage, or by Desault bandage. One fracture was treated with open reduction and internal fixation because of significant displacement of the central fragment and deformity of the shoulder. All cases healed without functional sequelae, but seven of the nine patients treated conservatively had visible deformity of the affected shoulder. Havranek recommends open reduction for cosmetic reasons if displacement of the central metaphyseal fragment results in shortening of the clavicle and deformity of the shoulder. Wilkes and Hoffer, on the other hand, reported 38 clavicular fractures in children with head injuries, all of which healed without immobilization and exhibited excellent remodeling. All patients recovered complete range of motion of the shoulder. Two lateral fractures resulted in "double clavicles," one of which required surgery for removal of a tender bony prominence.

Fractures of the midshaft of the clavicle rarely require surgical treatment, and open reduction has even been reported to increase the incidence of delayed union and nonunion. A fracture tenting the skin can be reduced beneath the trapezius muscle with a towel clip, with the patient under general or local anesthesia. Congenital pseudarthrosis of the clavicle (Chapter 2) should not be confused with fracture. Be-

sides debridement of an open fracture, the only indication for surgery in a midshaft clavicular fracture in a child is associated vascular injury, which must be treated immediately.

Fractures of the proximal or medial third of the clavicle are difficult to diagnosis. A lordotic roentgenographic view, shot at 40 degrees cephalad as described by Rockwood (1984), is helpful in differentiating between a sternoclavicular dislocation, which is rare in children, and a Salter-Harris type I or II fracture of the proximal clavicular physis, which is common. Because the medial clavicular physis usually does not fuse until ages 20 to 24 years, most injuries thought to be sternoclavicular dislocations in children and young adults actually are Salter-Harris types I and II fractures of the proximal clavicle (Fig. 16-122). A "knot" usually appears 2 weeks after injury at the medial end of the clavicle. These fractures should be treated conservatively; reduction is easily obtained but cannot be maintained. These fractures will remodel and leave only a small anterior prominence. Surgical treatment is not justified, and numerous complications have been reported when surgery is performed for this benign injury.

In true dislocations of the sternoclavicular joint the 40-degree cephalad supine roentgenogram will confirm absence of a proximal fracture or physeal separation and dislocation of the entire clavicle. In anterior dislocations, on the Rockwood view, the clavicle is cephalad compared with the contralateral uninvolved medial end. In posterior dislocations, which are extremely rare, the clavicle is caudad to the contralateral uninvolved medial end of the clavicle. Acute dislocations usually can be treated nonsurgically, but interposition of the joint capsule or ligaments may impede reduction. Heinig recommends, in adults, closed reduction of acute anterior dislocations after the hematoma is infiltrated by means of meticulous sterile technique with the patient under local anesthesia. Any late instability or deformity may be treated by ligament reconstruction or resection of the medial end of the clavicle. Internal fixation with transarticular pins should be avoided, because several deaths have been reported as a result of migration of pins or wires into the heart, pulmonary artery, innominate artery, or aorta. Surgical treatment should be reserved for irreducible posterior sternoclavicular dislocations.

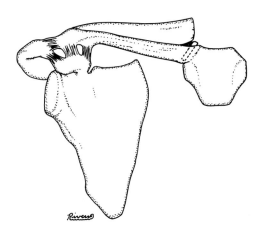

Fig. 16-122 Injury shown is Salter-Harris type I epiphyseal separation of medial clavicle rather than dislocation of sternoclavicular joint. (Redrawn from Rockwood CA, Jr. In Rockwood CA, Jr, Wilkins KE, and King RE, editors: Fractures in children, Philadelphia, 1984, JB Lippincott Co.)

ACROMIOCLAVICULAR DISLOCATIONS

Acromioclavicular injuries in children are of five types, according to Rockwood (1984) (Fig. 16-123). A type I injury is a contusion of the joint insufficient to rupture the acromioclavicular or coracoclavicular ligaments. A type II injury damages the acromioclavicular ligament but not the coracoclavicular ligament, and a partial periosteal sleeve (tube) tear also occurs. In a type III injury the acromioclavicular ligament is completely ruptured, but the coracoclavicular ligaments are intact and still attached to the periosteum; the clavicle is unstable and displaced superiorly through a rent in the periosteal tube (pseudodislocation) (Fig. 16-124). A type IV injury is identical to type III except that the clavicle is displaced posteriorly as well as superiorly. Type V is a severe injury in which the acromioclavicular ligament is disrupted and, although the coracoclavicular ligaments still are attached to the periosteal sleeve, the clavicle is unstable, with its lateral end buried in the trapezius and deltoid muscles or, having pierced the muscle, is under the skin of the posterior aspect of the shoulder. In many types III, IV, and V dislocations, there is an unrecognized fracture of the distal clavicle, with the acromioclavicular and coracoclavicular ligaments remaining intact and attached to the empty periosteal tube or to the most distal fragment. According to Rockwood (1984), types I, II, and III acromioclavicular separations, even with fracture of the distal third of the clavicle, can be treated nonsurgically in children and adolescents up to 16 years of age. For type IV dislocations Rockwood recommends closed reduction with the patient under general anesthesia; if this is unsuccessful, open reduction is performed, fixed with an extraarticular coracoclavicular lag screw if the reduction is unstable. Open reduction and internal fixation are recommended for the rare type V fracture. Falstie-Jensen and Mikkelsen recommend surgical treatment of types IV and V lesions because of the possibility of a total rupture of the coracoclavicular ligaments and periosteal damage that can be assessed only at surgery. According to them, although new bone will form from the periosteal envelope, the lateral end of the clavicle, if not treated surgically, will become Y-shaped, unsightly, and uncomfortable.

In types IV and V acromioclavicular dislocations, it is important to disengage the distal clavicle from the trapezius and deltoid muscles and replace it in the periosteal tube; if this cannot be accomplished by closed methods, surgery is indicated. The periosteal tube should be repaired and the deltoid-trapezius muscle fascia should be imbricated superiorly over the clavicle. If repair is unstable, internal fixation is required by either acromioclavicular or coracoclavicular fixation.

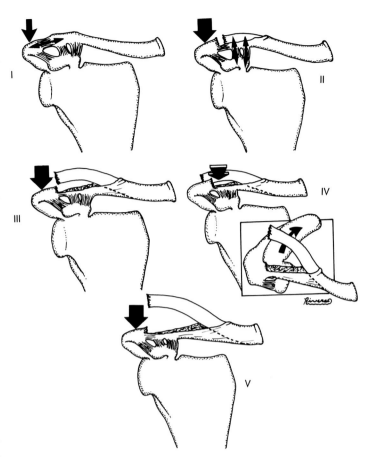

Fig. 16-123 Five types of acromioclavicular separation occurring in children (see text). Acromioclavicular and coracoclavicular ligaments are attached to periosteal tube even though distal end of clavicle is significantly displaced in types III, IV, and V. (Redrawn from Dameron TB and Rockwood CA, Jr. In Rockwood CA, Jr, Wilkins KE, and King RE, editors: Fractures in children, Philadelphia, 1984, JB Lippincott Co.)

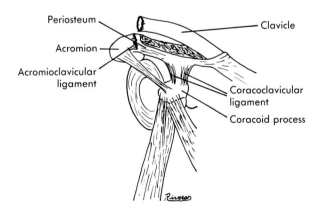

Fig. 16-124 Acromioclavicular and coracoclavicular ligaments remain attached to periosteal tube even when clavicle is displaced significantly (pseudodislocation). (From Falstie-Jensen S and Mikkelsen P: J Bone Joint Surg 64B:368, 1982.)

FRACTURES OF THE SHAFT AND PROXIMAL END OF THE HUMERUS

Fractures of the midshaft of the humerus in children always unite. Treatment in a hanging arm cast keeps shortening, angulation, and rotary deformity to a minimum, and open reduction almost never is indicated. The only indication for surgery in these fractures is the disappearance of previously present radial nerve function after reduction of a fracture at the junction of the middle and distal thirds of the humerus. This indicates that the nerve probably is trapped between the fracture fragments, and exploration of the nerve and internal fixation of the fracture are necessary.

Most fractures of the proximal humerus are epiphyseal, usually a Salter-Harris type II fracture. Salter-Harris type I fractures are more common in younger children, and types III and IV are rare (Fig. 16-125). Severe fracture or epiphyseal injury in a young child should arouse suspicion of child abuse. Neer and Horowitz classified proximal humeral epiphyseal fractures according to the amount of displacement (Fig. 16-126): a grade I fracture is displaced less than 5 mm and the most severe, grade IV fracture, is to-

tally displaced. Salter-Harris types I and II fractures of the proximal humerus rarely require surgical treatment (Fig. 16-127). Dameron and Reibel listed eleven ways to treat displaced Salter-Harris types I and II fractures in this area; most are conservative, but percutaneous pinning and open reduction and internal fixation are included. Closed reduction may be necessary if the fracture is severely displaced; reduction is maintained by some form of traction or percutaneous pinning with image intensification. Open reduction is indicated if the distal fragment is buttonholed completely through the deltoid muscle and is impinging against the skin and cannot be repositioned by closed methods. Open reduction should be done through a short deltoid-splitting approach, with care taken not to damage the axillary nerve, or through a short deltopectoral approach. The shaft is reduced through the split deltoid muscle and the fracture is pinned percutaneously. Open reduction also may be indicated for displaced Salter-Harris types III and IV fractures, interposition of the biceps tendon in the fracture site, or fracture-dislocation. These fractures should be treated as Neer types III or IV fractures in adults.

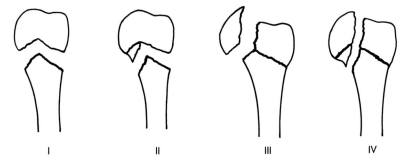

Fig. 16-125 Salter-Harris classification of proximal humeral epiphyseal injuries. Types I and II are extremely common; types III and IV are extremely rare. (Redrawn from Dameron TB and Rockwood CA, Jr. In Rockwood CA, Jr, Wilkins KE, and King RE, editors: Fractures in children, Philadelphia, 1984: JB Lippincott Co.)

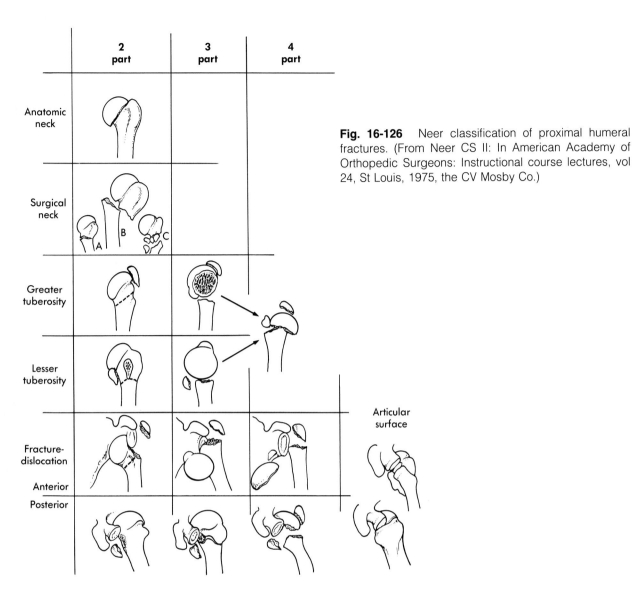

Fig. 16-126   Neer classification of proximal humeral fractures. (From Neer CS II: In American Academy of Orthopedic Surgeons: Instructional course lectures, vol 24, St Louis, 1975, the CV Mosby Co.)

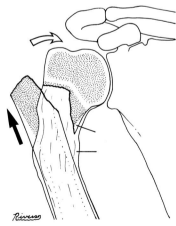

Fig. 16-127   Remodeling potential of proximal humeral epiphyseal fracture because of periosteal sleeve. (Redrawn from Ogden JA: Skeletal injury in the child, Philadelphia, 1982, Lea & Febiger.)

Closed reduction casting or percutaneous pinning

▶ *Technique (Sherk and Probst).* With the patient supine on an image intensifier table and using image intensification, manipulate the distal fragment into slight external rotation, 90 degrees of flexion, and 70 degrees of abduction. This will bring the fragments together satisfactorily. This maneuver should push the upper part of the shaft back through the rent in the deltoid muscle and anterior periosteum and correct the anterior angulation. Have an assistant support the proximal fragment to help achieve and maintain the reduction. Test for stability by bringing the distal fragment down out of flexion and abduction. If the reduction remains stable, apply a Velpeau dressing to be worn for 4 or 5 weeks until union is sufficient to permit gentle shoulder motion. If the fracture becomes redisplaced immediately after reduction, repeat the reduction maneuver and keep the arm supported in the salute position. Apply either a spica cast or skin traction in this position. As an alternative, drill one or two smooth Steinmann pins through the lateral shaft in a proximal direction into the humeral head to maintain the reduction. Cut the pins beneath the skin to be removed at 3 to 4 weeks (Fig. 16-128). Immobilize the arm in the neutral position.

Open reduction also may be indicated for (1) the rare displaced Salter-Harris types III and IV fractures, (2) interposition of the biceps tendon in the fracture site, and (3) fracture-dislocations. Open reduction and internal fixation of Salter-Harris type III or IV fractures, as well as biceps interposition and fracture-dislocations, are similar to the surgical procedures necessary for Neer types III or IV fractures in the adult.

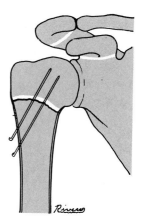

Fig. 16-128 Closed reduction and percutaneous pinning of proximal epiphyseal separation. Two wires cross physis. (Redrawn from Megerl F. In Weber BG, Brunner C, and Freuler F: Treatment of fractures in children and adolescents, Berlin, 1980, Springer-Verlag.)

FRACTURES OF THE DISTAL HUMERUS

Fractures of the distal humerus in children are most often supracondylar or involve a single condyle. Boyd and Altenburg found that of 713 fractures in patients 12 years old or younger, approximately 65% were supracondylar and about 25% were condylar (Table 16-3). Because the fragment consists mainly of cartilage, roentgenograms may be misleading and the fragment may appear smaller than its actual size and even significant displacement may not be appreciated. Arthrography has been suggested by several authors as a means of discerning injury patterns before complete ossification of the elbow. Hansen et al concluded that arthrographic examination to outline the cartilaginous structures around the distal humerus may be the only nonsurgical means of establishing the correct diagnosis and proper treatment of elbow injuries in children. Yates and Sullivan found that after arthrogram the original diagnosis and the treatment were altered in almost 20% of their patients. The injury pattern most often diagnosed was lateral condylar fracture. They recommend arthrography as particularly useful in condylar fractures and periarticular fractures in which anatomic alignment cannot be ascertained from plain roentgenograms, but they note that the need for arthrography should be infrequent when proper roentgenograms, including comparison views, are obtained.

Treatment of fractures of the distal humerus in children is complicated by several factors. Strong flexor and extensor muscle groups attached to the separated medial and lateral condyles, respectively, often rotate and displace the involved condyle by their pull. Even if closed reduction is obtained, this rotational pull on the fragment often redisplaces the fracture. Accurate alignment of the fracture surfaces and the physis may be difficult, even with wide exposure of the fracture site. After reduction, some type of internal fixation is needed because even the slightest tension on the muscles will displace the fragment. Smooth Kirschner wires used for internal fixation usually should be removed after 4 to 6 weeks. It often is necessary for pins to pass through the physis and although in theory this may cause growth disturbance, it rarely does.

Complications from incorrect diagnosis and inadequate treatment are numerous. Nonunion is most common after fracture of a single condyle. Malunion, or disturbances in the carrying angle of the elbow, may result from either nonunion or physeal growth disturbance. Cubitus varus deformity after supracondylar fracture most often results from malunion. Cubitus valgus deformity is most common after lateral condylar fractures, usually from nonunion. Physeal growth disturbances most often are the result of a Salter-Harris type III or IV physeal injury and may cause cubitus varus or cubitus valgus deformity. Avascular necrosis of the condyle is relatively uncommon. Acute compromise of either the neural or circulatory status is not uncommon after fractures around the elbow in children, but most are transient and lead to no permanent sequelae when adequate treatment is promptly instituted. The most serious of vascular complications is Volkmann's contracture, which results in an ugly deformity that often renders the hand and forearm practically useless.

Damage to nerves and impairment of circulation should be suspected in all fractures around the elbow in children, especially supracondylar fractures. If the patient can bend the fingers with the metacarpophalangeal joint extended and can appose the thumb to the little finger, the three major nerve trunks are intact. The sensory distribution of these nerves also should be tested. When circulation is impaired, the radial pulse is diminished or absent, the capillary circulation is sluggish, and swelling, cyanosis, and paresthesia or anesthesia of the hand and fingers occurs. Testing of the nerves and vessels should be repeated after treatment, and close and frequent observation of the neurocirculatory status in the hand is imperative; any impairment requires immediate attention.

Table 16-3 Elbow fractures in children

	No. cases	Percentage
Supracondylar fractures	465	65.4
Condylar fractures		25.3
Lateral condyle	124	
Medial epicondyle	33	
Medial condyle	23	
Fractures of neck of radius	34	4.7
Monteggia fractures	16	2.2
Olecranon fractures	12	1.6
T-condylar fractures	6	0.8
TOTAL	713	100.0

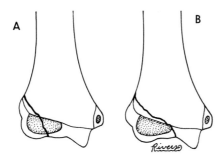

Fig. 16-129 Lateral humeral condylar fractures. **A,** Milch type I fracture, which is a Salter-Harris type IV epiphyseal fracture. **B,** Milch type II fracture, which is Salter-Harris type II epiphyseal fracture. (Redrawn from Milch H: J Trauma 4:592, 1964.)

Lateral Condylar Fractures

Fractures of the lateral condyle of the humerus are the most common distal humeral epiphyseal fracture, more common than fracture of the medial epicondyle or medial condyle or fracture-separation of the entire distal epiphysis. Most of these fractures occur when the child is approximately 6 years of age. Milch classified lateral condylar fractures into two basic types. In type I fractures, which are rare, the fracture line courses laterally to the trochlea through and into the capitellar-trochlear groove, producing a true Salter-Harris type IV fracture that frequently is stable (Fig. 16-129). Roentgenograms usually reveal a small, wafer-shaped bony metaphyseal fragment, and stress roentgenograms are helpful to determine motion at the fracture site, implying instability. In the more common type II fractures the fracture line extends into the area of the trochlea and produces inherent instability of the elbow because of the ability of the distal fragment and the forearm not only to angulate but to translate into a lateral position. Several authors have argued that the Milch type II fracture actually is a Salter-Harris type II fracture rather than a type IV epiphyseal injury. Lateral condylar fractures also have been classified according to the amount of displacement: undisplaced, moderately displaced, and completely displaced and rotated (Fig. 16-130). Badelon et al proposed a roentgenographic classification that includes four types (Fig. 16-131): type I, nondisplaced fracture visible on only one roentgenographic view; type II, visible fracture line with minimal displacement; type III, displacement of more than 2 mm on all roentgenographic views; and type IV, very serious displacement with complete separation of fracture edges.

Regardless of classification, most treatment recommendations are based on the amount of displacement of the fracture, which often is difficult to determine. Badelon et al report that the amount of displacement always is underestimated on roentgenograms. Varus and valgus stress roentgenograms are helpful to determine fracture stability and the presence of an intact cartilaginous hinge. If when the fracture is stressed, displacement occurs, then the hinge probably is not intact and the fracture is unstable; open reduction and internal reduction are indicated. Conversely, if when the fracture is stressed, no displacement occurs, cast immobilization alone may be justified (Fig. 16-132). Beaty and Wood recommend close observation with serial casting and roentgenograms for 6 to 8 weeks for undisplaced fractures, and they report one seemingly undisplaced fracture that became completely displaced 1 week after casting and required open reduction and internal fixation.

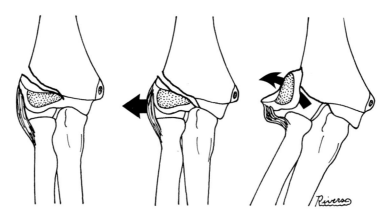

Fig. 16-130 Different stages of displacement of lateral condylar fracture: undisplaced, moderately displaced, and completely displaced and rotated. (Redrawn from Jakob R et al: J Bone Joint Surg 57B:430, 1975.)

A

B

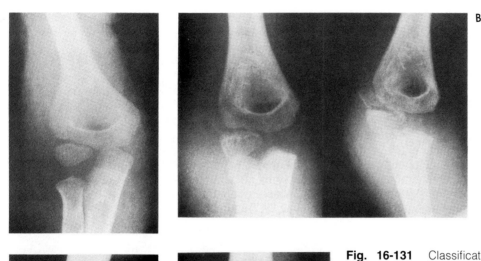

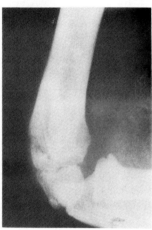

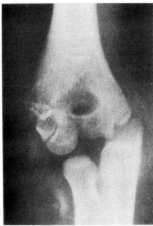

C

D

Fig. 16-131 Classification of lateral humeral condyle fractures according to amount of displacement. **A,** Type I, nondisplaced fracture. **B,** Type II, visible fracture line with minimal displacement (distinguished by slide of lateral cortex). **C,** Type III, displacement of more than 2 mm. **D,** Type IV, complete separation of fracture edges. (From Badelon O et al: J Pediatr Orthop 8:31, 1988.)

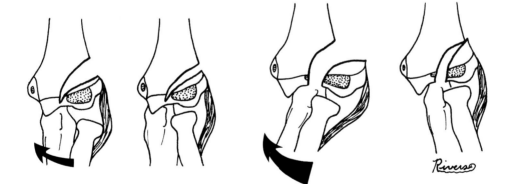

Fig. 16-132 Distal hinge in lateral condylar fracture, implying stability; if hinge is absent, then fracture is unstable. (Redrawn from Wilkins KE. In Rockwood CA, Jr, Wilkins KE, and King RE: Fractures in children, Philadelphia, 1984, JB Lippincott Co.)

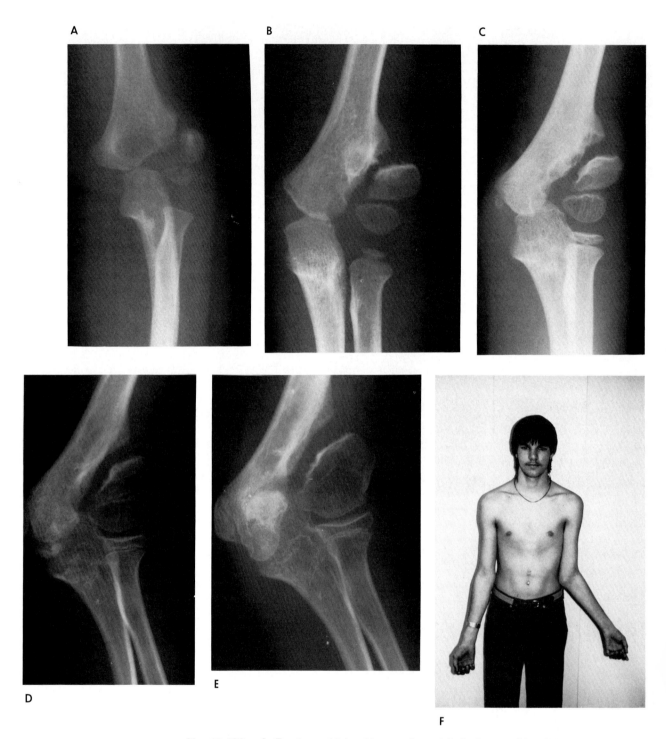

A B C

D E

F

Fig. 16-133   **A,** Fracture of lateral humeral condyle in 5-year-old child, treated with observation only. **B,** One year after fracture: established nonunion. **C,** Three years after fracture: capitellum and condyle appear to be migrating proximally. **D,** Five years after fracture: established cubitus valgus in addition to the nonunion. **E,** Ten years after fracture: severe cubitus valgus deformity; patient suffered mild ulnar nerve symptoms. **F,** Eleven years after fracture: patient has unsightly cubitus valgus deformity.

Open Reduction and Internal Fixation

Most authors agree that open reduction and internal fixation are necessary for any amount of displacement. Speed found results from closed treatment so unsatisfactory that he termed this a "fracture of necessity," indicating that open reduction and internal fixation were always required. Beaty and Wood, in a review of 53 fractures of the lateral condyle in children, reported union in all 32 patients treated with open reduction and internal fixation and four nonunions (28.5%) in 14 patients treated by closed methods. Four patients with unrecognized and untreated fractures had nonunions at long-term follow-up (Fig. 16-133), with cubitus valgus deformity, weakness, loss of elbow motion, and occasional pain; three had tardy ulnar nerve palsy. Badelon et al reported excellent results in 10 type I (undisplaced) fractures treated with casting (7) and percutaneous pinning (3), but poorer results in types II, III, and IV fractures treated with closed methods. They recommend open reduction and internal fixation for all but strictly nondisplaced (type I) fractures.

Open reduction most often is performed through a lateral approach, replacing the fragment without significant dissection and fixing it with pins or screws. Various methods of internal fixation have been suggested, including suture fixation, which is inadequate; smooth pin fixation, preferably with two pins either through the epiphysis or metaphyseal spike; and screw fixation, preferably through the metaphyseal area. Conner and Smith reported the use of a Glasgow screw through the physis and epiphysis without growth disturbance (Fig. 16-134), and Speed noted little difficulty with cubitus valgus caused by premature physeal closure when he used screws through the epiphysis. Excision of the fragment was once recommended, but most authors now agree that malunion or nonunion is preferable to this treatment.

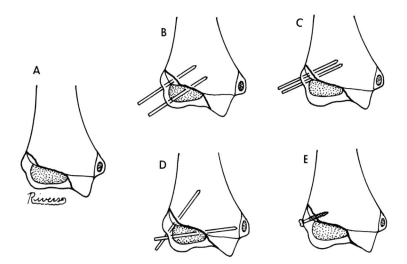

Fig. 16-134   Different methods of fixation of lateral condylar fractures. **A,** Fracture pattern. **B,** Parallel pins. **C,** Parallel pins through metaphysis only. **D,** Crossed pin fixation. **E,** Cancellous screw fixation. (Redrawn from Wadsworth TG: Clin Orthop 85:127, 1972.)

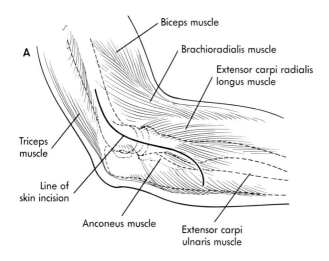

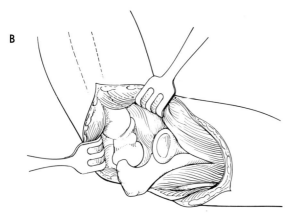

Fig. 16-135 Kocher lateral J approach to elbow joint. **A,** Skin incision. **B,** Approach has been completed, and elbow joint has been dislocated.

▶ *Technique.* Expose the elbow through a Kocher lateral J approach (Fig. 16-135). Carry the dissection down to the lateral humeral condyle. Expose both posterior and anterior surfaces of the joint by separating the fibers of the common extensor muscle mass. Limit soft tissue detachment to only that necessary to expose the fragment, the fracture, and the joint. The displacement and the size of the fragment are always greater than is apparent on the roentgenograms because much of the fragment is cartilaginous. The fragment usually is rotated as well as displaced. Irrigate the joint to remove blood clots and debris, reduce the articular surface accurately, and confirm the reduction by observing the articular surface, particularly at the trochlear ridge. Hold the position with a small tenaculum, bone holder, or towel clip. When a large metaphyseal fragment is present, insert two smooth Kirschner wires across it into the medial portion of the metaphysis; if necessary for secure fixation, insert the wires across the physis. When the epiphyseal portion is quite small, insert two smooth Kirschner wires across the condyle, across the physis, and into the humeral metaphysis. Direct the wires at an angle of 45 to 60 degrees; check the reduction and the position of the internal fixation by roentgenograms before closing the wound. Cut off the ends of the wires beneath the skin, but leave them long enough to allow easy removal (Fig. 16-136). Place the arm in a posterior plaster splint with the elbow flexed 90 degrees.

▶ *Postoperative management.* Immobilization should continue for approximately 6 to 12 weeks. At the end of that time the pins can be removed if union is progressing. Gentle active motion of the elbow is then usually resumed intermittently out of the splint. The splint is not removed permanently until the roentgenograms show solid union. These fractures are notorious for late and delayed union (Flynn and Richards), and some require immobilization with intermittent range-of-motion exercises for as long as 12 weeks.

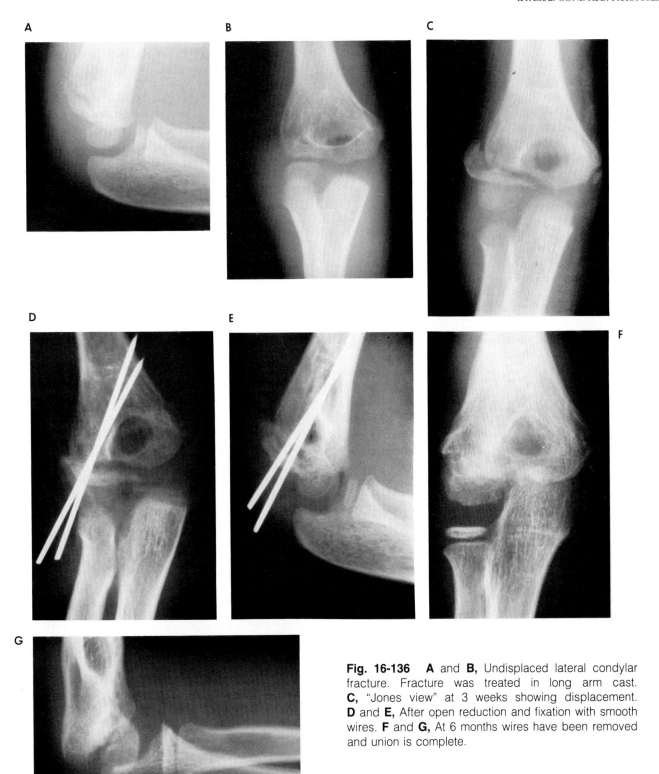

Fig. 16-136   A and **B,** Undisplaced lateral condylar fracture. Fracture was treated in long arm cast. **C,** "Jones view" at 3 weeks showing displacement. **D** and **E,** After open reduction and fixation with smooth wires. **F** and **G,** At 6 months wires have been removed and union is complete.

Nonunion or Delayed Union of Minimally Displaced Fractures

The most frequent and serious complication of lateral condylar fractures is nonunion, with resultant cubitus valgus. Nonunion must be distinguished from delayed union. Several authors have reported delay in union resulting from inadequate external immobilization or inadequate internal fixation. Flynn and Richards noted that immobilization of even minimally displaced fractures for at least 12 weeks often is necessary. Badelon et al recommend a minimum of 6 weeks of immobilization after open reduction. If union is not obtained in 12 weeks, Flynn and Richards recommend using a small wedge-shaped bone graft across the metaphyseal fragment, with or without supplemental smooth pin fixation. Jeffery used bone grafting with supplemental screw fixation. If the elbow appears to be stable and is not painful and the only roentgenographic abnormality is a lucent line with no motion of the fracture fragment on stress views, then observation and prolonged immobilization may be justified. If motion is present or a nonunion appears imminent, however, early operation is indicated.

▲ *Technique (Flynn and Richards; Jeffery).* Expose the fracture as described for open reduction and internal fixation. Limit soft tissue dissection to only that necessary to expose the fragment and the nonunion. Through the distal limb of the incision, expose the proximal ulna and take a "peg" bone graft from it 2.5 to 3 cm long, depending on the age of the child and the size of the lateral condylar fragment. Expose the fragment carefully, but do not disturb the fibrous union. Do not attempt to freshen the fracture fragments. Identify the physis, either visually or roentgenographically, but do not disturb it. Drill a hole for the peg graft through the metaphyseal portion of the condylar fragment and into the metaphysis of the proximal fragment, taking special care to avoid the physis. Insert the peg graft into the hole, and impact it soundly across the fibrous union. If desired, use an iliac cancellous bone graft instead (Jeffery). Insert a heavy pin, cancellous screw, or army screw adjacent to the graft. If the fragment is small, the fixation may, by necessity, have to cross the physis. Try to draw the condylar fragment firmly against the metaphysis. Penetration of the opposite cortex of the humerus may be necessary.

▲ *Postoperative management.* The limb is immobilized in plaster with the elbow at 90 degrees of flexion and the forearm in neutral rotation for 12 weeks. The pin or screw can then be removed, and active exercise is begun.

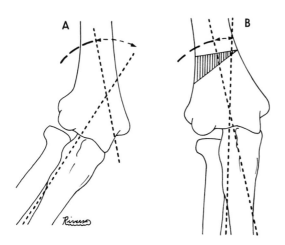

Fig. 16-137 **A,** Correction of cubitus valgus caused by nonunion of lateral humeral condyle. **B,** Opening wedge osteotomy laterally to restore alignment. (Redrawn from Milch H: Clin Orthop 6:120, 1955.)

Established nonunion with cubitus valgus. Cubitus valgus appears to result from nonunion and proximal migration of the lateral condyle, usually after displaced fractures, rather than from premature closure of the capitellar physis. Wilkins noted the similarity of this nonunion to nonunions in other areas of the skeleton such as the carpal scaphoid, in which significant displacement of the proximal fragment allows the cartilaginous articular surface of the distal fragment to come in contact with the bony surface of the proximal fragment and prevents union. Milch designed two osteotomies for nonunion in this area. In early nonunion of Milch type I fractures (Salter-Harris type IV), there is little lateral displacement and only minimal cubitus valgus. A closing wedge medial osteotomy as described by Speed or an opening wedge lateral osteotomy as described by Milch is recommended for these nonunions (Fig. 16-137). Autogenous bone graft and internal fixation with smooth pins should be performed. In Milch type II fractures there is significant lateral displacement of the fragment and some rotation, and a simple opening wedge lateral osteotomy results in an unacceptable medial prominence and unacceptable alignment of the distal humerus and forearm (Fig. 16-138, *A* and *B*). Milch recommends opening wedge displacement osteotomy (Fig. 16-138, *C* and *D*) for these nonunions. If the nonunion and cubitus valgus deformity have resulted in tardy ulnar nerve palsy, the angular deformity should be corrected and the palsy observed; if the angular deformity is minimal, anterior transposition of the nerve is indicated.

◣ *Technique (Milch).* For type II (Milch) cubitus valgus deformity an extensive osteotomy is necessary.

Place the patient in the prone position with the forearm supported on an arm board. Use a posterior muscle splitting incision, exposing the lower end of the humerus, but do not open the elbow joint. Split the fibers of the triceps muscle, retract them, and identify the ulnar nerve. When indicated for treatment of tardy ulnar nerve palsy, detach the flexor group of muscles from the medial epicondyle and transplant the nerve anteriorly. Now reattach the flexor muscles. As a landmark, note the upper limit of the condylar fragment. Perform a simple transverse osteotomy at the level of the intersection of the forearm axis with the lateral cortex of the humerus (Fig. 16-138, *A* and *B*). Notch the inferior surface of the proximal fragment to receive the apex of the superior surface of the distal fragment, which is moved laterally (Fig. 16-138, *C* and *D*). Adduct the distal fragment until the excessive angle of the abduction (valgus) has been reduced to the normal carrying angle, controlling the amount of correction by roentgenograms made with the extremity and the fragments in extension. When correction is satisfactory, fix the fragments by inserting two smooth crossed Kirschner wires, carefully flex the elbow, and immobilize it in plaster at 90 degrees.

◣ *Postoperative management.* The cast is left on for 6 to 12 weeks, depending on the age of the child and evidence of bony union. Then the wires are removed and motion is encouraged.

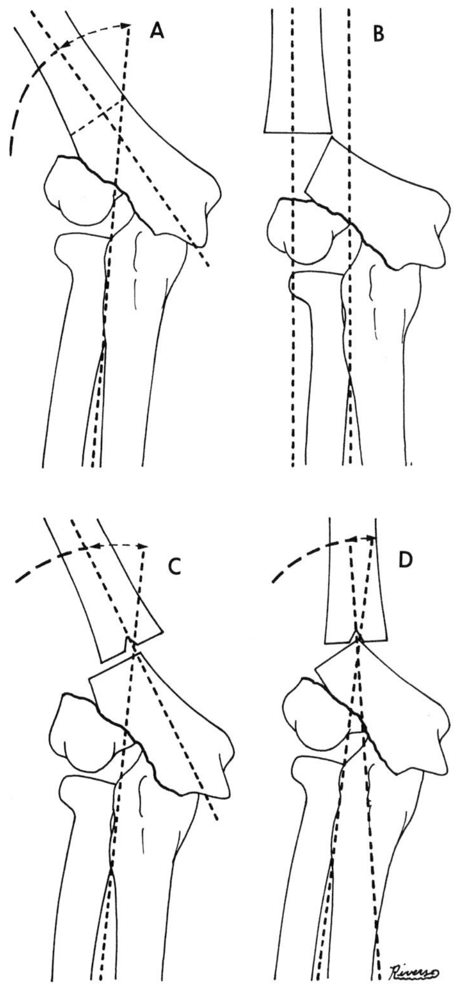

Fig. 16-138 **A** and **B,** Milch type II significantly displaced lateral condylar fracture, in which simple osteotomy would result in unacceptable alignment. **C** and **D,** Osteotomy with lateral displacement of distal humeral fragment, aligning arm satisfactorily with forearm. (Redrawn from Milch H: Clin Orthop 6:120, 1955.)

Medial Epicondylar Fractures

Medial epicondylar fractures constitute approximately 11% of injuries to the distal humerus. Most are acute avulsion injuries caused by overpull of the forearm flexor tendon or by the ulnar collateral ligament. These fractures may occur with dislocation of the elbow, and the fragment may become caught in the joint, preventing reduction of the dislocation Commonly cited indications for open reduction include (1) rotation and displacement of more than 1 cm because of the resulting weakness of the forearm flexors or cosmetic deformity, (2) persistent entrapment of a fracture fragment in the joint after reduction of elbow dislocation, (3) ulnar nerve dysfunction, and (4) valgus instability.

Displaced or Entrapped Medial Epicondyle

Displacement generally is considered significant only if distal displacement is more than 1 cm or the fragment is caught within the joint. Hines et al recommend surgical treatment of medial epicondylar fractures with rotation and displacement greater than 2 mm and reported 96% good results with operative treatment, noting decreased motion only in patients in whom arthrotomy was required for removal of an entrapped fracture fragment and in one patient with inadequate percutaneous pin fixation. If the fragment is trapped in the joint, the elbow almost always will remain dislocated because of the large size of the fragment and its attachment to the flexor muscles (Fig. 16-139). If the fragment is small, it may be difficult to see on the anteroposterior roentgenogram after successful reduction of the dislocation. The fragment may be overlapped by the distal humeral epiphysis or may be confused with one of the trochlear ossification centers. The medial epicondyle should be identified and its location noted after every elbow dislocation. Comparison anteroposterior and lateral roentgenograms of the opposite elbow may be helpful. According to Patrick, if the epicondyle can be seen on the lateral roentgenogram, then it is caught within the joint. If the fragment remains caught in the joint, closed reduction should be attempted with the arm supinated and stressed in valgus; passive dorsiflexion of the fingers may help put traction on the epiphysis (Fig. 16-140). If this is not successful, open reduction and removal of the fragment from the joint are required, with either excision or reduction and internal fixation of the fragment. Ulnar nerve paresthesias usually resolve with immediate accurate reduction of the fragment, and early transposition of the ulnar nerve usually is not warranted. Woods and Tullos recommend valgus stressing of the elbow to test stability. If the elbow is unstable, fixation of the collateral ligament and fragment is indicated, espe-

cially in high-performance athletes who significantly use their upper extremities.

For old dislocations with entrapment of the epicondyle within the joint, Patrick advises against removal of the fragment, but Fowles and Kassab reported increased flexion and relief of pain in six children with removal of the epicondyle from the joint and either reattachment to the humerus or excision. Ulnar nerve symptoms resolved after operation in two children, and two had ulnar nerve transposition.

▶ *Technique.* Begin a medial incision 7.5 cm long just distal to the elbow, and carry it proximally parallel to the medial surface of the humerus. If the fragment is entrapped within the elbow joint when the normal location of the medial epicondyle is exposed, only the raw surface of the condyle is seen; no loose fragment is visible. The ulnar nerve lies posteriorly. The medial capsule, the musculotendinous origin of the long flexor muscles, and the epicondyle are folded within the joint, covering the lower part of the coronoid fossa and process. With a small tenaculum, remove the epicondyle with its soft tissue attachments from within the joint. Now consider the fragment simply as a displaced epicondylar fracture. Replace the epicondyle accurately, and fix it with a screw or Kirschner wire. If the fracture is old or the fragment small and this is not possible, excise the fragment and suture the flexor muscles to the distal humeral metaphysis. Transfer the ulnar nerve anteriorly if necessary (Fowles and Kassab). Suture the tear in the capsule, repair the oblique ligament (medial collateral) if necessary, suture the forearm muscles, close the wound, and apply a posterior plaster splint with the elbow flexed 90 degrees.

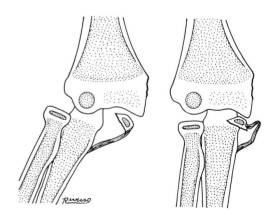

Fig. 16-139 Intraarticular displacement of medial epicondyle and entrapment within joint after reduction of dislocation of elbow. (Redrawn from Ogden JA: Skeletal injury in the child, Philadelphia, 1982, Lea & Febiger.)

▶ *Postoperative management.* The splint is worn for 4 weeks. Then the arm is supported by a sling permitting active motion of the elbow but preventing forced dorsiflexion of the wrist or supination of the forearm. At 6 weeks the wire or screw is removed and normal activities are resumed gradually.

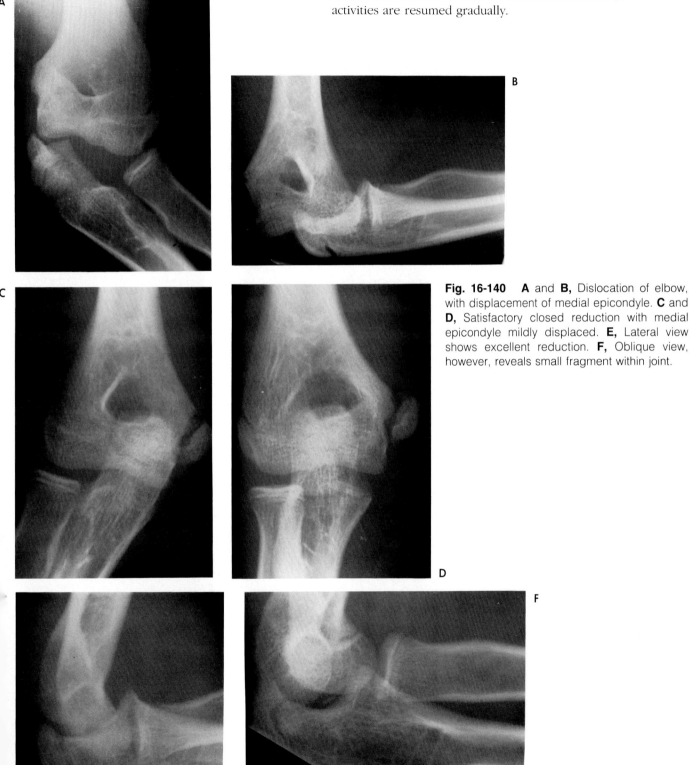

Fig. 16-140   A and **B,** Dislocation of elbow, with displacement of medial epicondyle. **C** and **D,** Satisfactory closed reduction with medial epicondyle mildly displaced. **E,** Lateral view shows excellent reduction. **F,** Oblique view, however, reveals small fragment within joint.

Medial Condylar Fractures

Fractures of the medial humeral condyle are among the least common injuries of the elbow, accounting for less than 1%. Kilfoyle described three types: type I, a greenstick or impacted fracture; type II, fracture through the humeral condyle into the joint with little or no displacement; and type III, intraarticular epiphyseal fracture with the medial condylar fragment displaced and rotated (Fig. 16-141). He recommended closed treatment of types I and II fractures, especially if nondisplaced. Nonunion of the medial condyle or formation of a bony bar, however, have been reported to occur after these fractures. Open reduction and internal fixation are recommended for all type III fractures.

Open Reduction and Internal Fixation

Fowles and Kassab described seven medial condylar fractures and recommended early diagnosis and accurate reduction and internal fixation of displaced fractures to avoid growth disturbance, articular roughening, and functional disability. Papavasiliou et al reported satisfactory results in 11 undisplaced fractures treated nonsurgically, 2 acute displaced fractures treated with percutaneous pinning, and 2 untreated fractures (2 years after injury) treated with supracondylar closing wedge valgus osteotomy fixed with Kirschner wires.

▲ *Technique.* Begin a medial incision just distal to the fractured condyle, and extend it proximally 7.5 cm parallel to the long axis of the humerus. Carry the dissection down to bone. Then isolate the ulnar nerve and retract it posteriorly. The capsule usually is ruptured widely and need not be incised for exposure of the fracture. Carefully examine the detached condyle, and remove all loose particles of bone. The fragment is surprisingly large, and often a part of the capitellum is included. Gently reduce the fracture, and hold it with a towel clip without disturbing the soft tissue attachments of the fragment. Restore the normal contour of the articular surfaces. Insert two smooth Kirschner wires through the condylar fragment and into the humerus in a proximal and lateral direction. Two wires are necessary to prevent rotation of the fragment. Use smooth Kirschner wires rather than screws because they are less likely to injure the physis. Before closing the incision, verify the position of the wires and the fragment by roentgenograms. Cut off the wires beneath the skin, leaving them long enough to allow easy removal. Close the wound and apply a plaster splint with the elbow flexed 90 degrees.

▲ *Postoperative management.* Postoperative management is the same as that described for fracture of the lateral condyle (p. 952).

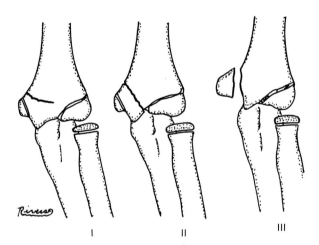

Fig. 16-141 Three types of medial condylar fractures described by Kilfoyle: type I, impacted; type II, epiphyseal and intraarticular; and type III, displacement of entire medial condyle. (Redrawn from Kilfoyle RM: Clin Orthop 41:43, 1965.)

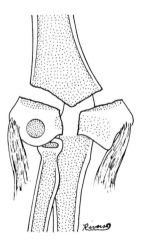

Fig. 16-142 T-condylar fracture of humerus. (Redrawn from Ogden JA: Skeletal injury in the child, Philadelphia, 1982, Lea & Febiger.)

Other Fractures of the Distal Humerus
Treatment

Other fractures of the distal humerus, such as fractures of the lateral epicondyle, usually do not require surgical treatment. The rare osteochondral fractures of the capitellum or trochlea, however, require arthrotomy or operative arthroscopy with either excision of the fragment or open reduction and internal fixation by pinning the intraarticular fragment.

Displaced T-condylar fractures (Fig. 16-142), also rare, require open reduction and internal fixation if they cause joint incongruity. Jarvis and D'Astous re-

ported satisfactory results using a posterior approach, splitting the triceps, and avoiding extensive dissection to prevent avascular necrosis of the trochlea. Osteotomy of the ulna occasionally may be necessary for adequate exposure. The condyles are secured to each other first with screws or Kirschner wires and then are fixed to the shaft with Kirschner wires or plates, depending on the age of the child (Fig. 16-143). Postoperatively, the arm is immobilized for only 1 to 3 weeks before an active range-of-motion exercise is begun.

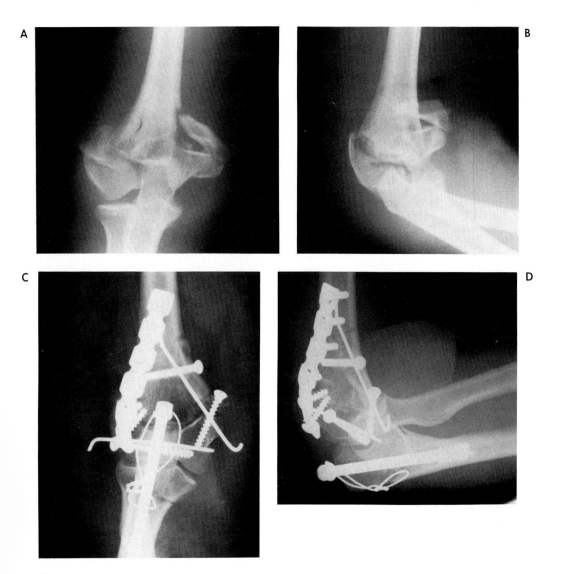

Fig. 16-143   A and **B,** Severely comminuted T-condylar fracture of elbow in 13-year-old child. **C** and **D,** After open reduction and internal fixation. Olecranon osteotomy was performed to expose intraarticular condylar fragments, which were fixed with cancellous screws; shaft fracture was fixed with contoured plate. Early motion was encouraged.

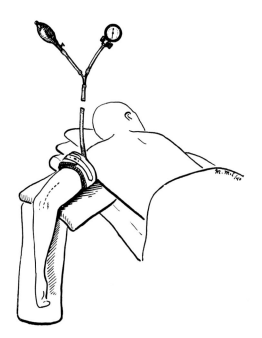

Fig. 16-144 Prone position with elbow flexed over arm board facilitates open reduction of fractures involving elbow joint and lower metaphyseal region of humerus. (From Van Gorder GW: J Bone Joint Surg 22:278, 1940.)

Open reduction and internal fixation

▶ *Technique.* Anesthetize the patient in the supine position, insert an endotracheal tube, and apply a pneumatic tourniquet. Then turn the patient prone, and support the abducted arm on a short arm board with the elbow at a right angle (Fig. 16-144). Expose the elbow posteriorly through an incision beginning 5 cm distal to the tip of the olecranon and extending proximally medial to the midline of the arm to 10 to 12 cm above the olecranon tip. Reflect the skin and subcutaneous tissue to either side carefully to expose the olecranon and triceps tendon. Expose the distal humerus through a posterior Campbell approach (Figs. 16-145 and 16-146) or a transolecranon approach. Isolate the ulnar nerve, and gently retract it from its bed with a Penrose drain or a moist tape. When the posterior Campbell approach is selected, raise a tongue of the triceps aponeurosis. Split the triceps muscle in the midline, and reflect the tissues from the lower humerus by subperiosteal dissection. Preserve soft tissue attachments to the fragments as much as possible, but some must be divided to obtain sufficient exposure. When a transolecranon approach is used, first drill a hole from the tip of the olecranon down the medullary canal. Then tap the hole with the tap to match a large AO cancellous

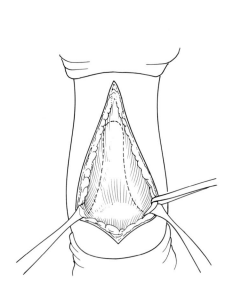

Fig. 16-145 Campbell posterior approach to elbow joint provides wide exposure for open reduction of T fractures of condyles. (Redrawn from Van Gorder, GW: J Bone Joint Surg 22:278, 1940.)

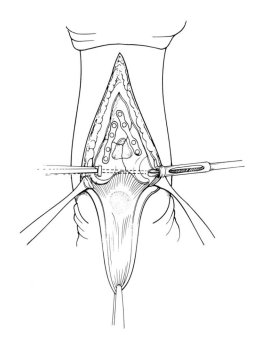

Fig. 16-146 Open reduction and internal fixation of T fracture of condyles with small plates. (Redrawn from Van Gorder GW: J Bone Joint Surg 22:278, 1940.)

screw 8 to 9 cm in length. Divide the olecranon transversely with an osteotome or oscillating saw approximately 2 cm from its tip. Reflect the olecranon and the attached triceps proximally to give excellent exposure of the posterior aspect of the lower end of the humerus.

Assemble the fragments of the distal humerus in three steps: (1) reduce and fix the condyles together, (2) if it is fractured, replace and fix the medial or lateral epicondylar ridge to the humeral metaphysis, and (3) fix the reassembled condyles to the humeral metaphysis.

Reduction and fixation of the condyles

Reduce the condyles, and hold them firmly with a bone-holding clamp. If necessary, fix small fragments temporarily one at a time with small Kirschner wires inserted with power equipment (Fig. 16-147, *A* to *C*). Insert malleolar or cancellous AO screws across the major fragments (Fig. 16-147, *D*). Then remove as many of the previously inserted Kirschner wires as possible and still maintain fixation. Rigid fixation of

the major fragments frequently stabilizes smaller condylar and articular fragments although on occasion small articular fragments may have to be discarded. When the bone is osteoporotic, use special washers to prevent the screw heads from sinking through the cortex. In normal bone, countersink screw heads to prevent excessive bulk outside the bone in and around the elbow joint.

Reduction and fixation of epicondylar ridge

Usually either the medial or lateral epicondylar ridge is fractured from the metaphysis. This must be accurately and firmly fixed to the proximal fragment because it forms one of the two buttresses to which the condyles must later be attached. Reduce the fragment, hold it with a bone-holding clamp, temporarily secure it with a Kirschner wire, and then with lag screws secure it to the metaphysis. When the site of the insertion of the screw is a sharp edge or ridge, nip out a small bit of the ridge with a rongeur before trying to place the screw. Finally, after the lag screws are inserted, remove the temporary Kirschner wire.

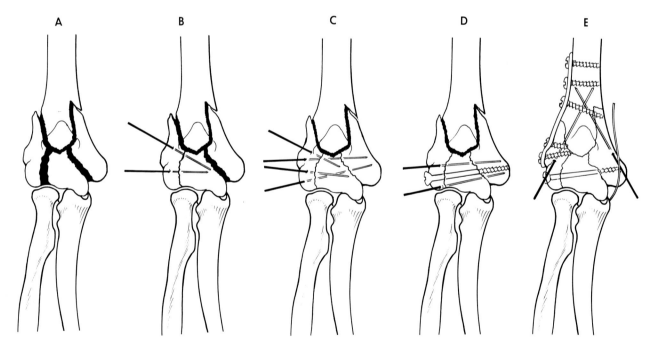

Fig. 16-147 Internal fixation for comminuted distal humeral fractures involving joint. **A,** Joint surface reconstruction is done first. **B** and **C,** Step-by-step reconstruction and preliminary fixation of joint fragments. **D,** Permanent fixation by cancellous screw. **E,** Fixation by plate and screws completed. Kirschner wires are then removed. (Redrawn from Schauwecker, F: The practice of osteosynthesis, Stuttgart, 1974, Georg Thieme Verlag.)

Reduction and fixation of reassembled condyles to metaphysis

After the reduction of the condyles, screws, threaded pins, or plates may be required to rigidly attach them to the metaphysis. If a screw can be placed obliquely through each epicondylar region to engage an intact opposite cortex, this is preferred. Occasionally the fracture extends so far up the shaft that screws alone will not provide adequate fixation. Do not depend on long narrow bone fragments to anchor major fixation devices. These fragments may break or the screws may pull out, and as a result the supracondylar element of the fracture may fall apart. Although excess metal is undesirable, a single contoured, double, or Y plate may be necessary to attach the epicondylar buttress to the proximal shaft (Fig. 16-147, *E*). Contour the plates for proper fit.

Take particular care in reassembling the condyles that the fixation device does not encroach on the olecranon or coronoid fossae. When encroachment occurs, some loss of flexion or extension of the elbow will result. Care also must be taken when the transverse condylar screws are inserted to be sure they do not penetrate or burrow under the articular cartilage of the trochlea. The trochlea is spool shaped and thus is wider peripherally than centrally. Transverse screws well within the anterior or posterior limit of the condyle may pass through the articular surface of the trochlea unless this anatomic consideration is remembered (Fig. 16-148). Thoroughly irrigate the joint of all debris. When using the posterior Campbell approach, repair the tongue defect in the triceps tendon with multiple interrupted sutures. With the transolecranon approach, reduce the proximal frag-

ment and insert a cancellous screw, using the previously drilled and tapped hole in the medullary canal. A transverse hole is drilled in the ulna distal to the osteotomy site, and a No. 20 wire is passed through this hole around the screw neck and tightened in a figure 8 manner.

▶ *Postoperative management.* A light posterior plaster splint is applied from the posterior axillary fold to the palm of the hand. The objectives of surgery are (1) to restore the articular surfaces and (2) to internally fix the fracture rigidly so that early motion can begin. If the patient's wound is satisfactorily healing at 7 days, the posterior plaster splint is removed periodically and gentle active and active assisted exercises are carried out. The posterior plaster splint is worn between exercise periods. By 3 weeks the posterior plaster splint can be removed and the arm is supported by a sling with active motion in the elbow as pain permits. Vigorous stretching by a therapist, forced motion whether active or passive, and manipulation while the patient is anesthetized are forbidden. Stretching and forced motion usually result in increased periarticular hemorrhage and fibrosis, increased joint irritability, and decreased rather than increased motion.

Triplane Fracture

Peterson described a triplane fracture of the distal humeral epiphysis that he believes to be the same fracture pattern that occurs in the ankle. If anatomic reduction cannot be obtained and maintained by closed methods, open reduction and internal fixation are indicated as in T-condylar fractures.

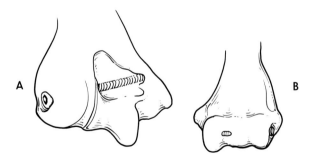

Fig. 16-148 Incorrect placement of screw across distal humerus. **A,** Transverse screw across condyles of distal humerus traversing olecranon fossa would markedly restrict elbow extension. **B,** Transverse screw across distal humeral condyles encroaches on articular surface of trochlea.

Supracondylar Fractures

Supracondylar fractures of the distal humerus account for 50% to 60% of elbow fractures in children. Despite its frequency, there is no general agreement on the treatment of this fracture, although all agree that anatomic reduction is essential to prevent cubitus varus or cubitus valgus deformity. Purely posterior displacement causes little deformity and purely horizontal rotation is compensated for at the shoulder joint. Coronal tilting may occur with opening of the lateral aspect of the fracture site, causing angulation into a varus position, or with impaction of the medial aspect of the fracture site, again resulting in cubitus varus (Fig. 16-149). Horizontal rotation predisposes to coronal tilting, and a combination of horizontal rotation, coronal tilting, and posterior angulation can result in a three-dimensional cubitus varus deformity (Fig. 16-150). By a mechanism not completely understood, lateral tilting is reduced by pronation of the forearm that closes the fracture medially (Fig. 16-151).

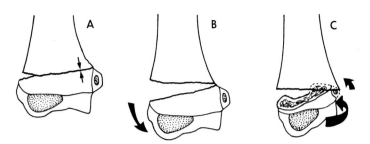

Fig. 16-149 Mechanism of coronal tilting. **A,** Impaction of fracture medially. **B,** Tilting of fracture laterally. **C,** Horizontal rotation. (Redrawn from Marion J et al: Rev Chir Orthop 48:337, 1962.)

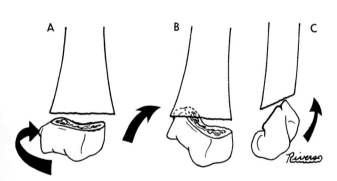

Fig. 16-150 Three static components that combine to produce cubitus varus. **A,** Horizontal rotation. **B,** Coronal tilting. **C,** Anterior angulation. (Redrawn from Wilkins KE. In Rockwood CA, Jr, Wilkins KE, and King RE: Fractures in children, Philadelphia, 1984, JB Lippincott Co.)

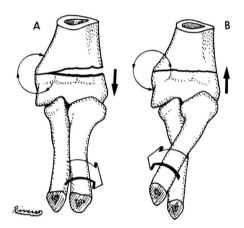

Fig. 16-151 Reduction of lateral tilt by pronation of forearm. **A,** Supination opening fracture laterally. **B,** Pronation closing fracture laterally. (Redrawn from Abraham E et al: Clin Orthop 171:309, 1982.)

Gartland classified supracondylar fractures into three types: type I, undisplaced; type II, displaced with intact posterior cortex; and type III, displaced with no cortical contact. His classification also notes whether the fracture is displaced posteromedially or posterolaterally. He made several observations related to treatment of these three types of fractures: (1) type I fractures can be treated satisfactorily with closed reduction and external fixation, such as a plaster cast; (2) type II displaced fractures are difficult to

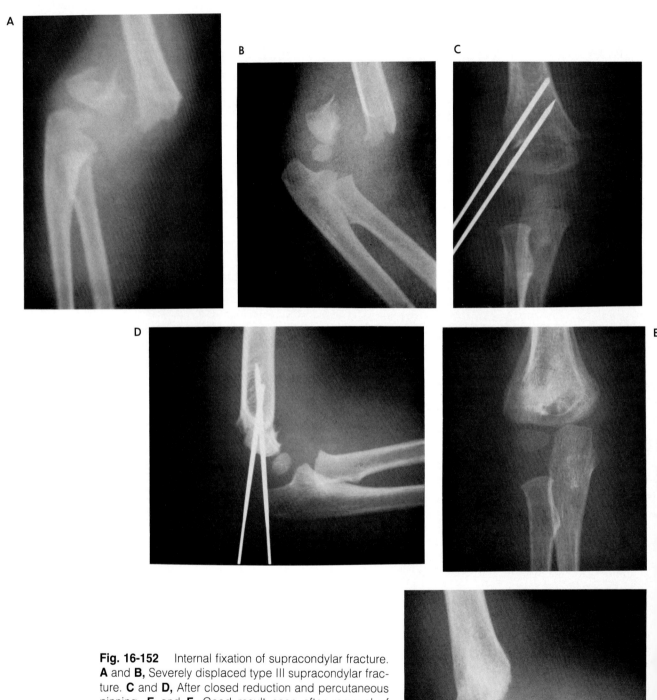

Fig. 16-152 Internal fixation of supracondylar fracture. **A** and **B,** Severely displaced type III supracondylar fracture. **C** and **D,** After closed reduction and percutaneous pinning. **E** and **F,** Good result soon after removal of pins.

reduce and hold by external methods; and (3) type III fractures are almost impossible to reduce and hold without some form of internal fixation (Fig. 16-152). Dameron listed four basic types of treatment: (1) side-arm skin traction, (2) overhead skeletal traction, (3) closed reduction and casting, with or without percutaneous pinning, and (4) open reduction and internal fixation.

Regardless of method the most important factor in treatment of these fractures seems to be obtaining satisfactory roentgenograms to determine adequate fracture reduction. Technically, the roentgenographic unit or image intensifier should be moved into the anteroposterior and lateral positions rather than moving the child's elbow and losing the reduction. The Jones anteroposterior view should be taken with the elbow flexed maximally, the cassette underneath the elbow, and the tube at a 90-degree angle to the cassette. Baumann's angle, offset at the fracture site, tilting, or angulation should be noted (Fig. 16-153). An anterior spike on the lateral view usually implies rotation rather than posterior displacement. A crescent sign, described by Marion et al, implies tilt either medially or laterally (Fig. 16-154).

Attempts have been made to correlate various roentgenographic measurements with adequate frac-ture reduction. Baumann's angle is the most frequently cited method of assessing fracture reduction and has been reported to correlate well with final carrying angle, not to change significantly from the time of initial reduction to final follow-up, and not to be obscured or invalidated by elbow flexion and pronation. The common formula is that a change of 5 degrees in Baumann's angle corresponds to a 2-degree change in the clinical carrying angle. Dodge found, however, that orientation of the roentgen beam more than 20 degrees from perpendicular in the cephalad-caudad direction invalidates the measurement. Webb and Sherman found Baumann's angle to correlate significantly with the carrying angle, but measurement inaccuracy increased in the very young child and the adolescent, and they recommended its use only in comparison with the normal elbow. Oppenheim et al believe that the humeral-ulnar-wrist angle is the most consistent and accurate method of approximating the true carrying angle. Webb and Sherman also found its accuracy rate higher than that of Baumann's angle. O'Brien et al, in an unpublished study, reported the metaphyseal-diaphyseal angle (Fig. 16-155) more accurate than Baumann's angle in determining the initial adequacy of reduction.

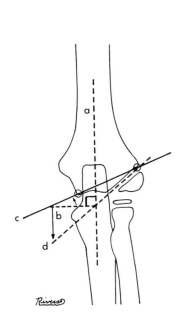

Fig. 16-153 Baumann's angle. Angle OC to OD should measure about 11 degrees. (Redrawn from Skolnic MD, Hall JE, and Micheli LJ: Orthopedics 3:395, 1980.)

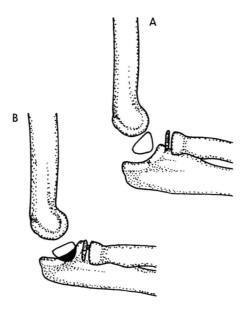

Fig. 16-154 Crescent sign. **A,** Normal lateral view of elbow. **B,** In varus deformity, part of ulna overlies distal humeral epiphyses, producing crescent sign. (Redrawn from Marion J et al: Rev Chir Orthop 48:337, 1962.)

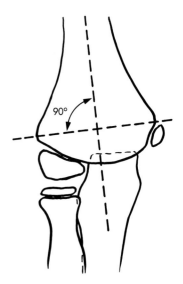

Fig. 16-155 Metaphyseal-diaphyseal angle. On anteroposterior roentgenogram, transverse line is drawn through metaphysis at widest point and longitudinal line is drawn through axis of diaphysis; angle is measured between lateral portion of metaphyseal line and proximal portion of diaphyseal line. (Courtesy Dr. RE Eilert.)

Nonsurgical Treatment

Closed reduction with splint or cast immobilization traditionally has been recommended for displaced supracondylar fractures, but loss of reduction and the necessity of repeated manipulations frequently have been reported to cause elbow stiffness and physeal damage. Pirone et al reported that, in displaced fractures, closed reduction and casting were associated with a lower percentage of good results and a higher percentage of early and late complications compared with skeletal traction, percutaneous pinning, and open reduction; they recommend that cast treatment be used only for undisplaced fractures. The criteria of Rang et al for closed reduction are easy reduction, stable fracture, minimal swelling, and no vascular compromise. Several authors have described reducing the fracture in extension and maintaining the reduction through use of the triceps bridge by holding the elbow in flexion if the pulse and vasculature tolerate it; an occasional author has mentioned holding the reduction by extension of the elbow. Bosanquet and Middleton reported good results with skin traction in full extension; they attributed the lack of cubitus varus or valgus deformity in their patients to good roentgenographic techniques. Skeletal traction by

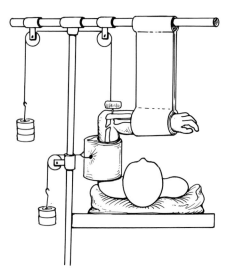

Fig. 16-156 Vertical traction as applied to patient with displaced supracondylar fracture of humerus. (Redrawn from Kramhøft M et al: Clin Orthop 221:215, 1987.)

means of either an olecranon pin or a screw applied with either side-arm or overhead positioning also has been widely recommended because of the advantages of increased mobility, decreased pain and swelling, and improved alignment (Fig. 16-156). Ippolito et al reported good results at long-term follow-up in 81% of nondisplaced and 78% of displaced fractures treated conservatively. Their treatment regimen included overhead skeletal traction for 2 to 10 days until reduction of the overriding fragments was obtained, further reduction of the fracture with the patient under general anesthesia, and application of a long plaster cast, including the traction bow, with the elbow in 90 degrees of flexion and the forearm pronated. The overhead traction position was maintained for another 2 to 3 days, after which the long plaster cast was connected to a shoulder-spica cast. After 2 weeks the traction bow was removed through a window in the cast; the cast was removed after an average of 4.5 weeks. The incidence of cubitus varus was 7.5% and of cubitus valgus, 5.6%, both of which occurred most frequently after displaced fractures. Spontaneous correction of the deformity occurred with growth in 3 patients with cubitus varus and in 13 with cubitus valgus. Kramhøft et al reported excellent or good results in 60 severely displaced supracondylar fractures with closed reduction and vertical skeletal traction with a screw in the olecranon. Eight fractures lost reduction and required reduction with the patients under general anesthesia. The length of hospitalization (average 2.6 weeks) was cited as the major disadvantage, which the authors believed was offset by the reduction in serious complications. Worlock and Colton reported the use of overhead olecranon traction by means of an olecranon screw and traction clip in 27 severely displaced supracondylar fractures; 22 children (81%) had excellent results and the other 5 had good results. Only 2 children (7%) had minimal cubitus varus deformities. The authors recommend this method as technically easy to perform and without significant complications. Pirone et al obtained equally good results in displaced fractures with overhead traction with an olecranon screw as with percutaneous pinning, and they recommend traction for the grossly swollen elbow in which the osseous landmarks are obscured and reduction is difficult or impossible.

Surgical Treatment

Percutaneous pinning. Closed reduction frequently is difficult not only to obtain but also to maintain because of the thinness of bone of the distal humerus between the coronoid and olecranon, where most supracondylar fractures occur. Percutaneous pinning techniques have been described by several authors and have become the treatment of choice for maintaining the closed reduction of displaced supracondylar fractures in children. Reported advantages of percutaneous pinning include decreased hospitalization time, better control of the distal fragment, and increased accuracy of reduction. Complications are rare—pin site infection, pin migration, and injury to the ulnar nerve from medial pinning—and seldom prevent a good result. In a study of 230 displaced extension-type fractures, Pirone et al found the best results were obtained with percutaneous wire fixation (78%). The number of pins required and the optimal position of the pins has been somewhat controversial. Danielsson and Pettersson noted a loss of reduction when only one pin was used. Swenson, Casiano, Flynn et al, and Pirone et al recommend two crossed pins, Arino et al recommend two lateral pins

(Fig. 16-157), Fowles and Kassab use one lateral oblique pin and a second vertical pin through the olecranon, and Haddad et al use two pins laterally and one medially. Herzenberg et al, in animal studies, found that medial and lateral pin fixation provides more inherent stability than lateral pinning alone. Graves and Beaty reported good results in 61 of 64 children (95%) with type III supracondylar fractures treated with closed reduction and percutaneous pinning. Of the three children with unsatisfactory results, two fractures had been fixed in a varus position with medial and lateral pins, and one fracture fixed in good alignment with two lateral pins had lost fixation and position postoperatively. They recommend medial and lateral pinning for added stability but note that if bony landmarks cannot be palpated because of edema or if injury to the ulnar nerve with a medial pin is of concern, then lateral pinning may be preferred. Aronson and Prager reported excellent or good results in 20 patients with displaced supracondylar fractures fixed with two lateral percutaneous pins. They emphasize the importance of correcting any rotational deformity of the distal fragment before the fracture is pinned.

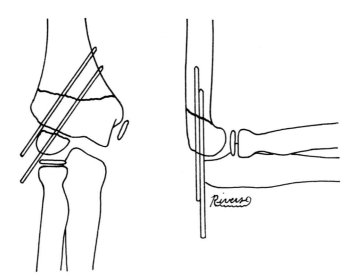

Fig. 16-157   Pinning of supracondylar fracture with two lateral pins inserted parallel crossing fracture site and opposite medial cortex. (Redrawn from Arino VL et al: J Bone Joint Surg 59A:914, 1977.)

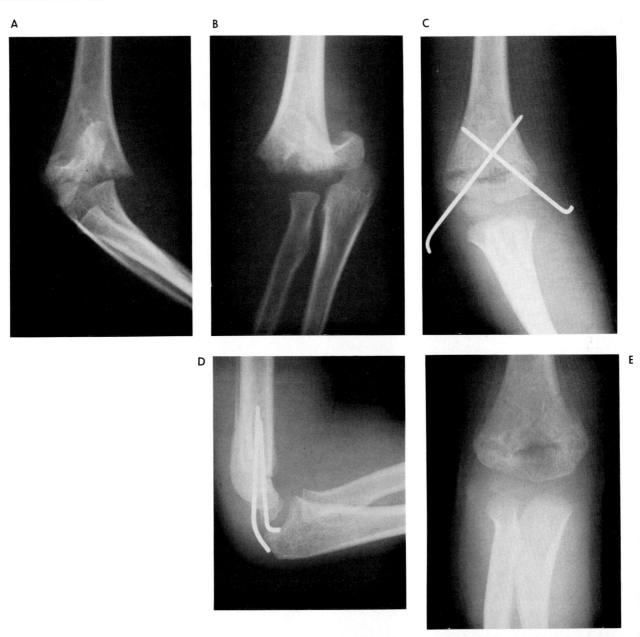

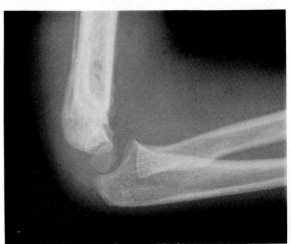

Fig. 16-158 Percutaneous cross pinning of supracondylar fracture. **A** and **B,** Severely displaced supracondylar fracture treated initially by olecranon skeletal traction because of severe swelling. **C** and **D,** Later treated by closed reduction and crossed pins. **E** and **F,** Good result shortly after pin removal.

Pins should be angulated superiorly approximately 40 degrees and posteriorly 10 degrees and must continue into the opposite cortex to provide solid fixation. The pins must be placed right at the medial epicondyle or slightly above it, never distal to the medial epicondyle. Smooth pins are preferred (Fig. 16-158). Some authors have advocated placing the patient in the prone position with the elbow flexed rather than in the standard supine position; although the prone position does provide easier accessibility for pin placement, orientation of the fragments with image intensification is more difficult than in the supine position. The ultimate result depends on the accuracy of the reduction rather than pin placement, and an unsatisfactory reduction held with percutaneous pins will have an unsatisfactory outcome. A small degree of residual cubitus varus has been reported in as many as 21% of fractures treated with percutaneous pinning, primarily because a poor position was accepted at the time of pinning. Aronson and Prager evaluate the quality of reduction by measuring Baumann's angle after reduction; they accept the reduction if Baumann's angle of the fractured extremity is within 4 degrees of that of the normal extremity.

Closed reduction and percutaneous pinning

▶ *Technique.* Place the patient prone or supine on a fracture table. Prepare and drape the elbow. Then outline the posterior triangle of the elbow joint—the medial and lateral epicondyles and the olecranon. Reduce the fracture by applying longitudinal traction, extending the fracture, and manipulating with the thumbs to correct lateral tilt, medial impaction, or posterior displacement. Flex the elbow to neutral. Crisscross two smooth Steinmann pins through the condyles and metaphysis, one to exit above the medial epicondyle and one to exit above the lateral epicondyle. Angle the medial pin 40 degrees from the axis of the humeral shaft, and direct it 10 degrees posteriorly, carefully avoiding the ulnar nerve (Fig. 16-159). After engagement of the shaft, use an image

intensifier to make sure the pin engages the opposite lateral cortex proximally. Repeat the procedure for the lateral pin. Cut the pins off beneath the skin, and bend their ends so they will not migrate proximally but can be retrieved easily in the office. Check and note the radial pulse.

▶ *Postoperative management.* A long-arm posterior plaster splint is worn for 3 weeks. Ulnar, radial, and median nerve function should be checked after anesthesia. The pins are removed at 3 weeks, and another posterior splint is applied. At 4 weeks intermittent active range-of-motion exercises are started at home; they should be taught by the physical therapist to the child and the parent, with instructions for the child to carry out the active range-of-motion program. Passive motion or forceful manipulative motion must be avoided in children because they will decrease the range of motion and frighten the child.

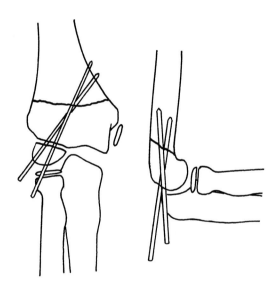

Fig. 16-159 Pinning of supracondylar fracture with divergent pins crossing fracture site and opposite cortex.

Closed reduction and percutaneous pinning, modified

▶ *Technique (Aronson and Prager).* Position the patient supine, and use image intensification to determine the direction of displacement and the status of the soft tissues of the fractured extremity. Supinate and pronate the forearm to tighten the lateral and medial soft tissue hinges, respectively; flex and extend the elbow to tighten the posterior and anterior hinges, respectively. For the rare flexion supracondylar fracture with anterior displacement of the distal fragment, extend the elbow to achieve satisfactory closed reduction.

For the more common extension type of supracondylar fracture, with countertraction on the humerus, apply traction to the forearm and examine the fracture with fluoroscopy (Fig. 16-160). Pronate or supinate the forearm to rotate the distal fragment into correct rotational alignment with the proximal fragment. Translate the distal fragment in a similar manner to correct medial or lateral displacement. While maintaining traction and precise forearm rotation, gently flex the elbow. Place gentle pressure on the olecranon as the elbow is flexed to correct posterior displacement of the distal fragment. As the elbow is flexed, the posterior soft tissue hinge becomes taut, correcting apex anterior angulation. Now maximally flex and pronate the elbow to lock the posterior and medial soft tissue hinges. Confirm the anteroposterior reduction by fluoroscopic examination, aiming the beam through the forearm and rotating the humerus from a medial to lateral position. Confirm lateral reduction by externally rotating the shoulder to obtain a lateral view of the elbow.

Maintain reduction while performing closed percutaneous pinning under image intensification to verify that the two lateral pins engage both fracture fragments (Fig. 16-161). After internal fixation, extend the elbow as far as possible without bending the pins. Compare the carrying angle with that of the normal extremity, and obtain true anteroposterior roentgenograms of both distal humeri to judge quality of reduction. Carefully position the arm with the medial and lateral epicondyles parallel to the cassette. Direct the roentgen beam to obtain a true anteroposterior view of the distal humerus. Further evaluate the quality of reduction by means of Baumann's angle (p. 965).

▶ *Postoperative management.* Postoperative management is the same as for fixation with crossed pins.

Open reduction and internal fixation. Open reduction and internal fixation of supracondylar fractures are indicated when closed reduction is unsatisfactory. Most authors agree that this is required in fewer than 5% to 10% of supracondylar fractures. Satisfactory closed reduction may not be possible in a type III displaced fracture with no cortical contact, a completely detached periosteum, and "puckering" or penetration of the skin by the fracture fragment. If the fragments cannot be reduced and held with percutaneous pinning, open reduction and internal fixation are indicated. If the elbow is so severely swollen that closed reduction cannot be maintained, olecranon traction may be used for several days, followed by closed or open reduction. Other indications for open reduction include open fractures that require irrigation and debridement and fractures complicated

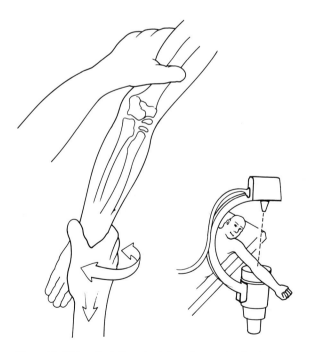

Fig. 16-160 Rotational deformity and displacement were evaluated under fluoroscopy. Anatomic correction of these deformities must be obtained before elbow is flexed. (Redrawn from Aronson DD and Prager BI: Clin Orthop 219:174, 1987.)

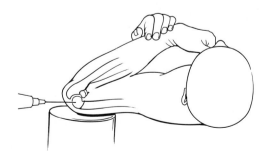

Fig. 16-161 Accurate position of pins ensured during procedure with aid of fluoroscopy. (Redrawn from Aronson DD and Prager BI: Clin Orthop 219:174, 1987.)

by vascular injury. Possible complications of open reduction include infection, vascular injury, myositis ossificans, excessive callus formation with residual stiffness, and decreased range of motion.

If open reduction and internal fixation are indicated, they should be performed after the swelling has decreased but no later than 5 days after injury because myositis ossificans seems to increase after that time. Open reduction has been described through lateral, posterior, medial, anterolateral, and antecubital approaches, but the lateral approach usually is preferred. Kekomäki et al, using an antecubital approach, and Danielsson and Pettersson, using a medial approach, reported good results with open reduction and internal fixation of severely displaced fractures that could not be reduced closed or had significant vascular injury. They also recommended fasciotomy at the time of open reduction. Gruber and Hudson also reported satisfactory results with open reduction and internal fixation of 31 difficult fractures. Pirone et al recommend a limited anterior approach to avoid opening uninjured tissue planes.

▶ *Technique.* Prepare and drape the arm in the usual fashion with the patient supine. Make a curved incision over the lateral humeral condyle, beginning about 2 cm distal to the olecranon, and carrying it proximally for about 6 cm above the condyle. Dissect the soft tissue, including the anconeus and common extensor origins, and retract these anteriorly and posteriorly respectively. Make sure the radial nerve is retracted posteriorly. A large hematoma may require evacuation before the fracture can be seen. Observe the supracondylar fragment, and note its alignment with the proximal fragment. Use a small curet to remove any hematoma at the fracture site. Note any interdigitations on the ends of the bone, and by matching them, reduce the fracture. Use two crossed Steinmann pins in a manner similar to that described for percutaneous pinning. Image intensification simplifies pin placement, as does an electric drill. Cut the pins just under the skin or leave them bent outside the skin for easy removal later. Close the incision in layers.

▶ *Postoperative management.* A posterior plaster splint is applied, and the radial pulse and neurologic function are checked after anesthesia. The pins are removed at 3 to 4 weeks, and an active, not passive, range-of-motion program is started.

Early Complications

Neurologic compromise associated with supracondylar fractures is reported to occur in from 3% to 22% of patients, usually a neurapraxia. Any of the peripheral nerves—medial, anterior intraosseous, radial, and ulnar—may be damaged, and mixed nerve lesions have been reported. Complete return of nerve function is usual, although this may require several months. Some authors recommend surgical exploration if nerve function has not returned within 6 to 8 weeks after reduction, whereas others recommend allowing a minimum of 2 months for resolution. Continued nerve palsies after fracture union may indicate nerve entrapment in the fracture callus.

Injury to the brachial artery occurs in as many as 10% of supracondylar fractures. Often the problem is corrected once the fracture is reduced and circulation returns to normal. Most authors recommend close observation of vascular status after reduction; if circulation does not return to normal (with the elbow flexed to less than 45 degrees) within about 5 minutes, consultation with a vascular surgeon is recommended and surgical exploration of the brachial artery may be necessary. Besides the clinical indications of capillary refill and pulse, Wenger and Moseley (Rang et al) recommend Doppler measurements or a pulse oximeter for evaluating circulation after reduction. Vasli reported the use of Doppler waveform analysis in which the Doppler equipment is connected to a spectrum analyzer, producing a picture of the velocity waveform that can be compared with the normal extremity and easily interpreted as normal or abnormal. Arteriogram generally is recommended if entrapment or severing of the artery is suspected. Rang does not perform open reduction even if the distal pulse is absent after reduction; he reports that the pulse usually returns within a week or two after fracture reduction, often quite suddenly. Unusually severe ischemic pain after reduction is an indication of vascular problems. Disappearance of the radial pulse with attempts at fracture reduction (not in an acute flexed position) implies interposition of the artery in the fracture site and necessitates surgical exploration.

Compartment syndrome is an uncommon, but serious, complication of supracondylar fractures. Compartment syndrome occurs as the result of hypoxic damage because of interruption of circulation to the muscle. Any evidence of compartment syndrome requires vascular consultation, compartment pressure measuring, and possibly fasciotomy. Moseley and Wilkins (Rang et al) recommend fasciotomy when there are clinical signs of compartment syndrome, such as undue pain and a palpable firmness in the forearm. Wilkins (Rang et al) points out that the morbidity associated with fasciotomy is minimal, whereas the morbidity associated with not treating the compartment syndrome is much greater. General indications for fasciotomy are (1) clinical signs such as demonstrable motor and/or sensory loss, (2) compartment pressures above 35 mm Hg (slit or wick) or above 40 mm Hg (needle), and (3) interrupted arterial circulation to the extremity for more than 4 hours.

Fasciotomy of the forearm. A number of techniques have been advocated for fasciotomy of the forearm, but the standard Henry approach (Fig. 16-162), as recommended by Eaton, Green, and Gelberman et al, most often is used. The forearm contains two compartments—superficial flexor compartment and deep flexor compartment—and both must be decompressed.

▶ *Technique (Rorabeck).* Begin the incision proximally at the level of the lacertus fibrosus, and extend it distally to the carpal tunnel with the forearm supinated (Fig. 16-162, *A*). Begin the skin incision medial to the biceps tendon, cross the elbow crease from medial to lateral, divide the lacertus fibrosus, and then follow the medial border of the brachioradialis muscle as far as the radial styloid process. Continue the incision distally across the wrist crease into the palm along the thenar crease. Incise the fascia that covers the superficial compartment from a point 2 cm proximal to the elbow crease to the palm. To gain access to the deep compartment, retract the brachioradialis and superficial radial nerve laterally and the flexor carpi radialis and radial artery medially (Fig. 16-162, *B*). The flexor pollicis longus and flexor digitorum profundus, as well as the pronator quadratus, muscles are now visible in the floor of the wound medially and the pronator teres laterally. Incise the fascia over each of these muscles to decompress the deep flexor compartment. Be sure to carry the incision into the palm to decompress the carpal tunnel as well. Inspect and identify each muscle belly in the superficial and deep compartments. Remove any muscle that is obviously necrotic, but do not resect any muscle with questionable viability because apparently ischemic muscle often regains its blood supply. Leave the skin and fascia open, and apply a single layer of nonadhesive dressing and a sterile bandage. Take care to ensure that the median nerve has soft tissue covering it.

▶ *Postoperative management.* Sterile saline-soaked gauze dressings are applied to the wound beginning on the third day after fasciotomy. Split-thickness skin graft or secondary wound closure is done on the seventh or eighth day.

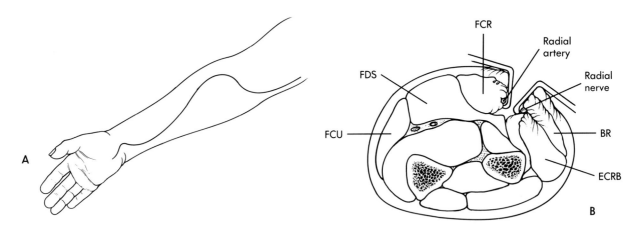

Fig. 16-162   A, Henry approach to volar aspect of forearm. **B,** Henry approach to superficial and deep compartments of forearm. *FCR,* Flexor carpi radialis; *BR,* brachioradialis; *ECRB,* extensor carpi radialis brevis; *FDS,* flexor digitorum superficialis; *FCU,* flexor carpi ulnaris. (Redrawn from Rorabeck CH: The American Academy of Orthopaedic Surgeons: Instructional course lectures, vol 32, St. Louis, 1983, The CV Mosby Co.)

Late Complications

Cubitus varus is the most common late sequela of supracondylar fractures, with reported incidences averaging 30%, ranging from 0 to as high as 60%. Cubitus valgus is rare and occurs more often from nonunion of lateral condylar fractures; an increase in valgus also is less cosmetically noticeable than varus deformity. Rotational malalignment may occur but is not usually a significant deformity. Several causes for cubitus varus have been suggested. Medial displacement and rotation of the distal fragment of the fracture were historically blamed for the deformity, but Smith proved in his experimental studies that medial tilting of the distal fragment was the most important cause of change in the carrying angle. He also showed that rotation of the distal fragment does not cause cubitus varus but is the single most important predisposing factor leading to medial tilt. LaBelle et al found medial tilting of the distal fragment the cause of deformity in all their patients with cubitus varus after supracondylar fracture. Growth disturbance in the distal humerus, especially overgrowth of the lateral condyle, also has been suggested as a cause.

Treatment. Cubitus varus is primarily a cosmetic deformity and rarely causes functional disability. Corrective osteotomy is indicated only after an adequate period of observation and only in those patients for whom the cosmetic deformity is unacceptable. The few reports in the literature of surgical correction of cubitus varus indicate a high complication rate and a high rate of unsatisfactory results, usually because of insufficient correction. Three basic types of osteotomies have been described for correction of cubitus varus deformity: lateral closing wedge osteotomy, medial opening wedge osteotomy with bone graft, and oblique osteotomy with derotation. King and Secor described the medial opening wedge osteotomy in 1951 but reported that disadvantages of this procedure include a gain in length of the extremity and some inherent instability. Lengthening the medial aspect of the humerus also may stretch and damage the ulnar nerve if it is not transposed anteriorly. Amspacher and Messenbaugh reported good results with an oblique osteotomy with cortical screw fixation, but this procedure attempts to correct a two-plane deformity with one osteotomy and requires rotation to correct the varus deformity.

The lateral closing wedge osteotomy is the easiest, safest, and inherently most stable osteotomy. The primary differences in techniques of lateral closing wedge osteotomy are the methods of fixation, including the use of a single screw, two screws and a wire attached between them, plate fixation, crossed Kirschner wires, and staples; some authors use no fixation. Crossed Kirschner wire fixation is the method most frequently reported in the literature, but reported complications include loosening of the fixation and recurrent deformity, pin tract infection, osteomyelitis, skin slough, nerve palsy, and, rarely, aneurysm of the brachial artery. DeRosa and Graziano reported good and excellent results with a step-cut technique of osteotomy fixed with a single cortical screw in 10 of 11 patients; the one patient with a poor result had persistent varus caused by unrecognized fracture of the cortical spike, which caused loss of fixation. The authors reported no ulnar or radial nerve injuries, infections, nonunions, or hypertrophic scars, and all patients retained preoperative ranges of motion. They concluded that osteotomy with one-screw fixation is a safe procedure with few complications, which can correct multiple planes of deformity (Fig. 16-163), but they emphasized the importance of careful preoperative planning and special attention to surgical detail.

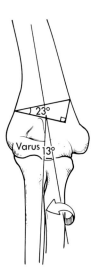

Fig. 16-163 Osteotomy designed to correct cubitus varus deformity of 13 degrees. Distal fragment may be rotated to correct additional deformity. (Redrawn from DeRosa GP and Graziano GP: Clin Orthop 236:160, 1988.)

Step-cut osteotomy

▲ *Technique (DeRosa and Graziano).* With the patient in a prone position and under tourniquet control, make a posterior approach to the distal humerus and reflect the triceps tendon, taking care to protect both the ulnar and radial nerves. Using the template constructed preoperatively, make a lateral closing wedge osteotomy in the metaphyseal region superior to the olecranon fossa. Place the apex of the template (angle to be corrected) medially, with the superior margin perpendicular to the humeral shaft. Join the inferior margin to the superior margin to outline the osteotomy (Fig. 16-164, *A*). Remove the osteotomy wedge leaving a lateral spike of bone on the distal fragment. Some trimming of the lateral shaft of the proximal fragment may be required for close approximation of the osteotomy. Temporarily fix the osteotomy with crossed Kirschner wires, and examine the arm for any remaining deformity. If necessary, correct rotational malalignment and hyperextension deformity at this time. Next place a cortical screw as a lag screw through the lateral spike into the proximal fragment and remove the Kirschner wires (Fig. 16-164, *B*). Close the wound in a routine manner, and apply a long-arm cast with the elbow in slight flexion and the forearm in full supination.

▲ *Postoperative management.* The cast is removed 4 weeks after surgery, and active range of motion exercises are begun. A posterior shell is used for protection between exercise periods until roentgenographic and clinical union is obtained.

French technique

French uses two parallel screws to secure the osteotomy (Fig. 16-165); the two screws are attached by a single figure-8 wire that is tightened for fixation. Bellemore et al reported superior results with fewer complications in children treated with a modified French technique (Fig. 16-166) compared with those with external fixation alone and those with Kirschner wire fixation.

▲ *Modified French technique (Bellemore, Barrett, et al).* Make a posterolateral incision, and split the triceps. Detach the triceps from its insertion, and reflect it proximally. Lift the middle two thirds of the muscle from the humerus subperiosteally, taking care to protect the neurovascular bundle. Remove a laterally based wedge of bone. Outline this wedge on the bone, ending just short of the medial cortex. Place one screw in the lateral cortex proximally above the proposed osteotomy, and another distally, below the proposed osteotomy, at an angle approximating that of the wedge to be resected. Then resect the wedge with an oscillating saw, leaving its apex intact at the medial cortex. Extend the elbow and close the wedge by fracturing the medial cortex, carefully retaining a periosteal hinge. Place the forearm in supination, and assess the carrying angle. If it is satisfactory, tighten a wire loop around the heads of the screws, which when tightened themselves will firmly appose the cut surfaces. If necessary, correct any rotational deformity at this time by offsetting the distal screw. Then derotate the distal fragment, correct for rotational deformity, and align it with the superior screw. Tighten the wires mentioned above.

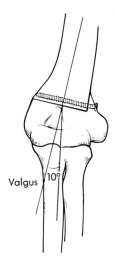

Fig. 16-164 Same site as shown in Fig. 16-163, after wedge removal and closure, screw is used for fixation. (Redrawn from DeRosa GP and Graziano GP: Clin Orthop 236:160, 1988.)

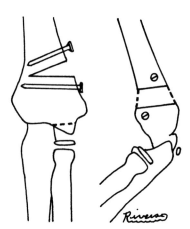

Fig. 16-165 French closing-wedge osteotomy using screw and wire fixation. (Redrawn from French PR: Lancet 2:439, 1959.)

◣ *Postoperative management.* The arm is flexed 90 degrees at the elbow with the forearm in neutral rotation in a posterior plastic splint for 3 weeks. An active mobilization program is started at that time.

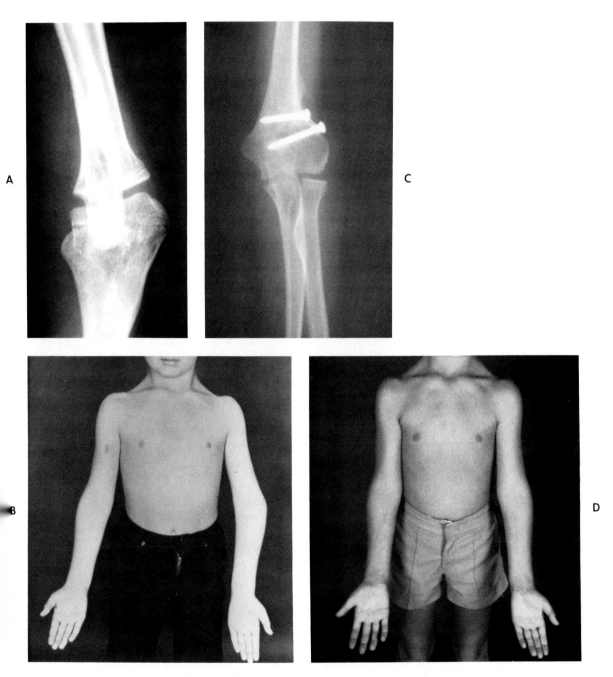

Fig. 16-166 **A** and **B,** Clinical roentgenogram and photograph of moderate cubitus varus secondary to supracondylar fracture. **C** and **D,** Clinical roentgenogram and photograph after French technique of supracondylar osteotomy. (From Bellemore MD et al: J Bone Joint Surg 66B:566, 1984.)

Separation of the Entire Distal Humeral Epiphysis

In younger children, because of the weakness of the physeal cartilage, the entire distal humeral epiphysis may separate from the humerus in the same area in which supracondylar fractures occur in older children (Fig. 16-167). DeLee et al classified these separations according to the age of the child and the degree of ossification of the lateral condylar epiphysis. Type A fractures occur in infants before the appearance of the secondary ossification center of the lateral condyle. These usually are Salter-Harris type I epiphyseal injuries, but they may be mistaken for elbow dislocations because of the lack of ossification of the epiphysis. According to Barrett et al, as well as others, these fractures can occur as a birth injury, but more important they can occur in this age-group because of child abuse. Type B fractures occur between the ages of 1 and 3 years, when the ossification center of the lateral condylar epiphysis is definitely present, and they may be either Salter-Harris type I or II epiphyseal fractures. Type C fractures occur in older children and produce a large metaphyseal fragment, usually displaced laterally but occasionally medially or posteriorly. Types A and B fractures are almost always displaced medially or posteromedially.

Separation of the entire epiphysis must be differentiated from dislocation of the elbow in the newborn and from a lateral condylar fracture (usually a Salter-Harris type IV epiphyseal separation) in older children (Fig. 16-168). On roentgenograms both the radial head and proximal ulna are displaced as a unit in relationship to the distal humerus (Fig. 16-169). If this displacement, usually posteromedial, persists, then the diagnosis of separation of the entire distal humeral epiphysis should be considered. In the older child in whom the lateral epiphysis is ossified, a constant relationship is maintained between the visible epiphysis and the radial head. Several authors, including Yates and Sullivan, Arkbarnia et al, and Hansen et al, recommend the use of arthrography as more accurate than standard roentgenography in diagnosing injuries of the elbow in young children because the cartilaginous ossification centers may not be visible on roentgenograms. They report that arthrographic examination, either single- or double-contrast, may confirm or change a diagnosis and may alter treatment in a number of children. Some children in their series believed to have condylar fractures actually had transverse epiphyseal fracture-separations (Salter-Harris type II) and several believed to have intraarticular fractures actually had supracondylar fractures. Some children originally considered for surgery were thus treated nonsurgically after accurate arthrographic diagnosis.

Because this separation is a Salter-Harris type I or II fracture and because it is in the plane of flexion and extension of the elbow, most will remodel without surgical treatment. Type A fractures in small children usually can be reduced satisfactorily and immobilized in a plaster splint. Type C fractures in older children generally can be reduced closed with the patient under general anesthesia. After satisfactory reduction a long-arm cast or posterior plaster splint should be applied if the fracture is stable; a pronated position should be used if the fracture is displaced medially. If the fracture is unstable after satisfactory closed reduction, smooth pins may be used to hold the reduction, similar to supracondylar fractures (p. 969). Holda et al recommend aggressive treatment of these separations because five of their seven patients with medially displaced fragments had mild cubitus varus deformities. They recommend open reduction, and internal fixation with pins when satisfactory closed reduction cannot be obtained and maintained. Mizuno et al also recommend open reduction and internal fixation with smooth pins if gentle closed reduction is not successful; however, they also recommend arthrograms to confirm the diagnosis because open reduction was performed in some of their patients as a result of confusion over the diagnosis.

Open Reduction and Internal Fixation

▲ *Technique (Mizuno et al).* Approach the distal humerus through a long posterior longitudinal incision. Carry the soft tissue dissection down to the subperiosteal area, and retract the ulnar nerve medially. Detach the triceps insertion with a cartilaginous piece of the olecranon, and reflect it posteriorly and superiorly to expose the fracture. Clean away any debris, including small hematomas and fracture fragments. Expose both fragments, and gently reduce the epiphyseal separation. Insert crossed Kirschner wires through the lateral and medial humeral condyles as for a supracondylar fracture (p. 969). Irrigate the wound copiously. Apply a posterior splint with the elbow at 90 degrees of flexion. Check the radial pulse.

▲ *Postoperative management.* Postoperative management is the same as for open reduction of supracondylar fractures (p. 971).

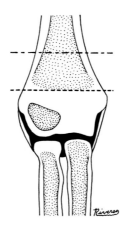

Fig. 16-167 Horizontal lines indicate area proximally where supracondylar fracture occurs, and distally where epiphyseal fracture-separation occurs in wide part of distal humerus in younger age group. (Redrawn from Mizuno K et al: J Bone Joint Surg 61A:570, 1979.)

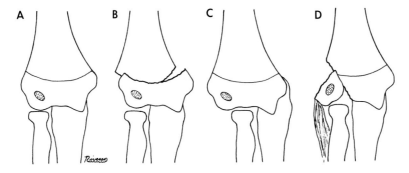

Fig. 16-168 Elbow injuries that may be confused clinically. **A,** Normal elbow before three centers of ossification appear. **B,** Separation of entire distal humeral epiphysis. **C,** Dislocation of elbow. **D,** Lateral condylar fracture. (Redrawn from Mizuno K et al: J Bone Joint Surg 61A:570, 1979.)

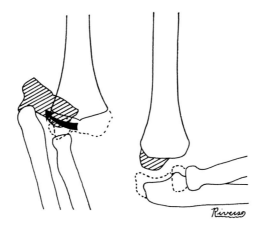

Fig. 16-169 Fracture-separation of entire distal humeral epiphysis displaced posteromedially. Note radial head and proximal ulna displacing as unit in relation to distal humerus. (Redrawn from Barrett WP et al: J Pediatr Orthop 4:618, 1984.)

ELBOW DISLOCATIONS
Acute Dislocations

Dislocation of the elbow in children is rare, accounting only for approximately 6% of all children's fractures and dislocations involving the elbow. In most large series of traumatic elbow dislocations, approximately half are reported to occur in persons younger than 20 years old. After review of three large series (those of Linscheid and Wheeler, Neviaser and Wickstrom, and Roberts), Wilkins concluded that 29% of all elbow dislocations occurred in patients between the ages of 10 and 20 years and 18% in patients younger than 10 years. Most pure dislocations are posterior, but they can occur anteriorly, medially, or laterally. Rarely, there is proximal radioulnar joint disruption (divergent dislocation) in either the anteroposterior or medial transverse plane.

Regardless of type, most elbow dislocations can be reduced closed. Open reduction is indicated when closed reduction cannot be obtained, when the dislocation is open or compound, or because of associated fractures. Arterial injuries that require surgical treatment usually are associated with open dislocations. Reduction usually is stable, but the elbow should be immobilized for about 6 weeks. Wilkins reported an 11% incidence of complications after elbow dislocation, including involvement of the three major nerves in the elbow area, myositis ossificans, recurrent dislocation, osteochondral fracture, and rarely an iatrogenic proximal radioulnar translocation after reduction (Fig. 16-170). Hallet noted that the median nerve may become trapped and block reduction, and several authors have reported median nerve entrapment after closed reduction. Proximal median nerve deficit, limited passive elbow motion, and an associated medial epicondyle avulsion after reduction of a posterior elbow dislocation should arouse suspicion of nerve entrapment. Immediate surgical exploration and release of the nerve are indicated.

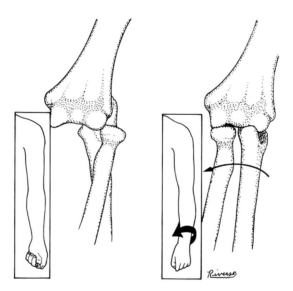

Fig. 16-170 Iatrogenic proximal radioulnar translocation following reduction. Ulna has become lodged in capitellotrochlear groove, and radius has been forced anterior to trochlea following hyperpronation reduction. (Redrawn from Harvey S and Tchélébi H: J Bone Joint Surg 61A:447, 1979.)

Chronic Recurrent Elbow Dislocation

Recurrent dislocations in children are rare, and most occur in adolescents. Opinions vary as to the need for surgical correction of asymptomatic chronic dislocations, but elbow deformity, limited range of motion, and chronic pain commonly are agreed to be indications for surgical treatment. Several authors, including Hassmann et al, Osborne and Cotterill, Symeonides et al, and Trias and Comeau, believe posterolateral instability is the most common posttraumatic lesion (Fig. 16-171) and recommend soft tissue repair and reconstruction on the lateral side of the elbow, reinforcement of this area, and reattachment of the lateral collateral ligament. The most frequently used reconstruction technique is that of Osborne and Cotterill. Other techniques advocated include reconstruction of the annular ligament, osteotomy of the ulna or radius, and ligament reconstruction combined with osteotomy.

▲ *Technique (Osborne and Cotterill).* Make a lateral longitudinal incision over the elbow beginning proximally at the lateral epicondylar ridge of the humerus and ending distally at the annular ligament. Open the elbow posterior to the lateral collateral ligament, and remove any fragments of bone from the posterolateral part of the capsule. Remove soft tissue, and roughen the bone at the lateral epicondyle and lateral side of the capitellum. With an awl, make one or two transverse holes through the lateral condyle as close to the articular surface of the humerus as possible (Fig. 16-172, *A*); then pass catgut sutures through these holes and through the posterolateral part of the capsule, and fix the capsule to the bone as tightly as possible (Fig. 16-172, *B*). If necessary, repair the medial part of the joint in the same way. Alternatively, the medial side of the joint can be tightened by a proximal advancement of the medial collateral ligament and medial epicondyle, with the epicondyle being fixed to the humerus with a screw.

▲ *Postoperative management.* A long-arm cast is applied with the elbow flexed 40 degrees. At 4 weeks the cast is removed, and active range-of-motion and strengthening exercises are begun. The elbow is maintained in a sling for 2 additional weeks.

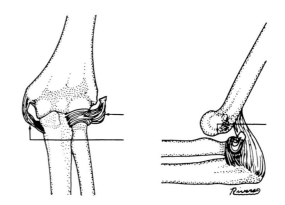

Fig. 16-171   Posterolateral elbow instability caused by lateral pocket defect in lateral condyle, torn lateral collateral ligament, and lax medial collateral ligament. (Redrawn from Osborne G and Cotterill P: J Bone Joint Surg 48B:340, 1966.)

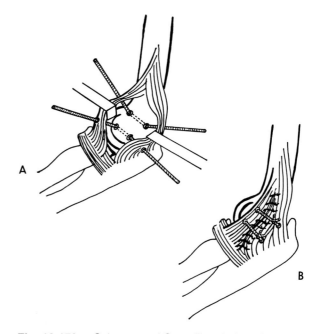

Fig. 16-172   Osborne and Cotterill technique for recurrent dislocation of elbow (see text). (From Osborne G and Cotterill P: J Bone Joint Surg 48B:340, 1966.)

Old Unreduced Elbow Dislocations

Speed (J.S.) noted that satisfactory function could be obtained by open reduction even in dislocations remaining unreduced for 3 months or longer and that results were better than after extensive arthroplasty procedures in immature patients. Fowles et al reported surgical treatment of 12 stiff elbows from 3 weeks to 3 years after unreduced dislocations, 11 of which had improved motion whereas one had a rigid myositis ossificans. They recommend surgical reduction as late as 3 years after injury and believe open reduction is always worth trying in a child.

Untreated (Chronic) Posterior Dislocation of Elbow in Children

▶ *Technique (Fowles et al).* Expose the elbow posteriorly through a Campbell posterolateral approach (p. 960). Free subperiosteally all muscle attachments from the distal humerus, both anteriorly and posteriorly. Release the attachments of the joint capsule around the humeral condyles. Expose the joint circumferentially, and detach the collateral ligaments from their proximal insertions. A fibrous ankylosis forms in most patients with the elbow in 30 to 60 degrees of flexion, and old articular fractures may be

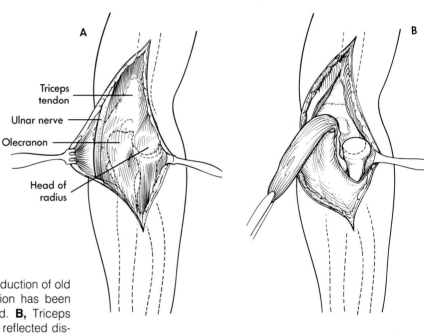

Triceps
tendon

Ulnar nerve

Olecranon

Head of
radius

Fig. 16-173   Speed technique of open reduction of old unreduced dislocation of elbow. **A,** Incision has been made and ulnar nerve has been isolated. **B,** Triceps aponeurosis has been dissected free and reflected distally. Triceps muscle has been incised longitudinally, and it and other muscles have been stripped subperiosteally from distal humerus. **C,** Lateral view of elbow to show extent of mobilization occasionally necessary before reduction becomes possible. **D,** Closure (see text).

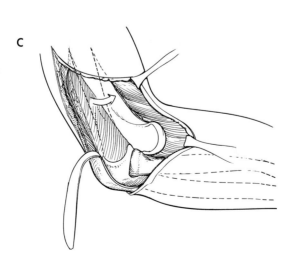

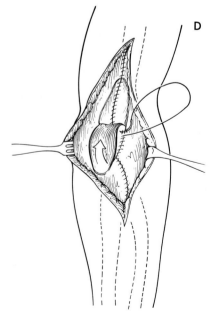

obscured by fibrous tissue within the joint. Release the thick, fibrotic, contracted capsule, and resect portions as necessary. Remove all the fibrous tissue from the joint, taking care to protect the underlying cartilage. Excise scar tissue carefully because it is often difficult to distinguish firm white scar from normal articular cartilage. Also remove subperiosteal new bone when it is an obstacle to reduction of the dislocation. If the triceps is tight, preventing reduction or limiting flexion to about 30 degrees after reduction, lengthen the muscle using Speed's V-Y muscle plasty (Fig. 16-173). Gently reduce the elbow. If the reduction is still difficult, release further the soft tissues proximally around the humerus and distally from the olecranon and the annular ligament until the elbow can be reduced without force. To avoid making the repair too tight do not reattach the ligaments to bone. If the ulnar nerve is tight or was compressed preoperatively, then transpose it anteriorly. Check the stability of the reduction manually at 90 degrees of flexion. If the joint redislocates easily, insert one or two Kirschner wires through the olecranon and into the humerus with the elbow flexed to 70 degrees.

▲ *Postoperative management.* Close the wound, and apply a long-arm cast with the forearm in neutral rotation. The cast and Kirschner wires are removed at 2 to 3 weeks. Active mobilization of the elbow is started slowly and is encouraged.

METAPHYSEAL AND EPIPHYSEAL OLECRANON FRACTURES

Purely epiphyseal fractures of the olecranon are extremely rare and are often confusing because of the complexity of the secondary ossification centers of the proximal ulna. The epiphysis fuses to the metaphysis at about age 14 years, but a sclerotic margin at the site of fusion may persist through adulthood and may be mistaken for a fracture (Fig. 16-174). Grantham and Kiernan, as well as Wilkins, classified epiphyseal fractures into two types (Fig. 16-175): a purely epiphyseal fracture and, in older children, a fracture in which a large metaphyseal fragment is attached to the epiphysis. Papavasiliou et al classified isolated fractures of the olecranon in children as intraarticular (group A) and extraarticular (group B). Included in the intraarticular fractures are simple crack fractures, simple fractures with minimal displacement, complete fractures of the olecranon involving the articular cartilage and with slight dorsal displacement of the proximal fragment, and grossly displaced fractures; a greenstick fracture is the only extraarticular fracture. They found that the fractures tended to be displaced in older children but not in younger children, which they attributed to the thicker articular cartilage in younger children. Canale and Graves classified 44 olecranon fractures in children as those with less than 5 mm of displacement, those with more than 5 mm of displacement, and open fractures.

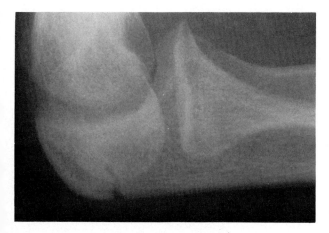

Fig. 16-174 Roentgenogram (lateral) of persistent delay of fusion of secondary ossification center, which can be confused with olecranon fracture.

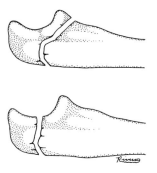

Fig. 16-175 Two types of olecranon epiphyseal fractures. Regardless of type, if displacement is significant, open reduction and internal fixation are probably indicated. (Redrawn from Wilkins KE. In Rockwood CA, Jr, Wilkins KE, and King RE, editors: Fractures in children, Philadelphia, 1984, JB Lippincott Co.)

Regardless of type, if significant displacement persists after attempts at closed reduction, open reduction and internal fixation with tension band wiring should be performed (Fig. 16-176). Matthews recommends open reduction and fixation for displacement of 4 mm or more, and Wilkins recommends palpation of the defect in the olecranon or flexion of the elbow to determine stability; if either suggests instability, he recommends open reduction and internal fixation with tension band wires secured over axial pins. Of the 15 isolated olecranon fractures in the series of Papavasiliou et al, 10 minimally displaced fractures were treated conservatively with excellent results, 4 grossly displaced fractures were treated surgically with some loss of extension, and 1 untreated fracture resulted in loss of extension and flexion.

In the 44 olecranon fractures reviewed by Canale and Graves, fractures with less than 5 mm of displacement were treated with a posterior plaster splint or long-arm cast until the fracture was not tender, then with a collar and cuff for a total of 3 to 4 weeks; good results were obtained in 28 of 30 patients. Of nine fractures with more than 5 mm of displacement treated with open reduction and tension band wiring, with or without axial fixation, or intrafragmentary screw fixation, seven had satisfactory results. Two open fractures treated with surgical debridement and irrigation and internal fixation had good results.

Metaphyseal fractures occur from either flexion or extension injuries. Extension injuries usually are associated with a valgus component after a shearing injury pattern. Closed reduction generally is successful, but if the reduction is unstable and the fracture is intraarticular, open reduction and internal fixaton with axial pins, tension band wires, or oblique screws may be necessary (Figs. 16-177 and 16-178). Open reduction and internal fixation with wires or screws, when necessary, should be performed as in adult olecranon fractures, although the deleterious effects on physeal growth are not currently unknown.

A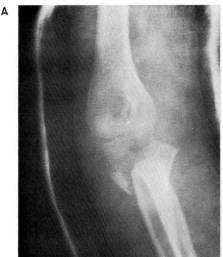

B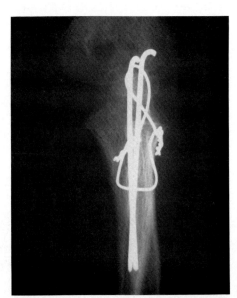

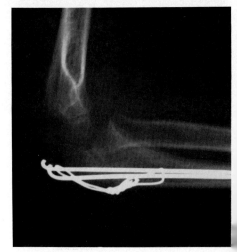

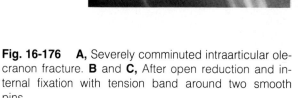

Fig. 16-176 **A,** Severely comminuted intraarticular olecranon fracture. **B** and **C,** After open reduction and internal fixation with tension band around two smooth pins.

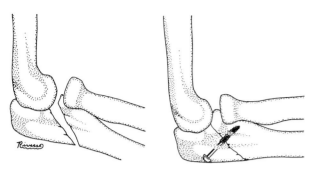

Fig. 16-177 Metaphyseal intraarticular olecranon fracture that is unstable and requires open reduction and internal fixation, here with oblique screw. (Redrawn from Wilkins KE. In Rockwood CA, Jr, Wilkins KE, and King RE, editors: Fractures in children, Philadelphia, 1984, JB Lippincott Co.)

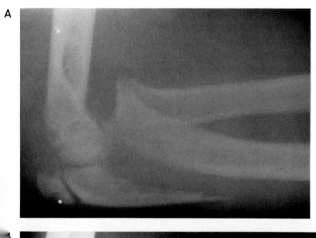

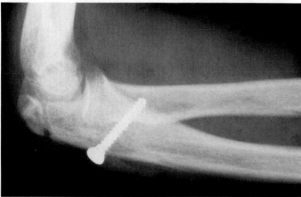

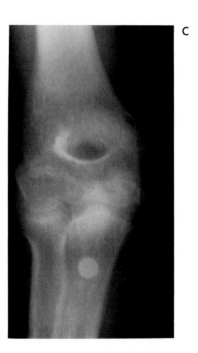

Fig. 16-178 Shearing intraarticular metaphyseal olecranon fracture, with displacement and instability. **A,** Before treatment. **B** and **C,** After open reduction and internal fixation with oblique cancellous screw.

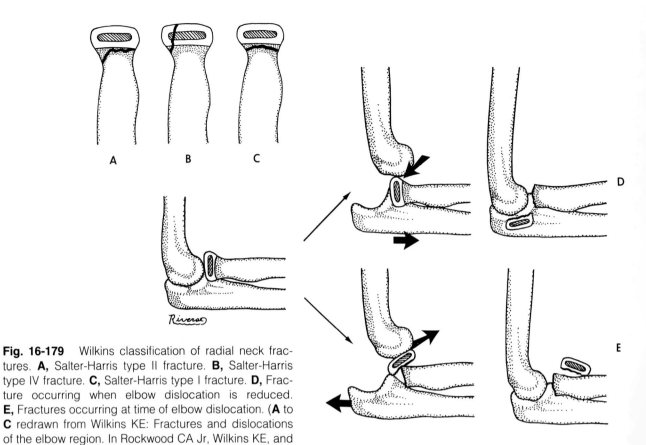

Fig. 16-179 Wilkins classification of radial neck fractures. **A,** Salter-Harris type II fracture. **B,** Salter-Harris type IV fracture. **C,** Salter-Harris type I fracture. **D,** Fracture occurring when elbow dislocation is reduced. **E,** Fractures occurring at time of elbow dislocation. (**A** to **C** redrawn from Wilkins KE: Fractures and dislocations of the elbow region. In Rockwood CA Jr, Wilkins KE, and King RE: Fractures in children, Philadelphia, 1984, JB Lippincott Co. **D** from Jeffery CC: J Bone Joint Surg 32B:314, 1950. **E** from Newman JH: Injury 9:114, 1977.)

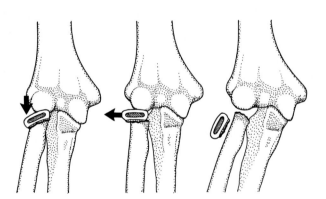

Fig. 16-180 Examples of angulation, translocation, and total displacement of radial neck fractures. (Redrawn from Wilkins KE. In Rockwood CA, Jr, Wilkins KE, and King RE: Fractures in children, Philadelphia, 1984, JB Lippincott Co.)

RADIAL HEAD AND NECK FRACTURES

Most fractures of the radial head and neck occur in children between the ages of 4 and 14 years, primarily because ossification of the radial head does not generally begin before the age of 5 years. The radial neck is fractured much more frequently than the radial head. Most radial neck fractures occur through the metaphysis, but they can occur through the physis, with a metaphyseal spike of bone producing a characteristic Salter-Harris type II epiphyseal injury. Most fractures of the epiphysis of the radial head are Salter-Harris type IV fractures.

Numerous classifications of radial neck fractures have been proposed, including those of Vostal, Newman, O'Brien, and Jeffrey. Wilkins combined the classifications of Jeffrey and Newman to produce a useful system: type A, Salter-Harris types I and II injuries of the proximal radial physis; type B, Salter-Harris type IV injuries of the proximal radial physis; type C, fractures involving only the proximal radial metaphysis; type D, fractures occurring when a dislocated elbow is reduced; and type E, fractures occurring in conjunction with the elbow dislocation (Fig. 16-179). Fractures also are defined as angulated, translocated (shifted), or totally displaced (Fig. 16-180). In elbow dislocations the proximal fragment may be loose in the joint or may be trapped and prevent reduction (Fig. 16-181).

Fig. 16-181 Dislocation of elbow and fracture of radial head. **A,** Posterior dislocation of elbow with suggestion of osteochondral fragment from radial head fracture. **B,** Oblique roentgenogram showing loose fragments of radial head entrapped within joint. **C** and **D,** After open reduction and excision of the loose fragment. Obvious ossification around both collateral ligaments and callus in area of radial head and neck are seen in **C.**

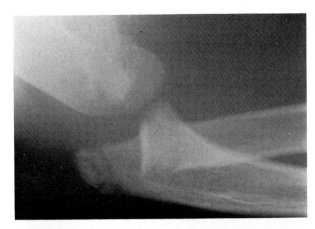
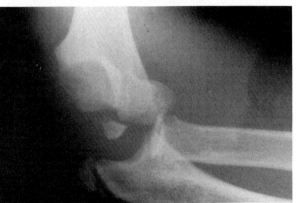
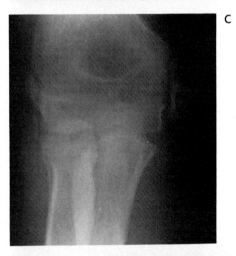
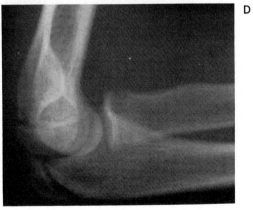

Closed reduction to an acceptable position (30 to 45 degrees of angulation) produces the most satisfactory results. Quite often, even a significantly angulated radial head and neck fracture can be reduced closed to an angle of less than 45 degrees. Tibone and Stoltz reported poorer results in older children with radial neck fractures and in children with other upper extremity injuries (usually on the medial aspect of the elbow). Steinberg et al reported that severely displaced fractures had better results with open reduction, but moderately displaced fractures did just as well with closed treatment. From their data

and review of the literature, they concluded that angulation of 30 degrees or less is compatible with a good result when treated with a cuff and collar. Pesudo et al suggested the use of a percutaneous pin and image intensification to manipulate and reduce the angulation of the fracture fragments. If satisfactory closed reduction (angulation less than 45 degrees) cannot be obtained, open reduction is indicated (Fig. 16-182). Fowles and Kassab reported 23 radial neck fractures, 15 of which with angulation of more than 60 degrees were treated with open reduction and internal fixation with transarticular Kirschner wires

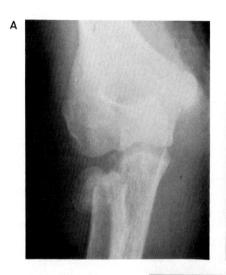
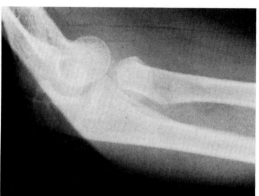
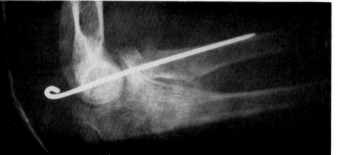
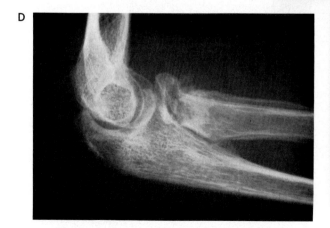
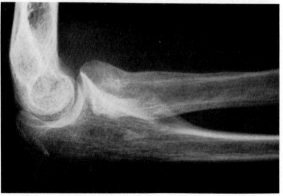

Fig. 16-182   Fracture of radial neck. **A** and **B,** Severely displaced fracture of radial neck. **C,** After failed closed reduction, open reduction and internal fixation with transcapitellar pin were done with good alignment of radial neck. **D,** Early pin removal was followed by delayed union. **E,** Complete healing of radial neck fracture after prolonged period in cast. Proximal radial physis closed with some persistent angulation. Range of motion is full.

through the humerus and radius. Because the Kirschner wires broke at the joint in two patients, they recommend avoiding the humerus by using oblique Kirschner wires. They found their worst results were in children with associated injuries of the same elbow treated with open reduction, but they believe this reflects the severity of the injury rather than the presence of associated lesions or the surgery itself.

Open reduction should be performed within 5 to 7 days of injury because myositis ossificans has been reported to occur more frequently after delayed surgical treatment. A lateral incision generally is used, and internal fixation is necessary; sutures in the periosteum do not provide adequate internal fixation. One or more oblique pins can be inserted across the fracture fragments (Fig. 16-183), although this is tech-

nically difficult. A large transcapitellar wire is easier to insert, but intraarticular breakage may occur. Wedge and Robertson reported equally good results with open reduction without internal fixation as with internal fixation.

Complications after open reduction include loss of motion, premature physeal closure, nonunion of the radial neck, avascular necrosis of the radial head, radioulnar synostosis, and injury to the posterior interosseous nerve. Unreduced fractures with angulation greater than 45 degrees usually result in significantly limited pronation and supination; after skeletal maturity the radial head may be excised, but this should not be done before skeletal maturity because it may result in proximal radioulnar synostosis, cubitus valgus, and radial deviation of the hand.

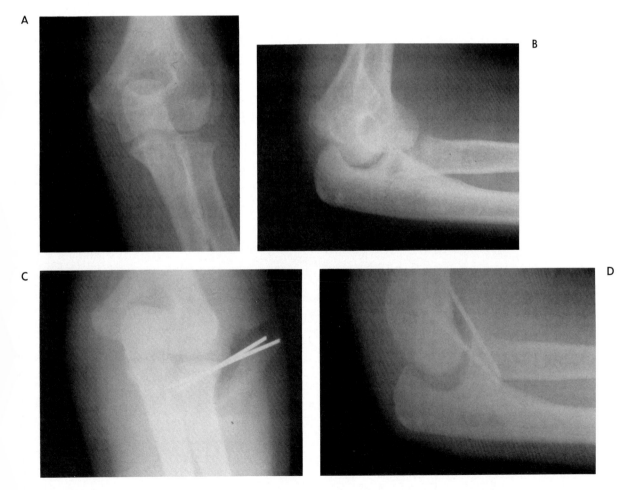

Fig. 16-183 Fixation of radial neck fracture with pins. **A** and **B,** Salter-Harris type III fracture of radial head and neck. **C** and **D,** After open reduction and internal fixation with smooth oblique pins inserted through epiphysis and metaphysis.

Closed and Open Reduction of Radial Neck Fractures

▲ *Technique.* Use a general anesthetic. Place the patient supine, and apply straight longitudinal traction. Use the Patterson manipulative technique described. Have an assistant hold the arm proximally, with one hand placed medially against the distal humerus, and apply straight longitudinal distal traction. Then apply a varus force to the forearm and digital pressure directly over the tilted radial head to complete the reduction. Hold the forearm in 90 degrees of flexion and in pronation (Fig. 16-184).

If this manipulation reduction is unsuccessful, the technique described by Pesudo et al can be tried. Have the assistant hold the arm with the shoulder abducted to 90 degrees and the forearm held in supination. With the use of an image intensifier and in a sterile operating field, introduce a Kirschner wire through the skin on the radial side of the elbow down to the angulated and displaced radial head and neck. Disimpact and push the radial head into anatomic position with the Kirschner wire. Remove the wire and flex the elbow to 90 degrees. Apply a cast in the neutral position, and leave it on for 4 to 6 weeks.

If these maneuvers are unsuccessful in reducing the fracture to less than 45 degrees of angulation, prepare for an open reduction. After preparing and draping the patient in the usual fashion, approach the fracture through a lateral approach (see p. 952). Remove any debris or torn annular ligament. Reduce the fracture gently. Secure the fixation with small Kirschner wires placed obliquely across fracture into the proximal radius. If this is impossible, then use a large transcapitellar pin across the joint and through the fracture site. If the annular ligament is torn, repair it. Close the incision in the standard fashion, holding the forearm in neutral rotation or in pronation and the elbow in 90 degrees of flexion, and apply a long-arm cast.

▲ *Postoperative management.* The pins are removed at approximately 3 to 6 weeks, but the cast is continued for 6 to 8 weeks because of the possibility of delayed union.

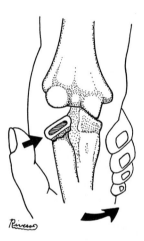

Fig. 16-184 Mechanism of reduction of radial neck fracture (see text). (Redrawn from Ogden JA: Skeletal injury in the child, Philadelphia, 1982, Lea & Febiger.)

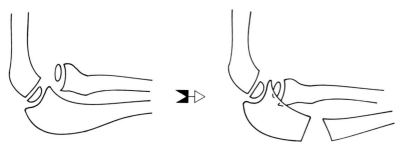

Fig. 16-185   Overcorrection with posterior convexity and elongation of ulna for anterior dislocation of radial head. (Redrawn from Hirayama T et al: J Bone Joint Surg 69B:639, 1987.)

Isolated Dislocations of the Radial Head

Isolated dislocations of the radial head are rare. Dislocations usually occur in conjunction with fractures of the ulna, but because of the plasticity of bone in children, acute isolated anterior dislocation, and more rarely lateral or posterior dislocation, can occur without fracture of the ulna. Vesely reported 17 isolated radial head dislocations, of which 13 were anterior, 3 lateral, and 1 posterior. Only 4 required open reduction. After closed reduction of an anterior dislocation, the forearm should be held in supination with the elbow flexed to 90 degrees; in posterior dislocation the forearm should be in pronation with the elbow at 90 degrees. Open reduction is indicated only when the dislocation has persisted for longer than 3 weeks or when closed reduction is not successful. Open reduction may be performed through the Boyd approach (p. 993), with repair of the annular ligament and fixation with a transcapitellar pin when necessary. In older children the reduction should be maintained for at least 3 weeks, after which the pin is removed and the cast is worn an additional 3 weeks. Complications of open reduction include redislocation and proximal radioulnar synostosis. Hirayama et al reported good results in nine chronic posttraumatic dislocations with osteotomy of the ulna, with overcorrection of the angular deformity and elongation of the bone. They believe the interosseous membrane of the forearm to be the most important structure in maintaining the corrected position of the radial head.

▶ *Technique (Hirayama et al).* After inflation of a pneumatic tourniquet on the upper portion of the arm, make a posterolateral skin incision extending from above the elbow to expose the joint and the proximal third of the ulna. Then excise the scar tissue around the radiohumeral and proximal radioulnar joints. If the ulna is angulated, perform a subperiosteal osteotomy of the ulna 5 cm below the olecranon. Distract the osteotomy by about 1 cm to elongate the ulna, and angulate it to produce overcorrection of the deformity. Correct anterior displacement of the radial head by posterior angulation of the ulna (Fig. 16-185) and lateral dislocation by medial angulation (Fig. 16-186). Hold the osteotomy with a metal plate bent to an angle of about 15 degrees. Be sure the repositioned radial head lies in the radial notch of the ulna to ensure proper spacing of the radiohumeral joint and to prevent excessive pressure on the radial head. Before wound closure, test the stability of the repositioned head by flexion, extension, pronation, and supination. Approximate the anconeus muscle, but do not repair the annular ligament. Apply a plaster splint with the elbow in 90 degrees of flexion and full supination.

▶ *Postoperative management.* Active movements are begun after 4 weeks.

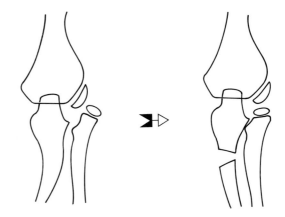

Fig. 16-186   Overcorrection with medial convexity and elongation of ulna for lateral dislocation of radial head. (Redrawn from Hirayama T et al: J Bone Joint Surg 69B:639, 1987.)

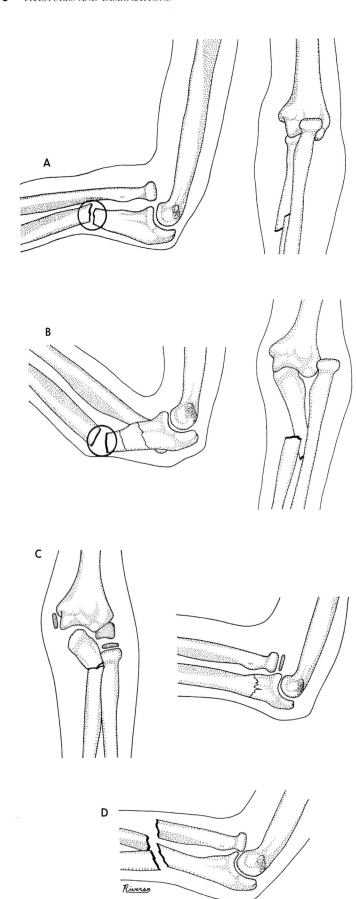

MONTEGGIA AND GALEAZZI FRACTURES

Dislocation of the radial or ulnar head frequently is associated with fracture of the forearm and, if not recognized and treated appropriately, can result in poor function. Monteggia described fractures of the radius or ulna with occult dislocation of the radial head proximally, and Galeazzi described an analogous dislocation of the ulnar head distally.

Monteggia Fracture

Bado described four types of Monteggia fractures in adults on the basis of the position of the radial head (Fig. 16-187): type I, anterior dislocation; type II, posterior dislocation; type III, lateral dislocation; and type IV, anterior dislocation with fracture of both the radius and ulna. He supplemented this classification with several unusual injuries that he called "equivalents" or Monteggia-like lesions (Fig. 16-188). More recently, several authors have suggested that, although this classification may relate to the mechanism of injury, it has no relationship to the treatment or results of these injuries in children. Wiley and Galey proposed a three-part classification of the disloca-

Fig. 16-187 Types of Monteggia fractures. **A,** Type I with anterior dislocation of radial head and anterior angulation of ulnar fracture. **B,** Type II with posterior dislocation of radial head and posterior angulation of ulnar fracture. **C,** Type III with lateral dislocation of radial head and lateral angulation of ulnar fracture. **D,** Rare type IV with fractures of radial and ulnar shafts and dislocation of radial head. (Redrawn from Bado JL: Clin Orthop 50:71, 1967.)

tion of the radial head associated with fracture of the proximal ulna: type I, anterior; type II, posterior; and type III, lateral. Letts et al suggested a more extensive classification system to include Monteggia equivalents in which there is bowing or greensticking of the ulna (Fig. 16-189). Olney and Menelaus, on the other hand, found the Bado classification applicable to children's fractures in their series of 102 Monteggia lesions. In 197 Monteggia lesions in children reported in the literature (Reckling, Bruce et al, Letts et al, Wiley and Galey, Olney and Menelaus), Bado type I lesions were by far the most common (59%), followed by type III lesions (26%). Types II (5%) and IV (1%) were rare. Olney and Menelaus found a type I equivalent (ulnar fracture associated with radial neck fracture or separation of the proximal radial epiphysis) in 14 of their 102 patients. In their report of 26 dislocations of the radial head associated with olecranon fracture, Theodorou et al found the dislocation to be lateral in 23 (58%), posterolateral in 13 (28%), anterolateral in 8 (17.4%), and anterior in 2 (4.3%); they had no posterior dislocations.

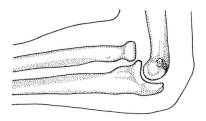

Fig. 16-188 Monteggia equivalent with isolated anterior dislocation of radial head. (Redrawn from Bado JL: Clin Orthop 50:71, 1967.)

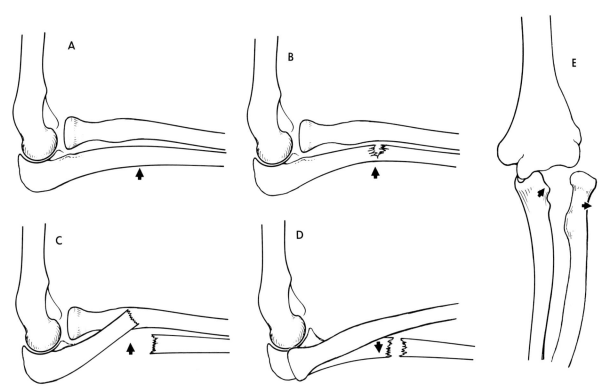

Fig. 16-189 Proposed classification of pediatric Monteggia fracture-dislocations. **A,** Anterior bend. **B,** Anterior greenstick. **C,** Anterior complete. **D,** Posterior. **E,** Lateral. (Redrawn from Letts M et al: J Bone Joint Surg 67B:724, 1985.)

Diagnosis of the Monteggia lesion is perhaps the most difficult aspect of treatment. Often roentgenograms of the elbow are not obtained or subtle dislocation or subluxation of the radial head is not recognized on roentgenograms. Theodorou et al reported that the correct diagnosis was missed in 15 of 46 children. They recommend that the distal forearm be included in the roentgenogram; in 26% of their patients the elbow dislocation was associated with a fracture of the lower end of the ipsilateral radius and ulna. On roentgenograms the radial head should always point through the middle of the capitellum in any position, especially on the lateral view. This can be confirmed by drawing a straight line through the radial head; in any position this line should pass through the center of the capitellum (Fig. 16-190).

Most Monteggia fractures can be treated by closed methods. If closed reduction is unsuccessful, interposition of the annular ligament or the capsule may be present, and open reduction may be necessary. Olney and Menelaus reported that most type I equivalent fractures associated with fracture of the proximal radius required open reduction and internal fixation, and some unstable type I fractures required fixation with an intramedullary wire or Rush pin after closed reduction. Wiley and Galey also used percutaneous intramedullary pinning for stabilization of the ulnar fracture. Letts et al recommend open reduction only

for adolescents in whom closed reduction is not successful or in whom the diagnosis has been delayed. Surgical treatment may consist of closed reduction of the radial head and open reduction of the ulnar fracture, or open reduction of both the radial head and ulnar fracture with internal fixation of the ulna. If open reduction of the radial head is performed, internal fixation of the proximal ulna with a plate and screws should be used only in older children. Stripping of the soft tissues, including the periosteum, should be minimal because myositis and synostosis are frequent in this area. In adolescents the ulna should be fixed with a plate or intramedullary nail at the time of radial head reduction. In younger children an intramedullary nail may be used for fixation if necessary. A single incision (Boyd approach) or two separate incisions may be used; King believes the use of two incisions decreases the likelihood of myositis or synostosis. Any material caught in the radiocapitellar articulation should be removed and the dislocation should be stabilized, preferably by repairing the annular ligament and flexing the elbow to 120 degrees. The radiocapitellar articulation may be held with a pin inserted across the radial head and neck into the capitellum, but this is technically demanding and results have not been uniformly satisfactory. Although the dangers of transcapitellar pinning are well known, when necessary a large, smooth pin as described by King can be used. Parents should be warned of the possibility of pin tract infection or breakage of the pin.

Open Reduction and Internal Fixation of Monteggia Fractures
Internal Fixation of the Ulna with Closed Reduction of Radial Head

▶ *Technique.* First attempt to reduce the dislocation of the radial head by traction on the forearm and countertraction on the arm followed by flexion of the elbow to 120 degrees. Check the reduction by roentgenograms; if it is satisfactory, proceed with the technique described here, but if not, carry out the technique described next. Make an incision along the subcutaneous border of the ulna to expose the fracture of this bone. Then fix the fracture by either a compression plate and screws or an intramedullary nail (p. 998). Next close the incision, and with the forearm in supination and the elbow flexed 120 degrees to prevent the redislocation of the radial head, apply a molded posterior plaster splint. Repeat the roentgenograms to confirm that the radial head has remained reduced.

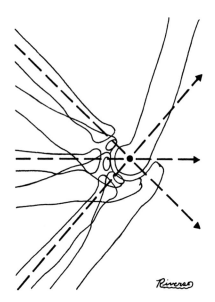

Fig. 16-190 Composite sketch to show radial head axis passing through center of capitellum in any position of flexion and extension. (Redrawn from Smith FM: Clin Orthop 50:7, 1967.)

▶ *Postoperative management.* At 2 weeks the posterior plaster splint is windowed or removed and the sutures are removed; during the first 4 to 6 weeks the elbow must be maintained at 110 to 120 degrees of flexion. Usually a long-arm cast is applied at 2 weeks. At 4 weeks the cast is removed and the extremity supported with a collar and cuff sling maintaining the elbow at 110 to 120 degrees. Gentle pronation and supination motions are permitted, but extension is not permitted below 90 degrees until 6 weeks after injury.

Open Reduction of Radial Head and Internal Fixation of Ulna

▶ *Technique (Speed and Boyd).* When reduction of the radial head is prevented by interposition of the annular ligament or capsule, expose both the fracture of the ulna and the dislocation of the radial head through the Boyd approach (Fig. 16-191, *A*). Next determine the status of the annular ligament. If the ligament is intact, incise and retract it to allow reduction of the radial head. More commonly it is torn or avulsed and displaced into the radial notch of the ulna. If it has been incised to allow reduction of the radial head or if it is not frayed too much, repair it with appropriate nonabsorbable sutures. If it cannot be repaired, reconstruct it as follows. Dissect from the muscles of the forearm a strip of fascia 1.3 cm wide and about 11.4 cm long. Leave the proximal end of the strip attached to the proximal end of the ulna where the deep fascia blends with the periosteum at the distal end of the triangular dorsal surface of the olecranon (Fig. 16-191, *B*). Pass the fascial strip posterior to the radial neck at a level distal to the radial notch of the ulna and proximal to the tuberosity of the radius and then around the neck of the radius. Now appose the fragments of the ulna and fix them rigidly. If the fracture is significantly comminuted, supplement the internal fixation with autogenous iliac bone, taking care that none is placed in the interosseous space. Now suture the new annular ligament about the radial neck (Fig. 16-191, *C*). It should be snug but not tight enough to erode the bone and restrict pronation and supination.

▶ *Postoperative management.* Postoperative management is the same as that described for this surgery with closed reduction of the radial head.

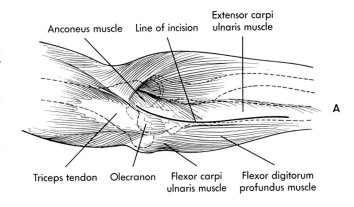

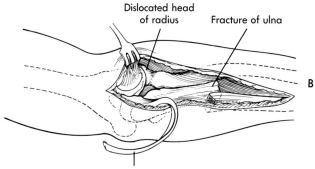

Strip of deep fascia reflected from forearm, leaving its base attached proximally to ulna

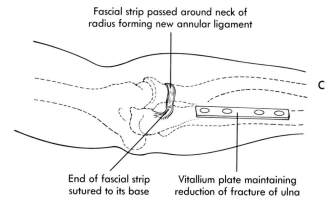

Fig. 16-191 Speed and Boyd procedure for Monteggia fracture-dislocations. **A,** Dislocations of head of radius and fracture of ulna exposed through one incision (Boyd). **B,** Exposure has been completed. Strip of deep fascia, its base level with radial neck, has been freed. **C,** Dislocation of proximal radius has been reduced, and new annular ligament has been sutured about radial neck. Fracture of ulna has been fixed with plate (intramedullary nail or compression plate would be more satisfactory). (Modified from Campbell WC and Smith H: Lewis practice of surgery, Hagerstown, Md, 1940, WF Prior Co, Inc.)

Complications

Complications reported in association with Monteggia fractures and their equivalents include posterior and anterior interosseous nerve lesions, vascular compromise, compartment syndrome, malunion, and proximal radioulnar synostosis. Most nerve injuries resolve within 3 to 6 months of injury. Varus angulation is the most common deformity at long-term follow-up, but as Ramsey and Pedersen noted, the deformity decreases with time and is not associated with redislocation of the radial head. Compartment syndrome and synostosis (cross-union) are discussed on p. 971 and p. 1000, respectively.

The treatment of undiagnosed radial head dislocation or chronic persistent radial head dislocation after Monteggia fracture historically has been radial head resection after skeletal maturity. Resection of the radial head in a skeletally immature child leads to angular deformity at both the elbow and the wrist, but Speed and Boyd found angular deformity and shortening in only 3 of 15 older children with radial head resection, neither of which produced significant functional limitations. According to more recent reports, satisfactory reduction of the radial head may be obtained as late as 6 months or more after traumatic dislocation. This generally requires osteotomy of the angulated ulna, followed by open reduction of the radial head, reconstruction of the annular ligament with fascia or other soft tissue, and stabilization of the radial head in normal position against the capitellum. Bell-Tawse, Lloyd-Roberts and Bucknill, and King all have described satisfactory results with late reduction of the radial head. Boyd used a slip of fascia from the extensor aponeurosis to reconstruct the torn or attenuated annular ligament (Fig. 16-191). Bell-Tawse used a central slip of the triceps fascia, and Lloyd-Roberts the lateral aspect of the triceps fascia attached distally. When the ulna is malunited, regardless of the amount of remodeling, osteotomy usually is necessary to "lengthen" the ulna and allow stable reduction of the radial head. When necessary in older children a transcapitellar pin may be used to hold the reduction (Fig. 16-192) and an intramedullary pin or compression plate to fix the osteotomy of the ulna. Internal fixation usually is not required in younger children.

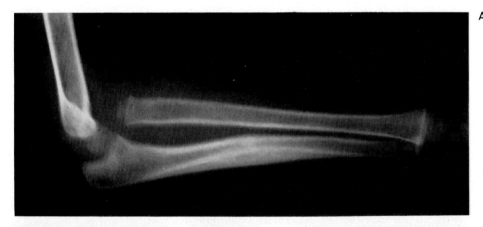

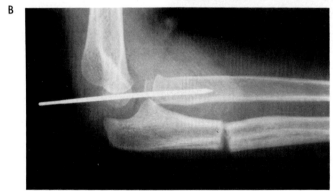
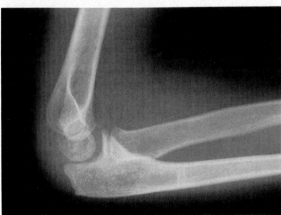

Fig. 16-192 Malunion of ulna and anterior dislocation of radial head. **A,** Before treatment. **B,** After Bell-Tawse procedure using triceps fascia, insertion of transcapitellar pin, and extension osteotomy of ulna. **C,** At 3 years after surgery, showing maintenance of radial head reduction. Sclerosis of radial head is worrisome.

Open Reduction of Old Monteggia Fracture in Children

▶ *Technique (Speed and Boyd).* Expose both the fracture of the ulna and the dislocation of the radial head through the Boyd approach (p. 993). If the ulna has united in malposition, make an osteotomy through the area of union and fix it internally with either a compression plate or an intramedullary nail. Reposition the head of the radius anatomically after removing any portion of the annular ligament that may be caught in the radiohumeral articulation. If the annular ligament cannot be repaired adequately, free a strip of fascia, 1.3 cm wide and approximately 11.5 cm long, from the muscles of the forearm, leaving it attached to the proximal ulna (see Fig. 16-192). Pass the fascial strip between the radial notch of the ulna and the tuberosity of the radius and around the neck of the radius. Fasten it to itself with interrupted nonabsorbable sutures. If the proximal radius is still unstable, fix it with a large, smooth, transarticular Steinmann pin as described in the next technique. Irrigate the wound and close it in layers. Keep the forearm slightly supinated, and apply a sterile dressing and a long-arm cast.

▶ *Postoperative management.* The parents should be warned about possible transcapitellar pin breakage and infection. The cast and pin are removed at 3 to 6 weeks, and range-of-motion exercises are begun.

▶ *Technique (Bell-Tawse; Lloyd-Roberts; King).* Place the patient supine on the operating table; prepare and drape the arm in the usual fashion on a hand table. Make a lateral longitudinal incision centered over the apex of the ulnar fracture, and carry the soft tissue dissection down to the malaligned fracture. Perform an osteotomy at the apex of the fracture. If the malunion is angulated anteriorly, pull the proximal fragment into hyperextension. In a young child, overriding of the fragments is acceptable. Now make a Boyd approach (p. 993). Carry the dissection down to the radial head and remove the capsule and remnant of annular ligament interposed in the joint, blocking reduction of the radial head against the capitellum. Now reduce the proximal radius. Free a central or lateral slip of the triceps fascia, as described by Bell-Tawse, Lloyd-Roberts, and King. This slip should be 8 cm long and 1 cm wide and is left attached distally to the ulna adjacent to the radial neck. Then pass the fascia from medially to laterally around the radial neck and through holes drilled in the ulna and suture it to itself (Fig. 16-193). Check the radial head reduction. Now introduce a large, smooth, Steinmann pin through the capitellum,

across the joint, and into the head and neck of the radius, as described by Lloyd-Roberts (Fig. 16-194). Bend its proximal end outside the skin. In older children when internal fixation is necessary, fix the ulna with a long intramedullary Steinmann pin or a compression plate. Apply a long-arm cast with the elbow in 90 degrees of flexion and the forearm in mild supination.

▶ *Postoperative management.* Postoperative management is the same as for the Speed and Boyd technique (p. 993).

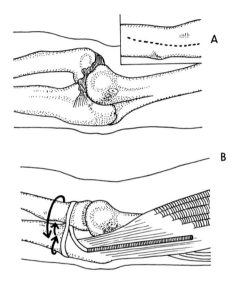

Fig. 16-193 Bell-Tawse procedure. **A,** Pathologic condition at radiohumeral joint. *Inset,* Skin incision. **B,** Use of fascial strip from triceps tendon to reconstruct annular ligament. (Redrawn from Bell-Tawse AJS: J Bone Joint Surg 47B:718, 1965.)

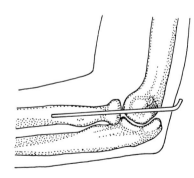

Fig. 16-194 Transcapitellar pin used after reduction of chronic dislocation of radial head. (Redrawn from Hurst LC and Dubrow EN: J Pediatr Orthop 3:227, 1983.)

Galeazzi Fracture-Dislocation

Galeazzi fracture-dislocations—fracture of the radius with disruption of the distal radioulnar joint—are rare in children. Walsh et al reported that fewer than 5% of all radial shaft fractures in children are associated with obvious disruption of the distal radioulnar joint. They divided their 41 fracture-dislocations into two groups: those with fracture in the distal third of the radius (Fig. 16-195, A) and those with fracture at the junction of the middle and distal thirds (Fig. 16-195, B); these two groups were further classified as anterior or posterior dislocations. Most fractures within the distal third of the radius were associated with anterior displacement of the radius; conversely, most fractures at the junction of the distal and middle third were associated with posterior displacement. Like Monteggia lesions, Galeazzi fracture-dislocations often are unrecognized; Walsh et al reported that in 41% of their patients the injury to the distal radioulnar joint was not initially recognized. Most of these injuries in children can be treated by closed reduction. Once the radius is restored to length and the angulation is corrected, the distal radioulnar joint will reduce and become stable. Mikic reported good re-

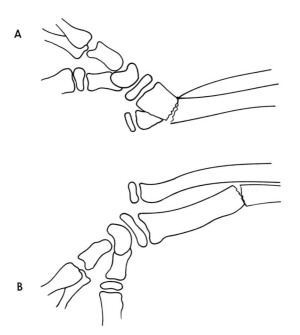

Fig. 16-195   **A,** Fracture-dislocation within distal third of forearm with posterior displacement of radius. **B,** Classic Galeazzi injury with radial fracture at junction of middle and distal thirds. Distal radius is anteriorly displaced. (Redrawn from Walsh HPJ et al: J Bone Joint Surg 69B:731, 1987.)

sults in 14 Galeazzi fractures in children treated conservatively, and Walsh et al reported excellent or good results in 36 of 39 (92%) fractures treated closed. All three poor results were in fractures of the distal third treated with below-elbow plaster casts. They recommend verifying relocation of the joint after reduction of the radial fracture and immobilization in an above-elbow cast with the forearm in supination. If closed reduction cannot be obtained, open reduction and internal fixation of the radius with a compression plate are indicated, especially in older children.

FOREARM FRACTURES

Forearm fractures are common in children, and most, regardless of level, do not require open reduction and internal fixation. Most authors agree that after closed reduction the arm should be placed in supination for proximal fractures, in neutral for fractures of the middle third, and in pronation for distal fractures. According to King the radial bicipital tuberosity proximally and the radial styloid distally are best seen in maximal supination, and he recommends that these two landmarks be aligned on the anteroposterior roentgenogram for proper rotational alignment.

Fractures of the Proximal Third of the Forearm

Fractures of the proximal third of the forearm are rare. Because of the possibility of radial head dislocation proximally and radioulnar dissociation distally, roentgenograms of the elbow and wrist joints always should be obtained in any forearm fracture. Holdsworth and Sloan noted that only 7% of both-bone forearm fractures were in the proximal third and did not recommend open reduction and internal fixation in children younger than 12 years. Because of the poor results in older children, however, surgical treatment may be indicated.

Fractures of the Middle Third of the Forearm

Fractures of the middle third of the forearm rarely require open reduction, especially in younger children. According to Weber et al the indications for surgical treatment are (1) open fracture, (2) fracture in an older child (shortly before skeletal maturity), (3) malunion, (4) irreducible fracture (because of soft tissue interposition), and (5) multiple refractures occurring over a short period of time. Nielson and Simonsen recommend open reduction and internal fixation in an older child when several attempts at closed reduction have failed. If open reduction is indicated, internal fixation should be used to prevent nonunion or recurrence of malposition. Vainionpää et al used small compression plates, one-third tubular plates, and intramedullary Kirschner wires for fixation in their 14 patients with severely displaced diaphyseal fractures of both bones of the forearm (Fig. 16-196). Ten patients had good results, and four had satisfactory results. The authors found better results in fractures of the distal third of the radius and ulna than in more proximal fractures, and they recommend open reduction and internal fixation for all severely displaced fractures of the forearm. Verstreken et al reported good results with intramedullary nailing of completely displaced shaft fractures in six children. They note that closed nailing through a distal approach avoids extensive dissection and allows immediate postoperative motion of the extremity. Compression plate fixation techniques may be used in older children as in adults, but the physis should be avoided.

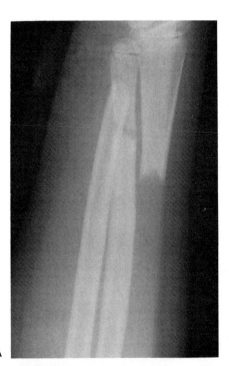
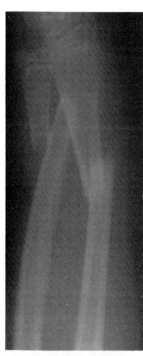

A

B

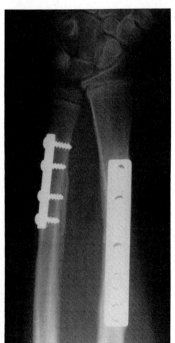
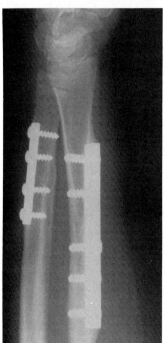

D

Fig. 16-196 Both-bone forearm fracture in older child with physes still open requiring open reduction. **A** and **B,** Before treatment. **C** and **D,** Fractures have healed after open reduction and internal fixation with compression plates.

Closed Intramedullary Nailing

▶ *Technique (Verstreken et al).* Place the child under general anesthesia in the decubitus position with the affected arm on a lateral table. Position a pneumatic tourniquet in case open reduction is required, but do not inflate it. Make a 1-cm longitudinal incision on the lateral side of the distal metaphysis of the less displaced bone (Fig. 16-197, *A*). Drill a hole in the bone with a brad awl, 1 cm proximal to the metaphysis, first perpendicularly and then obliquely toward the elbow. Depending on the bone diameter, choose a titanium blunted pin of the appropriate size. The pins range in size from 15 to 25/10 mm, and the proximal ends are bent at 30 degrees. Introduce the pin into the bone bent side first (Fig. 16-197, *B*) and push it, with a hammer if necessary, to the fracture site (Fig. 16-197, *C*). Reduce the fracture by external manipulation, and fix the pin in the proximal metaphysis (Fig. 16-197, *D*). Repeat the procedure for the other bone (Fig. 16-197, *E*). Bend the outer tip of the pins, and cut them 5 to 10 mm from the bone (Fig. 16-197, *F*). Use one or two stitches to close the skin.

▶ *Postoperative management.* Immediate motion is permitted, and discharge from the hospital usually is allowed on the first or second day after surgery. Sports are avoided for 2 months. Pins are removed by simple extraction after 3 months.

Fractures of the Distal Third of the Forearm

Fractures of the distal third account for approximately 75% of forearm fractures and almost never require open reduction and internal fixation. Most are dorsally displaced and in the plane of motion of the joint and will remodel satisfactorily if remodeling potential remains. Besides single or both-bone fractures, epiphyseal fractures of the distal radius and ulna occur, usually Salter-Harris types I or II, but these do not require surgery. Surgical treatment rarely is required for severely displaced fragments with soft tissue interposition, after failed closed reduction, or in open fractures. Lee et al reported premature closure of the distal radial physis after either epiphyseal compression injuries (Salter-Harris type V fractures) or repeated forceful attempts at reduction. They note that if the initial closed reduction achieves

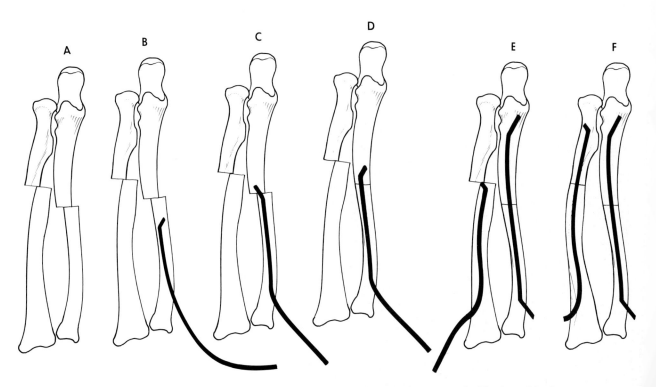

Fig. 16-197 Intramedullary nailing of both-bone forearm fractures. **A,** Displaced both-bone forearm fracture. **B,** Pin introduced into least displaced bone, bent side first. **C,** Pin advanced to fracture site. **D,** Fracture reduced by external manipulation and pin fixed in proximal metaphysis. **E,** Fracture of other bone reduced and fixed in same manner. **F,** Both pins in place.

apposition of more than 50%, repeated attempts at reduction should be avoided. Some open fractures, after irrigation and debridement, may be unstable and require some form of internal fixation. Smooth Steinmann pins can be used across the physis through the radial styloid. A metal plate, however small, should not be used in this area because of the possibility of damaging the physis. If the fragments are in good alignment, internal fixation is unneces-

sary. Satisfactory remodeling of angular deformities usually occurs, but remodeling will not correct rotational deformities. Some loss of pronation and supination may occur because of loss of the interosseous space if varus or valgus angulation persists (Fig. 16-198). Growth arrest of the distal ulnar and radial physes has been reported by several authors; this may be treated with ulnar lengthening, as described by Irani et al, or shortening, as described by Lee et al.

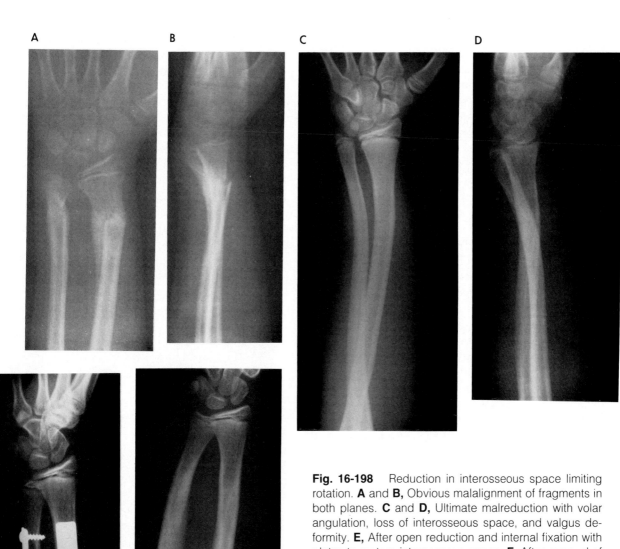

Fig. 16-198 Reduction in interosseous space limiting rotation. **A** and **B,** Obvious malalignment of fragments in both planes. **C** and **D,** Ultimate malreduction with volar angulation, loss of interosseous space, and valgus deformity. **E,** After open reduction and internal fixation with plates to restore interosseous space. **F,** After removal of plates and final healing: interosseous space and alignment are near normal.

Complications
Plastic Deformation

Because of the plastic nature of children's bone, the long bones frequently bend or bow rather than break. Most plastic deformities occur in the radius and ulna in children aged 2 to 15 years. In a review of reported series of plastic deformation of the forearm, Mabrey and Fitch found the ulna bowed in 83% of patients and the radius in 50%. In addition to the cosmetic deformity, bowing of one or both bones of the forearm may cause limitation of pronation and supination as the bowed bones encroach on the interosseous space. According to Borden physiologic remodeling in younger children eventually may permit full pronation and supination, but this is unlikely to occur in older children with uncorrected deformity. Sanders and Heckman described a method of closed reduction of plastic deformity of the forearm and reported an average correction of 85% of the angulation in eight patients. Their technique consists of applying a transversely directed force both proximally and distally to the apex of the bow with the apex placed over a rolled towel, usually with the patient under general anesthesia. Because the bowing occurred in more than one plane, sequential forces were applied to correct the deformity in both planes. Care was taken to avoid placing force over the epiphyses. With the application of a force of 20 to 32 kg the deformity gradually corrected over 2 to 3 minutes. If the other bone was fractured, it was then treated by whatever method would have been chosen had plastic deformation not occurred. A long-arm cast was applied with the elbow at 90 degrees of flexion and the forearm in full supination; the cast was worn from 6 to 8 weeks. Several important points must be remembered with this technique: (1) adequate anesthesia is essential; (2) the most deformed bone should be reduced first; (3) pressure is applied to the distal and proximal ends of the forearm, adjacent to but not directly over the epiphyses; and (4) force must be applied gradually to prevent fracture. The authors suggest reduction of any plastic deformity that prevents the reduction of a concomitant fracture or dislocation. Angulation of less than 20 degrees in young children usually will remodel satisfactorily, but they suggest consideration of reduction in children older than 4 years or any child with a deformity of more than 20 degrees, particularly if it limits pronation and supination. Mabrey and Fitch reported good results in 8 of 10 children treated with the technique of Sanders and Heckman.

Cross-Union

Cross-union is a rare complication of fractures of the forearm in children, but when both bones are united by a single callus, pronation and supination are impossible and the forearm may not be functional. Several factors have been suggested as contributing to the development of cross-union, including severe initial displacement, displacement after reduction, periosteal interposition, surgery, delayed surgery, remanipulation, excision of the radial head, and fractures of the radius and ulna at the same level. Vince and Miller reported 10 cross-unions in children and classified them according to location: type I, intraarticular in the distal third; type 2, nonarticular in the distal third or in the middle third; and type 3, in the proximal third. Type 3 cross-unions were the most frequent and occurred after mild injury and nonsurgical treatment, as well as after severe trauma; type 2 cross-unions consistently occurred after severe trauma, and there were no type 1 cross-unions. They concluded that the risk of cross-union is increased by surgical trauma to the soft tissue between the radius and ulna and that excision of the radial head alone was a greater risk factor than open reduction alone. Although their results after excision of the cross-union were not as good in children as in adults, they noted that delaying excision until the child is skeletally mature may preclude regaining full pronation and supination because of soft tissue contractures.

WRIST AND HAND FRACTURES, DISLOCATIONS, AND FRACTURE-DISLOCATIONS

Few injuries of the wrist and hand in children require surgical treatment, with the exception of fractures that involve a physis. These injuries must be anatomically reduced, for which open reduction sometimes is necessary. The time of physiologic closure of the physes should be noted in the phalanges and metacarpals because closure generally occurs earlier here than in other physes. Closure is earlier distally (phalanges) and later proximally (the distal radius), and once the physis has closed, a child's fracture can be treated as an adult's.

Distal Radial Fractures

The distal end of the radius is a common site of a torus fracture or a fracture involving the physis, most often a Salter-Harris type I or II fracture. The torus or buckle fracture is typically quite stable, heals with simple immobilization, and rarely results in complications. Premature closure of the distal radial physis is an uncommon complication usually encountered after repeated attempts at closed reduction of a type II fracture. Davis and Green reported premature closure in only 1 of 92 torus fractures of the distal radius. Lee et al described 10 patients with premature closure of the distal radial physis; 8 had type II fractures, 1 a type IV fracture, and 1 a type V fracture. Abram and Thompson attributed premature closure in one patient to an unrecognized type V physeal injury and recommend that patients with fractures adjacent to the distal radial physis, even if they do not directly involve it, be observed clinically and roentgenographically for at least 1 year to allow early recognition of premature physeal closure. Compartment syndrome, which is another rare complication after distal radial fracture in children, has been reported primarily in adults. Matthews described acute volar compartment syndrome in a 17-year-old and Santoro and Mara, in a 15-year-old, both with Salter-Harris type II fractures.

Carpal Fractures and Fracture-Dislocations

Injuries of the carpal bones have been considered rare in children, but Nafie found they constituted 3.9% (82 of 2102 fractures) of all fractures of the wrist in children and believes that many of these injuries are overlooked. The scaphoid was involved in 71 patients, the triquetrum in 5, the trapezium in 3, the hamate in 2, and the trapezoid in 1. The scaphoid is the largest bone in the proximal row of the carpus. Ossification begins between the ages of 5 and 6 years and is completed between the ages of 13 and 15 years. Before ossification the scaphoid is almost completely cartilaginous, accounting for the fewer scaphoid fractures in younger children. In Nafie's series, all patients with fracture of the scaphoid were 9 years old or older, and fractures of the waist of the scaphoid did not occur in any patient younger than 11 years. Fractures of the other carpal bones also occurred at about the time of complete ossification: triquetrum, between the ages of 12 and 13 years; trapezium and trapezoid, between 13 and 14 years; and hamate, 15 years. The correct diagnosis was made in 50% of patients before roentgenographic examination. The most common clinical signs of scaphoid fracture are dorsal swelling of the wrist, tenderness in the anatomic snuffbox and over the distal part of the radius, and painful dorsiflexion of the wrist and/or extension of the thumb. In 37% correct diagnosis was not made after initial roentgenograms. All but one of the fractures were treated with casting or splinting with good results. One scaphoid nonunion was discovered 18 months after injury when treatment was sought for a trivial wrist injury; union was obtained after autogenous cancellous bone grafting and Kirschner wire fixation. Vahvanen and Westerlund reviewed 108 scaphoid fractures in children, most of which were avulsions of the distal third of the scaphoid and all of which healed completely in a thumb spica cast. Painful nonunion of the proximal scaphoid, which is extremely rare in children, should be treated surgically if it limits function. A dorsal or volar approach may be used, and smooth pins should be used for internal fixation. Bipartite scaphoid has been described by Greene et al and others. Some have speculated that bipartite scaphoid may be an ununited waist fracture that has taken on the characteristics of a bipartite bone.

Metacarpal Fractures

Most fractures of the base or shaft of the metacarpals in children can be treated by closed reduction and observation. Normal rotation should be confirmed by the ability to flex the fingers into the palm. If malrotation persists, it will not remodel, and open reduction and internal fixation are indicated. Green notes that some multiple fractures of the metacarpal shaft in children require open reduction and internal fixation for stability. A significant intraarticular metacarpal head fracture also may require open reduction and internal fixation.

Most thumb metacarpal fractures occur at the base in the area of the physis rather than at the metacarpal head as in other metacarpals. Rarely, the thumb metacarpal may have physes at both the proximal and distal ends. Most physeal fractures in the thumb metacarpal are Salter-Harris type II injuries (Fig. 16-199) and can be treated by closed reduction without physeal arrest. Salter-Harris type III fractures (gamekeeper's thumb distally [Fig. 16-200] or Bennett's fracture proximally), however, are intraarticular and may result in a bony bridge if not treated properly. Closed reduction and percutaneous fixation or open reduction and internal fixation with smooth pins usually are indicated.

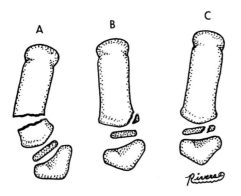

Fig. 16-199   Classification of thumb metacarpal fractures. **A,** Type A, metaphyseal fracture. **B,** Type B, Salter-Harris type II fracture. **C,** Type C, Salter-Harris type III fracture. (Redrawn from O'Brien ET. In Rockwood CA, Jr, Wilkins KE, and King RE, editors: Fractures in children, Philadelphia, 1984, JB Lippincott Co.)

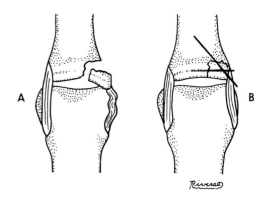

Fig. 16-200   Example of gamekeeper's thumb. **A,** Type III epiphyseal fracture. **B,** After open reduction and internal fixation with pins. (Redrawn from Wood VE: Orthop Clin North Am 7:527, 1976.)

Phalangeal Fractures

Phalangeal fractures probably are the most frequent hand fracture in children. Of 57 epiphyseal phalangeal fractures in children, Crick et al found 35 in the middle phalanx and 22 in the distal phalanx. Salter-Harris type III injuries were the most common (51%) and occurred primarily in older children (average age 13 years); type II fractures were the second most common (37%), and type I fractures were relatively uncommon (12%). Avulsion injuries of the distal phalanx and physis produce a Salter-Harris type I or II fracture (Fig. 16-201). Adequate closed reduction of type I fractures will produce satisfactory results. Type III fractures of the distal phalanx produce a "mallet" finger (Fig. 16-202), which usually can be treated with accurate closed reduction in young children; if this cannot be obtained and maintained, open reduction and internal fixation are indicated. Kirner congenital deformity (p. 322) should not be mistaken for a distal phalangeal fracture. Roentgenograms of the opposite hand will confirm the diagnosis. A large percentage of physeal separations occur in the middle and proximal phalanges, most commonly Salter-Harris type II. Type III fractures do occur, but type I and IV fractures are extremely rare in the physes (Fig. 16-203). Most type II fractures can be treated satisfactorily by closed methods. Type III fractures require anatomic reduction (Fig. 16-204); if this cannot be obtained closed, then open reduction and internal fixation are necessary (Fig. 16-205).

Diaphyseal fractures also occur in the phalanges, and most can be treated with closed reduction. Occasionally in older children, as in adults, the reduction cannot be maintained and internal fixation may be required as reported by Green and Anderson, Rang, and Coonrad and Pohlman.

Phalangeal neck fractures also usually can be treated by closed methods; open reduction is re-

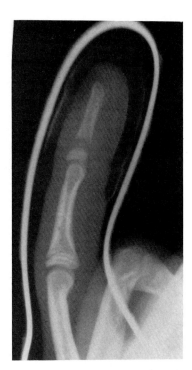

Fig. 16-201   Pediatric mallet finger after closed reduction and application of hyperextension splint.

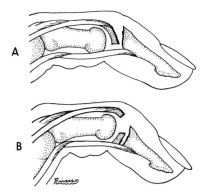

Fig. 16-202   Two types of mallet equivalent epiphyseal fractures in child. **A,** Salter-Harris type I fracture. **B,** Salter-Harris type III fracture. (Redrawn from Wood VE: Orthop Clin North Am 7:527, 1976.)

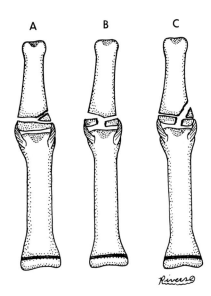

Fig. 16-203   Three types of epiphyseal fractures of the phalanges. **A,** Salter-Harris fracture type II. **B,** Type III fracture. **C,** Rare type IV fracture. (Redrawn from O'Brien, ET: Fractures of the hand and wrist. In Rockwood, CA, Jr, Wilkins, KE, and King, RE, editors: Fractures in children, Philadelphia, 1984, JB Lippincott Co.)

Fig. 16-204 Salter-Harris type III epiphyseal fracture. **A,** Satisfactory closed reduction. **B,** After healing.

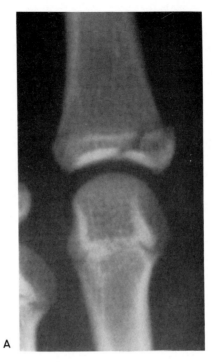
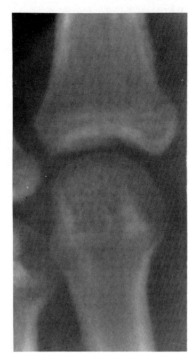

Fig. 16-205 Salter-Harris type III or IV fracture of proximal phalanx. **A,** Displacement of fracture. **B,** At time of open reduction and internal fixation with smooth pins across physis.

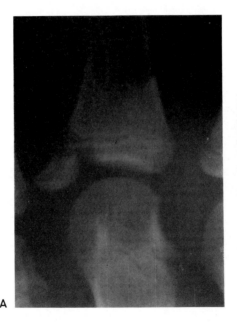
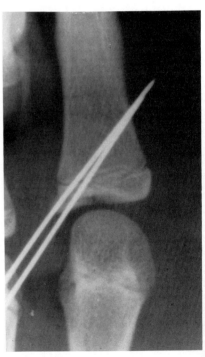

quired only if a severe angular deformity persists in an older child. Some degree of remodeling will occur in most younger children. Exceptions to this have been noted by Wood and by Dixon and Moon, who found that the volar plate can become interposed between the fracture fragments after rotation and angulation of the head fragment; this requires open reduction (Fig. 16-206).

Several types of intraarticular fractures of the phalanges can occur. Crick et al described four fracture patterns of interphalangeal joint fractures— transcondylar, unicondylar, avulsion, and supracondylar or shaft—and compared these to fractures produced by the same forces at the metacarpophalangeal joints (Fig. 16-207). They concluded that the collateral ligaments protect the epiphyses at the interphalangeal joints from stresses in the frontal (abduction/adduction) plane; instead, lateral bending forces produce fractures on the proximal side of the joint in this area. They also observed that angular deformities usually will correct in the sagittal plane when adequate growth remains, but not in the frontal plane; angular deformities did not occur in their patients whose fractures were treated surgically. Intraarticular fractures of the condyles and phalangeal neck fractures frequently resulted in permanent loss of motion at the interphalangeal joint in their patients.

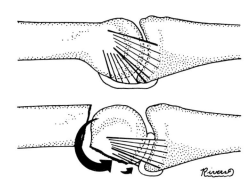

Fig. 16-206 Phalangeal neck fracture with interposition of volar plate. (Redrawn from Wood VE: Orthop Clin North Am 7:527, 1976.)

Fig. 16-207 Fracture patterns produced by lateral bending moments at interphalangeal and metacarpophalangeal joints. (Redrawn from Crick JC et al: J Orthop Trauma 1:318, 1987.)

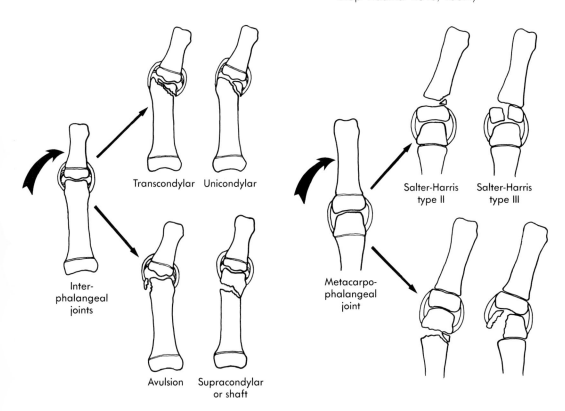

Open Reduction and Internal Fixation of Epiphyseal Fractures of Phalanges and Metacarpals

▶ *Technique.* Make a straight midlateral incision (Fig. 16-208) over the involved physis. After soft tissue dissection and retraction, mobilize the neurovascular structures and lateral bands. Now expose the physis, but take care not to damage it or the perichondral ring or periosteum overlying it. Carefully mobilize the fragments; clean out any small fragments or hematoma. With small hand surgery instruments, reduce the fracture anatomically. Make sure the reduction is satisfactory at both the physis and joint surface. Now with a power drill (low torque, high speed), transfix the fracture with two smooth parallel pins, preferably either in the metaphysis or epiphysis. Crossed pins and pins that cross the physis generally should be avoided, but sometimes small fracture fragments cannot be adequately transfixed and held oth-erwise. Cut off the pins beneath the skin, but leave them long enough to be removed easily in the office on an outpatient basis. Close the soft tissues appropriately, and apply a splint or cast.

▶ *Postoperative management.* The pins are removed at 4 weeks, and a range-of-motion exercise program is started at that time or shortly thereafter. This program should be taught to the parents and the patient and should concentrate on active range of motion only. (Passive range-of-motion exercises in the child cause the child to withdraw or guard against any motion at all.) The parents should be warned of the possibility of growth arrest with subsequent angular deformity. The parents also should be warned, according to O'Brien, of the possibility of avascular necrosis of the phalangeal or metacarpal heads after fractures in this area, which are similar to that in Freiberg's disease of the metatarsal heads.

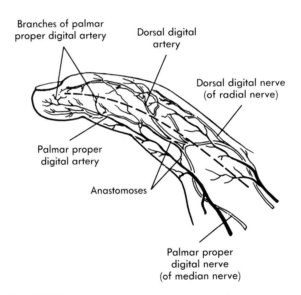

Fig. 16-208　Midlateral skin incision in finger extending from metacarpophalangeal joint to lateral edge of nail. To avoid flexor skin creases, it is placed slightly posterolateral. (Modified from McVay CB: Anson and McVay surgical anatomy, ed 6, Philadelphia, 1983, WB Saunders Co.)

Dislocations

Dislocations of the joints of the hand in children are even rarer than in adults, primarily because of the weakness of the physes that separate instead of the adjacent joint's becoming dislocated. Because of ligamentous laxity and the malleability of cartilage, however, dislocations can occur. Most dislocations occur in the proximal interphalangeal joint where the middle phalanx dislocates dorsally or laterally on the proximal phalanx. Dislocations of the distal interphalangeal joint are extremely rare. Fracture-dislocations also are uncommon, and open reduction and internal fixation are not indicated unless the dislocation is irreducible because of interposition of soft tissue structures such as the volar plate. Dislocations of the metacarpophalangeal joint usually occur at the thumb, usually are dorsal, and generally can be reduced by closed methods. If the dislocation is complex and complete, as described by Farabeuf, McLaughlin, and Green and Terry, with the volar plate interposed and the metacarpal encircled by the heads of the flexor pollicis brevis muscle, then open reduction usually is necessary (Fig. 16-209). The thumb metacarpal head also can be caught in a tight sling formed by the flexor pollicis brevis and adductor pollicis muscles, with the flexor pollicis longus muscle displaced ulnarward; this also requires open reduction.

O'Brien described a gamekeeper's thumb in children that results in ulnar instability of the thumb metacarpal either from rupture of the ulnar collateral ligament or a Salter-Harris type I or III epiphyseal fracture of the proximal phalanx. He recommends open reduction and internal fixation for the type III epiphyseal fracture (Fig. 16-210). Repair of ruptures of the ulnar collateral ligament of the thumb is as in adults.

Dislocation of the second metacarpophalangeal joint is common. Kaplan described the mechanism of this injury and noted that the metacarpal head is buttonholed through the palmar fascia with the flexor tendon on its ulnar side and the lumbrical muscles on the volar side. The volar plate is torn and turned dorsally to become caught between the metacarpal head and the base of the proximal phalanx. Closed reduction of this dislocation almost always fails, and open reduction usually is indicated.

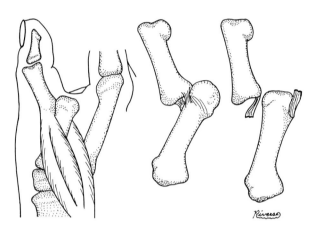

Fig. 16-209 Dislocation of metacarpophalangeal joint of thumb. (Redrawn from Wood VE: Orthop Clin North Am 7:527, 1976.)

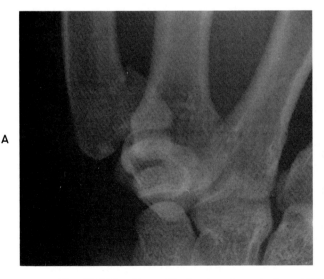
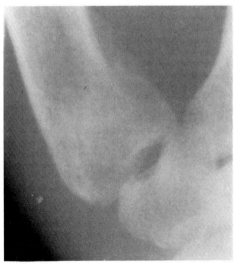

Fig. 16-210 Bennett's fracture in maturing child whose epiphyseal plate is essentially closed. **A,** Soon after injury. **B,** Early healing after treatment in abduction thumb spica cast.

Reduction of Thumb and Index Metacarpophalangeal Joint Dislocations
Open reduction of dorsal dislocation of metacarpophalangeal joint of thumb

▲ *Technique (Milford).* Make a transverse curved incision over the radial and volar aspects of the joint, exposing the articular surfaces of the phalanx and metacarpal. The base of the phalanx lies on the dorsal aspect of the head and neck of the metacarpal, and the head protrudes through the anterior capsule (Fig. 16-211). Disengage the flexor pollicis brevis muscle, releasing the head of the metacarpal. Flex the thumb and push the head through the rent in the capsule to complete the reduction.

▲ *Postoperative management.* The thumb is held in moderate flexion by a plaster splint. After 3 weeks the splint is removed and active motion is begun.

Open reduction of dislocation of metacarpophalangeal joints of fingers

▲ *Technique (Kaplan).* Begin the incision in the thenar crease of the hand at the radial base of the index finger and continue into the proximal crease of the hand (Fig. 16-212). To reduce the dislocation, divide all the constricting bands. Make the first incision to free the constriction of the cartilaginous plate (Fig. 16-213) parallel and radial to the vaginal ligament extending from the free edge of the torn ligament to the junction of the periosteum with the proximal phalanx. Be sure the incision penetrates the entire thickness of the plate. Division of the plate alone is not sufficient, however. Completely divide the transverse fibers of the taut natatory ligament, and make another longitudinal incision through the transverse fibers of the superficial transverse metacarpal ligament extending to the ulnar side of the first lumbrical muscle to release the constriction below the metacarpal head.

This triple incision frees the base of the proximal phalanx, which then returns to its normal place over the metacarpal head. This, in turn, permits the immediate replacement of the second metacarpal head in line with the other metacarpal heads, following which the flexor tendons, the vaginal ligament, and the nerves and vessels are restored to their normal positions. Close the wound in the usual manner, and immobilize the finger in functional position for about 1 week.

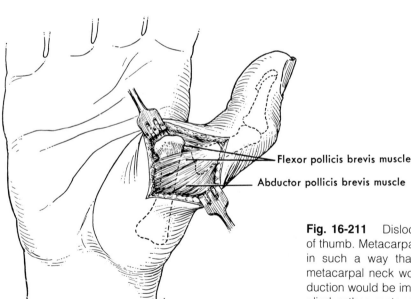

Flexor pollicis brevis muscle
Abductor pollicis brevis muscle

Fig. 16-211   Dislocation of metacarpophalangeal joint of thumb. Metacarpal head has penetrated joint capsule in such a way that were traction applied to thumb, metacarpal neck would be caught by capsule, and reduction would be impossible. Traction should not be applied; rather, metacarpal should be adducted and dislocated joint should be hyperextended while proximal end of proximal phalanx is pushed against and then over metacarpal head.

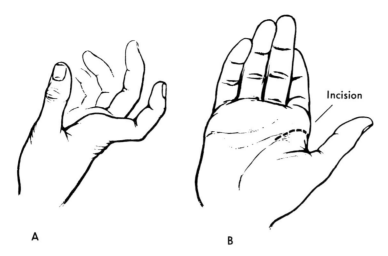

Fig. 16-212 Dislocation of second metacarpophalangeal joint. **A,** Deformity as seen from lateral side. **B,** Skin incision, *broken line*, used in open reduction. (From Kaplan EB: J Bone Joint Surg 39A:1081, 1957.)

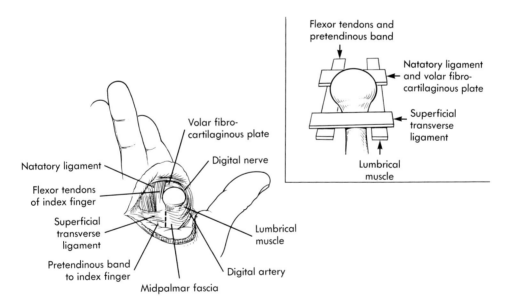

Fig. 16-213 Kaplan open reduction of dislocation of second metacarpophalangeal joint (see text). *Inset,* Diagram of four structures that surround and constrict metacarpal head. (Modified from Kaplan EB: J Bone Joint Surg 39A:1081, 1957.)

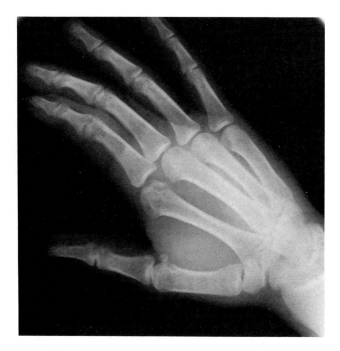

Fig. 16-214 Fracture of metacarpal head with irreducible dislocation. This fracture-dislocation of metacarpophalangeal joint of index finger is ideal for dorsal approach described by Becton et al since direct access to fracture area is provided.

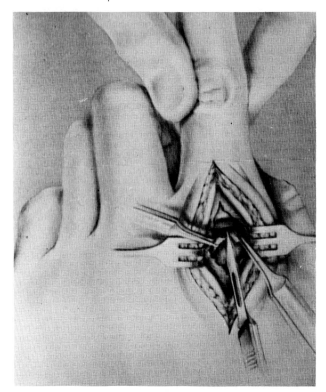

Fig. 16-215 Dorsal surgical approach to dislocated metacarpophalangeal joint. Volar plate that is caught over dorsal area of metacarpal head is incised longitudinally, and reduction is easily achieved. (From Becton JL et al: J Bone Joint Surg 57A:698, 1975.)

▶ *Technique (Becton et al).* Becton et al believe the dorsal approach has several advantages over the volar approach. The dorsal approach provides full exposure of the fibrocartilaginous volar ligament, which is the structure blocking reduction. The digital nerves are not as likely to be cut, and should there be an occult fracture of the metacarpal head, this can be reduced and fixed more easily (Fig. 16-214).

Over the metacarpophalangeal joint, make a 4 cm midline incision cutting the underlying extensor tendon and joint capsule as well. The fibrocartilaginous ligament may be difficult to identify because it is the same color as the articular cartilage, and its torn margin may not be visible. Make a small incision to ensure the tissue is in fact the fibrocartilaginous ligament; then complete the longitudinal incision (Fig. 16-215). Flex the wrist volarward to release the tension on the flexor tendons; then place traction on the finger and flex the metacarpophalangeal joint, reducing the dislocation. Observe to see if there is any free cartilage missing from the metacarpal head. This may be lodged in the joint. Suture the extensor tendon and skin, and splint the finger for 3 weeks.

REFERENCES

Epiphyseal injuries

Aitken AT: Fractures of the epiphysis, Clin Orthop 41:19, 1965.

Aitken AT and Magill HK: Fractures involving the distal femoral epiphyseal cartilage, J Bone Joint Surg 34A:96, 1952.

Birch JG, Herring JA, and Wenger DR: Surgical anatomy of selected physes, J Pediatr Orthop 4:224, 1984.

Blount WP: Fractures in children, Baltimore, 1955, Williams & Wilkins.

Blount WP: Unequal leg lengths. In The American Academy of Orthopaedic Surgeons: Instructional course lectures, vol 17, St Louis, 1960, The CV Mosby Co.

Boyd HB: Personal communication, 1975.

Bright RW: Operative correction of partial epiphyseal plate closure by osseous ridge resection and silicone rubber implant, J Bone Joint Surg 56A:655, 1974.

Bright RW: Partial growth arrest: identification, classification, and results of treatment, Orthop Trans 6:65, 1982 (abstract).

Canale ST, Russell RA, and Holcomb RL: Percutaneous epiphyseodesis: experimental study and preliminary clinical results, J Pediatr Orthop 6:150, 1986.

Carlson WO and Wenger DR: A mapping method to prepare for surgical excision of a partial physeal arrest, J Pediatr Orthop 4:232, 1984.

Chadwick CJ and Bentley G: The classification and prognosis of epiphyseal injuries, Injury 18:157, 1987.

Currey JD and Butler G: Mechanical properties of bone tissues in children, J Bone Joint Surg 57A:810, 1975.

Green WT and Anderson M: Experience with epiphyseal arrest in correcting discrepancies in length of the lower extremities in infantile paralysis, J Bone Joint Surg 29:659, 1947.

Green WT and Anderson M: Skeletal age in the control of limb growth. In The American Academy of Orthopaedic Surgeons: Instructional course lectures, vol 17, St Louis, 1960, The CV Mosby Co.

Gustilio RB et al: An analysis of 511 open fractures at Hennepin County General Hospital, J Bone Joint Surg 50A:830, 1968.

Holland CT: A radiologic note on injuries to the distal epiphyses of the radius and ulna, Proc R Soc Med 22:695, 1929.

Kling TF Jr, Bright RW, and Hensinger RN: Distal tibial physeal fractures in children that may require open reduction, J Bone Joint Surg 66A:647, 1984.

Langenskiöld A: An operation for partial closure of the epiphyseal plate in children and its experimental basis, J Bone Joint Surg 57B:325, 1975.

Langenskiöld A: Surgical treatment of partial closure of the growth plate, J Pediatr Orthop 1:3, 1981.

Morscher E and Jani L: Correction osteotomies in posttraumatic disturbances of growth-realignment: osteotomies after lesions of the growth cartilage. In Chapchal G, editor: Fractures in children, New York, 1981, Thieme-Stratton.

Moseley CF: A straight line graph for leg length discrepancies, J Bone Joint Surg 59A:171, 1977.

Moseley CF: A straight line graph for leg length discrepancies, Clin Orthop 136:33, 1978.

Ogden JA: Skeletal injury in the child, Philadelphia, 1982, Lea & Febiger.

Peterson HA: Partial growth arrest and its treatment, J Pediatr Orthop 4:246, 1984.

Peterson HA and Burkhart SS: Compression injury of the epiphyseal growth plate: fact or fiction? J Pediatr Orthop 1:377, 1981.

Phemister D: Operative assessment of longitudinal growth of bones in the treatment of deformities, J Bone Joint Surg 15:1, 1933.

Poland J: Traumatic separation of the epiphyses, London, 1898, Smith, Elder & Co.

Poland J: Traumatic separation of the epiphysis in general, Clin Orthop 41:7, 1965.

Rang M: The growth plate and its disorders, Baltimore, 1969, Williams & Wilkins.

Salter RB and Harris WR: Injuries involving the epiphyseal plate, J Bone Joint Surg 45A:587, 1963.

Tredwell SJ, Peteghem V, and Clough M: Pattern of forearm fractures in children, J Pediatr Orthop 4:604, 1984.

Wagner H: Surgical lengthening or shortening of the femur and tibia: techniques and indications. In Hungerford BS: Progress in orthopaedic surgery, Berlin, 1977, Springer-Verlag.

Weber BG: Fracture healing in the growing bone and in the mature skeleton. In Weber BG, Brunner CL, and Freuler F, editors: Treatment of fractures in children and adolescents, New York, 1980, Springer-Verlag.

Weber BG, Brunner C, and Freuler F, editors: Treatment of fractures in children and adolescents, New York, 1980, Springer-Verlag.

Open fractures

Fee NF, Dobranski A, and Bisla RS: Gas gangrene complicating open forearm fractures, J Bone Joint Surg 59A:135, 1977.

Reff RB: The use of external fixation devices in the management of severe lower-extremity trauma and pelvic injuries in children, Clin Orthop 188:21, 1984.

Tolo VT: External skeletal fixation in children's fractures, J Pediatr Orthop 3:435, 1983.

Foot fractures

Aitken AP and Poulson D: Dislocation of the tarsometatarsal joint, J Bone Joint Surg 45A:246, 1963.

Alexander AH and Lichtman DM: Surgical treatment of transchondral talar dome fractures (osteochondritis dissecans): long term followup, J Bone Joint Surg 62A:646, 1980.

Anderson LD: Injuries of the forefoot, Clin Orthop 122:18, 1977.

Berndt AL and Harty M: Transchondral fractures (osteochondritis dissecans) of the talus, J Bone Joint Surg 41A:988, 1959.

Bonnin JG: Dislocations and fracture—dislocations of the talus, Br J Surg 28:88, 1940.

Boyd HB and Knight RA: Fractures of the astragalus, South Med J 35:160, 1942.

Braddock GTF: Experimental epiphysial injury and Freiberg's disease, J Bone Joint Surg 41B:154, 1959.

Brand RA and Black H: *Pseudomonas* osteomyelitis following puncture wounds in children, J Bone Joint Surg 56A:1637, 1974.

Canale ST and Beaty JH: Injuries of the talus. In Hamilton WC, editor: Traumatic disorders of the ankle, New York, 1983, Springer-Verlag.

Canale ST and Belding RH: Osteochondral lesions of the talus, J Bone Joint Surg 62A:97, 1980.

Canale ST and Kelly FB Jr: Fractures of the neck of the talus: long term evaluation of 71 cases, J Bone Joint Surg 60A:143, 1978.

Cehner J: Fractures of the tarsal bones, metatarsals, and toes. In Weber BG, Brunner C, and Freuler F, editors: Treatment of fractures in children and adolescents, New York, 1980, Springer-Verlag.

Chapman HG and Galway HR: Os calcis fractures in childhood, J Bone Joint Surg 59B:510, 1977.

Childress HM: March foot in a seven year old child, J Bone Joint Surg 28:877, 1946.

Devas MB: Stress fractures in children, J Bone Joint Surg 45B:528, 1963.

Essex-Lopresti P: The mechanism, reduction technique, and results in fractures of the os calcis, Br J Surg 39:395, 1952.

Fitzgerald RH and Cowen JDE: Puncture wounds of the foot, Orthop Clin North Am 6:965, 1975.

Freiberg A: Infarction of the second metatarsal bone, Surg Gynecol Obstet 19:191, 1914.

Furnas DW: The cross-groin flap for coverage of foot and ankle defects in children, Plast Reconstr Surg 57:246, 1976.

Giannestras N and Sammarco GJ: Fractures and dislocations in the foot. In Rockwood C and Green D, editors: Fractures, Philadelphia, 1975, JB Lippincott Co.

Graham WP III et al: Injuries from rotary power lawnmowers, Am Fam Physician 13:75, 1976.

Gross RH: Fractures and dislocations of the foot. In Rockwood CA Jr, Wilkins KE, and King RE, editors: Fractures in children, Philadelphia, 1984, JB Lippincott Co.

Haliburton RA et al: The extra-osseous and intra-osseous blood supply of the talus, J Bone Joint Surg 40A:1115, 1958.

Harper MC and Ralston M: Isobutyl 2-cyanoacrylate as an osseous adhesive in the repair of osteochondral fractures, J Biomed Mater Res 17:167, 1983.

Hawkins LG: Fractures of the neck of the talus, J Bone Joint Surg 52A:991, 1970.

Johnson FG: Pediatric Lisfranc injury: bunk bed fracture, AJR 137:1041, 1981.

Jones R: Fracture of the base of the fifth metatarsal by indirect violence, Ann Surg 35:697, 1902.

Kavanaugh JH, Brower TD, and Mann RV: The Jones fracture revisited, J Bone Joint Surg 60A:776, 1978.

Karp MG: Köhler's disease of the tarsal scaphoid, J Bone Joint Surg 19:84, 1937.

King RE: Personal communication, 1986.

Lang AG and Peterson HA: Osteomyelitis following puncture wounds of the foot in children, J Trauma 16:993, 1976.

Letts RM and Gibeault D: Fractures of the neck of the talus in children, Foot Ankle 1:74, 1980.

Lyritis G: Developmental disorders of the proximal epiphysis of the hallux, Stereoradiology 10:250, 1983.

Marti R: Fractures of the talus and calcaneus. In Weber BG, Brunner C, and Freuler F, editors: Treatment of fracture in children and adolescents, New York, 1980, Springer-Verlag.

Matteri RE and Frymoyer JW: Fracture of the calcaneus in young children: report of three cases, J Bone Joint Surg 55A:1091, 1973.

McCullough CJ and Venugopal V: Osteochondritis dissecans of the talus: the natural history, Clin Orthop 144:264, 1979.

McKeever FM: Fractures of the neck of the astragalus, Arch Surg 46:720, 1943.

Mulfinger GL and Trueta J: The blood supply of the talus, J Bone Joint Surg 52B:160, 1970.

Parisien JS: Arthroscopic treatment of osteochondral lesions of the talus, Am J Sports Med 14:211, 1986.

Rowe CR et al: Fractures of the os calcis: a long-term follow-up study of 146 patients, JAMA 184:920, 1963.

Schmidt TL and Weiner DS: Calcaneal fractures in children: an evaluation of the nature of the injury in 56 children, Clin Orthop 171:150, 1982.

Smith GR et al: Subtle transchondral fractures of the talar dome: radiological perspective, Radiology 124:667, 1977.

Spak I: Fractures of the talus in children, Acta Chir Scand 107:553, 1954.

Stephens NA: Fracture dislocations of the talus in childhood: a report of two cases, Br J Surg 43:600, 1956.

Thomas HM: Calcaneal fracture in childhood, Br J Surg 56:664, 1969.

Trillat A et al: Tarsometatarsal fracture-dislocations, Rev Chir Orthop (suppl) 62:685, 1976.

Trott A: Fractures of the foot in children, Orthop Clin North Am 7:677, 1976.

Wells D and Oloff-Solomon J: Radiographic evaluation of transchondral dome fractures of the talus, J Foot Surg 26:186, 1987.

Wicks MH, Harbison JS, and Paterson DC: Tendon injuries about the foot and ankle in children, Aust N Z J Surg 50:158, 1980.

Wiley JJ: The mechanism of tarsometatarsal joint injuries, J Bone Joint Surg 53B:475, 1971.

Wiley JJ: Tarsometatarsal joint injuries in children, J Pediatr Orthop 1:255, 1981.

Yancey HA Jr: Lacerations of the plantar aspect of the foot, Clin Orthop 122:46, 1977.

Distal tibial and fibular epiphyseal fractures

Aitken AP: Fractures of the epiphyses, Clin Orthop 41:19, 1965.

Beaty JH and Linton RC: Medial malleolar fracture in a child: a case report, J Bone Joint Surg 70A:1254, 1988.

Bright RW: Operative correction of partial epiphyseal plate closure by osseous-bridge resection and silicone-rubber implant, J Bone Joint Surg 56A:655, 1974.

Carothers CO and Crenshaw AH: Clinical significance of a classification of epiphyseal injuries at the ankle, Am J Surg 89:879, 1955.

Cass JR and Peterson HA: Salter-Harris type IV injuries of the distal tibial epiphyseal growth plate, with emphasis on those involving the medial malleolus, J Bone Joint Surg 65A:1059, 1983.

Chadwick CJ: Spontaneous resolution of varus deformity of the ankle following adduction injury of the distal tibial epiphysis, J Bone Joint Surg 64A:774, 1982.

Chuinard EG and Peterson RE: Distraction-compression bone-graft arthrodesis of the ankle: a method especially applicable in children, J Bone Joint Surg 45A:481, 1963.

Cooperman DR: Spiegel PG, and Laros GS: Tibial fractures involving the ankle in children: the so-called triplane epiphyseal fracture, J Bone Joint Surg 60A:1040, 1978.

Crenshaw AH: Injuries of the distal tibial epiphysis, Clin Orthop 41:98, 1965.

Dale GG and Harris WR: Prognosis of epiphysial separation, J Bone Joint Surg 40B:116, 1958.

Denton JR and Fischer SJ: The medial triplane fracture: report of an unusual injury, J Trauma 21:991, 1981.

Dias LS and Giegerich CR: Fractures of the distal tibial epiphysis in adolescence, J Bone Joint Surg 65A:438, 1983.

Dias LS and Tachdjian MO: Physeal injuries of the ankle in children, Clin Orthop 136:230, 1978.

Friedenberg ZB: Reaction of the epiphysis to partial surgical resection, J Bone Joint Surg 39A:332, 1957.

Friedenberg ZB and Brashear R: Bone growth following partial resection of the epiphyseal cartilage, Am J Surg 91:362, 1956.

Grace DL: Irreducible fracture separations of the distal tibial epiphysis, J Bone Joint Surg 65B:160, 1983.

Hynes D and O'Brien T: Growth disturbance lines after injury of the distal tibial physis: their significance in prognosis, J Bone Joint Surg 70B:231, 1988.

Kärrholm J, Hansson LI, and Laurin S: Computed tomography of intraarticular supination-eversion fractures of the ankle in adolescents, J Pediatr Orthop 1:181, 1981.

Kärrholm J, Hansson LI, and Laurin S: Supination-eversion injuries of the ankle in children: a retrospective study of roentgenographic classification and treatment, J Pediatr Orthop 2:147, 1982.

Kärrholm LI, Hansson LI, and Laurin S: Pronation injuries of the ankle in children, Acta Orthop Scand 54:1, 1983.

Kärrholm J, Hansson LI, and Selvik G: Roentgen stereophotogrammetic analysis of growth pattern after supination-adduction ankle injuries in children, J Pediatr Orthop 2:271, 1982.

Kärrholm J, Hansson LI, and Selvik G: Roentgen stereophotogrammetric analysis of growth patterns after supination-eversion ankle injuries in children, J Pediatr Orthop 2:25, 1982.

Kleiger B and Barton J: Epiphyseal ankle fractures, Bull Hosp Jt Dis 25:240, 1964.

Kleiger B and Mankin HJ: Fracture of the lateral portion of the distal tibial epiphysis, J Bone Joint Surg 46A:25, 1964.

Kling TF, Bright RW, and Hensinger RM: Distal tibial physeal fractures in children that may require open reduction, J Bone Joint Surg 66A:647, 1984.

Langenskiöld A: Traumatic premature closure of the distal tibial epiphyseal plate, Acta Orthop Scand 38:520, 1967.

Langenskiöld A: An operation for partial closure of an epiphysial plate in children, and its experimental basis, J Bone Joint Surg 57B:325, 1975.

Letts RM: Hidden adolescent ankle fracture, J Pediatr Orthop 2:161, 1982.

Marmor L: An unusual fracture of the tibial epiphysis, Clin Orthop 73:132, 1970.

Mubarak SJ and Haegens AR: Diagnosis and management of compartment syndromes. In Moore JM, editor: AAOS Symposium on trauma to the leg and its sequelae, St Louis, 1981, The CV Mosby Co.

Peiro A et al: Triplane distal tibial epiphyseal fractures, Clin Orthop 160:196, 1981.

Peterson HA: Operative correction of post-fracture arrest of the epiphyseal plate: case report with a ten-year follow-up, J Bone Joint Surg 62A:1018, 1980.

Rang M: Children's fractures, ed 2, Philadelphia, 1983, JB Lipincott Co.

Roffman M, Moshel M, and Mendes DG: Bicycle spoke fracture, Clin Orthop 144:230, 1979.

Salter RB and Harris WR: Injuries involving the epiphyseal plate, J Bone Joint Surg 45A:587, 1963.

Shannak AO: Tibial fractures in children: follow-up study, J Pediatr Orthop 8:306, 1988.

Spiegel PG, Cooperman DR, and Laros GS: Epiphyseal fractures of the distal ends of the tibia and fibula: a retrospective study of 237 cases in children, J Bone Joint Surg 60A:1046, 1978.

Tillaux P: Traité l'anatomie topographique avec applications à la chirurgie, Paris, 1878, Asselin et Hozeau.

Weber BG and Sussenbach F: Malleolar fractures. In Weber BG et al, editors: Treatment of fractures in children and adolescents, Berlin, 1980, Springer-Verlag.

Wiley JJ: Tarsometatarsal joint injuries in children, J Pediatr Orthop 1:255, 1981.

Proximal tibial metaphyseal fractures

Aadalen R: Proximal tibial metaphyseal fractures in children, Minn Med, p 785, Nov 1979.

Bahnson DH and Lovell WW: Genu valgum following fractures of the proximal tibial metaphysis in children, Orthop Trans 4:306, 1980.

Balthazar DA and Pappas AM: Acquired valgus deformity of the tibia in children, J Pediatr Orthop 4:538, 1984.

Berkebile RD: Stress fracture of the tibia in children, Am J Roentgenol 91:588, 1964.

Bowen JR et al: Partial epiphysiodesis at the knee to correct angular deformity, Clin Orthop 198:184, 1985.

Coates R: Knock-knee deformity following upper tibial "greenstick" fractures, J Bone Joint Surg 59B:516, 1977.

Cozen L: Fracture of the proximal portion of the tibia in children followed by valgus deformity, Surg Gynecol Obstet 97:183, 1953.

Devas MB: Stress fractures in children, J Bone Joint Surg 45B:528, 1963.

Dunbar JS et al: Obscure tibial fracture of infants: the toddler's fracture, J Can Assoc Radiol 25:136, 1964.

Engh CA, Robinson RA, and Milgram J: Stress fractures in children, J Trauma 10:532, 1970.

Felman AH: Bicycle spoke fractures, J Pediatr 82:302, 1973.

Green NE: Tibial valga caused by asymmetrical overgrowth following a nondisplaced fracture of the proximal tibial metaphysis, J Pediatr Orthop 3:235, 1983.

Greiff J and Bergman F: Growth disturbance following fractures of the tibia in children, Acta Orthop Scand 51:315, 1980.

Haas LM and Staple TW: Arterial injuries associated with fractures of the proximal tibia following blunt trauma, South Med J 62:1439, 1969.

Hansen BA, Greiff J, and Bergmann F: Fractures of the tibia in children, Acta Orthop Scand 47:448, 1976.

Herring JA and Moseley C: Posttraumatic valgus deformity of the tibia, J Pediatr Orthop 1:435, 1981.

Houghton GR and Rooker GD: The role of the periosteum in the growth of long bones: an experimental study in the rabbit, J Bone Joint Surg 61B:218, 1979.

Izant RJ, Rothman BF, and Frankel V: Bicycle spoke injuries of the foot and ankle in children: an underestimated "minor" injury, J Pediatr Surg 4:654, 1969.

Jackson DW and Cozen L: Genu valgum as a complication of proximal tibial metaphyseal fractures in children, J Bone Joint Surg 53A:1571, 1971.

Jordan SE, Alonso JE, and Cook FF: The etiology of valgus angulation after metaphyseal fractures of the tibia in children, J Pediatr Orthop 7:450, 1987.

Karlström G, Lönnerholm T, and Olerud S: Cavus deformity of the foot after fracture of the tibial shaft, J Bone Joint Surg 57A:893, 1975.

Kelly RP and Whitesides TE Jr: Transfibular route for fasciotomy of the leg, J Bone Joint Surg 49A:1022, 1967.

Leach RE, Hammond G, and Stryker WS: Anterior tibial compartment syndrome, J Bone Joint Surg 49A:451, 1967.

Matin P: The appearance of bone scans following fractures, including immediate and long-term studies, J Nucl Med 20:1227, 1979.

Morton KS and Starr DE: Closure of the anterior portion of the upper tibial epiphysis as a complication of tibial-shaft fracture, J Bone Joint Surg 46A:570, 1964.

Ogden JA: Skeletal injury in the child, ed 2, Philadelphia, 1990, WB Saunders Co.

Parsch K, Manner G, and Dippe K: Genu valgum nach proximalen tibia—fraktur beim kind, Arch Orthop Unfallchir 90:289, 1977.

Pollen AG: Fractures and dislocations in children, Baltimore, 1973, The Williams & Wilkins Co.

Rang M: Children's fractures, ed 2, Philadelphia, 1983, JB Lippincott Co.

Reynolds DA: Growth changes in fractures of the long bones, J Bone Joint Surg 63B:83, 1981.

Robert M et al: Fractures of the proximal tibial metaphysis in children: review of a series of 25 cases, J Pediatr Orthop 7:444, 1987.

Salter RB and Best T: The pathogenesis and prevention of valgus deformity following fractures of the proximal metaphyseal region of the tibia in children, J Bone Joint Surg 55A:1324, 1973.

Skak SV: Valgus deformity following proximal tibial metaphyseal fracture in children, Acta Orthop Scand 53:141, 1982.

Skak SV, Jensen TT, and Poulsen TD: Fracture of the proximal metaphysis of the tibia in children, Injury 18:149, 1987.

Steel HH, Sandrow RE, and Sullivan PD: Complications of tibial osteotomy in children for genu varum or valgum, J Bone Joint Surg 53A:1629, 1971.

Taylor SL: Tibial overgrowth: a cause of genu valgum, J Bone Joint Surg 45A:659, 1963.

Visser JD and Veldhuizen AG: Valgus deformity after fracture of the proximal tibial metaphysis in childhood, Acta Orthop Scand 53:663, 1982.

Weber BG: Fibrous interposition causing valgus deformity after fracture of the upper tibial metaphysis in children, J Bone Joint Surg 59B:290, 1977.

Weber BG, Brunner C, and Freuler F, editors: Treatment of fractures in children and adolescents, Berlin, 1980, Springer-Verlag.

Whitesides TE Jr et al: Tissue pressure measurements as a determinant for the need of fasciotomy, Clin Orthop 113:43, 1975.

Willhoite DR and Moll JH: Early recognition and treatment of impending Volkmann's ischemia in the lower extremity, Arch Surg 100:11, 1970.

Zionts LE et al: Posttraumatic tibia valga: a case demonstrating asymmetric activity at the proximal growth plate on technetium bone scan, J Pediatr Orthop 7:458, 1987.

Proximal tibial and fibular epiphyseal fractures

Aitken AP: Fractures of the proximal tibial epiphyseal cartilage, Clin Orthop 41:92, 1965.

Aitken AP and Ingersoll RE: Fractures of the proximal tibial epiphyseal cartilage, J Bone Joint Surg 38B:787, 1956.

Blount WP: Fractures in children, Baltimore, 1955, The Williams & Wilkins Co.

Burkhart SS and Peterson HA: Fractures of the proximal tibial epiphysis, J Bone Joint Surg 61A:996, 1979.

Cozen L: Knock knee deformity after fracture of the proximal tibia in children, Orthopaedics 1:230, 1959.

Cozen L et al: Genu valgum after proximal tibial fractures in children, AJR 136:915, 1981.

Dal Monte A, Manes E, and Cammarota V: Post-traumatic genu valgum in children, Ital J Orthop Traumatol 9:5, 1983.

Gibson A: Separation of the upper epiphysis of the tibia, Ann Surg 77:485, 1923.

Gill JG, Chakrabarti HF, and Becker SJ: Fracture of the proximal tibial epiphysis, Injury 14:324, 1983.

Goss CM, editor: Gray's anatomy of the human body, ed 29, Philadelphia, 1973, Lea & Febiger.

Grant JCB: An atlas of anatomy, Baltimore, 1947, The Williams & Wilkins Co.

Harries TJ, Lichtman DM, and Lonon WD: Irreducible Salter-Harris II fracture of the proximal tibia, J Pediatr Orthop 3:92, 1983.

Herring JA and Moseley C: Posttraumatic valgus deformity of the tibia, J Pediatr Orthop 1:435, 1981.

Ippolito E and Pentimalli G: Post-traumatic valgus deformity of the knee in proximal tibial metaphyseal fractures in children, Ital J Orthop Traumatol 10:103, 1984.

Key JA and Conwell HE: The management of fractures, dislocations and sprains, ed 2, 1937, The CV Mosby Co.

McGuigan JA, O'Reilly MJG, and Nixon JR: Popliteal artery thrombosis resulting from disruption of the upper tibial epiphysis, Injury, 16:49, 1984.

Nicholson JT: Epiphyseal fractures about the knee. In The American Academy of Orthopaedic Surgeons: Instructional course lectures, vol 18, St. Louis, 1967, The CV Mosby Co.

Pappas AM, Anas P, and Toczylowski HM Jr: Asymmetrical arrest of the proximal tibial physis and genu recurvatum deformity, J Bone Joint Surg 66A:575, 1984.

Rang M: Children's fractures, ed 2, Philadelphia, 1983, JB Lippincott Co.

Resnick D and Niwayama G: Diagnosis of bone and joint disorders: with emphasis on articular abnormalities, Philadelphia, 1981, WB Saunders Co.

Salter RB and Harris WR: Injuries involving the epiphyseal plate, J Bone Joint Surg 45A:587, 1963.

Shelton WR and Canale ST: Fractures of the tibia through the proximal tibial epiphyseal cartilage, J Bone Joint Surg 61A:167, 1979.

Skak SB: Valgus deformity following proximal tibial metaphyseal fracture in children, Acta Orthop Scand 53:141, 1982.

Thompson GH and Gesler JW: Proximal tibial epiphyseal fracture in an infant, J Pediatr Orthop 4:185, 1984.

Visser JD and Veldhuizen AG: Valgus deformity after fracture of the proximal tibial metaphysis in childhood, Acta Orthop Scand 53:663, 1982.

Weber BG, Brunner Ch, and Freuler R, editors: Treatment of fractures in children and adolescents, Berlin, 1980, Springer-Verlag.

Welch PH and Wynne GF Jr: Proximal tibial epiphyseal fracture separation: case report, J Bone Joint Surg 45A:782, 1963.

Knee fractures and dislocations

Ahstrom JP: Osteochondral fracture in the knee joint associated with hypermobility and dislocation of the patella: report of eighteen cases, J Bone Joint Surg 47A:1491, 1965.

Aichroth PM: Osteochondral fractures and their relationship to osteochondritis dissecans of the knee, J Bone Joint Surg 53B:448, 1971.

Andersen PT: Congenital deformities of the knee joint in dislocation of the patella and achondroplasia, Acta Orthop Scand 28:27, 1958.

Bassett FH III: Acute dislocation of the patella, osteochondral fractures, and injuries to the extensor mechanism of the knee. In The American Academy of Orthopaedic Surgeons: Instructional course lectures, vol 25, St Louis, 1976, The CV Mosby Co.

Baxter MP and Wiley JJ: Fractures of the tibial spine in children: an evaluation of knee stability, J Bone Joint Surg 70B:228, 1988.

Belman DAJ and Neviaser RJ: Transverse fracture of the patella in a child, J Trauma 13:917, 1973.

Bensahel H and Sprung R: Les fractures de la rotule de l'enfant, J Chir 99:45, 1970.

Bernhang AM and Levine SA: Familial absence of the patella, J Bone Joint Surg 53A:1088, 1973.

Blount WP: Fractures of the patella. In Blount WP: Fractures in children, Baltimore, 1955, The Williams & Wilkins Co.

Bradley GW, Shives TC, and Samuelsom KM: Ligament injuries in the knees of children, J Bone Joint Surg 61A:588, 1979.

Cahuzac M et al: Les fractures de fatigue de la rotule chez l'infirme moteur d'origine cerebrale, Rev Chir Orthop 65:87, 1979.

Canale ST, Aust G, and Howard BC: Fractures of the patella in children, Unpublished manuscript, 1986.

Canale ST and Shelton WR: Fractures of the tibia through the proximal tibial epiphyseal cartilage, J Bone Joint Surg 61A:167, 1979.

Christie MJ and Dvonch VM: Tibial tuberosity avulsion fracture in adolescents, J Pediatr Orthop 1:391, 1981.

Clanton TO et al: Knee ligament injuries in children, J Bone Joint Surg 61A:1195, 1979.

Clawson K: Editorial comment on JH Levi and CR Coleman: fracture of the tibial tubercle, Am J Sports Med 4:262, 1976.

Cofield RH and Bryan RS: Acute dislocation of the patella: results of conservative treatment, J Trauma 17:526, 1977.

Coleman HM: Recurrent osteochondral fracture of the patella, J Bone Joint Surg 30B:153, 1948.

Crawford AH: Fractures about the knee in children, Orthop Clin North Am 7:639, 1976.

Crothers OD and Johnson JTH: Isolated acute dislocation of the proximal tibiofibular joint, J Bone Joint Surg 55A:181, 1973.

DeHaven KE and Collins HR: Diagnosis of internal derangement of the knee, J Bone Joint Surg 57A:802, 1975.

Delivannis SN: Avulsion of the tibial tuberosity: report of two cases, Injury 4:341, 1973.

Duncan JG and Souter WA: Hereditary onycho-osteodysplasia: the nail-patella syndrome, J Bone Joint Surg 45B:242, 1963.

Echeverria TS and Bersani FA: Acute fractures simulating a symptomatic bipartate patella, Am J Sports Med 8:48, 1980.

Ehrlich MG and Strain RE Jr: Epiphyseal injuries about the knee, Orthop Clin North Am 10:91, 1979.

Eilert R: Arthroscopy of the knee joint in children, Orthop Rev 5:61, 1976.

Fowler PJ: Meniscal lesions in the adolescent: the role of arthroscopy in the management of adolescent knee problems. In Kennedy JC, editor: The injured adolescent knee, Baltimore, 1979, The Williams & Wilkins Co.

Fowler PJ: The classification and early diagnosis of knee joint instability, Clin Orthop 147:15, 1980.

Fujikawa K, Iseki F, and Mikura Y: Partial resection of the discoid meniscus in the child's knee, J Bone Joint Surg 63B:391, 1981.

Fyfe IS and Jackson JP: Tibial intercondylar fractures in children: a review of the classification and the treatment of mal-union, Injury 13:165, 1981.

Gartland JJ and Benner JH: Traumatic dislocations in the lower extremity in children, Orthop Clin North Am 7:687, 1976.

George R: Bilateral bipartite patellae, Br J Surg 22:555, 1935.

Green WT Jr: Painful bipartite patellae: a report of three cases, Clin Orthop 110:197, 1975.

Griffin PP: The lower limb. In Lovell WW and Winter RB, editors: Pediatric orthopaedics, Philadelphia, 1978, JB Lippincott Co.

Griswold AS: Fractures of the patella, Clin Orthop 4:44, 1954.

Grönkvist H, Hirsch G, and Johansson L: Fracture of the anterior tibial spine in children, J Pediatr Orthop 4:465, 1984.

Hallopeau P: De certaines fractures de la rotule chez l'enfant, J Med (Paris) 42:927, 1923.

Hand WL, Hand CR, and Dunn AW: Avulsion fractures of the tibial tubercle, J Bone Joint Surg 53A:1579, 1971.

Hayes AG and Nageswar M: The adolescent painful knee: the value of arthroscopy in diagnosis, J Bone Joint Surg 59B:499, 1977.

Heckman JD and Alkire CC: Distal patellar pole fractures: a proposed common mechanism of injury, Am J Sports Med 12:424, 1984.

Helfet AJ: Disorders of the knee, Philadelphia, 1974, JB Lippincott Co.

Houghton GR and Ackroyd CE: Sleeve fractures of the patella in children: a report of three cases, J Bone Joint Surg 61B:165, 1979.

Hungerford DS and Barry M: Biomechanics of the patello-femoral joint, Clin Orthop 144:9, 1979.

Hyndman JC and Brown DC: Major ligamentous injuries of the knee in children, J Bone Joint Surg 61B:245, 1979.

Kaplan EB: Avulsion fracture of proximal tibial epiphysis: case report, Bull Hosp Jt Dis 24:119, 1963.

Kaye JJ and Freiberger RH: Fragmentation of the lower pole of the patella in spastic lower extremities, Radiology 101:97, 1971.

Kennedy JC: The injured adolescent knee, Baltimore, 1979, The Williams & Wilkins Co.

Lee HG: Avulsion fracture of the tibial attachments of the crucial ligaments: treatment by operative reduction, J Bone Joint Surg 19:460, 1937.

Letts M, Vincent N, and Gouw G: The "floating knee" in children, J Bone Joint Surg 68B:442, 1986.

McManus F, Rang M, and Heslin DJ: Acute dislocation of the patella in children: the natural history, Clin Orthop 139:88, 1979.

Medlar RC and Lyne ED: Sinding-Larsen-Johansson disease: its etiology and natural history, J Bone Joint Surg 60A:1113, 1978.

Meyers MH and Harvey JP Jr: Traumatic dislocation of the knee joint: a study of eighteen cases, J Bone Joint Surg 53A:16, 1971.

Meyers MH and McKeever FM: Fracture of the intercondylar eminence of the tibia, J Bone Joint Surg 41A:209, 1959.

Meyers MH and McKeever FM: Follow-up notes: fracture of the intercondylar eminence of the tibia, J Bone Joint Surg 52A:167, 1970.

Morrissy RT et al: Arthroscopy of the knee in children, Clin Orthop 162:103, 1982.

Nathan PA and Cole SC: Discoid meniscus: a clinical and pathologic study, Clin Orthop 64:107, 1969.

Ogden JA: Subluxation and dissociation of the proximal tibiofibular joint, J Bone Joint Surg 56A:145, 1974.

Ogden JA: Subluxation of the proximal tibiofibular joint, Clin Orthop 101:192, 1974.

Ogden JA: Development and growth of the musculoskeletal system. In Albright JA and Brand RA, editors: The scientific basis of orthopaedics, New York, 1979, Appleton-Century-Crofts.

Ogden JA: Skeletal injury in the child, Philadelphia, 1982, Lea & Febiger.

Ogden JA, Hempton RF, and Southwick WO: Development of the tibial tuberosity, Anat Rec 182:431, 1975.

Ogden JA and Southwick WO: Osgood-Schlatter's disease and tibial tuberosity development, Clin Orthop 116:180, 1976.

Ogden JA, Tross RB, and Murphy MJ: Fractures of the tibial tuberosity in adolescents, J Bone Joint Surg 62A:205, 1980.

Osgood RB: Lesions of the tibial tubercle occurring during adolescence, Boston Med Surg J 148:114, 1903.

Peterson L and Stener B: Distal disinsertion of the patellar ligament combined with avulsion fractures at the medial and lateral margins of the patella, Acta Orthop Scand 47:680, 1976.

Pollen AG: Fractures and dislocations in children, Baltimore, 1973, The Williams & Wilkins Co.

Pringle JH: Avulsion of the spine of the tibia, Ann Surg 46:169, 1907.

Rang M: Children's fractures, ed 2, Philadelphia, 1983, JB Lipincott Co.

Roberts JM: Avulsion fractures of the proximal tibial epiphysis in the injured adolescent knee. In Kennedy JC, editor: The injured adolescent knee, Baltimore, 1979, The Williams & Wilkins Co.

Roberts JM: Fractures and dislocations of the knee. In Rockwood CA Jr, Wilkins KE, and King RE, editors: Fractures in children, Philadelphia, 1984, JB Lippincott Co.

Roberts JM and Lovell WW: Fractures of the intercondylar eminence of tibia, J Bone Joint Surg 52A:827, 1970.

Rorabeck CH and Bobechko WP: Acute dislocation of the patella with osteochondral fracture: review of eighteen cases, J Bone Joint Surg 58B:237, 1976.

Rosenthal RK and Levine DB: Fragmentation of the distal pole of the patella in spastic cerebral palsy, J Bone Joint Surg 59A:934, 1977.

Schlatter C: Verletzungen des Schnabelförmigen Fortsatzes der Oberen Tibiaepiphyse, Beitr Klin Chir 38:874, 1903.

Scott JE and Taor WS: The "small patella" syndrome, J Bone Joint Surg 61B:172, 1979.

Sijbrandij S: Instability of the proximal tibiofibular joint, Acta Orthop Scand 49:621, 1978.

Sinding-Larsen MF: A hitherto unknown affection of the patella in children, Acta Radiol 1:171, 1922.

Smillie IS: Injuries of the knee joint, ed 5, Edinburgh, 1978, Churchill-Livingstone.

Tapper EM and Hoover NW: Late results after meniscectomy, J Bone Joint Surg 51A:517, 1969.

Tibone JE and Lombardo SJ: Bilateral fractures of the inferior pole of the patella in a basketball player, Am J Sports Med 9:215, 1981.

Vahvanen V and Aalto K: Meniscectomy in children, Acta Orthop Scand 50:791, 1979.

Von Vinz H: Operative Behandlung von Knochenbruchen bei Kindern, Zentralb Chir 97:1377, 1972.

Watson-Jones R: Fractures and joint injuries, vol 2, Baltimore, 1955, The Williams & Wilkins Co.

Weber MJ et al: Efficacy of various forms of fixation of transverse fractures of the patella, J Bone Joint Surg 62A:215, 1980.

Zaman M and Leonard MA: Meniscectomy in children: a study of fifty-nine knees, J Bone Joint Surg 60B:436, 1978.

Femoral fractures

Abbott LC and Gill GG: Valgus deformity of the knee resulting from injury to the lower femoral epiphysis, J Bone Joint Surg 24:97, 1942.

Aitken AP and Magill HK: Fractures involving the distal femoral epiphyseal cartilage, J Bone Joint Surg 34A:96, 1952.

Allen B, Kant A, and Emery F: Displaced fractures of the femoral diaphysis in children, J Trauma 17:8, 1977.

Anderson M and Green W: Lengths of the femur and the tibia, Am J Dis Child 75:279, 1948.

Anderson WA: The significance of femoral fractures in children, Ann Emerg Med 11:174, 1982.

Aronson DD, Singer RM, and Higgins RF: Skeletal traction for fractures of the femoral shaft in children: a long-term study, J Bone Joint Surg, 69A:1435, 1987.

Banagale RC and Kuhns LR: Traumatic separation of the distal femoral epiphysis in a newborn, J Pediatr Orthop 3:3, 1983.

Bassett FH III and Goldner JL: Fractures involving the distal femoral epiphyseal growth line, South Med J 55:545, 1962.

Blount W: Fractures in children, Baltimore, 1955, The Williams & Wilkins Co.

Brashear HR Jr: Epiphyseal fractures of the lower extremity, South Med J 51:845, 1958.

Brashear HR Jr: Epiphyseal fractures, J Bone Joint Surg 41A:1055, 1959.

Bright RW: Operative correction of partial epiphyseal plate closure by osseous-bridge resection and silicone-rubber implant, J Bone Joint Surg 56A:655, 1974.

Brouwer KJ, Molenaar JC, and Van Linge B: Rotational deformities after femoral shaft fractures in childhood, Acta Orthop Scand 52:81, 1981.

Brower KJ: Torsional deformities after fractures of the femoral shaft in childhood, Acta Orthop Scand Suppl 52, 1981.

Burton V and Fordyce A: Immobilization of femoral shaft fractures in children aged 2-10 years, Injury 4:47, 1972.

Canale ST et al: Acute osteomyelitis following closed fractures, J Bone Joint Surg 57A:415, 1975.

Cassebaum WH and Patterson AH: Fractures of the distal femoral epiphysis, Clin Orthop 41:79, 1965.

Cheng JCY and Cheung SSC: Modified functional bracing in the ambulatory treatment of femoral shaft fractures in children, J Pediatr Orthop 9:457, 1989.

Childress H: Distal femoral 90-90 traction for shaft fractures of the femur in children, Orthop Rev 8:45, 1979.

Clement DA and Colton CL: Overgrowth of the femur after femoral fractures in childhood, J Bone Joint Surg 68B:534, 1986.

Crawford AH: Fractures about the knee in children, Orthop Clin North Am 7:639, 1976.

Czitrom AA, Salter RB, and Willis RB: Fractures involving the distal femoral epiphyseal plate of the femur, Int Orthop 4:269, 1981.

Dameron T and Thompson H: Femoral-shaft fractures in children: treatment by closed reduction and double pica cast immobilization, J Bone Joint Surg 41A:1201, 1959.

Dehne E and Immermann E: Dislocation of the hip combined with fracture of the shaft of the femur on the same side, J Bone Joint Surg 33A:731, 1951.

Edvardsen P and Syversen S: Overgrowth of the femur after fracture of the shaft in childhood, J Bone Joint Surg 58B:339, 1976.

Ehrlich MG and Strain RE Jr: Epiphyseal injuries about the knee, Orthop Clin North Am 10:91, 1979.

Fardon D: Fracture of the neck and shaft of same femur, J Bone Joint Surg 52A:797, 1970.

Fein LH et al: Closed flexible intramedullary nailing of adolescent femoral shaft fractures, J Orthop Trauma 3:133, 1989.

Fry K, Hoffer M, and Brink J: Femoral shaft fractures in brain injured children, J Trauma 16:371, 1976.

Gibson J: Multiple injuries: the management of the patient with a fractured femur and a head injury, J Bone Joint Surg 42B:425, 1960.

Green WT and Anderson M: Epiphyseal arrest for the correction of discrepancies in length of the lower extremities, J Bone Joint Surg 39A:853, 1957.

Griffin PP: Fractures of the femoral diaphysis in children, Orthop Clin North Am 7:633, 1976.

Griffin PP, Anderson M, and Green WT: Fractures of the shaft of the femur in children, Orthop Clin North Am 3:213, 1972.

Gross RH and Stranger M: Causative factors responsible for femoral fracture in infants and young children, J Pediatr Orthop 3:341, 1983.

Gupta RC, Varma AN, and Mittal KK: Treatment of femoral diaphyseal fractures in children by strapping, Injury 12:234, 1980.

Guttmann GG and Simon R: Three-point fixation walking spica cast: an alternative to early or immediate casting of femoral shaft fractures in children, J Pediatr Orthop 8:699, 1988.

Helal B and Skevis XX: Unrecognized dislocation of the hip in fractures of the femoral shaft, J Bone Joint Surg 49B:293, 1967.

Henderson OL et al: Early casting of femoral shaft fractures in children, J Pediatr Orthop 4:16, 1984.

Herndon WA et al: Management of femoral shaft fractures in the adolescent, J Pediatr Orthop 9:29, 1989.

Hoffer M et al: The orthopaedic management of brain-injured children, J Bone Joint Surg 53A:567, 1971.

Holmes SJ, Sedgwick DM, and Scobie WG: Domiciliary gallow traction for femoral shaft fractures in young children, J Bone Joint Surg 65B:288, 1983.

Hougaard K: Femoral shaft fractures in children: a prospective study of the overgrowth phenomenon, Injury 20:170, 1989.

Humberger F and Eyring E: Proximal tibial 90-90 traction in treatment of children with femoral shaft fractures, J Bone Joint Surg 51A:499, 1969.

Irani R, Nicholson J, and Chung S: Long-term results in the treatment of femoral-shaft fractures in young children by immediate spica immobilization, J Bone Joint Surg 58A:945, 1976.

Kennedy JC, editor: The injured adolescent knee, Baltimore, 1979, The Williams & Wilkins Co.

Kirby RM, Winquist RA, and Hansen ST Jr: Femoral shaft fractures in adolescents, comparison between traction plus cast treatment and closed intramedullary nailing, J Pediatr Orthop 1:193, 1981.

Langenskiöld A: An operation for partial closure of an epiphyseal plate in children and its experimental basis, J Bone Joint Surg 57B:325, 1975.

Lansche WE, Mishkin MR, and Stamp WG: The management of

complications of femoral shaft fractures in children, South Med J 56:1001, 1963.

Larson RL: Epiphyseal injuries in the adolescent athlete, Orthop Clin North Am 4:839, 1973.

Lee W and Veal J: The Russell extension method in the treatment of fractures of the femur, Surg Gynecol Obstet 56:492, 1933.

Ligier JN et al: Elastic stable intramedullary nailing of femoral shaft fractures in children, J Bone Joint Surg 70B:74, 1988.

Lombardo SJ and Harvey JP Jr: Fractures of the distal femoral epiphysis: factors influencing prognosis—a review of thirty-four cases, J Bone Joint Surg 59A:742, 1977.

Makela EA et al: The effect of trauma to the lower femoral epiphyseal plate: an experimental study in rabbits, J Bone Joint Surg 70B:187, 1988.

Mann DC, Weddington J, and Davenport K: Closed Enders nailing of femoral shaft fractures in adolescents, J Pediatr Orthop 6:651, 1986.

Meals R: Overgrowth of the femur following fractures in children: influence of handedness, J Bone Joint Surg 61A:381, 1979.

Miller P and Welch M: The hazards of tibial pin replacement in 90-90 skeletal traction, Clin Orthop 135:97, 1978.

Moseley CF: A straight-line graph for leg-length discrepancies, J Bone Joint Surg 59A:174, 1977.

Mubarak SJ and Carroll N: Volkmann's contracture in children: aetiology and prevention, J Bone Joint Surg 61B:285, 1979.

Mubarak SJ et al: The wick catheter technique for measurement of intramuscular pressure, J Bone Joint Surg 58A:1016, 1976.

Neer CS II: Separation of the lower femoral epiphysis, Am J Surg 99:756, 1960.

Neer CS II and Cadman E: Treatment of fractures of the femoral shaft in children, JAMA 163:634, 1957.

Noah PR: The bulky boot, Orthop Rev 9(9): 131, 1981.

Patterson WJ: Separation of the lower femoral epiphysis, Can Med Assoc J 21:301, 1929.

Peterson CA and Peterson HA: Analysis of the incidence of injuries to the epiphyseal growth plate, J Trauma 12:275, 1972.

Peterson E and Haase J: Unstable fractures in children with acute, severe brain injury, Acta Orthop Scand 45:321, 1974.

Peterson HA and Burkhart SS: Compression injury of the epiphyseal growth plate: fact or fiction? J Pediatr Orthop 1:377, 1981.

Rang M: The growth plate and its disorders, Baltimore, 1969, The Williams & Wilkins Co.

Rang M: Children's fractures, ed 2, Philadelphia, 1983, JB Lippincott Co.

Riseborough EJ, Barrett IR, and Shapiro F: Growth disturbances following distal femoral epiphyseal fracture-separations, J Bone Joint Surg 65A:885, 1983.

Roberts JM: Fracture separation of the distal femoral epiphysis, J Bone Joint Surg 55A:1324, 1973.

Rosenberg NM, Vraneisch P, and Bottenfield G: Fractured femurs in pediatric patients, Ann Emerg Med 11:84, 1982.

Roser L: Initial spica cast for femoral shaft fractures in children. Northwest Med, p 1012, 1969.

Ryan JR: 90-90 skeletal femoral traction for femoral shaft fractures in children, J Trauma 21:46, 1981.

Salter RB, Czitrom A, and Willis RB: Fractures involving the distal femoral epiphyseal plate. Quoted in Kennedy JC, editor: Injury to the adolescent knee, Baltimore. 1979, The Williams & Wilkins Co.

Salter RB and Harris WR: Injuries involving the epiphyseal plate, J Bone Joint Surg 45A:587, 1963.

Saxer U: Fractures of the shaft of the femur. In Weber BG, Brunner C, and Frueler F, editors: Treatment of fractures in children and adolescents, New York, 1980, Springer-Verlag.

Schonk J: Comparative follow-up study of conservative and surgical treatment of femoral shaft fractures in children, Arch Chir Neerl 30:231, 1978.

Scott J, Wardlaw D, and McLauchlan J: Cast bracing of femoral shaft fractures in children: a preliminary report, J Pediatr Orthop 1:199, 1981.

Shapiro F: Fractures of the femoral shaft in children: the overgrowth phenomenon, Acta Orthop Scand 52:649, 1981.

Smith JB: Knee problems in children, Pediatr Clin North Am 24:841, 1977.

Staheli L: Femoral and tibial growth following femoral shaft fracture in childhood, Clin Orthop 55:159, 1967.

Staheli L: Fever following trauma in childhood, JAMA 199:503, 1967.

Staheli L and Sheridan G: Early spica cast management of femoral shaft fractures in young children, Clin Orthop 126:162, 1977.

Stephens DC, Louis DS, and Louis E: Traumatic separation of the distal femoral epiphyseal cartilage plate, J Bone Joint Surg 56A:1383, 1974.

Strauss E, Nelson JM, and Abdelwahab IF: Fracture of the lateral femoral condyle: a case report, Bull Hosp Jt Dis Orthop Inst 44:87, 1984.

Tachdjian MO: Pediatric orthopedics, Philadelphia, 1972, WB Saunders Co.

Thompson GH, Wilber JH, and Marcus RE: Internal fixation of fractures in children and adolescents: a comparative analysis, Clin Orthop 188:10, 1984.

Valdiserri L, Marchiodi L, and Rubbini L: Küntscher nailing in the treatment of femoral fractures in children: is it completely contraindicated? Ital J Orthop Traumatol 9:293, 1983.

Van Meter J and Branick R: Bilateral genu recurvatum after skeletal traction, J Bone Joint Surg 62A:837, 1980.

Viljanto J, Kiviluoto H, and Paananen M: Remodelling after femoral shaft fracture in children, Acta Chir Scand 141:360, 1975.

Wagner H: Surgical lengthening or shortening of femur and tibia: technique and indications, Prog Orthop Surg 1:71, 1977.

Watson-Jones R: Fractures and joint injuries, ed 4, Edinburgh, 1955-56, E & S Livingstone.

Weber B: Fracture of the femoral shaft in childhood, Injury 1:65, 1969.

Weber BG, Brunner C, and Freuler F, editors: Treatment of fractures in children and adolescents, New York, 1980, Springer-Verlag.

Ziv I, Blackburn N, and Rang M: Femoral intramedullary nailing in growing child, J Trauma 24:432, 1984.

Ziv I and Rang M: Treatment of femoral fracture in the child with head injury, J Bone Joint Surg 65B:184, 1983.

Hip fractures and dislocations

Anderson M, Green WT, and Messner MB: Growth and prediction of growth in the lower extremity, J Bone Joint Surg 45A:1, 1963.

Asher MA: Dislocations of the upper extremity in children, Orthop Clin North Am 7:583, 1976.

Barquet A: Traumatic hip dislocation in childhood: a report of 26 cases and a review of the literature, Acta Orthop Scand 50:549, 1979.

Barquet A: Recurrent traumatic dislocation of the hip in childhood, J Trauma 20:1003, 1980

Barquet A: Traumatic dislocation of the hip in childhood, Injury 13:435, 1982.

Bennet GC et al: Dislocation of the hip in trisomy 21, J Bone Joint Surg 64B:289, 1982.

Blickenstaff LD and Morris JM: Fatigue fracture of the femoral neck, J Bone Joint Surg 48A:1031, 1966.

Boitzy A: Fractures of the proximal femur. In Weber BG, Brunner Ch, and Freuler F, editors: Treatment of fractures in children and adolescents, Berlin, 1980, Springer-Verlag.

Brav EA: Traumatic dislocations of the hip: army experience and results over a twelve-year period, J Bone Joint Surg 44A:1115, 1962.

Brooks E and Rosman M: Central fracture dislocation of the hip in the child, J Trauma 28:1590, 1988.

Bunnell WP and Webster DA: Late reduction of bilateral traumatic hip dislocation in a child, Clin Orthop 147:160, 1980.

Byram G and Wickstrom J: Traumatic dislocation of the hip in children, South Med J 60:805, 1967.

Calandruccio RA and Anderson WE III: Post-fracture avascular necrosis of the femoral head: correlation of experimental and clinical studies, Clin Orthop 152:49, 1980.

Calandruccio RA and Belding, RH: Stress fractures of the femoral neck, Unpublished manuscript, 1986.

Canale ST and Bourland WL: Fracture of the neck and intertrochanteric region of the femur in children, J Bone Joint Surg 59A:431, 1977.

Canale ST and Manugian AH: Irreducible traumatic dislocations of the hip, J Bone Joint Surg 61A:7, 1979.

Carrell B and Carrell WB: Fractures of the neck of the femur in children with particular reference to aseptic necrosis, J Bone Joint Surg 23:225, 1941.

Choyce CC: Traumatic dislocation of the hip in childhood and relation to pseudocoxalgia, Br J Surg 12:52, 1924.

Chung SMK: The aterial supply of the developing proximal end of the human femur, J Bone Joint Surg 58A:961, 1976.

Colonna PC: Fracture of the neck of the femur in childhood: a report of six cases, Ann Surg 88:902, 1928.

Colonna PC: Fractures of the neck of the femur in children, Am J Surg 6:793, 1929.

Compere EL, Garrison M, and Fahey JJ: Deformities of the femur resulting from arrestment of growth of the capital and greater trochanteric epiphyses, J Bone Joint Surg 22:909, 1940.

Craig CL: Hip injuries in children and adolescents, Orthop Clin North Am 11:743, 1980.

Currey JD and Butler G: Mechanical properties of bone tissue in children, J Bone Joint Surg 57A:810, 1975.

DePalma A: Management of fractures and dislocations, Philadelphia, 1970, WB Saunders Co.

Devas MD: Stress fractures of the femoral neck, J Bone Joint Surg 47B:728, 1965.

Durbin FC: Avascular necrosis complicating undisplaced fractures of the neck of the femur in children, J Bone Joint Surg 41B:758, 1959.

Epstein HC: Traumatic dislocation of the hip, Baltimore, 1980, The Williams & Wilkins Co.

Ernst J: Stress fractures of the neck of the femur, J Trauma 4:71, 1964.

Fiddian J and Grace DL: Traumatic dislocation of the hip in adolescence with separation of the capital femoral epiphysis, J Bone Joint Surg 65B:148, 1983.

Fordyce AJW: Open reduction of traumatic dislocation of the hip in a child: case report and review of the literature, Br J Surg 58:705, 1971.

Freeman GE Jr: Traumatic dislocation of the hip in children: a report of 7 cases and a review of the literature, J Bone Joint Surg 43A:401, 1961.

Funk FJ: Traumatic dislocation of the hip in children: factors affecting prognosis and treatment, J Bone Joint Surg 44A:1135, 1962.

Gartland JJ and Brenner JH: Traumatic dislocations in the lower extremity in children, Orthop Clin North Am 7:687, 1976.

Gaul RW: Recurrent traumatic dislocation of the hip in children, Clin Orthop 90:107, 1973.

Gerber C, Lehmann A, and Ganz R: Femoral neck fractures in children: experience in 7 Swiss AO hospitals, Orthop Trans 9:474, 1985 (abstract).

Glass A and Powell HDW: Traumatic dislocation of the hip in children, J Bone Joint Surg 43B29, :1961.

Godfrey JD: Trauma in children, J Bone Joint Surg 46A:422, 1964.

Gupta RC and Shravat BP: Reduction of neglected traumatic dislocation of the hip by heavy traction, J Bone Joint Surg 59A:249, 1977.

Haliburton RA, Brockenshire FA, and Barber JR: Avascular necrosis of the femoral capital epiphysis after traumatic dislocation of the hip in children, J Bone Joint Surg 43B:43, 1961.

Harper MC and Canale ST: Angulation osteotomy: a trigonometric analysis, Clin Orthop 166:173, 1982.

Harper MC, Canale ST, and Cobb RM: Proximal femoral osteotomy: a trigonometric analysis of effect on leg length, J Pediatr Orthop 3:341, 1983.

Heiser JM and Oppenheim WL: Fracture of the hip in children, Clin Orthop 149:177, 1980.

Helal B and Skevis X: Unrecognized dislocation of the hip in fractures of the femoral shaft, J Bone Joint Surg 49B:293, 1967.

Ingram AJ and Bachynski B: Fractures of the hip in children: treatment and results, J Bone Joint Surg 35A:867, 1953.

Ingram AJ and Turner TC: Bilateral traumatic posterior dislocation of the hip complicated by bilateral fracture of the femoral shaft, J Bone Joint Surg 36A:1249, 1954.

Kay SP and Hall JE: Fracture of the femoral neck in children and its complications, Clin Orthop 80:53, 1971.

Key JA and Conwell HE: Management of fractures, dislocations and sprains, St Louis, 1951, The CV Mosby Co.

Lam SF: Fractures of the neck of the femur in children, J Bone Joint Surg 53A:1165, 1971.

Langenskiöld A and Salenius P: Epiphyseodesis of the greater trochanter, Acta Orthop Scand 38:199, 1967.

Laurent LE: Growth disturbances of the proximal end of the femur in the light of animal experiments, Acta Orthop Scand 28:255, 1959.

Libri R et al: Traumatic dislocation of the hip in children and adolescents, Ital J Orthop Traumatol 12:61, 1986.

Libshitz HI and Edeiken BS: Radiotherapy changes of the pediatric hip, Am J Roentgenol 137:585, 1981.

Lindseth RE and Rosene HA Jr: Traumatic separation of the upper femoral epiphysis in a newborn infant, J Bone Joint Surg 53A:1641, 1971.

MacFarlane IJA: Survey of traumatic dislocation of the hip in children, J Bone Joint Surg 58B:267, 1976.

Malgaigne JF: Treatise on fractures, Philadelphia, 1859, JB Lippincott Co.

Mason M: Traumatic dislocation of the hip in childhood, J Bone Joint Surg 36B:630, 1954.

Mass DP, Spiegel PG, and Laros GS: Dislocation of the hip with traumatic separation of the capital femoral epiphysis: report of case with successful outcome, Clin Orthop 146:184, 1980.

McDougall A: Fractures of the neck of the femur in childhood, J Bone Joint Surg 43B:16, 1961.

Miller WE: Fractures of the hip in children from birth to adolescence, Clin Orthop 92:155, 1973.

Morgan JD and Somerville EW: Normal and abnormal growth at the upper end of the femur, J Bone Joint Surg 42B:264, 1960.

Morrissy R: Hip fractures in children, Clin Orthop 152:202, 1980.

Mosley CF: A straight line graph for leg length discrepancies, J Bone Joint Surg 59B:116, 1977.

Neilsen PT and Thaarup P: An unusual course of femoral head necrosis complicating an intertrochanteric fracture in a child, Clin Orthop 183:79, 1984.

Ogden JA: Changing patterns of proximal femoral vascularity, J Bone Joint Surg 56A:941, 1974.

Ogden JA et al: Proximal femoral epipysiolysis in the neonate, J Pediatr Orthop 4:285, 1984.

Osaka AI et al: The pathogenesis of Perthes' disease, J Bone Joint Surg 58B:453, 1976.

Pearson DE and Mann RJ: Traumatic hip dislocation in children, Clin Orthop 92:189, 1973.

Petrini A and Grassi G: Long-term results in traumatic dislocation of the hip in children, Ital J Orthop Traumatol 9:225, 1983.

Pförringer W and Rosemeyer B: Fractures of the hip in children and adolescents, Acta Orthop Scand 51:91, 1980.

Piggot J: Traumatic dislocation of the hip in childhood, J Bone Joint Surg 43B:38, 1961.

Quinlan WR, Brady PG, and Regan BS: Fractures of the neck of the femur in childhood, Injury 11:242, 1980.

Rang M: Children's fractures, ed 2, Philadelphia, 1983, JB Lippincott Co.

Ratliff AHC: Fractures of the neck of the femur in children, J Bone Joint Surg 44B:528, 1962.

Ratliff AHC: Traumatic separation of the upper femoral epiphysis in children, J Bone Joint Surg 50B:757, 1968.

Ratliff AHC: Complications after fractures of the femoral neck in children and their treatment, J Bone Joint Surg 52B:175, 1970.

Schlansky J and Miller P: Traumatic hip dislocation in children, J Bone Joint Surg 55A:1057, 1973.

Stewart MJ and Milford LW: Fracture-dislocation of the hip, J Bone Joint Surg 36A:315, 1954.

Stimson LA: Fractures and dislocations, Philadelphia, 1917, Lea & Febiger.

Swiontkowski MF and Winquist RA: Displaced hip fractures in children and adolescents, J Trauma 26:384, 1986.

Theodorou SD, Ierodiaconou MN, and Mitsou A: Obstetrical fracture separation of upper femoral epiphysis, Acta Orthop Scand 53:239, 1982.

Trueta J: The normal vascular anatomy of the human femoral head during growth, J Bone Joint Surg 39B:358, 1957.

Wadsworth TG: Traumatic dislocation of the hip with fracture of the shaft of the ipsilateral femur, J Bone Joint Surg 43B:47, 1961.

Watson-Jones R: Fractures and joint injuries, Baltimore, 1957, The Williams & Wilkins Co.

Weber BG, Brunner C, and Freuler F: Treatment of fractures in children and adolescents, New York, 1980, Springer-Verlag.

Wilson DW: Traumatic dislocation of the hip in children: a report of four cases, J Trauma 6:739, 1966.

Wolfgang GL: Stress fracture of the femoral neck in a patient with open capital femoral epiphyses, J Bone Joint Surg 59A:680, 1977.

Wojtowycz M, Starshak RJ, and Sty JR: Neonatal proximal femoral epiphysiolysis, Radiology 136:647, 1980.

Slipped capital femoral epiphysis

Aadalen RJ et al: Acute slipped capital femoral epiphysis, J Bone Joint Surg 56A:1473, 1974.

Asnis SE: The Asnis guided screw system technique manual, Rutherford, NJ, 1984, Howmedica, Inc.

Asnis SE: Personal communication, 1985.

Aufranc OE, Jones WN, and Turner RH: Slipped capital femoral epiphysis, JAMA 198:546, 1966.

Barash HL, Galante JO, and Ray RD: Acute slipped capital femoral epiphysis: a report of nine cases, Clin Orthop 79:96, 1971.

Bassett FH III and Azuma H: Evaluation of venous drainage from the capital femoral epiphysis, Surg Forum 16:445, 1965.

Bennet GC, Koreska J, and Rang M: Pin placement in slipped capital femoral epiphysis, J Pediatr Orthop 4:574, 1984.

Bianco AJ: Treatment of mild slipping of the capital femoral epiphysis, J Bone Joint Surg 47A:387, 1965.

Bloom ML and Crawford AH: Slipped capital femoral epiphysis: an assessment of treatment modalities, Orthopedics 8:36, 1985.

Boyd HB: Personal communication, 1970.

Boyd HB: Treatment of acute slipped upper femoral epiphysis. In The American Academy of Orthopaedic Surgeons: Instructional course lectures, vol 21, St Louis, 1972, The CV Mosby Co.

Boyd HB, Ingram AJ, and Bourkhard HO: The treatment of slipped femoral epiphysis, South Med J 42:551, 1949.

Boyer W, Mickelson MR, and Ponseti IV: Slipped capital femoral epiphysis: long term follow-up study of 121 patients, J Bone Joint Surg 63A:85, 1981.

Broughton NS et al: Open reduction of the severely slipped upper femoral epiphysis, J Bone Joint Surg 70B:435, 1988.

Canale ST: Problems and complications of slipped capital femoral epiphysis. In The American Academy of Orthopaedic Surgeons: Instructional course lectures, vol 38, 1989, The CV Mosby Co.

Carney BT and Weinstein SL: Long-term follow-up of slipped capital femoral epiphysis, Orthop Trans 12:698, 1988 (abstract).

Carney BT, Weinstein SL, and Noble J: Long-term follow-up of slipped capital femoral epiphysis. Paper presented at the annual meeting of The American Academy of Orthopaedic Surgeons, Atlanta, Feb 6, 1988.

Casey BH, Hamilton HW, and Bobechko WP: Reduction of acutely slipped upper femoral epiphysis, J Bone Joint Surg 54B:607, 1972.

Chiroff RT, Sears EA, and Slaughter WH III: Slipped capital femoral epiphyses and parathyroid adenoma: case report, J Bone Joint Surg 56A:1063, 1974.

Clark CR, Southwick WO, and Ogden JA: Anatomic aspects of slipped capital femoral epiphysis and correction by biplane osteotomy. In The American Academy of Orthopaedic Surgeons: Instructional course lectures, vol 29, 1980, The CV Mosby Co.

Compere CL: Correction of deformity and prevention of aseptic necrosis in late cases of slipped femoral epiphysis, J Bone Joint Surg 32A:351, 1950.

Cowell HR: The significance of early diagnosis and treatment of slipping of the capital femoral epiphysis, Clin Orthop 48:89, 1966.

Crawford AH: Current concepts review: slipped capital femoral epiphysis, J Bone Joint Surg 70A:1422, 1988.

Crawford AH: The role of osteotomy in the treatment of slipped capital femoral epiphysis. In The American Academy of Orthopaedic Surgeons: Instructional course lectures, vol 38, 1989, The CV Mosby Co.

Cruess RL: The pathology of acute necrosis of cartilage in slipping of the capital femoral epiphysis: a report of two cases with pathological sections, J Bone Joint Surg 45A:1013, 1963.

DePalma AF, Danyo JJ, and Stose WG: Slipping of the upper femoral epiphysis, Clin Orthop 37:167, 1964.

Derian PS: Extremity fractures in children. I. Epiphyseal injuries, Postgrad Med 48:171, 1970.

Duncan JW and Lovell WW: Anterior slip of the capital femoral epiphysis: report of a case and discussion, Clin Orthop 110:171, 1975.

Dunn DM: The treatment of adolescent slipping of the upper femoral epiphysis, J Bone Joint Surg 46B:621, 1964.

Fahey JJ and O'Brien ET: Acute slipped capital femoral epiphysis: review of the literature and report of ten cases, J Bone Joint Surg 47A:1105, 1965.

Fairbank JT: Manipulative reduction in slipped upper femoral epiphysis, J Bone Joint Surg 51B:252, 1969.

Ferguson AB and Howorth MB: Slipping of upper femoral epiphysis: a study of seventy cases, JAMA 97:1867, 1931.

Fish JB: Cuneiform osteotomy in treatment of slipped capital femoral epiphysis, NY State J Med 72:2633, 1972.

Fish JB: Cuneiform osteotomy of the femoral neck in the treatment of slipped capital femoral epiphysis, J Bone Joint Surg 66A:1153, 1984.

Gage JR et al: Complications after cuneiform osteotomy for moderately or severely slipped capital femoral epiphysis, J Bone Joint Surg 60B:157, 1978.

Griffith MJ: Slipping of the capital femoral epiphysis, Ann Roy Coll Surg Engl 58:34, 1976.

Hall JE: The results of treatment of slipped femoral epiphysis, J Bone Joint Surg 39B:659, 1957.

Harris ED Jr, DiBona DR, and Krane SM: Collagenases in human synovial fluid, J Clin Invest 48:2104, 1969.

Harris WR: The endocrine basis for slipping of the upper femoral epiphysis: an experimental study, J Bone Joint Surg 32B:5, 1950.

Herndon CH: Treatment of minimally slipped upper femoral epiphysis. In The American Academy of Orthopaedic Surgeons: Instructional course lectures, vol 21, St Louis, 1972, The CV Mosby Co.

Herndon CH: Treatment of severely slipped upper femoral epiphysis by means of osteoplasty and epiphyseodesis. In The American Academy of Orthopaedic Surgeons: Instructional course lectures, vol 21, St Louis, 1972, The CV Mosby Co.

Herndon CH, Heyman CH, and Bell DM: Treatment of slipped capital femoral epiphysis by epiphyseodesis and osteoplasty of the femoral neck: a report of further experiences, J Bone Joint Surg 45A:999, 1963.

Herndon JH and Aufranc OE: Avascular necrosis of the femoral head in the adult: a review of its incidence in a variety of conditions, Clin Orthop 86:43, 1972.

Heyerman W and Weiner D: Slipped epiphysis associated with hypothyroidism, J Pediatr Orthop 4:569, 1984.

Heyman CH: Treatment of slipping of the upper femoral epiphysis: a study of results of 42 cases, Surg Gynecol Obstet 89:559, 1949.

Heyman CH and Herndon CH: Epiphyseodesis for early slipping of the upper femoral epiphysis, J Bone Joint Surg 36A:539, 1954.

Heyman CH, Herndon CH, and Strong JM: Slipped femoral epiphysis with severe displacement: a conservative operative treatment, J Bone Joint Surg 39A:293, 1957.

Hiertonn T: Wedge osteotomy in advanced femoral epiphysiolysis, Acta Orthop Scand 25:44, 1955-1956.

Hillman JW and Barrow JA III: Hormone treatment of early separation of epiphysis, J Bone Joint Surg 45A:1777, 1963.

Howorth MB: Coxa plana, J Bone Joint Surg 30A:601, 1948.

Howorth MB: Slipping of the upper femoral epiphysis. In The American Academy of Orthopaedic Surgeons: Instructional course lectures, vol 8, Ann Arbor, Mich, 1951, JW Edwards Co.

Howorth MB: The bone-pegging operation: for slipping of the capital femoral epiphysis, Clin Orthop 48:79, 1966.

Howorth MB: History: slipping of the capital femoral epiphysis, Clin Orthop 48:11, 1966.

Howorth MB: Pathology: slipping of the capital femoral epiphysis, Clin Orthop 48:33, 1966.

Howorth MB: Treatment: slipping of the capital femoral epiphysis, Clin Orthop 48:53, 1966.

Ingram AJ et al: Chondrolysis complicating slipped capital femoral epiphysis, Clin Orthop 165:99, 1982.

Jacobs B: A note on the diagnosis of early adolescent coxa vara (slipped epiphysis), Br J Radiol 35:619, 1962.

Jacobs B: Chondrolysis of the hip: objectives of study and historical background, Personal communication, June 1975.

Jacobs B and Wilson PD: The treatment of slipping of the upper femoral epiphysis: a follow-up study of 300 cases, Arch Orthop Unfallchir 56:349, 1964.

Johnson CE II and Hernandez AA: Prophylactic pinning in upper slipped capital femoral epiphysis, Orthopaedics 7:1502, 1984.

Joplin RJ: Slipped capital femoral epiphysis: the still unsolved adolescent hip lesion, JAMA 188:379, 1964.

Joyce JJ III and Grant BD: Early diagnosis of slipping of the upper femoral epiphysis, JAMA 188:1049, 1964.

Kelsey JL, Acheson RM, and Keggi KJ: The body build of patients with slipped capital femoral epiphysis, Am J Dis Child 124:276, 1972.

Kelsey JL, Keggi KJ, and Southwick WO: The incidence and distribution of slipped capital femoral epiphysis in Connecticut and Southwestern United States, J Bone Joint Surg 52A:1203, 1970.

King D: Slipping capital femoral epiphysis, Clin Orthop 48:71, 1966.

Kramer WG, Craig WA, and Noel S: Compensating osteotomy of the base of the femoral neck for slipped capital femoral epiphysis, J Bone Joint Surg 58A:796, 1976.

Lehman WB et al: The problem of in situ pinning of slipped capital femoral epiphysis, Orthop Trans 6:380, 1982 (abstract).

Lehman WB et al: A method of evaluating possible pin penetration in slipped capital femoral epiphysis using a cannulated internal fixation device, Clin Orthop 186:65, 1984.

Lindstrom N: Surgical treatment of epiphyseolysis capitis femoris, Acta Orthop Scand 28:131, 1958-1959.

Lowe HG: Avascular necrosis after slipping of the upper femoral epiphysis, J Bone Joint Surg 43B:688, 1961.

Lowe HG: Necrosis of articular cartilage after slipping of the capital femoral epiphysis: report of six cases with recovery, J Bone Joint Surg 52B:108, 1970.

Lunceford EM Jr: The use of multiple adjustable Moore nail fixation in slipping of the capital femoral epiphysis, Clin Orthop 48:95, 1966.

Lyden JP: Personal communication, 1985.

MacEwen GD: Advantages and disadvantages of pin fixation in slipped capital femoral epiphysis. In The American Academy of Orthopaedic Surgeons: Instructional course lectures, vol 29, St Louis, 1980, The CV Mosby Co.

Martin PH: Slipped epiphysis in the adolescent hip: a reconsideration of open reduction, J Bone Joint Surg 30A:9, 1948.

Maurer D and Larsen I: Acute necrosis of cartilage of the slipped capital femoral epiphysis, J Bone Joint Surg 52A:39, 1970.

Melby A, Hoyt W, and Weiner D: Treatment of chronic slipped capital femoral epiphysis by bone graft epiphysiodesis, J Bone Joint Surg 62A:119, 1980.

Menche D and Lehman WB: In situ pinning of slipped capital femoral epiphysis, Orthop Rev 9:129, 1982.

Morrissy RT: Principles of in situ fixation in chronic slipped capital femoral epiphysis. In The American Academy of Orthopaedic Surgeons: Instructional course lectures, vol 38, 1989, The CV Mosby Co.

Morrissy RT: Slipped capital femoral epiphysis technique of percutaneous in situ fixation, J Pediatr Orthop 10:347, 1990.

Nishiyama K, Sakamaki T, and Ishii Y: Follow-up study of the subcapital wedge osteotomy for severe chronic slipped capital femoral epiphysis, J Pediatr Orthop 9:412, 1989.

O'Beirne J et al: Slipped upper femoral epiphysis: internal fixation using single central pins, J Pediatr Orthop 9:304, 1989.

O'Brien ET and Fahey JJ: Remodeling of the femoral neck after in-situ pinning for a slipped capital femoral epiphysis, J Bone Joint Surg 59A:62, 1977.

Ordenberg G, Hansson IL, and Sandström S: Slipped capital femoral epiphysis in southern Sweden: long-term result with closed reduction and hip plaster spica, Clin Orthop 220:148, 1987.

O'Reilly DE: Acute traumatic separation of the capital femoral epiphysis, South Med J 64:847, 1971.

Orofino C, Innis JJ, and Lowrey CW: Slipped capital femoral epiphysis in Negroes: a study of ninety-five cases, J Bone Joint Surg 42A:1079, 1960.

Pearl AJ, Woodward B, and Kelly RP: Cuneiform osteotomy in the treatment of slipped capital femoral epiphysis, J Bone Joint Surg 43A:947, 1961.

Pedrini-Mille A et al: Chemical studies on the ground substance of human epiphyseal-plate cartilage, J Bone Joint Surg 49A:1628, 1967.

Ponseti IV and Barta CK: Evaluation of treatment of slipping of the capital femoral epiphysis, Surg Gynecol Obstet 86:87, 1948.

Ponseti IV and McClintock R: The pathology of slipping of the upper femoral epiphysis, J Bone Joint Surg 38A:71, 1956.

Rao JP, Francis AM, and Siwek CW: The treatment of chronic slipped capital femoral epiphysis by biplane osteotomy, J Bone Joint Surg 66A:1169, 1984.

Richards BS and Coleman SS: Subluxation of the femoral head in coxa plana, J Bone Joint Surg 69A:1312, 1987.

Roberts JM: Personal communication, 1986.

Rooks MD and Schmitt EW: The accuracy of subchondral placement of Knowles pins in slipped capital femoral epiphysis, Orthop Trans 8:45, 1984 (abstract).

Rooks MD, Schmitt EW, and Drvaric DM: Unrecognized pin penetration in slipped capital femoral epiphysis, Clin Orthop 234:82, 1988.

Roy DR and Crawford AH: Idiopathic chondrolysis of the hip: management by subtotal capsulectomy and aggressive rehabilitation, J Pediatr Orthop 8:203, 1988.

Salvati EA, Robinson JH Jr, and O'Down TJ: Southwick osteotomy for severe chronic slipped capital femoral epiphysis: results and complications, J Bone Joint Surg 62A:561, 1980.

Shaw JA: Preventing unrecognized penetration into the hip joint, Orthop Rev 13:122, 1984.

Singh S and Petrie JG: Slipped epiphyses in chondro-osteodystrophy: report of one case, J Bone Joint Surg 45A:1025, 1963.

Sørensen KH: Slipped upper femoral epiphysis: clinical study on aetiology, Acta Orthop Scand 39:499, 1968.

Southwick WO: Osteotomy through the lesser trochanter for slipped capital femoral epiphysis, J Bone Joint Surg 49A:807, 1967.

Southwick WO: Compression fixation after biplane intertrochanteric osteotomy for slipped capital femoral epiphysis: a technical improvement, J Bone Joint Surg 55A:1218, 1973.

Staheli LT: Fractures of the shaft of the femur. In Rockwood CA, Wilkins KE, and King RE, editors: Fractures in children, Philadelphia, 1984, JB Lippincott Co.

Steele HH: Non-operative treatment of slipped capital femoral epiphysis, Orthop Trans 5:7, 1981.

Stern MB, Murphy JL, and Miller DS: Slipped capital femoral epiphysis in Negroes, J Int Coll Surg 42:539, 1964.

Sugioka Y: Transtrochanteric anterior rotational osteotomy of the femoral head in the treatment of osteonecrosis affecting the hip: a new osteotomy operation, Clin Orthop 130:191, 1978.

Szypryt EP, Clement DA, and Colton CL: Open reduction or epiphysiodesis for slipped upper femoral epiphysis: a comparison of Dunn's operation and the Heyman-Herndon procedure, J Bone Joint Surg 69B:737, 1987.

Tillema DA and Golding JSR: Chondrolysis following slipped capital femoral epiphysis in Jamaica, J Bone Joint Surg 53A:1528, 1971.

Ulin R: Slipped proximal femoral epiphyses, Clin Orthop 41:64, 1965.

Volz RG and Martin MD: Illusory biplane radiographic images, Radiology 122:695, 1977.

Walters R and Simon SR: Joint destruction: a sequel of unrecognized pin penetration in patients with slipped capital femoral epiphysis of the hip. In Proceedings of the 8th Open Scientific Meeting of The Hip Society, St Louis, 1980, The CV Mosby Co.

Weiner DS, Weiner SD, and Melby A: Anterolateral approach to the hip for bone graft epiphysiodesis in the treatment of slipped capital femoral epiphysis, J Pediatr Orthop 8:349, 1988.

Weiner DS et al: A 30 year experience with bone graft epiphysiodesis in the treatment of slipped capital femoral epiphysis, J Pediatr Orthop 4:145, 1984.

Weinstein SL, Morrissy RT, and Crawford AH: Slipped capital femoral epiphysis. In The American Academy of Orthopaedic Surgeons: Instructional course lectures, vol 33, St Louis, 1984, The CV Mosby Co.

Wiberg G: Surgical treatment of slipped epiphysis with special reference to wedge osteotomy of the femoral neck, Clin Orthop 48:139, 1966.

Williams CS and Wickstrom J: Analysis of end-result studies in slipped capital femoral epiphysis, J La State Med Soc 116:425, 1964.

Wilson PD, Jacobs B, and Schecter L: Slipped capital femoral epiphysis: an end-result study, J Bone Joint Surg 47A:1128, 1965.

Zahrawi FB et al: Comparative study of pinning in situ and open epiphysiodesis in 105 patients with slipped capital femoral epiphysis, Clin Orthop 177:160, 1983.

Pelvic and acetabular fractures

Alonzo JE and Horowitz M: Use of the AO-ASIF external fixator in children, J Pediatr Orthop 7:594, 1987.

Altenberg AR: Acetabular labrum tears: cause of hip pain and degenerative arthritis, South Med J 70:174, 1977.

Baker WJ and Graf EC: The management of the urinary tract in fractures of the bony pelvis. In The American Academy of Orthopaedic Surgeons: Instructional course lectures, vol 11, Ann Arbor, Mich, 1954, JW Edwards Co.

Behrens F: External skeletal fixation. Part A: Introduction to external skeletal fixation. In The American Academy of Orthopaedic Surgeons: Instructional course lectures, vol 30, St Louis, 1981, The CV Mosby Co.

Behrens F: External skeletal fixation. Part H: Complications of external skeletal fixation. In The American Academy of Orthopaedic Surgeons: Instructional course lectures, vol 30, 1981, The CV Mosby Co.

Blair W and Hansen C: Traumatic closure of triradiate cartilage, J Bone Joint Surg 61A:144, 1979.

Bonnin JG: Sacral fractures and injuries to the cauda equina, J Bone Joint Surg 27:113, 1945.

Bryan WJ and Tullos HS: Pediatric pelvic fractures: a review of fifty-two patients, J Trauma 19:799, 1979.

Bucholz RW, Ezaki M, and Ogden JA: Injury to the acetabular triradiate physeal cartilage, J Bone Joint Surg 64A:600, 1982.

Carruthers FW and Logue RM: Treatment of fractures of the pelvis and their complications. In The American Academy of Orthopaedic Surgeons: Instructional course lectures, vol 10, Ann Arbor, Mich, 1953, JW Edwards Co.

Dommisse GF: Diametric fractures of the pelvis, J Bone Joint Surg 42B:432, 1960.

Dunn AW, and Morris HD: Fractures and dislocations of the pelvis, J Bone Joint Surg 50A:1639, 1968.

Eichenholtz SN and Stark RM: Central acetabular fractures, J Bone Joint Surg 46A:695, 1964.

Fernbach SK and Wilkinson RH: Avulsion injuries to the pelvis and proximal femur, Am J Radiol 137:581, 1981.

Gepstein R, Weiss RE, and Hallel T: Acetabular dysplasia and hip dislocation after selective premature fusion of the triradiate cartilage: an experimental study in rabbits, J Bone Joint Surg 66B:334, 1984.

Gertzbein SD and Chenoweth DR: Occult injuries of the pelvic ring, Clin Orthop 128:202, 1977.

Hall BB, Klassen RA, and Ilstrup DM: Pelvic fractures in children: a long-term follow-up study, Unpublished manuscript, 1983.

Haller JA Jr and Garrett R: A new philosophy of pediatric splenic surgery: save our spleens, Surg Rounds 3:23, 1980.

Harris WR et al: Avulsion of lumbar roots complicating fracture of the pelvis, J Bone Joint Surg 55A:1436, 1973.

Harrison TJ: The influence of the femoral head on pelvic growth and acetabular form in the rat, J Anat 95:12, 1961.

Hauser CW and Perry JF Jr: Massive hemorrhage from pelvic fractures, Minn Med 49:285, 1966.

Heeg M, Klasen HJ, and Visser JD: Acetabular fractures in children and adolescents, J Bone Joint Surg 71B:418, 1989.

Heeg M, Visser JD, and Oostvogel HJM: Injuries of the acetabular triradiate cartilage and sacroiliac joint, J Bone Joint Surg 70B:34, 1988.

Jones DB: March fracture of the interior pubic ramus: report of three cases, Radiology 41:586, 1943.

Judet R, Judet J, and Letournel E: Fractures of the acetabulum: classification and surgical approaches for open reduction, J Bone Joint Surg 46A:1615, 1964.

Kane WJ: Fractures of the pelvis. In Rockwood CA Jr and Green DP, editors: Fractures, Philadelphia, 1975, JB Lippincott Co.

Kelly J: Ischial epiphysitis, J Bone Joint Surg 45A:435, 1963.

Key JA and Conwell HE: Management of fractures, dislocations, and sprains, St Louis, 1951, The CV Mosby Co.

Lam CR: Nerve injury in fractures of the pelvis, Ann Surg 104:945, 1936.

McDonald GA: Pelvic disruptions in children, Clin Orthop 151:130, 1980.

Mears DC and Fu F: External fixation in pelvic fractures, Orthop Clin North Am 11:465, 1980.

Milch H: Avulsion fracture of the tuberosity of the ischium, J Bone Joint Surg 8:832, 1926.

Milch H: Ischio-acetabular (Walther's) fracture, Bull Hosp Jt Dis 16:7, 1955.

Morgenstern L: Conservation of the injured spleen, Surg Rounds 3:13, 1980.

Patterson FP: The cause of death in fractures of the pelvis, J Trauma 13:849, 1973.

Peltier LF: Complications associated with fractures of the pelvis, J Bone Joint Surg 47A:1060, 1965.

Ponseti IV: Growth and development of the acetabulum in the normal child, J Bone Joint Surg 60A:575, 1978.

Quinby WC Jr: Fractures of the pelvis and associated injuries in children, J Pediatr Surg 1:353, 1966.

Rankin LM: Fractures of the pelvis, Ann Surg 106:266, 1937.

Reed MH: Pelvic fractures in children, J Can Assoc Radiol 27:255, 1976.

Reff RB: The use of external fixation devices in the management of severe lower extremity trauma and pelvic injuries in children, Clin Orthop 188:21, 1984.

Rodrigues KF: Injury of the acetabular epiphysis, Injury 4:258, 1973.

Rowe CR and Lowell JD: Prognosis of fractures of the acetabulum, J Bone Joint Surg 43A:30, 1961.

Scuderi G and Bronson MJ: Triradiate cartilage injury: report of two cases and review of the literature, Clin Orthop 217:179, 1987.

Selakovich W and Love L: Stress fractures of the pubic ramus, J Bone Joint Surg 36A:573, 1954.

Slatis P: External fixation of double vertical fractures with a trapezoid compression frame, Injury 10:142, 1978.

Slatis P and Karaharj U: External fixation of the pelvic girdle with a trapezoid compression frame, Injury 7:53, 1975.

Sullivan CR: Fractures of the pelvis. In The American Academy of Orthopaedic Surgery: Instructional course lectures, vol 18, Ann Arbor, Mich, 1961, JW Edwards Co.

Tachdjian MO: Fractures of the pelvis. In Tachdjian MO: Pediatric orthopaedics, Philadelphia, 1973, WB Saunders Co.

Tile M: Fractures of the acetabulum, Orthop Clin North Am 11:481, 1980.

Tile M: Pelvic fractures: operative versus nonoperative treatment, Orthop Clin North Am 11:423, 1980.

Tolo VT: External skeletal fixation in children's fractures, J Pediatr Orthop 3:432, 1983.

Torode I and Zieg D: Pelvic fractures in children, J Pediatr Orthop 5:76, 1985.

Watts HG: Fractures of the pelvis in children, Orthop Clin North Am 7:615, 1976.

Spine fractures and dislocations

Amstutz HC and Carey EJ: Skeletal manifestation and treatment of Gaucher's disease, J Bone Joint Surg 48A:670, 1966.

Anderson LD and D'Alonzo RT: Fractures of the odontoid process of the axis, J Bone Joint Surg 56A:1663, 1974.

Babcock JL: Spinal injuries in children, Pediatr Clin North Am 22:487, 1975.

Bailey DK: The normal cervical spine in infants and children, Radiology 59:712, 1952.

Baker DR and McHollick W: Spondyloschisis and spondylolisthesis in children, J Bone Joint Surg 38A:933, 1956.

Blasier RD and LaMont RL: Chance fracture in a child: a case report with nonoperative treatment, J Pediatr Orthop 5:92, 1985.

Bohlman HH: Acute fractures and dislocations of the cervical spine, J Bone Joint Surg 61A:1119, 1979.

Bohlman HH and Davis DD: The pathology of fatal craniospinal injuries. In Brinkhous KM, editor: Accident pathology, Proceedings of an International Conference, Washington, DC, 1968, US Government Printing Office.

Bradford DS et al: Scheuermann's kyphosis and roundback deformity, J Bone Joint Surg 56A:740, 1974.

Bulos S: Herniated intervertebral lumbar disc in the teenager, J Bone Joint Surg 55B:273, 1973.

Caffey J: Pediatric x-ray diagnosis, Chicago, 1967, Year Book Medical Publishers, Inc.

Caffey J: The whiplash shaken infant syndrome, Pediatrics 54:396, 1974.

Campbell J and Bonnett C: Spinal cord injury in children, Clin Orthop 112:114, 1975.

Cattell HS and Filtzer DL: Pseudosubluxation and other normal variations in the cervical spine in children, J Bone Joint Surg 47A:1295, 1965.

Cullen JC: Spinal lesions in battered babies, J Bone Joint Surg 57B:364, 1975.

Davis D et al: The pathological findings in fatal craniospinal injuries, J Neurosurg 34:603, 1971.

Dickson RA and Leatherman KD: Spinal injuries in child abuse: case report, J Trauma 18:811, 1978.

Edmonson AS: The spine. In Edmonson AS and Crenshaw AH, editors: Campbell's operative orthopaedics, ed 6, St Louis, 1980, The CV Mosby Co.

Fielding JW: Cineroentgenography of the normal cervical spine, J Bone Joint Surg 39A:1281, 1957.

Fielding JW: Normal and selected abnormal motion of the cervical spine from the second cervical vertebra to the seventh cervical vertebra based on cineroentgenography, J Bone Joint Surg 46A:1779, 1964.

Fielding JW: Selected observations on the cervical spine in the child. In Ahstrom JP Jr, editor: Current practice in orthopaedic surgery, vol 5, St Louis, 1973, The CV Mosby Co.

Fielding JW: Fractures of the spine. Part I. Injuries of the cervical spine. In Rockwood CA Jr, Wilkins KE, and King RE: Fractures in children, Philadelphia, 1984, JB Lippincott Co.

Fielding JW et al: Tears of the transverse ligament of the atlas: a clinical and biomechanical study, J Bone Joint Surg 56A:1683, 1974.

Fielding JW and Hawkins RJ: Roentgenographic diagnosis of the injured neck. In The American Academy of Orthopaedic Surgeons: Instructional course lectures, vol 25, St Louis, 1976, The CV Mosby Co.

Fielding JW, Hensinger RN, and Hawkins RJ: Os odontoideum, J Bone Joint Surg 62A:376, 1980.

Flesh JR et al: Harrington instrumentation and spine fusion for unstable fractures and fracture-dislocations of the thoracic and lumbar spine, J Bone Joint Surg 59A:143, 1977.

Griffiths SC: Fracture of the odontoid process in children, J Pediatr Surg 7:680, 1972.

Grisel P: Enucleation de l' atlas et torticolis nasopharyngien, Presse Med 38:50, 1930.

Henrys P et al: Clinical review of cervical spine injuries in children, Clin Orthop 129:172, 1977.

Hensinger RN: Fractures of the spine. Part II. Fractures of the thoracic and lumbar spine. In Rockwood CA Jr, Wilkins KE, and King RE: Fractures in children, Philadelphia, 1984, JB Lippincott Co.

Hensinger RN, Lang JR, and MacEwen GD: Surgical management of spondylolisthesis in children and adolescents, Spine 1:207, 1976.

Herzenberg JE et al: Emergency transport and position of young children who have an injury of the cervical spine. The standard backboard may be hazardous, J Bone Joint Surg 71A:15, 1989.

Hess JH, Bronstein IP, and Abelson SM: Atlantoaxial dislocations unassociated with trauma and secondary to inflammatory foci of the neck, Am J Dis Child 49:1137, 1935.

Hohl M and Baker HR: The atlanto-axial joint: roentgenographic and anatomical study of normal and abnormal motion, J Bone Joint Surg 46A:1739, 1964.

Horal J, Nachemson A, and Scheller S: Clinical and radiological long term follow-up of vertebral-fractures in children, Acta Orthop Scand 43:491, 1972.

Hubbard DD: Injuries of the spine in children and adolescents, Clin Orthop 100:56, 1974.

Hubbard DD: Fractures of the dorsal and lumbar spine, Orthop Clin North Am 7:605, 1976.

Hunter GA: Non-traumatic displacement of the atlanto-axial joint, J Bone Joint Surg 50B:44, 1968.

Glasauer FE and Caves HC: Biomechanical fractures of traumatic paraplegia in infancy, J Trauma 13:166, 1973.

Jackson DW, Wiltse LL, and Cirincione RJ: Spondylolysis in the female gymnast, Clin Orthop 117:68, 1976.

Jackson RW: Surgical stabilization of the spine, Paraplegia 13:71, 1975.

Jones ET and Hensinger RN: Spinal deformity in idiopathic juvenile osteoporosis, Spine 6:1, 1981.

Keller RH: Traumatic displacement of the cartilaginous vertebral rim: a sign of intervertebral disc prolapse, Radiology 110:21, 1974.

Kewalramani LS and Tori JA: Spinal cord trauma in children: neurologic patterns, radiologic features, and pathomechanics of injury, Spine 5:11, 1980.

Kilfoyle RM, Foley JJ, and Norton PL: Spine and pelvic deformity in childhood and adolescent paraplegia: a study of 104 cases, J Bone Joint Surg 47A:659, 1965.

Kogutt MS, Swischuk LE, and Fagan GJ: Patterns of injury and significance of uncommon fractures in the battered child syndrome, Am J Roentgenol Radium Ther Nucl Med 121:143, 1974.

Lancourt JE, Dickson JH, and Carter RE: Paralytic spinal deformity following traumatic spinal-cord injury in children and adolescents, J Bone Joint Surg 63A:47, 1981.

Lowrey JJ: Dislocated lumbar vertebral epiphysis in adolescent children: report of three cases, J Neurosurg 38:232, 1973.

Marar BC and Balachandran N: Non-traumatic atlanto-axial dislocation in children, Clin Orthop 92:220, 1973.

Mayfield JK, Erkkila JC, and Winter RB: Spine deformity subsequent to acquired childhood spinal cord injury, Orthop Trans 3:281, 1979.

McRae DL: The significance of abnormalities of the cervical spine, Am J Roentgenol 84:3, 1960.

Melzak J: Paraplegia among children, Lancet 2:45, 1969.

Micheli LJ: Low back pain in the adolescent: differential diagnosis, Am J Sports Med 7:362, 1979.

Nachemson A: Fracture of the odontoid process of the axis: a clinical study based on 26 cases, Acta Orthop Scand 29:185, 1960.

Odom JA, Brown CW, and Messner DG: Tubing injuries, J Bone Joint Surg 58A:733, 1976.

Parke WW and Schiff DCM: The applied anatomy of the interverte-bral disc, Orthop Clin North Am 2:309, 1971.

Rogers WA: Treatment of fracture-dislocation of the cervical spine, J Bone Joint Surg 24:245, 1942.

Scheuermann HW: The classic. Kyphosis dorsalis juvenilis, Z Ortho Chir 41:305, 1921.

Schiff DCM and Parke WW: The arterial blood supply of the odon-toid process (dens), Anat Rec 172:399, 1972.

Sherk HH and Nicholson JT: Rotary atlanto-axial dislocation associ-ated with ossiculum terminale and mongolism, J Bone Joint Surg 51A:957, 1969.

Sherk HH, Nicholson JT, and Chung SMK: Fractures of the odon-toid process in young children, J Bone Joint Surg 60A:921, 1978.

Sherk HH, Schut L, and Lane J: Fractures and dislocations of the cervical spine in children, Orthop Clin North Am 7:593, 1976.

Sullivan CR, Bruwer AJ, and Harris LE: Hypermobility of the cervi-cal spine in children: a pitfall in the diagnosis of cervical dislo-cation, Am J Surg 95:636, 1958.

Turner RH and Bianco AJ Jr: Spondylolysis and spondylolisthesis in children and teen-agers, J Bone Joint Surg 53A:1298, 1971.

Werne S: Spontaneous atlas dislocation, Acta Orthop Scand 25:32, 1955.

Wholey MH, Bruwer AJ, and Baker HL: The lateral roentgenogram of the neck, Radiology 71:350, 1958.

Wiltse LL: Spondylolisthesis in children, Clin Orthop 21:156, 1961.

Wiltse LL, Newman PH, and Macnab I: Classification of spondyloly-sis and spondylolisthesis, Clin Orthop 117:23, 1976.

Wiltse LL, Widell EH, and Jackson DW: Fatigue fracture: the basic lesion in isthmic spondylolisthesis, J Bone Joint Surg 57A:17, 1975.

Wynne-Davies R and Scott JHS: Inheritance and spondylolisthesis: a radiographic family survey, J Bone Joint Surg 61B:301, 1979.

Fractures and dislocations of the shaft and epiphysis of the clavicle, acromioclavicular dislocations, and fractures of the shaft and proximal end of the humerus

Aitken AP: Fractures of the proximal humeral epiphysis, Surg Clin North Am 43:1573, 1963.

Alldred AJ: Congenital pseudarthrosis of the clavicle, J Bone Joint Surg 45B:312, 1963.

Asher MA: Dislocations of the upper extremity in children, Orthop Clin North Am 7:583, 1976.

Aufranc OE, Jones WN, and Bierbaum BE: Epiphyseal fracture of the proximal humerus, JAMA 207:727, 1969.

Aufranc OE, Jones WN, and Butler JE: Epiphyseal fracture of the proximal humerus, JAMA 213:1476, 1970.

Bowen A: Plastic bowing of the clavicle in children, J Bone Joint Surg 65A:403, 1983.

Cahill BR, Tullos HS, and Fain RH: Little league shoulder, Am J Sports Med 2:150, 1974.

Campbell J and Almond HGA: Fracture-separation of the proximal humeral epiphysis, J Bone Joint Surg 59A:262, 1977.

Cozen L: Congenital dislocation of the shoulder and other anoma-lies, Arch Surg 35:956, 1937.

Dameron TB and Reibel DB: Fractures involving the proximal hu-meral epiphyseal plate, J Bone Joint Surg 51A:289, 1969.

Edmonson AS and Crenshaw AH: Campbell's operative ortho-paedics, vol 2, ed 6, St Louis, 1980, The CV Mosby Co.

Eidman DK, Siff SJ, and Tullos HS: Acromioclavicular lesions in children, Am J Sports Med 9:150, 1981.

Fairbanks HAT: Cranio-cleido dysostosis, J Bone Joint Surg 31B:608, 1949.

Falstie-Jensen S and Mikkelsen P: Pseudodislocation of the acromi-oclavicular joint, J Bone Joint Surg 64B:368, 1982.

Frosch L: Congenital subluxation of shoulder, Klin Wochenschr 4:701, 1925.

Gardner E and Gray DJ: Prenatal development of the human shoul-der and acromioclavicular joints, Am J Anat 92:219, 1953.

Ghormley RK, Black JR, and Cherry JH: Ununited fractures of the clavicle, Am J Surg 51:343, 1941.

Gibson DA and Carroll N: Congenital pseudarthrosis of the clavi-cle, J Bone Joint Surg 52B:629, 1970.

Green NE and Wheelhouse WW: Anterior subglenoid dislocation of the shoulder in an infant following pneumococcal meningitis, Clin Orthop 135:125, 1978.

Greig DM: True congenital dislocation of the shoulder, Edinburgh Med J 30:157, 1923.

Haliburton RA, Barber JR, and Fraser RL: Pseudodislocation: an un-usual birth injury, Can J Surg 10:455, 1967.

Havranek P: Injuries of the distal clavicular physis in children, J Pe-diatr Orthop 9:213, 1989.

Heck CC Jr: Anterior dislocation of the glenohumeral joint in a child, J Trauma 21:174, 1981.

Heinig CF: Retrosternal dislocation of the clavicle: early recogni-tion, x-ray diagnosis, and management, J Bone Joint Surg 50A:830, 1968.

Hohl JC: Fractures of the humerus in children, Orthop Clin North Am 7:557, 1976.

Holstein A and Lewis GB: Fractures of the humerus with radial nerve paralysis, J Bone Joint Surg 45A:1382, 1963.

Howard FM and Shafer SJ: Injuries to the clavicle with neurovascu-lar complications: a study of fourteen cases, J Bone Joint Surg 47A:1335, 1965.

Jablon M, Sutker A, and Post M: Irreducible fractures of the middle-third of the clavicle, J Bone Joint Surg 61A:296, 1979.

Jeffery CC: Fracture separation of the upper humeral epiphysis, Surg Gynecol Obstet 96:205, 1953.

Katznelson A, Nerubay J, and Oliver S: Dynamic fixation of the avulsed clavicle, J Trauma 16:841, 1976.

Lloyd-Roberts GC: Orthopoaedics in infancy and childhood, Lon-don, 1971, Butterworth.

Lloyd-Roberts GC, Apley AG, and Owen R: Reflections upon the aetiology of congenital pseudarthrosis of the clavicle, J Bone Joint Surg 57B:24, 1975.

McClure JG and Raney B: Anomalies of the scapula, Clin Orthop 110:22, 1975.

Moseley HF: The clavicle: its anatomy and function, Clin Orthop 58:17, 1968.

Neer CS II: Fractures of the distal third of the clavicle, Clin Orthop 58:43, 1968.

Neer CS II and Horowitz BS: Fractures of the proximal humeral epiphyseal plate, Clin Orthop 41:24, 1965.

Nicastro JF and Adair DM: Fracture dislocation of the shoulder in a 32 month old, J Pediatr Orthop 2:427, 1982.

Nilsson S and Svartholm F: Fracture of the upper end of the hu-merus in children, Acta Chir Scand 130:433, 1965.

Penn I: The vascular complications of fractures of the clavicle, J Trauma 4:819, 1964.

Peterson CA and Peterson HA: Analysis of the incidence of injuries to the epiphyseal growth plate, J Trauma 12:275, 1972.

Pollen AG: Fractures and dislocations in children, Baltimore, 1973, The Williams & Wilkins Co.

Rockwood CA: Dislocations of the sternoclavicular joint. In The American Academy of Orthopaedic Surgeons: Instructional course lectures, vol 24, St Louis, 1975, The CV Mosby Co.

Rockwood CA Jr: Fractures of the outer clavicle in children and adults, J Bone Joint Surg 64B:642, 1982.

Rockwood CA Jr: Fractures and dislocations of the shoulder. Part III. Fractures and dislocations of the ends of the clavicle, scapula, and glenohumeral joint. In Rockwood CA Jr, Wilkins KE, and King RE, editors: Fractures in children, Philadelphia, 1984, JB Lippincott Co.

Rockwood CA Jr and Green DP: Fractures, vol 1, Philadelphia, 1975, JB Lippincott Co.

Rowe CR: Prognosis in dislocation of the shoulder, J Bone Joint Surg 38A:957, 1956.

Rowe CR: Anterior dislocation of the shoulder: prognosis and treatment, Surg Clin North Am 43:1609, 1963.

Rowe CR, Pierce DS, and Clark JG: Voluntary dislocation of the shoulder, J Bone Joint Surg 55A:445, 1973.

Samilson RL: Congenital and developmental anomalies of the shoulder girdle, Orthop Clin North Am 11:219, 1980.

Sherk HH and Probst C: Fractures of the proximal humeral epiphysis, Orthop Clin North Am 6:401, 1975.

Visser JO and Rietberg M: Interposition of the tendon of the long head of biceps in fracture separation of the proximal humeral epiphysis, Neth J Surg 32:12, 1980.

Wagner KT and Lyne ED: Adolescent traumatic dislocations of the shoulder with open epiphysis, J Pediatr Orthop 3:61, 1983.

Wall JJ: Congenital pseudarthrosis of the clavicle, J Bone Joint Surg 52A:1003, 1970.

Wickstrom J: Birth injuries of the brachial plexus: treatment of defects in the shoulder, Clin Orthop 23:187, 1962.

Wilkes JA and Hoffer MM: Clavicle fractures in head-injured children, J Orthop Trauma 1:55, 1987.

Williams DJ: The mechanisms producing fracture separation of the proximal humeral epiphysis, J Bone Joint Surg 63B:102, 1981.

Zenni EJ, Krieg JK, and Rosen MJ: Open reduction and internal fixation of clavicular fractures, J Bone Joint Surg 63A:147, 1981.

Lateral condylar fractures

Badelon O et al: Lateral humeral condylar fractures in children: a report of 47 cases, J Pediatr Orthop 8:31, 1988.

Badger GF: Fractures of the lateral condyle of the humerus, J Bone Joint Surg 36B:147, 1954.

Beaty JH and Wood AB: Lateral condylar fractures: long-term results. Paper presented at the meeting of The American Academy of Orthopaedic Surgeons, Las Vegas, Jan 18, 1985.

Blount WP: Unusual fractures in children. In The American Academy of Orthopaedic Surgeons: Instructional course lectures, vol 7, Ann Arbor, Mich, 1954, JW Edwards Co.

Blount WP, Schalz I, and Cassidy RH: Fractures of the elbow in children, JAMA 146:699, 1951.

Boyd HB: Fractures about the elbow in children, Surg Gynecol Obstet 89:775, 1949.

Bright RW: Physeal fractures. In Rockwood CA Jr, King RE, and Wilkins KE, editors: Fractures in children, vol 3, Philadelphia, 1984, JB Lippincott Co.

Conner AN and Smith MG: Displaced fractures of the lateral humeral condyle in children, J Bone Joint Surg 52B:460, 1970

Crabbe WA: Treatment of fracture separation of the capitular epiphysis, J Bone Joint Surg 45B:722, 1963.

Fahey JJ: Fractures of the elbow in children. In The American Academy of Orthopaedic Surgeons: Instructional course lectures, vol 17, Ann Arbor, Mich, 1960, JW Edwards Co.

Flynn JC and Richards JF: Non-union of minimally displaced fractures of the lateral condyle of the humerus in children, J Bone Joint Surg 53A:1096, 1971.

Fontanelta P, Mackenzie A, and Rossman M: Missing and malunited fractures of the lateral humeral condyle in children, J Trauma 18:329, 1978.

Hardacre JA et al: Fractures of the lateral condyle of the humerus in children, J Bone Joint Surg 53A:1083, 1971.

Ingersoll R: Fractures of the humeral condyles in children, Clin Orthop 41:32, 1965.

Jakob R et al: Observations concerning fractures of the lateral humeral condyles in children, J Bone Joint Surg 57B:430, 1975.

Jeffery CC: Nonunion of the epiphysis of the lateral condyle of the humerus, J Bone Joint Surg 40B:396, 1958.

Jones KG: Percutaneous pin fixation of fractures of the lower end of humerus, Clin Orthop 50:53, 1967.

Kini M: Fractures of the lateral condyle of the lower end of the humerus with complications, J Bone Joint Surg 24:270, 1942.

Marcus NW and Agins HJ: Articular cartilage sleeve fracture of the lateral humeral condyle, J Pediatr Orthop 4:620, 1984.

Marion J et al: Les fractures de l'extremité inferieure de l'humerus chez l'enfant, Rev Clin Orthop 48:337, 1962.

Milch H: Treatment of humeral cubitus valgus, Clin Orthop 6:120, 1955.

Milch H: Fracture of external humeral condyle, JAMA 160:641, 1956.

Milch H: Fractures and fracture-dislocations of humeral condyles, J Trauma 4:592, 1964.

Rang M: Children's fractures, ed 2, Philadelphia, 1983, JB Lippincott Co.

Salter RB and Harris WR: Injuries involving the epiphyseal plate, J Bone Joint Surg 45A:587, 1963.

Sharp IK: Fractures of the lateral humeral condyle in children, Acta Orthop Belg 31:811, 1965.

Sharrard WJW: Pediatric orthopaedics and fractures, Oxford, UK, 1971, Blackwell Scientific Publications, Ltd.

Smith FM: Children's elbow injuries: fractures and dislocations, J Orthop 50:7, 1967.

Smith FM and Joyce JJ: Fracture of lateral condyle of the humerus in children, Am J Surg 87:324, 1954.

Speed JS: Surgical treatment of condylar fractures of the humerus. In The American Academy of Orthopaedic Surgeons: Instructional course lectures, vol 7, Ann Arbor, Mich, 1950, JW Edwards Co.

Speed JS and Macey HB: Fractures of the humeral condyles in children, J Bone Joint Surg 15:903, 1933.

Tachdjian MO: Pediatric orthopedics, Philadelphia, 1972, WB Saunders Co.

Wadsworth TG: Premature epiphyseal fusion after injury of the capitulum, J Bone Joint Surg 46B:46, 1964.

Wadsworth TG: Injuries of the capitular epiphysis, Clin Orthop 85:127, 1972.

Weber BG, Brunner C, and Freuler F: Treatment of fractures in children and adolescents, Berlin, 1980, Springer-Verlag.

Wilkins KE: Fractures and dislocations of the elbow region. In Rockwood CA Jr, Wilkins KE, and King RE: Fractures in children, Philadelphia, 1984, JB Lippincott Co.

Zeier FG: Lateral condylar fracture and its many complications, Orthop Rev 10:49, 1981.

Medial epicondylar and medial condylar fractures

Aitken AP and Childress HM: Intra-articular displacement of the internal epicondyle following dislocation, J Bone Joint Surg 20:161, 1938.

Beghin JL, Bucholz RW, and Wenger DR: Intercondylar fractures of the humerus in young children, J Bone Joint Surg 64A:1083, 1982.

Blount WP: Unusual fractures in children. In The American Academy of Orthopaedic Surgeons: Instructional course lectures, vol 7, Ann Arbor, Mich, 1954, JW Edwards Co.

Blount WP: Fractures in children, Baltimore, 1955, The Williams & Wilkins Co.

Brodeur AE, Silberstein MJ, and Graviss ER: Radiology of the pediatric elbow, Boston, 1981, GK Hall Medical Publisher.

Burnstein SM, King JD, and Sanderson RA: Fractures of the medial epicondyle of the humerus, Contemp Orthop 3:7, July 1981.

Chacha PB: Fractures of the medial condyle of the humerus with rotational displacement, J Bone Joint Surg 52A:1453, 1970.

Chapchal G, editor: Fractures in children, New York, 1981, Thieme-Stratton.

Chessare JW et al: Injuries of the medial epicondylar ossification center of the humerus, Am J Roentgenol 129:49, 1977.

Cothay PM: Injury to the lower medial epiphysis of the humerus before development of the ossific center: report of a case, J Bone Joint Surg 49B:766, 1967.

Dangles C, Tylkowski C, and Pankovich AM: Epicondylotrochlear fracture of the humerus before the appearance of the ossification center, Clin Orthop 171:161, 1982.

Dunlop J: Traumatic separation of medial epicondyle of the humerus in adolescence, J Bone Joint Surg 17:577, 1935.

El Ghawabi MH: Fracture of the medial condyle of the humerus, J Bone Joint Surg 57A:677, 1975.

Eppright RH and Wilkins KE: Fractures and dislocations of the elbow. In Rockwood CA and Green DP, editors: Fractures, vol 1, Philadelphia, 1975, JB Lippincott Co.

Fahey JJ Fractures of the elbow in children, In The American Academy of Orthopaedic Surgeons: Instructional course lectures, vol 17, Ann Arbor, Mich, 1960, JW Edwards Co.

Fahey JJ and O'Brien E: Fracture-separation of the medial humeral condyle in a child confused with fracture of the medial epicondyle, J Bone Joint Surg 53A:1102, 1971.

Fowles JV and Kassab M: Displaced fractures of the medial humeral condyle in children, J Bone Joint Surg 62A:1159, 1980.

Fowles JV, Kassab MT, and Moula T: Untreated intra-articular entrapment of the medial humeral epicondyle, J Bone Joint Surg 66B:562, 1984.

Grant IR and Miller JS: Osteochondral fracture of the trochlea associated with fracture dislocation of the elbow, Injury 6:257, 1975.

Hines RF, Herndon WA, and Evans JP: Operative treatment of medial epicondyle fractures in children, Clin Orthop 223:170, 1987.

Holmberg L: Fractures in the distal end of the humerus in children, Acta Chir Scand Suppl 103,1945.

Ingersoll RE: Fractures of the humeral condyles in children, Clin Orthop 41:32, 1965.

Jarvis JD and D'Astous JL: Pediatric T-supracondylar fracture, J Pediatr Orthop 4:697, 1984.

Johansson O: Capsular and ligament injuries of the elbow joint, Acta Chir Scand Suppl 287, 1962.

Johansson J and Rosman M: Fracture of the capitulum humeri in children: a rare diagnosis, often misdiagnosed, Clin Orthop 146:157, 1980.

Kilfoyle FM: Fractures of the medial condyle and epicondyle of the elbow in children, Clin Orthop 41:43, 1965.

Maylahn DJ and Fahey JJ: Fracture of the elbow in children, JAMA 166:220, 1958.

Milch H: Fractures and fracture-dislocations of humeral condyles, J Trauma 4:592, 1964.

Ogden JA: Skeletal injury in the child, Philadelphia, 1982, Lea & Febiger.

Papavasiliou V, Nenopoulos S, and Venturis T: Fractures of the medial condyle of the humerus in childhood, J Pediatr Orthop 7:421, 1987.

Patrick J: Fracture of the medial epicondyle with displacement into the elbow joint, J Bone Joint Surg 28:143, 1946.

Peterson HA: Triplane fracture of the distal humeral epiphysis, J Pediatr Orthop 3:81, 1983.

Pollen AG: Fractures and dislocations in children, Baltimore, 1973, The Williams & Wilkins Co.

Rang M: Children's fractures, ed 2, Philadelphia, 1983, JB Lippincott Co.

Schwab GH et al: Biomechanics of elbow instability: the role of the medial colleteral ligament, Clin Orthop 146:42, 1980.

Silberstein JJ, Brodeur AE, and Graviss ER: Some vagaries of the lateral epicondyle, J Bone Joint Surg 64A:444, 1982.

Silberstein JJ et al: Some vagaries of the medial epicondyle, J Bone Joint Surg 63A:524, 1981.

Smith FM: Medial epicondyle injuries, JAMA 142:396, 1950.

Varma BP and Srivastava TP: Fractures of the medial condyle of the humerus in children: a report of 4 cases, including the late sequelae, Injury 4:171, 1972.

Watson-Jones R: Fractures and joint injuries, ed 3, Baltimore, 1946, The Williams & Wilkins Co.

Watson-Jones R: Fractures and joint injuries, ed 4, Baltimore, 1960, The Williams & Wilkins Co.

Whipple TL, Evans JP, and Urbaniak JR: Irreducible dislocation of a finger joint in a child, J Bone Joint Surg 62A:832, 1980.

Wood VE: Fractures of the hand in children, Orthop Clin North Am 7:527, 1976.

Woods GM and Tullos HG: Elbow instability and medial epicondyle fracture, Am J Sports Med 5:23, 1977.

Supracondylar fractures

Abe M: Arthrography of the elbow joint; its diagnostic value for the traumatic lesions of the elbow in children, J Jpn Orthop Assoc 53:1721, 1979.

Abraham E et al: Experimental hyperextension supracondylar fractures in monkeys, Clin Orthop 171:309, 1982.

Allen PD and Gramse AE: Transcondylar fractures of the humerus treated by Dunlop traction, Am J Surg 67:217, 1945.

Amspacher JC and Messenbaugh JF Jr: Supracondylar osteotomy of the humerus for correction of rotational and angular deformities of the elbow, South Med J 57:846, 1964.

Arino VL et al: Percutaneous fixation of supracondylar fractures of the humerus in children, J Bone Joint Surg 59A:914, 1977.

Arkbarnia BA et al: Arthrography for pediatric elbow injury diagnoses, Orthop Today 4(9):6, 1984.

Arnold JA, Nasca RJ, and Nelson CL: Supracondylar fractures of the humerus, J Bone Joint Surg 59A:589, 1977.

Aronson DD and Prager BI: Supracondylar fractures of the humerus in children: a modified technique for closed pinning, Clin Orthop 219:174, 1987.

Ashurst APC: An anatomical and surgical study of fractures of the lower end of the humerus, Philadelphia, 1910, Lea & Febiger.

Barrett WP, Almquist EA, and Staheli LT: Fracture separation of the distal humeral epiphysis in the newborn, J Pediatr Orthop 4:617, 1984.

Basom WC: Supracondylar and transcondylar fractures in children, Clin Orthop 1:43, 1953.

Beals RK: The normal carrying angle of the elbow, Clin Orthop 119:194, 1976.

Bellemore MC et al: Supracondylar osteotomy of the humerus with correction of cubitus varus, J Bone Joint Surg 66B:566, 1984.

Blount WP: Fractures in children. In The American Academy of Orthopaedic Surgeons: Instructional course lectures, vol 7, Ann Arbor, Mich, 1950, JW Edwards Co.

Blount WP: Unusual fractures in children. In The American Academy of Orthopaedic Surgeons: Instructional course lectures, vol 11, Ann Arbor, Mich, 1954, JW Edwards Co.

Bosanquet JS and Middleton RW: The reduction of supracondylar fractures of the humerus in children treated by traction-in-extension, Injury 14:373, 1983.

Bowman JM and Weiner GS: Neonatal fracture separation of the distal humeral chondral epiphysis: case report, Orthopaedics 3:875, 1980.

Boyd HB and Altenberg AR: Fractures about the elbow in children, Arch Surg 49:213, 1944.

Bright RW: Epiphyseal-plate cartilage: a biochemical and histological analysis of failure modes, J Bone Joint Surg 56A:688, 1974.

Carcassonne M, Bergoin M, and Hornung H: Result of operative treatment of severe supracondylar fractures of the elbow in children, J Pediatr Surg 7:676, 1972.

Carlson CS and Rosman MA: Cubitus varus: a new and simple technique for correction, J Pediatr Orthop 2:199, 1982.

Casiano E: Reduction and fixation by pinning "banderillero," Milit Med 125:262, 1961.

Chand K: Epiphyseal separation of the distal humeral epiphysis in an infant, J Trauma 14:521, 1974.

D'Ambrosia RD: Supracondylar fractures of the humerus: prevention of cubitus varus, J Bone Joint Surg 54A:60, 1972.

Dameron TB: Transverse fractures of the distal humerus in children. In The American Academy of Orthopaedic Surgeons: Instructional course lectures, vol 30, St Louis, 1981. The CV Mosby Co.

Danielsson L and Pettersson H: Open reduction and pin fixation of severely displaced supracondylar fractures of the humerus in children, Acta Orthop Scand 51:249, 1980.

DeLee JC et al: Fracture-separation of the distal humerus epiphysis, J Bone Joint Surg 62A:46, 1980.

DeRosa GP and Graziano GP: A new osteotomy for cubitus varus, Clin Orthop 236:160, 1988.

Dodge HS: Displaced supracondylar fractures of the humerus in children: treatment by Dunlop's traction, J Bone Joint Surg 54A:1408, 1972.

Dowd GSE and Hopcroft PW: Varus deformity in supracondylar fractures of the humerus in children, Injury 10:297, 1978.

Downs DM and Wirth CR: Fracture of the distal humeral chondral epiphysis in the neonate, Clin Orthop 169:155, 1982.

Eaton RG and Green WT: Epimysiotomy and fasciotomy in the treatment of Volkmann's ischemic contracture, Orthop Clin North Am 3:175, 1972.

El-Ahwany MD: Supracondylar fractures of the humerus in children with a note on the surgical correction of late cubitus varus, Injury 6:45, 1974.

El-Sharkawi H and Fattah HA: Treatment of displaced supracondylar fractures of the humerus in children in full extension and supination, J Bone Joint Surg 47B:273, 1965.

Elstrom JA, Pankovich AM, and Kassab M: Irreducible supracondylar fracture of the humerus in children, J Bone Joint Surg 57A:680, 1975.

Flynn JC, Matthews JG, and Benoit RL: Blind pinning of displaced supracondylar fractures of the humerus in children, J Bone Joint Surg 56A:263, 1974.

Fowles JV and Kassab MT: Displaced supracondylar fractures of the elbow in children, J Bone Joint Surg 56B:490, 1974.

French PR: Varus deformity of elbow following supracondylar fractures of the humerus in children, Lancet 2:439, 1959.

Fuller DJ and McCullough CJ: Malunited fractures of the forearm in children, J Bone Joint Surg 64B:364, 1982.

Gartland JJ: Management of supracondylar fractures of the humerus in children, Surg Gynecol Obstet 109:145, 1959.

Gelberman RH et al: Compartment syndromes of the forearm: diagnosis and treatment, Clin Orthop 161:252, 1981.

Graham HA: Supracondylar fractures of the elbow in children. I. Clin Orthop 54:85, 1967.

Graham HA: Supracondylar fractures of the elbow in children. II. Clin Orthop 54:93, 1967.

Graves SC and Beaty JH: Supracondylar fractures of the humerus in children: treatment by closed reduction and percutaneous pinning. Paper presented at the 56th annual meeting of The American Academy of Orthopaedic Surgeons, Las Vegas, Feb 11, 1989.

Griffin PP: Supracondylar fractures of the humerus, Pediatr Clin North Am 22:477, 1975.

Gruber MA and Hudson OC: Supracondylar fracture of the humerus in childhood, J Bone Joint Surg 46A:1245, 1964.

Haddad RJ, Saer JK, and Riordan DC: Percutaneous pinning of displaced supracondylar fractures of the elbow in children, Clin Orthop 71:112, 1970.

Hansen PE, Barnes DA, and Tullos HS: Arthroscopic diagnosis of an injury pattern in the distal humerus of an infant, J Pediatr Orthop 2:569, 1982.

Herzenberg JE et al: Biomechanical testing of pin fixation in pediatric supracondylar elbow fractures. Paper presented at the 55th annual meeting of The American Academy of Orthopaedic Surgeons, Atlanta, Feb 5, 1988.

Holda ME, Manoli A, and LaMont RL, Epiphyseal separation of the distal end of the humerus with medial displacement, J Bone Joint Surg 62A:52, 1980.

Ippolito E, Caterini R, and Scola E: Supracondylar fractures of the humerus in children: analysis at maturity of fifty-three patients treated conservatively, J Bone Joint Surg 68A:333, 1986.

Jones KG: Percutaneous pin fixation of fractures of the lower end of the humerus, Clin Orthop 50:53, 1967.

Kamal AS and Austin RT: Dislocation of the median nerve and brachial artery in supracondylar fractures of the humerus, Injury 12:161, 1980.

Kaplan SS and Reckling FW: Fracture separation of the lower humeral epiphysis with medial displacement, J Bone Joint Surg 53A:1105, 1971.

Kekomäki M et al: Operative reduction and fixation of difficult supracondylar extension fracture, J Pediatr Orthop 4:13, 1984.

King D and Secor C: Bow elbow (cubitus varus), J Bone Joint Surg 33A:572, 1951.

Kramhøft M, Keller IL, and Solgaard S: Displaced supracondylar fractures of the humerus in children, Clin Orthop 221:215, 1987.

Kristensen JL and Vibild O: Supracondylar fractures of the humerus in children, Acta Orthop Scand 47:375, 1976.

LaBelle H et al: Cubitus varus deformity following supracondylar fractures of the humerus in children, J Pediatr Orthop 2:539, 1982.

Langenskiöld A and Kivilaakso R: Varus and valgus deformity of the elbow following supracondylar fracture of the humerus, Acta Orthop Scand 38:313, 1967.

Liddell WA: Neurovascular complications in widely displaced supracondylar fractures of the humerus, J Bone Joint Surg 49B:806, 1967.

Macafee AL: Infantile supracondylar fracture, J Bone Joint Surg 49B:768, 1967.

Marion J et al: Les fractures de l'extrémité inferieure de l'humerus chez l'enfant, Rev Chir Orthop 48:337, 1962.

Marmor L and Bechtol CO: Fracture separation of the lower humeral epiphysis, J Bone Joint Surg 42A:333, 1960.

Mauer I, Kolovos D, and Loscos R: Epiphysiolysis of the distal humerus in a newborn, Bull Hosp Jt Dis 28:109, 1967.

Menon TJ: Fracture separation of the lower humeral epiphysis due to birth injury: a case report, Injury 14:168, 1982.

Micheli LS, Hall JE, and Skolnick MD: Supracondylar fractures of the humerus in children, Orthopedics 3:395, 1980.

Miller HG and Wilkins KE: The supracondylar fracture of the humerus in children: an analysis of complications, Unpublished manuscript, 1979.

Mizuno K, Hirohata K, and Kashiwagi D: Fracture-separation of the distal humeral epiphysis in young children, J Bone Joint Surg 61A:570, 1979.

Mubarak SJ and Hargens AR: Compartment syndromes and Volkmann's contracture, Philadelphia, 1981, WB Saunders Co.

Norell HG: Roentgenologic visualization of extracapsular fat: its importance in the diagnosis of traumatic injuries to the elbow, Acta Radiol 42:205, 1954.

O'Brien WR et al: The metaphyseal-diaphyseal angle as a guide to treating supracondylar fractures of the humerus in children. Presented at the 54th annual meeting of The American Academy of Orthopaedic Surgeons, San Francisco, Jan 23, 1987.

Oppenheim GE Jr et al: Supracondylar humeral osteotomy for traumatic childhood cubitus varus deformity, Clin Orthop 188:34, 1984.

Ormandy L: Olecranon screw for skeletal traction of the humerus, Am J Surg 127:615, 1974.

Palmer EE et al: Supracondylar fracture of the humerus in children, J Bone Joint Surg 60A:653, 1978.

Peiro A et al: Fracture-separation of the lower humeral epiphysis in young children, Acta Orthop Scand 52:295, 1981.

Peterson CA and Peterson HA: Analysis of the incidence of injuries to the epiphyseal growth plate, J Trauma 12:275, 1972.

Pirone AM, Graham HK, and Krajbich JI: Management of displaced extension-type supracondylar fractures of the humerus in children, J Bone Joint Surg 70A:641, 1988.

Prietto CA: Supracondylar fractures of the humerus: a comparative study of Dunlop's traction versus percutaneous pinning, J Bone Joint Surg 61A:425, 1979.

Ramsey RH and Griz J: Immediate open reduction and internal fixation of severely displaced supracondylar fractures of the humerus in children, Clin Orthop 90:131, 1973.

Rang M et al: Symposium: management of displaced supracondylar fractures of the humerus, Contemp Orthop 18:497, 1989.

Rogers LF: Fractures and dislocations of the elbow, Semin Roentgenol 13:97, 1978.

Rogers LF and Rockwood CA: Separation of the entire distal humeral epiphysis, Radiology 106:393, 1973.

Rogers LF et al: Plastic bowing, torus, and greenstick supracondylar fractures of the humerus: radiographic clues to obscure fractures of the elbow in children, Radiology 128:145, 1978.

Rorabeck CH: A practical approach to compartment syndromes. Part III: Management. In The American Academy of Orthopaedic Surgeons: Instructional course lectures, vol 33, St Louis, 1983, The CV Mosby Co.

Shifrin PG, Gehring HW, and Iglesias LJ: Open reduction and internal fixation of displaced supracondylar fractures of the humerus in children, Orthop Clin North Am 7:573, 1976.

Silberstein MJ et al: Some vagaries of the capitellum, J Bone Joint Surg 61A:244, 1979.

Skolnick MD, Hall JE, and Micheli LJ: Supracondylar fractures of the humerus in children, Orthopedics 3:395, 1980.

Smith FM: Children's elbow injuries: fractures and dislocations, Clin Orthop 50:7, 1967.

Smith L: Deformity following supracondylar fractures of the humerus, J Bone Joint Surg 42A:235, 1960.

Spinner M and Schreiber SN: Anterior interosseous nerve paralysis as a complication of supracondylar fractures of the humerus in children, J Bone Joint Surg 51A:1584, 1969.

Stanitski CL and Micheli LS: Simultaneous ipsilateral fractures of the arm and forearm in children, Clin Orthop 153:218, 1980.

Swenson AL: The treatment of supracondylar fractures of the humerus by Kirschner wire transfixion, J Bone Joint Surg 30A:993, 1948.

Symeonides PP et al: Recurrent dislocation of the elbow, J Bone Joint Surg 57A:1084, 1975.

Thorndike A and Dimmler CL: Fractures of the forearm and elbow in children: an analysis of three hundred and sixty-four consecutive cases, N Engl J Med 225:475, 1941.

Vasli LR: Diagnosis of vascular injury in children with supracondylar fractures of the humerus, Injury 19:11, 1988.

Webb AJ and Sherman FC: Supracondylar fractures of the humerus in children, J Pediatr Orthop 9:315, 1989.

Weber BG, Brunner C, and Freuler F: Treatment of fractures in children and adolescents, Berlin, 1980, Springer-Verlag.

Weiland AJ et al: Surgical treatment of displaced supracondylar fractures of the humerus in children, J Bone Joint Surg 60A:657, 1978.

Worlock PH and Colton C: Severely displaced supracondylar fractures of the humerus in children: a simple method of treatment, J Pediatr Orthop 7:49, 1987.

Yates C and Sullivan JA: Arthrography for pediatric elbow injury diagnosis, Orthop Today 4:9, 1984.

Yates C and Sullivan JA: Arthrographic diagnosis of elbow injuries in children, J Pediatr Orthop 7:54, 1987.

Elbow dislocations, metaphyseal and epiphyseal olecranon fractures, and radial head and neck fractures

Almquist EE, Gordon LH, and Blue AI: Congenital dislocation of the head of the radius, J Bone Joint Surg 51A1118, 1969.

Angelov A: A new method for treatment of the dislocated radial neck fracture in children. In Chapchal G, editor: Fractures in children, New York, 1981, Thieme-Stratton.

Beverly HC and Fearn CB: Anterior interosseous nerve plasy and dislocation of the elbow, Injury 16:126, 1984.

Blatz DJ: Anterior dislocation of the elbow, Orthop Rev 10:129, 1981.

Blount WP: Fractures in children. In The American Academy of Orthopaedic Surgeons: Instructional course lectures, vol 7, Ann Arbor, Mich, 1950, JB Edwards Co.

Blount WP: Fracture of the elbow in children, JAMA 146:699, 1951.

Blount WP: Fractures in children, Baltimore, 1955, The Williams & Wilkins Co.

Brodeur AE, Silberstein MJ, and Graviss ER: Radiology of the pediatric elbow, Boston, 1981, GK Hall, Medical Publisher.

Canale ST and Graves S: Olecronan fractures in children. Paper presented at The American Orthopedic Association Residents' Conference, Washington, DC, Nov 3-4, 1989.

DeLee JC: Transverse divergent dislocation of the elbow in a child, J Bone Joint Surg 63A:322, 1981.

Dougall AJ: Severe fracture of the neck of the radius in children, J R Coll Surg Edinb 14:220, 1969.

Durig M, Gauer EF, and Müller W: Die Operative Behandlung der Resdivierenden und Traumatischen Luxation des Ellenbogengelenkes nach Osborne und Cotterill, Arch Orthop Trauma Surg 86:141, 1976.

Evans E: Pronation injuries of the forearm with special attention to the anterior Monteggia fracture: clinical experimental study, J Bone Joint Surg 31B:578, 1949.

Fahey JJ: Fractures of the elbow in children. In The American Academy of Orthopaedic Surgeons: Instructional course lectures, Ann Arbor, Mich, 1960, JB Edwards Co.

Fielding JW: Radio-ulnar union following displacement of the proximal radial epiphysis, J Bone Joint Surg 46A:1277, 1964.

Fowles JV and Kassab MT: Observations concerning radial neck fractures in children, J Pediatr Orthop 6:51, 1986.

Fowles JV, Kassab MT, and Moula T: Untreated posterior dislocation of the elbow in children, J Bone Joint Surg 66A:921, 1984.

Galbraith KA and McCullough CJ: Acute nerve injury as a complication of closed fractures or dislocations of the elbow, Injury 11:159, 1979.

Gaston SR, Smith FM, and Boab OD: Epiphyseal injuries of the radial head and neck, Am J Surg 85:266, 1953.

Grant IR and Miller JH: Osteochondral fracture of the trochlea associated with fracture-dislocation of the elbow, Injury 6:257, 1975.

Grantham SA and Kiernan HA: Displaced olecranon fractures in children, J Trauma 15:197, 1975.

Hallet J: Entrapment of the median nerve after dislocation of the elbow, J Bone Joint Surg 63B:408, 1981.

Hamilton W and Parkes JC II: Isolated dislocation of the radial head without fracture of the ulna, Clin Orthop 97:94, 1973.

Harvey S and Tchélébi, H: Proximal radio-ulnar translocation: a case report, J Bone Joint Surg 61A:447, 1979.

Hassmann GC, Brunn F, and Neer CS II: Recurrent dislocation of the elbow, J Bone Joint Surg 57A:1080, 1975.

Henderson RS and Robertson IM: Open dislocation of the elbow with rupture of the brachial artery, J Bone Joint Surg 34B:636, 1952.

Hennig K and Franke D: Posterior displacement of brachial artery following closed elbow dislocation, J Trauma 20:96, 1980.

Henrikson B: Isolated fracture of the proximal end of the radius in children, Acta Orthop Scand 40:246, 1969.

Hirayama T et al: Operation for chronic dislocation of the radial head in children: reduction by osteotomy of the ulna, J Bone Joint Surg 69B:639, 1987.

Hume AC: Anterior dislocation of the head of the radius associated with undisplaced fracture of the olecranon in children, J Bone Joint Surg 39B:508, 1957.

Jacobs RL: Recurrent dislocation of the elbow joint, Clin Orthop 74:151, 1971.

Jakob R et al: Observations concerning fractures of the lateral humeral condyle in children, J Bone Joint Surg 57B:430, 1975.

Jeffery CC: Fracture of the head of the radius in children, J Bone Joint Surg 32B:314, 1950.

Johansson O: Capsular and ligament injuries of the elbow joint: a clinical arthrographic study, Acta Chir Scand Suppl 287, 1962.

Jones ERW and Esah M: Displaced fracture of the neck of the radius in children, J Bone Joint Surg 53B:429, 1971.

Kapel O: Operation for habitual dislocation of the elbow, J Bone Joint Surg 33A:707, 1951.

Kilburn P, Sweeney JG, and Silk FF: Three cases of compound posterior dislocation of the elbow with rupture of the brachial artery, J Bone Joint Surg 44B:119, 1962.

King T: Recurrent dislocation of the elbow, J Bone Joint Surg 35B:50, 1953.

Krishnamoorthy S, Bose K, and Wong KP: Treatment of old unreduced dislocation of the elbow, Injury 8:39, 1976.

Larsen LJ, Schottstaedt ER, and Bost FC: Multiple congenital dislocations associated with characteristic facial abnormality, J Pediatr 37:574, 1950.

Lewis RW and Thibodeau AA: Deformity of the wrist following resection of the radial head, Surg Gynecol Obstet 64:1079, 1937.

Lindhan S and Hugasson C: Significance of associated lesions including dislocation of fracture of the neck of the radius in children, Acta Orthop Scand 50:79, 1979.

Linscheid RL and Wheeler DK: Elbow dislocations, JAMA 194:113, 1965.

Lloyd-Roberts GC and Bucknill TM: Anterior dislocation of the radial head in children, J Bone Joint Surg 59B:402, 1977.

MacSween WA: Transposition of radius and ulna associated with dislocation of the elbow in a child, Injury 10:314, 1978.

Mannerfelt L: Median nerve entrapment after dislocation of the elbow, J Bone Joint Surg 50B:152, 1968.

Manske PR: Unreduced isolated radial head dislocation in a child, Orthopedics 5:1327, 1982.

Mantle JA: Recurrent posterior dislocation of the elbow, J Bone Joint Surg 48B:590, 1966.

Mardam-Bey T and Ger E: Congenital radial head dislocation, J Hand Surg 4:316, 1979.

Matev I: A radiological sign of entrapment of the median nerve in the elbow joint after posterior dislocation, J Bone Joint Surg 58B:353, 1976.

Matthews JG: Fractures of the olecranon in children, Injury 12:207, 1980.

McFarland B: Congenital dislocation of the head of the radius, Br J Surg 24:41, 1936.

Milch H: Bilateral recurrent dislocation of the ulna at the elbow, J Bone Joint Surg 18:777, 1936.

Neviaser JS and Wickstrom JK: Dislocation of the elbow: a retrospective study of 115 patients, South Med J 70:172, 1977.

Neviaser RJ and LeFevre GW: Irreducible isolated dislocation of the radial head, Clin Orthop 80:72, 1971.

Newell RLM: Olecranon fractures in children, Injury 7:33, 1975.

Newman JH: Displaced radial neck fractures in children, Injury 9:114, 1977.

O'Brien PI: Injuries involving the radial epiphysis, Clin Orthop 41:51, 1965.

Osborne G and Cotterill P: Recurrent dislocation of the elbow, J Bone Joint Surg 48B:340, 1966.

Papavasiliou VA, Beslikas TA, and Nenopoulos S: Isolated fractures of the olecranon in children, Injury 18:100, 1987.

Parvin RW: Closed reduction of common shoulder and elbow dislocations without anesthesia, Arch Surg 75:972, 1957.

Patterson RF: Treatment of displaced transverse fractures of the neck of the radius in children, J Bone Joint Surg 16:695, 1934.

Pesudo JV, Aracil J, and Barcelo M: Leverage method in displaced fractures of the radial neck, Clin Orthop 169:215, 1982.

Poland J: A practical treatise on traumatic separation of the epiphyses, London 1898, Smith, Elder & Co.

Pollen AG: Fractures and dislocations in children, Baltimore, 1973, The Williams & Wilkins Co.

Pritchard DJ, Linscheid RL, and Svien HJ: Intraarticular median nerve entrapment with dislocation of the elbow, Clin Orthop 90:100, 1973.

Rang M: Children's fractures, ed 2, Philadelphia, 1983, JB Lippincott Co.

Reichenheim PP: Transplantation of the biceps tendon as a treatment of recurrent dislocation of the elbow, Br J Surg 35:201, 1947.

Roberts PH: Dislocation of the elbow, Br J Surg 56:806, 1969.

Schubert JJ: Dislocation of the radial head in the newborn infant, J Bone Joint Surg 47A:1019, 1965.

Schwab GH et al: Biomechanics of elbow instability: the role of the medial collateral ligament, Clin Orthop 146:42, 1980.

Scullion JE: Delayed union following fracture of neck of the radius in children, Unpublished manuscript, 1981.

Silberstein MJ et al: Some vagaries of the olecranon, J Bone Joint Surg 63A:722, 1981.

Smith FM: Children's elbow injuries: fractures and dislocation, Clin Orthop 50:7, 1967.

Speed JS: An operation for unreduced posterior dislocation of the elbow, South Med J 18:193, 1925.

Speed JS and Boyd HB: Fractures about the elbow, Am J Surg 38:727, 1937.

Speed K: Fracture of the head of the radius, Am J Surg 38:157, 1924.

Steinberg EL et al: Radial head and neck fractures in children, J Pediatr Orthop 8:35, 1988.

Stelling FH and Cote RH: Traumatic dislocation of head of radius in children, JAMA 160:732, 1956.

Støren G: Traumatic dislocation of the radial head as an isolated lesion in children, Acta Chir Scand 116:114, 1959.

Symeonides PP et al: Recurrent dislocation of the elbow, J Bone Joint Surg 57A:1084, 1975.

Tachdjian MO: Pediatric orthopedics, Philadelphia, 1972, WB Saunders Co.

Thompson HC and Garcia A: Myostitis ossificans: aftermath of elbow injuries, Clin Orthop 50:129, 1967.

Tibone JE and Stoltz M: Fracture of the radial head and neck in children, J Bone Joint Surg 63A:100, 1981.

Trias A and Comeau Y: Recurrent dislocation of the elbow in children, Clin Orthop 100:74, 1974.

Vahvanen V: Fracture of the radial neck in children, Acta Orthop Scand 49:32, 1978.

Vesely DG: Isolated traumatic dislocations of the radial head in children, Clin Orthop 50:31, 1967.

Vostal O: Fracture of the neck of the radius in children, Acta Chir Traumatol Cech 37:294, 1970.

Wedge JH and Robertson DE: Displaced fractures of the neck of the radius, J Bone Joint Surg 64B:256, 1982.

Wheeler DK and Linscheid RL: Fracture-dislocations of the elbow, Clin Orthop 50:95, 1967.

Wiley JJ, Pegington J, and Horwich JP: Traumatic dislocation of the radius at the elbow, J Bone Joint Surg 56B:501, 1974.

Wilkins KE: Fractures and dislocations of the elbow region. In Rockwood CA Jr, Wilkins KE, and King RE, editors: Fractures in children, Philadelphia, 1984, JB Lippincott Co.

Wirth CJ and Keyl W: Fractures of dislocations of the radial head. In Chapchal G, editor: Fractures in children, New York, 1981, Thieme-Stratton.

Wood SK: Reversal of the radial head during reduction of fractures of the neck of the radius in children, J Bone Joint Surg 51B:707, 1969.

Zimmerman H: Fractures of the elbow. In Weber BG, Brunner C, and Freuler F, editors: Treatment of fractures in children and adolescent. New York, 1980, Springer-Verlag.

Monteggia and Galeazzi fractures

Bado JL: The Monteggia lesion, Springfield, Ill, 1962, Charles C Thomas, Publisher.

Bado JL: The Monteggia lesion, Clin Orthop 50:71, 1967.

Barquet A and Caresani J: Fracture of the shaft of ulna and radius with associated dislocation of the radial head, Injury 12:471, 1980.

Bell-Tawse AJS: The treatment of malunited anterior Monteggia fractures in children, J Bone Joint Surg 47B:718, 1965.

Boyd HB: Surgical exposure of the ulna and proximal third of the radius through one incision, Surg Gynecol Obstet 71:86, 1940.

Boyd HB and Boals JC: The Monteggia lesion: a review of 159 cases, Clin Orthop 66:94, 1969.

Bruce HE, Harvey JP Jr, and Wilson JC Jr: Monteggia fractures, J Bone Joint Surg 56A:1563, 1974.

Bryan RS: Monteggia fractures of the forearm, J Trauma 11:992, 1971.

Evans E: Pronation injuries of the forearm with special attention to the anterior Monteggia fracture: clinical experimental study, J Bone Joint Surg 31B:578, 1949.

Fahmy NRM: Unusual Monteggia lesions in children, Injury 12:399, 1980.

Galeazzi R: Di una particulare sindrome: traumatica delle scheletro dell avambraccio, Attie Mem Soc Lombardi di Chir 2:12, 1934.

Hurst LC and Dubrow EN: Surgical treatment of symptomatic chronic radial head dislocation: a neglected Monteggia fracture, J Pediatr Orthop 3:227, 1983.

Jessing P: Monteggia lesions and their complicating nerve damage, Acta Orthop Scand 46:601, 1975.

King RE: Fractures of the shafts of the radius and ulna. In Rockwood CA Jr, Wilkins KE, and King RE, editors: Fractures in children, Philadelphia, 1984, JB Lippincott Co.

Letts M, Locht R, and Weins J: Monteggia fracture-dislocations in children, J Bone Joint Surg 67B:724, 1985.

Lichter RL and Jacobsen T: Tardy palsy of posterior interosseous nerve with a Monteggia fracture, J Bone Joint Surg 57A:124, 1975.

Lloyd-Roberts GC and Bucknill TM: Anterior dislocation of the radial head in children, J Bone Joint Surg 59B:402, 1977.

May V and Mauck W: Dislocation of the radial head with associated fracture of the ulna, South Med J 54:1255, 1961.

Mikic ZD: Galeazzi fracture-dislocation, J Bone Joint Surg 57A:107, 1975.

Monteggia AB: Instit Chirurg 5:130, 1814.

Olney BW and Menelaus MB: Monteggia and equivalent lesions in childhood, J Pediatr Orthop 9:219, 1989.

Peiro A, Andres F, and Fernandez-Esteve F: Acute Monteggia lesions in children, J Bone Joint Surg 59A:92, 1977.

Penrose JH: The Monteggia fracture with posterior dislocation of the radial head, J Bone Joint Surg 33B:65, 1951.

Ramsey RH and Pedersen HE: The Monteggia fracture-dislocation in children, JAMA 182:115, 1962.

Reckling FW: Unstable fracture-dislocations of the forearm (Monteggia and Galeazzi lesions), J Bone Joint Surg 64A:857, 1982.

Speed JS and Boyd HB: Treatment of fractures of the ulna with dislocation of the head of the radius (Monteggia fracture), JAMA 115:1900, 1940.

Spinner M, Freundlich BD, and Teicher J: Posterior interosseous nerve palsy as a complication of Monteggia fractures in children, Clin Orthop 58:141, 1968.

Stein F, Grabias SL, and Deffer PA: Nerve injuries complicating Monteggia lesions, J Bone Joint Surg 53A:1432, 1971.

Theodorou SD, Ierodiaconou MN, and Roussis N: Fracture of the upper end of the ulna associated with dislocation of the head of the radius in children, Clin Orthop 22:240, 1988.

Thompson HA and Hamilton AT: Monteggia fracture: internal fixation of fractured ulna with intramedullary pin, Am J Surg 79:579, 1950.

Walsh HPJ, McLaren CAN, and Owen R: Galeazzi fractures in children, J Bone Joint Surg 69B:730, 1987.

Wiley JJ and Galey JP: Monteggia injuries in children, J Bone Joint Surg 67B:728, 1985.

Forearm fractures

Aitken AP: The end results of the fractured distal radial epiphysis, J Bone Joint Surg 17:302, 1935.

Albert SM, Wohl MA, and Rechtman AM: Treatment of the disrupted radio-ulnar joint, J Bone Joint Surg 45A:1373, 1963.

Almquist EE, Gordon LH, and Blue AI: Congenital dislocation of the head of the radius, J Bone Joint Surg 51A:1118, 1969.

Alpar EK et al: Midshaft fractures of forearm bones in children, Injury 13:153, 1981.

Arunachalam VSP and Griffiths JC: Fracture recurrence in children, Injury 7:37, 1975.

Beekman F and Sullivan JE: Some observations on fractures of long bones in children, Am J Surg 51:722, 1941.

Blount WP: Fractures of the forearm in children, Pediatr Clin North Am 2:1097, 1955.

Blount WP: Forearm fractures in children, Clin Orthop 51:93, 1967.

Borden S: Roentgen recognition of acute plastic bowing of the forearm in children, Am J Roentgenol 125:524, 1975.

Bucknill TM: The elbow joint, Proc R Soc Med 70:620, 1977.

Caravias DE: Some observations on congenital dislocation of the head of the radius, J Bone Joint Surg 39B:86, 1957.

Carr CR and Tracy HW: Management of fractures of the distal forearm in children, South Med J 57:540, 1964.

Catterall A: Fractures in children. In Wilson JN, editor: Watson-Jones fractures and joint injuries, ed 5, Edinburgh, 1976, Churchill-Livingstone.

Cooper RR: Management of common forearm fractures in children, J Iowa Med Soc 54:689, 1964.

Corbett CH: Anterior dislocation of the radius and its recurrence, Br J Surg 19:155, 1931.

Currey JD and Butler G: The mechanical properties of bone tissue in children, J Bone Joint Surg 57A:810, 1975.

Dameron TB: Traumatic dislocation of the distal radio-ulnar joint, Clin Orthop 83:55, 1972.

Daruwalla JS: A study of radioulnar movements following fracture of the forearm in children, Clin Orthop 139:114, 1979.

Davis DR and Green DP: Forearm fractures in children: pitfalls and complications, Clin Orthop 120:172, 1976.

Derian PS: Extremity fractures in children: upper extremity, Postgrad Med 48:132, 1970.

Evans EM: Rotational deformity in the treatment of fractures of both bones of the forearm, J Bone Joint Surg 27:373, 1945.

Evans EM: Fractures of the radius and ulna, J Bone Joint Surg 33B:548, 1951.

Fee NF, Dobranski A, and Bisla RS: Gas gangrene complicating open forearm fractures: report of five cases, J Bone Joint Surg 59A:135, 1977.

Fernandez DL: Conservative treatment of forearm fractures in children. In Chapchal G, editor: Fractures in children, New York, 1981, Thieme-Stratton.

Friberg KSI: Remodeling after distal forearm fractures in children. I. The effect of residual angulation on the spatial orientation of the epiphyseal plates, Acta Orthop Scand 50:537, 1979.

Friberg KSI: Remodeling after distal forearm fractures in children. II. The final orientation of the distal and proximal epiphyseal plates of the radius, Acta Orthop Scand 50:731, 1979.

Friberg KSI: Remodeling after distal forearm fractures in children. III. Correction of residual angulation in fractures of the radius, Acta Orthop Scand 50:741, 1979.

Fuller DJ and McCullough CJ: Malunited fractures of the forearm in children, J Bone Joint Surg 64B:364, 1982.

Gandhi RK et al: Spontaneous correction of deformity following fractures of the forearm in children, Br J Surg 50:5, 1962.

Glatzer RL et al: Fractures of both bones of the distal forearm in children, Bull Hosp Jt Dis 28:14, 1967.

Hamilton W and Parkes JC II: Isolated dislocation of the radial head without fracture of the ulna, Clin Orthop 97:94, 1973.

Hanlon CR and Estes WL: Fractures in childhood: a statistical analysis, Am J Surg 87:312, 1954.

Heipel KG and Freehafer AD: Isolated traumatic dislocation of the distal ulna or radioulnar joint, J Bone Joint Surg 44A:1387, 1962.

Hogstrom H, Milsson BE, and Willner S: Correction with growth following diaphyseal forearm fracture, Acta Orthop Scand 47:229, 1976.

Holdsworth BJ and Sloan JP: Proximal forearm fractures in children: residual disability, Injury 14:174, 1982.

Hughston JC: Fractures of the forearm in children, J Bone Joint Surg 44A:1667, 1962.

Irani RN et al: Ulnar lengthening for negative ulnar variance in hereditary multiple exostoses, Orthop Trans 6:350, 1982.

King RE: Fractures of the shafts of the radius and ulna. In Rockwood CA Jr, Wilkins KE, and King RE, editors: Fractures in children, Philadelphia 1984, JB Lippincott Co.

Knight RA and Purvis GD: Fractures of both bones of the forearm in adults, J Bone Joint Surg 31A:155, 1949.

Lee SB, Esterhai JL, and Das M: Fracture of the distal radial epiphysis, Clin Orthop 185:90, 1984.

Mabrey JD and Fitch RD: Plastic deformation in pediatric fractures: mechanism and treatment, J Pediatr Orthop 9:310, 1989.

Mardam-Bey T and Ger E: Congenital radial head dislocation, J Hand Surg 4:316, 1979.

McFarland B: Congenital dislocation of the head of the radius, Br J Surg 24:41, 1936.

Milch H: Roentgenographic diagnosis of torsional deformities in tubular bones, Surgery 15:440, 1944.

Miller JH and Osterkamp JA: Scintigraphy in scale plastic bowing of the forearm, Radiology 142:742, 1982.

Müller J, Roth B, and Willenegger H: Long-term results of epiphyseal fractures to the distal radius treated by percutaneous wire fixation. In Chapchal G, editor: Fractures in children, New York, 1981, Thieme-Stratton.

Nelson CA, Buchanan JR, and Harrison CS: Distal ulnar growth arrest, J Hand Surg 9A:164, 1984.

Neviaser RJ and LeFevre GW: Irreducible isolated dislocation of the radial head, Clin Orthop 80:72, 1971.

Nielson AB and Simonsen O: Displaced forearm fractures in children treated with plates, Injury 15:393, 1984.

Nilsson BE and Obrant K: The range of motion following fracture of the shaft of the forearm in children, Acta Orthop Scand 48:600, 1977.

Ogden JA: Skeletal injury in the child, Philadelphia, 1982, Lea & Febiger.

Onne L and Sandblom P: Late results in fractures of the forearm in children, Acta Chir Scand 98:549, 1949.

Patrick J: A study of supination and pronation with special reference to the treatment of forearm fractures, J Bone Joint Surg 28:737, 1946.

Pollen AG: Fractures and dislocations in children, Baltimore, 1973, The Williams & Wilkins Co.

Rang MC: Children's fractures, ed 2, Philadelphia, 1983, JB Lippincott Co.

Reed MH: Fractures and dislocations of the extremities in children, J Trauma 17:351, 1977.

Rose-Innes AP: Anterior dislocation of the ulna at the inferio radioulnar joint, J Bone Joint Surg 42B:515, 1960.

Rydholm V and Nilsson JE: Traumatic bowing of the forearm, Clin Orthop 139:121, 1979.

Salter RB and Harris WR: Injuries involving the epiphyseal plate, J Bone Joint Surg 45A:587, 1963.

Sanders WE and Heckman JD: Traumatic plastic deformation of the radius and ulna, Clin Orthop 188:58, 1984.

Sharrard WJW: Paediatric orthopaedics and fractures, vol 2, London, 1979, Blackwell Scientific Publications.

Smith FM: Children's elbow injuries: fractures and dislocations, Clin Orthop 50:7, 1967.

Stanitski CL and Micheli LJ: Simultaneous ipsilateral fractures of the arm and forearm in children, Clin Orthop 153:218, 1980.

Stelling FH and Cote RH: Traumatic dislocation of head of the radius in children, JAMA 160:732, 1956.

Støren G: Traumatic dislocation of the radial head as an isolated lesion in children, Acta Chir Scand 116:114, 1959.

Stühmer KG: Fractures of the distal forearm. In Weber BG, Bruner C, and Freuler F, editors: Treatment of fractures in children and adolescents, New York, 1980, Springer-Verlag.

Tachdjian M: Pediatric orthopaedics, vol 2, Philadelphia, 1972, WB Saunders Co.

Thomas EM, Tuson KWR, and Browne TSH: Fractures of the radius and ulna in children, Injury 7:120, 1975.

Thompson JL: Acute plastic bowing of bone, J Bone Joint Surg 64B:123, 1982.

Treadwell SJ, van Peteghem K, and Clough MP: Pattern of forearm fractures in children, J Pediatr Orthop 4:604, 1984.

Vainionpää S et al: Internal fixation of forearm fractures in children, Acta Orthop Scand 58:121, 1987.

Verstreken L, Delronge G, and Lamoureux J: Shaft forearm fractures in children: intramedullary nailing with immediate motion: a preliminary report, J Pediatr Orthop 8:450, 1988.

Vesely DG: Isolated traumatic dislocations of the radial head in children, Clin Orthop 50:31, 1967.

Vince KG and Miller JE: Cross-union complicating fracture of the forearm. II. Children. J Bone Joint Surg 69A:654, 1987.

Weber BG, Brunner C, and Frueler F, editors: Treatment of fractures in children and adolescents, New York, 1980, Springer-Verlag.

Wiley JJ, Pegington J, and Horwich JP: Traumatic dislocation of the radius at the elbow, J Bone Joint Surg 56B:501, 1974.

Wolfe JS and Eyring EJ: Median nerve entrapment within a greenstick fracture, J Bone Joint Surg 56A:1270, 1974.

Wrist and hand fractures, dislocations, and fracture-dislocations

Abram LJ and Thompson GH: Deformity after premature closure of the distal radial physis following a torus fracture with a physeal compression injury: report of a case, J Bone Joint Surg 69A:1450, 1987.

Baldwin LW et al: Metacarpophalangeal joint dislocations of the fingers: a comparison of the pathological anatomy of index and little finger dislocations, J Bone Joint Surg 49A:1587, 1967.

Barton NJ: Fractures of the phalanges of the hand in children, Hand 2:134, 1979.

Becton JL et al: A simplified technique for treating complex dislocation of the index metacarpophalangeal joint, J Bone Joint Surg 57A:698, 1975.

Beekman F and Sullivan JE: Some observations on fractures of long bones in children, Am J Surg 51:722, 1941.

Bloem JJAM: The treatment and prognosis of uncomplicated dislocated fractures of the metacarpals and phalanges, Arch Chir Neerl 23:55, 1971.

Blount WP: Fractures in children, Baltimore, 1955, The Williams & Wilkins Co.

Brundy M: Fractures of the carpal scaphoid in children, Br J Surg 56:523, 1969.

Burman M: Irreducible hyperextension dislocation of the metacarpophalangeal joint in a finger, Bull Hosp Jt Dis 14:290, 1953.

Coonrad RW and Pohlman MH: Impacted fractures in the proximal portion of the proximal phalanx of the finger, J Bone Joint Surg 51A:1291, 1969.

Cowen NJ and Kranik AD: An irreducible juxtaepiphyseal fracture of the proximal phalanx: report of a case, Clin Orthop 110:42, 1975.

Crick JC, Franco RS, and Conner JJ: Fractures about the interphalangeal joints in children, J Orthop Trauma 1:318, 1988.

Cullen JC: Thiemann's disease. Osteochondrosis juvenilis of the basal epiphyses of the phalanges of the hand: report of two cases, J Bone Joint Surg 52B:532, 1970.

Cunningham DM and Schwartz G: Dorsal dislocation of the index metacarpophalangeal joint, Plast Reconstr Surg 56:654, 1975.

Dameron TB: Traumatic dislocation of the distal radioulnar joint, Clin Orthop 83:55, 1972.

Davis DR and Green DP: Forearm fractures in children: pitfalls and complications, Clin Orthop 120:172, 1976.

Dixon GL Jr and Moon NF: Rotational supracondylar fractures of the proximal phalanx in children, Clin Orthop 83:151, 1972.

Dykes RG: Kirner's deformity of the little finger, J Bone Joint Surg 60B:58, 1978.

Eaton RG: Joint injuries of the hand, Springfield, Ill, 1971, Charles C Thomas, Publisher.

Engber WD and Clancy WG: Traumatic avulsion of the fingernail associated with injury to the phalangeal epiphyseal plate, J Bone Joint Surg 60A:713, 1978.

Farabeuf LHF (as quoted by Barnard HL): Dorsal dislocation of the first phalanx of the little finger. Reduction by Farabeuf's dorsal incision, Lancet 1:88, 1901.

Flynn JE: Problems with trauma to the hand, J Bone Joint Surg 35A:132, 1953.

Gamble JG and Simmons SC: Bilateral scaphoid fractures in a child, Clin Orthop 162:125, 1982.

Gelberman RH, Szabo RM, and Mortensen WW: Carpal tunnel pressures and wrist position in patients with Colles' fractures, J Trauma 24:747, 1984.

Gerard FM: Post-traumatic carpal instability in a young child, J Bone Joint Surg 62A:131, 1980.

Green DP: Hand injuries in children, Pediatr Clin North Am 24:903, 1977.

Green DP and Anderson JR: Closed reduction and percutaneous pin fixation of fractures phalanges, J Bone Joint Surg 55A:1651, 1973.

Green DP and Terry GC: Complex dislocation of the metacarpophalangeal joint, J Bone Joint Surg 55A:1480, 1973.

Greene MH, Hadied AM, and LaMont RL: Scaphoid fractures in children, J Hand Surg 9A:536, 1984.

Greene WB and Anderson WJ: Simultaneous fractures of the scaphoid and radius in a child: case report, J Pediatr Orthop 2:191, 1982.

Griffiths JC: Bennett's fracture in childhood, Br J Clin Pract 20:582, 1966.

Gruelich WW and Pyle SI: Radiographic atlas of skeletal development of the hand and wrist, ed 2, Palo Alto, Calif, 1959, Stanford University Press.

Grundy M: Fractures of the carpal scaphoid in children, Br J Surg 56:523, 1969.

Hakstian RW: Cold-induced digital epiphyseal necrosis in childhood, Can J Surg 15:158, 1972.

Hanlon CR and Estes WL: Fractures in childhood: a statistical analysis, Am J Surg 87:312, 1954.

Hardin CA and Robinson DW: Coverage problems in the treatment of wringer injuries, J Bone Joint Surg 36A:292, 1954.

Hunt JC, Watts HB, and Glasgow JD: Dorsal dislocation of the metacarpophalangeal joint of the index finger with particular reference to open dislocation, J Bone Joint Surg 49A:1572, 1967.

Kaplan EB: Dorsal dislocation of the metacarpophalangeal joint of the index finger, J Bone Joint Surg 39A:1081, 1957.

Kleinman WB and Grantham SA: Multiple volar carpometacarpal joint dislocation. Case report of traumatic volar dislocation of the medial four carpometacarpal joints in a child and review of the literature, J Hand Surg 3:377, 1978.

Lee MLH: Intra-articular and peri-articular fractures of the phalanges, J Bone Joint Surg 45B:103, 1963.

Lee SB, Esterhai JL, and Das M: Fracture of the distal radial epiphysis, Clin Orthop 185:90, 1984.

Leonard MH: Open reduction of fractures of the neck of the proximal phalanx in children, Clin Orthop 116:176, 1976.

Leonard MH and Dubravcik P: Management of fractured fingers in the child, Clin Orthop 73:160, 1970.

Lipscomb PR and Janes JM: Twenty-year follow-up of an unreduced dislocation of the first metacarpophalangeal joint in a child, J Bone Joint Surg 51A:1216, 1969.

Matthews LS: Acute volar compartment syndrome secondary to distal radius fracture in an athlete, Am J Sports Med 11:6, 1983.

Maxted MJ and Owen R: Two cases of non-union of carpal scaphoid fractures in children, Injury 13:441, 1982.

McCue FX et al: Athletic injuries of the proximal interphalangeal joint requiring surgical treatment, J Bone Joint Surg 52A:937, 1970.

McLaughlin HL: Complex locked dislocation of the metacarpal phalangeal joints, J Trauma 5:683, 1965.

Milch H: So-called dislocation of the lower end of the ulna, Ann Surg 116:282, 1942.

Milford L: The hand. Dislocations and ligamentous injuries. In Crenshaw AH, editor: Campbell's operative orthopaedics, ed 7, St Louis, 1987, The CV Mosby Co.

Murphy AF and Stark HH: Closed dislocation of the metacarpophalangeal joint of the index finger, J Bone Joint Surg 49A:1579, 1967.

Müssbichler H: Injuries of the carpal scaphoid in children, Acta Radiol 56:361, 1961.

Nafie SAA: Fractures of the carpal bones in children, Injury 18:117, 1987.

O'Brien ET: Fractures of the hand and wrist region. In Rockwood CA Jr, Wilkins KE, and King RE, editors: Fractures in children, Philadelphia, 1984, JB Lippincott Co.

Peiro A et al: Trans-scaphoid perilunate dislocation in a child: a case report, Acta Orthop Scand 52:31, 1981.

Pick RY and Segal D: Carpal scaphoid fracture and non-union in an eight-year-old child: report of a case, J Bone Joint Surg 65A:1188, 1983.

Rang M: Children's fractures, ed 2, Philadelphia, 1983, JB Lippincott Co.

Rasmussen LB: Kirner's deformity: juvenile spontaneous incurving of the terminal phalanx of the fifth finger, Acta Orthop Scand 52:35, 1981.

Salter RB and Harris WR: Injuries involving the epiphyseal plate, J Bone Joint Surg 45A:587, 1963.

Santoro V and Mara J: Compartmental syndrome complicating Salter-Harris type II distal radius fracture, Clin Orthop 223:226, 1988.

Segmüller G and Schöenberger F: Fractures of the hand. In Weber BG, Bruner C, and Freuler F, editors: Treatment of fractures in children and adolescents, New York, 1980, Springer-Verlag.

Seymour N: Juxtaepiphyseal fracture of the terminal phalanx of the finger, J Bone Joint Surg 48B:347, 1966.

Sharrard WJW: Paediatric orthopaedics and fractures, Oxford, UK, 1971, Blackwell Scientific Publications.

Southcott R and Rosman MA: Nonunion of carpal scaphoid fractures in children, J Bone Joint Surg 59B:20, 1977.

Stark HH: Troublesome fractures and dislocations of the hand. In The American Academy of Orthopaedic Surgeons: Instructional course lectures, vol 19, St Louis, 1970, The CV Mosby Co.

Stühmer KG: Fractures of the distal forearm. In Weber BG, Bruner C, and Freuler F, editors: Treatment of fractures in children and adolescents, New York, 1980, Springer-Verlag.

Tsuge K: Treatment of established Volkmann's contracture, J Bone Joint Surg 57A:925, 1975.

Vahvanen V and Westerlund M: Fracture of the carpal scaphoid in children: a clinical and roentgenographical study of 108 cases, Acta Orthop Scand 51:909, 1980.

Weber BG, Brunner C, and Feuler F, editors: Treatment of fractures in children and adolescents, New York, 1980, Springer-Verlag.

Wood VE: Fractures of the hand in children, Orthop Clin North Am 7:527, 1976.

Woods GM and Tullos HG: Elbow instability and medial epicondyle fracture, Am J Sports Med 5:23, 1977.

Zimmerman H: Fractures of the elbow. In Weber BG, Brunner C, and Feuler F, editors: Treatment of fractures in children and adolescents, New York, 1980, Springer-Verlag.

17 Rheumatologic Diseases

CHARLES T. PRICE

The spectrum of rheumatic disease in children is broad and includes the more common forms of juvenile arthritis and ankylosing spondylitis, as well as the much less common forms of rheumatic fever, Lyme disease, gout, systemic lupus erythematosus, dermatomyositis, scleroderma, and the vasculitides. The most difficult aspect of these conditions is differentiating them from other inflammatory conditions and among themselves.

JUVENILE RHEUMATOID ARTHRITIS

Juvenile rheumatoid arthritis (JRA) is a generalized systemic disease of which arthritis is only one manifestation. It is one of the more common chronic illnesses in children and a leading cause of disability and blindness. The incidence of juvenile rheumatoid arthritis is about 6 to 8 children per 100,000 of the population under 15 years of age. Calabro and Marchesano estimated that 250,000 children in the United States have JRA. It is estimated that approximately 5% of all cases of rheumatoid arthritis begin in childhood. The average age of onset is 6 years, with increased incidences between the ages of 1 and 4 years and 9 and 14 years. Girls are affected at least twice as often as boys.

The cause and pathogenesis of JRA are unknown. A number of etiologic factors have been suggested, including infection, autoimmunity, trauma, psychologic stress, and heredity. Immunodeficiency has been implicated because of the frequent occurrence of chronic arthritis in children with selective IgA deficiency, agammaglobulinemia, or heterozygous C2 complement component deficiency. The onset of JRA often follows trauma, although trauma to a joint may serve only as a localizing factor, and many patients report periods of psychologic stress within 4 to 6 weeks before the onset of symptoms of JRA. Although no definitive link has been established, there are increasing data that indicate a hereditary basis of the pathogenesis of JRA.

Because children may not be able to directly communicate symptoms of morning stiffness, stiffness after inactivity, or night pain as do adults with rheumatoid arthritis, the most obvious signs of JRA at presentation may be increased irritability, guarding of the joints, or refusal to walk. Fatigue and low-grade fever are also common. Anorexia, weight loss, and failure to grow are seen in many children.

Depending on the clinical signs and symptoms during the first 4 to 6 months of illness, JRA is classified into three distinct types. Polyarthritis begins in five or more joints, usually the knees, ankles, wrists, elbows, or small joints of the hands and feet. Monoarticular arthritis occurs in four or fewer joints, quite often in only a single joint, usually the knee. Systemic disease is characterized by daily spiking fevers greater than 39° C and the appearance of a characteristic erythematous nonpruritic rash, primarily on the trunk; there is usually leukocytosis and prominent involvement of viscera, including lymphadenopathy, hepatosplenomegaly, and pericarditis.

Polyarthritis occurs in approximately half of all children with JRA. The onset may be acute but is often insidious, with gradual development of joint involvement, usually of the large, rapidly growing joints of the knees, wrists, elbows, and ankles. The pattern of joint involvement is usually symmetric. The joints are swollen, with soft tissue inflammation, edema, and synovial effusion (Fig. 17-1). Many patients do not complain of pain, but the joints may be tender or painful with motion. Synovial cysts are uncommon in JRA, but when they occur in the popliteal space they may dissect into the calf (Baker's cyst). The terminal interphalangeal joints are affected in approximately 10% of children, with radial deviation at the metacarpophalangeal joints more frequent than ulnar drift. Involvement of the apophyseal joints of the spine is common. The cervical spine is rarely involved initially, but becomes involved in half of all children with polyarthritis. Scoliosis is increased as much as 30 times in children with JRA. Systemic manifestations in polyarthritis are usually not as acute or persistent as in children with systemic disease. Low-grade fever and slight to moderate hepatosplenomegaly and lymphadenopathy may be present.

Monoarticular arthritis (involvement of four or fewer joints) occurs in one third of children with JRA,

usually involving the knees, ankles, or wrists. In about half of these children, the disease begins in only one joint, usually the knee. The hips are usually spared. Pain on motion and local tenderness are usually minimal, but there is limitation of motion and some degree of flexion deformity of affected joints. Extraarticular manifestations are unusual. A recent study of 32 children with monoarticular arthritis found persistent muscle atrophy and leg length discrepancy long after resolution of the arthritis. Children under the age of 3 years at disease onset had significantly more atrophy and bone overgrowth than children whose disease began after 3 years of age.

Systemic disease occurs in 10% to 20% of patients. In this form, severe constitutional symptoms precede the development of overt arthritis. A hallmark of this form of the disease is a high, spiking fever, which in combination with the rheumatoid rash is virtually diagnostic. The daily or twice-daily temperature elevations rise to 39° C or higher, with a rapid return to the baseline fever; this characteristically occurs in the late afternoon or evening. The rash accompanying this intermittent fever is most commonly seen on the trunk and proximal extremities (Fig. 17-2), although it may occur on the face, palms, or soles. The lesions are of short duration in any specific location and tend to be migratory. The individual lesions are salmon-pink, discrete, maculopapular, circular or circinate,

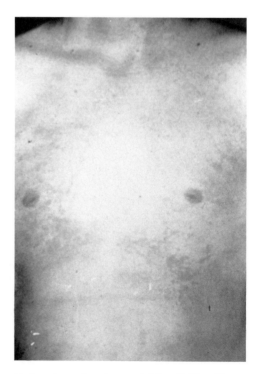

Fig. 17-2 Juvenile rheumatoid arthritis. Rheumatoid rash on trunk of 11-year-old boy with systemic disease.

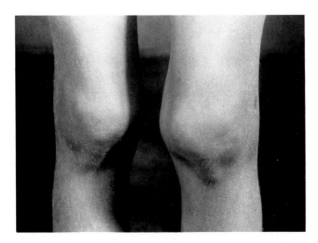

Fig. 17-1 Juvenile rheumatoid arthritis. Bilateral synovial knee effusion in 9-year-old boy.

and nonurticarial. Each macule may be surrounded by a zone of pallor and larger lesions may show central clearing. This rheumatoid rash occurs in 50% to 75% of children with systemic rheumatoid disease; it occasionally occurs in children with polyarthritis, but rarely in those with monoarticular arthritis. Because of its brief duration and appearance late in the day, during the episodes of fever, the rash is often missed by the physician.

Systemic onset of JRA is also accompanied by visceral lesions such as hepatosplenomegaly, lymphadenopathy, and pericarditis. Hepatic disease is most common at or near the onset of the disease and regresses with time. Enlargement of the spleen, which occurs in about 25% of patients, is generally most prominent during the first year of illness.

Other extraarticular manifestations of JRA include myocarditis, diffuse interstitial pulmonary fibrosis, central nervous system disease, tenosynovitis, myositis, subcutaneous rheumatoid nodules, chronic uveitis, and growth retardation. Myocarditis is less common than pericarditis but may produce cardiac enlargement or failure. Pulmonary hemosiderosis as the first manifestation of disease is rare, and pulmonary rheumatoid nodules have not been noted. Although central nervous system involvement has been described in children with JRA, it is often related to the presence of other factors such as viral infection, fever, embolism, or other systemic disease. Tenosynovitis and myositis are manifestations of active disease, and inflammation of the tendon sheaths develops principally over the dorsum of the wrist and around the ankle. Subcutaneous rheumatoid nodules occur in only 5% to 10% of patients and typically are seen in children with polyarthritis, usually overlying the periosteum of the olecranon. Chronic uveitis is one

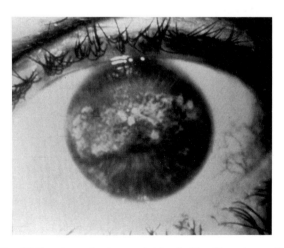

Fig. 17-3 Juvenile rheumatoid arthritis. Chronic uveitis in 8-year-old girl with monoarticular disease and positive ANA test.

of the most devastating complications of JRA (Fig. 17-3), leading to blindness in many cases. It is most likely to occur in young girls with early onset of the disease and with limited joint disease who have antinuclear antibody positivity. It occurs in over one fifth of children with monoarticular arthritis. Routine ophthalmologic examination is recommended at the time of diagnosis and should be repeated frequently during the first years of the disease. Secondary growth deformities are frequent in children with limited joint disease involving the knee and occasionally result in leg length discrepancies, with the involved leg growing longer. Early during active disease, development of the ossification centers or physes may be accelerated; later, premature fusion of the involved bones may result. Involvement of the metatarsals and metacarpals is characteristic, resulting in small hands or feet.

In general, most children with monoarticular JRA recover without serious impairment. A small percentage have recurrence of arthritis as adults. Children with systemic onset are most prone to develop life-threatening and sometimes fatal complications. The child most at risk to develop severe functional disability is the one with polyarthritis of late age of onset, early involvement of the small joints of the hands or feet, rapid appearance of joint erosions, unremitting inflammatory activity, prominent systemic manifestations, rheumatoid factor seropositivity, and subcutaneous nodules.

Pathology

JRA is characterized by many of the same histologic findings as adult rheumatoid arthritis, including villous hypertrophy of the synovium, hyperplasia of the synovial lining layer, edematous and hyperemic subsynovial tissues, prominent vascular endothelial hyperplasia, and infiltration of lymphocytes and plasma cells. Pannus formation may result, and the articular cartilage and contiguous bone may become progressively eroded and destroyed. End-stage disease is characterized by deformity, subluxation, and fibrous or bony ankylosis.

Laboratory Testing

Many children develop a normocytic, hypochromic anemia during active periods of the disease. Leukocytosis is also common with active disease, especially in children with systemic onset. Thrombocytosis is seen in severe disease. The erythrocyte sedimentation rate is useful for following a child with active disease and occasionally in monitoring therapeutic efficacy; it has the disadvantage of reflecting any form of infection or inflammation. Increases in serum levels of the immunoglobulins also correlate with disease activity. Ex-

Table 17-1 Synovial fluid characteristics of childhood monoarticular arthritis

Childhood arthritis	Gross appearance	Mucin clot	Average white cell count (range)	Neutrophils %	Glucose difference* (mg/dl)
Traumatic	Clear to hemorrhagic	Good	<5000	<50	<10
Rheumatoid	Clear to opalescent	Good to poor	20,000 (1500-100,000)	50-90	10-25
Infectious	Cloudy or turbid	Poor	100,000 (25,000-250,000)	>90	>50

From Calabro JJ, Parrino GR, and Marchesano JM: Bull Rheum Dis 21:615, 1970.
*Of paired levels found simultaneously in blood and synovial fluid specimens.

treme degrees of hypergammaglobulinemia are seen in the most severe cases; levels return toward normal with the patient's improvement. Viral antibody titers may be increased in some children. Testing for rheumatoid factor is positive less often in children than in adults; overall, only 20% of children with JRA are seropositive. Rheumatoid factor tends to be present in the child in whom the onset of JRA occurred at a later age. Tests for antinuclear antibodies are more useful diagnostically than latex agglutination and are positive in approximately 40% of children with JRA. Synovial fluid examination reveals typical inflammatory fluid (Table 17-1).

Differential Diagnosis

The diagnosis of JRA is often made by exclusion: other more common types of arthritis in children must be ruled out, as well as other rheumatic and connective tissue diseases (see box below).

DIAGNOSTIC CRITERIA FOR THE CLASSIFICATION OF JUVENILE RHEUMATOID ARTHRITIS

1. Age of onset less than 16 years
2. Arthritis in one or more joints defined as swelling or effusion, or by the presence of two or more of the following signs: limitation of motion, tenderness or pain on motion, and increased heat
3. Duration of disease, 6 weeks to 3 months
4. Type of onset of disease during the first 4 to 6 months classified as
   a. Polyarthritis—5 joints or more
   b. Monoarthritis—4 joints or fewer
   c. Systemic disease—intermittent fever, rheumatoid rash, arthritis, visceral disease
5. Exclusion of other rheumatic diseases

Modified from Brewer EJ Jr, et al: Bull Rheum Dis 23:712, 1972.

Rheumatic fever is much more likely than JRA to be acute and involve the large joints in a migratory fashion. It rarely, if ever, occurs in children younger than 5 years of age. The fever pattern is more sustained; rash, if present, is erythema marginatum rather than the evanescent macular rash of JRA. Muscle wasting, contractures, ankylosis, and chronic fusiform enlargement of joints, characteristic of late JRA, do not occur in rheumatic fever.

Polyarthralgia, monoarticular arthritis, or both may be initial symptoms of leukemia. Other similar conditions to be differentiated from JRA include hemophilic arthritis, viral synovitis, dactylitis of sickle cell anemia, traumatic arthritis, the arthritis of immunodeficiency, HLA-B27 spondylarthropathies, pigmented villonodular synovitis, synovial hemangioma, and connective tissue diseases such as systemic lupus erythematosus, scleroderma, and mixed connective tissue disease.

Roentgenographic Findings

Early roentgenographic changes generally include soft tissue swelling around the joints, juxtaarticular osteoporosis, and periosteal new bone formation. Marked bony overgrowth caused by enlargement of the epiphyses may occur at the interphalangeal joints, as may widening of the phalanges from periosteal new bone apposition. Marginal erosion and narrowing of the cartilaginous space may occur in disease of long duration, generally not before 2 years of active disease (Fig. 17-4). Atlantoaxial subluxation is the most characteristic change in the cervical spine. Fractures related to the generalized osteoporosis are frequent in young children, particularly those with severe disease, immobilization, or corticosteroid therapy, and characteristically occur in the metaphyseal or supracondylar area of the femur or as vertebral compression fractures. Premature physeal closure may slow growth, or accelerated physeal development may increase the length of long bones (Fig. 17-5).

Treatment
Nonoperative Treatment

Nonoperative treatment of JRA consists of general measures, such as rest and drug therapy, and local measures, such as physical therapy and splinting, to protect and preserve the involved joints. Aspirin is the most effective agent for control of pain, stiffness, and spasm. Enteric-coated or buffered aspirin is pre-

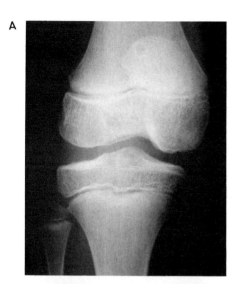

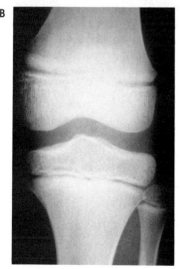

scribed in a dosage to achieve a blood salicylate level of 20 to 25 mg/dl 2 to 3 hours after a dose; salicylate levels should be monitored periodically to prevent chronic salicylate intoxication. Several nonsteroidal antiinflammatory drugs are available, but only tolmetin and naproxen have been approved for use in children. The majority of children with JRA require only aspirin or nonsteroidal antiinflammatory drugs, but one of the antirheumatic drugs may be considered for the child with polyarthritis unresponsive to a 6-month regimen of rest and aspirin or nonsteroidal antiinflammatory drugs. Corticosteroids are reserved for patients with serious systemic involvement that may be life threatening. Although bed rest is important in the acute phase of the disease, it may be detrimental if prolonged; local rest and protection of the involved joint or joints are preferable. Resting night splints may be fitted early to prevent wrist and finger contractures, flexion contracture of the knee, or equinus of the foot. If splints are used during the day, they should be removed twice daily for range of motion exercises. Physical therapy training and modalities such as radiant heat, hydrotherapy, gentle massage, and gentle range-of-motion exercises should be employed to limit impairment, prevent deformity, improve muscle strength, relieve stiffness and discomfort, and protect joints from overuse or misuse.

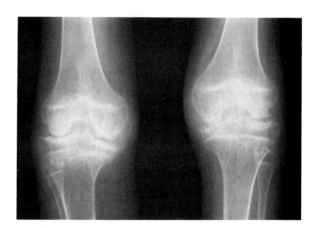

Fig. 17-4 Juvenile rheumatoid arthritis. **A,** Early roentgenographic findings in right knee of 9-year-old boy with monoarticular disease: marginal erosions, irregular subchondral margins, and mild joint space narrowing. **B,** Normal left knee.

Fig. 17-5 Juvenile rheumatoid arthritis. Premature closure of physes of distal femur and proximal tibia with severe joint space narrowing and destruction.

Operative Treatment

Surgical procedures in the patient with JRA may be performed for diagnosis, to relieve pain, to correct joint contractures or severe angulatory deformities, or to improve or maintain joint motion. Synovial biopsy and arthroscopy are often valuable diagnostic tools. Synovial biopsy showing chronic rheumatoid-type synovitis can help differentiate JRA from other disorders. Arthroscopy, especially of the knee, is sometimes done to determine if knee pain and persistent synovitis is due to JRA or some other knee pathology. It may also help to determine the necessity and timing of synovectomy.

Reconstructive surgery in patients with JRA may be classified into five general categories: soft-tissue procedures, osteotomy, arthrodesis, joint excision, and arthroplasty. Often combinations of these procedures are necessary to relieve pain and correct deformity.

Soft tissue procedures. Soft tissue procedures are indicated when contractures are too severe for nonoperative treatment such as splinting, bracing, or therapy. In the upper extremity, soft tissue procedures are most often indicated in the fingers and hands, and in the lower extremity, to correct flexion deformity of the knee or hip or equinus deformity of the foot.

Synovectomy has been a controversial but effective form of treatment of JRA for many years. The objective of synovectomy is to remove hyperplastic synovium from the joint before the development of pannus and articular cartilage and ligamentous destruction. Ideal indications for synovectomy include involvement of one or only a few joints, the hyperplastic "wet" type of rheumatoid synovitis, failure to respond to an adequate trial of nonoperative treatment, and no roentgenographic evidence of articular cartilage destruction. Few patients, however, meet all these criteria, and the decision to perform synovectomy requires astute clinical judgement. In children with monoarticular joint involvment, it is particularly difficult, since at least half of these children will recover or at least improve to the point of minimal impairment. If synovectomy is delayed until roentgenographic evidence of articular cartilage destruction is present, its effectiveness is greatly diminished. Determining what is an adequate trial of nonoperative treatment is also difficult. Severe pain, significant loss of motion, and development of contractures, despite several months of nonoperative treatment, are relative indications for synovectomy. Synovectomy is not effective in children with multiple joint involvement in the acute inflammatory phase and particularly not in those with systemic disease. The technique for open synovectomy is described on p. 396. Arthroscopic synovectomy has been suggested as an alternative to open synovectomy.

Osteotomy. Osteotomies are most commonly performed to correct severe angulatory deformities, particularly genu valgum and genu varum (pp. 367 to 369), when the involved joint is essentially ankylosed and relatively painless. The objective of osteotomy is to convert a painless, stiff joint in a poor functional position into a stiff joint in a good functional position.

Arthrodesis. Arthrodesis is reserved for irreversibly damaged joints unsuited for arthroplasty, such as the wrist, ankle, foot, and occasionally the fingers. Arthrodesis of the cervical spine (p. 443) is indicated when significant instability produces pain or neurologic impairment.

Joint excision. In the severely painful, contracted joint unsuited for arthroplasty, excision of one of the articular surfaces is occasionally indicated at skeletal maturity. Excision of the metatarsal heads (the Hoffman procedure) is sometimes indicated in older adolescents for severe metatarsalgia and clawing of the toes. Excision of the distal ulna, the lateral end of the clavicle, and the head of the radius may be performed to relieve pain and improve range of motion.

Arthroplasty. Surgical replacement of damaged joint surfaces is performed for the sequelae of JRA rather than for the active disease. The severe degenerative arthritis resulting from destruction of the articular cartilage by the inflammatory process, particularly in patients with multiple and bilateral joint destruction, often leaves no other choice but arthroplasty. The young age of these patients, however, should raise concern about the useful life of these mechanical devices and the operative risks associated with such an extensive procedure. The young adult with severe multiple joint involvement and sedentary activity level may be the best candidate.

Treatment of specific joints
Foot and ankle

Equinus deformity of the foot and varus of the hindfoot are the most frequent and difficult problems in patients with JRA. The best treatment is prevention with splinting before deformity occurs. Occasionally, early mild deformity can be corrected by manipulation and casting in the corrected position for several weeks. Severe equinovarus deformity that prevents ambulation may require triple arthrodesis or ankle arthrodesis.

Knee

Flexion contracture of the knee and genu valgum can usually be prevented by early splinting and traction, but a fixed contracture of more than 10 to 15 degrees requires more aggressive treatment. Posterior subluxation of the tibia on the femur is a major problem when correcting a fixed flexion contracture of the knee, because undue extension force on the knee may damage the anterior aspect of the proximal tibial physis, resulting in physeal arrest and recurvatum deformity of the tibia. Moderate flexion contracture associated with posterior subluxation may be treated with skeletal traction. If traction is ineffective,

surgery is indicated. Arthrotomy is performed, sectioning the anterior cruciate ligament if necessary and all intraarticular adhesions, along with hamstring lengthening and posterior capsulotomy. The patient is placed in 90-90 traction (p. 408), and careful longitudinal traction combined with anterior traction of the proximal tibia is instituted. Severe knee flexion contractures (greater than 20 degrees) may be corrected by supracondylar femoral osteotomy (p. 30). Following wound healing, an orthosis is worn. Total knee arthroplasty may be appropriate for severe bony destruction (Fig. 17-6).

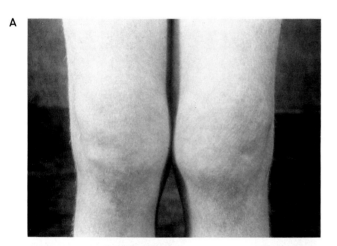

A

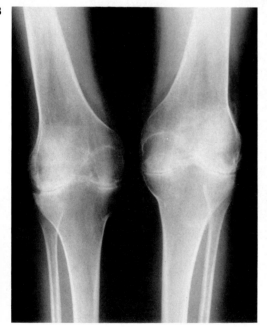

B

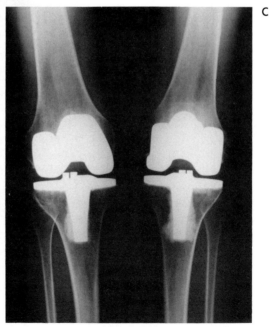

C

Fig. 17-6 Juvenile rheumatoid arthritis. Polyarticular involvement in 19-year-old man who required bilateral total knee arthroplasty. **A,** Preoperative clinical appearance. **B,** Preoperative roentgenographic appearance. **C,** Postoperative roentgenographic appearance.

Hip

Flexion contracture of the hip is usually associated with flexion contracture of the ipsilateral knee, and both deformities must be treated concurrently. Surgical release of the contracted hip flexors and joint capsule should be considered early, as should synovectomy if active synovitis persists. Destruction or abnormal development of the femoral head and acetabulum occurs in 30% to 50% of patients with JRA and is a major cause of disability. Harris and Baum, however, reported that of 35 patients with hip involvement, only 13 had required hip surgery at the latest follow-up. They also found knee involvement frequently associated with hip involvement; 24 knee procedures were performed in the 35 patients. Arthrodesis of the hip is still an effective procedure in the rare child with unilateral involvement, a normal spine, and essentially uninvolved knees. Total joint arthroplasty of the hip, knee, or both is occasionally appropriate in the young adult with severe sequelae of JRA (Fig. 17-7). Factors favoring this include severe, bilateral disease with functional impairment; an intelligent, motivated patient; and low demands on the joint arthroplasty related to the patient's life-style and activities. Again, the mechanical limitations of these implants must be considered.

Spine

Treatment of cervical spine involvement is discussed in Chapter 9.

Shoulder

Shoulder involvement is uncommon in JRA, and range-of-motion exercises usually prevent adduction contracture. Arthrodesis may be considered for the severely damaged, painful joint, but total joint replacement may be preferable if other joints in the extremity are functional, especially in the young adult.

Elbow

Limited pronation and supination of the elbow caused by destruction of the radiohumeral joint is often the first and most significant complaint (Fig. 17-8). Resection of the radial head should be considered if impairment is significant, if the degenerative process is confined to that portion of the elbow, if the wrist is functional, and if the physis has closed.

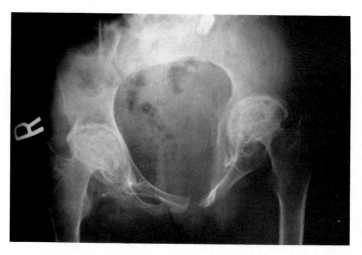

Fig. 17-7 Juvenile rheumatoid arthritis. Polyarticular disease in 16-year-old girl with severe bilateral hip involvement. Note deformity of femoral head and acetabulum (protrusio acetabuli).

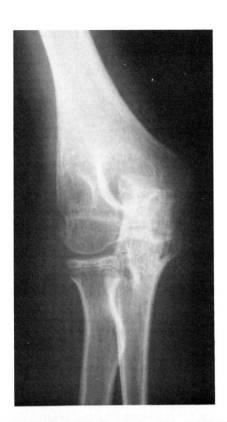

Hand and wrist

Hand and wrist problems are predominantly stiffness and deformity. Flexion deformity of the wrist and flexion contractures of the interphalangeal joints are the most frequent problems. Severe deformities may require soft tissue releases, synovectomy of the wrist or flexor and extensor tendon sheaths, capsulotomies of the metacarpophalangeal and interphalangeal joints, division of lateral band contractures, correction of boutonnière deformities, and occasional flexor and extensor tendon release. Arthroplasty of finger joints has not been successful in JRA because of the greater tendency in children toward stiff, contracted joints. In general, it is better to prevent deformity by early splinting. Wrist arthrodesis and joint replacement should be reserved for those patients in whom there is no other choice.

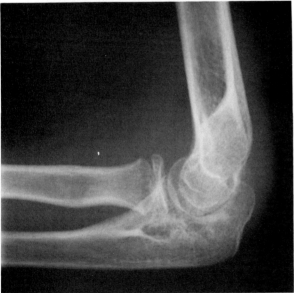

Fig. 17-8 Juvenile rheumatoid arthritis. Elbow involvement is evident by early narrowing of radiohumeral joint and cysts in subchondral bone of olecranon.

ANKYLOSING SPONDYLITIS

Ankylosing spondylitis is a systemic disease with a strong genetic basis. It generally begins in late adolescence or early adulthood, but may develop between the ages of 10 and 15 years. It occurs six times more frequently in males than in females. The presenting feature of ankylosing spondylitis is typically monoarticular peripheral arthritis, indistinguishable from JRA. The arthritis is usually asymmetric and occurs most frequently in the hips and knees. Heel pain is particularly suggestive of this condition. After the age of 7 to 10 years, the diagnosis is suggested by infrequent cervical spine involvement, seronegativity for rheumatoid factors or antinuclear antibodies, and a positive family history of similar disease.

The initial symptoms of ankylosing spondylitis are frequently those of sacroiliitis. Pain in the groin or buttock may be an early sign. Pain and stiffness in the lower back are usually worse in the morning upon arising and may cause awakening at night. Peripheral arthritis may precede the onset of spinal symptoms or occur at any point in the course of the disease. Initially, the back examination may be normal, but in time moderate to severe restriction of spinal motion, particularly extension, develops. Normal lumbar lordosis tends to become flattened by paravertebral muscle spasm. As the disease progresses, the inflammatory process gradually destroys the zygapophyseal joints, resulting in bony ankylosis. Ossification of the longitudinal ligaments and the annulus fibrosus results in the characteristic "bamboo-spine" roentgenographic appearance (Fig. 17-9).

In active disease, the erythrocyte sedimentation rate usually is elevated and mild anemia may be present. Tests for rheumatoid factor and antinuclear antibodies are rarely positive. About 90% of patients with ankylosing spondylitis test positive for the HLA B-27 antigen, in contrast to 8% of the normal Caucasian population. Although a positive test for HLA B-27 antigen is helpful for confirming a suspected diagnosis of ankylosing spondylitis, it should not be the sole diagnostic criterion because HLA B-27 occurs in the normal population and in other spondyloarthropathies.

The single most valuable diagnostic sign of ankylosing spondylitis is the roentgenographic appearance of early bilateral erosion and destruction of the sacroiliac joints (Fig. 17-10), with subsequent sclerosis and eventual obliteration of the joints because of ankylosis. In the early inflammatory stage, the sacroiliac joints may show only a subtle loss of the normally sharp, well-defined joint margins with subchondral erosion, causing the joint to appear wider than normal. However, because the sacroiliac joints normally appear widened in adolescents, definitive diagnosis cannot be made on roentgenographic appearance alone. Radioisotope scanning may be helpful when roentgenograms are not diagnostic.

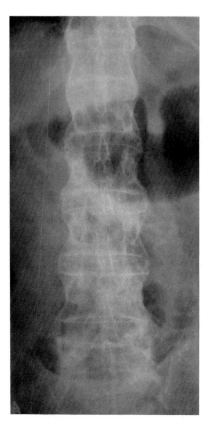

Fig. 17-9 Ankylosing spondylitis. "Bamboo spine"—ossification of longitudinal ligaments and annulus fibrosus.

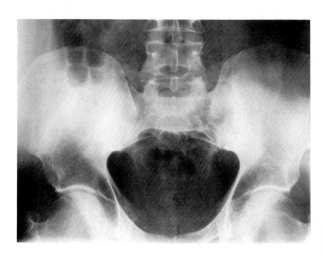

Fig. 17-10 Ankylosing spondylitis. Inferior erosion and superior fusion of sacroiliac joints.

In the thoracic and lumbar spine the earliest roentgenographic finding is a relative straightening of the spine caused by paravertebral muscle spasm. Lateral roentgenograms of the cervical, lower thoracic, and upper lumbar spine may show a "squared-off" appearance of the vertebral bodies resulting from loss of the normal concavity of their anterior surfaces. Later, bridging by new bone formation at the edges of the annulus fibrosus, ossification of the entire annulus and longitudinal ligaments, and obliteration of facet joints occur.

Treatment

There is no known cure for ankylosing spondylitis, so treatment is directed at controlling severe pain and spasm of the spinal muscles, controlling peripheral joint inflammation, and preventing late deformity of the spine. Aspirin and nonsteroidal antiinflammatory medications are usually sufficient to control pain and reduce inflammation. Proper rest and physical therapy are essential for maintaining posture, preserving range of motion, and preventing hip contractures. Bracing of the spine is indicated only occasionally in patients whose pain and spasm prevent control by active exercises. Surgical procedures on the spine are usually reserved for adults with severe flexion deformities.

LYME DISEASE

Lyme disease is caused by the spirochete *Borrelia burgdorferi* and is transmitted by the bite of the deer tick *(Ixodes dammini),* other ticks, deer flies, or mosquitoes. Typically the disease first appears in the summer, usually as a characteristic lesion of the skin, erythema chronicum migrans (ECM). Neurologic, cardiac, and articular manifestations may appear several weeks to years later. Monoarticular arthritis develops in approximately 50% of untreated patients, most commonly affecting large joints such as the hip, knee, shoulder, and elbow. Most episodes of Lyme arthritis last 7 days or less and tend to recur. In children, Lyme arthritis frequently occurs without the preceding ECM and may be mistaken for septic arthritis, reactive synovitis, or JRA. Approximately 10% of patients develop a severe erosive arthritis that is often associated with HLA-DR2.

Routine laboratory testing is usually nonspecific. The erythrocyte sedimentation rate is often elevated. Synovial fluid in patients with Lyme arthritis has a wide range of leukocyte counts, usually with a predominance of polymorphonuclear leukocytes. Specific serologic testing, using both indirect immunofluorescent assay and an enzyme-linked immunofluorescent assay, has been shown to be both sensitive and specific. Roentgenograms frequently show only joint effusion.

Steere et al reported that oral administration of antibiotics early in the disease can prevent or attenuate subsequent attacks of Lyme arthritis. The current recommendation for patients with early Lyme disease is oral tetracycline, 250 mg four times a day (20 to 50 mg/kg, up to 2 g/day), and in children younger than 8 years of age, phenoxymethyl penicillin, 50 mg/kg/day (maximum 2 g a day). Intravenous administration of penicillin has been shown to be particularly useful in patients with chronic or recurring arthritis.

GOUT

Gout in children is a congenital disturbance of uric acid metabolism inherited as an autosomal dominant trait. Deposition of uric acid in various mesenchymal tissues results in an inflammatory response. Manifestation of the condition usually occurs in adults and rarely in children. It has been estimated that fewer than 6% of adults with gout had symptoms before the age of 20 years. The clinical picture in children is similar to that in adults: acute, recurring attacks of severely painful arthritis and deposition of sodium urate (tophi) in the articular, periarticular, and subcutaneous tissues. The level of uric acid in the blood is usually elevated. Roentgenograms are generally normal in the early stages of the disease, but later, areas of bone erosion are evident.

Most children with gout can be treated medicinally, but in late stages of the disease, excision and curettage of the tophi may be indicated when they interfere with the function of tendons or joints, encroach on nerves, or threaten to cause skin necrosis and ulceration. In severe cases, amputation of the toes occasionally is necessary, as are partial resection of tendons, resection of joints, and arthroplasty or arthrodesis of painful joints.

RHEUMATIC FEVER

Rheumatic fever is an inflammatory disease that occurs as a delayed sequel to pharyngeal infection with group A streptococci. It involves primarily the heart, joints, central nervous system, skin, and subcutaneous tissues. Common clinical manifestations of the acute form are migratory polyarthritis, fever, and carditis. The acute phase is characterized by diffuse exudative and proliferative inflammatory reactions in the heart, joints, and skin. The characteristic feature of the joints in rheumatic fever is the swelling and edema of the articular and periarticular structures, with serous effusion into the joint space but without erosion of the joint surface or pannus formation. The arthritis of rheumatic fever usually involves the large joints, particularly the knees, ankles, elbows, and wrists. The hips are less commonly involved, and the spine is rarely affected. In the classic attack, several joints are involved in quick succession, each for a brief period of time. This migratory polyarthritis is accompanied by signs and symptoms of an acute febrile illness. Usually each joint remains inflamed for no more than a week before inflammation begins to subside, and it usually abates spontaneously in 2 to 3 weeks. Fewer than 5% of attacks persist for more than 6 months. Rheumatic fever never causes permanent joint deformities, with the very rare exception of the so-called Jaccoud type of deformity of the metacarpophalangeal joints. Its relationship with rheumatic fever is not clear. Diagnostic criteria for rheumatic fever include involvement of two or more joints, two minor manifestations such as fever and increase in erythrocyte sedimentation rate, and high titers of antistreptolysin O or some other streptococcal antibody.

Treatment is aimed at relieving pain and inflammation and eradicating the pharyngeal infection, and usually includes aspirin, nonsteroidal antiinflammatory drugs, and appropriate antibiotics. Bed rest is recommended for the first 3 weeks of illness, when carditis usually appears. Joint symptoms seldom require further treatment.

REFERENCES

Ansell BM and Swann M: The management of chronic arthritis of children, J Bone Joint Surg 65B:536, 1983.

Arden GP: Total hip replacement in juvenile chronic polyarthritis and ankylosing spondylitis, Orthop Dig 2:14, 1974.

Arden GP, Ansell BM, and Hunter MJ: Total hip replacement in juvenile chronic polyarthritis and ankylosing spondylitis, Clin Orthop 84:130, 1972.

Arnett FC, Bias WB, and Stevens MB: Juvenile-onset chronic arthritis: clinical and roentgenographic features of a unique HLA-B27 subset, Am J Med 69:369, 1980.

Arthritis Foundation Committee on Evaluation of Synovectomy: Multicenter evaluation of synovectomy in the treatment of rheumatoid arthritis: report of results at the end of 5 years, J Rheumatol 15:764, 1988.

Arthritis and Rheumatism Council and British Orthopaedic Association: Controlled trial of synovectomy of knee and MCP joints in rheumatoid arthritis, Ann Rheum Dis 35:437, 1976.

Barry PE and Stillman JS: Characteristics of juvenile rheumatoid arthritis: its medical and orthopedic management, Orthop Clin North Am 6:641, 1975.

Berens DL: Roentgen features of ankylosing spondylitis, Clin Orthop 74:21, 1971.

Bernstein B et al: Hip joint restoration in juvenile rheumatoid arthritis, Arthritis Rheum 20:1099, 1977.

Bernstein BH et al: Growth retardation in juvenile rheumatoid arthritis, Arthritis Rheum 20(suppl):212, 1977.

Blane CE, Ragsdale CG, and Hensinger RN: Late effects of JRA on the hip, J Pediatr Orthop 7:677, 1987.

Bianco AJ Jr and Peterson HA: Juvenile rheumatoid arthritis, Orthop Clin North Am 2:745, 1971.

Brattstrom M and Sundberg J: Juvenile rheumatoid gonarthritis. I. Clinical and roentgenological study, Acta Rheumat Scand 11:266, 1965.

Brewer EJ Jr: Juvenile rheumatoid arthritis, Philadelphia, 1970, WB Saunders Co.

Calabro JJ et al: Prognosis in juvenile rheumatoid arthritis: a fifteen-year followup of 100 patients, Arthritis Rheum 20:285, 1977.

Calabro JJ and Marchesano JM: Current concepts: juvenile rheumatoid arthritis, N Engl J Med 277:696, 1967.

Carmichael E and Chaplin DM: Total knee arthroplasty in juvenile rheumatoid arthritis, Clin Orthop 210:192, 1986.

Cassidy JT: Juvenile rheumatoid arthritis. In Kelly WN et al, editors: Textbook of Rheumatology, Philadelphia, 1981, WB Saunders Co.

Cassidy JT and Nelson AM: The frequency of juvenile arthritis, J Rheumatol 15:535, 1988.

Chandler HP et al: Total hip replacement in patients younger than 30 years old, J Bone Joint Surg 63A:1426, 1981.

Cleland LG, Treganza R, and Dobson P: Arthroscopic synovectomy: a prospective study, J Rheumatol 13(5):907, 1986.

Colville J and Raunio P: Total hip replacement in juvenile rheumatoid arthritis: analysis of 59 hips, Acta Orthop Scand 50:197, 1979.

Combe B, Krause E, and Sany J: Treatment of chronic knee synovitis with arthroscopic synovectomy after failure of intraarticular injection of radionuclide, Arthritis Rheum 32(1):10, 1989.

Culp RW et al: Lyme arthritis in children, J Bone Joint Surg 69A:96, 1987.

Eyring EJ, Longert A, and Bass JC: Synovectomy in juvenile rheumatoid arthritis: indications and short-term results, J Bone Joint Surg 53A:638, 1971.

Fried JA et al: The cervical spine in juvenile rheumatoid arthritis, Clin Orthop 179:102, 1983.

Goel KM and Shanks RA: Follow-up study of 100 cases of juvenile rheumatoid arthritis, Ann Rheum Dis 33:25, 1974.

Gondolph-Zink B et al: Semiarthroscopic synovectomy of the hip, Int Orthop 12(1):31, 1988.

Granberry WM: Soft-tissue release in children with juvenile rheumatoid arthritis, Arthritis Rheum 20:565, 1977.

Granberry WM: Synovectomy in juvenile rheumatoid arthritis, Arthritis Rheum 20:561, 1977.

Granberry WM and Brewer EJ Jr: Results of synovectomy in children with rheumatoid arthritis, Clin Orthop 101:120, 1974.

Granberry WM and Magnum GL: The hand in the child with juvenile rheumatoid arthritis, J Hand Surg 5:105, 1980.

Griffin PP, Tachdijian MO, and Green WT: Pauci-articular arthritis in children, JAMA 184:23, 1963.

Hanson V et al: Three subtypes of juvenile rheumatoid arthritis (correlations of age at onset, sex, and serologic factors), Arthritis Rheum 20(Suppl):184, 1977.

Hanson V et al: Prognosis of juvenile rheumatoid arthritis, Arthritis Rheum 20(suppl):279, 1977.

Harris CM and Baum J: Involvement of the hip in juvenile rheumatoid arthritis: a longitudinal study, J Bone Joint Surg 70A:821, 1988.

Haueisen DC, Weiner DS, and Weiner SD: The characterization of "transient synovitis of the hip" in children, J Pediatr Orthop 6:11, 1986.

Hensinger RN, DeVito PD, and Ragsdale CG: Changes in the cervical spine in juvenile rheumatoid arthritis, J Bone Joint Surg 68A:189, 1986.

Herold BC and Shulman ST: Poststreptococcal arthritis, Pediatr Infect Dis J 7:681, 1988.

Holgersson S et al: Arthroscopy of the hip in juvenile chronic arthritis, J Pediatr Orthop 1:273, 1981.

Jackson MA and Nelson JD: Etiology and medical management of acute suppurative bone and joint infections in pediatric patients, J Pediatr Orthop 2:313, 1982.

Jacobsen ST, Levinson JE, and Crawford AH: Late results of synovectomy in juvenile rheumatoid arthritis, J Bone Joint Surg 67A:8, 1983.

Kampner SL and Ferguson AB Jr: Efficacy of synovectomy in juvenile rheumatoid arthritis, Clin Orthop 88:94, 1972.

Kaufer H et al: Symposium: lower extremity joint reconstruction in very young patients, Contemp Orthop 12:79, 1986.

Kay J et al: Synovial fluid eosinophilia in Lyme disease, Arthritis Rheum 31(11):1384, 1988.

Klassen RA, Parlasca RJ, and Bianco AJ Jr: Total joint arthroplasty in children and adolescents, Mayo Clinic Proc 54:579, 1979.

Klein KS et al: Long term follow-up of arthroscopic synovectomy for chronic hemophilic synovitis, Arthroscopy 3(4):231, 1987.

Klein W et al: Arthroscopic synovectomy of the knee joint: indication, technique, and follow-up results, Arthroscopy 4(2):63, 1988.

Lachiewicz PF et al: Total hip arthroplasty in juvenile rheumatoid arthritis: two to eleven-year results, J Bone Joint Surg 68A:502, April 1986.

Laurin CA et al: Long-term results of synovectomy of the knee in rheumatoid patients, J Bone Joint Surg 56A:521, 1974.

Lawson JP and Steere AC: Lyme arthritis: radiologic findings, Radiology 154:37, 1985.

Liang MH and Cullen KE: Evaluation of outcomes in total joint arthroplasty for rheumatoid arthritis, Clin Orthop 182:41, 1984.

McAnarney ER et al: Psychological problems of children with chronic juvenile arthritis, Pediatrics 53:523, 1974.

McCollum DE, Nunley JA, and Harrelson JM: Bone-grafting in total hip replacement for acetabular protrusion, J Bone Joint Surg 62A:1065, 1980.

McMaster M: Synovectomy of the knee in juvenile rheumatoid arthritis, J Bone Joint Surg 54B(2):263, 1972.

Mogensen B et al: Synovectomy of the hip in juvenile chronic arthritis, J Bone Joint Surg 64B(3):295, 1982.

Mogensen B et al: Total hip replacement in juvenile chronic arthritis, Acta Orthop Scand 54:422, 1983.

Petty RE and Malleson P: Spondyloarthropathies of childhood, Pediatr Clin North Am 33:1079, 1986.

Petty RE and Tingle AJ: Arthritis and viral infection, J Pediatr 113:948, 1988.

Ranawat CS, Dorr LD, and Inglis AE: Total hip arthroplasty in protrusio acetabuli of rheumatoid arthritis, J Bone Joint Surg 62A:1059, 1980.

Rosenberg AM: Uveitis associated with juvenile rheumatoid arthritis, Semin Arthritis Rheum 16:158, 1987.

Ruddlesdin C et al: Total hip replacement in children with juvenile chronic arthritis, J Bone Joint Surg 68B(2):218, 1986.

Sarokhan AJ et al: Total knee arthroplasty in juvenile rheumatoid arthritis, J Bone Joint Surg 65A(8):1071, 1983.

Schaller JG: Arthritis in children, Pediatr Clin North Am 33(6):1565, 1986.

Schaller JG: Chronic arthritis in children: juvenile rheumatoid arthritis, Clin Orthop 182:79, 1984.

Schaller JG: The seronegative spondylarthropathies of childhood. Clin Orthop 143:76, 1979.

Scott RD, Sarokhan AJ, and Dalziel R: Total hip and total knee arthroplasty in juvenile rheumatoid arthritis, Clin Orthop 182:90, 1984.

Scott RD and Sledge CB: The surgery of juvenile rheumatoid arthritis. In Kelly WN et al, editors: Textbook of Rheumatology, Philadelphia, 1981, WB Saunders Co.

Simon S, Whiffen J, and Shapiro F: Leg-length discrepancies in monoarticular and pauci-articular juvenile rheumatoid arthritis, J Bone Joint Surg 63A:209, 1981.

Smythe H: Therapy of the spondylarthropathies, Clin Orthop 143:84, 1979.

Stechenberg BW: Lyme disease: the latest great imitator, Pediatr Infect Dis J 7:402, 1988.

Steere, AC et al: Longitudinal assessment of the clinical and epidemiological features of Lyme disease in a defined population, J Infect Dis 154:295, 1986.

Steere AC, Schoen RT, and Taylor E: The clinical evaluation of Lyme arthritis, Ann Intern Med 107:725, 1987.

Stiehm ER: Nonsteroidal anti-inflammatory drugs in pediatric patients, AJDC 142:1281, 1988 (editorial).

Still GF: On a form of chronic joint disease in children, Med Chir Trans 80:45, 1897.

Stockley I, Bell MJ, and Sharrard WJW: The role of expanding intramedullary rods in osteogenesis imperfecta, J Bone Joint Surg 71B(3):422, 1989.

18 Bone and Joint Infections

JAMES R. KASSER

Musculoskeletal infections remain common orthopaedic problems even though, with the advent of antibiotic therapy, mortality and morbidity have dropped precipitously. Prompt, accurate diagnosis allowing early definitive treatment ensures optimal results in all musculoskeletal infections. A combination of medical and surgical treatment is often required for musculoskeletal infections in children. Although antibiotic therapy is fairly standard for all musculoskeletal infections, depending on the infecting organism, the indications and techniques of surgery may differ depending on the disease, the location of the infection, and the particular patient.

ANTIBIOTIC THERAPY

Since sulfonamides and penicillin were introduced in the 1930s, treatment of bone and joint infections has changed dramatically. The continuing change in bacterial sensitivity and the spectrum of infecting organisms has been accompanied by a rapid and continual development of new antibiotics. This dynamic relationship between infecting organisms and the drugs necessary to eradicate them makes a definitive listing of antibiotic therapy impossible. The recommendations in the box at right are made on the basis of the most current information based on the age of the patient and the sensitivities of the infecting organism. Regional bacterial sensitivities and local conditions may dictate different standards, and consultation with the infectious disease service or specialists in the area may be advised for determining the most appropriate antibiotic therapy.

Intravenous antibiotic therapy is the appropriate treatment for initial management of most bone and joint infections. For suspected musculoskeletal sepsis in a newborn, oxacillin and gentamicin are commonly used. Between the ages of 6 months and 4 years, the probability of *Haemophilus influenzae* infection rises significantly and initial antibiotics are cephalexin or oxacillin and chloramphenicol. For children older than 4 years, oxacillin is appropriate initially unless clinical history or Gram staining indicates the probability of some infecting organism other than *Staphylococcus aureus*. Initial antibiotic therapy should be confirmed or amended by Gram stain and culture of aspirated fluid. Table 18-1 lists suggested dosages for commonly used antibiotics.

PRINCIPLES OF ANTIBIOTIC THERAPY

1. Make a specific bacteriologic diagnosis, if possible, using blood, bone, tissue, or synovial fluid cultures.
2. Use the narrowest spectrum drug available for the specific infection.
3. Monitor the patient carefully for secondary foci of infection, such as meningitis, endocarditis, or associated bone and joint infections.
4. Be aware of complications related to particular antibiotics, such as bone marrow suppression, renal toxicity, and hepatic toxicity.
5. Convert from in-hospital intravenous administration of antibiotics to outpatient intravenous administration or oral administration when appropriate.

The duration of antibiotic therapy in musculoskel-etal sepsis remains controversial, with general recommendations ranging from 3 to 6 weeks depending on the chronicity of the infection and the response of the patient to therapy.

Depending on the infection, the patient and family, and the preferences of the physician, conversion from in-hospital intravenous administration to in-hospital oral administration or outpatient intravenous or oral administration may be indicated. Nelson was an early advocate of oral administration of antibiotics in nosocomial infections to decrease cost and improve care. Although high-dose oral antibiotic therapy achieves a lower peak serum concentration than intravenous administration, it is sufficiently high for treatment of most infections. Nelson's series, as well as a small controlled series of patients with osteomyelitis reported by Kolyvas, supports the efficacy of oral antibiotic therapy. After response to intravenous therapy, the appropriate dose of oral antibiotics (Table 18-1) should be prescribed for the compliant patient and family, and the clinical progress of the pa-tient should be followed carefully. Increasing pain or swelling, recurrence of fever, or an increase in erythrocyte sedimentation rate indicates a need for an immediate return to intravenous therapy and reassessment of treatment. Biologic assay of serum antibiotic concentration (bactericidal level) has been recommended to monitor the efficacy of oral therapy. Gastrointestinal intolerance or inability of the patient to accept the drug makes oral therapy inadvisable. Whether oral therapy is continued with the patient in the hospital or as an outpatient depends on social and parental factors.

Outpatient or home intravenous therapy has recently become quite popular. In the standard program, a nurse maintains the intravenous catheter and the parents administer the drugs. Because of the time required for administration of each dose of antibiotic, drugs with a dosing interval more frequent than every 8 hours should not be prescribed for this method. New, long-acting drugs such as ceftriaxone may allow 24-hour dose intervals.

Table 18-1 Dosages for antibiotics used for therapy of bone and joint infections*

Drug	Dosage (mg/kg/day)	Interval between doses (hours)	Route
Amikacin	15-20	8-12	IV, IM
Amoxicillin	100	6	PO
Ampicillin	150	6	IV, IM, or PO
Carbenicillin	400-600	4-6	IV
Cefaclor	150	6	PO
Cefamandole	120	6	IV, IM
Cefazolin	75	8	IV
Ceftriaxone	75-100	12-24	IV, IM
Cefuroxime	75-100	6-8	IV
Cephalexin	100	6	PO
Cephalothin	150	4-6	IV
Chloramphenicol	75	6	IV, PO
Clindamycin	30	8	IV, PO
Cloxacillin	100	6	PO
Dicloxacillin	75	6	PO
Gentamicin	6 (children), 7.5 (infants)	8	IV, IM
Methicillin	200	6	IV
Nafcillin	150	6	IV, PO
Oxacillin	150	6	IV, PO
Penicillin	100 (150,000 U)	4-6	IV, PO
Ticarcillin	200-300	4-6	IV
Vancomycin	40	6	IV

*The following antibiotics are *not* recommended: (1) erythromycin—contributes to low synovial fluid levels; (2) ciprofloxacin—an oral antipseudomonas antibiotic, not approved for use in children.

ACUTE SEPTIC ARTHRITIS

Septic arthritis occurs twice as frequently as osteomyelitis during infancy and early childhood; in later childhood and adolescence, the overall frequency of musculoskeletal infection decreases and the occurrences of osteomyelitis and septic arthritis become nearly equal. The typical patient with septic arthritis is febrile (38° to 40° C) with a painful, swollen joint and only occasionally a history of acute trauma. The most commonly involved joints are the hip and knee, with the shoulder, elbow, ankle, and wrist much less often involved (Table 18-2). Physical findings include restriction of joint motion, joint effusion, and diffuse tenderness around the involved joint. Adjacent swelling along a long bone is generally indicative of a contiguous focus of osteomyelitis, but diffuse swelling may occur with long-standing septic arthritis. The differential diagnosis of septic arthritis usually includes reactive transient synovitis, migratory arthralgia, juvenile rheumatoid arthritis, hemophilic "arthritis," pigmented villonodular synovitis, and trauma. Early roentgenograms may reveal joint space widening (Fig. 18-1), soft tissue swelling, effusion, or an osseous lesion 7 to 10 days after onset. Technetium bone scanning may be helpful, but it is very nonspecific: the scan may show either normal, increased, or decreased uptake. In general, however, there is increased uptake on both sides of the involved joint.

Initial laboratory evaluation should include white blood cell count and erythrocyte sedimentation rate. The erythrocyte sedimentation rate, though nonspecific, is elevated to greater than 50 mm/hr in over 90% of patients with septic arthritis. If *H. influenzae* infection is suspected, antibody detection by latex fixation of serum and urine is helpful. If juvenile rheumatoid arthritis is suspected, testing for antinuclear antibodies (ANAs) and rheumatoid factor is indicated.

The definitive diagnostic test for septic arthritis is needle aspiration of the joint. Testing of the synovial fluid specimen should include white blood cell count with cell differential, Gram stain, aerobic and anaerobic cultures, and glucose and lactate measurement. Synovial fluid from most patients with septic arthritis has a white blood cell count between 50,000 and 200,000, with more than 75% polymorphonuclear cells. Gram staining provides a presumptive diagnosis in approximately 30% of patients with septic arthritis, and positive cultures are obtained in about two thirds of patients. Glucose and lactate measurements help determine whether the arthritis is truly septic or reactive; in septic arthritis glucose is decreased and lactate is elevated. Depending on the clinical setting, further studies to identify microbacteria, fungi, viruses, chlamydia, and spirochetes may be indicated.

Infecting organisms may invade the joint by the hematogenous route, by direct extension from an adjacent osteomyelitis, or by direct introduction through a wound. The most common bacteria in septic arthritis in children are *S. aureus, H. influenzae,* and streptococci (Table 18-3). *S. aureus* is the most common agent in neonates and children older than 4 years; in children between the ages of 6 months and 2 years, *H. influenzae* predominates. Streptococci of various types, including pneumococci, are the next most common, with group B pathogens predominating in neonates and group A β-hemolytic pathogens more prevalent in older infants and children. Significant numbers of patients with septic arthritis caused by other organisms have been reported: *Neisseria gonorrhoeae, Neisseria meningitidis, Escherichia coli, Pseudomonas, Klebsiella,* and *Salmonella* have all been implicated.

Table 18-2 Frequency and distribution of septic arthritis

Joints	No.	%
Knee	213	41
Hip	116	23
Ankle	70	14
Elbow	64	12
Wrist	22	4
Shoulder	18	4
Interphalangeal	4	
Metatarsal	3	
Sacroiliac	2	
Metacarpal	1	
Acromioclavicular	1	

From Jackson MA and Nelson JD: J Pediatr Orthop 2:313, 1982.

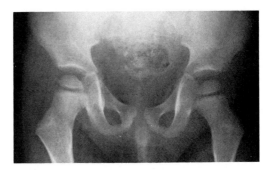

Fig. 18-1 Acute septic arthritis of left hip in 4-year-old boy. Note early widening of joint space medially.

The goal of treatment of joint sepsis is prevention of destruction of articular cartilage and retention of motion, strength, and function. The inflammatory response caused by the infecting organism, possibly coupled with chondrocyte activity, is responsible for cartilage degradation. Elimination of the organism through antibiotic therapy and joint drainage is appropriate treatment. Immediate decisions about drainage of the joint and antibiotics must be made on the basis of the white blood cell count and Gram stain of synovial fluid and the gross appearance of the joint. Parenteral antibiotic therapy is indicated for patients with suspected septic arthritis, and drug selection can often be guided by the Gram-stained smear of synovial fluid. When Gram staining is negative or equivocal, antibiotics should be based on the most frequent pathogens for the patient's age group. Nafcillin or other antistaphylococcal penicillin is appropriate in the child older than 5 years. For the younger child, and especially those younger than 2 years of age, coverage for both *S. aureus* and *H. influenzae* should be initiated. Although cefamandole affords single-dose coverage of both pathogens, recent reports have described the development of meningitis during therapy with this drug, so cefamandole should be used only if meningitis has been excluded, and the patient should be carefully watched.

Table 18-3 Organisms causing septic arthritis and osteomyelitis

	Arthritis			Osteomyelitis		
Bacteria	**Newborn (14 patients) (4%)**	**1 mo to 5 yr (337 patients) (70%)**	**Over 5 yr (120 patients) (26%)**	**Newborn (13 patients) (5%)**	**1 mo to 5 yr (142 patients) (50%)**	**Over 5 yr (121 patients) (45%)**
S. aureus	5/14 (36%)	37/337 (11%)	39/120 (33%)	7/13 (54%)	70/142 (49%)	86/121 (71%)
H. influenzae	1/14 (7%)	103/337 (31%)	1/120 (1%)	1/13 (8%)	7/142 (5%)	0/121
Streptococci						
Group A/Other	0/14	20/337 (6%)	10/120 (18%)	0/13	15/142 (11%)	8/121 (7%)
Group B	3/14 (21%)	6/337 (2%)	0/120	0/13	3/142 (2%)	0/121
Pneumococci	0/14	13/337 (4%)	1/120 (1%)	0/13	5/142 (4%)	0/121
N. gonorrhoeae	1/14 (7%)	7/337 (2%)	8/120 (7%)	0/13	0/142	0/121
N. meningitidis	0/14	9/337 (3%)	1/120 (1%)	0/13	0/142	0/121
Pseudomonas aeruginosa	1/14 (7%)	6/337 (2%)	3/120 (3%)	0/13	2/142 (1%)	2/121 (1%)
E. coli, Klebsiella sp., *Enterobacter* sp.	2/14 (14%)	5/337 (2%)	4/120 (3%)	0/13	2/142 (1%)	1/121 (1%)
Salmonella sp.	0/14	4/337 (1%)	0/120	1/13 (8%)	2/142 (1%)	1/121
Other	1/14 (7%)	9/337 (3%)	6/120 (5%)	1/13 (8%)	12/142 (8%)	3/121 (3%)
Unknown	0/14	118/337 (35%)	41/120 (34%)	3/13 (23%)	24/142 (17%)	21/121 (17%)

From Jackson MA and Nelson JD: J Pediatr Orthop 2:313, 1982.

Principles and Techniques of Joint Aspiration

In general, the child is sedated with intramuscular or monitored intravenous injection. The chosen sedative is supplemented with a dermal injection of 1% lidocaine (Xylocaine) in cooperative patients; the joint should not be anesthetized with lidocaine. Fluoroscopy is beneficial both for locating the site of aspiration and for documenting satisfactory arthrocentesis, especially in the hip. If no fluid is obtained, the joint should be washed with saline and the saline specimen sent for culture. Radiopaque dye (1 to 2 ml) may be injected after aspiration so that a roentgenographic record of the procedure may be obtained.

Necessary equipment for arthrocentesis includes a 20-gauge or larger needle, povidone-iodine (Betadine) or alcohol, sterile drapes, gauze, gloves, and a 10-cc syringe. An assistant is necessary to ensure that the patient remains still during the procedure. With the patient appropriately sedated, the portion of the extremity to be aspirated is prepared and draped to create a small sterile field. It is imperative that arthrocentesis be regarded as a sterile procedure.

Aspiration of Hip Joint

The anterior and medial approaches can be accomplished with equal ease. The choice of technique depends on the position in which the patient is most comfortable and the preference of the surgeon.

▲ *Technique (anterior approach)*. Extend the hip as much as the patient will tolerate, with the leg held in neutral position. The hip joint lies about midway between the pubic tubercle and the anterosuperior iliac spine. Insert the needle just lateral to this point and just proximal to the level of the greater trochanter. Palpate the femoral artery and be certain the insertion site is at least 1.5 cm lateral. Document needle insertion by image intensification or roentgenogram. Aim the needle approximately 20 degrees medially; roentgenographically, the needle is directed toward the upper portion of the femoral neck just distal to the femoral physis (Fig. 18-2). Because the hip joint extends inferiorly to the capsular insertion at the intertrochanteric line, a needle directed at the cartilaginous space between the femoral head and acetabulum is blocked by the acetabular labrum and the anterolateral cartilaginous extension of the ilium.

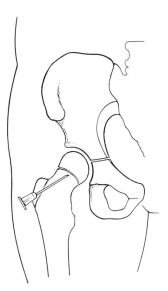

Fig. 18-2 Aspiration of hip through anterior approach, with bevel of needle directed toward physis of proximal femur.

▲ *Technique (adductor medial approach)*. Position the patient with the hip in full abduction and 60 to 90 degrees of flexion. Prepare and drape the medial aspect of the proximal thigh; drape the perineum out of the field. Insert the needle dorsal to the adductor longus tendon and just lateral to its insertion into the pubis. Advance the needle towards the ipsilateral axilla until the femoral neck is encountered. Roentgenographically, the needle should be directed at the upper portion of the femoral neck.

Aspiration of Sacroiliac Joint

Aspiration of the sacroiliac joint is occasionally done as part of the differential diagnosis of hip infection. Culture and sensitivity testing of the joint aspirate establishes the response of the infecting organism to appropriate antibiotics.

▲ *Technique (posterior approach)*. Position the patient supine and prepare and drape the area in a routine manner. With image intensification control, introduce an 18-gauge spinal needle in the midline at the level of the sacroiliac joint at a 45-degree angle with the transverse plane and a 30-degree angle with the sagittal plane. Pass the needle laterally and distally at these angles, using the image intensifier to guide it into the sacroiliac joint 0.5 cm from its most inferior margin.

Aspiration of Knee

▲ *Technique (superolateral approach).* Position the patient with the knee extended as much as possible. Prepare and drape the entire knee circumferentially. Palpate the superolateral corner of the patella; a significant effusion should be present in the suprapatellar pouch. Insert the needle under the superolateral corner of the patella (Fig. 18-3). Applying pressure over the suprapatellar pouch and medial joint with the sterile, gloved, nonaspirating hand may facilitate the procedure by distending the lateral suprapatellar pouch.

A medial approach may be made at the same level, but the vastus medialis muscle must be penetrated and the opposite leg will be in the way during the procedure, a particularly bothersome problem in an agitated pediatric patient.

▲ *Technique (inferolateral approach).* Position the patient with the knee in 70 to 90 degrees of flexion to pull the patellar fat pad distally away from the femoral condyles. Palpate the patellar tendon and joint line, and insert the needle 1 cm lateral to the patellar tendon and 1 cm above the joint line, aiming for the center of the femoral notch.

Aspiration of Ankle

▲ *Technique (anterolateral approach).* Position the patient with the ankle and foot in a neutral position. Insert the needle just anterior to the fibula, proximal to the sinus tarsi at the level of the joint line as confirmed by image intensification. Direct the needle toward the medial malleolus to enter the joint anteriorly (Fig. 18-4).

▲ *Technique (anteromedial approach).* Position the patient as above. Insert the needle at the anterosuperior aspect of the medial malleolus, at the level of the tibiotalar joint, just medial to the anterior tibial tendon. Direct the needle towards the posterolateral corner of the tibiotalar joint.

Aspiration of Shoulder

▲ *Technique (anterolateral approach).* Position the patient with the shoulder in slight external rotation, with the humerus resting in neutral position. Palpate the acromion, coracoid, and lesser tuberosity. Insert the needle just inferior and lateral to the coracoid process, directed straight posteriorly. A more inferior insertion of the needle places the neurovascular bundle at risk.

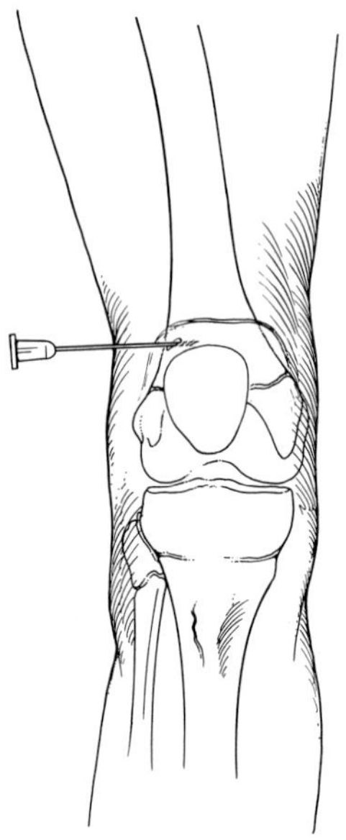

Fig. 18-3 Aspiration of knee through superolateral approach in suprapatellar pouch.

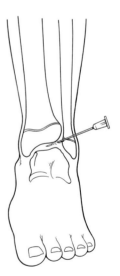

Fig. 18-4 Aspiration of ankle through anterolateral approach, puncture wound located between capsule of tibia and fibula.

Aspiration of Elbow

▶ *Technique (lateral approach).* Position the patient with the elbow flexed 70 to 90 degrees. Palpate the radiocapitellar joint and insert the needle just posterior to the radiocapitellar articulation (Fig. 18-5). The radial nerve falls further forward with elbow flexion.

▶ *Technique (posterior approach).* Approach the elbow through the anconeus triangle—the space between the capitellum, radial head, and olecranon; this space swells when there is significant elbow effusion. With the elbow flexed 90 degrees, insert the needle through the center of this triangle, directed toward the coronoid process of the ulna anteriorly.

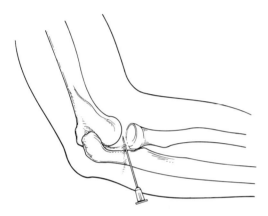

Fig. 18-5 Aspiration of elbow through lateral approach, penetrating anconeus muscle and anterolateral capsule.

Aspiration of Wrist

▶ *Technique (dorsal approach).* Palpate the radial styloid, Lister's tubercle, and the extensor pollicis longus tendon that courses around Lister's tubercle. Keeping the wrist palmar-flexed about 15 degrees, insert the needle in the fourth dorsal compartment, which contains the digital extensors (Fig. 18-6).

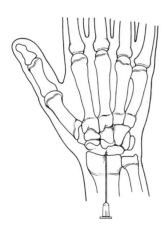

Fig. 18-6 Aspiration of wrist through dorsal approach at radiocarpal joint.

Drainage of the Septic Joint

Once the diagnosis of septic arthritis has been confirmed, immediate treatment is mandatory. The best method of draining a septic joint remains controversial. Multiple aspirations, arthroscopic drainage, and arthrotomy have all been reported to obtain satisfactory results. The choice of technique depends on the chronicity of the infection, the joint involved, and the patient's response to medical therapy. Since most antibiotics achieve a high synovial fluid concentration when administered parenterally or orally, there is no need for direct instillation of antibiotics into the joint. Although inflow and outflow catheter drainage systems may have a role in the treatment of a serious chronic infection (p. 1062), their usefulness in acute septic arthritis is limited. Surgical drainage of the joint with a closed, suction system remains the standard therapy for septic arthritis. A small window of capsule is removed, a small Penrose drain is inserted, and the capsule is left open for all septic joints. The drain is removed 24 to 72 hours after surgery, as decreased drainage indicates. In general, except for the shoulder and sacroiliac joint, cast immobilization of the joint should be maintained for 2 to 3 weeks until the wound heals. The wound is managed with either primary or primary-delayed closure.

In a 1975 report, Goldenberg suggested that multiple aspirations of the knee joint were superior to surgical drainage, and this technique may be satisfactory for the superficial joints (knee, ankle, wrist, and elbow) in patients with low white blood cell counts and less virulent organisms. For some patients, however, multiple aspirations may be more traumatic than a single surgical procedure. The techniques for multiple aspirations are the same as those described for diagnostic arthrocentesis. The joint is irrigated with sterile saline or Ringer's lactate at each aspiration. Comparison of the white cell count of the initial aspirate to that obtained at repeated aspirations should indicate a sharp decrease in white blood cells. If a large effusion persists, or if white cell counts greater than 10,000 remain after 48 hours, then joint drainage by arthroscopy or arthrotomy is advisable. The majority of septic joints in children should be treated with irrigation and drainage. Factors to be considered include the particular joint involved, the virulence of the infecting organism, the white blood cell count of the joint aspirate, and the systemic signs of the infection.

Hip

Because of the possibility of catastrophic sequelae of infection, such as necrosis of the femoral head, subluxation of the hip, and growth deformity, drainage of the septic hip joint requires a more aggressive approach; multiple aspirations are not indicated for treatment of the septic hip joint. The tenuous blood supply to the femoral head, as well as the transphyseal proximal femoral vasculature of infancy, places the femoral head at great risk for septic necrosis. Factors indicating a poor prognosis include age younger than 1 year, symptoms lasting more than 4 days before treatment, and associated osteomyelitis of the proximal femur (Fig. 18-7). Prompt surgical drainage, combined with appropriate antibiotic therapy, provides the best chance for successful treatment of septic arthritis of the hip. The approach chosen for surgical drainage of the hip joint depends on the preference and experience of the surgeon. The most common approaches are anterior and posterior. When the posterior approach is used, care must be taken to prevent injury to the posterior capsular retinacular vessels.

▲ *Technique (anterior approach).* Position the patient with a pad under the ipsilateral half of the sacrum and buttock, with the pelvis in a 30- to 45-degree oblique position. Prepare and drape the leg free. Make an oblique skin incision approximately 4 cm long in the skin creases 2 cm distal to the anterosuperior iliac spine, centering the skin incision directly distal to the anterosuperior iliac spine. Develop the interval between the tensor fascia femoris and the sartorius muscle from the anterosuperior iliac spine to a point over the intertrochanteric line; do not split the iliac apophysis. Take care not to injure the lateral femoral cutaneous nerve. Place retractors in this interval to expose the straight head of the rectus femoris muscle and pull it medially. Make a 1 cm window in the midportion of the anterior capsule of the hip joint, just distal to the reflected head of the rectus femoris muscle. Through this opening, irrigate the joint fully and place a drain. An alternative position for the capsulotomy is medial to the rectus femoris tendon, but insertion of the capsular-iliacus muscle in this area makes dissection more difficult. Leave the capsular incision open, loosely approximate the subcutaneous tissue, and either close the wound primarily or leave it open for delayed primary closure 48 to 72 hours after surgery.

If decompression is required for femoral osteomyelitis, the femoral neck can be drilled through this approach distal to the physis. Generally, the femoral neck should be drilled in children older than 18 to 24 months.

▲ *Postoperative management.* Bilateral long-leg casts with an abduction bar may be used, or a double spica cast if the hip is grossly unstable. The cast is removed 2 to 3 weeks after surgery when the wound is healed. Controlled range-of-motion exercises should be begun as soon as stability allows.

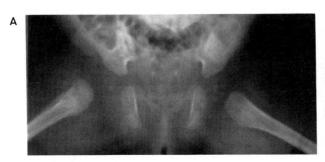
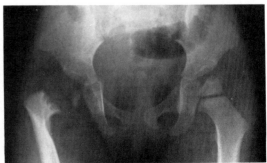

Fig. 18-7   A, Acute septic arthritis of right hip and osteomyelitis in proximal femur of 10-month-old girl after 14 days of symptoms. **B,** At age 4 years, extensive destruction of femoral head and neck.

▶ *Technique (posterior approach).* Place the patient in a lateral position. Prepare and drape the leg free. Make a skin incision extending from the greater trochanter to the posterosuperior iliac spine along the longitudinal axis of the femoral neck. Split the fibers of the gluteus maximus muscle longitudinally and retract them to expose the short external rotator muscles. If the inferior gluteal vessels are encountered, ligate them as needed. Identify and protect the sciatic nerve at the medial aspect of the dissection. If necessary for exposure, section the short external rotators, including the piriformis, gemellus superior, gemellus inferior, obturator internus, and obturator externus, from their attachments on the greater trochanter. Reflect these muscles medially to expose the posterior capsule. Make the capsulotomy near the pelvic attachment of the capsule longitudinally, taking care to protect the retinacular vessels coursing along the posterior aspect of the femoral neck. Irrigate the joint, insert drains, and leave the capsule open. When indicated, drill the femoral neck by making a small hole slightly posterior and distal to the greater trochanteric apophysis. If pus is encountered in the femoral neck, enlarge the hole to 1 cm to allow drainage. Close the skin loosely or leave open for delayed primary closure. Evaluate the stability of the hip to determine the need for postoperative immobilization. Generally, double spica cast immobilization is required after this approach.

▶ *Postoperative management.* Drains are removed 24 to 72 hours after surgery as decreased drainage indicates. Spica casting is continued for 2 to 3 weeks. Range-of-motion exercises are begun as soon as stability of the hip joint allows.

Sacroiliac Joint

Acute septic arthritis of the sacroiliac joint is uncommon in children but does occur. The area of infection can usually be identified by CT scan (Fig. 18-8). Surgical irrigation and drainage of the sacroiliac joint are indicated if aspiration reveals gross pus, if the child has acute symptoms of systemic infection, or if symptoms fail to respond to appropriate antibiotic treatment within 24 to 72 hours.

▶ *Technique (posterior approach).* Make an incision along the lateral lip of the posterior third of the iliac crest, extending it laterally and distally 5 to 8 cm from the posterosuperior iliac spine. Deepen the dissection down to the iliac crest, separate the lumbodorsal fascia from it, detach and reflect medially the aponeurosis of the sacrospinalis muscle together with the periosteum, and expose the posterior margin of the sacroiliac joint. Split the gluteus maximus muscle in line with its fibers, or incise its origin on the iliac crest, the aponeurosis of the sacrospinalis, and the sacrum, and reflect it laterally and distally to expose the posterior aspect of the ilium. Remove a small window of capsule from the joint for irrigation and drainage, insert a small Penrose drain, and leave the capsule open. Postoperative cast immobilization is not required. The drain is removed after 24 to 72 hours as drainage decreases.

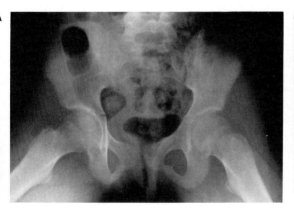
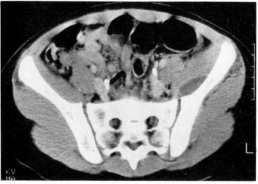

Fig. 18-8 **A,** Septic arthritis of left sacroiliac joint with retropsoas abscess. **B,** CT scan identifies lesion and shows widening and mild erosion of sacroiliac joint.

Knee

The knee is the second most commonly involved joint. In the neonatal period, distal femoral osteomyelitis may be associated with the septic arthritis, but this becomes less frequent as the child matures. Because the knee is a very superficial joint, easily accessible for aspiration, the technique of multiple aspirations (p. 1052) may be appropriate for early infection with a low white blood cell count by joint aspirate and less virulent organism. Arthroscopic drainage of the knee joint is also an alternative if multiple aspirations are ineffective or are not tolerated by the child. Arthroscopy also allows complete inspection of all compartments and removal of small debris in the knee joint. Currently, depending of the chronicity of the infection and the degree of soft tissue abscess, open surgical drainage is generally required (Fig. 18-9). An anterior approach is usually sufficient for drainage of all compartments of the knee, but multiple approaches may be necessary in severe infections.

▲ *Technique (anteromedial approach).* Make an incision extending from the superomedial aspect of the patella to the middle of the fat pad distally. Carry the dissection through the subcutaneous tissue. Incise the capsule and synovium longitudinally from just medial to the midpatella to the middle of the fat pad distally. Inspect the knee carefully and irrigate copiously. If any portion of the knee is inaccessible from this approach, a second incision anterolaterally, posterolaterally, or posteromedially may be necessary. Leave the capsule and synovium open, insert a drain, and loosely close the subcutaneous tissues. Close the skin or leave open for delayed primary closure. Alternatively, the anterolateral approach may be used with identical operative technique.

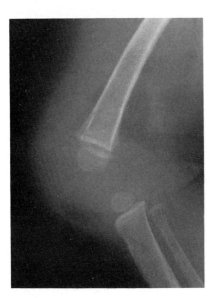

Fig. 18-9 Septic arthritis of knee in 2-year-old girl. Note large effusion and extensive soft tissue edema.

Ankle

Operative drainage of the ankle joint is best performed through an anteromedial or anterolateral approach. Guhl and Parisien have described arthroscopic approaches to the ankle joint (p. 792), and these may be appropriate for drainage of the early, less virulent septic arthritis. As in other joints following drainage, the capsule is left open, a small suction drain is inserted, and cast immobilization is used for 2 to 3 weeks after surgery.

▲ *Technique (anterolateral approach).* Make a longitudinal incision anterior to the lateral malleolus, lateral to the extensor tendons at the level of the ankle joint. Remove a window of joint capsule and irrigate the joint copiously.

▲ *Technique (anteromedial approach).* Make an incision just medial to the anterior tibial tendon at the level of the medial malleolus. Avoid dissection lateral to the anterior tibial tendon because of risk of injury to the neurovascular bundle. Identify the capsule at the level of the medial malleolus as it extends over the anterior neck of the talus. Remove a window of the capsule and irrigate the joint copiously.

Shoulder

The shoulders (Fig. 18-10) may be drained either through the more frequent anterior or less common posterior approach. The capsule is left open and a small drain is inserted. A collar and cuff or sling is generally used after shoulder drainage.

▲ *Technique (anterior approach).* Place the patient in a semisitting position and prepare and drape free the involved arm. Make a skin incision extending from the level of the acromion distally over the deltopectoral groove. Dissect a few fibers of the deltoid and retract these medially along with the cephalic vein. Identify the subscapularis tendon and divide the inferior one third of its muscle fibers to expose the anteroinferior aspect of the capsule. Do not incise the entire subscapularis tendon. Remove a 1-cm window of the capsule and irrigate the joint copiously. Open the tendon sheath over the long head of the biceps to confirm that pus or abscess formation is not retained in this area, since it can communicate with the shoulder joint. If a focus of osteomyelitis is suspected, the proximal humerus may be decompressed by drilling just anterior to the insertion of the pectoralis major muscle.

▲ *Technique (posterior approach).* Place the patient in the lateral decubitus position. Make an incision extending from the spine of the scapula distally to over the deltoid muscle laterally. Split the fibers of the posterior deltoid muscle, taking care to avoid the axillary nerve. Expose the external rotators and develop the interval between the infraspinatus and the teres minor muscles. Incise the capsule and irrigate the joint copiously.

Fig. 18-10   A, Septic arthritis of shoulder and osteomyelitis of proximal humerus in 14-month-old boy. **B,** Two years later. Note delay in ossification of proximal epiphysis and remodeling of humeral shaft.

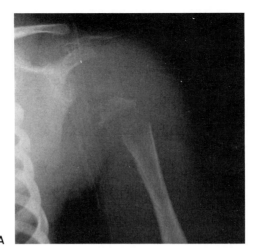

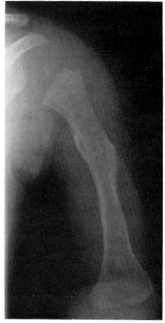

Elbow

The elbow joint may be drained through a medial, lateral, or posterior approach. The posterolateral approach is most commonly used. As in other joints, the capsule is left open, a small drain is inserted, and cast immobilization is used for 2 to 3 weeks after surgery.

▲ *Technique (lateral approach).* Make a short incision over the lateral epicondyle, extending 4 cm proximally and 2 cm distally. Separate the triceps from the extensor carpi radialis and brevis and extend this interval distally. With the elbow flexed and using careful anterior dissection adjacent to the capsule, retract distally the radial nerve, the brachioradialis, and the wrist extensors. Open the joint capsule and remove a small window of the capsule.

▲ *Technique (medial approach).* Make an incision over the medial epicondyle, extending 4 cm proximally and 2 cm distally. Identify the interval between the triceps and brachialis, and isolate and protect the ulnar nerve. Open the joint capsule both anteriorly and posteriorly and irrigate copiously.

▲ *Technique (posterolateral [anconeus] approach).* Make a skin incision over the posterolateral aspect of the elbow, extending along the humerus to the radial head and then curving posteriorly to the ulna. Identify the interval between the triceps and the brachioradialis and the wrist extensors. Follow this interval distally to identify the anconeus muscle. Expose the joint capsule between the extensor carpi radialis and the anconeus muscles. For further exposure of the joint, the interval between the anconeus and the extensor carpi ulnaris muscle may be developed distally, but this is usually not necessary for drainage. Open the joint capsule and remove a small window of the capsule. Drain and irrigate the joint.

Wrist

The wrist may be drained through a dorsal, medial, or lateral approach. The dorsal approach is the most versatile, but the medial or lateral approach may be appropriate when bony involvement dictates. The capsule is left open, a small drain is inserted, and cast immobilization is used for 2 to 3 weeks after surgery.

▲ *Technique (dorsal approach).* Make a longitudinal incision 4 cm long through the fourth dorsal compartment, between the extensor pollicis longus and the extensor indicis proprius tendons. Carry the dissection down through this compartment to the dorsal wrist capsule. Remove a small window of capsule and irrigate the joint.

▲ *Technique (medial approach).* Make an incision 5 cm long over the head of the ulna between the flexor and extensor carpi ulnaris tendons, taking care to avoid injuring the dorsal branch of the ulnar nerve. Expose the ulnar collateral ligament and synovium and incise them distal to the ulnar styloid. Do not detach the triangular fibrocartilage.

▲ *Technique (lateral approach).* Make a longitudinal incision 5 cm long between the abductor pollicis longus and extensor pollicis brevis tendons volarly and the extensor pollicis longus tendon dorsally. Deepen the incision into the anatomic snuffbox, taking care to prevent injury to the radial artery. Incise the radial collateral ligament and synovium and evacuate the joint. Irrigate the joint copiously.

ACUTE PYOGENIC OSTEOMYELITIS

Hematogenous bacterial osteomyelitis is a disease of childhood and, to a lesser degree, adolescence. The infection usually occurs in the metaphyses of long bones, and less frequently in the calcaneus, ilium, and vertebrae (Table 18-4). Osteomyelitis occurs most often in the metaphysis because of either mechanical or immunologic phenomenon. Morrissy and Haynes and Hobo documented a defect in phagocytosis in the end arterial loops in the metaphysis just beneath the physis. Others have suggested the possibility of precipitation of bacteria into the metaphysis with changes in the metaphyseal vascular pattern. Trauma is implicated in 30% to 40% of all patients with osteomyelitis. Once the infection is established, a septic infarct of bone occurs and the body attempts to isolate this focus of infection, forming an abscess. The pus spreads outward along the path of least resistance, into the subperiosteal space where rapid longitudinal spread may occur, limited by the perichondral ring at the physis. If the infection proceeds, extensive bone infarction (sequestration) occurs. Peri-osteal bone formation results in a shell of bone (involucrum) about the site of chronic bone infection. The epiphysis and physeal cartilage are spared until the end stage of the disease, except in the proximal femur and the proximal humerus.

Diagnosis

The diagnosis of osteomyelitis is based on clinical signs of swelling, tenderness, and fever; laboratory results of increased white blood cell count and erythrocyte sedimentation rate; and roentgenography, including bone scan and plain roentgenograms. Metaphyseal tenderness accompanying swelling in a febrile patient is highly suggestive of osteomyelitis, but fracture should be ruled out roentgenographically. Fever and elevation of white cell count are inconsistent signs. Usually the temperature is greater than 38° C, the white cell count is greater than 10,000, and the erythrocyte sedimentation rate is elevated. Although

Table 18-4 Distribution of hematogenous bacterial osteomyelitis

Bone	No. of patients
Femur	72
Tibia	62
Humerus	33
Fibula	14
Radius	12
Phalanx	11
Calcaneus	10
Ulna	6
Ischium	6
Metatarsal	5
Vertebrae	3
Ilium	4
Sacrum	3
Clavicle	2
Skull	2
Carpal bone	2
Rib	1
Pubis	1
Metacarpal	1
Cuboid	1
Cuneiform	1
Bone of pyriform aperture	1
Olecranon	1
Maxilla	1
Mandible	1
Scapula	1
Sternum	1

From Jackson MA and Nelson JD: J Pediatr Orthop 2:313, 1982.

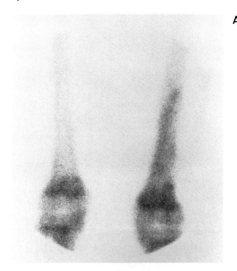

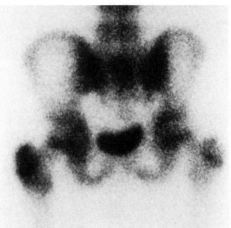

Fig. 18-11 **A,** Early signs of osteomyelitis in left distal femoral metaphysis and diaphysis on bone scan despite normal roentgenogram. **B,** Osteomyelitis of right greater trochanter in 12-year-old boy with normal roentgenogram.

there are no early roentgenographic changes in bone, soft tissue swelling with displacement of fat shadows is suggestive of osteomyelitis. Technetium bone scanning provides accurate early diagnosis with few false-negative or false-positive results. The bone scan is generally interpreted as indicative of a focus of osteomyelitis when there is increased uptake of the radionuclide (Fig. 18-11). Roentgenographic changes become apparent within 7 to 10 days (Fig. 18-12). If a septic infarct is present, an area of markedly decreased uptake may be indicative of a focus of infection; this occurs in about 5% of patients with osteomyelitis. White cell–labeled scans and gallium scans are occasionally useful for the diagnosis of osteomyelitis.

Aspiration, and possibly needle biopsy, of bone should be done before initiating antibiotic therapy. Although *S. aureus* accounts for most osteomyelitis, there is a wide variation in causative flora, mandating careful bacteriologic analysis for specific diagnosis and treatment. The bacteriologic spectrum of osteomyelitis is similar to that of septic arthritis (Table 18-3), except that *H. influenzae* rarely causes osteomyelitis. In an acutely ill child with suspected osteomyelitis, needle aspiration should not be delayed even if nuclear medicine evaluation has not been obtained. Several experimental studies indicate that metaphyseal aspiration does not cause an increased uptake of the radionuclide, giving a false-positive result.

▶ *Technique (aspiration of bone).* After appropriate sedation and dermal injection of lidocaine, identify the area of maximum tenderness, which usually corresponds to the area of increased uptake on the bone scan and to soft tissue swelling on plain roentgenograms. Place an 18- or 20-gauge needle of sufficient length through the soft tissue to bone so that the needle tip lies in the subperiosteal space. Aspirate any subperiosteal pus and document the presence of a subperiosteal abscess. Next penetrate the cortex and aspirate any blood or pus from the medullary cavity of the bone. The metaphyseal cortex compromised by infection allows easy penetration of the needle, but the denser diaphyseal cortex cannot be aspirated in this manner. A Craig biopsy needle may be used to provide pathologic tissue and better material for culture if aspiration with a needle is difficult.

Surgical Drainage of Acute Osteomyelitis

The indications for surgical drainage in early acute osteomyelitis are not always clear. After aspiration or needle biopsy and institution of antibiotic therapy, absolute indications are (1) subperiosteal abscess confirmed by aspiration or biopsy, (2) failure to respond promptly (within 24 to 72 hours) to antibiotic therapy, and (3) roentgenographic evidence of an abscess cavity in the bone. Beyond these absolute indications, each patient's clinical response to antibiotic therapy, along with laboratory and roentgenographic evaluations, determines the need for surgical intervention.

▶ *Technique.* Choose a safe approach through the soft tissues to the bone that avoids major neurovascular structures, since the wound may be left open after drainage. Incise the periosteum longitudinally, releasing any subperiosteal pus. In a very small bone, make a single drill hole through the cortex and enlarge it as needed with a curet. In a larger bone, use a drill and small osteotome to cut an oval cortical window (Fig. 18-13). Use a curet to enter the center of the medullary cavity. Avoid aggressive curettage because the risk of pathologic fracture increases significantly as the cancellous metaphyseal bone is removed. The rim of sclerotic bone that limits curettage in subacute osteomyelitis or Brodie's abscess is not encountered in acute osteomyelitis, and surgical restraint is mandatory. Leave the wound open with drains or packing in the bone and subperiosteal space, and use either delayed primary closure or closure by secondary intention. Cast immobilization should be continued for 6 to 12 weeks or longer as necessary after surgery for wound control, splinting of adjacent joints, and prevention of pathologic fracture.

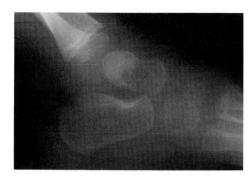

Fig. 18-12 Lytic changes apparent on roentgenogram 3 weeks after onset of osteomyelitis of talus.

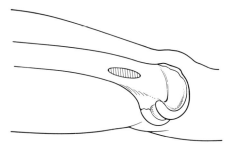

Fig. 18-13 For surgical drainage of acute osteomyelitis in larger bones, such as distal lateral femur, oval cortical window is made in metaphysis or diaphysis (see text).

SUBACUTE OSTEOMYELITIS

In a subacute infection, symptoms have persisted longer than 4 weeks before diagnosis. In a review of all types of osteomyelitis by Roberts et al, one third of patients had subacute infection. Patients are often afebrile and complain of bone pain. Roentgenograms reveal a lytic lesion with a surrounding area of reactive bone and adjacent periosteal reaction. Bone scanning is uniformly positive.

Brodie's abscess of bone is a lytic, geographically limited lesion with a rim of sclerotic bone (Fig. 18-14). The characteristic appearance is not always present, however, and lesions may appear very aggressive, with formation of a Codman triangle of reactive bone or may cross the physis into the epiphysis (Fig. 18-15). Biopsy for definitive diagnosis is always indicated and, although this may be done with a Craig biopsy needle, an open procedure with curettage of the lesion is usually performed. *S. aureus* is the most common organism causing Brodie's abscess. If a fungal cause or an unusual causative organism is suspected, the infectious disease service and bacteriology laboratory should be alerted to the need for special techniques. Neoplastic lesions are included in the differential diagnosis; Ewing's sarcoma, histiocytosis X, and osteosarcoma are primary bone tumors that may be confused with a Brodie's abscess. Cytologic evaluation of biopsy specimens should be included along with culture and sensitivity testing.

CHRONIC OSTEOMYELITIS

When septic infarction of bone is accompanied by a persistent focus of bacteria, chronic osteomyelitis may develop. Generally a septic focus of necrotic bone (sequestrum) is found and excision is necessary for resolution of the infection. The sequestrum may be documented on CT scan or tomogram (Fig. 18-16). Debridement should remove all devitalized bone, leaving only bleeding cortical and cancellous bone. Vital dyes have been used to determine the viability of remaining tissue; however, debridement of all nonbleeding bone, infected granulation tissue, and necrotic debris remains the standard treatment. Antibiotic therapy depends on the sensitivity of the bacteria present. Cultures of material from the superficial sinus tract are not accurate, and deep cultures are required for specificity. The use of vascularized tissue transfer in treating chronic osteomyelitis is somewhat controversial. Tissue coverage and added vascularity alone do not heal chronic osteomyelitis, especially if associated with a septic nonunion, although this is rare in children.

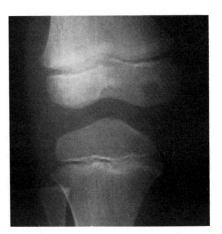

Fig. 18-15 Brodie's abscess in right distal femoral epiphysis of 3-year-old girl.

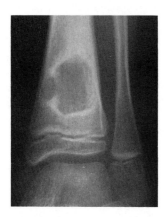

Fig. 18-14 Brodie's abscess in distal tibia of 9-year-old boy showing characteristic appearance of geographic, lytic lesion with rim of sclerotic bone.

Management of Septic Nonunion

The principles of management of septic nonunion are the same for all long bones: (1) debridement, (2) skeletal stabilization, (3) soft tissue coverage, and (4) bone grafting.

Debridement

The sinus tract, devitalized soft tissue, and all dead bone are excised and any sequestrum is removed.

Skeletal Stabilization

External skeletal fixation may vary from a uniplanar frame to the elaborate Ilizarov device. Whatever hardware is chosen should be placed with care to prevent injury to neurovascular structures. Since the primary goal of stabilization is union, sacrificing length in favor of stability and union is acceptable; however, when the limb length discrepancy is severe, an attempt may be made to gain both union and length simultaneously, as with the Ilizarov device. The primary goal of any procedure should be healing of the nonunion and resolution of the infection.

Soft Tissue Coverage

Following debridement and skeletal stabilization, additional soft tissue coverage may be required. Delayed primary closure, closure by secondary intention, and tissue transfer each plays a role in reducing or closing a soft tissue defect. In general, either a local flap or free tissue transfer is necessary to cover a significant defect.

Bone Grafting

Defects in bone may be filled with autogenous graft from the pelvis or free bone transfer of ilium, rib, or fibula, depending on the amount of tissue required and the skill of the surgeon. Vascularized bone transfer may be necessary for extensive bone loss. Young children have a remarkable ability to incorporate autografts over large segments (Fig. 18-17).

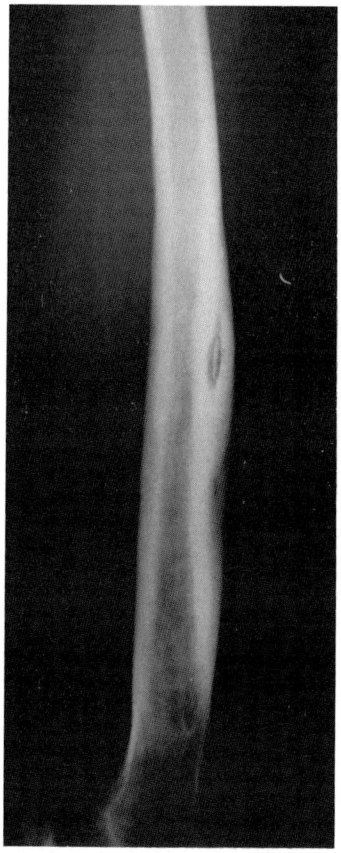

Fig. 18-16   Chronic osteomyelitis of left femur with sequestrum formation in anterior cortex seen on lateral roentgenogram.

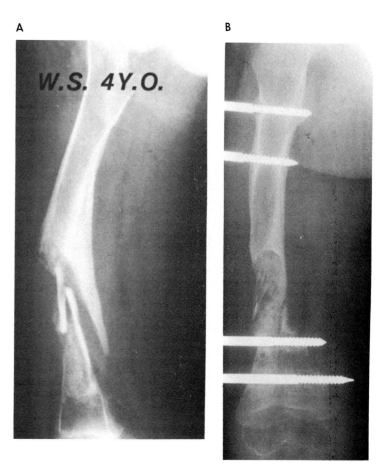

Fig. 18-17   **A,** Septic nonunion with segmental defect after chronic osteomyelitis of right distal femur in 4-year-old child. **B,** After debridement, reconstructive lengthening and bone grafting.

Inflow-Outflow Catheter System

Inflow-outflow wound irrigating systems are controversial. Parenteral antibiotic levels in bone and soft tissue are sufficiently high to treat most infections, and the accumulation of pus, exudate, and necrotic debris may be prevented by such a system. In chronic osteomyelitis and in large postoperative wound infections with hardware in place, inflow-outflow systems have been used with success to facilitate wound debridement and healing.

▲ *Technique.* Surgically debride the infected wound and continue sequential packing, irrigation, and debridement until a clean, granulating wound is obtained. Close the wound over an inflow-outflow catheter system consisting of two large-bore suction drainage tubes placed parallel deep in the wound. Approximate the subcutaneous tissue in a large wound with absorbable, interrupted sutures. Close the skin with nonabsorbable sutures in a watertight fashion. Instill the irrigant continuously at the rate of 50 cc/hr. Every 4 hours clamp the outflow catheter to distend the wound, leaving the clamp in place for 1 hour, or until the inflow stops or the wound becomes distended and painful. Then unclamp the outflow tube to flush the joint and remove any accumulated debris.

Saline may be used as an irrigant rather than an antibiotic solution because of the variable absorption of antibiotics through soft tissue. If an antibiotic is added to the irrigant, dosage should be adjusted appropriately, and antibiotic levels should be measured if there is a question of toxicity. The use of suction on the outflow tube often causes clogging, as does intermittent infusion. The length of treatment with this system depends on the status of the wound, the debris in the outflow catheter, and the ease of maintenance of the system; 3 weeks is usually the maximum.

CHRONIC RECURRENT MULTIFOCAL OSTEOMYELITIS

Chronic, recurrent, multifocal osteomyelitis is a clinical and roentgenographic syndrome of subacute, symmetric osteomyelitis. First described by Giedion et al in 1972, it is characterized by an insidious onset of pain over affected bones. The clinical course waxes and wanes over a period of months to years, with spontaneous resolution of lesions and symptoms the end result in all patients. Most commonly affected are the medial clavicle and the metaphyses of long bones, particularly the distal tibia. Vertebral involvement has been reported with associated vertebra plana. Patients have increased erythrocyte sedimentation rates and mild elevations in white blood cell count. Roentgenograms show generally lytic lesions surrounded by an area of sclerotic bone and a periosteal reaction indicative of the slow onset and less aggressive nature of the lesion (Fig. 18-18). Technetium bone scanning shows increased uptake in all lesions. Differential diagnoses include histiocytosis X, bacterial infection, and neoplasms, specifically leukemia, lymphoma, neuroblastoma, and rhabdomyosarcoma. These lesions are, by definition, culture negative. Pathologic evaluation shows either acute or chronic inflammation with granuloma formation, depending on the stage of the disease process. At least two biopsies should be taken, with attempts to culture all microorganisms, including bacteria, chlamydia, viruses, spirochetes, mycoplasmata, and fungi. Once the disease is clearly defined, antibiotic treatment is not indicated. Recurrent episodes of pain should be managed with antiinflammatory medication and splinting.

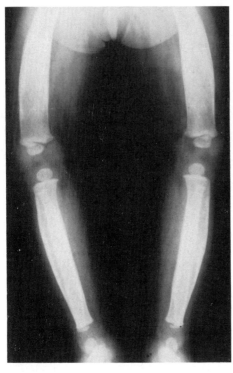

Fig. 18-18   Multifocal osteomyelitis of femur and tibia.

LONG-TERM CONSEQUENCES OF SEPTIC ARTHRITIS AND OSTEOMYELITIS

In general, if septic joints are treated promptly and correctly, serious sequelae are rare; however, they do occur, particularly in the hip. Long-term sequelae of septic arthritis include articular loss, varying from narrowing of the joint space to gross destruction of the articular cartilage; destruction of the epiphysis, particularly in the proximal femur and proximal humerus when septic arthritis is associated with osteomyelitis; and growth disturbance. After acute osteomyelitis, long-term sequelae include growth arrest or delay, chronic osteomyelitis, and pathologic fracture.

Destruction of the Femoral Head

After septic arthritis of the hip, the femoral head may be partially or completely destroyed. This destruction may be associated with pseudarthrosis of the femoral neck, septic necrosis of the femoral head, or joint space narrowing (Fig. 18-19). Treatment alternatives include observation, valgus osteotomy, trochanteric arthroplasty, Harmon or L'Episcopo reconstruction, and hip arthrodesis.

After septic arthritis, the destroyed femoral head does not always progress rapidly to pain and total disability and may function satisfactorily for many years. Adduction deformity may be managed with either soft tissue release or valgus osteotomy of the femur, as required. Advantages of observation are preservation of the abductor musculature for hip reconstruction in adulthood and avoidance of the complications of pain, subluxation, dislocation, and recurrent infection often associated with reconstructive procedures.

Partial destruction of the femoral head and proximal femoral growth arrest may cause overgrowth of the greater trochanter, and valgus osteotomy may be indicated. This osteotomy is designed to place the remaining, unaffected, inferior portion of the femoral head within the acetabulum, providing a normal articular cartilage surface for weight bearing. The valgus osteotomy (p. 166) also transfers the greater trochanter laterally and distally, improving the mechanical advantage of the hip abductor musculature.

Many authors recommend no treatment other than of the limb length discrepancy. If no portion of the femoral head remains for reconstruction, trochanteric arthroplasty may be indicated, although the results of this procedure are highly variable. If the acetabulum is deficient and the hip is unstable, pelvic osteotomy may also be required to maintain stability.

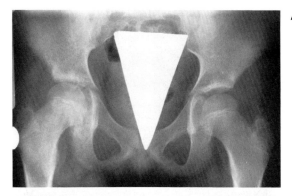
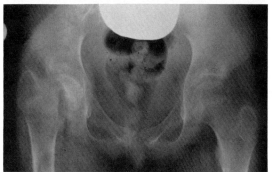

Fig. 18-19   **A,** Nine-year-old girl with septic arthritis of right hip of 5 days' duration before surgical drainage. **B,** Three months later, pathologic fracture of femoral neck with sequestration of avascular femoral head.

▶ *Technique (trochanteric arthroplasty).* Approach the hip through combined anterior iliofemoral and lateral incisions (p. 150). Open the hip capsule with asymmetric H-shaped incisions, with one short incision anteriorly along the pelvic insertion and a second parallel incision anterosuperiorly at the capsular insertion along the intertrochanteric line. Make a third incision between these two parallel incisions, along the axis of the femoral neck. Remove the fibrous contents of the acetabulum. Remove any remaining femoral head and neck and perform a femoral osteotomy at the level of the lesser trochanter. Remove the hip abductors from the greater trochanter and transfer them to the lateral femoral shaft. Place the cartilaginous greater trochanter within the acetabulum, performing any further capsular release necessary for reduction. Suture the capsule over the trochanter to maintain reduction.

Hip arthrodesis (p. 80) is indicated for relief of pain and correction of deformity when no other reconstructive procedure is possible.

Leg Length Discrepancy

Hematogenous osteomyelitis is a metaphyseal process that usually spares the adjacent physis, but occasionally growth in the affected limb is disturbed. This is particularly true in the infant's hip, where transphyseal vessels predispose to physeal destruction. Occasionally, the physes of the distal femur, proximal tibia, or distal tibia are affected, with partial or complete physeal arrest causing limb length discrepancy or angular growth deformity. When growth disturbance is suspected, a bony physeal bridge should be considered (Fig. 18-20). If initial roentgenograms do not show the bony bridge, tomograms should be obtained because a very small area of physeal bridging may produce significant growth disturbance and angular deformity. The technique for excision of bony bridge formation is described on p. 66. The appropriate treatment of leg length discrepancy after infection depends on the specific cause and the amount of the discrepancy. Methods for treating leg length discrepancy are discussed in Chapter 3.

OTHER INFECTIONS

Septic arthritis and osteomyelitis are by far the most common infections in children, but other infections do occur and must be promptly diagnosed and treated appropriately. Nail puncture wounds are common in children but are rarely complicated by infection. Some other relatively rare infections affecting children include gas gangrene, fungal infections, congenital syphilis, Lyme disease, cat scratch fever, and Caffey's disease.

Nail Puncture Wounds

Nail puncture wounds, particularly of the foot, are common in children and are seldom complicated by serious infection. If infection appears, usually 3 to 10 days after injury, there is a foreign body in the soft tissue or a bone or joint has been penetrated (Fig. 18-21). If roentgenograms confirm the presence of a foreign body or bone or joint injury acutely, surgical debridement is indicated. The most common infecting organisms in nail puncture wounds are *Pseudomonas* and *Staphylococcus*.

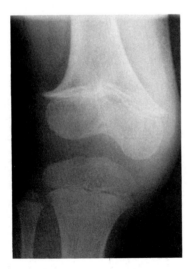

Fig. 18-20 Bony physeal bridge in right distal femoral physis after hematogenous osteomyelitis in 6-year-old girl.

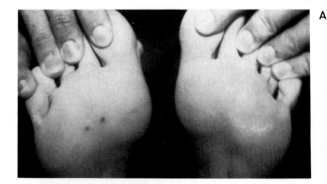

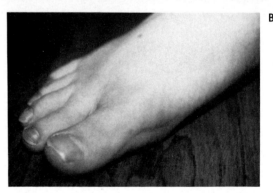

Fig. 18-21 A, Infection after nail puncture wound, plantar aspect of right foot. **B,** Clinical appearance 3 months after incision and drainage of metatarsophalangeal joint.

Gas Gangrene

Gas gangrene, though rare in children, is one of the most catastrophic problems in orthopaedic surgery. It is caused by infection with *Clostridium perfringens,* an anaerobic, gram-positive bacillus. Spores of *C. perfringens* are found in soil and in human and animal feces; they enter the body through an open injury, such as a grade III open fracture. The hallmark of this infection is myonecrosis with gas permeating the soft tissues, which gives the characteristic roentgenographic appearance. The skin is tense with crepitance on palpation, there is a rapid onset of increasing pain and swelling with a thin, hemorrhagic exudate and often purplish brown bullae, and the pulse is increased disproportionately to the temperature. Immediate roentgenographic confirmation should be obtained and clostridial infection should be assumed. *C. perfringens* elaborates a number of extracellular toxins, the most significant of which is α-toxin (a lecithinase), causing soft tissue destruction, hemolysis, and death. The combination of α-toxin and other extracellular toxins (collagenase, hyaluronidase, leukocidin, deoxyribonuclease, and fibrinolysis) leads to a rapid spread of the infection, resulting in high morbidity and mortality rates.

Treatment of gas gangrene is radical surgical debridement of all necrotic tissue and decompression of all fascial compartments. The area of debridement should extend beyond the area of necrotic and emphysematous tissue to normal tissue. All fascial planes are opened and left open. Amputation may be necessary as a lifesaving measure. Penicillin is the antibiotic of choice, but cephalosporin and clindamycin are also effective against this organism.

Because of its value in treating chronic osteomyelitis and other bone and joint infections, hyperbaric oxygen therapy has been advocated by some authors as the primary treatment of gas gangrene, but insufficient documentation is available to confirm its efficacy. Couch reported decreased morbidity and mortality in 54 patients with gas gangrene who were treated with hyperbaric oxygenation within 24 hours of diagnosis; it was especially effective when combined with surgical debridement and decompression. Hyperbaric oxygen should be used if available, but surgical debridement and decompression should not be delayed.

Polyvalent antitoxin has been used in the treatment of gas gangrene, but its effectiveness has not been firmly established.

Initial clostridial myonecrosis can be prevented by adequate debridement of high-risk wounds, leaving contaminated wounds open, and the use of appropriate antibiotic therapy. High-risk wounds include open fractures and severe crushing injuries, especially deep wounds involving the buttocks, thigh, and shoulder.

Fungal Bone and Joint Infections

Although fungal bone and joint infections are rare, they must be considered in differentiation of causative organisms. Special culturing techniques are required to identify fungal infecting agents, and the bacteriology laboratory should be notified if fungal infection is suspected. In general, fungal infections in children are associated with immune deficiencies, immunosuppression, intravenous catheters, prolonged antibiotic treatment, and steroid treatment. The fungi causing bone infections in children are most commonly *Candida, Aspergillus, Blastomyces, Coccidioides, Cryptococcus, Histoplasma, Brucella,* and *Sporothrix.*

Candida infection should be considered in the immunocompromised child. Neonatal septic arthritis or osteomyelitis may be caused by *Candida* infection in infants in the intensive care unit who are receiving broad-spectrum antibiotics and most of whom have umbilical catheters. Respiratory distress syndrome also places these infants at greater risk for severe infection. Multiple joints may be involved, but the knee is most commonly infected with a contiguous focus of osteomyelitis in the distal femur. Symptoms include tense, swollen, erythematous joints and pseudoparalysis. Aspiration of the joint confirms the diagnosis. Initial treatment should be medicinal, with amphotericin B and flucytosine. If synovial fluid evaluation does not document eradication of the organism and a decrease in synovial white cell count to less than 5000 within 24 to 48 hours of antibiotic therapy, surgical drainage is indicated.

Aspergillus infection is most common in patients with hematologic malignancies. The usual site of infection is the lungs, and disseminated aspergillosis is almost always fatal. Bone or joint infection with *Aspergillus* is extremely rare; Casscells reported a single patient with tibial osteomyelitis caused by *Aspergillus* organisms. Surgical drainage and antibiotic therapy with amphotericin B and 5-flucytosine, and sometimes rifampin, are generally recommended treatment methods.

Coccidioides organisms are endemic in the southwestern United States, primarily in the San Joaquin Valley of California. Infection occurs most frequently in the summer and fall and more often in adults than in children. Primary *Coccidioides* infection is a subclinical occurrence in 60% of patients; 40% have a flulike illness. The incubation period is 10 to 14 days. Arthritis and arthralgias may occur with the primary infection, but the fungus cannot be cultured from the joints at this stage of the infection. The primary focus of infection is pulmonary, and several weeks later the spread of the infection can be recognized. Because primary infections are frequently asymptomatic, some patients have disseminated coccidioidomycosis and often osteomyelitis. Coccidioidal arthritis should be differentiated from early reactive arthritis. Aspiration provides definitive diagnosis. Treatment includes therapeutic arthrocentesis with drainage and synovectomy. The use of amphotericin B is controversial when other systemic symptoms are not present, and there is no evidence to support its use in isolated bone and joint infections. When surgical procedures are performed, perioperative amphotericin B should be used to prevent spread of the disease. Oral ketoconazole, a new antifungal agent, may also be effective in treatment of this infection.

Cryptococcus neoformans is most prevalent in the urban environment, having been isolated from pigeon nests and roostings. Cryptococcosis is most common in patients over the age of 30 years. In their review of the literature and report of three patients with skeletal cryptococcosis, Chleboun and Nade stressed the high frequency of associated diseases, including sarcoidosis, histoplasmosis, tuberculosis, chronic rheumatoid heart disease, Hodgkin's disease, and leukemia. Skeletal lesions in cryptococcosis are osteolytic. Biopsy with curettage should be performed. Because osseous lesions have been reported to resolve after surgical treatment alone, the role of highly toxic drugs such as amphotericin B and flucytosine is controversial.

Infection with *Brucella* organisms produces a systemic illness known as undulant fever. With present techniques of pasteurization of diary products and practices of meat packing, the prevalence of this disease has greatly diminished. Patients usually have a history of daily spiking fevers for days or weeks, tender hepatosplenomegaly, arthralgias, and myalgias.

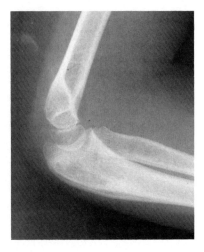

Fig. 18-22 *Brucella* osteomyelitis of olecranon in 9-year-old child.

Leukopenia or a leukemoid reaction may occur. Serologic diagnosis is made with a positive agglutinin reaction at serum dilutions of greater than 1 to 160, and blood cultures should be performed in all patients. *Brucella* organisms rarely cause arthritis or osteomyelitis, but sporadic cases have been reported (Fig. 18-22). Tetracycline is the antibiotic of choice, with streptomycin added in severe cases.

Congenital Syphilis

Congenital syphilis is transmitted from the mother to the unborn child at any stage of the disease: primary, secondary, or latent. The spirochete *Treponema pallidum* is transmitted into the fetal circulation across the placenta and becomes widely disseminated in the child. Prenatal death occurs in 25% to 30% of cases. Children with congenital syphilis have varying signs and symptoms. Signs of systemic illness are common, including hepatosplenomegaly, anemia, skin lesions, and hand and foot swelling. Skeletal lesions are present in approximately 70% of children; the classic "saber shin" deformity occurs in only 4% with late presentation. The primary roentgenographic finding is diffuse periosteal reaction over both long and flat bones, often with metaphyseal irregularity and lucency and increased density in the zones of provisional calcification. Localization of metaphyseal resorption to the medial proximal tibia produces Winberger's sign (Fig. 18-23). Patients older than 4 months may demonstrate Hutchinson's triad of tooth deformity with pointed or spiked incisors, interstitial keratitis, and eighth nerve deafness. Differential diagnoses include Caffey's disease, hypervitaminosis A, and abuse. The diagnostic blood test for syphilis is a positive VDRL (Venereal Disease Research Laboratory) test confirmed by an FTA (fluorescent treponemal antibody) test; because the VDRL frequently results in false-positive readings, confirmation by FTA is mandatory.

The ideal treatment of congenital syphilis is penicillin antibiotic therapy for the infected mother, but this is not always possible. The infected infant should be treated immediately with a single dose of 50,000 units/kg of benzathine penicillin.

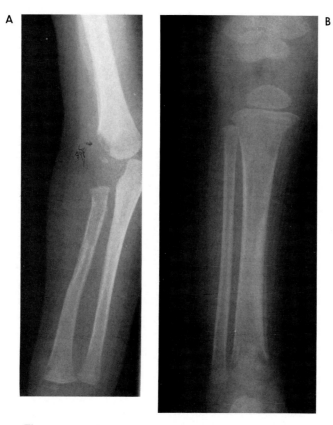

Fig. 18-23   Congenital syphilis. **A,** Elbow and forearm and, **B,** knee and tibia in 9-month-old girl. Note periosteal elevation and metaphyseal lytic lesions.

Lyme Disease

Lyme disease is a recently recognized condition in which a spirochete, *Borrelia burgdorferi,* is transmitted by the deer tick to a human, causing an infection whose prominent symptom is arthritis. The disease occurs most frequently in the summer, and most patients have characteristic skin lesions of erythema chronicum migrans; some, however, have no history of rash or recollection of a tick bite. Neurologic, cardiac, and articular manifestations of the infection appear later. Endemic areas of this infection include New England, the middle Atlantic states, Wisconsin, Minnesota, and California. The knee joint is most commonly involved, although multiple joints may be affected. Serologic testing confirms the diagnosis. Penicillin is the antibiotic of choice, administered either intravenously (20 million units/day) or orally (50 mg/kg/day). Steere reported a low rate of recurrence of infection after intravenous administration of penicillin, whereas Culp et al reported successful treatment with oral administration in only 23 of 33 patients—8 of the remaining 10 patients responded to subsequent intravenous therapy. Oral penicillin therapy should be instituted for a relatively acute septic arthritis; chronic septic arthritis or failure to respond to oral therapy mandates intravenous therapy. An alternative to penicillin therapy is tetracycline (30 mg/kg/day). Surgical intervention is rarely indicated in this disease.

Cat Scratch Fever

This is a nonbacterial, regional lymphadenitis of unknown cause. The disease occurs 3 to 30 days after a cat scratch, with symptoms usually appearing more than 12 days after the incident. Common symptoms include constitutional symptoms, fever, and regional lymphadenopathy, most commonly axillary adenopathy. Osseous lytic lesions distant from the area of involvement have been reported in association with this disease. Pathologic evaluation showed an inflamed lesion in all patients, and no organism could be cultured. Biopsy and curettage with specific antibiotic therapy has been the standard treatment of these associated bone lesions.

Tetanus

Although not an infection itself, tetanus occurs after infection with *Clostridium tetani.* The condition is actually caused by a toxin, tetanospasmin, which is elaborated by the bacillus. *C. tetani* is an anaerobic, spore-forming organism found in soil and in animal and human feces. In devitalized tissue, the spores germinate and produce the toxin that causes the disease. Over 80% of cases occur after a seemingly insignificant injury. The hallmark of tetanus is muscle spasms, with the presenting symptom being trismus in over 50% of patients. Restlessness, stiff neck, difficulty swallowing, and rigidity of abdominal and back muscles are also common symptoms. The generalized, sustained contraction of abdominal and back muscles produces the posture of opisthotonos. Prolonged trismus leads to the characteristic facial expression "risus sardonicus," the sardonic smile. The spasms are extremely painful and temperature may be elevated. Glottal and laryngeal spasms may necessitate tracheostomy. Dysphagia and hydrophobia are characteristic of this disease. The incubation period may be from 1 day to several months but is generally 3 to 20 days.

Treatment is directed at neutralization of the toxin and eradication of the infection. For suspected tetanus, antitoxin (human γ-globulin) should be administered intramuscularly (3000 to 6000 units). Repeat doses are not necessary. Penicillin should be given to treat the bacterial infection, but it will not affect the action of the toxin. Surgical debridement of the site of infection is necessary to remove the toxin. Diligent nursing care and support of respiration, fluid, and electrolytes are necessary. The death rate from this disease is 50%.

Tetanus is prevented by immunization with three doses of diphtheria-pertussis-tetanus (DPT) vaccine at 1-month intervals during infancy. A booster of 0.1 ml of tetanus toxoid should be administered before kindergarten; thereafter, a booster is required every 10 years. Any patient with a significant open wound should be given 0.1 ml of tetanus toxoid if the last booster was more than 10 years before or if immunization history is unknown. If the wound is contaminated and immunization history is unknown, antitoxin should be given as well.

Caffey's Disease

Infantile cortical hyperostosis was described by Caffey in 1945 as a self-limiting disease of early infancy characterized by irritability, soft tissue swelling and tenderness of the affected parts, and periosteal reaction on roentgenograms (Fig. 18-24). No infectious cause has been documented for this condition. Temperature may be elevated as high as 40° C. The most commonly involved bones are the skull, mandible, clavicle, scapulae, and ribs. Pathologically, there is thickened periosteum with lamellar reactive bone underneath. Early in the disease, inflammatory cells may be present. Usually the clinical presentation and roentgenographic appearance of this disease make biopsy unnecessary. Differential diagnoses include trauma, hypervitaminosis A, osteomyelitis, syphilis, parotitis, and malignancy. Laboratory evaluation is not helpful in the differential diagnosis because of the frequency of leukocytosis and elevated erythrocyte sedimentation rate. Long-term complications of Caffey's disease include synostosis of the ribs, radius and ulna, and tibia and fibula; facial asymmetry; long bone lesions; and cortical thinning. No specific treatment is required other than palliative measures.

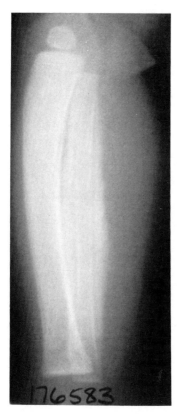

Fig. 18-24 Caffey's disease of right tibia and fibula in 3-month-old girl. Note diffuse periosteal reaction.

REFERENCES

Bacterial septic arthritis and osteomyelitis

Amundsen TR, Siegel MJ, and Siegel BA. Osteomyelitis and infarction in sickle cell hemoglobinopathies: differentiation by combined technetium and gallium scintigraphy, Radiology 153:807, 1984.

Andrew TA and Porter K: Primary subacute epiphyseal osteomyelitis: a report of three cases, J Pediatr Orthop 5:155, 1985.

Beaupré A and Carroll N: The three syndromes of iliac osteomyelitis in children, J Bone Joint Surg, 61A:1087, 1979.

Bjorksten B and Boquist L: Histopathological aspects of chronic recurrent multifocal osteomyelitis. J Bone Joint Surg, 62B:376, 1980.

Bliznak J: Emphysematous septic arthritis due to *Escherichia coli,* J Bone Joint Surg 58A:138, 1976.

Bogoch E, Thompson G and Salter RB: Foci of chronic circumscribed osteomyelitis (Brodie's abscess) that traverse the epiphyseal plate, J Pediatr Orthop 4:162, 1984.

Boston HC and Bianco AJ Jr, and Rhodes KH: Disk space infections in children, Orthop Clin North Am 6:953, 1975.

Brown T and Wilkinson RH: Chronic recurrent multifocal osteomyelitis, Radiology 166:493, 1988.

Canale ST et al: Does aspiration of bones and joints affect result of later bone scanning? J Pediatr Orthop 5:23, 1985.

Chacha PB: Suppurative arthritis of the hip joint in infancy, J Bone Joint Surg 53A:538, 1971.

Cleeland R and Squires E: Antimicrobial activity of ceftriaxone: a review, Am J Med 77:3, 1984.

Covey DC and Albright JA: Clinical significance of the sedimentation rate, J Bone Joint Surg 69A:148, 1989.

Coy JT et al: Pyogenic arthritis of the sacro-iliac joint: long-term follow up, J Bone Joint Surg 58A:845, 1976.

Davis JC et al: Chronic nonhematogeneous osteomyelitis treated with adjuvant hyperbaric oxygen, J Bone Joint Surg 68A:1210, 1986.

Duakles LM, Brotherton TS, and Feigin RD: Anaerobic infections in children: a prospective study, Pediatrics, 57:311, 1976.

Ebong WW: Pathologic fracture complicating long bone osteomyelitis in patients with sickle cell disease, J Pediatr Orthop 6:177, 1986.

Fitzgerald RH et al: Local muscle flaps in the treatment of chronic osteomyelitis, J Bone Joint Surg 67A:175, 1985.

Freeland AE, Sullivan DJ, and Westin GW: Greater trochanteric arthroplasty in children with loss of the femoral head, J Bone Joint Surg 62A:1351, 1980.

Gamble JG and Rinsky LA: Chronic recurrent multifocal osteomyelitis: a distinct clinical entity, J Pediatr Orthop 6:579, 1986.

Goldenberg DL et al: Treatment of septic arthritis: needle aspiration versus surgery, Arthritis and Rheum 18:83, 1975.

Goldstein WM, Gleason TF, and Barmada R: A comparison between arthrotomy and irrigation and multiple aspirations in the treatment of pyogenic arthritis, Orthopaedics 6:1309, 1983.

Green NS, Beauchamp RD, and Griffin PP: Primary subacute epiphyseal osteomyelitis, J Bone Joint Surg 63A:107, 1981.

Griebel M et al: Group A streptococcai postvaricella osteomyelitis, J Pediatr Orthop 5:101, 1985.

Guhl JF: New techniques for arthroscopic surgery of the ankle: a preliminary report, Orthopedics 9:261, 1986.

Hendrix RW, Lin PJP, Kane WJ: simplified aspiration or injection technique for the sacro-iliac joint, J Bone Joint Surg 64A:1249, 1982.

Herndon WA et al: Management of septic arthritis in children, J Pediatr Orthop 6:576, 1986.

Heydemann JS and Morrissy RT: Bone and joint sepsis in childhood problems in diagnosis, Orthop Trans 10:504, 1986.

Highland TR, LaMont RL: Osteomyelitis of the pelvis, J Bone Joint Surg 65A:230, 1983.

Hobo T: Fur pathogenese du akuten-hematogenen osteomyelitis: mit berucksichtigung du vital farbungslehre, Acta Scholar Med Univ Imp Kioto 4:1, 1921.

Howie DW et al: The technetium phosphate bone scan in the diagnosis of osteomyelitis in childhood, J Bone Joint Surg 65A:431, 1983.

Ivey M and Clark R: Arthroscopic debridement of the knee for septic arthritis, Clin Orthop 199:201, 1985.

Jackson MA and Nelson JD: Etiology and medical management of acute suppurative bone and joint infections in pediatric patients, J Pediatr Orthop 2:313, 1982.

Jones DC: "Cold" bone scan in acute osteomyelitis, J Bone Joint Surg 63B:7, 1981.

Kolyvas E et al: Oral antibiotic therapy of skeletal infections in children, Pediatrics 65:867, 1980.

Langenskiold A: Growth disturbance after osteomyelitis of the femoral condyles in infants, Acta Orthop Scand 55:1, 1984.

Lunseth PA and Heiple KG: Prognosis in septic arthritis of the hip in children, Clin Orthop 139:81, 1979.

McCoy JR, Morrissy RT and Siebert J: Clinical experience with the technetium 99 scan in children, Clin Orthop 154:175, 1981.

Mallouh A and Talab Y: Bone and joint infection in patients with sickle cell disease, J Pediatr Orthop 5:158, 1985.

May JW et al: Microvascular transfer of free tissue for closure of bone wounds of distal lower extremity, N Engl J Med 306:253, 1982.

Miskew DB, Block RA, and Witt PF: Aspiration of infected sacro-iliac joints, J Bone Joint Surg 61A:1071, 1979.

Morrey BF, Bianco AJ, and Rhodes KH: Septic arthritis in children. Orthop Clin North Am 6:923, 1975.

Morrey BF and Peterson HA: Hematogenous pyogenic osteomyelitis in children, Orthop Clin North Am 6:935, 1975.

McCloskey RV: Clinical and bacteriological efficacy of ceftriaxone in the United States, Am J Med 77:97, 1984.

Morrey BF, Bianco AJ, and Rhodes KH: Suppurative arthritis of the hip in children, J Bone Joint Surg 58A:388, 1976.

Morrissy RT and Haynes DW: Acute hematogenous osteomyelitis: a model with trauma as an etiology, J Pediatr Orthop 9:447, 1989.

Morrissy RT and Shore SL: Bone and joint sepsis, Pediatr Clin North Am 33:1551, 1986.

Nelson JD: Benefits and risks of sequential parenteral-oral cephalosporin therapy for suppurative bone and joint infections, J Pediatr Orthop 2:255, 1982.

Nelson JD, Howard JB and Shelton S: Oral antibiotic terapy for skeletal infections of children, J pediatr 92:131, 1978.

Nelson JD and Koontz WC: Septic arthritis in infants and children: a review of 117 cases, Pediatrics 92:131, 1978.

Oguachuba HN: Use of instillation-suction technique in the treatment of chronic osteomyelitis, Acta Orthop Scand 54:452, 1983.

Parisien JS: Diagnostic and surgical arthroscopy of the ankle: technique and indications, Bull Hosp Joint Dis 45:38, 1985.

Patterson DC: Acute suppurative arthritis in infancy and childhood, J Bone Joint Surg 52B:474, 1970.

Peltola H, Vahvanen V and Aalto K: Fever, C-reactive protein, and erythrocyte sedimentation rate in monitoring recovery from septic arthritis: a preliminary study, J Pediatr Orthop 4:170, 1984.

Perry J et al: Psoas abscess mimicking a septic hip: diagnosis by computed tomography, J Bone Joint Surg 67A:1281, 1985.

Prober CG and Yeager AS: Use of bactericoidal titer to assess adequacy of oral antibiotic therapy in acute osteomyelitis, J Pediatr 95:131, 1979.

Reilly JP et al: Disorders of the sacro-iliac joint in children, J Bone Joint Surg 70A:31, 1988.

Rosenbaum DM and Blumhagen JD: Acute epiphyseal osteomyelitis in children, Radiology 156:89, 1985.

Salter RB, Bell RS, and Keeley FW: The protective effect of continuous passive motion on living articular cartilage in acute septic arthritis,: and experimental investigation in to rabbit, Clin Orthop 159:223, 1981.

Scales PV, Hilty MD, and Sfakianakis GN: Bone scan patterns in acute osteomyelitis, Clin Orthop 153: 210, 1980.

Scales PV and Aronoff SC: Antimicrobial therapy of childhood skeletal infections, J Bone Joint Surg 66A:1487, 1984.

Skyhar MJ and Mubarak SJ: Arthroscopic treatment of septic knees in children, J Pediatr Orthop 7:647, 1987.

Smith RL et al: The effect of antibiotics on the destruction of cartilage in experimental infectious arthritis, J Bone Joint Surg 69A:1063, 1987.

Sorenson TS, Hedeboe J and Christensen ER: Primary epiphyseal osteomyelitis in children, J Bone Joint Surg 70B:818, 1988.

Sullivan JA, Vasileff T, and Leonard JT: An evaluation of nuclear scanning in orthopedic infections, J Pediatr Orthop 1:73, 1981.

Taylor AR and Mandsley RH: Instillation suction technique in chronic osteomyelitis, J Bone Joint Surg 52B:88-92, 1970.

Vaughn PA, Newman NM, and Rosman MA: Acute Hematogenous osteomyelitis in children, J Pediatr Orthop 7:652, 1987.

Weiland AJ, Moore JR, and Daniel RK: The efficacy of free tissue transfer in the treatment of osteomyelitis, J Bone Joint Surg 66A:181, 1984.

Wenger DR, Bobechko WP, and Gilday DL: The spectrum of intervertebral disk-space infection in children, J Bone Joint Surg 60A:100, 1978.

Whalen JL, Fitzgerald RH, and Morrissy RT: A histological study of acute hematogenous osteomyelitis following physeal injury in rabbits, J Bone Joint Surg 70A:1383, 1988.

Wilson TG and Patterson D: The technetium phosphate bone scan in the diagnosis of osteomyelitis in childhood, J Bone Joint Surg 65A:431, 1983.

Yu L et al: Chronic recurrent multifocal osteomyelitis, J Bone Joint Surg 71A:105, 1989.

Other infections and inflammatory conditions

Adams WG and Hindman SM: Cat scratch disease associated with an osteolytic lesion, J Pediatr 44:665, 1954.

Benach JL et al: Spirochetes isolcated from blood of two patients with lyme disease, N Engl J Med 308:740, 1983.

Burgdorfer W et al: Lyme disease: a tick borne spirochetosis? Science, 216:1317, 1982.

Busch LA and Parker RL: Brucellosis in the United States, J Infect Dis 125:289, 1972.

Carothers HA: Cat scratch disease: its natural history, JAMA 207:312, 1969.

Casscells SW: Aspergillus osteomyelitis of the tibia, J Bone Joint Surg 60A:994, 1978.

Chleboun J and Nades S: Skeletal cryptococcosis, J Bone Joint Surg 59A:509, 1977.

Collipp PJ and Koch R: Cat scratch disease associated with an osteolytic lesion, N Engl J Med 260:278, 1959.

Couch EP: Role of hyperbaric oxygenation in the treatment of gas gangrene: the USAF experience, J Bone Joint Surg 58A:737, 1976 (Abstract).

Cremin BJ et al: The lesions of congenital syphilis, Br J Radiol 43:333, 1979.

Culp RW et al: Lyme arthritis in children, J Bone Joint Surg 69A:96, 1987.

Dykes J, Segesman JK, and Birsner JW: Coccidioidomycosis of bone in children, Am J Dis Child 85:34, 1953.

Fitzgerald RH and Cowan JDE: Puncture wounds of the foot Orthop Clin North Am 6:965, 1975.

Green NE: Primary subacute epiphyseal osteomyelitis. In American Academy of Orthopaedic Surgeons: Instructional Course Lectures 32:37, 1983.

Green NE: *Pseudomonas* infections of the foot following puncture wounds. In American Academy of Orthopaedic Surgeons: Instructional Course Lectures 32:43, 1983.

Green NE and Bruno J: *Pseudomonas* infections of the foot after puncture wounds, South Med J 73:146, 1980.

Houston AN et al: Tetanus prophylaxis in the treatment of puncture wounds of patients in the deep South, J Trauma 2:439, 1962.

Jacobs RF et al: Management of *Pseudomonas* osteochondritis complicating puncture wounds of the foot, Pediatrics 69:432, 1982.

Lang AG and Peterson HA: Osteomyelitis following puncture wounds of the foot in children, J Trauma 16:993, 1976.

Miller EH and Semian DW: Gram-negative osteomy elitis following puncture wounds of the foot, J Bone Joint Surg 57A:535, 1975.

Morrissy RT and Shore SL: Bone and joint sepsis, Pediatr Clin North Am 33(6):1551, 1986.

Peebles TC et al: Tetanus-toxoid emergency boosters: a reappraisal, N Engl J Med 280:575, 1969.

Peterson HA: Hematogenous osteomyelitis in children. In American Academy of Orthopaedic Surgeons: Instructional Course Lectures 32:33, 1983.

Peterson HA: Fungal osteomyelitis in children. In American Academy of Orthopaedic Surgeons: Instructional Course Lectures, 32:46, 1983.

Pollock SF: Coccidioidal synovitis of the knee, J Bone Joint Surg 49A:1397, 1967.

Staheli LT, Church CC, and Ward BH: Infantile cortical hyperostosis (Caffey's disease), JAMA, 203:384, 1968.

Steere AC: Successful parenteral penicillin therapy for established Lyme arthritis, N Engl J Med 312:869, 1985.

Steere AC: Lyme disease, N Eng J Med 321:586, 1989.

Street L, Wilson WG, and Alva JD: Brucellosis in childhood, Pediatrics 55:416, 1975.

Svirsky-Fein, S et al: Neonatal osteomyelitis caused by *Candida Tropicalis,* J Bone Joint Surg 61A:455, 1979.

Weinstein L: Tetanus, N Engl J Med 289:1293, 1973.

Winter W et al: Coccidioidal arthritis and its treatment, J Bone Joint Surg 57A:1152, 1975.

19 Musculoskeletal Tumors

DEMPSEY S. SPRINGFIELD

DIAGNOSTIC TECHNIQUES

The majority of musculoskeletal tumors in children are benign, and many resolve spontaneously; other benign tumors may require only curettage or simple excision. Malignant neoplasms, however, demand early, aggressive, definitive treatment. Thus differentiating between benign and malignant lesions is mandatory. This differentiation begins with a thorough history. Initial complaints are usually pain, the presence of an unusual mass, impairment of an extremity, or incidental discovery of an abnormality on roentgenograms. Most benign tumors are painless, unless they cause some mechanical difficulty or pathologic fracture. Conversely, persistent pain is characteristic of malignant lesions. Physical examination should include a general evaluation, as well as careful examination of the affected part.

The roentgenographic appearance of the lesion often distinguishes a benign tumor from one that is malignant. Benign tumors usually have a clearly demarcated outline (Fig. 19-1). Central areas of rarefaction,

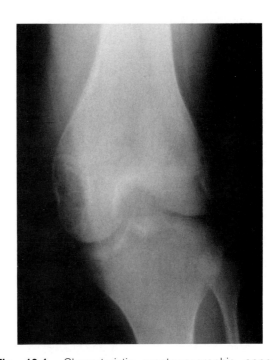

Fig. 19-1 Characteristic roentgenographic appearance of benign tumor (chondroblastoma). Note clearly demarcated outline of tumor.

with little or no reactive bone, may be present, or there may be a thin surrounding area of sclerosis. Primary malignant bone tumors are characterized by their massive size, irregular contours, and invasive bone destruction (Fig. 19-2); in many, a combination of destruction and new bone formation is present.

According to Enneking, clinical and roentgenographic evaluations identify as many as three fourths of all tumors as either obviously benign or clearly malignant. When clinical and roentgenographic findings do not adequately differentiate between a benign and malignant neoplasm, other diagnostic techniques are indicated.

Angiography is helpful in distinguishing benign from malignant lesions and is also useful for determining the soft tissue extent of a lesion. Most benign lesions show little or no neovascular reaction on angiogram. Angiography is generally not helpful in evaluating intraosseous tumors because cortical bone obscures fine vascular details. Only if detailed information concerning the vascular supply of a lesion is needed, or if embolization is a treatment possibility, will angiography be useful. Because of the possibility of complications, although slight, angiography is not ordinarily performed in patients younger than 3 years of age.

Although it has limited diagnostic capabilities, CT scanning aids in localizing the tumor in three dimensions. In benign tumors, the rim of intact cortical bone surrounding the lesion is clearly defined. The primary value of CT scanning is assessment of the intraosseous and extraosseous extent of the lesion and its relationship to major vessels and nerves (Fig. 19-3). Areas with a small anatomic cross section, such as the calf or forearm, are not evaluated as well by CT scanning as are larger structures. According to some authors, CT scans accurately reveal the extent of soft tissue tumors in 80% of patients. Jones and Kuhns, however, reported overestimation or underestimation of soft tissue extension in 11 of 25 children (44%) with CT scanning of tumors.

Radioisotopic scanning provides an overview of the skeleton for the detection of multiple lesions or skeletal metastases that is more sensitive and involves less radiation than conventional roentgenography; however, both false-negative and false-positive scans are possible. Areas of increased uptake should be correlated with clinical and roentgenographic findings (Fig. 19-4). Scanning can reveal roentgenographically occult activity and indicate whether the lesion is active or latent. Radioisotope scanning is also helpful in serially determining changes in activity. Most benign lesions are "cold" or show slightly increased uptake that correlates to the roentgenographic appearance; some aggressive benign lesions are "hot," and soft tissue lesions adjacent to bone frequently incite reactive bone not visible on roentgenograms but hot on the bone scan. Malignant lesions are generally

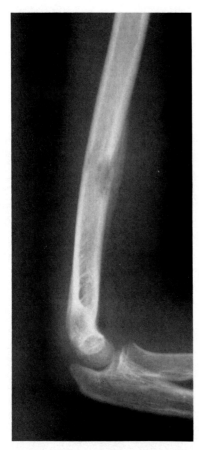

Fig. 19-2 Characteristic roentgenographic appearance of malignant tumor. Note irregular contour of lesion, invasive bone destruction, subperiosteal new bone formation, and absence of sclerotic rim.

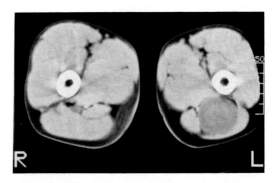

Fig. 19-3 CT scan of neurofibroma of posterior thigh compartment, showing exact size and location of lesion and its proximity to sciatic nerve.

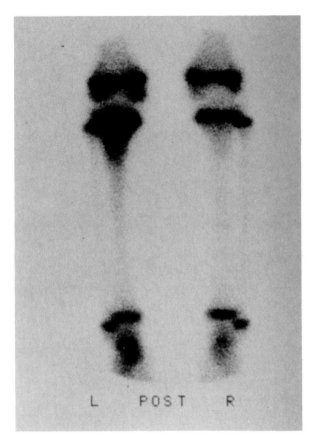

Fig. 19-4 Radioisotope scan showing increased uptake in area of lesion in proximal tibia.

quite hot, and the activity frequently extends well beyond roentgenographic margins.

Magnetic resonance imaging (MRI) is most valuable for further evaluation of lesions that are equivocal or obviously malignant. MRI provides more information about the extent of bone and soft tissue involvement and allows detection of subtle lesions that may be overlooked on roentgenograms (Fig. 19-5). Cohen et al, in a study of 139 children with tumors, reported that MRI was superior to CT in defining the size and extent of soft tissue tumor masses and the spread of bone sarcomas in bone marrow. In addition to using no radiation, MRI has the advantages of being noninvasive, painless, and well tolerated by older children.

Although recommended treatment of a specific tumor may be curettage, simple excision, or resection, the exact operation required must be individually designed for the specific clinical setting. No two tumors are identical. The skin incision, exposure, and tissue that must be removed are determined by the anatomic location and extent of the individual tumor. The general principles of treatment of musculoskeletal tumors are not meant to be definitive, but to provide guidelines for evaluation and planning for surgery.

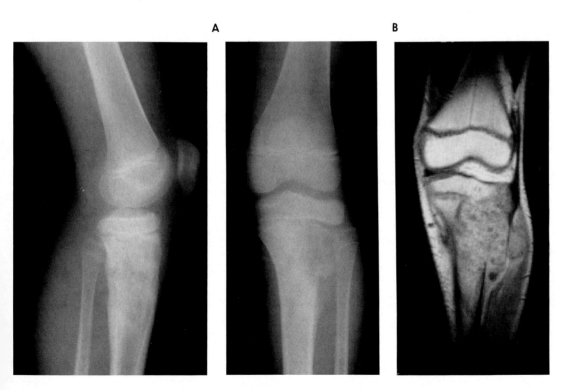

Fig. 19-5 **A,** Osteogenic sarcoma of proximal tibia on lateral and anteroposterior roentgenograms show lytic lesion. **B,** MRI showing skeletal and soft tissue extent of lesion.

Biopsy

The definitive diagnostic procedure remains biopsy, either needle or open. Biopsy should be performed only after complete clinical and roentgenographic evaluation and must be carefully planned. Biopsy through an incorrect anatomic plane can make later limb salvage procedures impossible. Ideally, the surgeon performing the biopsy should be prepared to perform the definitive surgery.

Needle

Needle biopsy may be appropriate for diagnostic confirmation when the tumor suspected is cytologically homogenous, can be diagnosed with limited tissue, and does not require immediate surgery; this group includes small, round-cell tumors, metastatic tumors, and typical osteosarcomas. Needle biopsy is more appropriate than incisional biopsy for some anatomic sites such as vertebral bodies because of the surgical exposure required for open biopsy. Needle aspirate biopsy should be planned as carefully as an open procedure, because the tract of the needle must be resected with the tumor if the lesion is malignant. Neurovascular structures should be avoided and the needle should not enter a joint.

Open

Most equivocal or suspected malignant musculoskeletal tumors should be biopsied by open technique to obtain adequate tissue for diagnosis. These tumors have considerable histologic variability, and the more tissue for evaluation, the better the chance for correct diagnosis. The biopsy incision must be positioned so that it can be included in tumor resection (Fig. 19-6). A longitudinal incision is usually preferable because transverse incisions are more difficult to include in resection and more uninvolved tissue is contaminated. Other precautions to prevent spread of the tumor include exposing the least possible amount of deep tissue, incising as few muscles as possible, avoiding neurovascular bundles, not opening joint capsules, and obtaining complete hemostasis before wound closure. A drain should be used unless the biopsy is very small and the superficial wound is completely dry before closure. Some authors object to the use of a tourniquet during open biopsy, but theoretic risks of tumor emboli have not been documented, and the advantage of a bloodless field seems to outweigh any potential disadvantages. Whenever possible, only the soft tissue (extraosseous) component of a bone tumor should be biopsied, to avoid the risk of pathologic fracture associated with bone biopsy. Because of the possibility of transplantation of tumor cells, instruments used for biopsy should not be used for resection or harvesting of bone grafts; separate instruments, gowns, gloves, and drapes should be used for each of these procedures.

TREATMENT
Surgical Margins

Enneking and associates defined four surgical margins in tumor treatment that describe, in oncologic terms, the extent of surgery: intralesional, marginal, wide, and radical (Fig. 19-7).

An *intralesional* surgical margin results from an operation that grossly enters the tumor. Incisional biopsy and curettage result in intralesional surgical margins. If the reactive rim of the lesion is removed, the surgical margin may be called an "extended" intralesional surgical margin. Only latent, inactive lesions (enchondroma, histiocytosis X, fibrous dysplasia, osteoid osteoma) should be treated with the standard intralesional surgical margin. Lesions that are benign but locally aggressive (aneurysmal bone cyst, giant cell tumor of bone, chondroblastoma, osteoblastoma) may be treated with an "extended" intralesional surgical margin. Benign synovial diseases (pigmented villonodular synovitis, synovial chondromatosis) are treated with an intralesional surgical margin.

A *marginal* surgical margin is obtained when the resection margin is the pseudocapsule of the tumor, as when the tumor is "shelled out." Most benign active tumors and all malignant tumors have microscopic disease extending into the pseudocapsule, and marginal excision leaves this microscopic tumor. A marginal surgical margin is suggested for benign, minimally active tumors (ganglion cysts, neurilemoma, myxoma, osteocartilaginous exostosis).

A *wide* surgical margin is obtained when the tumor

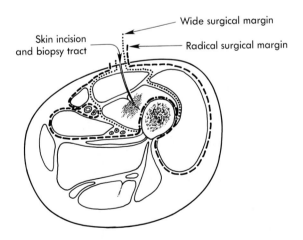

Fig. 19-6 Positioning of skin incision to include biopsy site in resection of soft tissue sarcoma in vastus intermedius muscle and outline of surgical margins.

is removed with a surrounding cuff of normal, uninvolved tissue; this is called "en bloc" resection by some. The amount of normal tissue excised is not defined, but 2 cm or a major fascial plane is probably the minimum safe distance between the tumor and the surgical margin; this distance should be greater in the direction of the tumor's growth. Sarcomas more often grow longitudinally (within muscles, between muscle planes, or within the medullary canal of bone) than tranversely across fascial boundaries that separate muscles or penetrate the periosteum; therefore the margin should be greater longitudinally than tranversely. As a general rule, whenever any portion of a muscle is involved with a sarcoma, it is better to excise the entire muscle, from origin to insertion. Intraosseous tumors usually extend longitudinally within the medullary canal of the bone further than transversely through the cortex and periosteum, as demonstrated by preoperative MRI. The bone margin, therefore, should be greater than the soft tissue margin and should be as wide as possible to reduce the risk of recurrence. A wide surgical margin is required for the most aggressive benign tumors (some giant

cell tumors of bone, an occasional chondroblastoma), recurrent benign tumors, low-to-medium-grade malignant tumors (chondrosarcoma, fibrosarcoma), and high-grade tumors that respond to adjuvant irradiation or chemotherapy (osteosarcoma, Ewing's sarcoma).

A *radical* surgical margin is obtained when the tumor and the compartment or compartments involved by the tumor are totally removed. Usually a radical surgical margin can be achieved only by amputation through or proximal to the joint, but some anatomic compartments can be resected without amputation. The anterior compartment of the thigh is the most common anatomic location suited to a radical surgical margin. A radical surgical margin is recommended for high-grade tumors that are not responsive to adjuvant irradiation or chemotherapy and for recurrent sarcomas, regardless of grade, unless adjuvant treatment is available. The incidence of local recurrence for high-grade tumors treated with a radical surgical margin is the lowest possible and is the standard against which less aggressive surgical resections must be measured.

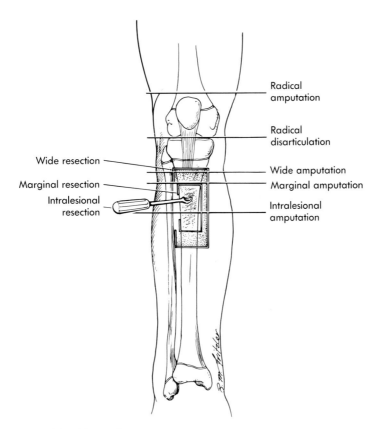

Fig. 19-7 Enneking description of surgical margins.

A   B

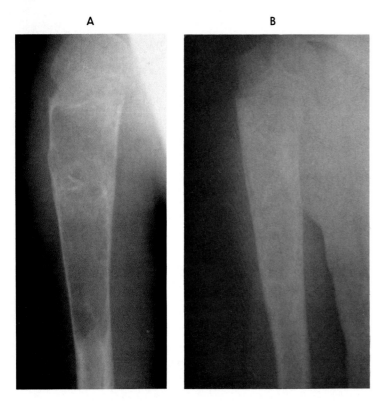

Fig. 19-8 **A,** Unicameral bone cyst in proximal humerus of 9-year-old boy. **B,** One year after injection of corticosteroids.

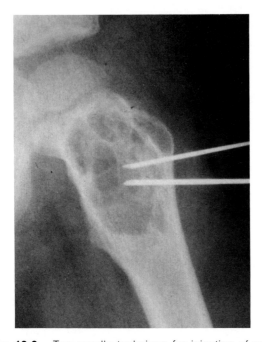

Fig. 19-9 Two-needle technique for injection of corticosteroid in unicameral bone cyst of left femoral neck.

Specific Procedures
Intralesional Corticosteroid Injection

Scaglietti introduced the concept of direct injection of bone lesions with corticosteroids. Since then, the treatment of unicameral bone cysts with intralesional injection of corticosteroids has become a popular method of stimulating the cyst to fill in with bone (Fig. 19-8). More than one injection may be necessary, and the injections are done at 6- to 8-week intervals. Although some authors report using as many as eight injections, three or four are usually sufficient to determine the effectiveness of treatment.

▶ *Technique.* With the patient under general anesthesia, prepare the skin directly over the cyst. With fluoroscopic control, pass percutaneously an 18- or 20-gauge spinal needle (with the stylet in place) directly to the thinnest portion of the cyst wall. Usually the needle can be easily pushed through the thinned cortex into the cyst—but if not, rotate the needle back and forth to drill the needle into the cyst until clear yellow or slightly bloody fluid is obtained. A Jamshidi needle may be used if the surrounding cortex does not permit passage of a spinal needle. If no fluid is obtained, discontinue the procedure and reconsider the diagnosis of unicameral bone cyst; incisional biopsy may be appropriate at this point. After the fluid has been aspirated, introduce a second needle into the cyst as far from the first as possible (Fig. 19-9). Inject a radiopaque dye into the cyst to confirm that the cyst is unicameral and will be filled by a single injection. If the cyst has more than one chamber, inject each separately. Then inject a corticosteroid (such as methylprednisolone) into the cyst. The optimal amount of corticosteroid has not been established, but the rule of thumb is 40 mg for a small cyst, 80 mg for a medium cyst, and 120 mg for a large cyst. Withdraw the needles and dress the injection sites.

Curettage

Curettage is the appropriate treatment for most skeletal tumors in children. The self-healing, benign lesions require only simple curettage through a small window in the bone. The more aggressive benign lesions with a tendency to recur require a more aggressive curettage with complete exposure of the lesion to achieve an extended intralesional margin. The surgical approach and exposure for an extended intralesional curettage depends on the site of the lesion and the specific tumor. The skin incision should be longitudinal, directly over the lesion, and long enough to provide complete exposure of enough bone to allow placement of a large window in the bone. When the curettage is performed for biopsy rather than definitive treatment, the incision should be small and should avoid the adjacent joint.

▶ *Technique.* After adequate surgical exposure, make a window in the bone and enlarge it so that there is no overhang of bone (Fig. 19-10). Curet all gross tumor and send it for pathologic evaluation. If the lesion is near the physis, curet to the adjacent subchondral bone, but protect the physis. If appropriate, fill the cavity with cancellous bone graft. For lesions large enough to compromise the mechanical stability of the involved bone, a cast may be applied until the lesion resolves and the graft has incorporated.

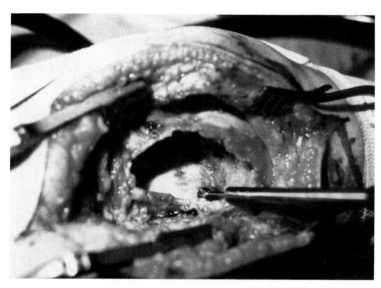

Fig. 19-10 Cortical window for curettage of lesion in right distal femur.

Wide Resection, Limb Salvage Wide Resection

Bone. Most bone tumors that require a wide surgical margin have an extraosseous soft tissue component that should not be exposed during the resection; the muscle covering is included in the resection. To achieve this, each operation must be tailored to the individual tumor and anatomic location. In the distal femur, for example, the vastus medialis or vastus lateralis muscle is often resected with the tumor. Diaphyseal femoral tumors usually require resection of the vastus intermedius muscle along with the femoral shaft. The deltoid muscle often must be resected with a tumor in the proximal humerus, and the popliteus muscle, with a tumor in the proximal tibia. If the muscle is invaded by the tumor, it should be resected from its origin to insertion.

Preoperative planning of limb salvage resection is important. First, the patient and family should be informed that limb salvage surgery is more complex than amputation, complications are more likely, recovery is longer, and postoperative levels of physical activity are lower. Not every patient is best treated with limb salvage resection; some would benefit more from amputation.

If limb salvage resection is chosen, two to four courses of multidrug chemotherapy are recommended before surgery. Most new chemotherapy protocols include preoperative (neoadjuvant) chemotherapy, and although preoperative chemotherapy has not been proven beneficial for all limb salvage operations, the delay in surgery is outweighed by the potential benefits.

To perform limb salvage resection, the level of bone transection must be carefully selected. Although the optimum amount of normal bone between the tumor and transection is not precisely defined, 5 cm is the recommended minimum, and as much bone should be removed as possible without compromising reconstruction. Thus, if the tumor involves the distal 7 cm of a bone, a minimum of 12 cm must be removed, but if an additional 5 to 10 cm can be removed without adversely affecting reconstruction, it should be resected. If, on the other hand, the additional bone resection would alter the reconstruction, only the minimum should be resected. If the minimum 5 cm of normal bone cannot be resected with the tumor, amputation is advised. Methods of reconstruction include arthrodesis with autograft or allograft, prosthetic replacement (Fig. 19-11), osteoarticular allograft, and rotationplasty. The reconstruction selected should be the one best suited for the particular patient and surgeon.

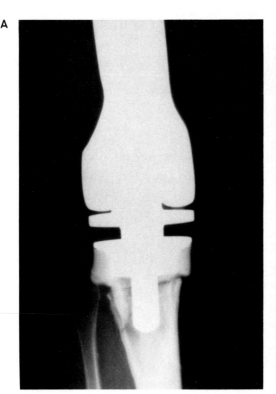 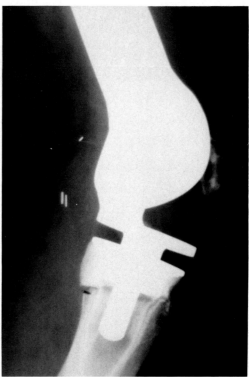

Fig. 19-11 Osteogenic sarcoma of distal femur in 17-year-old girl treated with limb salvage procedure and prosthetic replacement. **A,** Anteroposterior view; **B,** lateral view.

Because it is not feasible to describe planning and technique for every possible anatomic location and specific tumor, treatment of a common lesion, osteosarcoma of the distal femur, is described as an example.

▲ *Technique (wide resection of osteosarcoma of distal femur).* Prepare and drape the entire limb, including the hemipelvis, into the surgical field. Elevate the limb for 5 minutes and inflate a sterile tourniquet. Do not use a pressure wrap to exsanguinate the extremity because this increases the number of tumor cells entering the blood stream. Make a long, straight, anterior skin incision that includes the biopsy incision. Include the muscle directly over the tumor and a portion of the origin or insertion of any muscle attached to the distal femur with the bone and resected specimen. Do not expose the pseudocapsule of the tumor during the operation and strip the periosteum only from normal bone at the level of the planned transection. Open the knee joint; divide the collateral ligaments, cruciate ligaments, and posterior capsule; then distract the distal femur from the tibia. Identify the popliteal vessels and sciatic nerve in the popliteal fossa. The neurovascular bundle is the posterior margin of the resection. Ligate and divide the vessels off the distal femoral and popliteal arteries to the tumor. Turn back, laterally and medially, skin flaps and muscles that can be saved. Continue the dissection until the specimen is freed from the remainder of the extremity. Transect the muscles to be resected with the tumor at the level of bone transection. Finally, transect the bone and remove the specimen.

Curetted material from the canal of the femur is sent to the pathologist for evaluation of intramedullary extension proximal to the bone transection. The specimen should be carefully examined to determine the gross margin. If the surgical margin is inadequate, then appropriate additional tissue should be resected or the extremity amputated. Once the margin is determined to be adequate, the reconstruction of choice can be undertaken.

Wide resection of bone tumors in other anatomic sites is done in a similar fashion, but each procedure must be planned for the individual tumor. The reconstruction of the remaining defect varies depending on the preference of the patient and the available muscles. If only limited muscle resection is required, the reconstruction may include a moving joint (osteoarticular allograft, custom prosthetic arthroplasty, or a combination of the two), but if most of the muscles are resected, arthrodesis is recommended.

Soft tissue. The wide resection of a soft tissue tumor also requires resection of a cuff of normal tissue with the tumor and avoidance of exposing the tumor during the operation. Bone, nerves, or vessels immediately adjacent to the tumor must be resected with it. The entire muscle or muscles involved should be resected from origin to insertion. Resection of the entire muscle rather than resection of the belly of the muscle does not change function, but does improve local control of the tumor. Patients with major muscle resection function surprisingly well.

During the past decade the combination of surgery and irradiation, either before, during, or after surgery, has been shown to be effective in salvaging limbs that would otherwise require amputation. The most common application is to soft tissue sarcoma immediately adjacent to a major neurovascular bundle where a wide surgical margin would require removal of the neurovascular bundle. Before the use of adjuvant irradiation, resecting the tumor but saving the neurovascular bundle led to a high incidence of local recurrence, and amputation was advised. More recently, preoperative irradiation of approximately 55 Gy (5500 rads) has been recommended before resection without removal of the neurovascular bundle. This results in a marginal surgical margin because of the dissection between the tumor and adjacent neurovascular bundle, but the incidence of local recurrence has been low (less than 5%). Although the surgical margin at the neurovascular bundle is marginal other surgical margins should be wide.

The technique described as an example is wide resection of a soft tissue lesion in the vastus lateralis and vastus intermedius. Resection of soft tissue tumors involving other anatomic sites is modified depending on the muscles involved.

▲ *Technique (wide resection of vastus lateralis, vastus intermedius).* Position the patient supine on the operating table with the buttock on the involved side slightly elevated. Prepare and drape the lower extremity and hemipelvis. Make the skin incision as straight as possible, ellipsing the biopsy incision. Begin the incision at the anterior portion of the greater trochanter and extend it to the distal lateral femoral condyle. Split the tensor fasciae latae muscle in line with the skin incision. Anteriorly, separate the rectus femoris muscle from the vastus lateralis; posteriorly, release the posterior portion of the tensor fascia from the lateral fascial tissue that inserts onto the linea aspera. Identify the origins of the vastus lateralis and vastus intermedius and elevate them from the femur subperiosteally. Identify the profunda femoris artery and vein between the adductors and the medial aspect of the vastus intermedius; ligate and divide them if necessary. Posteriorly, along the linea aspera, a

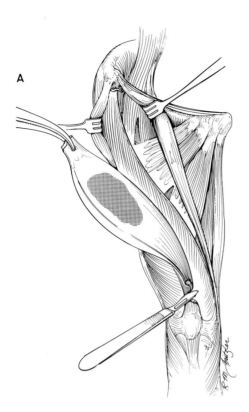

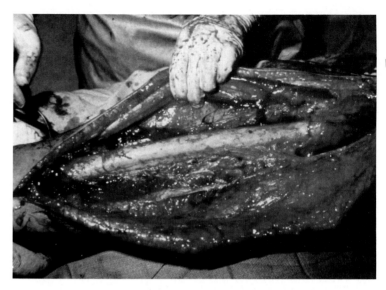

Fig. 19-12 **A,** Wide resection for malignant soft tissue tumor (*shaded area*) in rectus femoris. **B,** Intraoperative photograph showing extensive exposure necessary for resection of vastus lateralis and vastus intermedius.

large, deep vein drains multiple smaller perforating veins and will bleed profusely if not ligated or carefully preserved. Elevate the muscles being resected off the femur with a periosteal elevator from proximal to distal. Retract the superficial femoral vessels medially. Finally, transect the insertion of the vastus intermedius and vastus lateralis on the patellar extensor mechanism and remove the two muscles with the encased tumor (Fig. 19-12). Place drains in the depths of the wound. Close the tensor fasciae latae with interrupted sutures and close the skin. Apply a compression dressing with a plaster splint to immobilize the knee.

▶ *Postoperative management.* Ambulation on crutches is begun as soon as comfort permits. Quadriceps-setting exercises are encouraged as soon as tolerated. Gentle active motion of the knee is begun early, usually on the fourth or fifth day after surgery. Flexion of the knee is begun when the wound is healed and should be complete before physical therapy is discontinued.

Tikhoff-Linberg Resection

In 1928, Linberg described an interscapulothoracic resection of the shoulder girdle to replace forequarter amputation, noting that the operation had first been done by Professor Tikhoff. Linberg described removal of the scapula, clavicle, and proximal humerus en bloc, but suggested that variations could be

done as needed. The operation is now most commonly called a Tikhoff-Linberg resection and is most frequently used for management of tumors of the proximal humerus, especially osteosarcomas.

▶ *Technique.* Place the patient supine and rotated approximately 30 degrees with the affected side up. Prepare and drape the upper extremity and shoulder girdle, including the scapula. Begin the skin incision anteriorly over the clavicle as far medially as necessary depending on how much of the clavicle is to be resected (Fig. 19-13, *A*). Extend the incision laterally to the most medial aspect of the deltoid muscle, then distally along the deltopectoral groove continuing as far distally as necessary depending on how much of the humerus is to be resected. Continue the deltopectoral skin incision superiorly over the shoulder at the level of the acromioclavicular joint and distally to the tip of the scapula. The entire scapula can be resected through this incision, but if less scapula is to be resected, the posterior arm of the incision does not need to be so long. After the skin incision has been made, begin the deep dissection over the clavicle. Perform an osteotomy of the clavicle if only the lateral clavicle is resected or if the sternoclavicular joint is disarticulated (Fig. 19-13, *B*). Detach the origin of the pectoralis major from the clavicle and humerus, leaving a cuff of normal muscle with the specimen to obtain a wide surgical margin. Release the pectoralis minor from the coracoid and identify the neurovascular bundle. Usually the cora-cobrachialis can be saved. Detach it from the cora-coid and reflect it distally, taking care not to stretch the musculoskeletal nerve. Retract the neurovascular bundle medially and transect the insertions to the subscapularis and latissimus dorsi muscles on the hu-merus (with a cuff of normal tissue left attached) (Fig. 19-13, *B*). Most tumors treated with Tikhoff-Linberg resection are adjacent to the deltoid muscle, which should be entirely removed with the specimen. Ex-pose the humerus at least 5 cm distal to the most distal involvement of the tumor. Transect the biceps muscle through its muscle belly sufficiently distal to achieve a wide margin. Now develop the superior as-pect of the incision. Detach the trapezius muscle from the clavicle and spine of the scapula and reflect it medially. Identify the medial border of the scapula and detach the levator scapulae, rhomboid minor, and rhomboid major muscles from their insertions on the medial border of the scapula. Dissect the lat-eral skin from the deltoid muscle and retract it later-ally; identify the infraspinatous, teres major, and teres minor muscles. Now perform an osteotomy of the humerus so that the specimen is more mobile as the scapula is dissected from the chest. Lift the tip of the scapula off the chest and develop the interval be-tween the serratus anterior muscle on the chest wall and the subscapularis muscle on the scapula. Detach the scapular origins of the serratus anterior and lift the scapula further out of the wound. Laterally, divide the scapular origins of the medial head of the triceps muscle as far proximally as possible. Carefully protect the radial nerve during this part of the resection. Re-move the scapula, clavicle, and proximal humerus with the encased tumor (Fig. 19-13, *C*).

Various reconstructions of the extremity after a Tikhoff-Linberg have been suggested. If a limited ex-traarticular shoulder resection has been done and most of the scapula remains, shoulder arthrodesis is possible, but when the entire scapula has been re-moved a flail shoulder is the only reasonable option. The remaining humerus must be suspended from the chest wall or remaining clavicle, and the better the suspension, the better the final result. The best method is to suture the remaining muscles of the up-per arm to the remaining portions of the trapezius and pectoralis muscles, shortening the extremity 2 to 4 cm. If the remaining muscles will not support the distal humerus, some method must be found to keep the weight of the upper extremity from constantly pulling on the soft tissues. Dacron tape tied between the proximal humerus or rib may be used. Intramed-ullary rods or proximal humeral prostheses can be inserted to extend the proximal end of the humerus to make suspension easier.

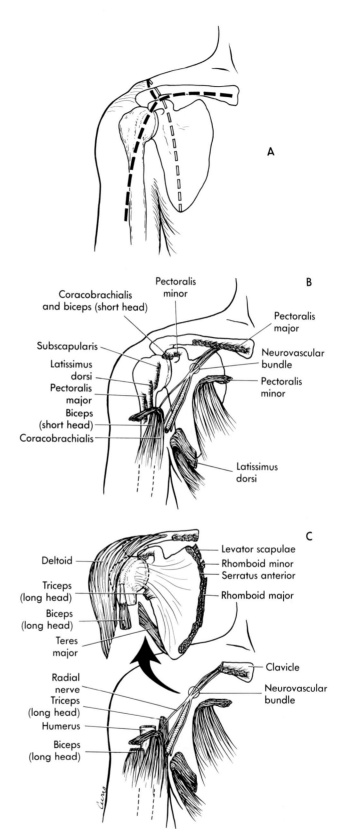

Fig. 19-13   Tikhoff-Linberg resection (see text). **A,** Skin incision over clavicle in deltopectoral groove. **B,** Osteot-omy of clavicle. **C,** Removal of scapula, clavicle, and proximal humerus with encased tumor.

▲ *Postoperative management.* The patient is immobilized in a sling for comfort, and range-of-motion exercises are begun for the shoulder, elbow, forearm, and wrist as soon as comfort allows. After 4 to 6 weeks, strengthening of the remaining shoulder muscles is begun.

Van Nes Rotationplasty

In patients younger than 10 years of age, resection of tumors in the distal femur removes the major physis of the lower extremity. In the past, above-knee amputation was performed even when the tumor could be safely resected without excision of the neurovascular bundle because there was no satisfactory method to manage the severe limb shortening resulting from distal femoral resection. More recently, however, two methods have been used to salvage limbs in these young patients. Prostheses that can be periodically lengthened have been reported for reconstruction of the extremity, but these are still in the developmental stage. The other method is based on an operation originally described by Borggreve for treatment of limb shortening and knee joint ankylosis caused by tuberculosis. It is generally called the Van Nes rotationplasty after Van Nes, who described its use for proximal femoral focal deficiency. This reconstruction is an excellent permanent solution for the young child with a tumor in the distal femur that requires wide resection. It allows more radical resection of the surrounding tissue than other types of limb salvage reconstruction because only the sciatic nerve must be saved and all surrounding muscle, femoral vessels, and skin can be resected. The middle portion of the femoral artery and vein adjacent to the tumor can be excised and these vessels anastomosed after the specimen has been removed and the extremity shortened.

The distal femoral epiphysis and proximal tibial epiphysis are resected with the tumor (extraarticular resection is recommended) and the distal tibial physis provides longitudinal growth in the location of the resected distal femoral epiphysis. To determine the appropriate length of the operated limb after reconstruction, the predicted growth of the unoperated distal femoral physis is calculated from standard growth charts and compared with the predicted growth of the distal tibial physis. The operated extremity initially should be longer than the unoperated extremity, with the difference in lengths expected to equalize with growth. After the proper length of the operated extremity is determined, the level of resection is selected. When growth is complete, the ideal is to have the axis of rotation of the operated ankle (now

the knee) at the level of the distal femoral condyle of the unoperated extremity. The tendency is to make the operated limb too long.

▲ *Technique (Van Nes rotationplasty).* Place the patient supine on the operating table. Prepare and drape the entire extremity, including the hemipelvis, in the operative field. Make two circumferential skin incisions connected by a posterior longitudinal incision (Fig. 19-14, *B*), with the proximal circumferential incision oblique and more proximal anteriorly and distal posteriorly. Make the distal circumferential incision oblique but with a greater line of angulation and the anterior portion of the incision more distal than the posterior portion. Make the distal skin incision over the proximal tibia and carry the dissection deep to the skin directly to bone. Through the connecting longitudinal incision, dissect the sciatic nerve and popliteal and femoral arteries and veins from the tissue of the distal thigh.

Identify the peroneal nerve where it is superficial to the fibula and trace it proximal and posterior to the biceps femoris and superficial to the lateral head of the gastrocnemius muscle to its origin from the common sciatic nerve. Medially, divide the fascia posterior to the pes anserinus at the level of the proximal tibial plateau to expose the medial head of the gastrocnemius. Divide the medial head of the gastrocnemius (leaving a small portion of its origin with the distal femur) and expose the popliteal artery and vein. Divide the lateral head of the gastrocnemius at the same level as the medial head, just distal to the joint line of the knee. Dissect the sciatic nerve and popliteal vessels from distal to proximal. Free the nerve the entire length of the resection specimen. If the vessels are to be resected with the tumor, do not dissect them out, but if they are to be saved, dissect them from the medial thigh.

To dissect the vessels, divide the gracilis, sartoris, semimembranous, and semitendinous muscles at the level of the adductor canal. Free the vessels from the canal by transecting the tendon of the adductor magnus where it is the superficial portion of the canal. Then dissect the femoral artery and vein from the adductor canal to the level of the proximal circumferential skin incision. If the vessels are on the pseudocapsule of the tumor, resect them with the tumor. If the vessels are to be resected, isolate them in the popliteal fossa and in the proximal anterior thigh. After the sciatic nerve has been completely freed and the soft tissue transected and just before cutting the tibia and femur, clamp and transect the vessels. They will be anastomosed after the distal leg has been rotated and shortened into its final position.

Once the sciatic nerve and femoral artery and vein have been dissected free from the thigh proximal to the level of the proximal circumferential incision, transect the muscles of the thigh at the level of the skin incision (Fig. 19-14, *C*). Expose the femur and select the level of transection. Before the femur is transected, make a mark in the anterior cortex of the bone proximal to the osteotomy site to be used as a rotational reference. After the femoral osteotomy has been made, make the proximal tibial osteotomy just distal to the tibial tubercle. Externally rotate the distal extremity and bring the distal femur and proximal tibia together to judge the length of the extremity (Fig. 19-14, *D*). If it is too long, remove additional bone from the femur. Expose the lateral aspect of the distal femur and medial aspect of the proximal tibia so that a six- to eight-hole compression plate can be applied for fixation. Position the externally rotated distal leg against the proximal femur with the axis of ankle flexion and extension in the anteroposterior plane of the extremity, and fix the two bones to-

gether with the compression plate. Use the mark in the anterior femur to determine the correct rotation. Coil the sciatic nerve and femoral artery and vein medially. Anastomose the vessels if they have been transected. Suture the transected quadriceps muscle to the gastrocnemius muscles, which are now anterior, and suture the hamstring muscles to the pretibial fascia. Leave large suction drains in the wound and close the subcutaneous tissue and skin (Fig. 19-14, *E*). Apply a compression dressing.

◢ *Postoperative management.* The patient is permitted to get up as soon as comfort allows. Active motion of the ankle (now the knee) joint is begun as soon as possible, usually the first day after surgery. Hip motion is also begun early. Once the wound has healed sufficiently, approximately 10 days after surgery, a temporary prosthesis, which includes a waist band with an external hip joint, is fitted. Once the osteotomy has healed, a permanent prosthesis without a hip joint is fitted. Plate removal after 1 to 2 years is optional.

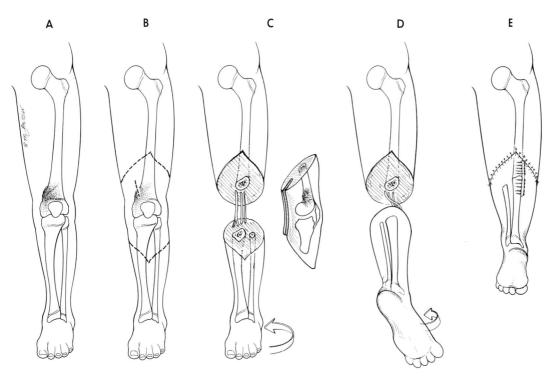

Fig. 19-14 Van Nes rotationplasty (see text). **A,** Preoperative view, lesion in distal femur. **B,** Circumferential skin incision, biopsy incision site. **C,** Transection of muscles of thigh and knee joint. **D,** Rotation of distal femur and proximal tibia. **E,** Closure after rotation and fixation.

Amputations

Amputations and disarticulations are standard operations that have been performed for centuries, and they are still important surgical procedures. Some patients whose tumors could be resected are better treated by amputation, and some tumors can be properly treated only by amputation of the extremity. Amputation should not be regarded as defeat, but as one of a number of alternatives for treatment of musculoskeletal tumors. The results are best with good preoperative planning, meticulous technique, and appropriate postoperative therapy.

Forequarter amputation. Forequarter amputation is used for tumors of the scapula, shoulder girdle, or proximal humerus that involve the neurovascular bundle. Patients are rarely able to use a functional prosthesis after this amputation, but many can use a cosmetic prosthesis. Postoperative physical therapy is directed at teaching the patient to function with only one upper extremity.

◣ *Technique.* Position the patient with the involved side rotated up at a 45-degree angle. The head of the operating table should be raised 30 degrees. Prepare and drape the upper arm, shoulder, chest to the midline, and upper back to the midline. Make the initial incision directly over and in the direction of the clavicle. Expose the midportion of the clavicle and resect a small segment so that the subclavian artery and vein can be identified. Ligate and divide these two vessels, then make the remainder of the skin incision. Curve the anterior incision distally from the incision over the clavicle along the deltopectoral groove into the axilla to the posterior axillary line (Fig. 19-15, *A*).

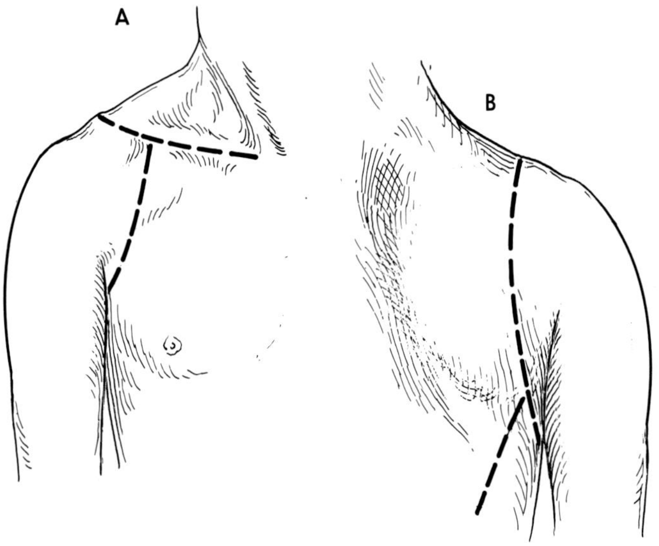

Fig. 19-15 Right forequarter amputation (see text). **A,** Anterior skin incision. **B,** Posterior skin incision.

Make the posterior portion of the skin incision over the shoulder at the acromioclavicular joint, then distally just medial to the lateral border of the scapula until it joins the anterior incision (Fig. 19-15, *B*). Make the posterior flap sufficiently large to cover the defect without tension. This is especially important in females, for tension of the closure will displace the breast laterally. Deepen the skin incisions to the deep fascia. Now complete the operation from posterior. Raise the posterior skin flap medially to the medial border of the scapula. It may be necessary to lengthen the inferior portion of the skin incision in the posterior axillary line to allow the posterior flap to be raised far enough medially. Along the inferior portions of the scapula, transect the rhomboid major and inferior trapezius muscles and then transect the rhomboid minor muscle, leaving a portion of normal muscle along the medial border of the scapula. More superiorly, transect the remainder of the trapezius and levator scapulae muscles from their insertions on the scapula to permit the scapula to be raised off the chest wall. Develop the plane between the subscapularis and serratus anterior muscles by blunt dissection. Now complete the most superior portion of the incision. From posteriorly, identify the divided subclavian vessels and brachial plexus, and transect the nerves. Transect the serratus anterior and pectoralis major and minor muscles, allowing the extremity to be removed from the body. Bury the nerves in muscle to reduce symptoms from neuromas that develop on the cut ends. Leave drains in the wound, and close the skin flaps.

◣ *Postoperative management.* The patient is allowed out of bed on the first day after surgery if symptoms permit. Physical therapy is begun immediately, and a cosmetic prosthetic shoulder is constructed before the patient leaves the hospital.

Hemipelvectomy. Hemipelvectomy, or hindquarter amputation, is required for tumors that involve the pelvis and sciatic nerve, with or without involvement of the iliac vessels. Preoperatively the patient's bowel should be gently cleansed with 2 days of a clear liquid diet and enemas.

◣ *Technique.* Position the patient on the operating table with the involved side rotated up 30 degrees. Place a Foley cathether in the urinary bladder. Prepare and drape the lower extremity and hemipelvis to the midline anteriorly and posteriorly. Make the initial skin incision over the iliac crest from the anterosuperior spine to approximately the midportion of the iliac crest (Fig. 19-16, *A*). Deepen this incision to expose the abdominal muscles at their attachment to the iliac crest. Transect the abdominal muscles off the iliac crest with a portion of their insertion left on the bone. Take care not to dissect between the iliacus muscle and the ilium, but rather enter the retroperitoneal space superficially to the iliacus muscle. Palpate the retroperitoneal space to be sure the tumor does not involve the bladder or bowels, then complete the skin incision, extending it posteriorly to the posterosuperior iliac spine. Just posterior to the anterosuperior iliac spine, curve the lateral aspect of the incision over the buttocks approximately half way between the sciatic notch and the greater trochanter, then posteriorly at the level of the buttock crease. Curve the medial aspect of the incision medially at the anterosuperior iliac spine along the inguinal ligament to join the posterior portion of the incision in the perineum (Fig. 19-16, *B*). Deepen the medial portion of the incision, lifting the inguinal ligament off the ilium and reflecting the abdominal muscles medially.

Identify the common iliac artery and vein in the retroperitoneal space; ligate and divide them. Transect the psoas and femoral nerves. Palpate and inspect the anterior portion of the sacroiliac joint. Transect the sciatic nerve and sacral nerve roots. Now raise a posterior flap. If the common iliac artery has been ligated, the gluteus maximus muscle has lost its blood supply and should be resected. A broad-based posterior skin flap will survive and be of sufficient length to cover the defect. Make this flap as broad as half the distance between the anterior iliac spine and the tip of the coccyx. Raise this posterior skin flap medially to the sacroiliac joint. Now direct attention to the pubis. Bluntly dissect the bladder from the posterior aspect of the pubis and identify the symphysis, which can be felt as a ridge along the posterior aspect of the pubis in the midline. Gently push an osteotome by hand through the symphysis, taking care not to damage the urethra, which is just inferior to the symphysis. Open the sacroiliac joint with an osteotome from anterior to posterior and abduct the lower extremity. Release the fascial attachments between the sacrum and ischium, particularly the sacrospinous and sacroischial ligaments, allowing the extremity with the hemipelvis to be distracted from the body. Release remaining soft tissue attachments and remove the specimen. Leave drains in the wound, and suture the posterior muscles and fascia to the abdominal muscles with interrupted nonabsorbable sutures. Close the subcutaneous tissue and skin in a routine fashion, and wrap the wound with an elastic bandage.

▶ *Postoperative management.* The patient is allowed out of bed as soon as possible, usually the second or third day after surgery. Crutch training is begun immediately, and the patient is encouraged to use crutches rather than a wheelchair. The Foley catheter is left in the urinary bladder for 4 to 7 days. Male pa-

tients usually have significant scrotal swelling and often a large hematoma; female patients have difficulty controlling their bladder sphincter in the immediate postoperative period.

Many patients with hemipelvectomy find a sitting prosthesis helpful in balance, and this can be used as soon as the wound is healed. Although few patients use a hemipelvectomy prosthesis for more than a few hours a day or for more than social occasions, they should be given this option.

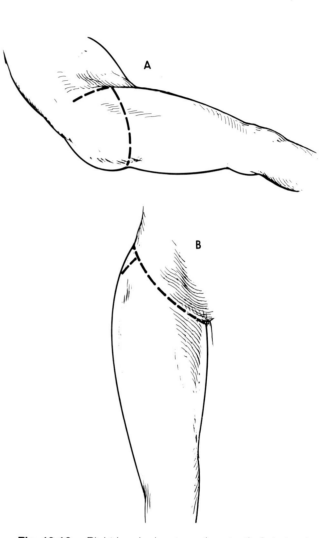

Fig. 19-16 Right hemipelvectomy (see text). **A,** Lateral view of skin incision. **B,** Anterior view of skin incision.

Transmedullary amputations. Amputations through the midportion of an extremity are called either an *above* or *below*-knee or -elbow amputation. The amputation is technically straightforward, and the principles are the same for each of the four locations. The below-knee amputation is often required for patients with vascular insufficiency in the foot and, because the posterior skin and soft tissue have a better blood supply than the anterior tissues, this amputation is usually done with a long posterior flap and no anterior flap. Adequate surgical margins are critical in tumor management and skin flaps are often determined by the site of the tumor, the biopsy incision, or both. Most children with musculoskeletal tumors have no vascular compromise, and the skin incision can be made to accommodate the tumor and preserve as much bone length as oncologically safe. When possible, skin flaps of equal lengths are preferred.

A wide amputation for high-grade bone sarcomas is appropriate, but there is an approximately 5% incidence of local recurrence. A radical amputation reduces the incidence of local recurrence, but probably does not increase the chances of survival. The safe distance between the tumor and the transection of the bone is controversial, but most agree that 5 cm is the minimum and more is better. For soft tissue sarcomas, the entire compartment involved by tumor should be resected rather than transecting the muscle. For example, a high-grade sarcoma in the anterior compartment of the upper arm that arises from the biceps muscle and is adjacent to the neurovascular bundle should be treated with an above-elbow amputation, but the entire anterior compartment of the upper arm should be resected with the specimen. Each amputation must be planned as carefully as each limb salvage resection.

All transmedullary amputations can be performed with this technique. The transverse anatomy of the extremity at the level of amputation should be reviewed preoperatively. "Bone caps" have been recommended over the transected bone ends in children, since overgrowth is occasionally a problem; it is more likely to occur in younger children. Revision may be necessary after several years of growth.

▲ *Technique.* A sterile tourniquet may be used during amputation. The level of bone transection is selected before surgery, based on the most proximal extent of the tumor.

Make the apex of the skin incision on the medial and lateral sides of the extremity to be amputated 1 to 2 cm proximal to the level of bone transection. Make the anterior and posterior flaps equal lengths if the tumor and biopsy incision permit, or as necessary to close the wound. Incise the skin and subcutaneous tissue to the level of the superficial fascia and allow them to retract slightly. Do not pull the skin from the deep fascia, for this reduces the blood supply to the skin. Transect the anterior fascia and muscle at the level of the retracted skin, beveling proximally to the level where the bone will be transected. With the tourniquet inflated it is not necessary to identify and ligate the vessels until the distal portion of the extremity has been removed. Transect the bone with a Gigli or power saw. Then transect the posterior muscles by beveling out to the the level of the skin. The muscles may be cut as a group rather than individually. Once the distal portion of the limb has been removed, identify and ligate the major artery and vein. Identify the major nerves and either bury them in muscle or gently retract and sharply cut them so that they retract into the stump. Release the tourniquet and obtain hemostasis with ligatures and cautery. Smooth the sharp bone edges with a rasp. Suture the anterior muscles to the posterior muscles to cover the end of the bone. Leave a large drain deep to the muscle adjacent to the bone. Close the superficial fascia, subcutaneous tissue, and skin, and apply a compressive dressing. If a trained prosthetist is available, an immediate-fit prosthesis can be applied.

▲ *Postoperative management.* Postoperative rehabilitation should include early ambulation with a temporary prosthesis, usually within the first week after surgery. Once the stump has matured, usually 2 to 3 weeks after surgery, an initial prosthesis is made and the physical therapy rehabilitation program is continued.

Specific Tumors

Obviously, the treatment of a specific tumor must be tailored to the anatomic site and extent of the lesion, and it is impossible to provide step-by-step instructions for the surgical treatment of all possible combinations of anatomic locations and extents. Instead, lesions have been categorized into groups with similar treatment methods, although the clinical setting of a particular tumor may alter the generally suggested treatment. When a tumor behaves more aggressively than expected, it must be treated as its behavior demands.

Observation

Nonossifying fibroma. Nonossifying fibroma probably represents faulty ossification rather than neoplasm, and occurs almost exclusively during childhood and adolescence. It has been estimated that roentgenographic evidence of this cortical defect may be found in approximately one third of growing children, most commonly in the femur and tibia. Most lesions are found incidentally when roentgenograms are made for unrelated reasons. The tumor begins in the metaphysis, near or at the physis, and appears to migrate toward the center of the bone as the epiphyseal region grows away from it. The inner boundary of the lesion is often demarcated by a thin or prominent scalloped line of sclerosis (Fig. 19-17). On gross examination, the lesion may be completely or partially yellow, depending on the lipid content, or may contain enough hemosiderin to make it distinctly brown. Microscopic examination reveals a dominant, cellular, fibroblastic connective-tissue background, with the cells arranged in whorled bundles.

Nonossifying fibromas very rarely require treatment, and the majority resolve by skeletal maturity. Occasionally, repeated pathologic fracture through a large lesion in the femur or tibia may necessitate curettage and bone grafting (Fig. 19-18).

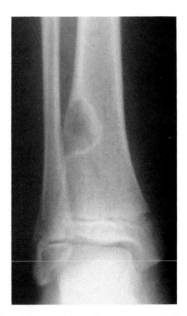

Fig. 19-17   Nonossifying fibroma in distal tibia of 10-year-old boy noted as "incidental finding." Note eccentric location and sclerotic rim.

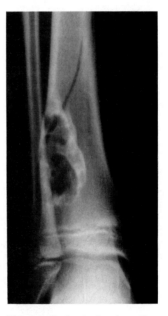

Fig. 19-18   Third pathologic fracture through nonossifying fibroma in distal tibia of 13-year-old boy.

Osteochondroma. Osteochondromas are cartilaginous lesions that arise from the surface of the bone probably secondary to an abnormality in the periphery of the physis. The cartilage grows out from the bone and undergoes enchondral ossification to produce a bony excrescence. Exostoses are common, accounting for 50% of benign bone tumors. Over half occur in patients younger than 20 years. Exostoses may occur in any bone, but are most common in the metaphyseal region of long bones. The distal femur, proximal humerus, and proximal tibia are the most frequent locations. Most exostoses are solitary, and patients with multiple lesions usually have a positive family history for multiple exostoses (multiple hereditable exostosis). Usually the patient first notices a hard, nontender mass fixed to the bone. A few patients have pain caused by irritation of an overlying muscle, but most are asymptomatic. Diagnosis is made from the clinical setting and roentgenographic appearance. The characteristic roentgenographic appearance of exostoses is a projection composed of cortex continuous with that of the underlying bone and a spongiosa, similarly continuous. This projection may have a broad base (Fig. 19-19, *A*) or may be distinctly pedunculated (Fig. 19-19, *B*). Sessile exostoses may be flat, whereas pedunculated ones are sometimes long and slender. All gradations between these exist. Many are cauliflower-shaped, with or without a stalk. Irregular zones of calcification may be present, and the affected bone is often abnormally wide at the level of the lesion.

On gross examination, the cartilage cap is ordinarily only 2 to 3 mm thick and has a smooth surface. The cartilage may be 1 cm or more thick in the actively growing benign exostosis of adolescence. Irregularity and thickening of the cap demand careful histologic study because of the possibility of secondary chondrosarcoma. The exostosis is covered by periosteum, which is continuous with that of the adjacent bone.

During childhood, excision of exostoses is indicated only for symptomatic irritation of an overlying structure, pressure on a nerve, or displacement of a major vascular bundle. Peterson has described surgical correction of specific deformities in children with multiple exostoses (Fig. 19-20). Shortening of the ulna with ulnar deviation of the carpus may be treated with ulnar lengthening and partial epiphysiodesis of the distal radius (Fig. 19-21). Valgus deformity of the knee or ankle may also be corrected by stapling or partial epiphysiodesis.

Malignant change rarely occurs in children and adolescents, but evaluation for suspected malignancy should be performed in the skeletally mature patient with a sudden increase in pain or growth of a known lesion. The risk of malignant changes has been reported to be less than 1% for solitary lesions and up to 10% for multiple exostoses.

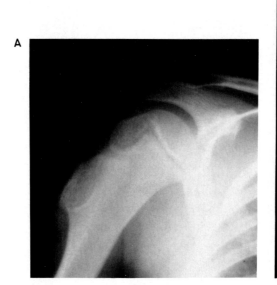
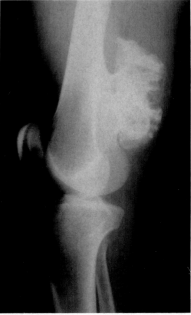

Fig. 19-19   Osteochondroma (exostosis). **A,** Broad-based lesion in proximal humerus of 6-year-old boy. **B,** Painful, pedunculated lesion in distal femur of 17-year-old boy.

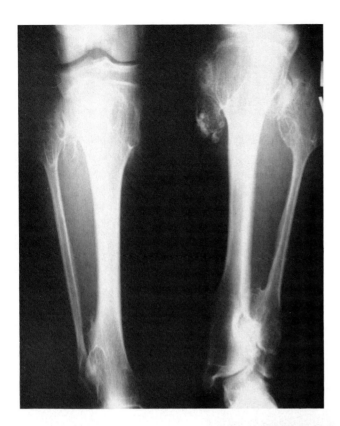

Fig. 19-20 Multiple osteochondromatosis of both tibiae and fibulae of 15-year-old girl. Note valgus deformity of left ankle.

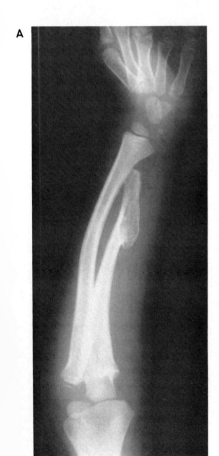

A

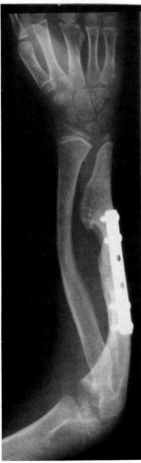

B

Fig. 19-21 **A,** Osteochondroma of distal ulna in 8-year-old boy with pseudo-Madelung deformity, subluxation of radial head. **B,** After ulnar lengthening.

Fibrous dysplasia. Fibrous dysplasia is a developmental abnormality rather than a true neoplasm. Most patients have a single lesion (monostotic), but multiple lesions (polyostotic) do occur. Fibrous dysplasia manifests itself early in life, usually before the age of 10 years. The single most common location is a rib, although any bone may be involved. Most patients are asymptomatic, although the dysplasia may produce defective growth, deformity, and pain in any bone (Fig. 19-22). Yellow or brown patches of cuta-

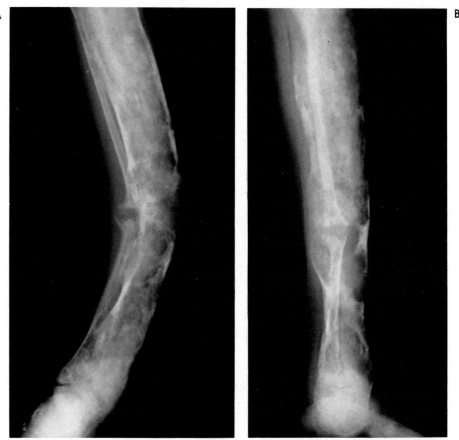

Fig. 19-22 Fibrous dysplasia producing severe defective growth and deformity of tibia in 18-year-old woman. **A,** Anteroposterior and, **B,** lateral views of right tibia.

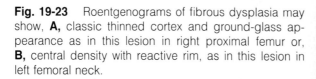

Fig. 19-23 Roentgenograms of fibrous dysplasia may show, **A,** classic thinned cortex and ground-glass appearance as in this lesion in right proximal femur or, **B,** central density with reactive rim, as in this lesion in left femoral neck.

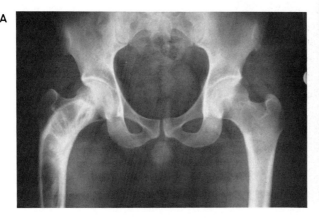

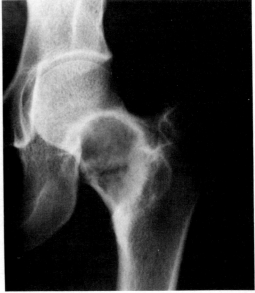

neous pigmentation may accompany the bone lesion. The roentgenographic appearance of fibrous dysplasia is extremely variable, but the classic form is a lesion in the medullary canal that blends with a thinned cortex and has a ground glass appearance (Fig. 19-23, *A*). Some lesions have a homogenous increased density, whereas others have decreased central density with a reactive rim (Fig. 19-23, *B*). Occasionally a lesion contains calcified cartilage. The gross appearance of the lesion is also variable, but most are well-defined and composed of dense fibrous tissue. Usually, enough small osteoid trabeculae are embedded in this fibrous tissue to impart a distinctly gritty quality. The major histologic feature is proliferation of fibroblasts that produce dense collagenous matrix. The fibroblastic cells may form a storiform or cartwheel arrangement. The fibrous element typically contains trabeculae of osteoid and bone, producing the "alphabet soup" appearance on low-power microscopy.

If the diagnosis is certain, observation is appropriate because the lesions commonly stop growing when the patient reaches puberty. Biopsy is indicated when the diagnosis cannot be made from clinical or roentgenographic findings. Recurrence is likely after curettage, although it is suggested if diagnostic biopsy is done. Weakened and deformed bones should be straightened, and internal fixation with bone grafting should be used to strengthen the dysplastic bone. Surgery is frequently required in the proximal femoral and tibial diaphyseal lesions. Surgical correction of deformities may not be indicated in patients with extensive involvement because the bones heal with fibrodysplastic bone.

Enchondroma. Enchondromas are benign cartilage tumors within the medullary canal; they consist of persistent normal cartilage that did not undergo enchondral ossification either from the original cartilaginous anlage or the physis. They account for 11% of all benign bone tumors, and almost half are found in the hands or feet, usually the phalanges (Fig. 19-24). Most enchondromas are asymptomatic and are found either when the patient sustains a pathologic fracture or when roentgenograms are made for an unrelated reason. Diagnosis of enchondroma can usually be made from the clinical setting and roentgenographic appearance of the lesion. Roentgenograms show a localized central region of rarefaction, usually metaphyseal with slight to prominent stippled or mottled calcification, especially in large tubular bones, or ossification may make the lesion radiopaque. The cortex is often expanded. Roentgenograms should be made of all long bones of the affected extremity to determine the presence of any other enchondromas. Enchondromas are seldom seen intact because, if

treated, most are curetted; however, specimens generally consist of fragments of bluish white hyaline cartilage containing foci of calcification. Histologically, the fragments may appear to be moderately cellular cartilage, but careful examination shows the nuclei to be small and fairly uniform in size.

If the diagnosis of enchondroma is obvious, observation is the treatment of choice. Many enchondromas in children resolve spontaneously and the risk of repeated pathologic fracture is small. The patient should be examined for evidence of other lesions or hemangioma. Clinical and roentgenographic examinations may be repeated every 3 months for a year, then yearly or when symptoms warrant. If the diagnosis is in question, thorough curettage and bone grafting are recommended. Pathologic fractures should be treated nonoperatively if possible. After the fracture has healed, the lesion can be curetted and bone grafted if there is risk of another pathologic fracture. The recurrence rate of enchondroma is low, and the risk of malignant degeneration is essentially nonexistent in children, except in patients with multiple enchondromas (Ollier disease) or with multiple enchondromas and hemangiomas (Maffucci syndrome), in whom the risk of developing a secondary chondrosarcoma ranges from 1% to 15%. Occasionally children with Ollier disease develop severe angular deformity or limb length discrepancy that requires treatment.

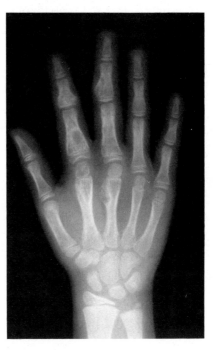

Fig. 19-24 Multiple enchondromatosis in metacarpals and phalanges of 6-year-old girl.

Hemangioma. Hemangiomas are the most common tumors in infancy and childhood, accounting for 7% of benign soft tissue tumors in all age groups. They are generally divided into two subgroups: capillary hemangiomas and cavernous hemangiomas. Capillary hemangiomas are more common, occurring in approximately 5% of all children, and usually appear within the first few weeks of life in the skin or subcutaneous tissue of the head or neck. They are elevated, red to purple in color, and composed of capillary-sized vessels lined with flattened endothelium. They may enlarge until the child is about 6 months old, then regress over the years; by the time the child is 7 years old, 75% to 95% have completely regressed. Small capillary hemangiomas in inconspicuous locations can probably be ignored, but rapidly enlarging lesions that threaten a vital structure or pose a cosmetic problem should be treated. Cavernous hemangiomas are less frequent and usually arise within muscles; they do not spontaneously regress. They are composed of large, dilated, blood-filled vessels lined by flattened endothelium. On a roentgenogram, large deep lesions appear as localized or diffuse nonhomogenous water density masses; calcification is common (Fig. 19-25). Cavernous hemangiomas that cause no symptoms can be left undisturbed, but if the lesion causes pain or restriction of motion because of

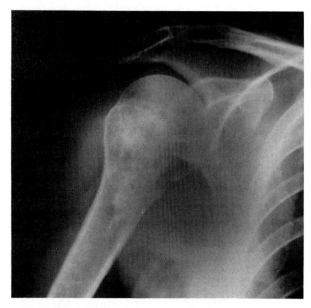

Fig. 19-25 Hemangioma of proximal humerus in 19-year-old woman.

pressure on neighboring structures, limited resection is indicated. Patients with hemangiomas may have intermittent pain, swelling, and erythema caused by local thrombophlebitis, and these can be treated with rest, elevation, and aspirin.

On surgical exposure, a hemangioma is likely to be blue and usually honeycombed in appearance. Bony trabeculae may be produced and give a "sunburst" effect. The histologic interpretation of vascular lesions of bone is complicated by the difficulty in knowing when a conglomeration of vascular channels is a hemangioma rather than a hamartomatous malformation. Most hemangiomas of bone are cavernous, although sometimes a capillary component is present.

Simple Curettage

Unicameral bone cyst. Unicameral bone cysts (or simple cysts) are relatively common benign lesions that apparently result from a disturbance of growth at the physis. The lesion usually becomes evident during the first two decades of life, and 80% occur between the ages of 3 and 14 years. Seventy percent involve the proximal femur or the humerus, and the lesions are twice as common in males as in females. Patients may have local pain, but most cysts are discovered only after pathologic fracture has occurred. Occasionally there is swelling in the region. On a roentgenogram, the unicameral bone cyst is seen as a lucency in the medullary portion of the shaft of the bone generally abutting the physis. The cortex ordinarily is eroded and thinned but is intact unless a pathologic fracture has occurred (Fig. 19-26). On roentgenogram, the unicameral bone cyst is seen as a lucency in the medullary portion of the shaft of the bone generally abutting the physis (Fig. 19-27). Typically, the involved bone shows only slight expansion, not exceeding that of the physis (Fig. 19-28).

On gross examination, the cystic cavity is filled with a clear or yellowish green fluid of low viscosity. The inner surface of the cyst wall frequently has ridges separating depressed zones, and sometimes the wall is covered by a layer of fleshy tissue 1 cm or more in thickness. Occasionally, partial or complete septa are seen, the latter type making the cyst multicameral. Histologically, the lining of the cyst may be merely a very thin layer of fibrous tissue. Thicker areas are composed of fibrogenic connective tissue, which often contains numerous benign giant cells, hemosiderin pigment, a few chronic inflammatory cells, and lipophages. The histologic and gross features may be modified by fracture.

Until recently, treatment of unicameral bone cysts consisted of curettage and bone grafting. However, in 1979, Scaglietti et al reported favorable results in 90%

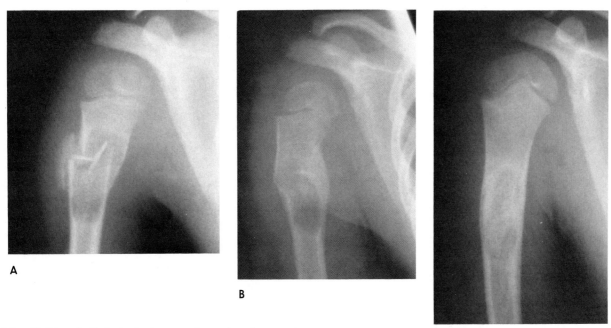

Fig. 19-26   A, Pathologic fracture through unicameral bone cyst in proximal humerus. **B,** Six months after fracture; site was injected with corticosteroid. **C,** One year after fracture.

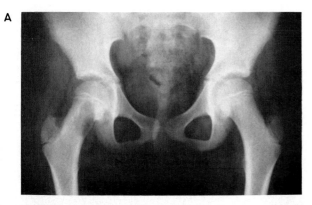

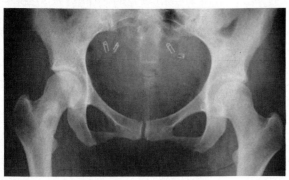

Fig. 19-27   A, Unicameral bone cyst in femoral neck abutting physis in 11-year-old girl before curettage, bone grafting, and immobilization in spica cast. **B,** Ten years after treatment.

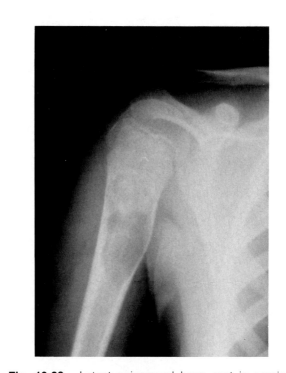

Fig. 19-28   Latent unicameral bone cyst in proximal humerus of 11-year-old boy with intact cortex.

of their patients with injection of methylprednisolone acetate. More recently, Oppenheim and Galleno compared the results of operative treatment and steroid injection in the management of unicameral bone cysts in 57 patients. They found that steroid injection resulted in lower morbidity, a lower recurrence rate, and lower cost than surgery. Some authors have suggested that drilling multiple holes into the lesion is therapeutic. Whatever the method of treatment chosen, the recurrence rate is higher in patients younger than 10 years of age with cysts in a juxtaphyseal location. The chance of permanent cure is good in patients who are older than 10 years of age in whom the cyst has been left behind by the growing physis. For large lesions in the femur or tibia with impending pathologic fracture, treatment with curettage and bone grafting, and possibly supplementary internal fixation, may be required.

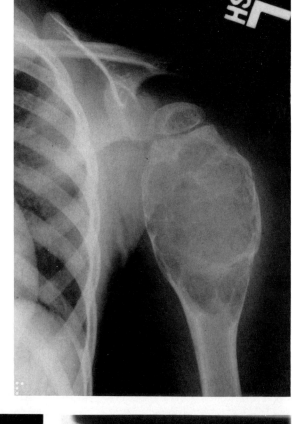

Fig. 19-29 A, Aneurysmal bone cyst in proximal humerus of 10-year-old girl. Note expansion and thinning of cortex. **B,** Immediately after curettage and bone grafting. **C,** Recurrence of lesion 2 years after surgery.

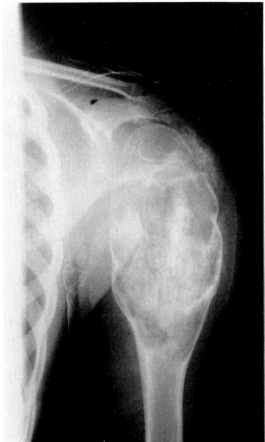

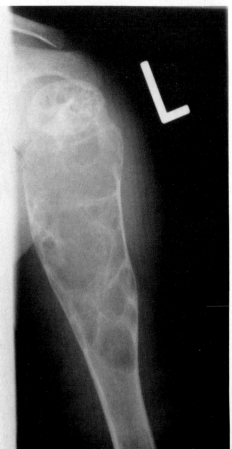

Aneurysmal bone cyst. Aneurysmal bone cysts are benign, usually solitary, expansile lesions of bone, accounting for approximately 10% of benign lesions. Eighty percent of primary aneurysmal bone cysts are diagnosed in patients between the ages of 10 and 20 years. More than half of these cysts arise in large tubular bones, and almost 30% arise in the spine. When in the spine, the lesion begins in the posterior elements but can extend into the vertebral body. Patients usually complain of mild pain, often associated with activity. The roentgenographic appearance is typical: the lesion is usually metaphyseal, eccentric, and radiolucent with an expanded and thinned cortex (Fig. 19-29). The periosteal reaction may be well developed or may suggest an aggressive tumor. Occasionally, the periosteal reaction associated with an aneurysmal bone cyst forms a Codman's triangle or "onionskinning."

On gross examination, anastomosing cavernomatous spaces ordinarily compose the bulk of the lesion. The spaces are usually filled with unclotted blood. The eggshell-thin layer of subperiosteal new bone, which delimits the lesion, is readily discernible. The essential histologic feature is the presence of the cavernomatous spaces, the walls of which lack the normal features of blood vessels. The solid portions of an aneurysmal bone cyst may be fibrous, but they usually contain a lacework of osteoid trabeculae. Benign giant cells are often present in large numbers. The histological features of aneurysmal bone cysts overlap those of simple bone cysts, making differentiation difficult or impossible.

Aneurysmal bone cysts are controlled in almost all patients with simple curettage. Most are large enough to require bone grafting. Allograft or internal fixation and grafting are occasionally recommended for extremely large lesions in young patients (Fig. 19-30).

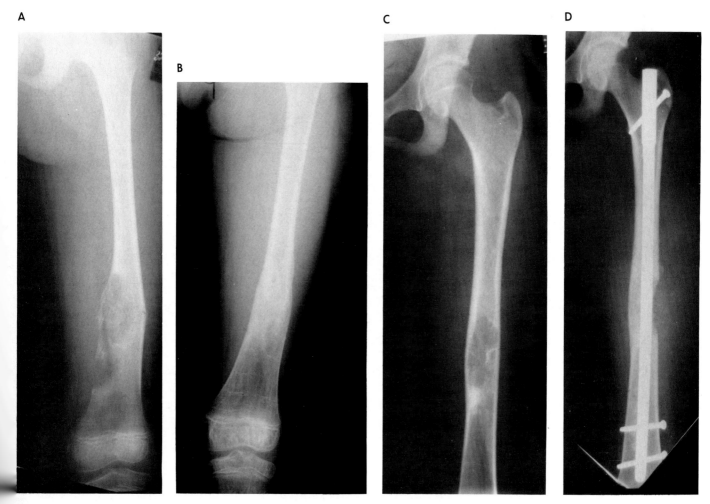

Fig. 19-30 **A,** Recurrent aneurysmal bone cyst in femur of 12-year-old girl. **B,** One year after curettage and grafting. **C,** Second recurrence 3 years after curettage and grafting. **D,** Repeat curettage and grafting, and fixation with Russell-Taylor interlocking nail.

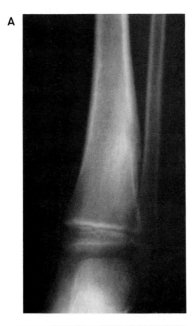

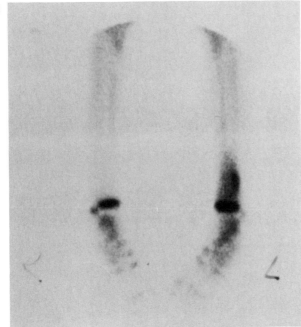

Fig. 19-31 **A,** Roentgenogram of osteoid osteoma in distal lateral tibia of 10-year-old boy. **B,** Radionuclide scan showing increased uptake in lesion and surrounding tibia.

Osteoid osteoma. Osteoid osteoma is a small, solitary, benign, painful lesion. It accounts for 11% of benign bone tumors and is three times more common in males than in females. Over 80% are diagnosed in patients between the ages of 5 and 24 years. Any bone may be involved, but the proximal femur and the spine are common locations. Osteoid osteoma is a unique lesion in that it can be diagnosed from the patient's pain pattern: constant, boring pain that is worse at night, is not related to activity, and is relieved by aspirin. The pain is often referred to the adjacent joint region. The lesion may be accompanied by swelling or occasional increased warmth of the overlying skin, but there is neither redness nor fever. When an extremity is involved, limping is common and flexion contractures may occur. Spinal lesions may produce painful scoliosis. The typical roentgenographic appearance is increased density of the cortex with a small central radiolucent nidus. The radiolucent nidus is the lesion and the surrounding density is reactive bone. Lesions in cortical bone generally produce periosteal reactive bone (Fig. 19-31, *A*). Osteoid osteomas in cancellous bone, especially in the femoral neck or tarsal bones, may produce little new periosteal reactive bone. Radionuclide scanning is usually positive and is valuable when plain roentgenograms are normal (Fig. 19-31, *B*). Tomograms or CT scans may be necessary to delineate the lesion completely.

On gross inspection, osteoid osteomas may be found in relatively nonsclerotic cancellous bone or buried in a large region of cortical sclerosis; the actual nidus, however, usually stands out as a discrete round or oval mass of tissue and is ordinarily redder than the surrounding bone. The nidus seldom exceeds 1 cm in greatest dimension, even when symptoms have been present for several years. Microscopic examination reveals a distinct demarcation between the nidus and the surrounding bone, which may be densely sclerotic but has no other typical features. The nidus consists of an interlacing network of osteoid trabeculae with a variable amount of mineralization, usually concentrated in the center of the nidus. The trabeculae are usually thin and arranged in a tangle of numerous anastomoses. Within the trabecular framework, instead of bone marrow elements, there is a somewhat vascular, fibrous connective tissue that contains variable numbers of benign giant cells.

The lesion is cured with curettage of the nidus, but all of the nidus must be removed. The nidus may be accurately located preoperatively with CT scanning identified intraoperatively by direct observation, biopsied, and then thoroughly curetted. No attempt should be made to remove all of the reactive bone.

Eosinophilic granuloma. Eosinophilic granuloma is a benign, nonneoplastic, lytic lesion of bone probably arising from the reticuloendothelial system. It is one of the disorders included in the spectrum of histiocytosis X; others are Hand-Schuller-Christian disease and Letterer-Siwe disease. Eosinophilic granulomas occur from infancy to the sixth decade of life, with a peak incidence between the ages of 5 and 10 years. Any bone may be be involved, but the skull is the single most common location. Patients with eosinophilic granuloma usually have a solitary painful focus and often a palpable or visible mass. When a lesion involves a vertebral body, it may cause total collapse of the body (vertebra plana). The roentgenographic appearance is a radiolucent destructive lesion with periosteal reaction (Fig. 19-32). Eosinophilic granuloma is often called the "great imitator"; the lesions are similar in appearance to Ewing's sarcoma, although eosinophilic granulomas are usually smaller.

The lesional tissue is soft and may be gray, pink, or yellow. A pathognomonic histologic feature is foci of proliferating histiocytic cell, frequently with ill-defined cytoplasmic boundaries and characteristically containing an oval or indented nucleus. Mitotic figures may be common, and varied numbers of eosinophils, lymphocytes, and neutrophils are nearly always present. Chronic osteomyelitis and eosinophilic granuloma are difficult to distinguish on review of frozen section, and suspected eosinophilic granulomas should always be cultured.

Incisional biopsy usually results in resolution of the lesion, but simple curettage is recommended at the time of biopsy. Successful treatment with direct corticosteroid injection has been reported, but too few reports are available for this to be recommended. Patients should be carefully evaluated for other lesions in the skeleton and other organs. Most patients who develop multiple bone lesions do so within 6 months of the original diagnosis.

Marginal Excision

Pigmented villonodular synovitis. Pigmented villonodular synovitis is an idiopathic condition of the synovial tissue that is rare in children and more common in young adults (before the age of 40 years). The knee joint is most commonly affected, followed by the hip joint. Other joints may be involved, including the small joints of the hand and foot and the ankle and elbow joints. The patient usually complains of swelling and discomfort in the affected joint. The symptoms gradually progress in severity over months to years. Physical examination shows an accumulation of fluid in the joint, and aspiration obtains a dark brown serosanguineous fluid. On a roentgenogram, bone involvement is usually manifested by the presence of a soft tissue mass associated with erosion of the adjacent bone or joint. The opened joint usually shows diffuse reddish brown to rust discoloration of the synovium with villous projections. This shaggy appearance of the synovium can be seen on an arthrogram or with arthroscopy and is virtually diagnostic. The microscopic pattern is diverse, with some areas demonstrating delicate, elongated villi and others with bulbous projections covered by synovial cells. Hemosiderin may be found in synovial cells and macrophages or lying free within the connective tissue proliferation and associated with multinucleated giant cells.

Initial treatment is synovectomy, but recurrence is frequent. Surgery should be repeated only for significant pain or erosion of bone.

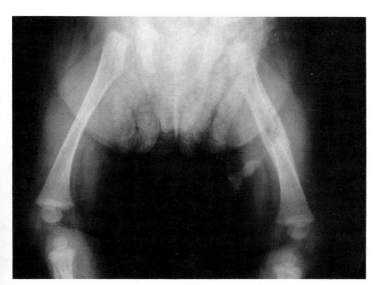

Fig. 19-32 Pathologic fracture through eosinophilic granuloma in proximal femur of 2-year-old child. Note lytic lesion and periosteal bone formation that mimics malignant lesion.

Synovial chondromatosis. In synovial chondromatosis the subliminal cells of the synovium produce cartilage that is then extruded into the joint; the cause of this benign process is not known. The patient is usually a young adult who complains of swelling, mild pain, and "locking" of the involved joint. Joint effusion is rare. The knee joint is the most commonly involved, followed by the elbow and hip joints. The roentgenographic appearance of the joint may be normal, but more often some of the cartilaginous loose bodies have central calcifications that appear on the roentgenogram as intraarticular densities. The synovium may be hyperemic, and in areas occupied by loose bodies may show thickening and villous projections. If the cartilaginous bodies have not been sequestrated, their attachment to the synovium may look like small, glistening, gray-white nodules. Often the entire synovium is involved and the nodules are so abundant that they appear to form a solid mass. Histologically, the loose bodies range from masses of cartilage to bodies in which there is a mixture of cartilage, bone, and occasionally fatty marrow. The nuclei of the chondrocytes are generally large and hyperchromatic. Double and triple nucleated cells are common.

Synovectomy and removal of loose bodies from the joint are the recommended treatment. Diffuse synovial lesions may recur because it is difficult to remove every vestige of them. The solitary chondroma rarely recurs after excision.

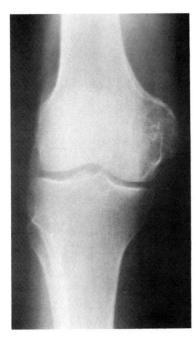

Fig. 19-33 Chondroblastoma in medial femoral condyle of 16-year-old girl.

Neurofibroma. Neurofibroma is a benign tumor of nerve that most commonly affects young adults. Most are superficial lesions of the skin or subcutaneous tissue and can occur anywhere over the body surface. Neurofibromas are usually solitary lesions, except in patients with von Recklinghausen disease. The lesions grow slowly and produce few symptoms, although some patients may have pain over the lesion. On gross examination, they are white-gray tumors without secondary degenerative changes. In major nerves, they expand the nerve in a fusiform fashion and normal nerve can be seen entering and exiting the mass. If the lesion remains confined by the epineurium, it possesses a true capsule; however, more commonly these tumors arise in small nerves and readily extend into soft tissue. Histologically, in its most characteristic form, neurofibroma contains interlacing bundles of elongated cells with wavy, dark-staining nuclei. The cells are intimately associated with wirelike strands of collagen, and small to moderate amounts of mucoid material separate the cells and collagen. The stroma of the tumor is dotted with occasional mast cells, lymphocytes, and rarely xanthoma cells.

When neurofibroma is not associated with an important nerve, marginal resection (including the nerve) is indicated. When a major nerve is involved, total resection is not appropriate unless the lesion continues to grow or exhibits signs of malignant degeneration. These lesions should be biopsied and observed, unless the patient's symptoms demand treatment.

Neurilemoma. Neurilemoma, also called a *schwannoma,* is a benign tumor of the nerve sheath seen most commonly in young adults. Neurilemoma may involve any nerve, but has a predilection for the head, neck, and flexor surfaces of the upper and lower extremities. Consequently, the spinal roots and the cervical, sympathetic, vagus, peroneal, and ulnar nerves are most commonly affected. Neurilemomas usually appear as painless, slow-growing masses. Direct palpation usually produces an electric-like shock (Tinel's sign). Pain and neurologic symptoms are uncommon unless the tumor becomes large. If a major motor or sensory nerve is involved, the patient may have physical signs of neurologic loss. When it involves small nerves, the tumor is freely movable except for a single point of deep attachment. In larger nerves, the tumor is movable except along the long axis of the nerve where the attachment restricts mobility.

Because these tumors arise within nerve sheaths, they are surrounded by a true capsule of epineurium. Tumors of small nerves may resemble neurofibromas in their fusiform shape; they often eclipse or obliterate the nerve of origin. In larger nerves the tumors are eccentric masses over which the nerve fibers are splayed. The tumors have a pink, white, or yellow appearance and usually measure less than 5 cm. Microscopically, neurilemomas are uninodular masses surrounded by fibrous capsules consisting of epineurium and residual nerve fibers.

At surgery, the neurilemoma is easily separated from the nerve, and marginal excision is curative. Recurrence is unusual, and malignant change is very rare.

Extended Curettage

Chondroblastoma. Chondroblastoma (Codman tumor) is a benign cartilage tumor that arises in the epiphyses. It accounts for less than 1% of all benign bone tumors. Chondroblastomas occur most frequently in adolescents and young adults. The proximal humerus is the most common location (20% of all lesions), but the distal femur, proximal tibia, and proximal femur frequently are involved. Pain in the adjacent joint is the most common symptom; joint effusion is usually present and range of motion may be reduced.

The roentgenographic appearance is diagnostic. The lesion is a radiolucency in the epiphyseal end of the bone, with a small focus of calcification. It appears to destroy bone and is often demarcated by a thin sclerotic margin (Fig. 19-33). Even though originating in the epiphysis, lesions may expand to involve the metaphysis. If the lesion becomes large, the bone may be deformed.

On gross examination, the lesion is small, grayish pink, and may contain zones of hemorrhage or necrosis. Although chondroblastomas often abut the articular cartilage of a joint, they rarely produce destruction of the cartilage. Histologically, the basic proliferating cells are considered to be chondroblasts, cells related to cartilage-forming connective tissue. The round or oval nucleus of the chondroblast is often indented or may have a longitudinal groove.

Extended curettage of the lesion that includes the reactive surrounding bone is curative in 90% of lesions, and recurrences can almost always be treated successfully with a second curettage. Rarely, wide resection is necessary for recurrences that invade the joint and for the occasional lesion in the pelvis.

Osteoblastoma. Osteoblastoma is a rare benign tumor often called a *giant osteoid osteoma* because of the similarity of their histologic appearances. Osteoblastoma accounts for less than 1% of primary tumors of bone and has a marked predilection for males. Over half of osteoblastomas occur in patients between the ages of 10 and 20 years, and 50% occur in the posterior elements of the spine. Pain, usually at the site of the tumor, is the primary symptom. Lower extremity lesions may cause limping. Involvement of the spinal cord or nerves may cause weakness or even paraplegia, and scoliosis is common with spinal lesions.

The roentgenographic appearance is a mixture of lucency and density (Fig. 19-34). The lesion tends to infiltrate the surrounding bone beyond its apparent margin. On gross examination, tumor tissue is hemorrhagic, granular, and friable because of its vascularity and osteoid component, which shows variable calcification. When the tumor bulges from and distorts the contour of the affected bone, the margins of the tumor are sharply defined.

Histologically, osteoblasts with regularly shaped nuclei containing little chromatin and often having abundant cytoplasm produce interlacing trabeculae or discrete small islands of osteoid or bone. Under low-power microscopy, an osteoblastoma appears loosely arranged because of the large number of capillaries between the trabeculae of bone. The edges of the osteoblastoma are sharp, with no tendency to permeate the surrounding normal bone.

Extended curettage or, if the lesion's location permits, wide resection is recommended. Recurrence is uncommon and malignant change is rare.

A
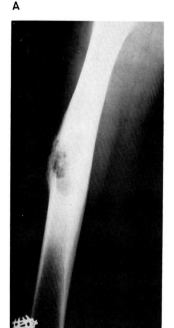

B
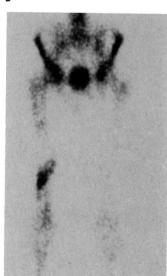

Fig. 19-34   A, Roentgenogram of osteoblastoma in femoral shaft of 17-year-old boy. **B,** Lesion is evident in bone scan with increased uptake in mid-diaphysis of femur.

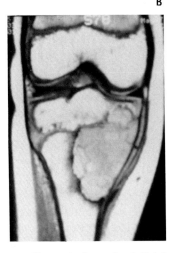

Fig. 19-35 **A,** Chondromyxofibroma of proximal tibial metaphysis and epiphysis in 9-year-old boy. **B,** MRI showing bony and soft tissue borders of lesion.

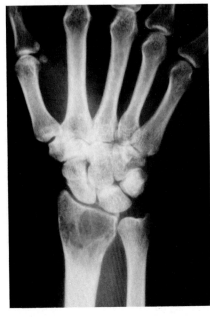

Fig. 19-36 Giant cell tumor of distal radius in 17-year-old girl.

Chondromyxofibroma. Chondromyxofibroma is an uncommon tumor probably of cartilaginous origin. It is twice as common in males as in females and is most frequently found in patients between the ages of 10 and 30 years. Most chondromyxofibromas involve the metaphyseal region of long bones; one third are in the tibia. A dull, aching pain is the most common symptom, and there may be local swelling.

The roentgenographic appearance is similar to that of an aneurysmal bone cyst: a radiolucent, eccentric lesion that destroys the cortex but is contained by a periosteal rim (Fig. 19-35). Occasionally, the bone is expanded by the lesion.

On gross examination, chondromyxofibroma may resemble hyaline cartilage or appear to be a somewhat translucent fibrous mass. A striking feature is the sharp delineation from the surrounding bone, a feature different from chondrosarcoma. The surface of the tumor is often distinctly lobulated, and the cavity from which it is enucleated is frequently characterized by corrugations corresponding to the tumor lobules. The name of the tumor indicates the variation of microscopic appearances, which may include myxomatous zones, fibrous zones, and fields with a distinctly chondroid appearance. A highly characteristic feature is an increased concentration of nuclei at the periphery of the lobules, but this should not be confused with the similar appearance of some chondrosarcomas.

The risk of recurrence after extended curettage is approximately 25%, and malignant transformation is rare.

Giant cell tumor of bone. Giant cell tumor of bone is a distinctive neoplasm of poorly differentiated cells. The multinucleated giant cells apparently result from fusion of the proliferating mononuclear cells. Giant cell tumors of bone are unusual in skeletally immature patients with growing physes and are most often found in patients between the ages of 18 and 45 years. The distal femur is the most common location, followed by the proximal tibia and distal radius (Fig. 19-36). Joint symptoms are common, including pain, swelling, giving way, and weakness. A hard, sometimes crepitant and painful mass is found in more than 80% of patients. Atrophy of the muscles from disuse may be present, as well as effusion in the adjacent joint or local heat and redness.

The roentgenographic appearance is diagnostic, but the lesion is often difficult to see, especially in the distal femur, where the patella covers the lesion on the anteroposterior view and the normal radiolucent appearance of the distal femur may obscure the lesion on the lateral view. Giant cell tumors are radiolucent, involve the metaphysis and epiphysis, and abut the subchondral bone. In patients with open physes, the lesion is usually in the metaphysis and may break through the cortex to form a soft tissue component (Fig. 19-37).

On gross examination, the tumor is characteristically soft, friable, and gray to red. The aggressive nature of giant cell tumors accounts for their usually immense size when they have been neglected. In skeletally mature patients, the tumor always extends to the articular cartilage, and its boundaries are only moderately well demarcated from adjacent bone and cartilage. Even in very large lesions, the periosteum is rarely breached. Histologically, the basic proliferating cell has a round-to-oval or even spindle-shaped nucleus, surrounded by an ill-defined cytoplasmic zone. Discernible intercellular substance is not being produced. Mitotic figures can be found in practically every lesion and may be numerous. The nuclei lack the hyperchromatism and variation in size and shape that are characteristic of sarcoma.

Patients with sufficient remaining bone and without displaced pathologic fracture should be treated with extended curettage. The key to successful curettage is a large opening in the bone so that the entire cavity can be adequately inspected. In skeletally mature patients, polymethylmethacrylate (PMMA) may be used to fill the defect left after curettage. Whether the PMMA is effective in killing tumor cells is not known, but it does improve the stability of the compromised articular surface. PMMA has not been shown to cause degenerative arthritis in the adjacent articular cartilage, and its removal does not appear necessary. Long-term follow-up of patients with giant cell tumors of bone is essential because malignant change has been reported to occur nearly 40 years after primary treatment. Several studies have reported recurrence rates of 50% and more and malignant change in as many as 10% of patients. Benign giant cell tumor of bone may metastasize to the lung, and routine periodic chest roentgenograms are recommended.

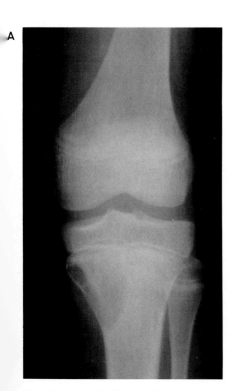
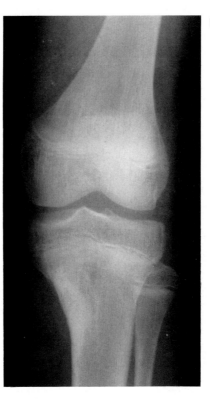

Fig. 19-37   A, Giant cell tumor of proximal tibial metaphysis in 10-year-old girl. **B,** One year after curettage and grafting.

Wide Resection

Osteosarcoma. Osteosarcomas are divided into two major types: conventional high-grade intramedullary osteosarcoma and juxtacortical osteosarcoma, which may be categorized as parosteal or periosteal.

Conventional high-grade osteosarcomas are more common and occur almost exclusively in adolescents and young adults; half occur in teenagers and three quarters in patients between the ages of 5 and 25 years. Most of these tumors arise in the distal femur or proximal tibia, with the proximal humerus, proximal femur, and pelvis the next three most common locations. Pain and occasionally loss of motion in the adjacent joint are frequent symptoms. A hard, usually

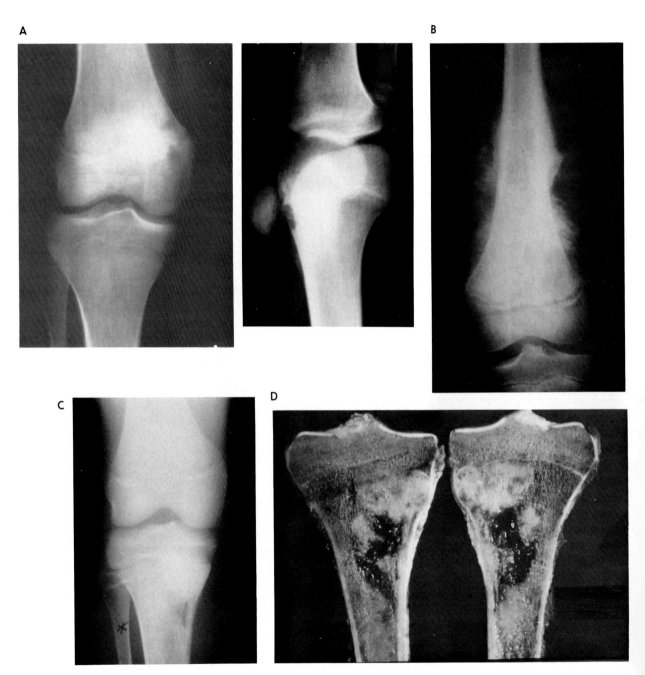

Fig. 19-38 Roentgenographic and gross characteristics of osteogenic sarcoma. **A,** Combination of bone destruction and new bone formation in distal femur of 18-year-old woman. **B,** "Sunburst" spicules of new bone formation in distal femur of 12-year-old boy. **C,** Lesion in right proximal tibia. **D,** Note necrosis, telangiectasia, and hemorrhage in cross-section of same lesion.

mildly tender mass can be palpated. Half of the patients have elevated serum alkaline phosphatase levels and one fourth, elevated serum lactate dehydrogenase levels.

The roentgenographic appearance varies from mainly radiolucent to radiodense, but most lesions are a combination of bone destruction and new bone formation (Fig. 19-38, *A*). There is usually cortical destruction, "fluffy" bone formation (Fig. 19-38, *B*), and periosteal reaction. Osteosarcomas vary from extremely soft, friable, granular masses to firm, fibrous lesions with foci or irregular ossification and variable amounts of chondroid material to densely sclerotic lesions. Nearly all have soft peripheral zones with areas of necrosis, cyst formation, telangiectasis, and hemorrhage (Fig. 19-38, *C* and *D*).

Histologically, osteosarcomas consist of a malignant stroma and malignant neoplastic osteoid and bone. The primary tissue seen may be osseous, cartilaginous, or fibrous, but all types contain malignant osteoid. The determination of malignancy of osteoid and bone is based on features of pleomorphism, hyperchromaticity, and bizarre mitoses of the osteoblasts around and within the osteoid and bone. In other areas of this lesion the sarcomatous stroma or the bone and osteoid may predominate, whereas in many lesions all three elements are seen. Malignant cartilage may be seen either in tiny foci or composing the bulk of the tumor.

The standard treatment is wide surgical resection and adjuvant chemotherapy. The use of preoperative (neoadjuvant) chemotherapy is being investigated and may increase the number of patients who can be successfully treated with limb salvage operations. Amputation is recommended when the major neurovascular bundle is next to the tumor or when the child has so much growth left in the adjacent physis that leg length discrepancy would be excessive. A radical surgical margin can be obtained with an above-knee amputation when the primary tumor is in the tibia. Lesions in the distal femur can be treated with a wide surgical margin with a high, above-knee amputation or with a radical surgical margin with a hip disarticulation. The incidence of local recurrence is slightly lower in patients treated with a radical surgical margin than in those treated with a wide surgical margin, but the overall survival rate is the same.

Juxtacortical osteosarcomas are malignant, bone-forming tumors arising from the surface of the bone without involvement of the medullary canal. These osteosarcomas usually occur in the second or third decade of life. The patient complains of a mild ache and often has noticed a hard mass fixed to the bone. Parosteal osteosarcomas often arise from the poste-rior distal femur or posterior proximal tibia and reduce knee flexion. They have the roentgenographic appearance of mature bone and are often confused with exostoses. Parosteal osteosarcomas attach to the cortex or periosteum and, unlike exostoses, do not communicate with the medullary canal (Fig. 19-39).

Periosteal osteosarcomas are less common than parosteal osteosarcomas. They occur most often in the proximal anterior tibia and are usually diaphyseal. The roentgenogram shows thin strands of bone radiating perpendicularly from the surface of the bone. Although chondroid differentiation usually dominates the histologic pattern of juxtacortical osteosarcomas, there is a condensation of pink matrix near the centers of the neoplastic lobules that has the quality of osteoid. Typical spicules of new bone, sometimes numerous, are almost always found near the underlying cortex. Juxtacortical osteosarcomas, both parosteal and periosteal, are treated with a wide surgical margin, and adjuvant chemotherapy is indicated only for tumors of a high histologic grade.

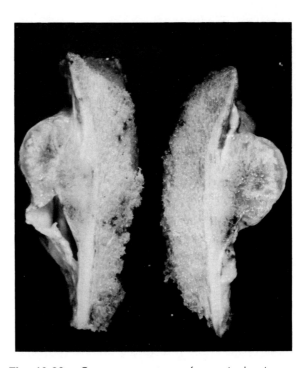

Fig. 19-39 Gross appearance of parosteal osteosarcoma. Note attachment to cortex and lack of communication with medullary canal.

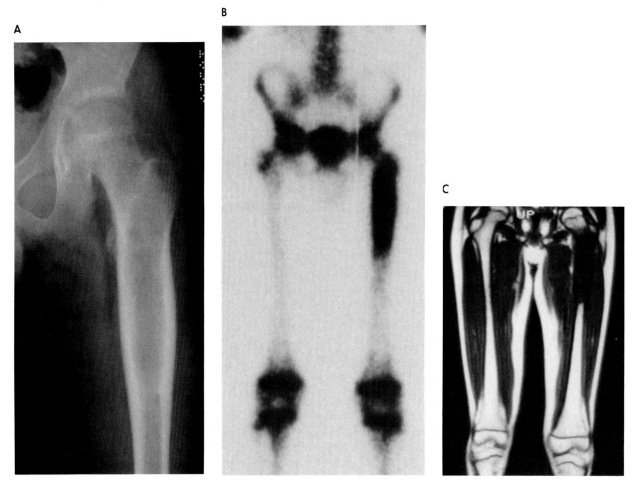

Fig. 19-40   Ewing's sarcoma in proximal femur of 12-year-old boy. **A,** Roentgenogram showing expansion of medullary canal and mild lateral "onionskin" effect. **B,** Bone scan with increased uptake in entire upper third of femur. **C,** MRI demonstrating lesion in proximal femoral metaphysis.

Ewing's sarcoma. Ewing's sarcoma is a small, round-cell sarcoma that is one of the most lethal of bone tumors. It accounts for slightly more than 6% of all malignant tumors. Ewing's sarcoma occurs most commonly in persons between the ages of 10 and 30 years, and two thirds of them occur in persons under the age of 20 years. Males are affected twice as often as females. Most Ewing's sarcomas are in the extremities, but any bone may be involved. The lower extremities and pelvis are the most common locations, followed by the spine, sacrum, and ribs. Pain and swelling are frequent symptoms. Most patients have a palpable tender mass, and some have dilated veins over the tumor. Many patients have elevated temperatures and increased erythrocyte sedimentation rates.

On a roentgenogram the extensive nature of the lesion is evident and often the entire shaft of a long bone is involved (Fig. 19-40). Lytic destruction is the most common roentgenographic finding, but there may be regions of density caused by new bone formation. Elevation of the periosteum produces characteristic multiple layers of new bone giving the "onionskin" appearance associated with Ewing's sarcoma.

Solid masses of viable tumor are characteristically gray-white, moist, glistening, and somewhat translucent. They may have an almost liquid consistency, which may mimic pus. Even with low-power magnification, Ewing's sarcoma is remarkably cellular, with little intercellular stroma. Under higher magnification, the cells are regular with round-to-oval nuclei. The cytoplasm surrounding these nuclei is slightly granular, and the outlines of the cells are indistinct. The nuclei themselves contain a rather finely dispersed chromatin that imparts a ground-glass appearance.

Multiagent chemotherapy has improved the 5-year survival rate from less than 10% to more than 40% in patients with Ewing's sarcoma. Surgical excision of the lesion, especially if it can be obtained without amputation, is becoming more important in treatment of Ewing's sarcomas. Lesions of the pelvis have the worst prognosis, and distal lesions have a better prognosis than proximal lesions.

Chondrosarcoma. Chondrosarcomas are very rare in children, occurring more commonly after the fifth decade of life. They constitute approximately 11% of malignant tumors in all ages. Most arise spontaneously (primary chondrosarcoma), but some are from a preexisting enchondroma or from the cap of an exostosis (secondary chondrosarcoma). The exact incidence of an osteochondroma or enchondroma undergoing malignant degeneration is not known but is estimated to be less than 1%. Patients with multiple hereditary osteochondromas or Ollier disease (multiple enchondromas) are at greater risk than those with a single lesion. Primary chondrosarcomas occur most commonly in the pelvis or proximal femur. Local swelling or pain, either alone or in combination, is the significant presenting symptom. If the mass is palpable, it is characteristically hard and may be painful.

The typical roentgenographic appearance is a radiolucent lesion with calcification and varying amounts of surrounding reactive bone. Central chondrosarcomas of the long bones often produce fusiform expansion of the shaft and thickening of the cortex. On gross examination the size of the lesion is most helpful in differentiating periosteal chondroma from chondrosarcoma. The former is almost always less than 3 cm in greatest dimension, and the latter is rarely less than 5 cm. Chondrosarcomas are characteristically composed of lobules that vary from a few millimeters to several centimeters in diameter. Chondrosarcomas produce a matrix substance that varies in consistency from that of a firm hyaline cartilage to that of mucus; a myxoid quality is strongly suggestive of malignancy. Chondrosarcomas are the most difficult of the malignant tumors to evaluate histologically. The criteria differentiating a low-grade chondrosarcoma from a chondroma are very subtle, and experience is necessary for accurate appraisal.

Chondrosarcoma is treated by surgical resection; chemotherapy and irradiation do not ordinarily play a role. A wide surgical margin is recommended for both primary and secondary chondrosarcomas, since these lesions have a pronounced propensity for local recurrence.

Adamantinoma. Adamantinoma is an uncommon lesion occurring almost exclusively in the tibia or mandible. Of all reported adamantinomas of the long bones, 90% have involved the tibia. Pain is the most common initial symptom, and a mass, which may be painful, is the only physical finding of consequence.

The characteristic roentgenographic appearance is multiple radiolucent lesions within the cortex surrounded by reactive bone (Fig. 19-41). The lesions may extend into the soft tissue, medullary canal, or both. Some of the lucent zones are small, entirely cortical, and similar to those seen in lesions of fibrous dysplasia. Typically, one of the lytic areas, usually in the midshaft, is the largest and most destructive-appearing, actually destroying the cortex.

On gross examination, most adamantinomas are clearly delimited peripherally, with lobulated contours. Most are gray or white and may contain spicules of bone and calcareous material. Various histologic patterns have been described, but all have an epithelial quality. A common pattern consists of neoplastic islands in which the peripheral cells, often columnar, are arranged in a palisaded fashion. In the

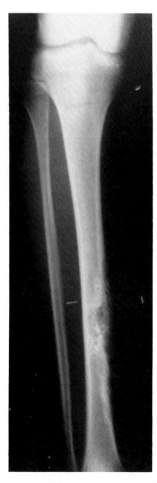

Fig. 19-41 Adamantinoma of tibia in 18-year-old patient.

centers of some of these islands, a stellate, reticulum-like appearance is seen. Even cyst formation may occur within these islands, and this basic pattern has prompted the use of the term *adamantinoma.* A second pattern consists of islands of cells resembling cutaneous basal cells. These cellular aggregates often show peripheral palisading of nuclei, and they ordinarily are disposed in a fibrous stoma. The appearance of this second pattern is similar to that of basal cell carcinoma of the skin.

Because adamantinoma, ossifying fibroma, and fibrous dysplasia may be present in the same patient, incisional biopsy of the wrong part of the lesion may give a false histologic picture. In children, a radiolucent lesion in the cortex of the tibia or fibula is more likely to be ossifying fibroma or fibrous dysplasia. If the clinical findings suggest adamantinoma (pain and progressive resorption of bone), the most aggressive portion of the lesion should be biopsied by either a very generous incisional or an excisional biopsy. Adamantinoma should be treated with a wide surgical margin. Frequent recurrence and metastasis have been reported after inadequate local excision.

Neuroblastoma. Neuroblastoma is made up of primitive neuroblasts and its cause is unknown. It is the third most common childhood malignancy, accounting for 10% to 12% of all malignancies in children. About one fourth of neuroblastomas are congenital, half are diagnosed by the age of 2 years, 90% are diagnosed by the age of 5 years, and only sporadic lesions occur during adolescence or adulthood. The peak incidence is at about 18 months of age.

Neuroblastomas may be found in the paramidline at any point between the base of the skull and the pelvis. Common locations include the retroperitoneum, mediastinum, cervical region, and sacral region. Symptoms depend on the age of the patient, the location of the lesion, and any associated clinical syndromes. Patients with neuroblastomas usually appear chronically ill, with nonspecific symptoms including fever, weight loss, gastrointestinal disturbances, and anemia. Fever and joint pain are common, often leading to a misdiagnosis of rheumatoid fever. In about half the patients a nodular fixed mass can be palpated, and approximately one third of newborns have blue-red cutaneous metastases.

On a roentgenogram, retroperitoneal lesions cause anterior, lateral, downward displacement of the kidneys. Calcification is present in 50% of lesions, typically consisting of finely stippled densities in the central portion of the tumor. Metastatic lesions commonly occur in bone, especially in the skull, femur, and humerus (Fig. 19-42).

Neuroblastomas are lobulated masses averaging 6 to 8 cm in diameter; they are intimately related to the adrenal gland or sympathetic chain. The most primitive tumors resemble the anlage of the developing sympathetic nervous system and adrenal medulla.

Treatment of neuroblastoma is complete excision of the lesion, with or without irradiation. A recent treatment protocol combines total body irradiation with high-dose chemotherapy and bone marrow transplant. The two most important prognostic factors are the age of the patient and clinical stage of the lesion. Children younger than 2 years of age have a better survival rate than those older than 2 years. Cervical, thoracic, and pelvic tumors have better prognoses than retroperitoneal and adrenal tumors.

Synovial cell sarcoma. Synovial cell sarcoma is a malignant soft tissue tumor and, although the name suggests that it is of synovial origin, it is very rarely found within a joint; it most commonly is found in the soft tissues not associated with synovial or tendon sheath tissue. Synovial cell sarcomas account for 10% of all soft tissue sarcomas and occur most often in patients between the ages of 15 and 35 years. Most (85% to 95%) synovial cell sarcomas occur in the extremities, where they tend to arise in the vicinity of large joints, especially the knee region. Approximately one third of synovial cell sarcomas affect the knee or distal thigh region. Next in frequency are the regions of the ankle and foot, elbow, upper arm, and shoulder. Most patients with synovial cell sarcomas complain of pain long before the tumor is found, occasionally for a year or more. The most typical physical finding is a palpable, deep-seated swelling or mass that is associated with pain in slightly more than 50% of patients.

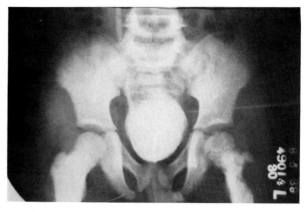

Fig. 19-42   Metastatic neuroblastoma in proximal left femur in 4-year-old child.

The majority of synovial cell sarcomas appear on roentgenograms as round or oval, more or less lobulated swellings or masses of moderated density, usually located close to a large joint. Calcifications or dystrophic ossifications are usually seen within the tumor (Fig. 19-43).

The gross appearance of the lesion varies considerably depending on the rate of growth and the location. Slow-growing lesions tend to be sharply circumscribed, round or multilobular, and completely or partially enclosed by a glistening pseudocapsule. Cyst formation may be prominent. Most lesions are firmly attached to surrounding tendons, tendon sheaths, or the exterior wall of the joint capsule. They are typically 3 to 5 cm in greatest dimension.

Microscopically, synovial cell sarcomas are com-

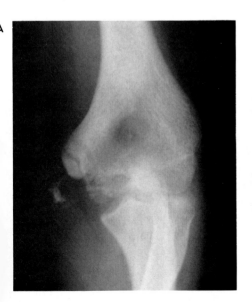
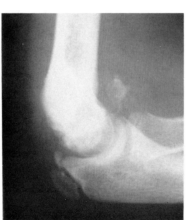

Fig. 19-43   Synovial cell sarcoma of left elbow of 11-year-old boy. **A,** Anteroposterior and, **B,** lateral views. Note calcification in lesion medial and anterior to joint.

posed of epithelial cells and fibrosarcoma-like spindle cells. The epithelial cells are characterized by large, round or oval, vesicular nuclei and abundant pale-staining cytoplasm with distinctly outlined cellular borders. The surrounding spindle cell or fibrous component, which is usually the most prominent feature of the tumor, consists mostly of well-oriented, rather plump, spindle-shaped cells of uniform appearance with scant and indistinct cytoplasm and oval dark-staining nuclei. Commonly the cellular portions of synovial sarcoma alternate with less cellular areas that are markedly altered by collagen deposition, myxoid change, and/or calcification. Mast cells are another typical feature of synovial cell sarcomas; they have no particular arrangement but are more numerous in the spindle cells than in the epithelial portions.

In the past, most patients with synovial cell sarcoma were treated with a radical surgical margin, which usually meant an amputation, but more recently limb-sparing wide surgical margins, with adjuvant irradiation, have been used. Small lesions within a muscle or between two muscles and not adjacent to bone or neurovascular bundles can be resected without adjuvant irradiation, but the entire muscle or muscles should be resected. Lesions in the hands or feet may require amputation, but even these can be treated with a combination of irradiation and limited surgery. Preoperative irradiation is suggested for lesions adjacent to bone or a neurovascular bundle. Adjuvant chemotherapy has not been shown to benefit patients with synovial cell sarcoma, but many new protocols are being investigated. Reported recurrence rates of synovial cell sarcoma vary from 28% to 49%. The most favorable prognosis is for the young patient with a small tumor (less than 5 cm) in a distal location.

REFERENCES

General

Dahlin DC: Bone tumors, ed 4, Springfield, IL, 1978, Charles C Thomas, Publisher.

Enneking WF: Musculoskeletal tumor surgery, New York, 1983, Churchill Livingston.

Enneking WF, Spanier SS, and Goodmen MA: A system for the surgical staging of musculoskeletal sarcomata, Clin Orthop 153:106, 1980.

Enzinger FM and Weiss SW: Soft tissue tumors, ed 2, St. Louis, 1988, The CV Mosby Co.

Hajdu SI: Pathology of soft tissue tumors Philadelphia, 1979, Lea & Febiger.

Hudson TM: Radiologic: pathologic correlation of musculoskeletal lesions, Baltimore, 1987, Williams & Wilkins.

Huvos AG: Bone tumors: diagnosis treatment and prognosis, Philadelphia, 1979, WB Saunders Co.

Jaffe H: Tumors and tumourous conditions of bones and joints, ed 2, Philadelphia, 1958, Lea & Febiger.

Lichlenstein L: Bone tumors, ed 5, St. Louis, 1977, The CV Mosby Co.

Russell WO et al: A clinical and pathological staging system for soft tissue sarcomas, Cancer 40:1562, 1977.

Diagnostic radiology

Aisen AM et al: MRI and CT evaluation of primary bone and soft tissue tumors, AJR 146:749, 1986.

American Academy of Orthopaedic Surgeons: Atlas of limb prosthetic, St. Louis, 1981, The CV Mosby Co.

Bohndorf K et al: Magnetic resonance imaging of primary tumours and tumour-like lesions of bone, Skeletal Radiol 15:511, 1986.

Chang AE et al: Evaluation of computed tomography in the detection of pulmonary metastases, Cancer 43:913, 1979.

Coffre C et al: Problems and pitfalls in the use of computer tomography for the local evaluation of long bone osteosarcoma: report on 30 cases, Skeletal Radiol 13:147, 1985.

Cohen MD et al: Efficacy of magnetic resonance imaging in 139 children with tumors, Arch Surg 121:522, 1986.

Finn HA et al: Scintigraphy with gallium-67 citrate in staging of soft tissue sarcomas of the extremity, J Bone Joint Surg 69A:886, 1987.

Gillespy T III et al: Staging of intraosseous extent of osteosarcoma: correlation of preoperative CT and MR imaging with pathologic macroslides, Radiology 167:765, 1988.

Heiken JP et al: CT of benign soft tissue masses of the extremities, Am J Roentgenol 142:575, 1984.

Hudson TM et al: Angiography in the management of musculoskeletal tumors, Surg Gynecol Obstet 141:11, 1975.

Hudson TM et al: The comparative value of bone scintigraphy and computed tomography in determining bone involvement by soft tissue sarcomas, J Bone Joint Surg 66A:1400, 1984.

Jones ET and Kuhns LR: Pitfalls in the use of computed tomography for musculoskeletal tumors in children, J Bone Joint Surg 63A:1297, 1981.

Kirchner PT and Simon MA: The clinical value of bone and galium scintigraphy for soft tissue sarcomas of the extremities, J Bone Joint Surg 66A:319, 1984.

Moon KL et al: Musculoskeletal applications of nuclear magnetic resonance, Radiology 147:161, 1983.

Pettersson H et al: Primary musculoskeletal tumors: examination with MR imaging compared with conventional modalities, Radiology 164:237, 1987.

Simon MA and Kirchner PT: Scintigraphic evaluation of primary bone tumors, J Bone Joint Surg 62A:75, 1980.

Sundaram M and McGuire MH: Computed tomography or magnetic resonance for evaluating solitary tumors or tumorlike lesions of bone? Skeletal Radiol 17:393, 1988.

Vilali M et al: Amputation and Prostheses, London, 1978, Bailliere Tindall.

Weinberger G and Levinsohn EM: Computed tomography in the evaluation of sarcomatous tumors of the thigh, Am J Roentgenol, 130:115, 1978.

Biopsy

Enneking WF: The issue of the biopsy, J Bone Joint Surg 64A:1119, 1982, (editorial).

Joyce MJ and Mankin HJ: Caveat arthoscopos: extra-articular lesions of bone simulating intra-articular pathology of the knee, J Bone Joint Surg 65A:239, 1983.

Mankin HJ, Lange TA, and Spanier SA: The hazards of biopsy in patients with malignant primary bone and soft tissue tumors, J Bone Joint Surg 64A:1121, 1982.

Simon MA: Biopsy of musculoskeletal tumors, J Bone Joint Surg 64A:1253, 1982.

Specific procedures

Borggreve: Kniegelensevatz durch das un der beinlangsasch un 180 degrees geduchte fusgelenk, Arch Orthop Unfall Chir 28:175, 1930.

Kotz R and Salzer M: Rotation-plasty for childhood osteosarcoma of the distal part of the femur, J Bone Joint Surg 64A:959, 1982.

Linberg BE: Interscapulo-thoracic resection for malignant tumors of the shoulder joint region, J Bone Joint Surg 10:344, 1928.

Marzhede G and Stener B: Function after removal of various hip and thigh muscles for extirpation of tumors, Acta Orthop Scand 52:373, 1981.

Van Nes CP: Rotation-plasty for congenital defects of the femur making use of the ankle of the shortened limb to control the knee joint of a prosthesis, J Bone Joint Surg 32B:12, 1950.

Amputations

Aitken GT: Overgrowth of the amputation stump, Inter-Clin Info Bull 1:1, 1962.

Lewis NM et al: The expandable prosthesis: an alternative to amputation for children with malignant bone tumors, AORN J 46:457, 1987.

Meyer LC and Sauer BW: The use of porous high density polyethelyn caps in the prevention of appositional bone growth in the juvenile amputee: a preliminary report, Inter-Clin Info Bull 14:1, 1975.

Romano RL and Burgess EM: Extremity growth and overgrowth following amputation in children, Inter-Clin Info Bull 5:11, 1966.

Swenson AB: Silicone-rubber implants to control the overgrowth phenomenon in the juvenile amputee, Inter-Clin Info Bull 11:5, 1972.

Nonossifying fibroma

Arata MA, Peterson HA, and Dahlin DC: Pathological fractures through non-ossifying fibromas, J Bone Joint Surg 63A:980, 1981.

Brower AC, Culver JE Jr, and Keats TE: Histological nature of the cortical irregularity of the medical posterior distal femoral metaphysic and children, Radiology 99:389, 1971.

Dunham WK et al: Developmental defects of the distal femoral metaphysics, J Bone Joint Surg 62A:801, 1980.

Osteochondroma

Hudson TM, Chew FS, and Manaster BJ: Scintigraphy of benign exostoses and exostotic chondrosarcomas, Am J Roentgenol 10:581, 1983.

Lange RH, Lange TA, and Rao BK: Correlative radiographic, scintographic, and histologic evaluation of exostoses, J Bone Joint Surg 66A:1454, 1984.

Shapiro F, Simons, and Glimcher MJ: Hereditary multiple exostoses, J Surg Joint Surg 61A:815, 1979.

Snearly WN and Peterson HA: Management of ankle deformities in multiple hereditary osteochondroma, J Pediatr Orthop 9:427, 1989.

Solomon L: Hereditary multiple exostosis, J Bone Joint Surg 45B:292, 1963.

Fibrous dysplasia

Albright F et al: Syndrome characterized by osteitis fibrosa disseminata, area of pigmentation and endocrine dysfunction, with precocious puberty in females, N Engl J Med 216:727, 1937.

Enneking WF and Gearen PF: Fibrous dysplasia of the femoral neck: treatment by cortical bone-grafting, J Bone Joint Surg 68A:1415, 1986.

Grabias SL and Campbell CJ: Fibrous dysplasia, Orthop Clin North Am 8:771, 1977.

Harris WH, Dudley HR Jr, and Barry RJ: The natural history of fibrous dysplasia: an orthopaedic, pathological, and roentgenographic study, J Bone Joint Surg 44A:207, 1962.

Henry A: Monostotic fibrous dysplasia, J Bone Joint Surg 51B:300, 1969.

Lichtenstein L: Polyostolic fibrous dysplasia, Arch Surg 36:874, 1938.

Stephenson RB et al: Fibrous dysplasia: an analysis of options for treatment, J Bone Joint Surg 69A:400, 1987.

Stewart MJ, Gilmer WS, and Edmondson AS: Fibrous dysplasia of bone, J Bone Joint Surg 44B:302, 1962.

Enchondroma

Bean WB: Dyschondroplasia and hemangiomata (Maffucci's syndrome), Arch Intern Med 95:767, 1955.

Bean WB: Dyschondroplasia and hemangiomata (Maffucci's syndrome) Part II, Arch Intern Med 102:544, 1958.

Lewis RJ and Ketcham AS: Maffucci's syndrome: functional and neoplastic significance: case report and review of the literature, J Bone Joint Surg 55A:1465, 1973.

Noble J and Lamb DW: Enchondromatra of bones of the hand: a review of 40 cases, Hand 6:275, 1974.

Ollier M: Exostoses osteogeniques multiples, Lyon Med 88:484, 1898.

Schwartz HS et al: The malignant potential of enchondromatosis, J Bone Joint Surg 69A:269, 1987.

Sun Te-ching et al: Chondrosarcoma in Maffucci's syndrome, J Bone Joint Surg 67A:1214, 1985.

Hemangioma

Allen PW and Enziner FM: Hemangiomas of skeletal muscle: an analysis of 89 cases, Cancer 29:8, 1972.

Johnson KW, Ghormley RK, and Dockerty MB: Hemangiomas of the extremities, Surg Gynecol Obstet 102:531, 1956.

Unicameral bone cyst

Campanacci M, Capanna R, and Picci P: Unicameral and aneursymal bone cysts, Clin Orthop 204:25, 1986.

Capanna R et al: Contrast examination as prognostic factor in the treatment of solitary bone cyst by cortisone injection, Skeletal Radiol 12:97, 1984.

Chigira M et al: The aetiology and treatment of simple bone cysts, J Bone Joint Surg 65B:633, 1983.

Cohen J: Unicameral bone cysts: a current synthesis of reported cases, Orthop Clin North Am 8:715, 1977.

Cohen J: Etiology of simple bone cysts, J Bone Joint Surg 52A:1493, 1970.

Kruls HSA: Pathological fractures in children due to solitary bone cyst, Reconstr Surg Traumatol, 17:113, 1979.

Neer CS II et al: Treatment of unicameral bone cyst: a follow-up study of 175 cases, J Bone Joint Surg 48A:731, 1966.

Oppenheim WL and Galleno H: Operative treatment versus steroid injection in the management of unicameral bone cysts, J Pediatr Orthop 4:1, 1984.

Scaglietti O: Sull'azione osteogenetica dell'acetato di prednisolone, Boll Soc Tosco-Umbra Chir 35:1, 1974.

Scaglietti O, Marchetti PG, and Bartolozzi P: Final results obtained in the treatment of bone cyst with methyprednisolone acetate (Depo-Medrol) and a discussion of results achieved in other bone lesions, Clin Orthop 165:33, 1982.

Aneurysmal bone cyst

Biesecker JL et al: Aneurysmal bone cysts, Cancer 26:615, 1970.

Capanna R et al: Aneurysmal bone cyst of the spine, J Bone Joint Surg 67A:527, 1985.

Hudson TM: Fluid levels in aneurysmal bone cyst: a CT feature, Am J Roentgenol 141:1001, 1984.

Lichtenstein L: Aneurysmal bone cysts, Cancer 3:279, 1950.

Martinez V and Sissons HA: Aneurysmal bone cyst: a review of 123 cases including primary lesions and those secondary to other bone pathology, Cancer 61:2291, 1988.

Tillman BP et al: Aneurysmal bone cyst: an analysis of ninety five cases, Mayo Clin Proc 43:478, 1968.

Osteoid osteoma and osteoblastoma

Ayla AG et al: Osteoid-osteoma: intraoperative tetracyline-fluorescence demonstration of the nidus, J Bone Joint Surg 68A:747, 1986.

Freiberger RH: Osteoid osteoma of the spine: a cause of backache and scoliosis in children and young adults, Radiology 75:232, 1960.

Ghelman B, Thompson FM, and Arnold WD: Intraoperative radio-active localization of an osteoid-osteoma, J Bone Joint Surg 63A:826, 1981.

Golding JSR: The natural history of osteoid osteoma with a report of twenty cases, J Bone Joint Surg 36B:218, 1954.

Healey JH and Ghelman B: Osteoid osteoma and osteoblastoma: current concepts and recent advances, Clin Orthop 204:76, 1986.

Herrlin K et al: Computed tomography in suspected osteoid osteomas of tubular bones, Skeletal Radiol 9:92, 1982.

Jaffe HL: "Osteoid osteoma": a benign osteoblastic tumor composed of osteoid and atypical bone, Arch Surg 31:709, 1935.

Keim HA and Reina EG: Osteoid osteoma as a cause of scoliosis, J Bone Joint Surg 57A:159, 1975.

Marsh BW et al: Benign osteoblastoma: range of manifestations, J Bone Joint Surg 57A 1, 1975.

McLeod RA, Dahlin DC, and Beabour JW: The spectrum of osteoblastoma, Am J Roentgenol 126:132, 1976.

Mobey E: The natural course of osteoid osteoma, J Bone Joint Surg 33A:166, 1951.

Norman A: Persistance or recurrence of pain: a sign of surgical failure in osteoid osteoma, Clin Orthop 130:263, 1978.

Pettine KA and Klassen RA: Osteoid-osteoma and osteoblastoma of the spine, J Bone Joint Surg 68A:354, 1986.

Rinsky LA et al: Intraoperative skeletal scintigraphy for localization of osteoid-osteoma in the spine: case report, J Bone Joint Surg 62A:143, 1980.

Schajuwicz F and Lemos C: Malignant osteoblastoma, J Bone Joint Surg 58B:202, 1976.

Sherman MD: Osteoid osteoma: review of the literature and report of 30 cases, J Bone Joint Surg 29A:918, 1947.

Sims FH, Dahlin DC, and Beabout JW: Osteoid-osteoma: diagnostic problem, J Bone Joint Surg 57A:154, 1975.

Smith FW and Gilday DL: Scintigraphic appearances of osteoid osteoma, Radiology 137:191, 1980.

Eosinophilic granuloma

Cohen M et al: Direct injection of methylprednisolone sodium succinate in the treatment of solitary eosinophilic granuloma of bone, Radiology 136:289, 1980.

Lichlenstein L: Histiocytosis X: integration of eosinophilic granuloma of bone, "Letterer-Siwe disease," and "Schaller-Christian disease" as related manifestation of a single nosologic entity, Arch Pathol 56:84, 1953.

Lieberman PH et al: Reappraisal of eosinophilic granuloma of bone: Hand Schuller Christian syndrome and Letterer-Siwe syndrome, Medicine 48:375, 1969.

Pigmented villonodular synovitis

Byers PD et al: The diagnosis and treatment of pigmented villonodular synovitis, J Bone Joint Surg 50B:290, 1968.

Flandry F and Hughston JC: Pigmented villonodular synovitis, J Bone Joint Surg 69A:942, 1987.

Granowitz SP, D'Antonio J, and Mankin HJ: The pathogenesis and long term end results of pigmented villonodular synovitis, Clin Orthop 114:335, 1976.

Chondroblastoma

Codman EA: Epiphyseal chondromatous giant cell tumors of the upper end of the humerus, Surg Gynecol Obstet 52:543, 1931.

Dahlin DC and Ivins JC: Benign chondroblastoma: a study of 125 cases, Cancer 30:401, 1972.

Green P and Whittaker RP: Benign chondroblastoma: case report with pulmonary metastasis, J Bone Joint Surg 57A:418, 1975.

Huvos AG and Marcove RC: Chondroblastoma of bone: a critical review, Clin Orthop 95:300, 1973.

Jaffe HJ and Lichtenstein L: Benign chondroblastoma of bone: a re-interpretation of the so-called calcifying or chondromatous giant cell tumor, Am J Pathol 18:969, 1942.

McLeon RA and Beabout JW: The roentgenographic features of chondroblastoma, Am J Roentgenol 118:464, 1973.

Springfield DS et al: Chondroblastoma: a review of seventy cases, J Bone Joint Surg 67A:748, 1985.

Giant cell tumor of bone

Campanacci M, Giunti A, and Olmi R: Giant cell tumors of bone: a study of 209 cases with long-term follow-up with 130, Ital J Orthop Traumatol 1:249, 1975.

Goldenberg RR, Campbell CJ, and Bonfiglio M: Giant-cell tumor of bone: an analysis of two hundred and eighteen cases, J Bone Joint Surg 52A:619, 1970.

Jaffe HL, Lichtenstein L, and Portis RB: Giant cell tumor of bone: its pathologic appearance, grading, supposed variants and treatment, Arch Pathol 30:993, 1940.

Marcove RC et al: Cryosurgery in the treatment of GCT of bone: 52 consecutive cases, Clin Orthop 134:275, 1978.

McDonald DJ et al: Giant-cell tumor of bone, J Bone Joint Surg 68A:235, 1986.

Persson BM and Wouters HW: Curettage and acrylic cementation in surgery of GCT of bone, Clin Orthop 120:125, 1976.

Picci P et al: Giant-cell tumor of bone in skeletally immature patients, J Bone Joint Surg 65A:486, 1983.

Osteosarcoma

Cortes EP et al: Amputation and adriamycin in primary osteosarcoma, N Engl J Med 291:998, 1974.

deSantos LA, Bernardino ME, and Murray JA: Computed tomography in the evaluation of osteosarcoma: experience with 25 cases, Am J Roentgenol 132:535, 1979.

Destouet JM, Guild LA, and Murphy WA: Computed tomography of long bone osteosarcoma, Radiology 131:439, 1979.

Eilber F et al: Adjuvant chemotherapy for osteosarcoma: a randomized prospective trial, J Clin Oncol 5:21, 1987.

Enneking WF and Springfield DS: Osteosarcoma, Orthop Clin North Am 8:785, 1977.

Hudson TM et al: Radiologic imaging of osteosarcoma: role in planning surgical treatment, Skeletal Radiol 10:137, 1983.

Jaffe N et al: Adjuvant methotrexate citrovorum factor treatment of osteosarcoma, N Engl J Med 291:994, 1974.

Jaffe N et al: High-dose methotrexate in osteogenic sarcoma: a 5-year experience, Cancer Treat Rep 62:259, 1978.

Link MP et al: The effect of adjuvant chemotherapy on relapse-free survival in patients with osteosarcoma of the extremity, New Engl J Med 134:1600, 1986.

Marcove RC: En bloc resection for osteogenic sarcoma, Cancer Treat Rep 62:225, 1978.

Marcove RC et al: Osteogenic sarcoma under age of twenty-one: a review of one hundred and forty five operative cases, J Bone Joint Surg 52A:411, 1970.

Matsuno T et al: Telangiectatic ostegenic sarcoma, Cancer 38:2538, 1976.

Rosen G et al: Preoperative chemotherapy for osteogenic sarcoma: selection of post operative adjuvant chemotherapy based on the response of the primary tumor to preoperative chemotherapy, Cancer 49:1221, 1982.

Rosen G et al: Chemotherapy, en bloc resection, and prosthetic bone replacement in the treatment of osteogenic sarcoma, Cancer 37:1, 1976.

Simon MA et al: Limb-salvage treatment versus amputation for osteosarcoma of the distal end of the femur, J Bone Joint Surg 68A:1331, 1986.

Springfield DS et al: Surgery for osteosarcoma, J Bone Joint Surg 70A:1124, 1988.

Sundaram M, McGuire MH, and Herbold DR: Magnetic resonance imaging of osteosarcoma, Skeletal Radiol 16:23, 1987.

Winzler K et al: Neoadjuvant chemotherapy for osteogenic sarcoma: results of a cooperative German/Austrian study, J Clin Oncol 2:617, 1984.

Ewing's sarcoma

Kissane JM et al: Ewings sarcoma of bone: clinicopathologic aspects of 303 cases from the intergroup Ewings sarcoma study, Hum Pathol 14:773, 1983.

Neff JR: Nonmetastatic Ewings sarcoma of bone: the role of surgical therapy, Clin Orthop 204:111, 1986.

Sherman RS and Soong KY: Ewing's sarcoma: its roentgen classification and diagnosis, Radiology 66:529, 1956.

Thomas PRM et al: The management of Ewing's sarcoma: role of radiotherapy in local tumor control, Cancer Treat Rep 68:703, 1984.

Juxtacortical osteosarcoma and chondrosarcoma

Ahuja SC et al: Juxtacortical (parosteal) oseogenic osteosacroma: histologic grading and prognosis, J Bone Joint Surg 59A:632, 1977.

Bertoni F et al: Periosteal chondrosarcoma and periosteal osteosarcoma: two distinct entities, J Bone Joint Surg 64B:370, 1982.

Campanacci M et al: Parosteal osteosarcoma, J Bone Joint Surg 66B:313, 1984.

deSantos LA et al: The radiographic spectrum of periosteal osteosarcoma, Radiology 127:123, 1978.

Geschickter CF and Copeland MM: Parosteal osteoma of bone: a new entity, Am Surg 133:790, 1951.

Schajowicz F: Juxtacortical chondrosarcoma, J Bone Joint Surg 59B:473, 1977.

Unni KK, Dahlin DC, and Beabout JW: Periosteal osteogenic sarcoma, Cancer 37:2476, 1976.

Synovial cell sarcoma

Cadman NL, Soule EH, and Kelly PJ: Synovial sarcoma: an analysis of 134 tumors, Cancer 18:613, 1965.

Crocker DW and Stout AP: Synovial sarcoma in children, Cancer 12:1123, 1959.

Lee SM, Hajdu SI, and Exelby PR: Synovial sarcoma in children, Surg Gynecol Obstet 138:701, 1974.

Varela-Duran J and Enzinger TM: Calcifying synovial sarcoma, Cancer 50:345, 1982.

Soft tissue sarcomas

Bowden L and Booker RJ: The principle and technique of resection of soft parts for sarcoma, Surgery 44:963, 1958.

Lindberg R et al: Conservative surgery and postoperative radiotherapy in 300 adults with soft tissue sarcomas, Cancer 47:2391, 1981.

Shiu MH et al: Surgical treatment of 297 soft tissue sarcomas of the lower extremity, Ann Surg 182:597, 1975.

Suit HD et al: Radiation and surgery in the treatment of primary sarcoma of soft tissue: preoperative, intraoperative and postoperative, Cancer 55:2659, 1985.

Suit HD et al: Preoperative radiation therapy for sarcomas of the soft tissues, Cancer 47:2269, 1981.

Suit HD and Russell WO: Radiation therapy of soft tissue sarcomas, Cancer 36:759, 1975.

Suit HD, Russell WO, and Martin RG: Management of patients with sarcoma of soft tissue in an extremity, Cancer 31:1247, 1973.

Index